CARDIAC PROBLEMS IN PREGNANCY

THIRD EDITION

CARDIAC PROBLEMS IN PREGNANCY

Diagnosis and Management of Maternal and Fetal Heart Disease

Third Edition

Edited by

URI ELKAYAM, M.D.

Professor of Medicine
Director, Heart Failure Program
University of Southern California School of Medicine
and
Physician in Charge
High Risk Obstetrical-Cardiology Clinic
Los Angeles County/University of Southern California
Medical Center
Los Angeles, California

NORBERT GLEICHER, M.D.

President
The Center for Human Reproduction
Chicago, Illinois
and
Clinical Professor of Obstetrics and Gynecology
University of Illinois at Chicago
Chicago, Illinois

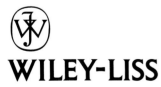

WILEY-LISS

A JOHN WILEY & SONS, INC., PUBLICATION

New York • Chichester • Weinheim • Brisbane • Singapore • Toronto

Library of Congress Cataloging-in-Publication Data:

Cardiac problems in pregnancy : diagnosis and management of maternal
    and fetal heart disease / edited by Uri Elkayam, Norbert Gleicher. — 3rd
    ed.
        p.   cm.
    Includes bibliographical references and index.
    ISBN 0-471-16358-9 (cloth : alk. paper)
    1. Heart diseases in pregnancy.   2. Fetal heart rate monitoring.
3. Fetal heart—Diseases.   I. Elkayam, Uri.   II. Gleicher, Norbert.
    [DNLM: 1. Pregnancy Complications, Cardiovascular—diagnosis.
2. Pregnancy Complications, Cardiovascular—therapy.   3. Heart
Diseases—in pregnancy.   4. Fetal Diseases.   WQ 244 C266 1998]
RG580.H4C37   1998
618.3–dc21
DNLM/DLC
for Library of Congress   97-18625
                                                     CIP

Printed in the United States of America.

10 9 8 7 6 5 4 3 2 1

We greatly appreciate the tolerance of our two families,
which allowed us to dedicate the time to complete this book.

Batia, Ifat, Jonathan, and Danielle Elkayam

Gabrielle, Anja, and Daliah Gleicher

CONTENTS

PREFACE

Like the two preceding editions, the third edition of this book aims to offer a comprehensive summary of available knowledge and, at the same time, to provide a very practical guide for diagnosis and treatment of heart disease during pregnancy in both mother and fetus. While the overall format of the first two editions has been maintained, the significant amount of new information published during the seven years since the publication of the second edition required a very extensive revision of that volume. No chapter in the book, therefore, escaped change, and in fact, over half of the chapters have been either added or substituted with a considerable change in authorship. New chapters in the third edition include cardiopulmonary imaging, prosthetic heart valves, acute myocardial infarction, Marfan syndrome, and pregnancy after cardiac transplantation. In addition, new chapters on the use of diuretics, vasodilators, and angiotensin converting enzyme inhibitors in pregnancy have been added.

Again, the editors' efforts in preparing this book were, to a large extent, dependent on the collaboration with a large number of cardiologists, obstetricians, surgeons, internists, and pharmacists who contributed their knowledge, clinical expertise, and time. Our special appreciation goes to Dr. Louis Buttino, who not only greatly contributed as an author to this new edition, but also actively participated in the editing process of the fetal section. We also gratefully acknowledge the assistance of Drs. Omar Rashid Wani and Ilyas Somer Karaalp, and Lorine Araiza in the preparation of the maternal section.

Finally, no book like this can be written without a large body of clinical experience. Such experience could not be obtained without the willingness of many patients to entrust the care of themselves and their fetuses to us and the other authors of this book. This book is, therefore, dedicated to them and all future patients with heart disease during pregnancy, adults or unborn. If this new edition will contribute to their care, we, the editors and authors, have achieved our goal.

Uri Elkayam, M.D.
Norbert Gleicher, M.D.

CONTRIBUTORS

Walid S. Alami, MD, Multiorgan Transplant Center, Houston, Texas

Page A.W. Anderson, MD, Duke University Medical Center, Durham, North Carolina

Syed W.H. Bokhari, MD, University of Southern California School of Medicine, Los Angeles, California

Michael D. Bork, DO, Oakwood Hospital and Medical Center, Dearborn, Michigan

Orestes Borrego, MD, Tampa General Hospital, Tampa, Florida

Michael A. Brodsky, MD, University of California Irvine Medical Center, Orange, California

Barbara K. Burton, MD, Center for Medicine and Reproductive Genetics, Chicago, Illinois

Louis Buttino, Jr., MD, Franciscan Medical Center, Dayton, Ohio

Steven E. Calvin, MD, University of Minnesota, Minneapolis, Minnesota

Alessandra Capponi, MD, Centro di Medicina Fetale, Clinica Ostetrica e Ginecologica, Universita di Roma "Tor Vergata", Rome, Italy

Luis J. Castro, MD, University of Southern California School of Medicine, Los Angeles, California

R.S. Chari, MD, University of Alberta Hospital, Maternal Fetal Medicine, Edmonton, Alberta, Canada

Harold Chen, MD, Louisiana State University Medical Center School of Medicine, Shreveport, Louisiana

Steven L. Clark, MD, University of Utah School of Medicine, Salt Lake City, Utah

Eytan Cohen, MD, Beilinson Campus Rabin Medical Center, Petah-Tikva, Israel

Robbin G. Cohen, MD, University of Southern California School of Medicine, Healthcare Consultation Center, Los Angeles, California

Patrick M. Colletti, MD, University of Southern California School of Medicine, Los Angeles, California

Jafna L. Cox, MD, FRCPC, Dalhousie University, Halifax, Nova Scotia, Canada

William Cusick, MD, Stamford Hospital, Stamford, Connecticut

John G. D'Alessio, MD, University of Tennessee, Memphis, Tennessee

Ravi Dave, MD, University of Southern California School of Medicine, Los Angeles, California

Diane Debich-Spicer, BS, Tampa General Hospital, Tampa, Florida

Greggory R. DeVore, MD, Obstetrics and Gynecology, Salt Lake City, Utah

Terrence Dillon, MD, Pediatric Cardiologists of Dayton, Inc., Beavercreek, Ohio

Shigeharu Doi, MD, Osaka University, Osaka, Japan

Ramin Ebrahimi, MD, University of California Irvine, Medical Center, Orange, California

James F.X. Egan, MD, University of Connecticut, Farmington, Connecticut

Uri Elkayam, MD, University of Southern California School of Medicine, Los Angeles County and University of Southern California Medical Center, Los Angeles, California

Mohammed R. Essop, MD, Division of Cardiology, University of the Witswatersrand, Baragwanath Hospital, Johannesburg, South Africa

A.Y. Frangieh, MD, University of Tennessee, Memphis, Tennessee

Yair Frenkel, MD, Sackler School of Medicine, Tel Aviv University, Sheba Medical Center, Tel Hashomer, Israel

William H. Frishman, MD, New York Medical College, Westchester County Medical Center, Valhalla, New York

Giovanni Gambuzza, MD, Artemisia Medical Centre, Rome, Italy

Moshe Garty, Tel Aviv University, Bellinson Campus Rabin Medical Center, Petah-Tikva, Israel

Eran Geller, MD, Stanford University School of Medicine, Palo Alto Veteran Administration Health Care System, Palo Alto, California

Enid Gilbert-Barness, University of South Florida, School of Medicine, Tampa, Florida

Jeffrey Ginsberg, MD, McMaster University, Hamilton Health Sciences Corporation, McMaster Division, Hamilton, Ontario, Canada

Claudio Giorlandino, MD, Artemisia Medical Centre, Rome, Italy

Norbert Gleicher, MD, Center for Human Reproduction, Chicago, Illinois

T. Murphy Goodwin, MD, Women's Hospital, Los Angeles, California

Nina L. Gotteiner, MD, Children's Hospital, Chicago, Illinois

Scott E. Gray, MD, Regional Perinatal Center, Springfield, Missouri

Tomoaki Ikeda, MD, Osaka University, Osaka, Japan

Afshan Hameed, MD, University of Southern California School of Medicine, Los Angeles, California

Earl C. Harrison, MD, University of Southern California School of Medicine, Los Angeles, California

Kristina Hoffman, PharmD, Moffit Cancer Hospital, Tampa, Florida

Agneta K. Hurst, PharmD, University of Southern California School of Pharmacy, Los Angeles, California

Toru Kanzaki, MD, Osaka University, Osaka, Japan

Steven S. Khan, MD, University of California School of Medicine, Cedars Sinai Medical Center, Los Angeles, California

Siri Linda Kjos, MD, University of Southern California School of Medicine, Women's and Children's Hospital, Los Angeles, California

Mark B. Lampert, MD, Mid West Medical Group, South Bend, Indiana

Roberto M. Lang, MD, The University of Chicago, Chicago, Illinois

Kai Lee, PhD, University of Southern California School of Medicine, Los Angeles, California

Richard V. Lee, MD, Children's Hospital of Buffalo, Buffalo, New York

Cyril Y. Leung, MD, University of California Irvine Medical Center, Orange, California

William McGehee, MD, University of Southern California School of Medicine, Los Angeles County/University of Southern California Medical Center, Los Angeles, California

Anilkumar Mehra, MD, University of Southern California School of Medicine, Los Angeles, California

Marla A. Mendelson, MD, Heart Disease Center, Northwestern University Medical School, Chicago, Illinois

Gladys Moriguchi Mitani, PharmD, University of Southern California School of Pharmacy, Los Angeles County/University of Southern California Medical Center, Los Angeles, California

Yuji Murata, MD, University of California Irvine Medical Center, Orange, California

David Niv, MD, Tel Aviv University, Tel Aviv Medical Center, Tel Aviv, Israel

Enrique Ostrzega, MD, University of Southern California School of Medicine, Los Angeles, California

Sueng-Dae Park, MD, Osaka University, Osaka, Japan

Athena Poppas, MD, Brown University School of Medicine, Rhode Island Hospital, Providence, Rhode Island

Jaya Ramanathan, MD, University of Tennessee College of Medicine, Memphis, Tennessee

William F. Rayburn, MD, University of Oklahoma Health Science Center, Oklahoma City, Oklahoma

Cheryl L. Reid, MD, University of California at Irvine, University of California Irvine Medical Center, Orange, California

Giuseppe Rizzo, MD, Centro di Medicina Fetale, Clinica Ostetrica e Ginecologica, Universita di Roma "Tor Vergata", Rome, Italy

Carlo Romanini, MD, Centro di Medicina Fetale, Clinica Ostetrica e Ginecologica, Universita di Roma "Tor Vergata", Rome, Italy

Karen Rosene-Montella, MD, Brown University School of Medicine, Women and Infant's and Rhode Island Hospitals, Providence, Rhode Island

Arie Roth, MD, Tel Aviv Medical Center, Tel Aviv, Israel

Valery Rudick, MD, Tel Aviv University, Tel Aviv Medical Center, Tel Aviv, Israel

John D. Rutherford, MB, ChB, FRACP, FACC, University of Texas, Dallas, Texas

Pinhas Sareli, MD, Division of Cardiology, University of the Witswatersrand, Baragwanath Hospital, Johannesburg, South Africa

Harold Schulman, MD, FACOG, Vero Beach, Florida

Avraham Shotan, MD, Heart Institute, Sheba Medical Center, Tel Hashomer, Israel

B.M. Sibai, MD, University of Tennessee, Memphis, Tennessee

Irving Steinberg, PharmD, University of Southern California Schools of Pharmacy and Medicine, Los Angeles County/University of Southern California Medical Center, Los Angeles, California

Carole A. Warnes, MD, Adult Congenital Heart Disease Clinic, Mayo Clinic, Rochester, Minnesota

Josef Widerhorn, MD, All Saints Episcopal Hopsital, Fort Worth, Texas, and University of North Texas Health Science Center at Fort Worth, Fort Worth, Texas

James B. Young, MD, Cleveland Clinic Foundation, Cleveland, Ohio

MATERNAL SECTION

PART I

PHYSIOLOGIC CHANGES DURING NORMAL PREGNANCY AND THE PUERPERIUM

1

HEMODYNAMICS AND CARDIAC FUNCTION DURING NORMAL PREGNANCY AND THE PUERPERIUM

URI ELKAYAM, MD, AND NORBERT GLEICHER, MD

INTRODUCTION

Pregnancy is associated with substantial physiologic changes that require adaptation of the cardiovascular system (Table 1.1). The development of newer and more accurate, noninvasive as well as invasive diagnostic modalities has improved the understanding of cardiac changes during pregnancy and allows better monitoring of such changes throughout pregnancy, labor and delivery, and the puerperium. The increased circulatory burden of pregnancy can unmask previously unrecognized heart disorders and rapidly worsen heart disease toward a potentially lethal situation. The recognition and management of cardiac illness in pregnancy is difficult at times. A comprehensive understanding of cardiocirculatory adaptation during pregnancy and the early postpartum period is essential for the appropriate management of pregnant patients with cardiovascular disorders; this chapter intends to provide the necessary background.

HEMODYNAMIC CHANGES DURING PREGNANCY

Blood Volume

One of the major cardiocirculatory changes during pregnancy relates to blood volume. Changes in blood volume were studied first by Miller et al in 1915[1] and since then by numerous investigators.[2-21] Although there has been general agreement that blood volume increases significantly during pregnancy, there has been disagreement about the magnitude of the increment and the pattern of change throughout pregnancy. The increase in blood volume starts as early as the 6th week of pregnancy. A rapid increase takes place until midpregnancy, when the volume continues to rise but at a much slower rate (Fig. 1.1).[7] Considerable individual variations in the degree of volume expansion during pregnancy, ranging from 20% to nearly 100% of nonpregnant values, have been reported.[6] One report[5] described a 33% increase in blood volume at 21–24 weeks of gestation, a progressive rise to a peak of 49% at 33–36 weeks, and a plateau for the last 8 weeks of pregnancy. Other investigators[10-13] suggested either a slight decrease or a slow increase in volume during the last several weeks before term. In general, most studies show a continuous blood volume increase up to a maximal value of about 50% above the nonpregnant state.[3-13] Expressed in milliliters per kilogram, the mean recorded blood volume ranged from 73 to 96 mL/kg.[1-3,5,7]

In addition to blood volume expansion a redistribution of this volume has been described during pregnancy.[21] Studies in the third gestational trimester showed an increase of both interstitial and plasma volume, with a greater proportion of the extracellular fluid volume lying intravascularly in normal pregnancy than in nonpregnant women.[20] An interesting observation was reported by Pritchard and Rowland,[6] who demonstrated that in spite of considerable variations between individuals in the intensity of hypervolemia, the same degree of hypervolemia usually develops during subsequent pregnancies of the same subject. Other investigators suggested that blood volume increments seem higher in multigravidas than in primigravidas and in multiple compared to single pregnancies.[14-17] In a recent report by Thomsen et al,[22] the development of blood volume during twin pregnancy, measured from 20th gestational week to term, paralleled that seen during sin-

Cardiac Problems in Pregnancy, Third Edition
Edited by Uri Elkayam, MD, and Norbert Gleicher, MD
Copyright © 1998 by Wiley-Liss, Inc. ISBN 0-471-16358-9

TABLE 1.1   Cardiocirculatory Changes During Normal Pregnancy

Parameter	Changes[a] at Various Times (weeks)					
	5	12	20	24	32	38
Heart rate	↑	↑↑↑	↑↑↑	↑↑↑	↑↑↑↑	↑↑↑↑
Systolic blood pressure	↔	↓	↓	↔	↑	↑↑
Diastolic blood pressure	↔	↓	↓↓	↓	↔	↑↑
Stroke volume	↑	↑↑↑↑↑	↑↑↑↑↑↑	↑↑↑↑↑↑	↑↑↑↑↑	↑↑↑↑↑
Cardiac output	↑↑	↑↑↑↑↑↑	↑↑↑↑↑↑↑	↑↑↑↑↑↑↑	↑↑↑↑↑↑↑	↑↑↑↑↑↑↑↑
Systemic vascular resistance	↓↓	↓↓↓↓↓	↓↓↓↓↓↓	↓↓↓↓↓↓	↓↓↓↓↓↓	↓↓↓↓↓
Left ventricular ejection fraction	↑	↑↑	↑↑	↑↑	↑	↑

[a]↑, ≤5%; ↑↑, 6–10%; ↑↑↑, 11–15%; ↑↑↑↑, 16–20%; ↑↑↑↑↑, 21–30%; ↑↑↑↑↑↑, >30%; ↑↑↑↑↑↑↑, >40%.

Source: Modified from Robson et al, *Am J Physiol* 1989;256:H1060–H1065.

gleton pregnancies, but values were significantly higher (Fig. 1.2), with a difference of approximately 20%. The rise in blood volume during pregnancy has important clinical implications. A significant direct correlation was found between total growth and birth weight and extent of plasma volume expansion.[4,9,17,18,20] In addition, intrauterine growth retardation,[23] small for gestational age babies, and preeclampsia,[21] have all been associated with reduced blood volume expansion. Such situations thus impose a substantially greater than normal demand on the cardiocirculatory system which, especially in the case of an associated heart disorder, may lead to rapid decompensation. The volume of the extracellular fluid space is determined by sodium and water accumulation.[21] Normal pregnancy is associated with accumulation of approximately 900 mmol of sodium, which must be a result of change in the factors promoting sodium excretion and retention.

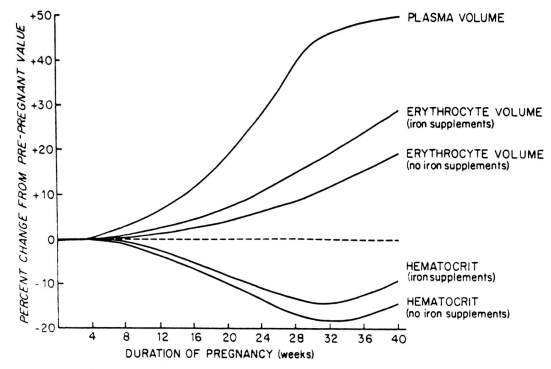

Figure 1.1   Changes in plasma volume, erythrocyte volume, and hematocrit during pregnancy. Increase in plasma volume is more rapid than increase in erythrocyte volume, causing the "physiological anemia of pregnancy," which can be partially corrected with iron supplements. (From Pitkin RM, *Clin Obstet Gynecol* 1976;19:489, with permission.)

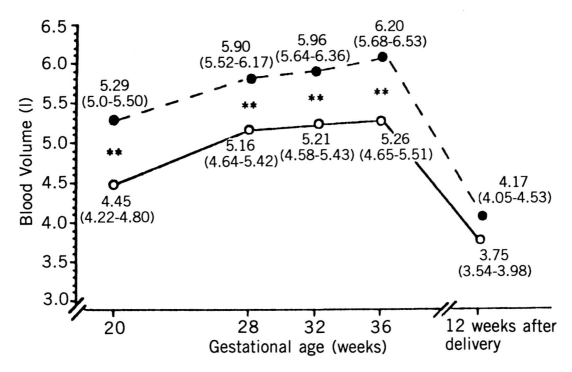

Figure 1.2   Changes in blood volume during twin pregnancy (solid circles, $N = 10$) and singleton pregnancy (open circles, $N = 40$). (From Thomson et al, *Acta Obstet Gynecol Scand* 1994;73:14–20, with permission.)

There is an increase in red blood cell mass during pregnancy that ranges from 17 to 40%.[8] However, since plasma volume increase is larger and more rapid, hemoglobin concentration falls during pregnancy, a situation that has been called the "physiologic anemia of pregnancy." Hematocrit levels can be as low as 33–38%, and hemoglobin levels can reach 11–12 g/100 mL.[16,24] The pattern of change in hematocrit is characterized by a gradual decrease until week 30, followed by a gradual increase afterward. Regular administration of iron is followed by a rise in hemoglobin concentration up to nonpregnancy levels and results in an increase in the oxygen-carrying capacity of the maternal blood.[25] Treatment with iron in the last trimester of gestation also results in a significant rise in hemoglobin.[26]

Mechanisms of Hypervolemia in Pregnancy   The mechanisms leading to hypervolemia in pregnancy are still not entirely understood and seem to be multifactorial (Fig. 1.3). Some of the changes in maternal plasma volume may be attributable to changes in fluid balance, mediated by the steroid hormones of pregnancy.[27] Estrogen promotes sodium retention both by direct renal action and by increased hepatic production of renin substrate.[21] Exogenous estrogen has been demonstrated to correct blood volume reduction following bilateral oophorectomy.[28] This role of estrogen is further supported by the increase in blood volume observed in other high estrogen conditions such as the use of oral contraceptives,[29] estradiol treatment in postmenopausal women,[30] estrogen treatment for prostatic carcinoma,[31] and stilbestrol therapy for carcinoma of the breast.[32]

Plasma levels of renin, which is produced during pregnancy not only in the kidneys but also the uterus and liver,[33] are elevated during gestation. This effect has been attributed to the action of estrogens.[34–36] The increase in renin, which stimulates aldosterone secretion, is associated with sodium retention and an increase in total body water.[37,38] Since primary hyperaldosteronism is also characterized by increased blood volume,[39] the importance of hyperaldosteronism in the genesis of hypervolemia in pregnancy appears to be confirmed.

In a recent review, Duvekot and Peeters[24] suggested a possible involvement of several other hormones in enhancing sodium retention during pregnancy. These hormones include desoxycorticosterone, prostaglandins, estrogens, prolactin, placental lactogen, growth hormone, and adrenocorticotrophic hormone. In addition, the upright and supine postures of the mother favor salt retention.[40] The effect of the uteroplacental unit, a large arteriovenous fistula, and the increased ureteral pressure secondary to partial obstruction may also be contributing to sodium retention.[40] The role of

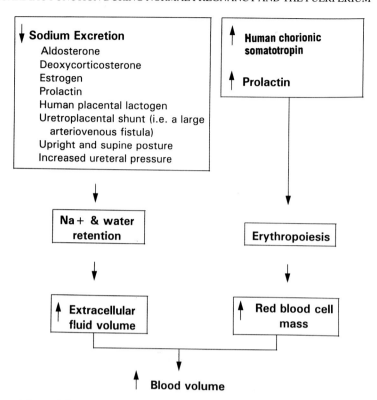

Figure 1.3   Potential mechanisms of hypervolemia during pregnancy.

atrial natriuretic factor (ANF) in mediating changes in fluid balance during gestation is still unclear. An increased level of ANF during the last trimester of pregnancy has been reported by some investigators,[41] while others found a decrease in its level during the same period.[22,42]

A fetus is not essential for the development of hypervolemia. A 50% increase in volume has also been reported with hydatidiform moles.[19] Chesley and Duffus[43] demonstrated that posture affects the evaluation of plasma volume in late pregnancy. Volume appears to decline in the supine position because the enlarged uterus occludes the inferior vena cava and traps blood in the legs.

Cardiac Output

One of the more significant hemodynamic phenomena during pregnancy is the change in cardiac output (CO). The first assessment of change in CO in pregnancy dates to 1915, when Lindhard[44] reported an increment of 50%. His study was followed by numerous investigations using various techniques for the measurement of CO, including the direct Fick principle,[43,45] dilution techniques,[46,48] impedance cardiography,[40] and, most recently, echocardiography[41,49–53] and Doppler techniques.[54]

It is generally agreed that CO begins to rise during the first trimester, probably around the 5th to 10th week of pregnancy. The peak increment in CO has been reported by most investigators between the 25th and 35th weeks of gestation.[48,49–54a] Robson et al,[49] who performed serial hemodynamic measurements in 13 women before conception and then at monthly intervals throughout pregnancy, showed a significant increase in CO by 5 weeks of gestation, with progressive increase until 24 weeks, by which time CO was increased 43–48% (Fig. 1.4). Cardiac output was then maintained until term. Similar results were also shown by Mabie et al.[51] These investigators, however, showed an increase in cardiac output even in late pregnancy, with a peak effect occurring at 38 weeks. Easterling et al[54] reported a steady rise in CO until 34 weeks, when it reached 40% above postpartum values. From 34 weeks until last determination prior to delivery, values varied between individuals, with an increase of ≥ 1.0 L/min in 29% of women and a ≥ 1.0 L/min fall in 9% of cases.

Cardiac output is the product of stroke volume and pulse rate. The rise in CO early in pregnancy is disproportionately greater than the increase in heart rate[49] and therefore is attributable mostly to the augmentation in stroke volume (Fig. 1.4). As pregnancy advances, heart rate increases and becomes a more predominant factor in increasing CO.[49,51] Stroke volume seems to increase gradually until the end of the second trimester; then it remains at the same level or shows a mild decrease during the third trimester.[49,51]

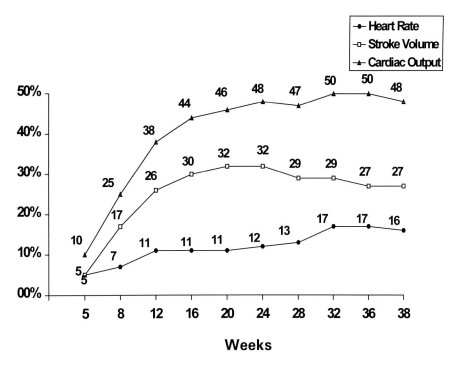

Figure 1.4   Percent changes of heart rate, stroke volume, and cardiac output measured in the lateral position throughout pregnancy compared to prepregnancy values. (Modified from Robson et al, *Am J Physiol* 1989;256:H1060–H1065.)

A unique and important hemodynamic phenomenon of pregnancy is the fluctuation in resting CO with changes in position.[55–57] Compression of the inferior vena cava by the enlarged gravid uterus in the supine position results in a decreased venous return to the heart and a significant decrease in CO (Fig. 1.5). The effect of maternal posture on CO was demonstrated by several investigators. A significant decrease (25–30%) in CO, when measured by dye dilution technique, was demonstrated in the supine position between the 38th and 40th weeks of pregnancy but not before the 24th week.[55–57] Since heart rate was not affected, it was concluded that positional decline in cardiac output was due to decreased stroke volume. Evaluation of hemodynamic changes during twin pregnancy has recently shown a significantly greater increase in CO compared to singleton pregnancy (approximately 15% at 24 weeks.)[50]

Effect of the Gravid Uterus on the Circulation

The hemodynamic effect of the gravid uterus was first alluded to in 1953 by Howard et al,[58] who showed an elevated pressure in the femoral vein of pregnant women. Radiologic studies have demonstrated an obstruction of the vena cava in approximately 90% of women who were studied in the supine position.[58–62] Lifting the uterus away from the vena cava during laparotomy resulted in a significant fall in caval pressure. The same effect was noted when a lateral recumbent position was assumed (Fig. 1.5).[59] The effect of changes in maternal posture was found to be diminished when the fetal head was engaged in the pelvis. This is probably because engagement restricts uterine mobility.[60] The remarkable degree of caval compression by the gravid uterus in late stages of pregnancy was demonstrated over 30 years ago, when Kerr et al[59,60] showed that caval pressures recorded in the supine position before delivery were comparable to pressures obtained by complete manual obstruction of the vena cava during surgery. These investigators also noted that a paravertebral, collateral circulation develops during pregnancy which permits blood from the legs and the pelvic organs to bypass the occluded inferior caval vein.[60] Simultaneous pressure recordings obtained by direct methods from different arteries have given highly persuasive evidence that the vascular compression exerted by the uterus involved not only the inferior vena cava but also the aorta and its branches.[61] In 1968 Bieniarz et al[62] used angiographic techniques and demonstrated an aortoiliac compression in late pregnancy. The aorta was found to be laterally displaced and, during uterine relaxation, less densely

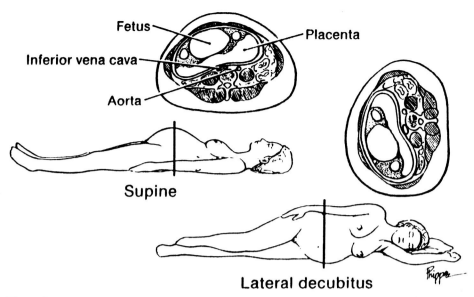

Figure 1.5   Venocaval compression of the inferior vena cava and abdominal aorta by the gravid uterus can lead to reduced venous return and thus to decreased cardiac output.

opacified at the region of lumbar lordosis (vertebrae L4 and L5). The aortic displacement was increased during uterine contractions, and the common iliac artery, crossing vertebrae L4 and L5, was transiently occluded. The right renal artery was found in some cases to be stretched, elongated, blurred, and less opaque at the point of crossing the convexity of the vertebra. Other aortic branches, such as the ovarian and lumbar arteries, were similarly blurred and less dense.

Supine Hypotensive Syndrome of Pregnancy

A posture-induced fall in cardiac output is normally followed by a compensatory increase in peripheral resistance, and therefore no significant change in systemic blood pressure or heart rate occurs.[59] Occasionally, however, a significant increase in heart rate and a fall in blood pressure can be seen, resulting in symptoms such as weakness, lightheadedness, nausea, dizziness, and even syncope.[59,61–66] This phenomenon, described as the "supine hypotensive syndrome of pregnancy,"[67] is usually relieved promptly when the supine position is abandoned.[64]

The incidence of the supine hypotensive syndrome ranges in different reports from 0.5% to 11.2%.[58–60,65] It has been widely assumed that this syndrome derives from acute occlusion of the inferior vena cava, owing to the pressure exerted by the pregnant uterus in the supine position (Fig. 1.5).[65] Supine caval occlusion is, however, a common occurrence in late pregnancy, being found regardless of whether the patient shows a tendency to develop the supine hypotensive syndrome. Ligation of the iliac veins in pregnant

and nonpregnant animals resulted in no major change in heart rate and blood pressure, confirming the assumption that the supine hypotensive syndrome is not caused solely by mechanical compression of the inferior vena cava.[66] Some investigators have proposed that women developing the supine hypotensive syndrome have poorly developed collateral systems of the paravertebral circulation, possibly associated with a strong tendency toward vasovagal attacks.[56]

A recent study by Pirhonen and Erkkola showed a significant increase in uterine artery systolic/diastolic ratio in the supine position in 10 healthy women 33–41 weeks pregnant who had signs of the supine hypotensive syndrome.[64] Two patients evidenced concomitantly a transient deceleration in the fetal heart rate. Hirabayashi et al,[67] who described a case of severe supine hypotensive syndrome in a parturient with breech presentation during cesarean section with poor response to left tilt, emphasized the importance of trying right tilt if left tilt is ineffective. It should be noted that although the supine hypotensive syndrome is usually recognizable by maternal symptoms, severe asymptomatic hypotension may occur.[65]

Heart Rate

Heart rate (HR) rises during pregnancy with a mean increase of about 10–20 beats per minute at term (Table 1.1, Fig. 1.3). Mean values vary from 78–89 beats per minute.[41,49,51] Twin pregnancies are associated with an earlier acceleration of the HR and a higher HR during pregnancy compared to singleton pregnancy.[50] The HR decreases slightly with a change from the supine to the lateral position.[68,69] The rise in HR is gradual with a peak at the third trimester.[49,51]

Systemic Arterial Blood Pressure

Rubler et al[70] demonstrated a lack of significant differences in blood pressure (BP) between nonpregnant women and women at different stages of pregnancy. However, most longitudinal studies observing the same group of women as they advance through pregnancy have demonstrated a slight fall of arterial BP.[24,49,51,71–73] The decrease in BP starts in the first trimester and reaches a peak in midpregnancy, when BP starts a gradual rise, reaching or exceeding prepregnancy levels (Table 1.1, Fig. 1.3) before term.[51,54] The magnitude of the change varies from study to study.

Several issues related to BP during pregnancy should be considered. First, the reliable measurement of the diastolic pressure has been complicated by the absence of a fifth Korotkoff sound in some women. This may be related to the hyperdynamic state of maternal circulation, which may cause the fifth Korotkoff sound to be heard even after complete deflation of the cuff.[74] At the same time, however, the fifth Korotkoff sound can be heard in most pregnant women and is more accurate than the fourth sound when compared to results obtained from invasive BP measurements.[75,76] The diastolic BP measured with the use of the fourth sound will be 5–13 mmHg higher than that measured using the fifth sound and may lead to an erroneous conclusion. The use of the fifth sound is therefore recommended for the measurement of diastolic BP during gestation.[77] The use of automated cuff measurement of BP may avoid many operator-dependent biases associated with measurement of BP by auscultation.[74,78] A second important issue is the patient's position, which may greatly influence levels of recorded BP during pregnancy. In general, blood pressures, both systolic and diastolic, are approximately 16 mmHg higher in the sitting position than in the recumbent position.[79] After midpregnancy, because of a potential of caval occlusion in the recumbent position, pressure should be measured in the lateral position. Systolic blood pressure is approximately 12 mmHg lower in the first trimester compared to postpartum values, while diastolic pressure decrease is slightly longer. Both increasing age and parity appear to be associated with higher systolic and diastolic blood pressures during pregnancy.[72,73] Hypertension in pregnancy is defined as increments in systolic and diastolic BP of ≥30 and ≥15 mmHg, respectively, or a diastolic pressure of ≥90 mmHg as measured on more than one occasion[80] (see Chapter 22).

Systemic Vascular Resistance

A significant fall in systemic vascular resistance (SVR) occurs during pregnancy (Table 1.1), resulting in a fall in blood pressure, mainly of the diastolic component, and a widening of pulse pressure. Clark et al[48] found SVR to be reduced to 21% between 36 and 38 weeks gestation, versus 11–13 weeks postpartum in 10 normal primiparous patients.[49] Robson et al,[49] who performed serial hemodynamic measurements throughout pregnancy, showed a gradual fall in SVR starting as early as 5 weeks gestation (9%), with a maximum decrease at 20 weeks (34%). Values of SVR remained constant between the 20th and 32nd weeks, with a slight increase seen from week 32 until term. Systemic vascular resistance during the 38 weeks was still 27% lower than preconception values. Similar findings were described by Easterling et al,[54] who performed serial evaluations from the 10th week of gestation to the early postpartum period.

The mechanisms for decreased systemic vascular resistance in pregnancy are not clear. The administration of oral contraceptives containing both estrogen and progestational compounds results in a fall in SVR.[81] Administration of estrogen and prolactin to animals has produced significant effects on vascular resistance.[82,83]

On the basis of the foregoing observations, it seems likely that there is a relationship between changes in SVR during pregnancy and hormonal activity. In addition, increased levels of circulating prostaglandins PGE_2 and PGI_2 may lead to direct vasodilation.[84,85] Prostacyclin also may be responsible for attenuation of the vasoconstrictor effect of angiotensin II described during pregnancy. Resistance to the pressor effect of angiotensin and noradrenaline may also contribute to a fall in SVR.[86,87] Suggested mechanisms for this phenomenon include receptor down-regulation[88] and counterregulatory effects of vasodilating prostaglandins.[89] Recent evidence suggests that nitric oxide (NO) may also be related to gestational vasodilation.[90] Increased production of NO has been suggested by documented increased in the urinary excretion of its derivatives NO_2/NO_3 under basal condition in the pregnant rats.

Regional Blood Flow (Table 1.2)

Uterine Blood Flow   A significant increase in uterine blood flow occurs during normal human pregnancy. Earlier studies using electromagnetic flowmeters have shown a rise of uterine blood flow from approximately 50 mL/min at the 10th week of gestation to around 200 mL/min at the 28th week and to 500 mL/min at term.[91,92] Later studies using placental scintigraphy suggested that uterine flow may, in the lateral position, rise to a high of 1200 mL/min at 37 weeks of gestation. The rise in uterine blood flow is made possible by a progressive fall in vascular resistance. Recent use of Doppler technology has allowed the demonstration of changes in vascular resistance, which are reflected by changes in uterine blood flow velocity and waveform.[93–97]

These studies have confirmed an increase in blood velocity concomitant to a fall in impedance to flow in the uteroplacental circulation.[93] The characteristic increase in diastolic uteroplacental blood flow occurs as early as in the 5th week of gestation.[94] Compared to nonpregnant values, there is an increase in iliac artery flow and a decrease in external

TABLE 1.2   Changes in Regional Blood Flow During Normal Pregnancy

Organ	Change[a]	Comments
Uterus	↑	Progressive rise from 50 mL/min at 10 weeks up to 1200 mL/min at 37 weeks
Kidneys	↑	30–80% increase accompanied by 50% increase in glomerular filtration rate, returns to nonpregnant state at term
Extremities	↑	Increased flow to the hands higher than to the legs
Skin	↑	Results in warm skin, clammy hands, vascular spiders, palm erythema, and nasal congestion
Liver	↔	
Brain	↔	
Breast	↑	Indirect evidence, may cause continuous murmurs
Coronary arteries	?	Data not available

[a]↑, increase; ↔, no significant change.

iliac artery flow, suggesting redistribution of pelvic blood flow as a cause for pregnancy associated rise in uterus artery flow.[97] Changes in uteroplacental vascular resistance and blood flow continue until 24–25 weeks and remain unchanged thereafter.[98] The low placental vascular resistance has been attributed to a lack of nervous influences and an increased level of vasodilators such as prostacyclin and nitric oxide. In addition, it has been suggested that an increase in the activity of the enzyme Na^+/K^+-ATPase in placental smooth muscle and endothelial cells causes stabilization of smooth muscle cell membranes and thus contributes to maintenance of low vascular resistance.[99]

Experiments with animals have shown a correlation between fetal size and uteroplacental blood flow.[100,101] A marked increase in blood flow in a patient with a twin pregnancy described by Metcalfe et al[92] suggests a similar relationship in humans. Because of the increase in intramural pressure, uterine blood flow falls significantly during contractions. Animal studies have shown a decrease in uterine blood flow during exercise, due to diversion of blood to skeletal muscles.[99,102] A recent study by Erkkola et al demonstrated an association of strenuous exercise with a substantial increase (30%) in uterine artery impedance, which directly correlated to the increase of heart rate. These findings support animal studies that showed a fall in uterine blood flow during heavy exercise.[103]

Renal Blood Flow   Renal blood flow increases markedly during normal pregnancy. In the early stages of gestation, renal blood flow increases gradually and significantly and in midpregnancy is 60–80% above the nonpregnant state. In the third trimester, it is increased approximately 50%.[40,104,105]

Concomitantly, there is an increase in glomerular filtration rate (GFR) throughout pregnancy.[106] Between 9 and 11 weeks, GFR reaches a peak of 50% higher than the nonpregnant level which is sustained until the end of pregnancy (Fig. 1.6).[24,106–108] With progression of pregnancy, renal blood flow becomes very sensitive to change in body position. While flow increase may be preserved in the lateral position, it is lower in the supine, sitting, or upright position.[105]

Changes in renal flow during pregnancy are believed to be mediated by steroid hormones.[109] A study by Gallery et al[110] showed no significant effect of prostacyclin on renal flow and GFR in spite of central hemodynamic effects. This observation suggests that changes in renal hemodynamics during pregnancy are not caused by prostacyclin.

Extremities Flow   Blood flow through the hands rises progressively from the early weeks of pregnancy until delivery.[111] The flow subsides during the puerperium and returns to nonpregnant levels over several weeks. Significant elevation can still be present by the 6th week postpartum. Blood flow to the legs and feet shows similar, though less striking, changes. In addition, in the last part of pregnancy, blood flow to the legs may fall as a result of the aortic and vena caval compression by the large uterus. The flow is somewhat higher in twin pregnancy after the 30th week of gestation than in single pregnancies.

Skin Perfusion   A significant increase in skin perfusion has been found during pregnancy.[112] Specifically, there is a slow but steady rise up to 18–20 weeks of gestation, followed by a sharp and substantial rise between the 20th and 30th weeks, and no significant change thereafter. The increase in skin per-

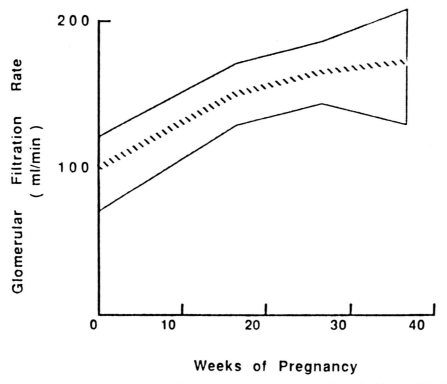

Figure 1.6 Changes in glomerular filtration rate during pregnancy. (From Davidson and Dunlop, *Semin Nephrol* 1984;4:198–207, with permission.)

fusion was maintained for at least one week postpartum. Increased blood flow in the skin causes a considerable increase in skin temperature,[113] manifested clinically by typically warm skin and clammy hands.

Microscopic examination of the nail bed reveals capillary dilatation in most pregnant women.[23] Vascular spiders and palm erythema are seen during pregnancy in about 60% of white women and are an additional sign of vasodilation.[114] Another area in which blood flow increases during pregnancy is the membrane of the nasal mucosae. This explains the common finding of nasal congestion in pregnancy.[115]

Mammary Blood Flow   Mammary blood flow has not been measured directly in humans. However, indirect estimations by plethysmography and thermometry suggested a progressive increase of flow during pregnancy, reaching a peak in the early postpartum period.[116] The augmented mammary flow is evidenced by engorgement of the breasts, starting early in pregnancy, and dilatation of the veins in the surface of the breasts, which is usually accompanied by the sensations of heat and tingling. Increased mammary blood flow can be accompanied by a continuous murmur (Chapter 2).

Flow to Other Organs   Early studies showed no significant changes in hepatic and cerebral blood flow during pregnan-

cy.[117,118] The effect of pregnancy on coronary blood flow is still unknown. An increase due to the augmentation in cardiac output is likely, however.

Oxygen Consumption

Oxygen consumption, commonly estimated by measurement of oxygen extracted by the lungs over a given time period, reflects the rate of the body's metabolism. In pregnancy, there is a progressive increase in resting oxygen consumption, with a peak increase of 20–30% near term.[119] The rise in oxygen consumption can be attributed to the increased metabolic needs of the mother and her growing fetus. A very obvious discrepancy between the dynamics of change in cardiac output and oxygen consumption during pregnancy has been reported. While most of the increase in cardiac output occurs during the early part of pregnancy, with a peak increase around the 20th week, oxygen consumption shows a gradual rise throughout pregnancy, reaching its peak near term. It has been suggested that this discrepancy supports reproductive needs. A rapid increase in cardiac output that is proportionally greater than the rise in oxygen consumption, especially in early gestation, results in the flow of well-oxygenated blood to the uterus when it is most needed for organogenesis, before the fetoplacental circulation is fully developed.[120]

The continuous increase in oxygen consumption in the later phases of pregnancy, when cardiac output increase is slow and small, results in a widening of the arterial venous oxygen difference to nonpregnant levels. The arterial venous oxygen difference is, therefore, small in early pregnancy, increases gradually throughout pregnancy, and reaches nonpregnant levels in the latter part of gestation.

Cardiac Function During Pregnancy

Katz et al[71] utilized echocardiography to serially evaluate left ventricular response to the chronic volume overload state of pregnancy. In spite of a progressive increase in left ventricular dimensions and volume, no significant change could be found in several indices of left ventricular systolic function, including ejection fraction, percent fractional shortening, and mean normalized rate of internal diameter shortening. Left ventricular volume overload also did not result in thickening of the left ventricular walls. Rubler et al[70] reported an increase in left ventricular myocardial contractility, measured echocardiographically during pregnancy. These authors found an increased velocity of myocardial circumferential fiber shortening and posterior wall slope during pregnancy. More recently, several other investigators have used echocardiography for the assessment of left ventricular systolic function in pregnancy. Capeless et al[53] performed serial echocardiographical evaluations before conception and then at 8, 16, and 24 weeks gestation in eight women with normal pregnancies. The study, performed in the left lateral recumbent position, demonstrated increases in left ventricular ejection fraction from 61 ± 2% before pregnancy to 64 ± 2% at 8 weeks, 66 ± 2% at 16 weeks, and 64 ± 2% at 24 weeks. These changes were not statistically significant. Robson et al[49] performed serial echocardiographic evaluations in 13 normal women prior to and then throughout pregnancy. Left ventricular ejection fraction increased gradually and reached its maximum at the 20th gestational week and then decreased gradually to almost prepregnancy values at 38 weeks (Table 1.1). Similar findings were described by the same investigators in a group of patients with twin pregnancies.[50] Mabie et al[51] studied 18 normal pregnancies and found a significant increase in left ventricular fractional shortening during pregnancy, reaching its peak at 20–23 weeks and thereafter remaining constant. In contrast, Clark et al[48] performed invasive hemodynamic monitoring using a pulmonary artery catheter at 36–38 weeks of gestation. These investigators found no difference in the level of left ventricular filling pressure and left ventricular stroke work index compared to 11–13 weeks postpartum.

In summary, the majority of studies have demonstrated a gradual improvement in left ventricular systolic function starting early in pregnancy, progressing gradually until the 20th week of gestation, and then remaining constant until the end of pregnancy. Since left ventricular systolic function directly correlates with changes in systemic vascular resistance, improvement in systolic function is most likely a result of left ventricular afterload reduction.

CARDIOCIRCULATORY CHANGES DURING LABOR AND DELIVERY

Significant hemodynamic changes observed during labor and delivery can be attributed in large part to pain and anxiety.[121,122] Uterine contractions that are followed by a significant increase of 300–500 mL in central blood volume also contribute to the important circulatory changes.[123,124]

In spite of important differences in methodology and techniques of determination, significant increases in cardiac output during labor have been reported consistently.[123–125] Henricks and Quilligan[121] in 1956 used the pulse pressure method to evaluate cardiac output in 47 women in various stages of labor. They noted a 31% rise in cardiac output over the relaxed state between uterine contractions. Other studies, in which the dye dilution technique was used, confirmed their results.[123,125,126] Recent investigations using Doppler and cross-sectional echocardiography of the pulmonary valve showed an increase in cardiac output from a prelabor mean value of 6.99 to 7.88 L/min at cervical dilatation of 8 cm or greater as a result of augmentation of both stroke volume and heart rate.[127] Cardiac output augmentation increased progressively during labor: 17% at 3 cm or less, 23% at 4–7 cm, and 34% at 8 cm or more. Smaller increments in cardiac output were reported by Lee et al[128] during contractions in women laboring under epidural anesthesia. A cumulative increase in cardiac output between contractions, demonstrated by serial measurements throughout labor, was most obvious in the late stage of labor and in prolonged labor. In the lateral position, cardiac output between contractions is higher than in the supine position, and the increase during contractions is smaller.[129] Cardiac output increase was smaller in patients receiving caudal analgesia than in women treated with local anesthesia.

It has been postulated that squeezing of the uterus during contractions results in an increase in circulating blood volume and venous return to the heart and is, therefore, the major mechanism behind the increasing cardiac output. The increase of pulmonary arterial venous oxygen difference during each uterine contraction also suggests a sudden flow of blood from the maternal uterine vascular bed into the systemic circulation.[130] Henricks and Quilligan[121] have demonstrated clearly that pain and anxiety alone have a significant hemodynamic effect that is associated with a 50–61% increase in cardiac output. Since the increase of cardiac output during contraction was found to be accompanied by a rise in blood pressure and pulse rate, some investigators suggested that increased sympathetic tone due to pain, anxiety, and muscular activity was the major cause for the increased cardiac output during contraction, and that squeezing of blood from the uterus was of only secondary importance.[123]

The reported effect of uterine contraction on heart rate is variable. Robson et al[127] found a tachycardic response to contractions, with a peak increase of 19% at cervical dilatation of ≧8 cm in the left semilateral position. Other investigators also reported an increase in heart rate following uterine contraction. However, the increase was found to be smaller.[123,131,132] These data are at variance with the results of Kjeldsen,[133] who showed no significant change in heart rate during contractions, and those of Ueland and Hansen,[129] who demonstrated that uterine contractions were almost invariably accompanied by slowing of the heart rate. A similar decrease in heart rate during uterine contraction, observed by Henricks,[134] was thought to be a result of baroreceptor stimulation. The discrepancy in reported heart rate responses to uterine contractions may be explained in terms of the differences in position and forms of sedation used during labor.[123] Different results have also been assumed to reflect the very significant variations of individual heart rate responses to uterine contraction.[133] Lee et al[128] showed a smaller increase in cardiac output during contractions in women laboring under epidural anesthesia.

Both the systolic and diastolic blood pressures increase during uterine contractions.[121–127] The elevation of blood pressure was shown to precede the uterine contraction by 5–8 seconds. Blood pressure returned to resting levels when the contraction subsided. Cunningham[125] confirmed these findings and also showed a progressive increase in blood pressure with a peak in the second stage of labor. Since the peripheral resistance changes only slightly during labor, the increase in blood pressure is attributed to the rise in cardiac output.[123] Redistribution of maternal cardiac output to the upper part of the peripheral circulation after compression of the distal aorta and the common iliac artery has also been suggested to play a role in the elevation of systemic pressures as measured in the arm.[63]

The hemodynamic effect of uterine contractions is less pronounced in lateral recumbency than in the supine position.[133] The effect on cardiac output of an ineffective uterine contraction is unpredictable and inconsistent.[121,124] Oxygen consumption increases about threefold during uterine contraction. Its mean value increases gradually to levels 100% higher than measured prior to labor.[135]

Hemodynamic changes during labor are markedly influenced by the form of anesthesia or analgesia employed (Chapter 24). Ueland and Hansen[124] demonstrated substantial differences between women receiving local and paracervical block anesthetics and others who received caudal anesthesia. In general, caudal anesthesia does not affect the hemodynamic changes due to uterine contractions. The decrease in pain and apprehension abolishes, however, the progressive rise in cardiac output that is seen between contractions and limits the absolute increase of cardiac output at delivery. Both caudal and local anesthesia failed to alter significantly the cardiovascular response to uterine contractions. These forms of anesthesia have been shown to be safe in patients with severe heart disease. In the supine position, contractions of the uterus increase cardiac output approximately 15–20% regardless of either stage of labor or method of analgesia.[136]

When local anesthesia is used, tachycardia may develop during the second stage of labor and can be accentuated by uterine contractions. Both the systolic and diastolic blood pressures show a mild gradual rise during the first stage of labor and a significant increase during the second stage. These changes are associated with a progressive increase in stroke volume toward a peak immediately following delivery. In contrast, caudal anesthesia is associated with no significant change in heart rate, and both the diastolic and systolic blood pressures are maintained constant throughout labor and delivery. The stroke volume is also maintained throughout labor but rises rapidly after delivery. No difference could be found between local and caudal anesthesia with regard to mean blood volume loss during delivery.[124]

HEMODYNAMIC EFFECTS OF CESAREAN SECTION

More stable hemodynamics were noted in normal pregnant women undergoing cesarean section under epidural anesthesia without epinephrine.[139] The administration of anesthesia was followed by only minor hemodynamic changes. Blood pressure showed a moderate decline after induction of anesthesia, but then remained constant throughout the surgical procedure. There were no significant changes in heart rate, cardiac output, or stroke volume. Following delivery, cardiac output showed a relatively mild increase (25% above control values), and there was no change in heart rate.

In summary maternal hemodynamics during cesarean section can be significantly affected by anesthesia. The marked fluctuations with subarachnoid block anesthesia may not be tolerated by a patient with heart disease. Balanced anesthesia with thiopentol, nitrous oxide, and succinylcholine, and epidural anesthesia without epinephrine, are associated with smaller hemodynamic fluctuations and therefore should be preferred in patients with limited cardiac reserves.

HEMODYNAMIC CHANGES POSTPARTUM

In spite of the external hemorrhage associated with delivery, cardiac output is significantly higher 1–2 hours postpartum than prior to the initiation of contractions.[123,124] An increase in cardiac output of 60–80% occurs immediately after delivery, followed by a rapid decrease within 10 minutes to values approaching those found 1 hour postpartum. The high cardiac output state following delivery is probably the result of the shift of blood from the emptied uterus into the systemic circulation ("autotransfusion") and a decrease in caval compression, allowing an increased venous return to the heart. The placental separation, per se, was not found to cause any further hemodynamic changes. The increase in cardiac output was reported to remain almost unchanged for days and even weeks postpartum.[13] Robson et al,[127] however, found returns of heart rate and cardiac output (measured by the Doppler technique) to prelabor values by one hour after delivery and of mean blood pressure and stroke volume by 24 hours after delivery. A 10% loss of blood volume was noted 1–10 hours postpartum in patient delivering vaginally.[9,126] Cesarean section was associated with a more significant loss of 17–29%. No change in hematocrit was noted, however, in either group. After vaginal delivery, a steady decline in blood volume was seen over the next several days. In the surgically delivered group, blood volume remained stable from one hour to several days after the operation. When studied after the third postpartum day, the blood volumes in both groups were found to be 10% lower than the predelivery values.[129]

Robson et al[140,141] performed two investigations using a Doppler and M-mode echocardiography with the aim of studying hemodynamic changes during the puerperium in healthy women with uncomplicated singleton pregnancies. The patients were studied at 38 weeks gestation and then at 48 hours and 2, 6, 12, and 24 weeks after delivery (Fig. 1.7). There was a 13% decrease in heart rate at 48 hours and a 21% decrease at 2 weeks after delivery, with no further change after that period. Stroke volume increased 10% 48 hours following delivery and was decreased 8–10% 2 weeks postpartum, with further significant decrease (17–19%) occurring 24 weeks postpartum. Change in cardiac output was not reported at 48 hours but showed a significant decrease (27–29%) by 2 weeks after delivery with a gradual decline to a maximum decrease of 32–34% at 24 weeks.

End diastolic dimension of the left ventricle measured by M-mode echocardiogram did not change between 38 weeks of pregnancy and 48 hours postdelivery but declined slightly (4%) at 24 weeks postpartum (Table 1.3). There was no change in left ventricular end systolic dimension. Left atrial dimension decreased 11% and left ventricular wall thickness and mass decreased significantly (16 and 23%, respectively) at 24 weeks while left ventricular ejection fraction peak LV dD/dt (rate of change of dimension) and mean V_{cf} (rate of circumferential fiber shortening) showed a significant fall following pregnancy. Both systemic blood pressures demonstrated a small but a statistically significant increase 24 hours postpartum when compared to 38 weeks gestation.

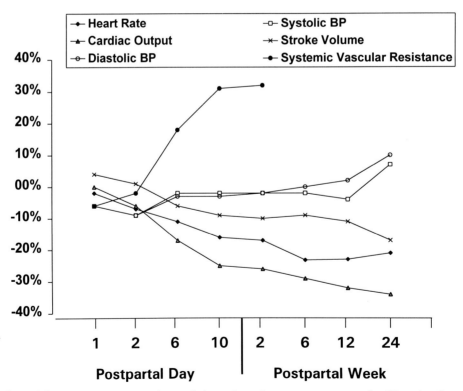

Figure 1.7   Percent postpartum changes in hemodynamic parameters compared to 38 weeks of gestation. (From Robson et al, *Br J Obstet Gynaecol* 1987;94:1028–1035, with permission.)

**TABLE 1.3   Values of Echocardiographic Parameters
at 38 Weeks of Gestation and Postpartum**

Parameter	Pregnancy: 38 Weeks	Postnatal Weeks			
		2	6	12	24
End systolic dimension (cm)	3.22	3.30	3.23	3.22	3.17
End diastolic dimension (cm)	4.86	4.75	4.72	4.68	4.17
LA dimension (cm)	3.74	3.42	3.45	3.36	3.33
Total LV thickness (cm)	2.01	1.97	1.94	1.81	1.69
LV mass (g)	203	191	182	167	157
Ejection fraction (%)	70	67	68	67	67
Mean V_{cf} (diam/s)	1.27	1.09	1.08	1.05	1.07

Abbreviations: LA, left atrial; LV, left ventricular; V_{cf}, velocity of circumferential shortening.
(From Robson et al., *Br J Obstet Gynaecol* 1987; 1028–1035, with permission.)

In 10 women who experienced postpartum hemorrhage,[142] stroke volume was significantly lower and heart rate significantly higher compared to control group, during the first 48 hours following delivery. Blood pressure and cardiac output were not significantly different from values in the control group.

Although cesarean sections are often performed to avoid the marked hemodynamic alterations associated with labor, this mode of delivery should not be selected for that reason alone. Since the surgical procedure and some of the anesthetic techniques are also associated with major hemodynamic changes. Ueland et al,[137–139] as a part of an overall investigation of the maternal cardiovascular response to labor and delivery, reported the effect of cesarean section under various anesthetic agents. Ueland et al[137] also studied the effect of subarachnoid block anesthesia on maternal cardiodynamics in 12 women undergoing cesarean sections for obstetric reasons. Between 5 and 10 minutes following the administration of the spinal anesthetic, the investigators observed a significant decrease in stroke volume and cardiac output, associated with a marked increase in heart rate and a decline in blood pressure. Hemodynamic changes did not correlate with either the dose or the level of anesthesia. The hypotension did not seem to have a deleterious effect on the newborn infant and could be completely reversed by turning the patient on her side. The authors concluded that cesarean section under spinal anesthesia is associated with significant cardiovascular changes, and they recommended that this form of anesthesia not be used in patients with heart disease.

The hemodynamic fluctuations were found to be significantly smaller when cesarean section was performed under thiopentol, nitrous oxide, and succinylcholine anesthesia.[138] Cardiac output did not change significantly, whereas the heart rate increased slightly and diastolic pressure increased moderately. Delivery was followed by some increase in stroke volume and cardiac output, accompanied by a slight decrease in heart rate and blood pressure.

REFERENCES

1. Miller JR, Keith NM, Rownreel LG. Plasma and blood volume in pregnancy. *JAMA* 1915;65:779–782.

2. Dieckmann WJ, Wegner CR. The blood in normal pregnancy. I. Blood and plasma. *Arch Intern Med* 1934;53:71–86.

3. Berlin NI, Goetsch C, Hyde GM, Parsons RJ. The blood volume in pregnancy as determined by P-32-labelled red blood cells. *Surg Gynecol Obstet* 1953;97:173–176.

4. Hytten FE, Pfaintin DB. Increase in plasma volume during normal pregnancy. *J Obstet Gynaecol Br Commonw* 1963;70:402–407.

5. Rovinsky JJ, Jaffin H. Cardiovascular hemodynamics in pregnancy. I. Blood and plasma volumes in multiple pregnancies. *Am J Obstet Gynecol* 1965;93:1–15.

6. Pritchard JA, Rowland RC. Blood volume changes in pregnancy and the puerperium. III. Whole body and large vessel hematocrits in pregnant and nonpregnant women. *Am J Obstet Gynecol* 1964;88:391–395.

7. Lund CJ, Donovan JC. Blood volume during pregnancy. *Am J Obstet Gynecol* 1967;98:393–403.

8. Chesley LC. Plasma and red cell volumes during pregnancy. *Am J Obstet Gynecol* 1972;112:440–450.

9. Ueland K. Maternal cardiovascular dynamics. VII. Intrapartum blood volume changes. *Am J Obstet Gynecol* 1976;126:671–677.

10. Thomson KJ, Hirsheimer A, Gibson JC, Evans WA Jr. Studies on the circulation in pregnancy. III. Blood volume changes in normal pregnant women. *Am J Obstet Gynecol* 1938;36:48–59.

11. Roscoe MH, Donaldson GMM. The blood in pregnancy. II. The blood volume, cell volume and haemoglobin mass. *J Obstet Gynaecol Br Emp* 1946;53:527–538.

12. McLennan CE, Thouin LG. Blood volume in pregnancy. A critical review and preliminary report of result with a new technique. *Am J Obstet Gynecol* 1948;55:189–200.

13. Caton WL, Roby CC, Reid DE, Gibson JG. Plasma volume and extravascular fluid volume during pregnancy and the puerperium. *Am J Obstet Gynecol* 1949;57:471–481.

14. Adams JQ. Cardiovascular physiology in normal pregnancy: studies with the dye dilution technique. *Am J Obstet Gynecol* 1954;67:741–759.

15. Rovinsky JJ. Blood volume and the hemodynamics of pregnancy. In: Philipp EE, Parnes J, Newton M, eds. *Scientific Foundation of Obstetrics and Gynaecology.* Philadelphia: FA Davis; 1970:332–340.

16. Hytten FE, Thomson AM. Maternal physiological adjustments. In: Assali NS, ed. *Biology of Gestation.* New York: Academic Press; 1968:449.

17. Pirani BBK, Campbell DM, MacGillivary I. Plasma volume in normal first pregnancy. *J Obstet Gynaecol Br Commonw* 1973;80:884–887.

18. Goodlin RC, Dobry CA, Anderson JC, Woods RE. Clinical signs of normal plasma volume expansion during pregnancy. *Am J Obstet Gynecol* 1983;145:1001–1007.

19. Pritchard JA. Changes in the blood volume during pregnancy and delivery. *Anesthesiology* 1965;26:393–399.

20. Brown MA, Zammit VC, Mitar DM. Extracellular fluid volumes in pregnancy induced hypertension. *J Hypertension* 1992;10:61–68.

21. Brown MA, Gallery ED. Volume homeostasis in normal pregnancy and preeclampsia: physiology and clinical implications. *Baillieres Clin Obstet Gynecol* 1994;8:287–310.

22. Thomsen JK, Fogh-Andersen N, Jaszczak P. Atrial natriuretic peptide, blood volume, aldosterone, and sodium excretion during twin pregnancy. *Acta Obstet Gynecol Scand* 1994;73:14–20.

23. Salas SP, Rosso P, Espinoza R, Robert, JA, Valdes G, Donoso E. Maternal plasma volume expansion and hormonal changes in women with idiopathic fetal growth retardation. *Obstet Gynecol* 1993;81:1029–1033.

24. Duvekot JJ, Peeters LLH. Renal hemodynamics and volume hemostasis in pregnancy. *Obstet Gynecol Survey* 1994;49:830–839.

25. Butler EB. The effect of iron and folic acid on red cell and plasma volume in pregnancy. *J Obstet Gynaecol Br Commonw* 1968;75:497–510.

26. Pritchard JA. Anemias complicating pregnancy and the puerperium. In: Committee on Maternal Nutrition/Food and Nutrition Board, National Research Council, eds. *Maternal Nutrition and the Course of Pregnancy.* Washington, DC: National Academy of Sciences–National Research Council; 1970;74.

27. Longo LD, Maternal blood volume and cardiac output during pregnancy: a hypothesis of endocrinologic control. *Am J Physiol* 1983;245:R720–R729.

28. Friedlander M, Laskey N, Silbert. Effect of estrogenic substance on blood volume. *Endocrinology* 1936;20:329–332.

29. Walters WA, Lim YL. Haemodynamic changes in women taking oral contraceptives. *J Obstet Gynaecol Br Commonw* 1970;77:1007–1012.

30. Luotola H, Pyorala T, Lahteenmaki P, Toivanen J. Haemodynamic and hormonal effects of short-term oestradiol treatment in post-menopausal women. *Maturitas* 1979;1:287–294.

31. Varenhorst E, Karlberg BE, Wallentin L, Wranne B. Effects of oestrogens, orchidectomy and cyproterone acetate on salt and water metabolism in carcinoma of the prostate. *Eur Urol* 1981;7:231–236.

32. Bateman JC. A study of blood volume and anemia in cancer patients. *Blood* 1951;6:639–651.

33. Broughton Pipkin F. The renin–angiotensin system in normal and hypertensive pregnancies. In: Rubin PC, ed. *Handbook of Hypertension, 10, Hypertension in Pregnancy.* Amsterdam: Elsevier; 1988; 118–167.

34. Crane MG, Harris JJ. Plasma renin activity and aldosterone excretion rate in normal subjects. II. Effect of oral contraceptive agents. *J Clin Endocrinol Metab* 1969;29:558–562.

35. Hsueh WA, Luetscher JA, Carlson EJ, Grislis G, Fraze E, McHargue A. Changes in active and inactive renin throughout pregnancy. *J Clin Endocrinol Metab* 1982;54:1010–1016.

36. Tapia HR, Johnson CE, Strong CG. Effect of oral contraceptive therapy on the renin–angiotensin system in normotensive and hypertensive women. *J Obstet Gynecol* 1973; 41:643–649.

37. Seitchik J. Total body water and total body density of pregnant women. *J Obstet Gynecol* 1967;29:155–166.

38. Preedy JRK, Aitken EH. The effect of estrogen on water and electrolyte metabolism. I. The normal. *J Clin Invest* 1956; 35:423–429.

39. Biglier EG, Forsham PH. Studies on the expanded extracellular fluid and the responses to various stimuli in primary aldosteronism. *Am J Med* 1961;30:564–576.

40. Dafnis E, Sabatini S. The effect of pregnancy on renal function: physiology and pathophysiology. *Am J Med Sci* 1992;303:184–205.

41. Fournier A, Gregoire I, El-Esper N, Lalau JD, Westeel PF, Makdassi R, Fievet P. Atrial natriuretic factors in pregnancy and pregnancy-induced hypertension. *Can J Physiol Pharmacol* 1991;69:1601–1608.

42. Thomsen JK, Fogh-Andersen N, Jaszczak P, Giese J. Atrial natriuretic peptide (ANP) decrease during normal pregnancy as related to hemodynamic changes and volume regulation. *Acta Obstet Gynecol Scand* 1993;72:103–110.

43. Chesley LC, Duffus GM. Posture and apparent plasma volume in late pregnancy. *J Obstet Gynaecol Br Commonw* 1971;78:406–412.

44. Lindhard J. Über das Minutenvolumen des Herzens bei Ruhe und bei Muskelarbeit. *Pfluegers Arch* 1915;161:233–383.

45. Bader RA, Bader MG, Rose DJ, Braunwald E. Hemodynamics at rest and during exercise in normal pregnancy as studied by cardiac catheterization. *J Clin Invest* 1955;34:1524–1536.

46. Walters WAW, MacGregor WG, Hills M. Cardiac output at rest during pregnancy and the puerperium. *Clin Sci* 1966;30:1–11.

47. Lees MM, Taylor SH, Scott DB, Kerr MG. A study of cardiac output at rest throughout pregnancy. *J Obstet Gynaecol Br Commonw* 1967;74:319–328.

48. Clark SL, Cotton DB, Lee W, Bishop C, Hill T, Southwick J, Pivarnik J, Spillman T, DeVore GR, Phelan J, Hankins GDV, Benedetti TJ, Tolley D. Central hemodynamic assessment of normal term pregnancy. *Am J Obstet Gynecol* 1989;161:1439–1442.

49. Robson SC, Hunter S, Boys RJ, Dunlop W. Serial study of factors influencing changes in cardiac output during human pregnancy. *Am J Physiol* 1989;256:H1060–H1065.

50. Robson SC, Hunter S, Boys RJ, Dunlop W. Hemodynamic changes during twin pregnancy: A Doppler and M-mode echocardiographic study 1989;161:1273–1278.

51. Mabie WC, DiSessa TG, Crocker LG, Sibai BM, Arheart KL. A longitudinal study of cardiac output in normal human pregnancy. *Am J Obstet Gynecol* 1994;170:849–856.

52. Vered Z, Poler SM, Gibson P, Wlody D, Perez JE. Noninvasive detection of the morphologic and hemodynamic changes during normal pregnancy. *Clin Cardiol* 1991;14:327–334.

53. Capeless EL, Clapp JF. Cardiovascular changes in early phase of pregnancy. *Am J Obstet Gynecol* 1989;161:1449–1453.

54. Easterling TR, Benedetti TJ, Schmucker BC, Millard SP. Maternal hemodynamics in normal and preeclamptic pregnancies: a longitudinal study. *Obstet Gynecol* 1990;76:1061–1069.

55. Ueland K, Novy MJ, Peterson EN, Metcalfe J. Maternal cardiovascular dynamics. IV. The influence of gestational age on the maternal cardiovascular response to posture and exercise. *Am J Obstet Gynecol* 1969;104:856–864.

56. Kerr MG. Cardiovascular dynamics in pregnancy and labour. *Br Med Bull* 1968;24:19–24.

57. Lees HM, Taylor SH, Scott BD, Kerr MG. The circulatory effect of recumbent postural change in late pregnancy. *Clin Sci* 1967;32:453–465.

58. Howard BK, Goodson JH, Mengert WF. Supine hypotensive syndrome in late pregnancy. *Obstet Gynecol* 1953;1:371–377.

59. Kerr MG. The mechanical effects of the gravid uterus in late pregnancy. *J Obstet Gynaecol Br Commonw* 1965;72:513–529.

60. Kerr MG, Scott DB, Samuel E. Studies of the inferior vena cava in late pregnancy. *Br Med J* 1964;1:532–533.

61. Bieniarz J, Mapueda E, Caldeyro-Barcia R. Compression of aorta by the uterus in late human pregnancy. I. Variations between femoral and brachial artery pressure with changes from hypertension to hypotension. *Am J Obstet Gynecol* 1966;95:795–808.

62. Bieniarz J, Crottongini JJ, Curuchet E, Romero-Salinas G, Yoshida T, Poseiro JJ, Caldeyro-Barcia R. Aortocaval compression by the uterus in late human pregnancy. II. An angiographic study. *Am J Obstet Gynecol* 1968;100:203–217.

63. Holmes F. Incidence of the supine hypotensive syndrome in late pregnancy. A clinical study in 500 subjects. *J Obstet Gynaecol Br Emp* 1960;67:254–258.

64. Pirhonen JP, Erkkola RU. Uterine and umbilical flow velocity waveforms in the supine hypotensive syndrome. *Obstet Gynecol* 1990;76:176–179.

65. Kinsella SM, Lohmann G. Supine hypotensive syndrome. *Obstet Gynecol* 1994;83:774–788.

66. Abitol MM. Inferior vena cava compression in the pregnant dog. *Am J Obstet Gynecol* 1978;130:194–198.

67. Hirabayashi Y, Saitoh K, Fukuda H, Shimizu R. An unusual supine hypotensive syndrome during cesarean section: the importance of trying right tilt if there is a poor response to left tilt. *MASUI* 1994;43:1590–1592.

68. Kim YI, Chandra P, Marx GF. Successful management of severe aortocaval compression in twin pregnancy. *Obstet Gynecol* 1975;46:362–364.

69. Ueland K, Metcalfe J. Circulatory changes in pregnancy. *Clin Obstet Gynecol* 1975;18:41–50.

70. Rubler S, Prabodhkumar MD, Pinto ER. Cardiac size and performance during pregnancy: estimates with echocardiography. *Clin Obstet Gynecol* 1977;40:534–540.

71. Katz R, Karliner JS, Resnik R. Effects of a natural volume overload state (pregnancy) on left ventricular performance in normal human subjects. *Circulation* 1978;58:434–441.

72. Christianson RE. Studies on blood pressure during pregnancy. I. Influence on parity and age. *Am J Obstet Gynecol* 1976;125:509–513.

73. MacGillivray I. Hypertension in pregnancy and its consequences. *J Obstet Gynaecol Br Commonw* 1961;68:557–569.

74. Lee W. Cardiorespiratory alterations during normal pregnancy. *Crit Care Clin* 1991;7:763–775.

75. Shenan A, Gupta M, Halligan A, Taylor DJ, deSwiet M. Lack of reproducibility in pregnancy of Korotkoff phase IV as measured by mercury sphygmomanometry. *Lancet* 1996;347:139–142.

76. Brown MA, Recter L, Smith B, Buddle ML, Morris R, Whitworth JA. Measuring blood pressure in pregnant women: a comparison of direct and indirect methods. *Am J Obstet Gynecol* 1994;171:661–667.

77. Blank SG, Helseth G, Pickering TG, West JE, August P. How should diastolic blood pressure be defined during pregnancy? *Hypertension* 1994;24:234–240.

78. Sherman AH, Kissane J, deSwiet M. Validation of the Spacelab 90207 ambulatory blood pressure monitor for use in pregnancy. *Br J Obstet Gynaecol* 1993;100:904–908.

79. Easterling TR. Cardiovascular physiology of the normal pregnancy. In: Gleicher N, ed. *Principles and Practice of Medical Therapy in Pregnancy,* 3rd ed. Norwalk: CT: Appleton & Lange; 1992; p. 762–766.

80. Lindheimer MD. Hypertension in pregnancy. *Hypertension* 1993;22:127–137.

81. Walters WAW, Lim YL. Cardiovascular dynamics in women receiving oral contraceptive therapy. *Lancet* 1969;2:879–881.

82. Griess FC, Anderson SG. Effect of ovarian hormones on the uterine vascular bed. *Am J Obstet Gynecol* 1970;107:829–836.

83. Bryant EE, Douglas BH, Ashburn AD. Circulatory changes following prolactin administration. *Am J Obstet Gynecol* 1973;115:53–57.

84. Gerber JG, Payne NA, Murphy RC, Nies AS. Prostacyclin produced by the pregnant uterus in the dog may act as a circulating vasodepressor substance. *J Clin Invest* 1981;67: 632–636.

85. Van Assche FA. The role of prostacyclin and thromboxane in pregnancy. *Verh K Acad Geneeskd Belg* 1990;52:105–125.

86. Schrier RW, Briner VA. Peripheral arterial vasodilation hypothesis of sodium and water retention in pregnancy: implications for pathogenesis of preeclampsia–eclampsia. *Obstet Gynecol* 1991;77:632–639.

87. Allen R, Castro L, Arora C, Krakow D, Huang S, Platt L. Endothelium-derived relaxing factor inhibition and the pressor response to norepinephrine in the pregnant rat. *Obstet Gynecol* 1994;83:92–96.

88. Brown GP, Venuto RC. Angiotensin II receptor alterations during pregnancy in rabbits. *Am J Physiol* 1986;251: E58–E64.

89. Paller MS. Mechanisms of decreased pressor responsiveness to ANG II, NE and vasopressin in pregnant rats. *Am J Physiol* 1984;247:H100–H108.

90. Podjarny E, Mandelbaum A, Bernheim J. Does nitric oxide play a role in normal pregnancy and pregnancy-induced hypertension? *Nephrol Dial Transplant* 1994;9:1527–1540.

91. Assali NS, Rauramo L, Peltonen T. Measurement of uterine blood flow and uterine metabolism. VIII. Uterine and fetal blood flow and oxygen consumption in early human pregnancy. *Am J Obstet Gynecol* 1960;79:86–98.

92. Metcalfe J, Romney SL, Ramsey LH, Reid DE, Barwell CS. Estimation of uterine blood flow in normal human pregnancy at term. *J Clin Invest* 1955;34:1632–1638.

93. Jurkovic D, Jauniaux E, Kurjak A, Hustin J, Campbell S, Nicolaides KH. Transvaginal color Doppler assessment of the uteroplacental circulation in early pregnancy. *Obstet Gynecol* 1991;77:365–369.

94. Jaffe R, Warsof SL. Transvaginal color Doppler imaging in the assessment of uteroplacental blood flow in the normal first-trimester pregnancy. *Am J Obstet Gynecol* 1991; 164:781–785.

95. Kaminopetros P, Higueras MT, Nicolaides KH. Doppler study of uterine artery blood flow; comparison of findings in the first and second trimesters of pregnancy. *Fetal Diagn Ther* 1991;6:58–64.

96. Bewley S, Cooper P, Campbell S. Doppler Investigation of uteroplacental blood flow resistance in the second trimester: a screening study for pre-eclampsia and intrauterine growth retardation. *Br J Obstet Gynaecol* 1991;98:871–879.

97. Palmer SU, Zamudio S, Coffin C, Parker S, Stamm E, Moore LG. Quantitative estimation of human uterine artery blood flow and pelvic blood flow redistribution in pregnancy. *Obstet Gynecol* 1992;80:1000–1006.

98. Kofinas AD, Espeland MA, Penry M, Swain M, Hatjis C. Uteroplacental Doppler flow velocity waveform indices in normal pregnancy: a statistical exercise and the development of appropriate reference values. *Am J Perinatol* 1992;9: 94–101.

99. Boura ALA, Walters WAW, Read MA, Leitch IM. Autacoids and control of human placental blood flow. *Clin Exp Pharmacol Physiol* 1994;21:737–748.

100. Ferris TF, Stein JH, Kauffman J. Uterine blood flow and uterine renin secretion. *J Clin Invest* 1972;51:2827–2833.

101. Myers SA, Sparks JW, Makowski EC. Relationship between placental blood flow and placental and fetal size in guinea pig. *Am J Physiol* 1982;243:H404–H409.

102. Hohimer AR, Bissonnette JM, Metcalfe J, McKean TA. Effect of exercise on uterine blood flow in the pregnant pygmy goat. *Am J Physiol* 1984;246:H207–H212.

103. Erkkola RNC, Pirhonen JP, Kivijarvi AK. Flow velocity waveform in uterine and umbilical arteries during submaximal bicycle exercise in normal pregnancy. *Obstet Gynecol* 1992;79:611–615.

104. Nunlap W. Serial changes in renal hemodynamics during normal human pregnancy. *Br J Obstet Gynaecol* 1981;88:1–9.

105. Lindheimer MD, Katz AI. The kidney in pregnancy. In: Brenner RM, Rector FC, eds. *The Kidney.* 4th ed. Philadelphia: WB Saunders; 1988;1253.

106. Duvekot JJ, Cheriex EC, Pieters FA, Menheere PP, Peeters LH. Early-pregnancy change in hemodynamics and volume homeostasis are consecutive adjustments triggered by a primary fall in systemic vascular tone. *Am J Obstet Gynecol* 1993;169:1382–1392.

107. Krutzen E, Olofsson P, Back SE, Nilsson-Ehle P. Glomerular filtration rate in pregnancy: a study in normal subjects and in patients with hypertension, preeclampsia, and diabetes. *Scand J Clin Lab Invest* 1992;52:387–392.

108. Davidson JM, Dunlop W. Changes in renal hemodynamics and tubular function induced by normal human pregnancy. *Semin Nephrol* 1984;4:198–207.

109. Fainstat T. Ureteral dilatation in pregnancy: a review. *Obstet Gynecol Survey* 1963;18:845–860.

110. Gallery ED, Ross M, Grigg R, Bean C. Are the renal functional changes of human pregnancy caused by prostacyclin? *Prostaglandins* 1985;30:1019–1029.

111. Ginsburg J, Duncan SLB. Peripheral blood flow in normal pregnancy. *Cardiovasc Res* 1967;1:132–137.

112. Katz M, Sokal MM. Skin perfusion in pregnancy. *Am J Obstet Gynecol* 1980;137:30–33.

113. Beinder E, Huch A, Huch R. Peripheral skin temperature and microcirculatory reactivity during pregnancy. A study with thermography. *J Perinatal Med* 1990;18:383–390.

114. Bean WB, Dexter MW, Cogswell RC. Vascular changes of skin in pregnancy. *Surg Gynecol Obstet* 1949;88:739–752.

115. Fabricant ND. Sexual functions and the nose. *Am J Med Sci* 1960;239:498–502.

116. Pickles VR. Blood flow estimations as indices of mammary activity. *J Obstet Gynaecol Br Emp* 1953;60:301–311.

117. Munnell EW, Taylor HC Jr. Liver blood flow in pregnancy. Hepatic vein catheterization. *J Clin Invest* 1947;26:952–956.

118. McCall ML. Cerebral blood flow and metabolism in toxemias of pregnancy. *Surg Gynecol Obstet* 1949;89:715–721.

119. Elkus R, Popovich J. Respiratory physiology in pregnancy. *Clin Chest Med* 1992;13:555–565.

120. Metcalfe J, Ueland K. The heart and pregnancy. In: Hurst JW, Logue RB, Schlant RC, Wegner NR, eds. *The Heart Arteries and Veins.* New York: McGraw-Hill; 1978:1721–1734.

121. Henricks CH, Quilligan EJ. Cardiac output during labor. *Am J Obstet Gynecol* 1956;71:953–972.

122. Burch GE. Heart disease and pregnancy. *Am Heart J* 1977;93:104–116.

123. Adams JG, Alexander AM. Alterations in cardiovascular physiology during labor. *Am Obstet Gynecol* 1958;12: 542–549.

124. Ueland K, Hansen JM. Maternal cardiovascular dynamics. III. Labor and delivery under local and caudal analgesia. *Am J Obstet Gynecol* 1969;103:8–18.

125. Cunningham I. Cardiovascular physiology of labor and delivery. *J Obstet Gynaecol Br Commonw* 1966;73:498–503.

126. Hansen JM, Ueland K. The influence of caudal analgesia on cardiovascular dynamics during normal labor and delivery. *Acta Anaesthesiol Scand* 1966;23(suppl):449–452.

127. Robson C, Dunlop W, Boys RJ, Hunter S. Cardiac output during labour. *Br Med J* 1987;295:1169–1172.

128. Lee W, Rokey R, Cotton DB, et al. Maternal hemodynamic effects of uterine contractions by M-mode and pulsed-Doppler echocardiography. *Am J Obstet Gynecol* 1989;161:974–977.

129. Ueland K, Hansen JM. Maternal cardiovascular dynamics. II. Posture and uterine contractions. *Am J Obstet Gynecol.* 1969;103:1–7.

130. Hamilton HFH. Blood viscosity in pregnancy. *J Obstet Gynaecol Br Emp* 1950;57:530–538.

131. Rose DJ, Bader ME, Bader Ra, Braunwald E. Catheterization studies of cardiac hemodynamics in normal and pregnant women with reference to left ventricular work. *Am J Obstet Gynecol* 1956;72:233–246.

132. Goeltner E, Quade C. Intrathorakaler Venendruck, Pulse und atmung während der Eröffnungswehen. *Gynaecologia* 1967;163:235–240.

133. Kjeldsen J. Hemodynamic investigations during labor and delivery. *Acta Obstet Gynecol Scand* 1979;89(suppl):10–252.

134. Henricks CH. The hemodynamics of uterine contraction. *Am J Obstet Gynecol* 1958;76:969–981.

135. Wult KH, Kunzel W, Lehmann V. Clinical aspects of placental gas exchange. In: Longo LD, Bartels H, eds. *Respiratory Gas Exchange and Blood Flow in the Placenta.* Bethesda, MD: US Department of Health, Education and Welfare; 1972:505–521. US Dept of Health, Education and Welfare publication NIH 73-36.

136. Midwall J, Jaffin H, Herman MB, Kupersmith J. Shunt flow and pulmonary hemodynamics during labor and delivery in Eisenmenger's syndrome. *Am J Cardiol* 1978;42:299–303.

137. Ueland K, Gills RE, Hansen JM. Maternal cardiovascular dynamics. I. Cesarean section under subarachnoid block anesthesia. *Am J Obstet Gynecol* 1968;100:42–54.

138. Ueland K, Hansen J, Eng M, Kalappa R, Parer JT. Maternal cardiovascular dynamics. V. Cesarean section under thiopental, nitrous oxide, and succinylcholine anesthesia. *Am J Obstet Gynecol* 1970;108:615–622.

139. Ueland K, Akamatsu TJ, Eng M, Bonica JJ, Hansen JM. Maternal cardiovascular dynamics. VI. Cesarean section under epidural anesthesia without epinephrine. *Am J Obstet Gynecol* 1972;114:775–780.

140. Robson SC, Dunlop, W. Hemodynamic changes during the early puerperium. *Br Med J* 1987;294:1065.

141. Robson SC, Hunter S, Moore M, Dunlop W. Hemodynamic changes during the puerperium: a Doppler and M-mode echocardiographic study. *Br J Obstet Gynaecol* 1987;94:1028–1035.

142. Robson SC, Boys RJ, Hunter S, Dunlop W. Maternal hemodynamics after normal delivery and delivery complicated by postpartum hemorrhage. *Obstet Gynecol* 1989;74:234–299.

PART II

CARDIAC EVALUATION OF THE PREGNANT WOMAN

2

CARDIAC EVALUATION DURING PREGNANCY

URI ELKAYAM, MD, AND NORBERT GLEICHER, MD

INTRODUCTION

The evaluation of cardiac disease in pregnancy may be complicated by the normal anatomical and functional changes of the cardiovascular system. Such changes may result in signs and symptoms that can either simulate or obscure heart disease. It is therefore imperative in many cases to use additional diagnostic tools to obtain objective and reliable information about cardiac status. The selection of such tools should be influenced by their diagnostic yield as well as by the potential risk to the fetus.

HISTORY AND PHYSICAL EXAMINATION (TABLE 2.1)

Symptoms

Reduction in exercise tolerance and tiredness are the most commonly found symptoms during pregnancy and are most probably related to increased body weight and anemia of pregnancy. Lightheadedness, or even syncopal episodes, can occur in the later phases of gestation, presumably because mechanical compression of the enlarged uterus on the inferior vena cava results in decreased venous return to the heart and in a fall in cardiac output (Chapter 1). Palpitations are a common complaint during pregnancy; they are probably due to the hyperdynamic circulation of pregnancy and are usually not associated with cardiac arrhythmias.[1–3] Similarly common is dyspnea, which occurs in about half of women before the 19th week of gestation and in as many as 76% of women by 31 weeks.[2] Orthopnea is occasionally seen, especially in the later stages of pregnancy, and is probably due to mechanical pressure of the enlarged uterus on the diaphragm.

Physical Signs

Hyperventilation is a common phenomenon in pregnancy and can be misinterpreted as dyspnea.[3] The mechanism of hyperventilation may be associated with elevated progesterone and its effect on the respiratory center.[2,3] Occasional findings of basilar rales may further simulate a picture of congestive heart failure. In normal pregnancy, pulmonary basilar rales are caused by basal compression of the lungs and atelectasis secondary to enlargement of the uterus and increased abdominal pressure. The higher position of the diaphragm during pregnancy displaces the heart toward a more horizontal position (Fig. 2.1). A left ventricular impulse is usually easily palpated, diffuse, brisk, and unsustained and may be displaced to the left. A right ventricular impulse at the mid- to lower left sternal border can usually be palpated, as can the pulmonary trunk (second left intercostal space), mimicking findings typical for pulmonary hypertension. The systemic arterial pulse is usually full, becomes sharp and jerky between the 12th and 15th weeks of gestation, and maintains this quality until about 1 week after delivery. The pulse is often collapsing in character and associated with capillary pulsation; it can simulate the findings of aortic regurgitation, but the reduction in diastolic blood pressure is smaller.

The jugular veins appear somewhat distended from about the 20th week of pregnancy. The venous pulsation in the neck is more easily seen, with clear definition of prominent A and V peaks and brisk X and Y descents.[4]

Edema of the ankles and legs is a common finding in late pregnancy. The incidence of this phenomenon increases with age. The formation of edema can be attributed to fall in colloid osmotic pressure of the plasma and the concomitant increase in femoral venous pressure in the legs. An increase in capillary permeability during pregnancy has also been sug-

Cardiac Problems in Pregnancy, Third Edition
Edited by Uri Elkayam, MD, and Norbert Gleicher, MD
Copyright © 1998 by Wiley-Liss, Inc. ISBN 0-471-16358-9

TABLE 2.1   Cardiac Symptoms and Findings During Normal Pregnancy

SYMPTOMS

Decreased exercise capacity
Tiredness
Dyspnea
Orthopnea
Palpitations
Lightheadedness
Syncope

PHYSICAL FINDINGS

Inspection
   Hyperventilation
   Peripheral edema
   Distended neck veins with prominent A and V waves and brisk X and Y descents
   Capillary pulsation
Precordial palpation
   Brisk, diffuse, and displaced left ventricular impulse
   Palpable right ventricular impulse
   Palpable pulmonary trunk impulse
Auscultation
   Pulmonary basilary rales
   Increased first heart sound with exaggerated splitting
   Exaggerated splitting of second heart sound
   Midsystolic ejection-type murmurs at the lower left sternal edge and/or over the pulmonary area
     radiating to suprasternal notch and more to the left then right side of neck
   Continuous murmurs (cervical venous hum, mammary souffle)
   Diastolic murmurs (rare)

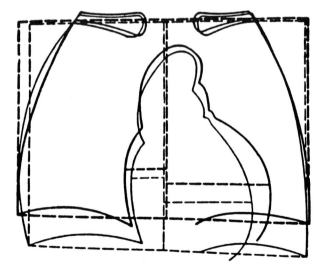

Figure 2.1 Changes in cardiac outline seen on chest X-ray during normal pregnancy. Heavy lines represent the position of the heart during pregnancy, while the lighter lines represent the nonpregnant state. (From Klaften and Palugyay, *Arch Gynaekol* 1927;131:347, with permission.)

gested as a contributing factor to the edema formation but was not convincingly proven.[6]

Auscultatory Findings

Heart Sounds   The first heart sound shows an increased loudness of both components, starting at the 12th–20th weeks of gestation, and remains loud up to about the 32nd week, when the intensity diminishes in some of the cases. The first sound returns to normal 2–4 weeks postpartum.[7,8] In addition to the increased intensity, the first sound demonstrates an exaggerated splitting, which is maximal in the third to fifth left intercostal space, close to the sternum, and is also audible in the pulmonary area, down the left sternal edge, and at the apex. The amplitude of the second, or tricuspid, element of the first heart sound increases on inspiration and decreases on expiration. The cause for the changes in the quality of the first heart sound in pregnancy is not entirely clear. Cutforth and MacDonald[7] suggested that the increased plasma volume is a major contributing factor, Perloff[4] proposed an accentuation of the intensity of the first heart sound due to tachycardia and a hyperkinetic left ventricle during pregnancy.

There is no change in the character of the second heart sound during the first 30 weeks of pregnancy. At late pregnancy, however, the second sound is often increased, and when the patient is examined in the lateral position, it exhibits wide splitting. Compression of the inferior vena cava by the uterus and the lack of free diaphragmatic movement have been suggested as the mechanism responsible for the normal or even less than normal splitting of the second sound when patients are examined in the supine position.[7]

A high incidence of a third heart sound was reported in pregnancy 30 years ago.[7,8] In our experience, however, such a sound is rare in healthy women during gestation. A fourth heart sound was found by phonocardiographic studies in 16% of pregnant women during early pregnancy (15th–22nd week) but is rarely detected on auscultation.

Systolic Murmurs   As a result of the hyperkinetic circulation during pregnancy, the incidence of innocent systolic murmurs is high and was found in 96% of the cases reported by Cutforth and MacDonald[7] (Fig. 2.2). The characteristic murmur is midsystolic, grade 1-2/6, and is best heard at the lower left sternal edge and over the pulmonary area and radiating to the suprasternal notch and more to the left side than to the right side of the neck. The murmur represents audible vibrations due to the ejection of blood from the right ventricle into the pulmonary trunk and/or from the left ventricle into the brachiocephalic arteries at the point of branching from the aortic arch. The murmur is best heard with the patient in the supine position and the diaphragm firmly applied to the chest wall. Mishra et al[9] used echocardiography to examine the significance of a heart murmur in 103 pregnant women who were referred for cardiac opinion. The echocardiogram and Doppler results were normal in all 79 women who had a soft or short ejection systolic murmur. Three of 15 women who had loud or long ejection systolic murmur had abnormalities (one patient had mitral valve prolapse with mild mitral regurgitation; the second, nonobstructive hypertrophic cardiomyopathy; the third, mild aortic stenosis due to bicuspid aortic valve). All seven patients who had diastolic, pansystolic, or late systolic murmurs or abnormal electrocardiograms had abnormalities (three ventricular septal defects,

one atrial septal defect with rheumatic mitral regurgitation, one mitral valve prolapse with mild mitral regurgitation, one nonobstructive hypertrophic cardiomyopathy). The study showed that echocardiography is not needed in patients with a typical flow murmur of pregnancy but is useful in distinguishing between a functional and an organic murmur in cases of murmurs that are louder or longer or associated with other auscultatory or electrocardiographic abnormalities.

Diastolic Murmurs   A soft, medium- to high-pitched diastolic murmur has been reported in some normal pregnant women. The murmur can be best heard at the lower left sternal edge and over the pulmonary area and may resemble the early diastolic murmurs of pulmonary or aortic insufficiency, or stenosis of the mitral or tricuspid valves. The murmurs are thought to be due to increased flow through the tricuspid or mitral valve or to a physiologic dilatation of the pulmonary artery during pregnancy.[10,11] In our experience, however, the occurrence of a diastolic murmur in a healthy pregnant woman is rare.

Continuous Murmurs   A cervical venous hum is the most common innocent continuous murmur in children; it is also found frequently in nonpregnant women and is present in almost all pregnant women.[4,11] The venous hum is heard maximally over the supraclavicular fossa just lateral to the sternocleidomastoid muscle. It is more prominent on the right side and radiates only rarely below the clavicle. The mammary souffle (Fig. 2.2) is sometimes heard during late pregnancy and the early postpartum period, especially in lactating women, and is thought to be due to increased flow in the mammary vessels.[11] The mammary souffle can be either systolic or continuous.[11–15] The continuous murmur is always louder in systole. The murmur is maximally heard at the second left or right intercostal space; but it can be louder at the third or fourth intercostal space and is occasionally bilateral. It can also be heard over the breast during the later phase of gestation and during the postpartum period in lactating women. The murmur is best heard when the patient is examined in the supine position and can be modified or obliterated in the upright position or when the stethoscope is pressed

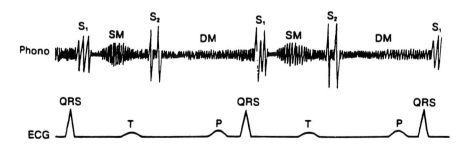

Figure 2.2   Phonocardiographic recording of a mammary souffle, a continuous murmur occasionally heard in pregnant women near term or during lactation. (From Tilkian and Conover, *Understanding Heart Sounds and Murmurs,* 2nd ed. Philadelphia: WB Saunders 1984, with permission.)

harder against the skin.[11] It is characterized by a significant day-to-day-or even beat-to-beat-variation, and disappears after termination of lactation.[4]

The differential diagnosis for the continuous mammary souffle is a patent ductus arteriosus or arterial venous fistula of the chest wall.[11,15] While the mammary souffle generally peaks earlier than the second heart sound, the ductus murmur usually peaks after the second heart sound. The ductus murmur also is not obliterated by local compression. In addition, murmurs of ductus arteriosus and arterial venous fistula can be differentiated from the mammary souffle by the absence of day-to-day and/or beat-to-beat variations and/or their persistence after the end of lactation.[12]

There is still controversy in regard to the origin of the mammary souffle. Although Hurst and coworkers[10] suggested a venous origin to this continuous murmur, other investigators[13,15] postulated that the mammary souffle is arterial in origin. Tabatznik and coworkers[13] suggested that the junction of the internal mammary artery and the intercostal systems were the most likely points of formation. Perloff[11] suggested that the delay in onset, the systolic accentuation, the relatively high frequency, and persistence during the Valsalva maneuver are in accord with arterial origin.

CHEST X-RAY

The radiation dose associated with a routine chest X-ray examination is minimal: The average dose to the skin in the primary beam is 70–150 mrad, while the estimated dose to the uterus is 0.2–43.0 mrad.[16] In spite of the small amount of radiation, this diagnostic test should not be used casually during pregnancy because of the potential adverse biological effects of any amount of radiation. When chest radiography is performed, the pelvic area should be shielded by protective lead material.

Changes seen on chest films in normal pregnancy may simulate cardiac disease and should be interpreted with caution[17,18] (Table 2.2). Straightening of the left upper cardiac border because of prominence of the pulmonary conus is often seen. The heart may seem enlarged because of its horizontal positioning secondary to the elevated diaphragm (Fig. 2.1). In addition, an increase in lung markings may simulate a pattern of flow redistribution typically seen with increased pulmonary venous pressure due to left ventricular failure or mitral valve disease. Pleural effusion is often found early

TABLE 2.2 Chest X-Ray Findings During Normal Pregnancy

Straightening of the left upper cardiac border
Horizontal position of the heart
Increased lung marking
Small pleural effusion in early postpartum period

postpartum.[18,19] It is usually small and bilateral, resorbing 1–2 weeks after delivery.

ELECTROCARDIOGRAPHIC CHANGES

The change in position of the maternal heart in relation to the chest wall as a result of elevation of the diaphragm is reflected in the surface electrocardiogram (Table 2.3). A gradual shift of the QRS axis to the left in the frontal plane was reported by some investigators with advancing pregnancy.[4] Others described a normal distribution of the frontal plane QRS and T-wave axis in 50 pregnant women at late pregnancy.[2] No significant shift of axis was found during the maximum distention at full term. In some cases in which shifting occurred, it was mostly a slight rightward movement. A small Q wave and an inversion of the P wave in lead III, both usually abolished by inspiration, are occasionally seen, and increased R/S ratio in leads V_2 and V_1 is not uncommon. Transient ST-segment and T-wave changes may also be seen during normal pregnancy.[20] Oram and Holt[21] found sagging of the ST segment with a depression of up to 1 mm associated with isoelectric or low voltage T waves in the same leads in 14 of 100 normal pregnant women. Left-sided precordial leads were mainly affected, and similar changes were found in only 6% of healthy nonpregnant women. Szekely and Snaith[22] showed that ST-segment and T-wave changes may recur in the same patient during subsequent pregnancies. Copeland and Stern[23] reported findings of type I (Wenckebach), second-degree atrioventricular (AV) block in pregnant women who were otherwise healthy. The incidence, however, was very small (6 cases of 26,000 electrocardiograms studied.)[23] The similar finding of multiple transient episodes of type I, second-degree AV block in 2 of 50 young, nonpregnant women without apparent heart disease[24] suggests that the relationship between pregnancy and the development of the block is doubtful. Increased susceptibility to arrhythmias during pregnancy can be manifested by frequent findings of sinus tachycardia and premature beats both supraventricular and ventricular[1,25] (Chapter 13).

Electrocardiographic changes have been described in healthy pregnant women receiving ritodrine tocolysis.[26-28]

TABLE 2.3 Electrocardiographic Findings During Normal Pregnancy

QRS-axis deviation
Small Q wave and inverted P wave in lead III
  (abolished by inspiration)
ST-segment and T-wave changes (ritodrine tocolysis,
  cesarean section)
Frequent sinus tachycardia
Higher incidence of arrhythmias
Increase R/S ratio in leads V_2 and V_1

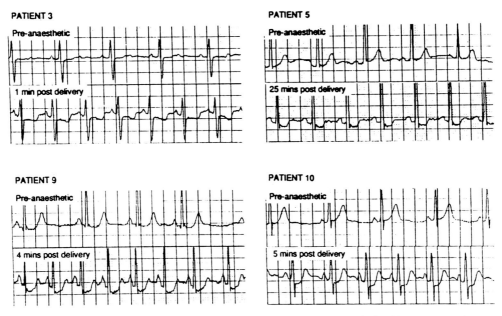

Figure 2.3 ST-segment depression associated with cesarean section in healthy women. These changes were not associated with ventricular wall motion abnormalities. (From McLintic et al, *Anesth Analg* 1992;74:51–56, with permission.)

Sinus tachycardia has been reported in almost all patients; in addition, high incidence of ST-segment depression, T-wave flattening, and prolongation of QT interval were observed. ST segment depression was found to be related to the degree of maternal tachycardia and the level of hypokalemia and hyperglycemia that occur during early ritodrine tocolysis.[28]

Several reports have described electrocardiographic changes during cesarean section (Fig. 2.3). In the majority of patients, ST-segment depressions mimicking myocardial ischemia were recorded. The majority of changes were reported to occur between induction of anesthesia and end of surgery[29] or early post surgery. They are transient, and are seen most commonly in leads I, AVL, and V_5.[29–35] Concomitant use of Echocardiographic evaluation failed to detect regional wall motion abnormality during the appearance of electrocardiographic changes,[31,33] suggesting that ST-segment depression seen during cesarean section is not a result of myocardial ischemia,[31,32,34] a conclusion that is supported by lack of change in plasma level of myocardial specific creatine kinase.[34] Similar electrocardiographic changes have been documented with various anesthetic techniques. The incidence, however, may be somewhat higher with the use of epidural versus spinal or general anesthesia.[33]

An early study (1970) of maternal electrocardiograms recorded during labor and delivery described high incidence of arrhythmias,[36] which included atrial and ventricular premature beats, sinus bradycardia and tachycardia, episodes of sinus arrest, paroxysmal supraventricular tachycardia, and aberrant ventricular conduction. A recent study by Mathew et

al[33] reported a high incidence of ST-segment depression on Holter monitoring in patients undergoing cesarean section but failed to find such changes during vaginal delivery in 22 women. Increased incidence of arrhythmias has been documented in normal pregnancies (Chapter 13). Shotan et al[1] demonstrated a high incidence of atrial and ventricular premature beats in a group of pregnant women, referred for investigation of a heart murmur, in whom organic heart disease was excluded. A significant reduction in the number of ventricular premature beats was seen in nine healthy women when Holter monitoring was repeated postpartum.[1] An increased susceptibility to paroxysmal supraventricular tachycardia during normal pregnancies has also been demonstrated,[37] and paroxysmal ventricular tachycardia has been reported in several cases with apparently normal heart.[38]

DOPPLER ECHOCARDIOGRAPHY

Both maternal and fetal echocardiography measurements are safe for use during pregnancy.[39] A recent study by Stoddard et al[40] described the safe use of transesophageal echocardiography in pregnant women.[39] The procedure was performed in 10 patients between 5 and 31 weeks of gestation. Midazolam in a dose ranging from 1.0 to 4.0 mg was used for sedation, and the probe insertion time ranged between 6 and 21 minutes. The procedure was found to be safe and well tolerated, without evidence of adverse effect to the fetus.

TABLE 2.4 Doppler and Electrocardiographic Findings During Normal Pregnancy

Slightly increased systolic and diastolic left ventricular
   dimensions (when patient examined in the lateral position)
Unchanged or slightly improved left ventricular systolic function
Moderate increase in size of right atrium, right ventricle, and
   left atrium
Progressive dilation of pulmonary, tricuspid, and mitral valve
   annuli
Functional pulmonary, tricuspid, and mitral regurgitation
Small pericardial effusion

A small but significant increase in the size of cardiac chambers has been seen during normal pregnancy (Table 2.4). Several measurements in 13 women before conception and then at monthly intervals throughout pregnancy were performed by Robson et al[41] (Table 2.5). These investigators reported a 7% increase in left ventricular diastolic dimension and a 4% in end systolic dimension, while left atrial dimension increased a maximum of 16% and ejection fraction 6%.

The maximum increase was seen during the third trimester. A prospective study by Campos et al[11,42] demonstrated a progressive increase in all four cardiac chamber dimensions (Table 2.6), with 19% average increase at term of right atrium, 18% of right ventricle, 12% of left atrium, and 6% of left ventricle. No change was noted in the thickness of left ventricular walls; because of increase in end diastolic dimension, however, there was a significant increase in left ventricular myocardial mass. Similar data have been described by other investigators.[43,44] In addition to these changes, early and progressive dilatation of pulmonary, tricuspid, and mitral annuli has been reported[11,42] (Table 2.7). These changes have been found to be associated with a progressive increase in multivalvular regurgitation. Maximum regurgitation was seen at term (mitral, 28% of patients; tricuspid, 94%; pulmonary, 94%; aortic, 0%) (Fig. 2.4). A repeat study 3–6 weeks postpartum still revealed a significant prevalence of tricuspid (83%) and pulmonary (67%) regurgitation. A recent study by Sadaniantz et al[44] demonstrated an increase in the mitral valve A wave, which was interpreted as a reflection of change in left ventricular filling during pregnancy.

TABLE 2.5 Changes in Echocardiographic Parameters During Normal Pregnancy

Parameter	Preconception	Gestational Week									
		5	8	12	16	20	24	28	32	36	38
End systolic dimension (cm)	2.9	2.9	2.8	2.9	2.9	2.9	2.9	2.9	2.9	3.0	3.0
End diastolic dimension (cm)	4.5	4.5	4.6	4.7	4.7	4.7	4.8	4.8	4.8	4.8	4.8
Left artial dimension (cm)	3.1	3.1	3.3	3.3	3.3	3.4	3.5	3.6	3.6	3.6	3.6
Total left ventricular thickness (cm)	1.5	1.5	1.5	1.6	1.6	1.7	1.7	1.7	1.8	1.8	1.9
Left ventricular mass (g)	120	124	127	137	141	149	157	165	166	179	183
Ejection fraction (%)	72	74	76	76	77	77	77	76	76	74	74

Source: Modified from Robson et al, *Am J Physiol* 1989;250:H1060–H1065.

TABLE 2.6 Cardiac Chamber Dimensions (mm) During Normal Pregnancy and Puerperium

Chamber	Pregnant Women (n = 18)					Control (n = 18)
	8th–12th Week	20th–24th Week	30th–34th Week	36th–40th Week	Puerperium	
LV	41 ± 3	43 ± 2	43 ± 2	44 ± 2	42 ± 2	40 ± 3
LA	30 ± 2	31 ± 2	33 ± 2	33 ± 3	30 ± 3	28 ± 2
RV	30 ± 2	32 ± 2	35 ± 3	35 ± 2	31 ± 2	28 ± 3
RA	43 ± 2	47 ± 2	51 ± 3	51 ± 3	47 ± 3	44 ± 4

Abbreviations: LA, left atrium; LV, left ventricle; RA, right atrium; RV, right ventricle.

Source: Reproduced with permission from Campos O, *Echocardiography* 1996;13:135–145.

TABLE 2.7   Valve Annular Diameters (mm) in Normal Pregnancy and Puerperium

	Pregnant Women ($n = 18$)					
Valve	8th–12th Week	20th–24th Week	30th–34th Week	36th–40th Week	Puerperium	Control ($n = 18$)
Mitral	22 ± 1	23 ± 1	24 ± 1	24 ± 1	22 ± 1	20 ± 1
Tricuspid	22 ± 2	23 ± 1	25 ± 1	25 ± 1	22 ± 1	20 ± 1
Pulmonary	20 ± 2	22 ± 2	25 ± 2	25 ± 2	23 ± 2	21 ± 2
Aortic	18 ± 1	17 ± 1	18 ± 1	18 ± 1	18 ± 1	18 ± 1

Source: Reproduced with permission from Campos O, *Echocardiography* 1996;13:135–145.

Prevalence of silent pericardial effusion, mostly small, has been reported during normal pregnancy.[45–47] A recent study in 52 normal pregnant women described the finding of pericardial effusion in 15% of the cases during the first trimester, 19% during the second, and 44% during the third trimester and was completely resolved 6 weeks postdelivery.[47] The frequency of effusion in primigravidas was higher than that in multigravidas (69 vs. 36%, < 0.023). In addition, higher frequency was found in women who gained more than 12 kg during their pregnancy.

STRESS TEST

An exercise test is extremely useful for establishing the diagnosis of ischemic heart disease and for assessing the functional capacity of patients in whom heart disease is known or suspected. There is only little information, however, regarding the efficacy and safety of diagnostic stress test during pregnancy. Fetal bradycardia has been described during maximal exercise or the recovery period.[48–50] The presence of fetal bradycardia may reflect marked fetal hypoxia,[51] acidosis, or severe hyperthermia.[52] Because of these findings, and until there is more information regarding the safety of maximal exercise during pregnancy, the use of submaximal exercise tests (approximately 70% of maximal predicted heart rate) with fetal monitoring is recommended when exercise testing is needed during gestation. The safety of a submaximal exercise during pregnancy has been demonstrated by several investigators.[49,53–55] Van Doorn et al[55] performed a longitudinal study in 33 healthy women during pregnancy and the postpartum period. The exercise electrocardiogram demonstrated depression of the ST segment in 12% of women in the absence of clinical signs of ischemia. The incidence of these changes, however, was not affected by the pregnancy.

The measurement of maximal oxygen consumtion during exercise is superior to the functional assessment based on symptoms in the objective evaluation of cardiac reserve.[56] A

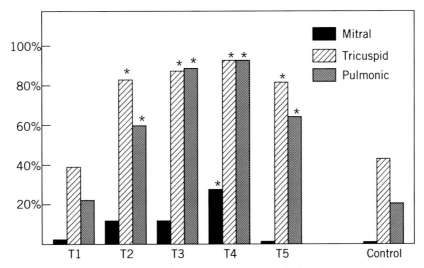

Figure 2.4   Prevalence of physiological valvular regurgitation during pregnancy and puerperium. (Reproduced from Campos et al, *Int J Cardiol* 1993;40:265–272, with permission.)

recent evaluation by Lotgering et al[57] has demonstrated that maximal oxygen consumption was unaffected by pregnancy. The results of this study suggest therefore that prepregnancy values of maximum oxygen consumption can be used as a baseline for assessment of change in maximal aerobic exercise in patients with heart disease during gestation.

RADIONUCLIDE TECHNIQUES

Myocardial perfusion scans and radionuclide ventriculography are noninvasive techniques that provide high quality information on cardiac function during systole and diastole, coronary perfusion, and intracardiac shunts. These techniques, however, are associated with a small degree of radiation to the fetus and should be used with caution during pregnancy (Chapter 3). The dose of radiation estimated to reach the fetus from commonly used radiopharmaceuticals is less then one rad for thallium-201 and technetium-99m-labeled *sestamibii* and between 1 and 2 rads for technetium-99m-labeled red blood cells. This small dose is unlikely to increase the incidence of malformation even when received at the period critical for the induction of any specific type of maldevelopment. Because of the low incidence of coronary artery disease in women in childbearing age and the usefulness of other noninvasive tools such as echocardiography and the Doppler technique in the diagnosis and assessment of other forms of heart disease, the need to use radionuclide techniques for cardiac workup during pregnancy is extremely remote. When the results of such testing are nevertheless required, the procedure should be avoided if possible during the first trimester of pregnancy.

PULMONARY ARTERY CATHETERIZATION

The use of a balloon flotation pulmonary artery catheter allows the measurement of right atrial, right ventricular, and pulmonary artery pressures at the bedside. The inflation of the balloon at the tip of the catheter results in occlusion of a small pulmonary artery branch, allowing the measurement of pulmonary artery wedge pressure, which correlates well with left ventricular end diastolic pressure. In addition, the pulmonary artery catheter allows the determination of cardiac output by the thermodilution technique, the measurement of oxygen saturation in the mixed venous blood, and both atrial and ventricular pacing. The ability to pass the catheter under pressure monitoring alone, without the need for fluoroscopy, makes this tool especially attractive for use during pregnancy. Accumulated experience with this technique in recent years has shown its value in the management of high risk patients during pregnancy, labor, and delivery and in the postpartum period.[58] Continuous hemodynamic monitoring in the peripartum period allows early recognition and imme-

diate correction of hemodynamic problems. We therefore recommend the insertion of a pulmonary artery catheter at the early stage of labor in any cardiac patient who has been symptomatic during pregnancy and/or has documented cardiac dysfunction, moderate or severe valvular stenosis, symptomatic valvular regurgitation, most symptomatic congenital cardiac malformations, known pulmonary hypertension, uncontrolled systemic hypertension, known ischemic heart disease, hypoxemia, oliguria, and hemodynamic instability. Because of the significant hemodynamic changes that occur postpartum, hemodynamic monitoring may need to be continued in the puerperium to assure hemodynamic stability.

CARDIAC CATHETERIZATION

Cardiac catheterization may be indicated in rare instances of cardiac decompensation during pregnancy when sufficient information cannot be obtained by noninvasive techniques. This diagnostic procedure is the only technique that enables direct visualization of the coronary circulation, and it may be needed for the assessment of valvular disease, especially when surgery is considered. With the combined use of fluoroscopy and cineangiography, this technique may be associated with the largest X-ray dose of any examination in diagnostic radiology (Chapter 3) (standard fluoroscopy is associated with a skin dose of 1–2 rads/min, and the use of cineangiography could deliver 5–10 rads/min. The adverse effect of radiation is linearly proportional to the absorbed dose. The risks and the nature of side effects vary with the developmental stage of the fetus. These risks include resorption or death of the embryo, congenital malformations, and as previously discussed, cancer induction and potential genetic changes.[59] Radiation during the 1st gestational week is associated with high likelihood of absorption or resorption of the preimplanted blastocyst, whereas exposure to radiation during the 2nd–6th weeks of pregnancy is associated with increased risk of teratogenic effects. Radiation between the 7th and 15th weeks of gestation may affect developing brain cells and may lead to alterations in neurologic function or behavior, as well as mental retardation. An association between childhood cancer and intrauterine exposure to radiation is likely.[60] The risk seems to be cumulative, and its incidence has been reported to be influenced by the magnitude of radiation during the entire pregnancy, although risk may be higher when radiation exposure occurs during the first trimester.

Because of the potential risk to the fetus, cardiac catheterization should be used only when information cannot be obtained by alternative noninvasive methods. If possible, the procedure should be performed after the period of major organogenesis (>12 weeks after last menses). The fetus should be appropriately shielded,[61] and exposure to radiation should be kept to a minimum. In addition, Jackson et al[62] have reported technical difficulty in puncturing the femoral artery, which is overlain by the distended femoral vein during pregnancy. For this reason, and to minimize radiation to the abdomen, the brachial rather than the femoral approach may be preferred. Only the absolute minimum time exposure should be used to answer the specific questions asked. A radiologist should be consulted for the careful selection of technical exposure factor and filtration and collimation of the radiation beam to anatomical areas of interest.

REFERENCES

1. Shotan A, Ostrzega E, Mehra A, Johnson JV, Elkayam U. Incidence of arrhythmias in normal pregnancy and relation to palpitations, dizziness and syncope. *Am J Cardiol,* 1997; 79:1061–1064.
2. Zeldis SM. Dyspnea during pregnancy. Distinguishing cardiac from pulmonary causes. *Clin Chest Med* 1992;13:567–585.
3. Tenholder MF, South-Paul JE. Dyspnea in pregnancy. *Chest* 1989;96:381–388.
4. Perloff JK. Pregnancy and cardiovascular disease. In: Braunwald E, ed. *Heart Disease.* 3rd ed. Philadelphia: WB Saunders; 1988;1848–1869.
5. Robertson EG. Increased erythrocyte fragility in association with osmotic changes in pregnancy serum. *J Reprod Fertil* 1968;16:323–324.
6. Sptez S. Capillary filtration during normal pregnancy. *Acta Obstet Gynecol Scand* 1965;44:227–242.
7. Cutforth R, MacDonald MB. Heart sounds and murmurs in pregnancy. *Am Heart J* 1966;71:741–747.
8. O'Rourke RA, Ewy GA, Marcus FI. Cardiac auscultation in pregnancy. *Med Ann DC* 1970;39:92–94.
9. Mishra M, Chambers JB, Jakson G. Murmurs in pregnancy: an audit of echocardiography. *Br Med J* 1992;304:1413–1414.
10. Hurst JW, Staton J, Hubbard D. Precordial murmurs during pregnancy and lactation. *N Engl J Med* 1958;259:515–517.
11. Perloff JK. *The Clinical Recognition of Congenital Heart Disease.* 4th ed. Philadelphia: WB Saunders; 1994;15–18.
11. Campos O. Doppler echocardiography during pregnancy: physiological and abnormal findings. *Echocardiography* 1996; 13:135–146.
12. Szekely P, Julian DG. Heart disease and pregnancy. *Curr Probl Cardiol* 1979;4:1–74.
13. Tabatznik B, Randall TW, Hersch C. The mammary souffle of pregnancy and lactation. *Circulation* 1960;22:1069–1073.
14. Tilkian AG, Conover MB. *Understanding Heart Sounds and Murmurs.* 2nd ed. Philadelphia: WB Saunders; 1984.
15. Scott JT, Murphy JED. Mammary souffle: report of two cases of simulation patent ductus arteriosus. *Circulation* 1958;18: 1038–1043.
16. Wagner CK, Leser RG, Saldana LR. *Exposure of the Pregnant Patient to Diagnostic Radiation. A Guide to Medical Management.* Philadelphia: JB Lippincott; 1985;52.
17. Klaften E, Palugyay J. Vergleichende Untersuchungen über Lage und Ausdehnung von Herz und Lunge in der Schwanger schaft und im Wochenblatt. *Arch Gynaekol* 1927;131:347.
18. Fidler JL, Patz EF, Ravin CE. Cardiopulmonary complications of pregnancy: radiographic findings. *Am J Roentgenol* 1993; 161:937–942.
19. Austin JHM. Postpartum pleural effusion. *Ann Intern Med* 1983;98:555–556.
20. Boyle DM, Lloyd-Jones RL. The electrocardiographic ST segment pregnancy. *J Obstet Gynecol Br Commonw* 1966;73:986–987.
21. Oram S, Holt M. Innocent depression of the ST segment and flattening of the T-wave during pregnancy. *J Obstet Gynaecol Br Commonw* 1961;68:765–770.
22. Szekely P, Snaith L. *Heart Disease and Pregnancy.* Edinburgh: Churchill Livingstone; 1974.
23. Copeland GD, Stern TN. Wenckebach periods in pregnancy and puerperium. *Am Heart J* 1958;52:291–298.
24. Sobotka PA, Mayer JH, Bauernfeind RA, Kanakis C, Rosen KM. Arrhythmias documented by 24-hr continuous ambulatory electrocardiographic monitoring in young women without apparent heart disease. *Am Heart J* 1981;101:753–759.
25. Widerhorn J, Rahimtoola SH, Elkayam U. Cardiac rhythm disorders. In: Gleicher N, ed. *Principles and Practice of Medical Therapy in Pregnancy.* 2nd ed. Norwalk, CT: Appleton & Lange 1992;135.
26. Hadi HA, Albazzaz SJ. Cardiac isoenzyme and electrocardiographic changes during ritodrine tocolysis. *Am J Obstet Gynecol* 1989;161:318–321.
27. Hendricks SK, Katz M. Effects of ritodrine tocolysis on cardiac isoenzyme and electrocardiography. *Am J Obstet Gynecol* 1990;163:699–701.
28. Faidley CK, Dix PM, Morgan MA, Schechter E. Electrocardiographic abnormalities during ritodrine administration. *South Med J* 1990;83:503–506.
29. Kleinman B. Electrocardiographic changes during cesarean section. *Anesthesiology* 1993;78:997–998.
30. Palmer CM, Norris MC, Giudici MC, Leighton BL, DeSimone CA. Incidence of electrocardiographic changes during cesarean delivery under regional anesthesia. *Anesth Analg* 1990;70: 36–43.
31. McLintic AJ, Pringle SD, Lilley S, Houston AB, Thorburn J. Electrocardiographic changes during cesarean section under regional anesthesia. *Anesth Analg* 1992;74:51–56.
32. Palmer CM. What do electrocardiographic and echocardiographic changes during cesarean section mean? *Anesth Analg* 1993;76:457.
33. Mathew JP, Fleisher LA, Rinehouse JA, Sevarino FB, Sinatra RS, Nelson AH, Prokop EK, Rosenbaum SH. ST segment depression during labor and delivery. *Anesthesiology* 1992; 77:635–641.
34. Zakowski MI, Ramanathan S, Baratta JB, Cziner D, Goldstein MJ, Kronzon I, Turndorf H. Electrocardiographic changes during cesarean section is cause for concern? *Anesth Analg* 1993;76:162–167.

35. Eisenach JC, Tuttle R, Stein A. Is ST segment depression of the electrocardiogram during cesarean section merely due to cardiac sympathetic block? *Anesth Analg* 1994;78:287–292.

36. Upshaw CB Jr. A study of maternal electrocardiograms recorded during labor and delivery. *Am J Obstet Gynecol* 1970; 107:17–27.

37. Elkayam U, Goodwin TM. Adenosine therapy for supraventricular tachycardia during pregnancy. *Am J Cardiol* 1995; 75:521–523.

38. Brodsky M, Doria R, Allen B, Sato D, Thomas G, Sada M. New onset ventricular tachycardia during pregnancy. *Am Heart J* 1992;123:933–941.

39. Bioeffects Committee of the American Institute of Ultrasound in Medicine. *J Ultrasound Med Biol* 1983;2:R14.

40. Stoddard MF, Longaker RA, Vuocolo LM, Dawkins PR. Transesophageal echocardiography in the pregnant patient. *Am Heart J* 1992;124:785–787.

41. Robson SC, Hunter S, Boys RJ, Dunlop W. Serial study of factors influencing changes in cardiac output during human pregnancy. *Am J Physiol* 1989;256:H1060–H1065.

42. Campos O, Andrade JL, Bocanegra J. Ambrose JA, Carvalho AC, Harada K, Martinez EE. Physiologic multivalvular regurgitation during pregnancy: a longitudinal Doppler echocardiographic study. *Int J Cardiol* 1993;40:265–272.

43. Vered Z, Poler SM, Gibson P, Wlody D, Perez JE. Noninvasive detection of the morphologic and hemodynamic changes during normal pregnancy. *Clin Cardiol* 1991;14:327–334.

44. Sadaniantz A, Kocheril AG, Emaus SP, Garber CE, Parisi A. Cardiovascular changes in pregnancy evaluated by two-dimensional and Doppler echocardiography. *J Am Soc Echocardiogr.* 1992;5:253–258.

45. Haiat R, Halphen C. Silent pericardial effusion in late pregnancy: a new entity. *Cardiovasc Intervent Radiol* 1984;7: 267–269.

46. Enein M, Aziz A, Zina A, Kassem M, El-Tabbakh G. Echocardiography of the pericardium in pregnancy. *Obstet Gynecol* 1987;69:851–853.

47. Abduljabbar HS, Marzouki KM, Zawawi TH, Khan AS. Pericardial effusion in normal pregnant women. *Acta Obstet Gynecol Scand* 1991;70:291–294.

48. Artal R, Romem Y, Paul RH, Wiswell R. Fetal bradycardia induced by maternal exercise. *Lancet* 1984;2:258–260.

49. Carpenter MW, Sady SP, Hoegsberg B, Sady MA, Haydon B, Cullinane EM, Couston DR, Thompson PD. Fetal heart rate response to maternal exertion. *JAMA* 1988;259:3006–3009.

50. Veille JC, Bacevice AE, Wilson B, Janos J, Hellerstein HK: Umbilical artery waveform during bicycle exercise in normal pregnancy. *Obstet Gynecol* 1989;73:957–960.

51. Bracero LA, Schulman H, Baxi LV. Fetal heart rate characteristics that provide confidence in the diagnosis of fetal well-being. *Clin Obstet Gynecol* 1986;29:3–11.

52. Bell R, O'Neill M. Exercise and pregnancy: a review. *Birth* 1994;21:85–95.

53. Sorenson KE, Borlum KG. Fetal heart function in response to short-term maternal exercise. *Br J Obstet Gynaecol* 1986;93: 310–313.

54. Erkkola RU, Pirhonen JP, Kivijarvi AK. Flow velocity waveforms in uterine and umbilical arteries during submaximal bicycle exercise in normal pregnancy. *Obstet Gynecol* 1992; 79:611–615.

55. Van-Doorn MB, Lotgering FK, Struijk C, Pool, J. Wallenburg HC. Maternal and fetal cardiovascular responses to strenuous bicycle exercise. *Am J Obstet Gynecol* 1992;166:854–859.

56. Haywood MP, Cumming DV, Pattison CW. Physiology and clinical applications of cardiopulmonary exercise testing. *Br J Hosp Med* 1995;53:275–282.

57. Lotgering FK, Van Doorn MB, Struijk JP, Wallenburg HC. Maximal aerobic exercise in pregnant women: heart rate, O_2 consumption, CO_2 production and ventilation. *J Appl Physiol* 1991;70:1016–1023.

58. American College of Obstetricians and Gynecologists. Invasive hemodynamic monitoring in obstetrics and gynecology. *Int J Gynecol Obstet* 1993;42:199–205. ACOG technical bulletin 175, December 1992.

59. Medical radiation exposure of pregnant and potentially pregnant women. Recommendations of the National Council on Radiation Protection and Measurements. Washington, DC: NCRPM; 1977.

60. Wakeford R. The risk of childhood cancer from intrauterine and preconceptional exposure to ionizing radiation. *Environ Health Perspect* 1995;103:1018–1025.

61. Instrumentation and monitoring methods for radiation protection: Recommendation of the National Council on Radiation Protection and Measurements. Washington, DC: NCRPM; 1978.

62. Jackson A. Gillespie JE, Beards SC, Whittaker SL. Technical difficulty of femoral artery puncture in late pregnancy. *Eur J Radiol* 1993;17:113–114.

3

CARDIOVASCULAR IMAGING IN THE PREGNANT PATIENT

PATRICK M. COLLETTI, MD, AND KAI LEE, PHD

INTRODUCTION

Cardiac imaging has become a mainstay in the evaluation of patients with suspected cardiovascular abnormalities. In the pregnant patient, however, special considerations must be made regarding the use of ionizing radiation, radiopharmaceuticals, and contrast agents. Special consideration for the use of magnetic resonance imaging in the pregnant patient is also necessary. Often the clinical situation is unclear and the true risk/benefit ratio unknown. This chapter offers some basic guidelines regarding the use of cardiac imaging in the pregnant patient.

RADIATION

The classical unit for radiation absorbed dose is the rad. One rad equals 100 ergs of absorbed energy per gram of tissue for any type of radiation. The currently used term for radiation absorbed dose is the gray (Gy), but in this chapter we retain the more familiar rad units, which still are found in much of the literature. One gray equals 100 rads. A subdivision of a rad is the millirad (1 mrad = 0.001 rad). The amount of radiation absorbed by the chest surface with a typical posterior/anterior view is between 15 and 25 millirads per exposure, depending on the technique used. Other imaging procedures can give a higher or lower radiation dose to the area being examined.

The deposited radiation is primarily due to the X-ray energy absorbed by the photoelectric effect. For the purposes of this discussion, the majority of the radiation dose to the chest region is due to primary radiation coming directly from the X-ray machine, while radiation to the fetus is due to secondary radiation that has been redirected or scattered by Compton interactions with tissue in the chest. These scattered photons may then interact in the tissues of the fetus, with the potential for energy deposition within the fetal tissues. Only a small portion of the primary radiation is scattered in the direction of the fetus and then absorbed by the fetal tissue. Typically, the amount of radiation that scatters to the uterus and is absorbed by the embryo or fetus is less than 5% of the radiation absorbed by tissues directly in the X-ray beam. For example, if a chest PA radiograph delivered 20 mrad to the directly exposed areas in the chest, scatter radiation absorbed at the level of the uterus would be considerably less than 1 mrad. While multiple technical factors, including the kilovolts (peak) and milliamperes used for the exposure and the patient's body habitus would be important, the stage of fetal development is of even greater significance. A 4000 g term fetus would obviously be positioned to receive much greater scatter radiation from cardiac imaging than a 3 mm embryo.[1]

Irradiation of the embryo during the first 10 days postconception would most likely either have no effect or result in resorption of the embryo. Irradiation during the period of organ formation, days 10–50, can cause teratogenesis and congenital malformations. Brief irradiation such as that related to diagnostic imaging might possibly cause discrete tissues to be affected if there is any change at all. It is impossible to separate radiation-induced congenital abnormalities from naturally occurring abnormalities, which may be seen in 4–6% of all fetuses. Irradiation after the completion of

Cardiac Problems in Pregnancy, Third Edition
Edited by Uri Elkayam, MD, and Norbert Gleicher, MD
Copyright © 1998 by Wiley-Liss, Inc. ISBN 0-471-16358-9

organogenesis (beyond 50 days) would most likely cause intrauterine growth retardation if there was any effect at all. Again, it is difficult to prove cause and effect because 4% of human fetuses may spontaneously show intrauterine growth retardation. The risk of abnormal outcome associated with 1 rad exposure may be approximated at 0.003%. This is thousands of times smaller than the spontaneous risks of abortion, malformation, or genetic disease.[2] Possible fetal effects of radiation are listed in Table 3.1.

The currently accepted maximum whole-body radiation dose to a pregnant radiation worker is less than 500 mrad during an entire pregnancy.[3] The 500 mrad is whole-body dose, not just dose to chest. The risk of such a small amount of exposure to radiation is difficult to demonstrate in any meaningful fashion.

Current recommendations[4] regarding intrauterine radiation exposure are as follows:

1. With less than 5 rads, the patient can be reassured of very low likelihood of a problem.
2. With 5–10 rads, the patient would be counseled regarding the low risk of a problem.
3. With 10–15 rads during the first 6 weeks, individual considerations for termination of pregnancy are made.
4. With more than 15 rads, termination of pregnancy is usually recommended.

While a routine chest radiograph should give extremely low amounts of radiation to the pregnancy, procedures utilizing fluoroscopy and cine techniques obviously can give rather large radiation doses to the thorax, with proportion-

ately large scattered radiation doses in the direction of the fetus. Standard fluoroscopy would deliver 1–2 rads/min to the chest, and high level fluoroscopy or cine could deliver as much as 5–10 rads/min to the chest. Thus, 10 minutes of high level fluoroscopy of the chest would give a maximum exposure to the embryo or fetus of considerably less than 10 rads. One would expect that a relatively straightforward cardiac catheterization examination using primarily low level fluoroscopy would result in a fetal exposure of less than 1 rad. A very difficult examination with multiple interventions could easily yield a fetal radiation dose of 5–10 rads.

Methods of reducing fetal radiation exposure from X-ray examinations include the use of high speed film–screen combinations, X-ray beam collimation, and reduced fluoroscopy and cine time during cardiac catheterizations. Avoidance of direct irradiation to the fetus is essential.

Having the patient wear a lead apron during radiographic procedures is of little help in reducing fetal radiation exposure, which is primarily due to Compton-scattered photons. In fact, there is a theoretical risk of increased secondary radiation emitted from the lead shield by photons that otherwise would not have interacted with the body.

NUCLEAR MEDICINE PROCEDURES

Unlike cardiac catheterization, radiation to the embryo and fetus from nuclear medicine procedures is primarily due to distribution of the radiopharmaceutical to the bladder or the placenta, or directly across the placental barrier to the fetus. The most commonly used radiopharmaceuticals in cardiac nuclear medicine are thallium-201 chloride, technetium-99m sestamibi, and technetium-99m-labeled red blood cells.

Thallium-201 chloride ordinarily distributes throughout the body according to regional perfusion and sodium/potassium pump function. A significant portion of the agent is excreted by glomerular filtration, and the bladder may receive approximately 1 rad of radiation. Obviously, the bladder is well positioned to allow radiopharmaceuticals in the urine to irradiate the pregnant uterus. In addition, the placenta is extremely vascular and would be expected to contain a considerable amount of activity. Substances of molecular weight less than 10,000 will readily cross the placental barrier. Thus, one would expect a portion of the thallium-201 to cross the placental barrier and be available for direct intracellular radiation within the conceptus. Even so, it is likely that fetal dose is considerably less than 1 rad per examination.

Technetium-99m-labeled sestamibi also distributes according to regional perfusion. Sestamibi is taken up into cells by a mechanism different from that of thallium-201. The sestamibi may be found primarily within mitochondria. A smaller amount of sestamibi lie within the bladder and placenta, as compared to thallium-201. Sestamibi may be found in much larger quantities in the liver. Because of the relatively low

TABLE 3.1   In Utero Radiation Effects

Post conception Time (days)	Phase	Possible Effects
1–9	Preimplantation	Most likely effect is death; malformation unlikely (18–50 rads?)
10–12	Implantation	Death less likely Malformation still unlikely Growth retardation possible. (10–50 rads?)
13–50	Organogenesis	Fetal anomalies Growth retardation (>25 rads)
51–280	Fetal growth	Intrauterine growth retardation Central nervous system abnormalities Possible increased incidence of cancer or leukemia (>1 rad)

molecular weight of sestamibi, a small amount would be expected to cross the placental barrier. The amount of radiation reaching the conceptus should be less than 1 rad.

Cardiac function studies with technetium-99m-labeled red blood cells might be expected to distribute throughout the vascular pool, and thus the placenta would be expected to have a large amount of activity. Only a small amount of free technetium would be available to enter the bladder or to directly cross the placental barrier. It would be very unlikely for the fetus to receive more radiation than that received by the placenta, which should be between 1 and 2 rads.

Occasionally, the possibility of thromboembolic disease and pulmonary embolism must be considered during pregnancy. Peripheral contrast radiographic venography should be achievable, with a fetal radiation exposure of less than 0.5 rad, if special care is made not to irradiate the pelvis more than is necessary to evaluate the pelvic veins by a single radiograph.[5] Pulmonary scintigraphy with technetium-macroaggregated albumin will generally give most of the radiation exposure to the maternal lungs and urinary tract, depending on the residence time of the particles in the pulmonary microvasculature. The majority of the activity is trapped in the lungs, although there may be a significant amount of activity in the urinary tract, which could receive one rad. It is unlikely that significant amounts of activity will cross the placental barrier, and thus γ radiation emitted from the lungs and urinary tract and perhaps to a lesser extent from the placenta would be expected to give a fetal radiation dose of less than 0.05 rad.[6] Factors affecting fetal exposure from radiopharmaceuticals are listed in Table 3.2.

CARDIOVASCULAR MAGNETIC RESONANCE IMAGING

Although magnetic resonance imaging poses no known risks to the developing embryo or fetus, two recent studies have suggested that some changes may occur in animals that experience typical clinical MRI exposures to static magnetic field, dynamic magnetic fields, and radiofrequency energy.[7] While there is considerable experience in magnetic resonance imaging in pregnant humans, obviously safety cannot

TABLE 3.2 Factors Affecting Fetal Radiation Doses with Diagnostic Nuclear Medicine Procedures

Physical Factors	Physiological Factors
Isotopic half-life	Physiologic half-life
γ Energy	Percentage crossing placenta
Percent β decay	Maternal and fetal distribution
Amount needed for adequate study	Competitive inhibition by nonradioactive isotopes
	Maternal hydration

be proven.[8] Currently, the U.S. Food & Drug Administration recommends prudence in imaging pregnant patients with magnetic resonance techniques. Special considerations should be made to avoid any unnecessary magnetic resonance imaging examinations during the first trimester.

CONTRAST AGENTS

Commonly used radiographic iodinated contrast agents readily cross the placental barrier, and this statement applies to both ionic and nonionic contrast agents. There is considerable experience in intravenous urography in pregnant patients and no additional risks have been identified, although the general risks of iodinated contrast agents (e.g., vomiting, bronchiospasm, vasovagal reaction, shock, seizure) must always be considered, along with the potential long-term risk of renal failure. Overall, the pregnancy does not appear to affect these risks significantly.

Gadolinium-containing contrast agents used in magnetic resonance imaging readily cross the placental barrier, and while safety has not been determined, it is unlikely that a single exposure to gadolinium-containing contrast agent would cause significant fetal risk.

CARDIAC ULTRASOUND

Despite considerable study of potential embryo and fetal injury by sonography, including Doppler sonography, it is extremely unlikely that cardiac or peripheral vascular examinations with ultrasound could create any risk at all for the fetus. Thus, echocardiography and ultrasound peripheral vascular studies should be considered safe for the pregnant patient.

RECOMMENDATIONS

The following guidelines are proposed regarding the use of cardiovascular imaging in the pregnant patient:

1. Echocardiography, including Doppler and color Doppler studies, should be considered safe in the pregnant patient and should be the initial mode of examination in the majority of cases.

2. The amount of radiation to the fetus from chest radiography is extremely small and probably should be considered safe, hence usable when appropriate.

3. Cardiac nuclear medicine studies, including thallium-201 and technetium-99m sestamibi myocardial scintigraphy and technetium-99m-labeled red blood cell cardiac function studies, would be expected to convey less than one rad to the conceptus. These radionuclides may be used when absolutely necessary. Lung scanning

should not be avoided for reasons of perceived radiation if pulmonary embolism is a serious clinical possibility. The minimal effective radiopharmaceutical dose should be used in the pregnant patient. Increased fluid intake and frequent voiding should be encouraged.

4. While the risk of magnetic resonance for cardiovascular imaging should be quite small, and such techniques may be used in the rare case that echocardiography is inconclusive, it may be best to avoid MRI in the first trimester if possible. Because a chest examination by means of computerized tomography may deliver up to one rad to the fetus by scatter radiation, MRI should be preferable in pregnancy.

5. Cardiac catheterization and interventional procedures may typically yield fetal exposures of less than one rad. It is well to bear in mind that difficult examinations with multiple interventions and the use of high level fluoroscopy and multiple cine views could easily yield a fetal radiation dose of 5–10 rads.

6. It is advisable to consult with the patient prior to performing studies involving ionizing radiation during pregnancy. Potential risks or lack of knowledge of risk should be discussed.

7. A health physicist with expertise in radiation dosimetry may be required to give a best estimate of the amount of radiation to be given to the conceptus. Generally, termination of pregnancy is not recommended for fetal doses less than 5 rads. With 10–15 rads, especially during the first 6 weeks, many experts suggest termination of pregnancy if possible. With greater than 15 rads, nearly all recommend termination.

8. One must bear in mind that the overall risk of these low levels of radiation is extremely minimal and cannot be documented, especially since abnormal outcomes may occur spontaneously.

REFERENCES

1. Ragozzino MW, Breckle R, Hill LM, Gray JE. Average fetal depth in utero: data for estimation of fetal absorbed radiation dose. *Radiology* 1986;158(2):513–515.

2. Brent RI. The effect of embryonic and fetal exposure to x-ray, microwaves, and ultrasound: counseling the pregnant and nonpregnant patient about these risks. *Semin Oncol* 1989;16(5): 347–368.

2a. Stovall M, Blackwell CR, Cunditt J, Novac DH, Palta JR, Wagner LK, Webster EW, Shalek RJ. Fetal dose from radiotherapy with photon beams: report of AAPM rediation therapy committee task group No. 36. *Med Phys* 1995; 22:63–82.

3. NCRP Report No. 91. Recommendations on limits for exposure to ionizing radiation. Washington, DC: National Commission on Radiation Protection, 1987.

4. NCRP Report No. 54. Medical radiation exposure of pregnant and potentially pregnant women. Washington, DC: National Commission on Radiation Protection, 1977.

5. Ginsberg JS, Hirsh J, Rainbow AJ, Coates G. Risks to the fetus of radiologic procedures used in the diagnosis of maternal venous thrombolic disease. *Thromb Haemostasis* 1989;61(2): 189–196.

6. Marcus CS, Mason GR, Kuperus JH, Mena I. Pulmonary imaging in pregnancy. Maternal risk and fetal dosimetry. *Clin Nuclear Med* 1985;10(1):1–4.

7. Kanal E. Pregnancy and the safety of magnetic resonance imaging. *MRI Clin North Am* 1994;2(2):309–317.

8. Colletti PM, Sylvestre PB. Magnetic resonance imaging in pregnancy. *MRI Clin North AM* 1994;2(2):291–307.

9. Kameyama Y, Imouye M. Irradiation injury top the developing nervous system: mechanisms of neuronal injury. *Neurotoxicology* 1994; 15:75–80.

10. Doll R, Wakeford R. Risk of childhood cancer from fetal irradiation. *Br J Radiol* 1997; 70:130–139.

PART III

CARDIAC DISORDERS AND PREGNANCY

4

CONGENITAL HEART DISEASE AND PREGNANCY

CAROLE A. WARNES, MD, AND URI ELKAYAM, MD

INTRODUCTION

Enormous changes in the care of patients with congenital heart disease (CHD) have led to increasing numbers of adult survivors reaching childbearing age.[1] Although pregnancy may be carried out safely and successfully in many women with CHD, the condition may be associated with increased risk in some patients.

GENERAL CONSIDERATIONS

Preconception Evaluation and Counseling

The management of patients with CHD should begin prior to conception. A careful cardiac examination and a functional evaluation is needed to determine the likelihood of the patient's being able to tolerate the increased load of pregnancy. Elevated pulmonary artery pressure, depressed ventricular function, cyanosis, and impaired functional capacity are predictors for maternal and fetal complications and should be diagnosed prior to pregnancy. Preconception evaluation should, therefore, include physical examination and careful history, chest X-ray, 12-lead electrocardiogram, echocardiogram, Doppler study, and, if indicated, cardiac catheterization. In patients with a history of impaired functional capacity, exercise testing with measurement of oxygen consumption is helpful for objective assessment of functional classification. The anticipated risk of pregnancy should be carefully assessed and discussed with the potential mother, by both the cardiologist and the obstetrician. An important consideration is the statistical risk that the baby may inherit some form of congenital heart disease. In anticipation for

pregnancy, any drugs that may be potentially teratogenic should be discontinued. Antepartum and peripartum care must be planned carefully based on the type of maternal defect and family history, and should include guidance on the need for prophylactic antibiotic and anticoagulation therapy.

Maternal Outcome

Maternal outcome is determined by the nature of the CHD, the presence and severity of pulmonary hypertension, cyanosis and right and left ventricular dysfunction, functional capacity of the patient, and the history of prior surgical repairs.[2] In the mother who is at a New York Heart Association (NYHA) functional class I-II, maternal mortality is approximately 0.4%. When the functional class is III-IV, maternal mortality approaches 7%. For this reason, NYHA functional class clearly needs to be determined when patients come in for prepregnancy counseling.[3]

Because of the hemodynamic changes that take place during pregnancy, including an increase in plasma volume, increased cardiac output, and fall in peripheral resistance (Chapter 1), stenotic lesions (e.g., aortic stenosis) are less well tolerated than regurgitant lesions. The fall in peripheral resistance tends to exaggerate a gradient across the aortic valve but could improve lesions such as mitral regurgitation by unloading the left ventricle, helping to offset the burden imposed by the increased volume. Thus, the individual anomaly and hemodynamics need to be considered prior to conception.

Shime et al[4] reported the deterioration of functional capacity and development of heart failure in as many as 47% of patients with cyanotic heart disease and in only 13% of pa-

Cardiac Problems in Pregnancy, Third Edition
Edited by Uri Elkayam, MD, and Norbert Gleicher, MD
Copyright © 1998 by Wiley-Liss, Inc. ISBN 0-471-16358-9

tients with acyanotic congenital heart disease. Surgical repair improves the outcome of pregnancy in women with cyanotic heart disease.

When increased risk of complications and mortality for both the mother and the fetus can be predicted, pregnancy should be considered contraindicated. If pregnancy occurs in a high risk patient, an early termination is recommended unless there is a method available to deal safely with the hemodynamic anomaly (e.g., surgery, balloon valvuloplasty). Such measures may be considered if continuation of pregnancy is desired by the patient and her family and the risk associated with potential operative intervention is well understood. The care of a high risk patient requires a multidisciplinary approach involving experienced cardiologists, obstetricians, and anesthesiologists, to minimize risks to the mother and the fetus.

Fetal Outcome

Fetal outcome depends on presence of maternal cyanosis, maternal functional capacity, and maternal lesions that may reduce blood supply to the uterus (e.g., coarctation). Cyanosis is a recognized handicap to fetal growth[5] and is associated with an increased incidence of first-trimester spontaneous abortion. In addition, infants born to cyanotic mothers demonstrate a low birth weight for gestational age and prematurity. Early observations[5,6] showed a relation between degree of cyanosis and maternal hemoglobin and the incidence of spontaneous abortion and fetal growth restriction. No infant survived if the mother's hemoglobin exceeded 18 mg/dL. For these reasons, surgical correction of cyanosis before conception is recommended.

Incidence of Congenital Heart Disease in the Fetus   The incidence of CHD in the general population is in the range of 8/1000.[7] The reported incidence in the offspring of women with CHD ranges from 3.4 to 14.3%.[8–11] Dennis and Warren[8] reported a 3.4% recurrence of CHD in 308 patients with ventricular septal defect (VSD), pulmonary valvular or infundibular stenosis, or any combination thereof, including cases with tetralogy of Fallot. Emanuel et al[11] found CHD in 14.3% of 36 offspring of mothers with atrioventricular septal defect. The highest incidence has been reported by Whittemore et al, who evaluated prospectively over 25 years 236 women with cardiac defects and their 418 offspring[5] and retrospectively 191 men with CHD and their 419 children.[12] Of these 837 live children of 427 probands, 14.1% (118) had a CHD; 13.4% occurred in the maternal study and 14.8% in the paternal study. Included in these studies were 31 high-risk probands, 10 with genetic syndromes, and 21 who had an affected sibling. With removal of the high risk probands from the total study group, the risk of one affected parent having a child with a cardiac anomaly was 10.7%. The maternal study[5] reported a recurrence rate of 16.1%; after exclusion of high risk probands, the rate was 14.2%. These recurrence rates were higher than in many other studies such as the Second National Heart Study (NHS-2) of the Natural History of CHD Study, which examined the recurrence rate for CHD in relatives of patients with aortic stenosis, pulmonary stenosis, and ventricular septal defects.[13] Nora and Nora, who analyzed data on infants in the Baltimore/Washington area[14] in a population-based study of 4390 patients with CHD, found the prevalence of all CHD in the offspring to be 4.8/1000. In this group, however, 522 (12%) had a chromosomal abnormality, which was trisomy 21 in three-quarters of the patients. As in the study by Whittemore et al,[5] an elevated sibling risk was found in all diagnostic categories. The outflow lesion category was associated with the highest frequency rate of cardiac malformations in offsprings, with the highest rates in left-sided obstructions (6.7%) and in patent ductus arteriosus (7.9%). In Whittemore's study,[5] left-to-right shunting, mostly due to VSDs, was the most common cardiac anomaly. This defect showed spontaneous closure in almost half the patients. Coarctation of the aorta and aortic stenosis in the mother were associated with the highest incidence rate (20% of CHD in newborns). Other authors have been unable to duplicate the high recurrence of rates of CHD reported by Whittemore. The wide variation in the reported incidence probably relates to many factors, such as sample size, ascertainment bias, and extent of diagnostic workup for CHD in the offspring.

In summary, the offspring of mothers with CHD appear to bear an increased risk of cardiac defects, which varies between 4 and 8%, depending on the individual defect. If there is a genetic syndrome or a family history of a cardiac anomaly, the risk may be higher. For any mother with CHD, fetal cardiac echocardiography may be performed as early as 18 weeks of gestation to determine whether the fetus carries any significant cardiac anomaly.

Peripartum Management

Since abrupt hemodynamic changes are associated with labor and delivery, it is important to have a coordinated approach among anesthesiologists, cardiologists, and obstetricians. Vaginal delivery is preferable and safer for most patients with CHD, and cesarean section is indicated only for obstetric reasons. Patients who are at high risk should be admitted around the time of labor and delivery for induction and hemodynamic monitoring. Blood should be cross-matched in case blood loss occurs around delivery or postpartum. Hemodynamic evaluation and monitoring by means of a ˚Swan–Ganz catheter is advisable whenever the measurement of left ventricular filling pressure and thermodilution cardiac output can help in the management of the patient. This procedure is not useful in most patients with right ventricular outflow obstruction and low pulmonary artery pressures and in patients with right-to-left shunt. In patients with the Eisenmenger syndrome, continuous or frequent monitoring of systemic blood pressure and blood oxygen saturation is recommended. Measurement of left ventricular filling pressure in these patients does not provide important information, and intracardiac shunt makes measurement of cardiac output by thermodilution impossible. In addition, the insertion of a Swan–Ganz catheter in such patients is associated with a higher incidence of complications.[15]

Particular attention should be paid to analgesia and anesthesia, and the mode of anesthesia should be established jointly by the anesthesiologist, cardiologist, and obstetrician (see also Chapter 24). Hypotension should be avoided in particular in patients who may be dependent on the preload and in patients with intracardiac shunts. Maternal and fetal electrocardiographic monitoring should be performed continuously. Finally, the second stage of labor should be kept fairly short. If labor is not progressing smoothly, a facilitated delivery via vacuum extraction or forceps may be indicated. Women who are dependent on preload should be delivered in the left lateral position, to prevent the fetus from compressing the inferior vena cava and to ensure the maintenance of venous return.

Finally, consideration needs to be given to the prevention of infective endocarditis in patients with susceptible cardiac lesions. The American Heart Association guidelines suggest that antibiotic prophylaxis for an *uncomplicated* delivery is unnecessary. The many deliveries accomplished with an episiotomy, however, probably qualify as "complicated," and patients are at risk of contracting endocarditis by this route. The risk, however, appears to be small, and indeed Sugrue et al[16] reported an incidence of 0.9% in 2165 women with rheumatic heart disease or CHD, and Marquis[17] found no case of endocarditis after normal delivery in more than 1750 cardiac patients during a 25-year period. Nonetheless, endocarditis after delivery has been reported;[18,19] and despite the American Heart Association's recommendations,[20] antibiotic prophylaxis is a common practice in many hospitals, including the author's. We give prophylaxis to every patient with CHD except those patients with an isolated secundum atrial septal defect, repaired septal defects 6 months after surgery and no residua, and those with a successfully ligated patent ductus arteriosus.

Atrial Septal Defect (ASD)

Secundum ASD is the most common cardiac defect seen with pregnancy. Physical examination usually reveals a parasternal right ventricular lift and an ejection systolic murmur at the second left intercostal space. This murmur is never more than grade 3/6 and relates to the increased flow across the pulmonary valve. The second hart sound is widely split and fixed, and if the shunt is more than 2.5:1, a tricuspid diastolic flow rumble may also be heard at the left sternal edge.[21] The diagnosis during pregnancy may be missed, since the mur-

mur caused by the ASD may be mistaken for the physiological murmur of pregnancy (see Chapter 2). The electrocardiogram frequently shows partial right bundle branch block with right-axis deviation, and sometimes right ventricular hypertrophy. The chest X-ray shows a prominent pulmonary artery with a pulmonary plethora, and the heart may be enlarged, with a right ventricular contour and a prominent right atrium. Transthoracic echocardiography and color Doppler can usually easily confirm the diagnosis.[22] Atrial arrhythmias may occur with a secundum atrial septal defect, but usually do not occur until the fourth decade of life. Pulmonary hypertension also tends to occur after the fourth or fifth decade.[23] Less common types of atrial septal defect include the primum ASD and the sinus venosus ASD. The primum ASD consists of a defect in the lower part of the atrial septum (atrioventricular septal defect) and is usually associated with a cleft mitral valve, which is variably regurgitant. When there is significant mitral regurgitation, patients often present earlier in life, and atrial arrhythmias are also more common. A sinus venosus atrial septal defect is a defect in the superior portion of the septum, commonly associated with an anomalous pulmonary vein, frequently the right upper pulmonary vein. Presentation is usually the same as for a secundum atrial septal defect. Since a defect in the superior portion of the septum may be missed by transthoracic echocardiography, transesophageal echocardiography may be necessary to confirm the diagnosis.

The vast majority of patients with an isolated ASD will have a successful and uncomplicated pregnancy.[24] Women with a large defect, however, having a significant left-to-right shunt, may develop congestive failure during pregnancy, which may be exacerbated by atrial arrhythmias.[2,4] In a review published several years ago, Metcalfe et al[24] revealed one case of maternal death in 219 pregnancies in 113 women with ASD. One of the major concerns when a patient with ASD becomes pregnant is the development of peripheral venous thrombosis and subsequent paradoxical embolus.[25] Attention should therefore be paid to leg care, particularly around the time of delivery. If necessary, compressive stockings or leg squeezers may be used, and early mobilization is recommended. To try to help prevent clot formation, a baby aspirin once daily is recommended after the first trimester, to the end of pregnancy. If congestive failure occurs during pregnancy despite good medical therapy, surgical closure should be considered. The management of atrial arrhythmias is discussed in detail in Chapter 13.

The recurrence risk of ASD in the offspring has been reported to be approximately 2.5%.[26] With primum ASD, however, Emanuel et al[11] reported an incidence of CHD in 14.3% of the offspring of 36 mothers. The majority of these offspring also had an ostium primum defect and similar abnormalities in the mitral valve.

Bacterial endocarditis does not occur in patients with an isolated ostium secundum ASD, and prophylactic antibiotic treatment is not necessary. For those with a primum ASD, however, since there is an abnormality of the atrioventricular valves, we recommend that endocarditis prophylaxis be given. The rare patient with ASD who has severe pulmonary hypertension and Eisenmenger's syndrome should be advised against pregnancy (see following discussion on Eisenmenger's syndrome). Delivery is usually vaginal, and cesarean section delivery is reserved for obstetrical indications.

Ventricular Septal Defect (VSD)

Isolated VSD is a common cardiac malformation in childhood, but many such defects have closed by adulthood.[21] The clinical picture is determined by the size and the site of the defect. Physical examination of the patient with a VSD often reveals a holosystolic thrill at the left sternal edge associated with a holosystolic murmur maximally heard at the third or fourth left intercostal space. If the defect is in the muscular septum, the murmur may stop partway through systole. The electrocardiogram may be normal, but left ventricular hypertrophy suggests a larger left-to-right shunt, and right ventricular hypertrophy suggests elevated pulmonary pressures. The chest X-ray film usually shows an enlarged left ventricle and left atrium and pulmonary plethora. The diagnosis can easily be confirmed by transthoracic echocardiography.[21] At preconception counseling, left ventricular size and function and pulmonary artery pressure should be determined noninvasively.

Women with VSD usually tolerate pregnancy very well. Early reports described congestive heart failure and even death in some patients with VSD during pregnancy.[24] Later reports by Whittemore et al[2] (1982) indicated no death in a group of 50 patients with VSD, where there were 98 pregnancies with 80% live-born infants. This report confirmed the occurrence of heart failure and arrhythmias in some patients, especially those with impaired functional capacity prior to pregnancy. The incidence of recurrence of a VSD in the offspring of mothers has been reported to be 4% by one study[26] and 11% in another.[2] Pregnancy following closure of an uncomplicated VSD is usually unremarkable, provided there are no important residua, such as left ventricular dysfunction, aortic regurgitation, or pulmonary hypertension. Endocarditis prophylaxis should be given around the time of delivery, and delivery is usually vaginal.

Patent Ductus Arteriosus (PDA)

Patent ductus arteriosus is one of the most common congenital cardiovascular anomalies, occurring with a female/male ratio of 2:1.[3,4] Most cases are diagnosed and surgically corrected in early childhood. In the adult with PDA, physical examination usually reveals normal palpation or a slightly hyperdynamic left ventricle. The pulse pressure is usually wide, and a continuous murmur ("machinery murmur") is heard

maximally in the second intercostal space. The murmur typically envelops the second heart sound. In cases of a larger PDA with the development of pulmonary hypertension, the diastolic part of the murmur may be absent, and indeed the systolic murmur may be virtually inaudible.[21] Other signs of pulmonary hypertension are a right ventricular heave and a palpable P_2. There may be an ejection click from the dilated pulmonary artery and a diastolic murmur of pulmonary regurgitation. If reverse shunting occurs, cyanosis and clubbing may be present in the lower extremities. In cases of a PDA, the electrocardiogram may be normal, or it may show left ventricular hypertrophy. The chest X-ray may be normal with a small PDA, although with a large shunt or older patient, the film may show an enlarged left ventricle with enlargement of the pulmonary artery and increased pulmonary vascularity. The color Doppler echocardiogram can facilitate diagnosis by permitting visualization of continuous flow in the pulmonary artery. Pulmonary artery pressure can also be estimated.

Most patients with a small PDA tolerate pregnancy without significant difficulty except for the risk of infective endarteritis during delivery, but if there is a significant shunt, they may develop congestive heart failure.[1,27] No mortality was reported by Szekely and Snaith[28] or by Metcalfe et al,[24] who reviewed large series of unoperated patients. Whittemore et al[2] reported 42 patients with surgically corrected PDA who had 105 pregnancies that were mostly uneventful and without mortality. A few patients developed arrhythmias and hypertension, and 11% of live-born infants had CHD. The risk of recurrence of a PDA in the offspring of a mother with the same anomaly was estimated to be 4%.

If left ventricular dysfunction is present at the onset, patients may develop congestive heart failure and should be treated with digoxin and diuretics. Ideally, surgical closure of a PDA should be performed prior to gestation. Mode of delivery is vaginal in the majority of patients. Endocarditis prophylaxis should be given for delivery, and hemodynamic monitoring is recommended in symptomatic patients and in patients with a large shunt or echocardiographic evidence for left ventricular systolic dysfunction.

Aortic Stenosis (AS)

Congenital obstruction of the left ventricular outflow can be valvular, supravalvular, or subvalvular. The bicuspid aortic valve is the most common congenital cardiac malformation, but it is much more common in males than females; hence the incidence in pregnancy is low.[21] Most young women with congenital AS are asymptomatic. Severe aortic stenosis, however, may be associated with symptoms of fatigue, exercise intolerance, syncope, or angina pectoris.

On physical examination, there may be a slow rate of rise of the carotid arterial pulse, and severe stenosis may be associated with a systolic thrill or shudder. Apical palpation may reveal a sustained impulse of left ventricular hypertrophy, and there may be an additional presystolic pulsation. Auscultation often reveals an aortic ejection click followed by a systolic ejection murmur, loudest at the left sternal edge or the second right intercostal space and radiates to the neck. With increasing severity of stenosis, the murmur becomes longer and late peaking, and prolongation of left ventricular ejection may lead to paradoxical splitting of the second heart sound. The aortic component of the second heart sound may be audible in young patients when the valve is still pliable, but audibility diminishes when the valve begins to calcify. A fourth heart sound is common as a result of reduced left ventricular compliance. The chest X-ray usually shows a normal or slightly enlarged left ventricle, as well as post-stenotic dilatation of the ascending aorta. The diagnosis is easily confirmed by two-dimensional echocardiography and Doppler,[21] which provide additional information regarding thickness and calcification of the valve, pressure gradient across the valve, valve area, degree of left ventricular hypertrophy, systolic and diastolic function of the left ventricle, and involvement of other valves.

Ideally, women with severe AS should be counseled before pregnancy and should undergo either a balloon or surgical valvotomy if the anatomy is appropriate, or valve replacement. The potential risk associated with this condition during pregnancy is reflected by an early report by Arias and Pineda,[29] who reviewed the English literature until 1978 and reported 38 pregnancies in 23 women with a maternal mortality of 17% and a fetal mortality of 32%. In their 1982 study, Whittemore et al[2] cited 59 pregnancies in 27 women with left heart obstruction, including AS and coarctation of the aorta without maternal death; but 6 women developed hypertension, 5 developed congestive heart failure, 2 had angina, and 1 an arrhythmia. More recently, Lao et al[30] reported a retrospective review of 25 pregnancies in 13 patients with congenital AS who delivered between 1976 to 1992. The aortic valve area ranged between 0.7 and 2.0 cm² and the peak pressure gradient across the aortic valve between 30 and 125 mmHg. Thirty-eight percent of the patients had other, corrected congenital heart malformations (including coarctation of the aorta in 31%, PDA in 15%, ASD in 8%, VSD in 8%). Fifty-four percent of the patients had also mild to moderate aortic regurgitation, and two of the patients had had surgical commissurotomy of the aortic valve many years (11 and 23, respectively) prior to pregnancy. Clinical deterioration was reported in 8 of the 25 pregnancies. Three of the patients had severe AS (aortic valve area < 0.7 cm²); one had two uneventful pregnancies while the other two showed deterioration of symptoms necessitating a percutaneous balloon valvuloplasty at 16 weeks of gestation in one patient and a therapeutic abortion at 13 weeks in the other. Other reports have also described clinical deterioration of patients with AS and the need to correct the valve either with percutaneous balloon technique or with surgery during pregnancy. Ben Ami[31] described a patient who required aortic valve replace-

ment during the 29th week of gestation as a result of fatigue, shortness of breath with mild exertion, and syncope, after lack of improvement with nonspecified medical therapy and bed rest. Surgery was associated with prolonged fetal bradycardia and loss of beat-to-beat variability, which returned to normal at the end of the procedure. Balloon valvuloplasty was reported in five patients with congenital AS.[32–35] The procedure was performed in the second trimester in four cases and in the third trimester in one. Valve area was 0.5 cm² in one patient, 0.7 cm² in two patients, and was not reported in two patients, who had pressure gradients across the aortic valve of 128 and 123 mmHg, respectively. Clinical improvement and normal fetal outcome was reported following the procedure in all patients.

In summary, most cases of AS are tolerated well during pregnancy. Severe AS (valve area < 1.0 cm²), however, can be associated with maternal morbidity and even mortality during pregnancy and in the peripartum period. With early diagnosis, close follow-up, avoidance of excessive exertion, and bed rest where appropriate, pregnancy may be safely carried out. Particularly important is hemodynamic monitoring during labor and delivery,[31] with maintenance of preload and avoidance of any anesthesia that would induce vasodilatation and hypotension. In patients with severe AS who demonstrate clinical deterioration that does not respond to medical therapy prior to fetal maturity, percutaneous balloon valvuloplasty is a viable therapeutic option, as is surgical valve replacement during pregnancy. Based on limited experience, balloon valvuloplasty appears to be associated with a smaller risk of fetal loss than aortic valve replacement during pregnancy.[37] Valvuloplasty should, therefore, be considered when the aortic valve anatomy is appropriate (i.e., a mobile valve without any calcification and little or no aortic regurgitation). Since both procedures carry risk to the fetus (radiation with valvuloplasty, increased fetal wastage with surgery), and since complaints associated with pregnancy itself may mimic cardiac disease, symptoms should be carefully evaluated and their relation to the underlying disease clearly established before these procedures are performed. Appropriate lead shielding to the fetus should be provided, and attempts should be made to minimize the use of radiation when valvuloplasty is performed. When fetal maturity can be established, repair or replaement of the mother's aortic valve should be done after the delivery.

Seventy-eight percent of the pregnancies reported by Whittemore et al[2] resulted in live-born infants, but 20% of the newborns had cardiac defects and 12% had an obstructive defect. The majority of anomalies occurred in the offspring of patients without surgical repair. Mother–child defect concordance was estimated by Nora and Nora to be 4% in women with congenital AS.[36] Most patients with aortic stenosis can safely undergo vaginal delivery, with cesarean section preserved for hemodynamically unstable patients or those presenting obstetrical indications.

Coarctation of the Aorta

Coarctation of the aorta is a narrowing of the aorta, usually just distal to the left subclavian artery, and is associated with systemic hypertension above the coarctation and reduced blood pressure below. The most common associated anomaly is a bicuspid aortic valve, and sometimes a ventricular septal defect is present. Coarctation is also associated with cerebral aneurysms.[21]

Physical examination reveals higher systolic blood pressure in the arms than in the legs, and diminished and delayed femoral pulses. Left ventricular impulse is forceful and sustained as a result of left ventricular hypertrophy and outflow obstruction, and on auscultation there is commonly an ejection click, either from a bicuspid aortic valve or dilatation of the ascending aorta. A systolic murmur is heard in the second left intercostal space, and occasionally there may be palpable and audible collaterals, producing a continuous murmur over the interscapular area. An S_4 is frequently present, the result of left ventricular hypertrophy and abnormal relaxation.[21] The electrocardiogram may show left ventricular hypertrophy. The chest X-ray usually shows normal left ventricular size. The ascending aorta may be dilated with a "figure 3" sign along the left mediastinal border formed by the ascending aorta, the indentation, and then the poststenotic dilatation. Rib notching is often seen secondary to dilated intercostal vessels. The diagnosis can usually be confirmed by two-dimensional echocardiography[21] and magnetic resonance imaging,[38] which demonstrates the site of coarctation and indicates whether it is discrete or tubular. Doppler velocities down the descending aorta may also help predict the gradient, although such determinations can be difficult in adult patients.[21]

Exacerbation of systemic hypertension may occur in patients with unoperated coarctation during pregnancy and there is an increased risk of aortic dissection and rupture due to a weakening of the arterial walls mediated by hormonal changes.[1] In addition, congestive heart failure and angina pectoris can occur, as well as cerebral hemorrhage from rupture of an aneurysm of the circle of Willis.[1,39]

Early studies reported high maternal mortality, ranging from 3 to 9%.[40–43] The majority of maternal deaths occurred before labor and delivery. With modern medical management and proper control of systemic hypertension, however, pregnancy is usually safe to the mother with uncomplicated coarctation,[44–46] although severe hypertension congestive failure may occur as well as aortic dissection.[2,4,47] Connolly et al[46] recently reported the outcome of 37 pregnancies in 15 patients with unoperated coarctation of the thoracic aorta seen at the Mayo Clinic from 1980 to 1994. Thirty-three pregnancies resulted in live births; four had spontaneous miscarriages. In addition, 22 patients had 41 successful and two unsuccessful pregnancies after coarctation surgery. There were no pregnancy-related maternal deaths. Hyper-

tension was seen during pregnancy in 9 patients (5 unoperated and 4 operated); 3 of them had premature deliveries; their offspring had CHD. There was no maternal death reported and hypertension was seen in 9 patients (5 unoperated and 4 operated).

Experience at the University of Southern California in approximately 30 pregnancies in patients with unoperated coarctation of the aorta seen in the last 15 years has been similar. Two of the patients, however, had major complications. One, who presented at the 22nd week of gestation with pulmonary edema, had severe aortic stenosis. This patient was treated medically for 10 weeks and, after a fetal maturation, delivered uneventfully by cesarean section. The birth was followed by successful aortic valve replacement, but the patient died 10 days later of cardiac arrhythmia. A second patient had an uneventful pregnancy and died suddenly at 37 weeks from dissection of the ascending aorta a few minutes after experiencing severe chest pain.

In early studies, fetal mortality was reported to be as high as 13–25%.[40–43] Connolly et al reported spontaneous abortion in four pregnancies in unoperated patients and one neonatal death and fetal loss in two out of 41 pregnancies in patients after surgical correction of the coarctation.[46] Although placental blood flow may be reduced,[47] birth weights were reported to be normal by Connolly et al,[46] and there was no significant difference between cases prior to and after surgery (3.3 ± 0.6 vs. 3.4 ± 0.5 kg).

The mainstays of treatment during pregnancy should be limitation of physical activity and the control of blood pressure, ideally with β-adrenergic blocking agents,[38] to reduce the shear stress on the arterial wall and minimize the small but real risk of aortic dissection. Systolic blood pressure should be maintained at less then 140 mmHg. At the same time, however, excessive reduction of blood pressure is not recommended, since it may result in a reduction of placental blood flow that could affect the fetus. Because of potential increase in blood pressure during labor and transient hypertension at the time of delivery, some authors have recommended cesarean section. Most patients, however, can be safely delivered vaginally, usually with epidural anesthesia. If the second stage progresses slowly, it may be necessary to use low outlet forceps or vacuum extraction to shorten the second stage. Beta blockers should be continued throughout delivery. Since there is an increased risk of aortic dissection following correction of aortic coarctation with balloon angioplasty,[48] cesarean section may be safer in such patients. Most aortic ruptures during pregnancy occur prior to labor and delivery, and death during or immediately after labor and delivery is rare. Surgical correction of coarctation during pregnancy has been successful[48] but is not recommended unless major complications develop (e.g., aortic dissection, uncontrollable hypertension, heart failure that does not respond to medical therapy). Since risk of dissection is increased during gestation (Chapter 17), balloon angioplasty for correction of aortic coarctation is not recommended during pregnancy or in women of childbearing age. Because of the potential risk of endocarditis in patients with coarctation, antibiotic prophylaxis around the time of delivery is recommended.

Pulmonary Stenosis (PS)

Congenital obstruction to the right ventricular outflow tract is most commonly seen at the valvular level but can also occur at the subvalvular or supravalvular level. The majority of patients with valvular PS are asymptomatic, and symptoms of fatigue and dyspnea usually appear only in cases of severe stenosis, as a consequence of decreased cardiac output.

Physical examination reveals a prominent A wave in the jugular venous pulse and a right ventricular parasternal lift. In severe stenosis, there may be a systolic thrill in the second left intercostal space.[21] When the valve is mobile, an ejection click will precede a systolic murmur, which gets longer and peaks later with increasing stenosis. As the obstruction becomes more severe, the pulmonary component of the second heart sound becomes softer and delayed, and in severe stenosis will be completely absent. In severe cases, the electrocardiogram will show right ventricular hypertrophy. The chest X-ray usually shows a normal heart size, enlargement of the main and left pulmonary artery secondary to poststenotic dilatation, and in severe cases, reduced pulmonary vascularity. Two-dimensional echocardiography and Doppler will reliably make the diagnosis, measure the pressure gradient across the pulmonic valve, and determine right ventricular systolic pressure from the tricuspid regurgitant velocity.

Isolated PS, even when severe, is usually well tolerated during pregnancy. If there is an associated patent foramen ovale or small atrial septal defect, patients may become cyanotic owing to right-to-left shunting. In most patients, even with severe PS, right ventricular function is maintained until advanced age. Early reports by Neilson et al[49] described 11 patients with PS who had 26 pregnancies. There were four spontaneous abortions; one patient with severe stenosis had right heart failure during her first pregnancy, and after valvotomy, three uneventful pregnancies. Whittemore et al[2] described 46 pregnancies in 24 women with PS; 78% of the pregnancies resulted in live-born infants, but 19% of the infants had cardiac defects. These investigators estimated the risk of inheriting PS from a mother with this entity to be 3.5%. Most of the reports of pregnancies complicated by PS were published more than 25 years ago[27] and indicated occasional congestive heart failure. Our unpublished experience in the last 15 years indicates that with proper medical management, pregnancy can usually be brought to term with favorable maternal and fetal outcome. In the rare case of right ventricular failure or in a patient with intracardiac shunt at either the atrial or ventricular level with cyanosis, pulmonary balloon valvotomy can be performed during pregnancy, with lead shielding of the mother's abdomen to protect the fetus

from radiation.[1] Ideally, however, balloon valvuloplasty, which is now the procedure of choice for isolated pulmonary valve stenosis,[50] should be performed before pregnancy. Vaginal delivery will be tolerated in the majority of patients with PS.

Tetralogy of Fallot

Tetralogy of Fallot is the most common cyanotic congenital heart disease in children and adults[21] and is the most common cyanotic congenital lesion in pregnancy. Classically, tetralogy of Fallot has four anatomic abnormalities: (1) pulmonary stenosis, which usually is infundibular, but there can be associated valvular and supravalvular stenosis; (2) a large ventricular septal defect that sits immediately beneath the aortic valve; (3) dextroposition of the aorta, which overrides the ventricular septal defect; and (4) right ventricular hypertrophy. The latter is a consequence of the PS. The clinical spectrum varies widely, and adult patients with unrepaired tetralogy have varying degrees of cyanosis and clubbing, depending on the degree of PS. Death in unoperated tetralogy of Fallot is commonly from arrhythmia, ventricular failure (often secondary to aortic regurgitation), bacterial endocarditis (usually on the aortic valve), and cerebrovascular accidents. There is usually a right ventricular heave, and with severe PS, there may be a systolic thrill at the left sternal edge associated with a long systolic murmur due to the outflow obstruction. The second heart sound is single and may be palpable, as the aorta is closer than usual to the chest wall. Frequently, there is an associated aortic regurgitation, since the aortic cusps prolapse into the VSD and the aorta itself is dilated. The electrocardiogram usually shows right ventricular hypertrophy. The chest radiograph will show right ventricular enlargement with a narrow pulmonary pedicle. Twenty-five percent of cases will have a right aortic arch. Diagnosis is easily made from two-dimensional echocardiography, and Doppler can determine the degree of PS, VSD, and aortic regurgitation.[22]

The hemodynamic changes during pregnancy may lead to clinical deterioration and both maternal and fetal complications. The fall in peripheral vascular resistance can exaggerate right-to-left shunt and cause worsening of cyanosis. In addition, the increased volume load of pregnancy may exaggerate both right and left ventricular dysfunction and precipitate heart failure. Labor and delivery are particularly important, since any hypotension will also exaggerate the right-to-left shunt, with worsening of cyanosis and possible cardiac arrhythmias. Pregnancy in surgically untreated women with tetralogy of Fallot was reported in early studies to have a maternal mortality of more than 4%.[28] The presence and degree of maternal hypoxia, as judged by the maternal hematocrit, correlate with an increased rate of spontaneous abortion. As many as 80% of pregnancies of women whose hematocrit is greater than 65% are likely to end in spontaneous abortion. In addition, cyanosis may result in premature delivery and low birth weight for gestational age.[51,52]

Presbitero et al[18] reported a retrospective review of 46 pregnancies in 21 cyanotic patients with tetralogy of Fallot or pulmonary atresia. Patients who had undergone surgical repair and were no longer cyanotic were specifically excluded. There were 46 pregnancies and 15 live births (9 premature), 26 spontaneous abortions and 5 stillbirths. Eight patients had cardiovascular complications, including one cerebral infarct. Peripartum bacterial endocarditis occurred in 2 patients, both with palliated tetralogy. Neither had antibiotic prophylaxis during labor, and one subsequently died with massive hemoptysis and a ruptured aneurysm at the site of her shunt.

Relief of cyanosis by reparative operation reduces the risk of pregnancy considerably. Most patients with good repair can anticipate a successful pregnancy. At preconception counseling, however, they should be carefully assessed in terms of functional capacity and should have a physical examination and an echocardiogram to determine the presence or absence of residual lesions. These include residual VSD, PS, or regurgitation, aortic regurgitation, and ventricular dysfunction. Patients who have had shunt procedures to improve cyanosis may develop pulmonary hypertension, and the presence of this condition should also be assessed prior to pregnancy. Metcalfe et al[24] reported on 40 pregnancies in 18 women with surgically repaired tetralogy. Five of the pregnancies were interrupted, and an equal number ended with a spontaneous abortion, but there was no maternal mortality or morbidity. Whittemore et al[2] found cardiac defects in 15% of infants born to women with cyanosis, and in 17% of acyanotic women. In contrast, Metcalfe et al[24] found congenital heart disease in only one of 30 infants born to women with surgically repaired tetralogy of Fallot. More recently, the incidence of tetralogy of Fallot in the newborn offspring of a woman with tetralogy of Fallot and a normal husband has been estimated to be 4%.[53]

Ebstein's Anomaly

Ebstein's anomaly is a relatively rare entity in which the tricuspid valve is malformed and displaced inferiorly into the right ventricle.[21] The hemodynamic abnormality is determined by the degree of displacement, severity of tricuspid regurgitation, right ventricular dysfunction, and the presence or absence of a patent foramen ovale or, atrial septal defect, which is present in about 50% of patients. Patients may also suffer from atrial fibrillation or supraventricular tachyarrhythmias, often associated with an accessory pathway (approximately 25% of cases). Symptoms can be severe, particularly in patients with cyanosis.

Physical examination may therefore reveal cyanosis (if there is an atrial communication), elevated venous pressure with prominent V waves due to tricuspid regurgitation. Pal-

pation may reveal a right parasternal lift consistent with right-sided volume overload. On auscultation, there is frequently a loud tricuspid component of the first sound from the large "sail-like" anterior leaflet and frequently one or more clicks from the abnormal tricuspid valve. A murmur of tricuspid regurgitation will be present at the lower left sternal border to varying degree. The electrocardiogram, if the patient is in sinus rhythm, demonstrates very large P waves, consistent with the right atrial enlargement. Right bundle branch block and preexcitation are frequently present, although there may be a prolonged P-R interval. The chest X-ray film may show the characteristic cardiac contour with a narrow pedicle and a globular cardiac silhouette from right atrial enlargement. Pulmonary vasculature is usually normal or decreased. The diagnosis is easily confirmed by two-dimensional echo–Doppler techniques.[22] Patients who are symptomatic with an increasing cardiothoracic ratio, particularly if they have an atrial communication and/or a bypass tract, should be considered for surgical repair. In many cases, if the tricuspid valve is not tethered, an excellent functional result can be obtained from valve repair and closure of the atrial septal defect if present.[54] For those with tethered valves, a tricuspid valve replacement may be necessary. Patients who have Ebstein's anomaly with or without repaired or replaced valve should be carefully evaluated prior to contemplating pregnancy. This evaluation should include a clinical exam, chest X-ray, echocardiogram, and functional testing to determine residual tricuspid regurgitation, right-sided function, the presence of any residual shunt, and cardiac reserve.

Several successful pregnancies have been reported in women with Ebstein's anomaly. Donnelly et al[55] reported 12 women with Ebstein's anomaly who had 36 infants, none of whom had congenital heart disease, and there were no pregnancy-related maternal deaths. Neonatal outcome was good, but there was an increased risk of prematurity and dysmaturity in the babies born to cyanotic mothers. The largest series to date was published in 1994 by Connolly and Warnes,[56] who reported 44 women with 111 pregnancies resulting in 85 live births (76%). Ten patients had had cardiac repair, 20 had an interatrial communication at the time of pregnancy, and 16 of them were cyanosed. No serious pregnancy-related maternal complications occurred. There were 19 spontaneous abortions, 7 therapeutic abortions, 2 early neonatal deaths, and 23 premature deliveries. The incidence of CHD was 6% (5 of 83) in the offspring. In this study, the offspring of 28 men were also evaluated, and the incidence of congenital heart disease was 1% (1 of 75). This study concluded that pregnancy in women with Ebstein's anomaly is well tolerated but is associated with an increased risk of prematurity, fetal loss, and CHD. In addition, a significantly lower birth weight was found in the offspring of cyanotic versus acyanotic women. The authors emphasized, however, that each case needs to be assessed individually prior to pregnancy, with particular attention to ventricular size and function, as well as presence of cyanosis, arrhythmias, and other congenital anomalies. Exercise stress testing may be helpful for evaluation of functional capacity for patients who require and are amenable to cardiac repair. Pregnancy may be well tolerated after tricuspid valve repair or replacement, and in patients with atrial septal defects, the risk of paradoxical embolus is obviated after repair. Antibiotic prophylaxis is advisable for labor and delivery, and most patients can be delivered vaginally.

COMPLEX CYANOTIC CHD

Tricuspid Atresia

Tricuspid atresia is characterized by an absent tricuspid valve orifice, hypoplasia of the right ventricle, and an obligatory atrial septal defect. The great arteries may be normally related or transposed. Several cases of tricuspid atresia have been reported in association with pregnancy, and a few cases of pregnancy leading to the delivery of surviving infants, who subsequently developed normally, have been described.[57–60] Patton et al[51] reported pregnancies in two patients with tricuspid atresia. The first patient, who had Potts' shunt (descending aorta to left pulmonary artery) and was in the NYHA functional class III, had cesarean section for fetal distress at 35 weeks and delivered a 1504 g, growth-retarded infant with a coarctation of the aorta. The second patient, who had AS in addition to ASD, VSD, and transposition of the great vessels, had had pulmonary banding as a child. She was at NYHA functional class III and has spontaneous delivery at 34 weeks of a 1680 g fetus.

Presbitero et al[18] reported 26 pregnancies in 10 patients with single ventricle and/or tricuspid atresia without maternal mortality. Live birth, however, occurred in only 31%. There is a strong relation between the level of arterial oxygen saturation and hemoglobin in the mother and the incidence of spontaneous abortion, premature delivery, growth retardation, and neonatal deaths. For patients with marked right atrial enlargement, there is an increased risk of atrial arrhythmias[18] and thrombus formation within the right atrium, which may lead to paradoxical embolus. The presence of pulmonary hypertension increases the risk of maternal death. For women who have had radical repair in the form of a Fontan operation, pregnancy may be carried out[61] with a favorable maternal outcome, provided there are no significant residual lesions. The risk of fetal loss, however, remains increased in these cases. The presence or absence of any obstruction to the Fontan circulation, should be carefully assessed prior to pregnancy, along with ventricular function. The majority of stable patients with tricuspid atresia can be delivered vaginally. Antibiotic prophylaxis is recommended for labor and delivery, as well as close monitoring of blood pressure and oxygen saturation.

Transposition of the Great Vessels

When the aorta arises from the morphologic right ventricle, and the pulmonary artery from the morphologic left ventricle, the result is two parallel and separate circulations, and there is a communication between the two circulations in the form of an ASD, VSD, or PDA. Ninety percent of all infants in whom the great vessels are transposed die within the first year unless surgical repair is accomplished. The development of reparative operations, however, allows the majority of infants to survive and reach childbearing age. The most common type of repair seen in women of reproductive age is the Mustard operation, which is an atrial baffle procedure designed to divert the vena caval blood to the mitral valve and left ventrical, hence out to the pulmonary artery.[62] In turn, pulmonary venous blood returns to the right ventricle and then out to the aorta. Thus, the circulation is restored to the normal direction, but the right ventricle is left to support the systemic circulation. This arrangement may maintain function for more than two decades, but ultimately the right ventricle begins to dilate and fails, with associated tricuspid regurgitation. Other problems include slow junctional rhythm and atrial arrhythmias for which patients may need medication or sometimes a pacemaker.[62]

There have been several reports of successful pregnancy in women with transposition of the great vessels after a Mustard procedure. Lynch-Salamon et al[63] reported pregnancies in 3 women who had had a Mustard operation in childhood. Two pregnancies were complicated by failure of the systemic (morphologic right) ventricle, and one by preterm labor. All three infants were healthy and were delivered vaginally between 34 and 39 weeks gestation. Labor was managed with antibiotic prophylaxis against endocarditis, hemodynamic assessment, epidural anesthesia, and low forceps delivery to avoid expulsive efforts in the second stage of delivery. Clarkson et al[64] reported 9 women with 15 pregnancies following a Mustard procedure. They were asymptomatic before pregnancy and remained so during each pregnancy. There were 12 live births, 2 spontaneous abortions, and 1 intrauterine death. None of the live-born infants had congenital heart disease. Lao et al[65] reported a retrospective review of 7 pregnancies in 4 patients with surgical correction of dextrotransposition of the great vessels. Three patients had the Mustard procedure and one patient had the Rastelli procedure (placement of a conduit from the right ventricle to the pulmonary artery to relieve PS and close the VSD in a way designed to divert the blood from the left ventricle to the aorta). One pregnancy in a patient with the Mustard procedure had to be terminated for reasons of functional deterioration; preterm delivery occurred in 3 other cases. There was no perinatal mortality or CHD in any of the fetuses.

Dellinger and Hadi[66] reported one case of successful pregnancy completion in a patient with transposition of the great arteries corrected by the Mustard operation. A full-term pregnancy was also reported by Rousseil et al[67] in a 24-year-old primigravida who had had the Mustard operation. This patient, however, developed signs and symptoms of moderate right ventricular failure and frequent episodes of accelerated junctional rhythm, treated successfully with digitalis and delivered by elective cesarean section under close hemodynamic monitoring. Magerian et al[68] have reported 5 pregnancies following the Mustard operation in 4 patients who were in NYHA functional class I or II prior to pregnancy. Two patients required hospitalization for control of supraventricular arrhythmias and a third patient had asymptomatic sinus bradycardia. Fetal growth restriction was seen in two cases; another women had two pregnancies that ended in preterm labor. There were, however, no neonatal or perinatal deaths, nor any significant morbidity. In summary, these reports demonstrate that pregnancy is relatively well tolerated in patients with good functional capacity after surgical correction of transposition of the great arteries either by the Mustard or the Rastelli procedure. Right ventricular failure, deterioration of functional capacity, and maternal arrhythmias may occur. Fetal outcome may be better than in other complex CHD,[18] but incidence of premature delivery and fetal growth restriction is high.

The critical determinant of whether pregnancy is advisable, however, is the degree of right ventricular dysfunction. Careful assessment of right ventricular dilatation and function, degree of tricuspid regurgitation, and any associated lesions should be performed prior to conception. The functional capacity of the patient should be determined by careful history taking and, if necessary, exercise testing. Pregnancy in patients with the Rastelli procedure is possible, provided ventricular function is adequate, there is no significant conduit obstruction, the right ventricular pressure is less than two-thirds of the systemic pressure, and there is no significant subaortic obstruction at the site of the VSD patch. Vaginal delivery is recommended for the stable patients, with antibiotic prophylaxis and hemodynamic monitoring.

Truncus Arteriosus

Truncus arteriosus is a condition in which a single large artery (the trunk) forms the outlet of both ventricles via a large semilunar valve above a large VSD.[21] This single artery gives rise to both the coronary and the pulmonary arteries. Many patients die in infancy or childhood from congestive heart failure. The rare patient who survives to adulthood usually has Eisenmenger physiology unless the pulmonary arteries are obstructed. Most patients who survive to childbearing age, however, had therefore had undergone surgical repair. For patients with Eisenmenger physiology, pregnancy is strongly contraindicated. After successful surgical repair, however, provided there is no significant elevation of the pulmonary artery pressure, and in the absence of other

significant hemodynamic abnormalities, pregnancy may be successfully undertaken.

Reports of pregnancy in patients with truncus arteriosus are rare. In 1951 Simon and Lustberg[69] described a patient with truncus arteriosus who had a successful pregnancy and full-term delivery of a normal infant. The mother died suddenly, however, from what was thought to be pulmonary infarction, on the third day postpartum. More recently, Perry[70] described a pregnancy in a 31-year-old woman with truncus arteriosus, repaired initially at age 13. Repair included closure of VSD and placement of a Dacron conduit plus aortic valve homograft. Nine years later, the patient's conduit was replaced again, the avitric homograft was replaced by a porcine aortic valve and a foramen ovale was closed. She had pulmonary hypertension and was in NYHA functional class II prior to pregnancy. The patient did well until 28 weeks of gestation, when she developed increasing exertional dyspnea which was improved after initiation of digitalis therapy. In her 36th gestational week, the patient delivered a newborn with a heart murmur that was not further investigated. For obstetrical reasons, delivery was by cesarean section.

Single Ventricle

This is a condition in which one ventricular chamber receives blood from both the mitral and tricuspid valves or from one large atrioventricular valve.[21] In 85% of such cases, the great arteries are transposed, and in almost half of cases, this anomaly is associated with PS. Patients without PS develop pulmonary hypertension and severe pulmonary vascular disease with Eisenmenger physiology. Pregnancy in these patients is contraindicated.

Successful pregnancies have been reported in patients with a single ventricle.[71–76] Fong et al[74] described a case of a 29-year-old parturient with a single ventricle and transposition of the great arteries, ventricular inversion, ASD, right atrioventricular valve atresia with arterial O_2 saturation of 86–88%, ventricular ejection fraction of 28%. She had a history of pregnancy 4 years earlier, complicated only by fetal growth retardation. In the 17th week, the reported pregnancy was complicated by retinal artery thromboembolism, which was treated with heparin. In the 36th week, owing to fetal distress, the patient delivered a 1845 g newborn by an emergency cesarean section. Summer et al[75] reported a pregnancy in a 31-year-old patient with a single ventricle. The patient, who had had pulmonary banding at age 14 and was at the NYHA functional class II, had an uncomplicated pregnancy and delivered by cesarean section under epidural anesthesia. Zavisca et al[76] reported on a patient with a single ventricle and pulmonary atresia with a Potts shunt (left descending aorta to left pulmonary artery). At 28 weeks, she developed severe congestive heart failure, which improved after therapy with oxygen, bed rest, digoxin, and diuretics. At

32 weeks, heart failure worsened and the patient delivered by cesarean section under opioid-based general anesthesia with good maternal as well as fetal outcome. Presbitero et al[18] reported 26 pregnancies in 10 patients with single-ventricle and/or tricuspid atresia without maternal mortality. Fetal outcome was poor, with only 31% live births.

In summary, successful pregnancies have been reported in women with a single ventricle. Such pregnancies, however, may be associated with severe maternal complications including congestive heart failure and thromboembolic events, and even death. High incidence of fetal loss, premature labor, and small-for-age babies should be anticipated in the majority of cases. Delivery by cesarean section is often required to resolve maternal or fetal distress. In the stable patient, however, delivery should be performed vaginally. Because of risk for endocarditis, antibiotic prophylaxis for labor and delivery is recommended.

Other recent reports on pregnancy in patients with complex cyanotic heart disease include a case of a 24-year-old patient with dextrocardia, sinus inversus, a double-outlet right ventricle, large VSD, and severe pulmonary stenosis.[77] At 32 weeks, the mother had increased cyanosis and shortness of breath, and at 33 weeks she delivered a 940 g fetus by an elective cesarean section because of severe intrauterine growth retardation. Walsh et al[78] described a successful pregnancy in a patient with double-inlet left ventricle postseptation, resection of subpulmonic obstruction, pulmonary valvotomy, and implantation of a pacemaker (due to postoperative development of complete atrioventricular block). The patient was asymptomatic prior to gestation and had a successful pregnancy, with a spontaneous vaginal delivery at 39 weeks of a healthy male infant.

In summary, although successful pregnancies have been reported in patients with complex cyanotic heart diseases, these conditions may be associated with the development of heart failure, cardiac arrhythmias, thromboembolic events, and endocarditis, and even death. In addition, there is a high incidence of spontaneous abortion, stillbirths, premature deliveries, and infants that are small for their gestational age, and cardiac as well as noncardiac congenital defects. Degree of cyanosis is a major factor determining the likelihood of delivering a healthy infant. Both right and left ventricular function need to be assessed carefully prior to any pregnancy, as well as pulmonary artery pressure and patient's functional capacity. If a significant maternal hazard is believed to exist, pregnancy should be prevented, and if it occurs, an early therapeutic abortion is indicated. Because of high risk of thromboembolic events, anticoagulation should be considered at least during the third trimester and one month postpartum. Antibiotic prophylaxis is recommended peripartum. In the stable patient, vaginal delivery is the procedure of choice. Cesarean section should be performed for obstetrical reasons and in the presence of maternal instability. Careful monitor-

ing by pulse oximetry is recommended to ensure adequate oxygenation. In case of vaginal delivery, the second stage should be kept fairly short, and if labor is not progressing promptly, it should be facilitated by either forceps or vacuum extraction.

EISENMENGER'S SYNDROME

Eisenmenger's syndrome is a general term used to describe severe pulmonary hypertension and pulmonary vascular obstructive disease secondary to a communication between the systemic and pulmonary circulation. This communication is most commonly a ventricular septal defect, atrial septal defect, and patent ductus arteriosus.[21,79] The pulmonary vascular disease causes right-to-left shunting, and the degree of pulmonary vascular obstructive disease determines the degree of cyanosis.

Because of the rarity of this condition and the common advice against pregnancy, clinical experience with Eisenmenger's syndrome in pregnancy is limited and anecdotal. No single institution has been able to amass enough experience to report statistically significant data based only on its own records. In 1979 Gleicher et al[80] presented a retrospective review of 70 pregnancies in 44 patients with adequate documentation of Eisenmenger's syndrome. Fifty-two percent of these patients died in connection with a pregnancy. Death of the mother resulted in 30% of all pregnancies. No statistically significant difference in maternal mortality could be found between first and subsequent pregnancies, indicating that a successful pregnancy in patients with Eisenmenger's syndrome could not be taken as a positive prediction for further pregnancies. In a review of the literature published after the report by Gleicher et al, we were able to find reports of 55 women with Eisenmenger's syndrome who had at least one pregnancy.[81–100] Reported maternal mortality in these patients was 39%. In addition, three of four who were managed by us died in connection with pregnancy. One suffered a pulmonary embolism near term and died several hours after cesarean section delivery. Another patient died one day postpartum, shortly after the development of an episode of hypoxemia and hypotension, and the third patient died 7 days postpartum. The fourth patient survived an episode of desaturation and hemodynamic instability secondary to proven pulmonary embolism. These data demonstrate the continuing hazard associated with pregnancy in patients with Eisenmenger.

The majority of deaths occurred in the early postpartum period, usually preceded by refractory hypoxemia. Although the cause for hypoxemia and death is not entirely clear, micro- and macropulmonary embolism are commonly found in many of these patients and may be related to increased coagulation.

Cesarean sections were found by Gleicher et al[80] to be associated with an extremely high maternal mortality. Nonetheless, the authors stressed that patients who require cesarean sections may represent a biased study group, indicating an already severely compromised situation. The widely cited belief that under almost any circumstances, patients with Eisenmenger's syndrome should be delivered vaginally rather than by cesarean section may be based on relatively poor data. Avila et al[100] recently reported delivery by cesarean section in 9 women with Eisenmenger's syndrome; 7 of these patients survived. The maternal probability of death was found to be significantly higher when any kind of delivery was compared to elective termination of pregnancy.[80] This observation led the authors to suggest that termination of pregnancy was indicated in all patients with Eisenmenger's syndrome. The reason for maternal risk relates significantly to the change in hemodynamics that occurs during pregnancy. The fall in systemic vascular resistance increases right-to-left shunt, reduces arterial oxygen saturation, and increases erythrocytosis. Conversely, bearing down during labor increases systemic vascular resistance and can depress cardiac output and induce syncope. In the setting of fixed pulmonary vascular resistance, all these hemodynamic changes are poorly tolerated. Sterilization may be a reasonable alternative, and this can be performed laparoscopically, ideally with cardiac anesthesia.

In addition to the risks to the mother, pregnancy is associated with poor fetal outcome. Only 26% of all pregnancies reported by Gleicher et al reached term.[80] At least 55% of all deliveries were premature, and at least 30% of all delivered infants showed evidence of intrauterine growth retardation. This number represented almost half of all newborns for whom available information allowed valid clinical evaluation. The total perinatal mortality for this group reached 28% and was found to be significantly associated with prematurity. More recent information demonstrates equally poor fetal outcome in women with Eisenmenger's syndrome.[92]

A patient with Eisenmenger's syndrome who becomes pregnant should be strongly advised to interrupt pregnancy. If the patient refuses, the following management strategy is recommended: careful follow-up by a cardiologist for early detection of any sign of symptomatic deterioration or hemodynamic instability. A coordinated and concerted approach is necessary between cardiologists, high risk obstetricians, and anesthesiologists to obtain optimum results. Excessive exertion should be avoided, to diminish cardiac demands. If episodes of dyspnea occur, oxygen may be administered.[94,101] There is very little evidence to suggest, however, that this therapy improves either fetal or maternal outcome. Congestive heart failure, if it develops, should be treated with digitalis and diuretics. Fetal well-being should be followed throughout pregnancy with routine antepartum testing, and fetal cardiac ultrasound should be performed at 18 weeks of gestation to evaluate the fetal heart. Although the value of he-

parin therapy has not been proven[102] because of the high incidence of documented pulmonary embolism, use of subcutaneous heparin at a dose adjusted to prolong activated partial thromboplastin time to 1.5–2.0 times normal (see Chapter 33) is recommended during the third trimester of pregnancy and at least one month postpartum. Premature delivery should be anticipated, and the patient should be hospitalized for any sign of premature uterine activity. Labor should proceed in accordance with an approach coordinated by the cardiologist, the obstetrician, and the anesthesiologist. In cases of elective induction, a prior evaluation of fetal lung maturity is recommended. Labor and delivery should occur in an intensive care unit[95] next to an available operating room with close monitoring of blood pressure, cardiac rate and rhythm, and arterial oxygen saturation. Insertion of a Swan–Ganz catheter has been shown to lead to instability due to arrhythmias and the apprehension associated with the procedure.[15] Since left ventricular failure is usually not the problem, and since cardiac output cannot be measured by the thermodilution method, the yield of this procedure is low. Epidural anesthesia represents the best method of anesthesia for these patients, however, it should be done gradually and carefully to avoid systemic hypotension. The second stage of labor should be kept short by means of either elective low forceps delivery or vacuum extraction.[91] Meticulous attention to leg care, including the use of thromboguards, is advisable because of the risk of venous thrombosis and paradoxical embolus. Because of the possibility of deteriorating hemodynamics and pulmonary embolism, a postpartum hospitalization of at least 2 weeks is suggested.

SUMMARY

Most patients with mild to moderate acyanotic CHD tolerate pregnancy, labor, and delivery well, and their management can be almost routine. Patients with more severe problems require frequent assessment and follow-up by the obstetrician and the cardiologist, who should work as a team. Management consists of limitation of physical activity when appropriate, avoidance of excessive weight gain, reduction of salt intake, immediate treatment of infection, use of diuretics to prevent fluid retention, close observation for signs or symptoms of early congestive heart failure with prompt treatment, and control of dysrhythmias with antiarrhythmic drugs known to be safe for the fetus (Chapter 30). Delivery by cesarean section is indicated only for obstetrical reasons and when there is cardiac instability in spite of medical therapy. The second stage of labor should be as short as possible. Patients with severe cyanotic CHD and reduced functional capacity or Eisenmenger's syndrome constitute a high risk group and should be advised against pregnancy or counseled for therapeutic abortion if pregnancy has occurred. It is critical that the patient understand the maternal and fetal risks associated with pregnancy. Corrective and palliative treatment improve maternal and fetal outcome. If total surgical correction has been performed without a significant residual, the tolerance of pregnancy is essentially normal. Sterilization is recommended in patients for whom pregnancy may be life-threatening due to severe cardiac disability that cannot be controlled by medical or surgical therapy. Cardiovascular surgery during pregnancy should be considered only in patients who are severely disabled and are not responding to optimal medical therapy. Anticoagulation during the third trimester and one month postpartum is recommended for patients with cyanotic heart disease and Eisenmenger's physiology. The use of prophylactic antibiotics at the time of delivery is indicated in most patients with CAD. Hemodynamic and electrocardiographic monitoring should be used in all high risk patients to identify and correct hemodynamic and electrical instability as soon as possible.

REFERENCES

1. Perloff JK. Congenital heart disease and pregnancy. *Clin Cardiol* 1994;17:579–587.

2. Whittemore R, Hobbins JC, Engle MA. Pregnancy and its outcome in women with and without surgical treatment of congenital heart disease. *Am J Cardiol* 1982;50:641–651.

3. Elkayam U, Gleicher N. Cardiac problems in pregnancy. I. Maternal aspects: the approach to the pregnant patient with heart disease. *JAMA* 1984;251:2338–2839.

4. Shime J, Mocarski EJM, Hastings D, Webb GD, McLaughlin PR. Congenital heart disease in pregnancy: short- and long-term implications. *Am J Obstet Gynecol* 1987;313–322.

5. Whittemore R. Congenital heart disease: its impact on pregnancy. *Hosp Pract* 1983;18:65–74.

6. Neill CA, Swanson S. Outcome of pregnancy in congenital heart disease. *Circulation* 1961;24:1003. Abstract.

7. Taussig HB. World survey of the common cardiac malformations: developmental error or genetic variant? *Am J Cardiol* 1982;50:544–559.

8. Dennis NR, Warren J. Risks to the offspring of patients with some common congenital heart defects. *J Med Genet* 1981;18:8–16.

9. Czeizel A, Pornoi A, Peterffy E, Tarcal B. Study of children of parents operated on for congenital cardiovascular malformations. *Br Heart J* 1982;47:290–293.

10. Rose V, Gold RJM, Lindsay G, Allen M. A possible increase in the incidence of congenital heart defects among the offspring of affected parents. *J Am College Cardiol* 1985;6:376–382.

11. Emanuel R, Somerville J, Inns A, Withers R. Evidence of congenital heart disease in the offspring of parents with atrioventricular defects. *Br Heart J* 1983;49:144–147.

12. Whittemore R, Wells JA, Castellsague X. A second-generation study of 427 probands with congenital heart defects and their 837 children. *J Am College Cardiol* 1994;23:1459–1467.

13. Driscoll DJ, Michels VV, Gersony WM, Hayes CJ, Keane JF, Kidd L, Pieroni DR, Rings LJ, Wolfe RR, Weidman WH. Occurrence risk for congenital heart defects in relatives of patients with aortic stenosis, pulmonary stenosis, or ventricular septal defect. *Circulation* 1993;87 (suppl I):I-114–1-120.

14. Nora JJ, Nora AH. Maternal transmission of congenital heart diseases, new recurrence risk figures, and the question of cytoplasmic inheritance and vulnerability to teratogens. *Am J Cardiol* 1987;59:459–463.

15. Devitt JH, Noble WH, Byrick RJ. A Swan–Ganz catheter related complication in a patient with Eisenmenger's syndrome. *Anesthesiology* 1982;57:335–337.

16. Sugrue D, Blake S, Troy P, MacDonald D. Antibiotic prophylaxis against infective endocarditis after normal delivery: is it necessary? *Br Heart J* 1980;44:499–502.

17. Marquis RM. Bacterial endocarditis following delivery in women with heart disease. In: Anguissola AB, Paddu V, eds. *Cardiologia d'Oggi.* Turin: Edizioni Medico Scientifiche;1975:278 pp.

18. Presbitero P, Somerville J, Stone S, Aruta E, Spiegelhalter D, Rabajoli F. Pregnancy in cyanotic congenital heart disease. Outcome of mother and fetus. *Circulation* 1994;89:2673–2676.

19. Lein JN, Stander RW. Subacute bacterial endocarditis following obstetric and gynecologic procedures. Report of eight cases. *Obstet Gynecol.* 1959;13:568–573.

20. Dajani AS, Taubert KA, Wilson W, Bolger AF, Bayer A, Ferrieri P, Gewitz MH, Shullman ST, Nouri S, Newburger JW, Hutto C, Pallasch TJ, Gage TW, Levison ME, Peter G, Zuccaro G. Prevention of bacterial endocarditis. Recommendations by the American Heart Association. *JAMA* 1997;277:1794–1801.

21. Perloff JK. *The Clinical Recognition of Congenital Heart Disease.* Philadelphia: WB Saunders; 1994.

22. Ryon T. Congenital heart disease. In Feigenbaum H, ed. *Echocardiography,* 5th ed. Philadelphia: Lea & Febiger; 1994;350–446. See also: Hausmaun D, Daniel WG, Mugge A, Ziemer G, Pearlman AS. Value of transesophageal color Doppler echocardiography for detection of different types of atrial septal defects in adults. *J Am Soc Echocardiogr* 1992;5:481–488.

23. Espino-Vela J, Alvarado-Toroa A. Natural history of atrial septal defect. *Cardiovasc Clin* 1971;2:103–125.

24. Metcalfe J, McAnulty JH, Ueland K. *Heart Disease and Pregnancy, Physiology and Management.* Boston: Little, Brown; 1986;223–264.

25. Loscalzo J. Paradoxical embolization: clinical presentation, diagnostic strategies and therapeutic options. *Am Heart J* 1986;112:141–145.

26. Nora JJ, McGill CW, McNamara DG. Empiric recurrence risks in common and uncommon congenital heart lesions. *Teratology* 1970;3:325–329.

27. Elkayam U, Gleicher N. Congenital heart disease and pregnancy. *Heart Failure* 1993;9:46–58.

28. Szekely P, Snaith L. *Heart Disease and Pregnancy.* London: Churchill Livingstone, 1974.

29. Arias F, Pineda J. Aortic stenosis and pregnancy. *J Reprod Med* 1978;4:229–232.

30. Lao TT, Sermer M, MaGee L, Farine D, Colman JM, et al. Congenital aortic stenosis. *Am J Obstet Gynecol* 1993;169:540–545.

31. Ben-Ami M, Battino S, Rosenfeld T, Marin G, Shalev E. Aortic valve replacement during pregnancy. A case report and review of the literature. *Acta Obstet Gynecol Scand* 1990;69(7–8):651–653.

32. McIvor RA. Percutaneous balloon aortic valvuloplasty during pregnancy. *Int J Cardiol* 1991;32:1–4.

33. Colclough GW, Ackerman WE, Walmsley PN. Epidural anesthesia for cesarean delivery in parturient with aortic stenosis. *Reg Anesth* 1991;16:62.

34. Banning AP, Pearson JF, Hall RJC. Role of balloon dilatation of the aortic valve in pregnant patients with severe aortic stenosis. *Br Heart J* 1993;70:544–545.

35. Lao TT, Adelman AG, Sermer M, Colman JM. Balloon valvuloplasty for congenital aortic stenosis in pregnancy. *Br J Obstet Gynaecol* 1993;100:1141–1142.

36. Nora JJ, Nora AH. The evolution of specific genetic and environmental counseling in congenital heart disease. *Circulation* 1978;57:205–213.

37. Bernal JM, Miralles PJ. Cardiac surgery with cardiopulmonary bypass during pregnancy. *Obstet Gynecol Survey* 1986;41:1–6.

38. Dizon-Tomson D, Magee KP, Twickler DM, Cox SM. Coarctation of the abdominal aorta in pregnancy: diagnosis by magnetic resonance imaging. *Obstet Gynecol* 1995;85:817–819.

39. Pitkin RM, Perloff JK, Koos BJ, Beall MH. Pregnancy and congenital heart disease. *Ann Intern Med* 1990;112:445–454.

40. Szekely P, Julian DG. Heart disease and pregnancy. *Curr Probl Cardiol* 1979;4:1–74.

41. Barash PG, Hobbins JC, Hook R, Stansel HC Jr, Whittemore R, Hehre FW. Management of coarctation of the aorta during pregnancy. *J Thorac Cardiovasc Surg* 1975;69:781–784.

42. Mortensen JD, Ellsworth HS. Coarctation of the aorta and pregnancy: obstetric and cardiovascular complications before and after surgical correction. *JAMA* 1965;191:596–598.

43. Deal K, Wooley CF. Coarctation of the aorta and pregnancy. *Ann Intern Med.* 1973;78:706–710.

44. Faclouach S, Azzouzi L, Tahiri A, Chrarbi PV. Aortic coarctation and pregnancy: à propos of 3 cases followed-up during a period of 10 years. *Ann Cardiol Angiol* 1994;45:262–265.

45. Zeira M, Zohar S. Pregnancy and delivery in women with coarctation of the aorta. *Harefuah* 1993;124:756–758.

46. Connolly HM, Ammash NM, Warnes CA. Pregnancy in women with coarctation of the aorta. *J Am College Cardiol* 1996;27(suppl A):43A. Abstract.

47. Kuperminc MJ, Lessing JB, Jaffer A, Vidne BA, Peyser MR. Fetomaternal blood flow measurements and management of combined coarctation and aneurysm of the thoracic aorta in pregnancy. *Acta Obstet Gynecol Scand* 1993;72:398–402.

48. Ritter SB. Coarctation and balloons: inflated or realistic? *J Am College Cardiol* 1989;13:696–699.

49. Neilson G, Galea EG, Blunt A. Congenital heart disease and pregnancy. *Med J Aust* 1970;1:1086–1088.

50. Stanger P, Cassidy SC, Girod DA, Kan JS, Lababidi Z, Shapiro SR. Balloon pulmonary valvuloplasty: results of the Valvuloplasty and Angioplasty of Congenital Anomalies Registry. *Am J Cardiol* 1990;65:775–783.

51. Patton DE, Lee W, Cotton DB, Miller J, Carpenter RJ Jr, Huhta J, Hankins G. Cyanotic maternal heart disease in pregnancy. *Obstet Gynecol Survey* 1990;45:594–600.

52. Larsen-Disney P, Price D, Meredith J. Undiagnosed maternal Fallot tetralogy presenting in pregnancy. *Aust N Z J Obstet Gynecol* 1992;32:169–171.

53. Zellars TM, Driscoll DJ, Michels VV. Prevalence of significant congenital heart defects in children of parents with Fallot's tetralogy. *Am J Cardiol* 1990;65:523–526.

54. Danielson GK, Driscoll DJ, Mair DD, Warnes CA, Oliver WC. Operative treatment of Ebstein's anomaly. *J Thorac Cardiovasc Surg* 1992;104:1195–1202.

55. Donnelly JE, Brown JM, Radford DJ. Pregnancy outcome and Ebstein's anomaly. *Br Heart J* 1991;66:368–371.

56. Connolly HM, Warnes CA. Ebstein's anomaly: outcome of pregnancy. *J Am College Cardiol* 1994;23:1194–1198.

57. Collins ML, Leal J, Thompson NJ. Tricuspid atresia and pregnancy. *Obstet Gynecol* 1977;50(suppl 1):72S–73S.

58. Cooke FN, Hernandez FA. Tricuspid atresia: a case report of a 51-year-old woman treated by an extracardiac shunt. *South Med J* 1959;52:1016–1018.

59. Taussig HB, Keinonen R, Momberger N, Kirk H. Long-term observations on the Blalock–Taussig operation. IV. Tricuspid atresia. *Johns Hopkins Med J* 1973;132:135–145.

60. Hatjis CG, Gibson M, Capeless EL, Auletta FJ, Anderson GG. Pregnancy in patients with tricuspid atresia. *Am J Obstet Gynecol.* 1983;145:114–115.

61. Canobbio M, Mair D. Pregnancy outcome following Fontan operation. *Circulation* 1993;88:1–290. Abstract.

62. Warnes CA, Somerville J. Transposition of the great arteries: results in adolescents and adults late after the Mustard procedure. *Br Heart J* 1987;58:148–155.

63. Lynch-Salamon DI, Maze SS, Combs CA. Pregnancy after Mustard repair for transposition of the great arteries. *Obstet Gynecol* 1993;82:676–679.

64. Clarkson PM, Wilson NJ, Neutze JM, North RA, Calder AL, Barratt-Boyes BG. Outcome of pregnancy after the Mustard operation for transposition of the great arteries with intact ventricular septum. *J Am College Cardiol* 1994;24:190–193.

65. Lao TT, Sermer M, Colman JM. Pregnancy following surgical correction for transposition of the great arteries. *Obstet Gynecol* 1994;83:665–668.

66. Dellinger EH, Hadi HA. Maternal transposition of the great arteries in pregnancy: a case report. *J Reprod Med* 1994;39:324–326.

67. Rousseil MP, Irion O, Beguim F, Jaques O, Adamic R, Lerch R, Friedli B, Rifat K. Successful term pregnancy after Mustard operation for transposition of the great arteries. *Eur J Obstet Gynecol Reprod Biol* 1995;59:111–113.

68. Megerian G, Bell JG, Huhta JC, BoHalico JN, Weimer S. Pregnancy outcome following Mustard procedure for transposition of the great arteries: a report of five cases and review of the literature. *Obstet Gynecol* 1994;83:512–516.

69. Simon DL, Lustberg A. A case of truncus arteriosus communis compatible with full-term pregnancy. *Am Heart J* 1951;42:617–623.

70. Perry CP. Childbirth after surgical repair of truncus arteriosus. *J Reprod Med* 1990;35:65–67.

71. Ahmed S, Hawes D, Dooley S, Faure E, Brunner EA. Intrathecal morphine in a patient with a single ventricle. *Anesthesiology* 1981;54:515–517.

72. Leibbrandt G, Munch U, Gander M. Two successful pregnancies in a patient with single ventricle and transposition of the great arteries. *Int J Cardiol* 1982;1:257–262.

73. Stiller RJ, Vintzileos AM, Nochimson DJ, Clement D, Campbell WA, Leach CN Jr. Single ventricle in pregnancy: case report and review of the literature. *Obstet Gynecol* 1984;64(suppl 3):185–205.

74. Fong J, Druzin M, Gimbel AA, Fisher J. Epidural anesthesia for labour and cesarean section in a parturient with a single ventricle and transposition of the great arteries. *Can J Anesth* 1990;37:680–684.

75. Summer D, Melville C, Smith CD, Hunt T, Kenney A. Successful pregnancy in a patient with a single ventricle. *Eur J Obstet Gynecol Reprod Biol* 1992;4:239–241.

76. Zavisca FG, Johnson MD, Holubec JT, Kao YJ, Racz GB. General anesthesia for cesarean section in a parturient with a single ventricle and pulmonary atresia. *J Clin Anesth* 1993;5:315–320.

77. Rowbottom SJ, Gin T, Cheung LD. General anesthesia for caesarean section in a patient with Douceted complex cyanotic heart disease. *J Anaesth Intensive Care* 1994;22:74–78.

78. Walsh, Savage R, Hess DB. Successful pregnancy in a patient with double inlet left ventricle treated with septation procedure. *South Med J* 1990;83:358–359.

79. Saha A, Balakrishnan KG, Jaiswal PK, Venkitachalam CG, Tharakan J, Titus T, Kutty R. Prognosis for patients with Eisenmenger syndrome of various etiology. *Int J Cardiol* 1994;45:199–207.

80. Gleicher N, Midwall J, Hochberger D, Jaffin H. Eisenmenger's syndrome and pregnancy. *Obstet Gynecol Survey* 1979;34:721–741.

81. Spinnato JA, Kraynack BJ, Cooper MW. Eisenmenger's syndrome in pregnancy: epidural anesthesia for elective cesarean section. *N Engl J Med* 1981;304:1215–1217.

82. Kubo N, Yokoyama K. Lumbar epidural and caudal anesthesia for vaginal delivery in Eisenmenger's syndrome. *MASUI* 1981;30:1388–1395.

83. Mukhtar AI, Halliday HL. Eisenmenger's syndrome in pregnancy: a possible cause of neonatal polycythemia and persistent fetal circulation. *Obstet Gynecol* 1982;60:651–652.

84. Blake P, Blake S, McDonald D. Pregnancy in patients with Eisenmenger's syndrome. *Irish Med J* 1983;76:308–309.

85. Furuya H, Okamura F, Ishida T, Chiba Y. General anesthesia for a cesarean section on the patient with Eisenmenger's syndrome. *MASUI* 1983;32:1269–1273.

86. Rusenberg B, Simon K, Peretz BA, Roguin N, Birkhahn HJ. Eisenmenger's syndrome in pregnancy. Controlled segmental epidural block for cesarean section. *Reg Anesth* 1984;7:131–133.

87. Lieber S, Dewilde PH, Huyghens L, Traey E, Gepts E. Eisenmenger's syndrome and pregnancy. *Acta Cardiol* 1985;40:421–424.

88. Ogura M, Suzukawa M, Tagami M, Inada Y, Toyooka H, Ohgami Y, Kinoshita K, Mizuno M. High-dose fentanyl anesthesia in a pregnant patient with Eisenmenger's syndrome. *MASUI* 1985;34:241–246.

89. Lieber S, Dewilde PH, Huyghens L, Traey E, Gepts E. Eisenmenger's syndrome and pregnancy. *Acta Cardiol* 1985;40:421–424.

90. Huyghe-de-Mahence A, André-Fouet X, Bernet D, Seligman G. Eisenmenger's syndrome and pregnancy: à propos of 2 spontaneous deliveries, one of which was fatal. *Ann Cardiol Angiol* 1985;34:547–549.

91. Robinson PN, Macleod UG. Location for delivery in a patient with Eisenmenger's syndrome. *Anesthesia* 1986;41:883–887. Letter.

92. Heytens L, Alexander JP. Maternal and neonatal death associated with Eisenmenger's syndrome. *Acta Anaesth Belg* 1986;37:45–51.

93. Maarek-Charbit M, Corone P. Eisenmenger's syndrome and pregnancy. *Arch Mal Coeur Vaiss* 1986;79:733–740.

94. Bitsch M, Johansen C, Wennevold A, Osler M. Eisenmenger's syndrome and pregnancy. *Eur J Obstet Gynecol Reprod Biol* 1988;28:69–74.

95. Cumba-Rochiquez MA, Yanez-Gonzalez AM, Gonzalez-Ruiz F. Epidural anesthesia for cesarean section in a patient with Eisenmenger's syndrome. *Rev Esp Anestesiol Reanim* 1989;36:45–47.

96. Gilman DH. Cesarean section in undiagnosed Eisenmenger's syndrome. *Anesthesia* 1991;46:371–373.

97. Atanassoff P, Alon E, Schmid ER, Pasch T. Epidural anesthesia for cesarean section in a patient with severe pulmonary hypertension. *Acta Anaesthesiol Scand* 190;34:75–77.

98. Antoine JM, Bonnardot JP, Vitoux B, Salat-Baroux J. Eisenmenger syndrome and pregnancy. à propos of a case. *J Gynecol Obstet Biol Reprod* 1991;20:79–82.

99. Corone S, Davido A, Lang T, Corone P. Outcome of patients with Eisenmenger syndrome. à propos of 62 cases followed up for an average of 16 years. *Arch Mal Coeur Vaiss* 1992;85:521–526.

100. Avila WS, Grinberg M, Snitcowsky R, Faccioli R, Da Luz PL, Bellotti G, Pileggi F. Maternal and fetal outcome in pregnant women with Eisenmenger's syndrome. *Eur Heart J* 1995;16:460–464.

101. Midwall J, Jaffin H, Herman MV, Kupersmith J. Shunt flow and pulmonary hemodynamics during labor and delivery in the Eisenmenger syndrome. *Am J Cardiol* 1978;42:299–303.

102. Pitts JA, Crosby WM, Basta LL. Eisenmenger's syndrome in pregnancy: does heparin prophylaxis improve the maternal mortality rate? *Am Heart J* 1977;93:321–326.

5

RHEUMATIC VALVULAR DISEASE AND PREGNANCY

Mohammed R. Essop, MD, and Pinhas Sareli, MD

INTRODUCTION

The management of cardiac disease during pregnancy poses a double challenge—primarily to ensure maternal survival, but at the same time to promote fetal well-being and to allow a gestational period sufficient to enable prediction of adequate fetal maturity for ex utero survival. Optimal management of these patients requires intimate knowledge both of physiologic cardiovascular changes that occur during pregnancy (Chapter 1) and of pharmacotherapy (Chapter 27–36), and a close liaison between the attending cardiologist and the obstetrician.

The high rate of teenage pregnancies combined with an endemic prevalence of rheumatic disease in developing countries results in cardiac disease being the most important comorbid state during pregnancy. Nevertheless, the vast majority of patients have an uneventful outcome. The major causes of maternal mortality at our hospital are still noncardiac, including thromboembolism, hypertensive disease, obstetric hemorrhage, and sepsis. In the United States, where patients with congenital cardiac disease who either desire pregnancy or are already pregnant contribute an increasing proportion of the pregnant cardiac load, rheumatic disease is not infrequent, especially in areas with dense immigrant populations.

Of crucial importance in the management of the pregnant cardiac population is the ability to identify those at greatest risk, so that appropriate surveillance and therapy can be instituted in these patients. Recent advances in the management of valvular disease include the use of β-adrenergic blocking agents for patients with mitral stenosis, vasodilators in those with mitral or aortic regurgitation, and interventional techniques including balloon valvuloplasty for mitral or aortic stenosis. The role of these therapies in the pregnant patient is as yet unclear, and while certain recommendations may be made, management of the individual patient should at all times be tempered by patient-related factors, the specific clinical context, and the experience and judgment of the attending medical staff.

ACUTE RHEUMATIC FEVER

Improvement in living standards and more widespread use of antimicrobial chemotherapy have resulted in a worldwide decline in the incidence of acute rheumatic fever. It has not been our experience that pregnant patients may be predisposed to acute rheumatic fever. On the contrary, despite reports published earlier,[1–6] and despite the high incidence of acute rheumatic fever in our population, we have rarely encountered this condition during pregnancy. The mean age at presentation is 13, ranging from 6 to 18 years. Although acute rheumatic carditis has been postulated as a mechanism for left ventricular dilatation and congestive heart failure, it has been our experience[7] and that of others[8] that heart failure rarely occurs in the absence of hemodynamically significant mitral or aortic regurgitation. In patients with active rheumatic carditis presenting with heart failure, we have observed functionally severe mitral regurgitation and its anatomic correlates of annular dilatation, chordal elongation, and leaflet prolapse sufficiently frequently[9] to regard these features as a pathoanatomic hallmark of the disease. Left ventricular systolic function is usually normal.[10] Milder episodes of acute rheumatic fever in the pregnant patient may be difficult to diagnose because of the presence of tachycardia, functional murmurs, and anemia. Nevertheless, the modified Duckett

Cardiac Problems in Pregnancy, Third Edition
Edited by Uri Elkayam, MD, and Norbert Gleicher, MD
Copyright © 1998 by Wiley-Liss, Inc. ISBN 0-471-16358-9

Jones criteria[11] should be applied in a similar manner to the nonpregnant patient, bearing in mind the limitation of these guidelines.

Acute rheumatic fever is managed similarly in pregnant and nonpregnant patients. Corticosteroids may be inappropriate in patients with severe episodes with heart failure, since in the vast majority of these patients symptoms are due to an incompetent mitral or aortic valve rather then myocardial failure. In those who do not respond to inotropic and vasodilator therapy, consideration should be given to surgical restoration of valvular competence to prevent maternal death. The results of mitral valve repair in the rheumatic population are clearly not as good as in patients with degenerative disease, and it is our belief that mitral valve replacement offers a better alternative. Milder degrees of acute rheumatic fever require only bed rest, treatment of streptococcal pharyngitis (preferably with penicillin), and correction of coexistent anemia and nutritional deficiency. Sulfonamides are best avoided because of potential hyperbilirubinemia and kernicterus in the newborn, although this was not the experience of Baskin et al.[12]

CHRONIC RHEUMATIC HEART DISEASE

Mitral Stenosis

Of all the rheumatic valvular lesions, mitral stenosis is not only the most frequent, it is also the one most likely to lead to a potentially serious outcome. Not infrequently, previously occult mitral stenosis is discovered for the first time during pregnancy. This is easily understood when one considers the interaction between the physiologic cardiovascular adjustments to pregnancy (Chapter 1) and the hemodynamics of mitral stenosis.

Pathophysiology The normal mitral valve area ranges between 4 and 6 cm^2. A considerable reduction in the valve area can occur without adverse consequences. Hemodynamically important stenosis occurs only when the valve area decreases to less than 2 cm^2. With increasing narrowing of the valve, there is a progressive rise in the diastolic gradient between the left atrium and ventricle, elevation in the mean left atrial or pulmonary capillary wedge pressure, and decrease in cardiac output. When mitral valve area is critically reduced—to about 1 cm^2—a large diastolic gradient is present even at rest, and any demand for increased cardiac output is accompanied by significant elevation of left atrial pressure and the development of pulmonary edema. In addition to mitral valve area, the mitral valve gradient and left atrial pressure depend on flow rate across the valve. Pregnancy imposes three major hemodynamic burdens on the heart: It increases cardiac output and heart rate, expands blood volume, and intensifies oxygen demand. Acting in combination, these factors result

in significantly adverse hemodynamics in patients with mitral stenosis. The greatest danger occurs during late pregnancy, labor, and the early postpartum period. This is logical, since the increase in blood volume, cardiac output, and heart rate in pregnancy is progressive to term. During labor, there is a further 10–15% increase in cardiac output, augmented during uterine contractions, which result in an autotransfusion of 300–500 mL of blood.[13] Immediately after delivery, there is an increase in preload and blood volume from the contracted uterus and release of aortocaval compression. The elevated cardiac output persists for several days postpartum and then gradually declines to normal levels over a 2-week period.[14]

Symptoms and Clinical Features Elevated left atrial pressures manifest as dyspnea, while inability to increase cardiac output presents as undue fatigue. On average, pregnancy may be predicted to result in a deterioration of one or two classes in the New York Heart Association (NYHA) functional status. Ankle edema due to right heart failure is sometimes inappropriately ascribed to preeclampsia. An elevated jugular venous pressure is a clue to the presence of right heart failure rather than preeclampsia. Mitral stenosis, usually easily recognized in pregnancy, is sometimes missed because the murmur is diastolic and submammary.[15] Sinus rhythm is usual in this age group.

Echocardiography Two-dimensional echocardiography with color flow mapping is easily performed and safe. It provides much information, including confirmation of the diagnosis and objective assessment of stenosis severity, presence of concomitant valve lesions, and suitability of the valve for a conservative procedure such as balloon or closed surgical mitral commissurotomy.

Prognosis Survival in the overall group of patients with uncorrected mitral stenosis depends greatly on symptoms. Thus, 10-year survival for patients in NYHA class I is 85%, in class II it is 50%, class III 20%, and class IV 0%.[16] Maternal mortality in patients who are minimally symptomatic is less than 1%.[17] Mortality in patients with more advanced symptoms (functional class III-IV) who have atrial fibrillation or significant pulmonary hypertension can be significantly higher, although improved medical and surgical management of these patients has resulted in favorable prognosis in most cases.[19] Likewise, perinatal mortality depends largely on maternal prepregnant symptomatic status, with no increase in mortality in minimally symptomatic mothers, 12% mortality in class III patients, and 30% mortality in class IV patients.[20]

Management The availability of new therapies has engendered some controversy even in the optimal management of the nonpregnant patient with mitral stenosis.[21] This controversy is compounded in the pregnant patient because of the need to consider the risks to the fetus of drug therapy, radiation exposure during percutaneous mitral balloon valvuloplasty, or anesthesia with or without cardiopulmonary bypass during surgical commissurotomy. For the clinician treating these patients, three groups of patients may be identified: the patient with known mitral stenosis who desires to become pregnant, the patient with well-compensated mitral stenosis who is already pregnant, and the patient who is in a critical hemodynamic state and usually in an advanced stage of pregnancy or early postpartum.

Patients with mitral stenosis contemplating pregnancy usually have a mobile noncalcific valve and should be offered either percutaneous balloon valvuloplasty or closed mitral valvotomy depending on local experience. This approach attenuates any anticipated deterioration in functional class and obviates the need for pharmacologic therapy during pregnancy. Careful judgment is required in the occasional patient with calcific mitral stenosis in whom the only therapeutic option is mitral valve replacement. If symptoms are minimal and adverse prognostic factors such as atrial fibrillation and pulmonary hypertension are absent, a policy of intensive medical therapy may be safer than mitral valve replacement. If mitral valve replacement prior to pregnancy is necessary, however, we agree with other authors[22] (Chapter 6) that bioprosthetic valves, selected to avoid the need for anticoagulation, are not a suitable alternative to metallic valves due to the accelerated degeneration of the former during pregnancy and the consequent need for repeat mitral valve surgery. The issues regarding anticoagulation in pregnancy are discussed in more detail in Chapter 33.

Optimal management of the already pregnant patient with compensated mitral stenosis requires careful assessment of the risk/benefit ratio to mother and fetus of standard pharmacologic therapy (diuretics and beta blockers) versus percutaneous balloon valvuloplasty. β-Adrenergic blockers are safe and well tolerated by both mother and fetus (see also Chapter 29); by reducing heart rate they significantly ameliorate the hemodynamics of mitral stenosis. Beta blockers may not only have a beneficial hemodynamic effect, but by inhibiting episodes of paroxysmal atrial fibrillation they may also prevent the formation of left atrial thrombi.[21] The vast majority of patients in our experience can be carried successfully through pregnancy and puerperium by the judicious use of these drugs combined with a diuretic for those with accompanying shortness of breath.

Since the first case reports in 1988 of mitral balloon valvuloplasty during pregnancy by Safian[23] and Palacios,[24] numerous publications have confirmed the technical feasibility and hemodynamic improvement following this procedure.[25–33] While percutaneous balloon valvuloplasty may be seen as an attractive alternative to medical therapy, two shortcomings make it difficult to recommend unconditionally. The first, severe mitral regurgitation is not specific to pregnancy,

has an incidence of about 8%,[34] and is largely unpredictable.[35] Of more specific relevance to pregnancy is the risk of fetal distress and irradiation during balloon valvuloplasty. Fetal bradycardia, observed in several studies, is usually transient with no apparent adverse effect.[27,31,33] Using film badge dosimeters, Lung et al were able to show that abdominal radiation was less than 0.2 mSv.[33] Although this is well below the 5 mSV radiation limit recommended for pregnant women,[36] the real long-term risk to the fetus of even such low radiation levels is as yet unknown. Based on these data, we would agree with Ribeiro et al that mitral balloon valvuloplasty should be attempted only in patients in whom symptoms are not adequately controlled on optimal medical therapy[37] or when close follow-up during pregnancy, labor, and delivery is not possible. Mitral balloon valvuloplasty is best done beyond 20 weeks of gestation, when irradiation risk to the fetus is less.[38] It should be performed by experienced physicians, with adequate abdominal and pelvic shielding, and in an abbreviated form (omitting left ventricular cineangiography and detailed pressure and shunt evaluations), to allow completion of the procedure in as short a time as possible. Where balloon valvuloplasty cannot be performed, closed mitral valvotomy is a suitable alternative.[39]

Pregnant patients with mitral stenosis who are in a critical hemodynamic state with pulmonary edema, hypotension, and right heart failure pose a considerable therapeutic challenge. In this situation maternal survival takes precedence. A rapid trial of intravenous diuretics, beta blockers if in sinus rhythm, digitalis for atrial fibrillation, and dc cardioversion if necessary should be instituted. Failure to achieve significant clinical improvement is an indication for urgent mechanical relief of mitral stenosis. The choice of balloon valvuloplasty, open or closed surgical commissurotomy, or mitral valve replacement should be dictated by echocardiographic valve characteristics and local expertise and should be performed as expeditiously as possible. A fetal mortality of about 10–30% may be expected during procedures requiring cardiopulmonary bypass (Chapter 23).[40]

Obstetric Considerations During Labor and Delivery

Vaginal delivery is the preferred method and may be allowed either in the recumbent or left lateral position. Cesarian section should be reserved for obstetric indications. Epidural anesthesia attenuates wide fluctuations in blood pressure and is recommended for patients with mitral stenosis. There is some evidence that it may also have a beneficial effect in lowering left atrial and pulmonary artery pressure.[41] The second stage of labor should be shortened as much as possible by performing an outlet forceps or vacuum extraction delivery.[42,43] Hemodynamic monitoring with a flotation balloon catheter in the pulmonary artery may be reserved for patients with more advanced disease. Tocolytic agents that are positively chronotropic may exacerbate the hemodynamics of mitral stenosis and are contraindicated for premature labor.[20]

If necessary, magnesium sulfate is preferable.[20] The question of infective endocarditis prophylaxis is discussed in Chapter 16.

Mitral Regurgitation

Compared to mitral stenosis, mitral regurgitation is not only much more infrequent during pregnancy but is also much better tolerated. The volume of mitral regurgitant flow depends not only on the regurgitant orifice size but also on the systolic gradient between the left ventricle and left atrium. Left ventricular systolic pressure in turn depends on systemic vascular resistance. Since both systemic blood pressure and vascular resistance decline during pregnancy, the volume of mitral regurgitant flow is reduced, with a proportionate increase in forward stroke volume.

Asymptomatic patients require no specific therapy, while those with symptoms of heart failure may be treated with diuretics and digitalis, like nonpregnant patients with mitral regurgitation. If vasodilator therapy is selected, hydralazine is preferable to angiotensin-converting enzyme inhibitors, since the safety of the latter during pregnancy has not been established.

Surgery is usually the definitive therapy for significant symptomatic mitral regurgitation and is preferably delayed until no further pregnancies are anticipated. Rarely is surgery advisable during pregnancy, bearing in mind a maternal mortality of 2–3% and fetal mortality of up to 30%.[20]

Aortic Stenosis

Rheumatic aortic stenosis is rare during pregnancy, probably reflecting a predilection of this condition for males and older patients. Inability to increase stroke volume in the presence of a pregnancy-induced decline in systemic vascular resistance may result in systemic hypotension with dizziness or syncope. Pulmonary congestion is unusual and is explained by markedly decreased left ventricular compliance related to concentric left ventricular hypertrophy. Data on aortic stenosis and pregnancy are limited to a single study,[44] which showed a maternal mortality of 17% and a fetal mortality of up to 32%. A maternal mortality of 40% was noted in patients having therapeutic abortion and may be due to hypovolemia related either to blood loss or vasodepressor mechanisms.

Asymptomatic patients should be carefully monitored throughout pregnancy to ensure adequate restriction of physical activity and maintenance of hemoglobin levels. Mechanical relief is the only therapeutic option in symptomatic patients with aortic stenosis. Although percutaneous aortic balloon dilatation in the elderly has fallen into disrepute because of the high incidence of recurrence, this therapy may have a bridging role in pregnant patients with symptomatic aortic stenosis. Experience in pregnancy is limited to a total of four patients,[45–47] all of whom had a congenital bicuspid aortic valve. The procedure was associated with a significant reduction in aortic valve gradient and successful outcome of pregnancy in all patients. Unlike congenital bicuspid valves, rheumatic aortic stenosis is often associated with some degree of insufficiency, and balloon valvuloplasty may be expected to exacerbate this. Nevertheless, we believe that balloon valvuloplasty in the occasional pregnant patient with predominant and severe symptomatic aortic stenosis of rheumatic etiology may be preferable to aortic valve replacement.

During labor, delivery, and the postpartum period, stringent measures to avoid blood loss or hypotension should be employed. Invasive monitoring with arterial and pulmonary flotation catheters may also be useful. As in patients with mitral stenosis, assisted vaginal delivery is preferable.

Aortic Regurgitation

Aortic regurgitation is seen more commonly than aortic stenosis in women of childbearing age. When it is due to rheumatic disease, concomitant mitral valve disease is almost invariable. As with mitral regurgitation, aortic regurgitation is well tolerated during pregnancy even when it is severe. Regurgitant volume is reduced during pregnancy because of both a decline in systemic vascular resistance, which results in a decrease in the diastolic aortic/left ventricular gradient, and an increase in heart rate, which shortens diastole and therefore the time for regurgitation. In nonpregnant patients with severe asymptomatic aortic regurgitation, vasodilator therapy using hydralazine[48] or nifedipine[49,50] has reduced left ventricular volumes, mass, and the need for surgery. We believe that vasodilator therapy in similar patients who are pregnant may be inappropriate because of the potential risks of drug therapy to the fetus and because pregnancy itself confers a hemodynamic advantage to these patients. In symptomatic patients, standard therapy including diuretics and digitalis is indicated. The value of vasodilator therapy in these patients is unknown. If deemed necessary, however, hydralazine should be preferred because of its well-established safety during pregnancy.

REFERENCES

1. Hibbard LT. Maternal mortality due to cardiac disease. *Clin Obstet Gynecol* 1975;18:27–36.
2. Clinch J. Chorea gravidarum. *Hosp Med* 1967;2:317.
3. Lewis BV, Parsons M. Chorea gravidarum. *Lancet* 1966;1:284–286.
4. Mendelson CL. *Cardiac Disease in Pregnancy.* Philadelphia: FA Davis; 1960;114.
5. Ueland K, Metcalf J. Acute rheumatic fever in pregnancy. *Am J Obstet Gynecol* 1966;95:586–587.
6. Beresford OD, Ram AN. Chorea gravidarum. *J Obstet Gynecol Br Emp* 1950;57:66.

7. Barlow JB, Marcus RH, Pocock WA, Barlow CW, Essop MR, Sareli P. Mechanisms and management of heart failure in active rheumatic carditis. *South Afr Med J* 1990;78:181–186.

8. Massel BF, Fyler DC, Roy SB. The clinical picture of rheumatic fever. Diagnosis, immediate prognosis, course and therapeutic implications. *Am J Cardiol* 1958;1:436–448.

9. Marcus RH, Sareli P, Pocock WA, Meyer TE, Magalhaes MP, Grieve T, Barlow JB. Functional anatomy of severe mitral regurgitation in active rheumatic carditis. *Am J Cardiol* 1989;63:577–584.

10. Essop MR, Wisenbaugh T, Sareli P. Evidence against a myocardial factor as the cause of left ventricular dilatation in active rheumatic carditis. *J Am College Cardiol* 1993;22:826–829.

11. Special Committee Report. Jones criteria (modified) for guidance in the diagnosis of rheumatic fever. *Circulation* 1956;13:617–620.

12. Baskin CG, Law S, Wenger NK. Sulfadiazine rheumatic fever prophylaxis during pregnancy: does it increase the risk of kernicterus in the newborn? *Cardiology* 1980;65:222–225.

13. Mashini IS, Albazzaz SJ, Fadel HE, Abdulla AM, Hadi HA, Harp R, Devoe LD. Serial noninvasive evaluation of cardiovascular hemodynamics during pregnancy. *Am J Obstet Gynecol* 1987;156:1208–1213.

14. Robson SC, Dunlop W, Hunter S. Hemodynamic changes during the early puerperium. *Br Med J* 1987;294:1065.

15. Oakley CM. Pregnancy in heart disease: pre-existing heart disease. *Cardiovasc Clin* 1989;19(3):57–80.

16. Carabello BA. Timing of surgery in mitral and aortic stenosis. *Cardio Clin* 1991;9(2):229–238.

17. Clark SL. Cardiac disease in pregnancy. *Crit Care Clin* 1991;7(4):777–797.

18. Szekely P, Snaith L. Atrial fibrillation and pregnancy. *Br Med J* 1961;5237:1407–1410.

19. Szekely P, Turner R, Snaith L. Pregnancy and the changing pattern of rheumatic heart disease. *Br Heart J* 1973;35:1293–1303.

20. Brady K, Duff P. Rheumatic heart disease in pregnancy. *Clin Obstet Gynaecol* 1989;32(1):21–40.

21. Essop MR. Relief of rheumatic mitral stenosis—when and how? *Am J Cardiol* 1994;73:85–87. Editorial.

22. Oakley CM. Anticoagulation and pregnancy. *Eur Heart J* 1995;16:1317–1319.

23. Safian RD, Berman AD, Sachs B, Diver DJ, Come PC, Baim DS, McKay L, Grossman W, McKay RG. Percutaneous mitral balloon valvuloplasty in a pregnant patient with mitral stenosis. *Cathet Cardiovasc Diagn* 1988;15:103–108.

24. Palacios IF, Block PC, Williams GT, Rediker DE, Dagget WM. Percutaneous mitral balloon valvotomy during pregnancy in a patient with severe mitral stenosis. *Cathet Cardiovasc Diagn* 1988;15:109–111.

25. Mangione JA, Zuhani MF, Del Castillo JM, Nogueira EA, Arie S. Percutaneous double balloon mitral valvotomy in pregnant women. *Am J Cardiol* 1989;64:99–102.

26. Smith R, Brender D, McCredie M. Percutaneous transluminal dilatation of the mitral valve in pregnancy. *Br Heart J* 1989;61:551–553.

27. Esteves CA, Ramos AIO, Braga SLN, Harrison JK, Sousa JEMR. Effectiveness of percutaneous balloon mitral valvotomy during pregnancy. *Am J Cardiol* 1991;68:930–934.

28. Ruzyllo W, Dabrowski M, Woroszylska M, Sadowska RS. Percutaneous mitral commissurotomy with the Inoue balloon for severe mitral stenosis during pregnancy. *J Heart Valve Dis* 1992;1:209–212.

29. Ben Farhat M, Maatouk F, Betbout F, Ayari M, Brahim H, Souissi M, Sghairi K, Gamra H. Percutaneous balloon mitral valvuloplasty in eight pregnant women with severe mitral stenosis. *Eur Heart J* 1992;13:1658–1664.

30. Ribeiro PA, Fawzi ME, Awad M, Dunn B, Duran CG. Balloon valvotomy for pregnant patients with severe pliable mitral stenosis using the Inoue technique with total abdominal and pelvic shielding. *Am Heart J* 1992;124:1558–1562.

31. Gangbar EW, Watson KR, Howard RJ, Chisolm RJ. Mitral balloon valvuloplasty in pregnancy: advantages of a unique balloon. *Cathet Cardiovasc Diagn* 1992;25:313–316.

32. Patel JJ, Mitha AS, Hassen F, Patel N, Naidu R, Chetty C, Pillay R. Percutaneous balloon mitral valvotomy in pregnant patients with tight pliable mitral stenosis. *Am Heart J* 1993;125:1106–1109.

33. Lung B, Cormier B, Elias J, Michel PL, Nallet O, Porte JM, Sananes S, Uzan S, Vahanian A, Acar J. Usefulness of percutaneous balloon commissurotomy for mitral stenosis during pregnancy. *Am J Cardiol* 1994;73:398–400.

34. Rothlisberger C, Essop MR, Skudicky D, Skoularigis J, Wisenbaugh T, Sareli P. Results of percutaneous balloon mitral valvotomy in young adults. *Am J Cardiol* 1993;72:73–77.

35. Essop MR, Wisenbaugh T, Skoularigis J, Middlemost S, Sareli P. Mitral regurgitation following mitral balloon valvotomy—differing mechanisms for severe versus mid–moderate lesions. *Circulation* 1991;84:1669–1679.

36. Wagner LK, Hayman LA. Pregnancy and women radiologists. *Radiology* 1982;145:559–562.

37. Ribeiro PA, Al Zaibag M. Mitral balloon valvotomy in pregnancy. *J Heart Valve Dis* 1992;1:206–208. Editorial.

38. Dekaban AS. Abnormalities in children exposed to X-radiation during various stages of gestation. Tentative timetable of radiation injury to the human fetus: part I. *J Nuclear Med* 1968;9:471–477.

39. Vosloo S, Reichart B. The feasibility of closed mitral valvotomy in pregnancy. *J Thorac Cardiovasc Surg* 1987;93:675–679.

40. Bernal JM, Miralles PJ. Cardiac surgery with cardiopulmonary bypass during pregnancy. *Obstet Gynecol Surg* 1986;41:1–6.

41. Hemmings GT, Whalley DG, O Connor PH. Invasive monitoring and anaesthetic management of a patient with mitral stenosis. *Can Anaesth Soc J* 1987;34:182–188.

42. Metcalf J, McAnulty JH, Ueland K, eds. *Burwell and Metcalf's Heart Disease and Pregnancy.* Boston: Little, Brown; 1986;55.

43. Pearse CS. Cardiac disease in pregnancy. In: Arias F, ed. *High Risk Pregnancy and Delivery.* St. Louis: CV Mosby; 1984;181.

44. Arias F, Pinada J. Aortic stenosis and pregnancy. *J Reprod Med* 1978;4:229–232.

45. Angel JL, Chapman C, Knuppel RA. Percutaneous balloon valvuloplasty in pregnancy. *Obstet Gynecol* 1988;3:438–440.

46. McIvor RA. Percutaneous balloon aortic valvuloplasty during pregnancy. *Int J Cardiol* 1991;32:1–4.

47. Banning AP, Pearson JF, Hall RJC. Role of balloon dilatation of the aortic valve in pregnant patients with severe aortic stenosis. *Br Heart J* 1993;70:544–545.

48. Greenberg BH, Massie B, Bristow JD, Cheitlin M, Siemienczuk D, Topic N, Wilson RA, Szlachcic J, Thomas D. Long-term vasodilator therapy of chronic aortic insufficiency: a randomized double-blinded, placebo-controlled clinical trial. *Circulation* 1988;78:92–103.

49. Scognamiglio R, Fasoli G, Ponchia A, Dalla-Volta S. Long-term nifedipine unloading therapy in asymptomatic patients with chronic severe aortic regurgitation. *J Am College Cardiol* 1990;16:424–429.

50. Scognamiglio R, Rahimtoola SH, Fasoli G, Nistri S, Dalla Volta S. Nifedipine in asymptomatic patients with severe aortic regurgitation and normal left ventricular function. *N Engl J Med* 1994;331:689–694.

6

PREGNANCY IN THE PATIENT WITH ARTIFICIAL HEART VALVE

Uri Elkayam, md, and Steven S. Khan, md

INTRODUCTION

Since 1960, more than a million prosthetic heart valves have been implanted in patients with native valvular disease.[1] A large number of these patients are women in the childbearing age, and many of them desire to have children.[2–16] Issues regarding prosthetic heart valves in the obstetric patient fall into three main categories: selection of the appropriate type of valve for a patient in the childbearing age who desires to become pregnant later, potential risk to the mother and fetus associated with pregnancy, and management during pregnancy of the patient with prosthetic heart valve.

SELECTION OF A PROSTHETIC VALVE IN WOMEN IN THE CHILDBEARING AGE

Heart valves are conveniently separated into two types: mechanical prostheses and tissue or bioprosthetic valves (Table 6.1).[1] The most widely used mechanical valves are currently the disk valves, and the most commonly used disk valve in the United States is the St. Jude Medical bileaflet prosthesis (Fig. 6.1). Other commonly implanted mechanical valves are the Medtronic–Hall tilting disk prosthesis (Fig. 6.2) and the Bjork–Shiley valve, a single tilting disk prosthesis (Fig. 6.3). The latter is no longer available in the United States but continues to be implanted in the rest of the world. The other main category of mechanical valves available consists of the caged ball valves. The Starr–Edwards valve, which consists of a rubber ball inside a metal cage, is the only model available in the United States (Fig. 6.4).

Tissue valves can be separated into three categories: xenografts, homografts, and autografts. Xenografts, or valves from another species, are currently the most commonly tissue valves implanted. Most of the information regarding pregnancy in women with bioprosthetic valves has been obtained in patients with xenografts. Porcine xenografts are made from pig heart valves mounted on plastic or wire stents such as the Hancock or Carpentier–Edwards porcine valves (Figs. 6.5 and 6.6). A relatively recent addition is the Carpentier–Edwards pericardial valve, which is made from bovine (cow) pericardial tissue and is currently available only for the aortic position. It appears to have excellent hemodynamics, even in the smaller valve sizes, and it appears to be at least as durable as current porcine valves.[3] No information, however, is available on pregnancy in patients with this valve. Homograft valves[4] are tissue valves obtained from a human donor. Homograft valves have excellent hemodynamics; their durability is at least comparable to porcine xenograft tissue valves; and they are more resistant to reinfection in patients with complicated aortic valve endocarditis.[5] Supply of these valves is limited by donor availability, and information regarding pregnancy in women with these valves is not available.

A third option for aortic valve replacement is the pulmonary autograft, also known as the Ross procedure.[17] The procedure consists of transplantation of the patient's own pulmonary valve to the aortic position and implantation of a pulmonary homograft in the pulmonary position. Although this procedure may represent an important alternative in the management of aortic valve disease in young women,[18] the long-term durability of the transplanted pulmonary valve in

Cardiac Problems in Pregnancy, Third Edition
Edited by Uri Elkayam, MD, and Norbert Gleicher, MD
Copyright © 1998 by Wiley-Liss, Inc. ISBN 0-471-16358-9

TABLE 6.1 Types of Prosthetic Heart Valve

Type	Model
MECHANICAL	
Caged ball	Starr–Edwards
Single tilting disk	Bjork–Shiley
	Medtronic–Hall
	Omnicarbon
Bileaflet tilting disk	St. Jude Medical
	Carbomedics
	Edwards–Duromedics
BIOPROSTHETIC	
Heterograft	Hancock
	Carpenter–Edwards
	Ionescu–Shiley
Homograft	

Source: Vongpatanasin et al, *N Engl J Med* 1996;335:407–416, with permission.

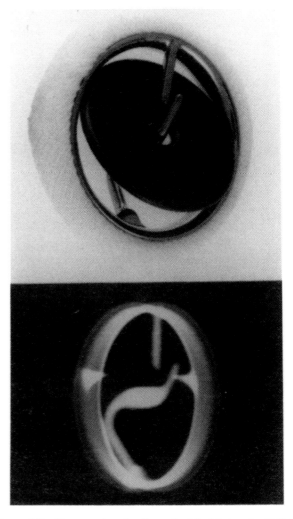

Figure 6.2 Photograph and radiograph of the Medtronic–Hall tilting disk prosthesis. (From Harrison EC et al, *Ann Emergency Med* 1988;17:194, with permission.)

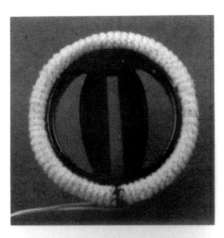

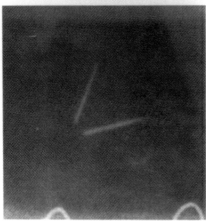

Figure 6.1 Photograph and radiograph of the St. Jude Medical imaged bileaflet prosthesis. (From Vongpatanasin et al, *N Engl J Med* 1996;335:407, with permission.)

the aortic position remains a major concern. We have not been able to find information on pregnancy in patients after the Ross procedure.

The advantages and disadvantages of tissue valves and mechanical valves[19–21] when used in the young female of childbearing age are summarized in outline form in Table 6.2. The primary areas of difference are durability, incidence of thromboembolism, risk of hemorrhage, hemodynamics, and fetal outcome. Since data comparing these valves in pregnant patients are sparse, relevant information obtained from the nonpregnant as well as the pregnant population will be discussed.

Durability

In younger patients, prosthetic valve durability is a major factor influencing the decision as to which type of valve to im-

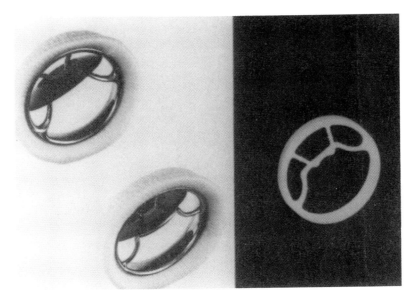

Figure 6.3   Photograph and radiograph of the Bjork–Shiley convex concave (top left) and spherical disk (bottom left) tilting disk prosthesis. (From Harrison EC et al, *Ann Emergency Med* 1988;17:194, with permission.)

plant. Mechanical valves are clearly more durable than tissue valves. Currently available, second-generation mechanical valves have an extremely low incidence of structural failure.[22] The experience with the St. Jude valve, for example, extends beyond 15 years with no significant incidence of mechanical valve failure.[23] In contrast, tissue valves have limited durability, with approximately a 30% incidence of valve deterioration at 10 years in the general population.[23-25] Data on tissue valve durability in younger patients suggest an even

higher failure rate. Craver et al[26] have reported dysfunction of bioprosthetic valves in 13% of patients ages 15–34 over 1.9 years compared to 2.9% in patients over 34 years ($p < 0.01$). Similarly, Jamieson et al[27] reported the greatest rate of deterioration in younger patients (27% freedom from deterioration at 10 years for patients less than 30 years of age, 77% for patients between 30 and 59 years of age, and 83% for patients over the age of 60). Figure 6.7 shows durability by age of the Hancock porcine valve in various age groups. In pa-

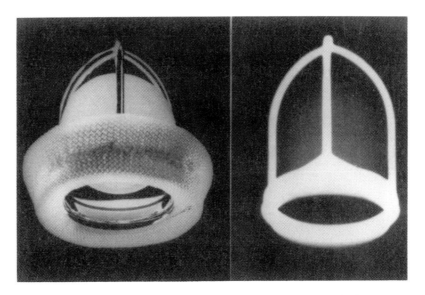

Figure 6.4   Photograph and radiograph of the Starr–Edwards caged ball prosthesis. (From Harrison EC et al, *Ann Emergency Med* 1988;17:194, with permission.)

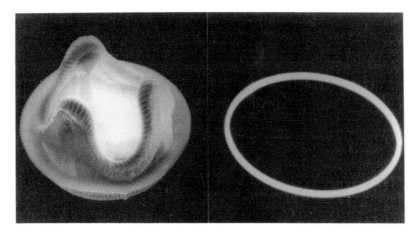

Figure 6.5   Photograph and radiograph of the Hancock porcine bioprosthesis. (From Harrison EC et al, *Ann Emergency Med* 1988;17:194, with permission.)

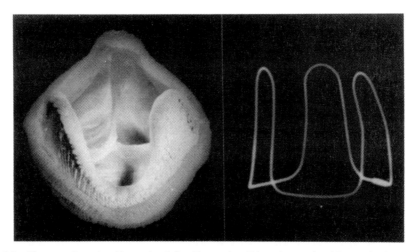

Figure 6.6   Photograph and radiograph of the Carpentier–Edwards porcine bioprosthesis. (From Harrison EC et al, *Ann Emergency Med* 1988;17:194, with permission.)

TABLE 6.2   Comparison of Advantages and Disadvantages of Tissue and Mechanical Valves

Property/Outcome	Tissue	Mechanical
Durability	Limited (10–12 years)	Indefinite
Thromboembolism	Low risk	High risk if not anticoagulated
Anticoagulation	Not needed after initial 3 months	Required indefinitely
Hemodynamics	Good, with exception of smallest valve sizes	Excellent
Accelerated deterioration during pregnancy	Yes	No
Fetal loss	No effect	Increased
Prematurity	Probably no effect	Increased
Small-for-date	Probably no effect	Increased

Actuarial Freedom from Prosthetic Valve Dysfunction: Overall and by Age Groups

(Includes structural valve deterioration and/or nonstructural dysfunction. Excludes paravalvular leak.)

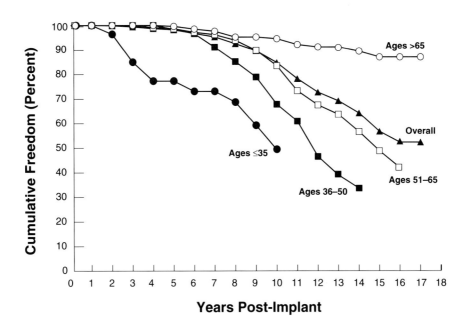

Key   Number At Risk

▲	Overall	762	670	644	608	584	553	508	461	403	355	294	227	183	140	101	61	37	18	7*
●	≤35 Years	31	28	26	22	20	19	17	17	15	12	10	7*	4	3	2	2	1	0	0
■	36-50 Years	76	71	66	62	61	59	55	47	42	36	30	26	19	15	12	6*	3	1	0
□	51-65 Years	276	242	232	224	217	209	194	182	163	149	123	93	78	60	42	25	15	7*	4
○	>65 Years	379	329	320	300	286	266	242	215	183	158	131	101	82	62	45	28	18	10	3*

*Actuarial estimates are not plotted where the number of patients at risk is less than 10.

Figure 6.7   Actuarial freedom from structural valve deterioration of the modified orifice aortic Hancock porcine valve. (Courtesy of Medtronic, Inc., © 1996.)

tients age 35 or younger, 77% of valves were free of structural failure at 5 years, 49% at 10 years, and only 25% at 15 years. These data indicate that at least half of the porcine tissue valves implanted in young women in the childbearing age can be expected to fail within 10 years after surgery. The Carpentier–Edwards pericardial valve has shown improved long-term durability in the aortic position. At an average follow-up of 5.5 years in 124 patients, 98% were free of reoperation at 9 years with no incidence of structural deterioration.[19] No information, however, is available regarding the durability of this valve in younger patients. Yacoub et al[28] recently summarized their 14-year experience with homografts for aortic valve replacement and reported increased risk for late valve degeneration in recipients younger than 30 years.

Recent reports have provided strong indication of a pregnancy-related accelerated deterioration of tissue valves (Table 6.3). Hanania et al[15] reported valve deterioration and need for reoperation for valve degeneration in 7 of 74 bioprostheses exposed to pregnancy, an average of 5.9 years after the initial operation. An even higher incidence of tissue valve failure was described by Kadri et al,[6] with valve deterioration occurring in 4 of 14 patients, and by Sbarouni et al,[14] who found valve deterioration in 17 of 49 women with bioprosthetic valves; 15 of the latter patients required valve replacement, 2 of them during pregnancy and 13 postpartum. Lee et al[13] reported tissue valve deterioration during pregnancy in only 4 out of 95 pregnancies in 57 women with tissue valves. However, the 10-year graft survival rate in the

TABLE 6.3   Evidence for Tissue/Valve Deterioration During Pregnancy

Ref: First Author	Number of Pregnancies	Number of Patients with Valve Deterioration	Comments
Kadri[6] (1989)	14	4 (29%)	
Born[11] (1992)	25	4 (16%)	2 maternal deaths
Sbarouni[14] (1993)	49	17 (35%)	2 operated during pregnancy and 15 shortly thereafter
Hanania[15] (1994)	74	7 (10%)	
Lee[13] (1994)	95	4 (4%)	10-year valve survival: 1 pregnancy, 55% 2 pregnancies, 17%
	257	36 (14%)	

porcine valve group was lower following two subsequent pregnancies (17%) than following one (55%), supporting the assertion of a degenerative effect of pregnancy on tissue valves.

Since women in the childbearing age with a bioprosthetic valve, especially those who become pregnant, are likely to need reoperation, the risk associated with such surgery needs to be considered during the selection of a prosthetic valve for a young woman. Overall operative mortality for valve reoperation recently reported has ranged from 5.0 to 21.3%,[29] with an average mortality of 10.6% for elective and emergency surgery combined and 6% for elective surgery. Since these figures include patients of all ages, it is feasible to suggest that the risks of reoperation in younger patients may be lower. This assumption is supported by the results of two recent studies. Piehler et al[30] reported a 6% mortality associated with reoperation on 2246 prosthetic valves in 1984 low risk patients [i.e., young age, low New York Heart Association (NYHA) functional class, etc.], with only 1.3% mortality associated with a first reoperation. Similarly, a mortality rate of 6.0% was reported by Jamieson et al[28] in 107 women 35 years or less undergoing rereplacement of bioprostheses.

In summary, currently available mechanical valves provide an excellent record of long-term durability in young patients of childbearing age. In contrast, current tissue valves are likely to deteriorate structurally after 10–12 years, with accelerated deterioration in younger patients (under age 30) and during pregnancy. A large number of women under the age of 35 receiving tissue valves should therefore expect to require valve rereplacement within 10 years, with an anticipated surgical mortality rate of approximately 6%.

Hemodynamics

Selection of a valve with better hemodynamic performance may result in a favorable effect on preservation of cardiac function, functional capacity, morbidity, and perhaps even long-term survival.[31–33]

The newer mechanical valves such as the St. Jude Medical and the Medtronic–Hall have consistently shown better hemodynamic performance than the Starr–Edwards ball valves and the standard porcine valves (Table 6.4). The latter valves (such as the Hancock or Carpentier–Edwards[34] porcine valve) have mediocre hemodynamics, especially in the smaller sizes (19–21 mm), because of the presence of muscle tissue in the septal leaflet of the porcine valve.[35–42] The greatest potential advantage of mechanical valves is, therefore, in patients with a small aortic root.[40–44] Homograft valves and the new Carpentier–Edwards pericardial valve also appear to have better hemodynamics than standard porcine valves.[45–48]

Thromboembolism and Hemorrhage

Thromboembolism and bleeding complications from anticoagulants remain the major disadvantages of mechanical valves. Although current designs of these valves have lower rates of thromboembolic events, the incidence remains high

TABLE 6.4   Effective Orifice Area for Various Prosthetic Valves

Valve Type	Eff. Orifice Area (cm^2)	
	Aortic	Mitral
Caged ball	1.2–1.6	1.4–3.1
Single tilting disk	1.5–2.1	1.9–3.2
Bileaflet tilting disk	2.4–3.2	2.8–3.4
Heterograft bioprosthesis	1.0–1.7	1.3–2.7
Homograft bioprosthesis	3.4–4.0	Not available

Source: Modified from Vongpatanasin et al, *N Engl J Med* 1996;335:407–416, with permission.

enough to require life-long anticoagulation. The thromboembolic event rate in a recent large series of patients with St. Jude valves[23] treated with anticoagulation averaged 1.3 episodes/100 patient-years, which was similar to the 1.9 episodes/100 patient-years reported for porcine aortic valves without anticoagulation.[49] Similarly, a comparison of older generation mechanical prosthesis[50] (Bjork–Shiley) and porcine (Hancock and Carpentier–Edwards) valves showed no significant difference in incidence of thromboembolic complications over time.[50,51] A recent meta-analysis by Cannegieter et al[52] of 13,088 patients with mechanical valves indicated a relationship between the risk of major embolism and the use of anticoagulation, as well as the type and location of the prosthesis. The incidence of major embolism was 0.8/100 patient-years for aortic valves, 1.3/100 patient-years for mitral valves, and 1.4/100 patient-years for patients with both aortic and mitral prosthetic valves. The rate of thromboembolism was 30–40% lower for bileaflet and tilting disk valves than for caged ball valves and for patients treated with oral anticoagulation (1.0/100 patient-years) compared to aspirin (1.4/100 patient-years). The combination of Coumadin and aspirin provided no additional benefit against thromboembolism over Coumadin alone.

Pregnancy has been associated with a significant increase in the incidence of thromboembolic events. Predisposing factors for thromboembolism during pregnancy have been older generation mechanical valves in the mitral position and the use of subcutaneous heparin rather than Coumadin for anticoagulation. Sbarouni et al[14] reported major thromboembolic events in 20 out of 151 pregnancies (13%) in 133 women with mechanical valves, and Hanania et al[15] reported 16 thromboembolic events in a group of 108 mechanical prostheses (15%).

Data on the rates of bleeding complications with mechanical and tissue valves are conflicting. The VA cooperative study found a significantly higher rate of fatal and nonfatal valve-related complications in patients randomized to a mechanical valve. These investigators found a 5-year probability of freedom from bleeding of 67% for aortic mechanical prostheses compared to 85% for aortic tissue valves. This high rate of bleeding complications may have been related to the high intensity of anticoagulation[53] in this study and increased patients' age.[54] Other studies have demonstrated an incidence of major bleeding in patients with mechanical heart valve prostheses treated with Coumadin of 1.4 per 100 patient-years[52] and the number of complications to be similar for the Bjork–Shiley, Hancock, and Carpentier–Edwards valves (1.0, 1.5, and 1.5 events/100 patient-years, respectively).

Bleeding complications during pregnancy have been more frequently observed in patients with mechanical valves than with tissue valves. Sbarouni et al[14] reported no bleeding complications in 57 pregnancies in women with bioprostheses and seven major bleeding complications requiring more

than two units of transfused blood in 124 pregnancies in women with mechanical valves (5%). Hemorrhagic complications have been reported in 2.5–17% of cases at the time of delivery or the puerperium both on heparin and on Coumadin.[12,14,16,55]

In summary, major contributing factors for thromboembolic events are a mechanical prosthesis, especially a caged ball valve, the mitral location, multiple prosthetic valves, and inadequate anticoagulation. The risk of thromboembolic events, both valve thrombosis and peripheral embolization, is similar in patients with bioprosthetic valves and patients with mechanical prosthesis who receive adequate anticoagulation. Pregnancy is associated with a significant increase in the risk of thromboembolic events. Available data suggest a low incidence of hemorrhagic complications in the nonpregnant population of patients with mechanical valves. This incidence, however, is higher than that observed in patients with tissue valves. Increased rate of hemorrhagic complications has been reported during pregnancy in patients treated with anticoagulation, especially at the time of delivery and the early postpartum period.

Survival

No survival information is available to reflect differences between tissue and mechanical valves in young patients. Available studies in the general population have failed to demonstrate a survival benefit of either mechanical or tissue heart valves.[49,50]

Fetal Outcome in Patients with Mechanical Versus Tissue Valves

Available information on fetal outcome in patients with prosthetic heart valves (Table 6.5) suggests an increased risk in patients with mechanical prostheses, most probably related to the mandatory use of anticoagulation in such patients. The majority of existing data demonstrate an increased incidence of fetal loss due to spontaneous abortion[11,13,15] and stillbirth[11,13,14] and, in addition, an increased incidence of prematurity,[11,14] low birth weight,[11] birth defects,[11,13,15] and neonatal mortality.[11,14]

Summary and Recommendations

The selection of a prosthetic valve for a woman of childbearing age who desires to become pregnant after surgery remains difficult. New-generation mechanical valves, which have excellent durability and a low risk of reoperation, provide a superior hemodynamic profile, especially in small sizes in the aortic position. However, their thrombogenicity and need for anticoagulation are associated with an increased risk of thromboembolism and bleeding during pregnancy. However, major thromboembolic events have been reported

TABLE 6.5 Fetal Outcome in Women with Prosthetic Mechanical (M) and Tissue (T) Valve(s)

Outcome	Born et al[11] (1992)		Sbarouni et al[14] (1993)		Lee et al[13] (1994)		Hanania et al[15] (1994)	
	M	T	M	T	M	T	M	T
Spontaneous abortions (%)	17.5	—	12	10	11	1[a]	17	7
Prematurity (%)	46.5	10.5[a]	24	7	6	8	14	
Low birth weight (%)	50	10.5[a]	NA	NA	9	11	NA	NA[b]
Stillbirth (%)	3.2		7	4	NA	NA	NA	NA
Neonatal mortality (%)	16.2		2		3	1.5	NA	NA
Birth defects (%)	12.1				4		1	2

[a] $p < 0.05$.

[b] Significantly higher birth weight in tissue valve group (2970 g vs. 2580 g, $p < 0.05$).

during gestation mostly in patients with older generation mechanical prostheses in the mitral position and in patients with suboptimal anticoagulation.[11,13–15] A relatively high incidence of valve thrombosis has been reported in such cases with a high maternal and fetal mortality. The use of anticoagulation is associated with an increased incidence of maternal and fetal bleeding complications and increased fetal loss.

The use of tissue valves is also associated with major limitations. There is still a relatively high rate of valve deterioration with approximately 30% of the patients requiring rereplacement of the valve within 10 years. The rate of valve deterioration is further accelerated in patients younger than 20 years and during pregnancy, with the result of an increased need for valve replacement, either during pregnancy or in the early postpartum period. Such surgery is associated with an average surgical mortality of 6%. Although recently developed pericardial valves may provide a better hemodynamic profile in the aortic position and possibly improved durability compared to porcine tissue valves, no information is available regarding their use in pregnancy. Similarly, no information is available regarding pregnancies in patients with homografts and in patients following the Ross procedure.

In patients who require chronic anticoagulation for reasons unrelated to their prosthetic valve (e.g., atrial fibrillation), the choice of a modern single or bileaflet mechanical valve makes good clinical sense because of the durability and reduced risk of thromboembolism of such devices. A tissue valve may be an equally good choice in patients who are not capable of or willing to participate in the close follow-up and stringent monitoring of anticoagulation required during pregnancy. Because of their durability, hemodynamic advantages, and, with careful anticoagulation, low risk of thromboembolic as well as bleeding complications, we recommend current-generation mechanical prostheses to all other patients who need valve replacement during their childbearing years who can and will cooperate in a close medical follow-up during pregnancy. These recommendations are not shared by all authors. Some investigators recommend the use of tissue valves to all patients who do not require anticoagulation

therapy for other reasons,[13,16] while Hanania et al[15] recommend a mechanical prosthesis only for the aortic valve or in the presence of atrial fibrillation.

RISKS ASSOCIATED WITH PREGNANCY IN WOMEN WITH PROSTHETIC HEART VALVES

Congestive Heart Failure

Increasing heart failure in women with prosthetic valves during pregnancy may be caused by an increased hemodynamic burden (Chapter 1) or by the occurrence of valve thrombosis or valve deterioration. Pregnancy is associated with important hemodynamic changes that may lead to cardiac decompensation in patients with prosthetic heart valves, especially those with systolic or diastolic left ventricular dysfunction. Numerous available reports describing experience in over 1000 pregnancies[2–16,55,56] in patients with one or more prosthetic heart valves have demonstrated that most patients who are asymptomatic or only mildly symptomatic (NYHA functional class I-II) tolerate the hemodynamic burden of pregnancy. However, decreased functional capacity and the need to initiate or increase medical therapy are not uncommon. Born et al[11] described deterioration of NYHA functional classification from I-II during the first trimester to III-IV in the second or third trimester in 18 of 60 cases. This change in clinical status was due to valve thrombosis, stenosis, or rupture of a bioprosthesis in five of the patients. Caruso et al[57] reported initiation of diuretic therapy in more than 50% of pregnancies in women who conceived after cardiac valve replacement. Salazar et al[55] described the development of pulmonary edema during the 13th week of pregnancy in a patient with a prosthetic mitral valve. Sbarouni et al[14] reported on death due to pulmonary edema in a patient who was NYHA class I prepregnancy, in whom no valve thrombosis could be found. Sareli et al[7] reported the development of pulmonary edema during labor in two patients who were hemodynamically stable before delivery.

In summary, patients with prosthetic valves may develop worsening heart failure during pregnancy and therefore require careful monitoring of fluid status and titration of diuretics.

Thromboembolic Events

Pregnancy is associated with an increased incidence of thromboembolic events that are due to a hypercoagulable state and possibly to changes in metabolism and clearance of heparin (Table 6.6).[58] The occurrence of thromboembolic complications seems to be related to the type and position of the prosthetic valve and to the anticoagulation regimen. Mechanical valves, especially older generation valves (Bjork–Shiley, Starr–Edwards) in the mitral position and use of subcutaneous heparin or aspirin rather than Coumadin have been shown to be associated with most major thromboembolic events. Sbarouni et al[14] conducted a retrospective survey on the outcome of pregnancy in women with artificial valves treated in major European centers. These investigators reported no thromboembolic complication in 63 pregnancies in 49 women with bioprostheses. In contrast, 151 pregnancies in 133 women with mechanical valves were associated with 13 cases of valve thrombosis, 4 of which were fatal. In addition, there were 8 major embolic events, 2 fatal (one associated with valve thrombosis); 12 of 13 thrombosed valves and all 8 major embolic events were associated with mitral valve prostheses. The only case of aortic valve thrombosis occurred in a patient who stopped her anticoagulation. Ten of 13 patients with thrombosed valves and 5 of 8 cases with major embolic events were treated with heparin.

Similar information was provided by the French Cooperative study[15] of 155 pregnancies in 103 women with valvular prostheses (95 mechanical, 60 bioprostheses, including 27 bivalvular prostheses). This study reported 16 thromboembolic events including 10 prosthetic valve thromboses requiring valve replacement in 4 cases and 6 systemic thromboemboli. These events occurred in 13 mitral, 2 aortic, and 1 pulmonic mechanical prostheses. Thromboembolic events were found to be four times more frequent in patients on heparin compared to patients on Coumadin. Out of 16 patients who had thromboembolic events, 14 had an old-generation prosthesis (Bjork–Shiley, 6; Starr–Edwards, 7; Omniscience, 1) and only two had a St. Jude valve, both of them in the mitral position. Salazar et al[55] followed prospectively

40 pregnancies in 37 women with prosthetic valves. These investigators reported two cases of fatal thrombosis of Bjork–Shiley valves, one in the mitral and the other in the aortic position, and one case of cerebral embolism in a patient with a Starr–Edwards mitral prosthesis. All three patients were treated with adjusted dose heparin (to maintain partial thromboplastin time at 1.5–2.5 times the control).

Born et al[11] published results of a prospective study evaluating the outcome of 60 pregnancies in 49 patients with prosthetic heart valves in Brazil. Patients were treated with oral anticoagulation for 34–37 weeks of gestation. Forty pregnancies occurred in women with mechanical valves (mostly Lillehei–Kaster and Starr–Edwards). Valve thrombosis was reported in 7.5% of patients with mechanical valves and in none during 25 pregnancies in patients with a bioprosthesis (Carpentier–Edwards, 6; dura mater, 6; bovine pericardium, 7; others, 6). Embolic episodes were seen in one patient in each group (2.5 and 5.0%, respectively). Sareli et al[7] prospectively followed 50 pregnancies in 49 patients with 62 valvular prostheses. Of the 60 mechanical valves, 46 were either Medtronic–Hall or St. Jude Medical. All patients received Coumadin either until 36 weeks or until labor. Although control of anticoagulation was poor, none of the patients developed thromboembolic complications. This observation supports the claims for improved safety of newer generation mechanical valves over the older devices.

In summary, recent information suggests an increase in risk of thromboembolic events during pregnancy in patients with prosthetic heart valves. This incidence varies between 10 and 15%, with approximately two-thirds of the reported cases presenting with valve thrombosis, which may be fatal. The incidence of thromboembolic complications is significantly higher in patients with mechanical compared to tissue valves. Thromboembolism has been reported mostly in patients with older generation mechanical valves (Starr–Edwards, Bjork–Shiley, etc.), in the mitral position, and in patients treated with subcutaneous heparin. The adequacy of anticoagulation in these cases has not been well documented.

Risk of Cardiovascular Drugs

Patients with prosthetic heart valves are often prescribed various cardiovascular medications for the treatment of heart failure, arrhythmias, and valve thrombosis. The risks to the

TABLE 6.6 Incidence of Major Thromboembolic Events During Pregnancy

Ref: First Author	Major TE Events	Valve Thrombosis	Death	Pregnancies	Patients
Born[11] (1992)	4 (10%)	3	0	40	NA
Sbarouni[14] (1993)	21 (14%)	13	6	151	133
Hanania[15] (1994)	22 (23%)	10	3	95	NA
Salazar[55] (1996)	3 (7.5%)	2	2	40	37

fetus associated with use of such therapy are described elsewhere in this book (Chapters 27–36).

Risk of Anticoagulation

The general topic of anticoagulation in pregnancy is discussed in detail in Chapter 33. The risks of anticoagulation during pregnancy in the patient with a prosthetic valve include teratogenic effects, an increased likelihood of fetal as well as maternal bleeding, increased fetal loss, and failure to prevent major maternal thromboembolic events.

Although the occurrence of teratogenic effects of Coumadin has been reported in one study in as many as 67% of newborns,[59] the majority of available studies indicate a lower incidence of approximately 5–10%.[7,11,12] As expected, bleeding complications both in the mother and in the fetus have been reported during pregnancy in women treated with anticoagulation. Sbarouni et al[14] reported seven major maternal bleeding complications (5 during pregnancy and two postpartum) in 132 cases that required more than two units of transfused blood and resulted in hysterectomy. Five of these cases were treated with heparin and two with Coumadin. Severe bleeding during delivery and puerperium has also been described by other investigators.[12,13,55] Salazar et al[55] described neonatal death due to cerebral hemorrhage in a case of premature labor (35 weeks) in a woman treated with oral anticoagulants.

There is a strong evidence for an important effect of anticoagulation on fetal outcome in patients with prosthetic valves. The French Cooperative study reported a significant difference in the rate of live-born children between mothers with mechanical valves (53%) and those with bioprostheses (80%, $p < 0.01$). Seven of the children were born prematurely, all of them to mothers treated with anticoagulants. The birth weight was over 400 g lower (2.6 kg vs. 3.0 kg) in the patients with mechanical prostheses ($p < 0.05$). Spontaneous abortions were more common in patients treated with anticoagulation (17%) than in those who were not (2%, $p < 0.02$). Sbarouni et al reported live birth in 83% of pregnancies in women with bioprostheses and 75% in patients with mechanical prostheses ($p = $ NS). The incidence of prematurity was significantly lower ($p < 0.05$) in patients with bioprostheses. Fetal outcome was most favorable in women receiving heparin for the first trimester followed by warfarin, compared to warfarin or heparin throughout. There was no difference in outcome between patients taking oral anticoagulants and patients treated with heparin for the first trimester and warfarin thereafter, except for lower incidence of prematurity ($p < 0.05$). Nor was there any difference in the outcome between patients taking warfarin throughout and patients on heparin throughout. Women taking heparin followed by warfarin were more likely to have a healthy baby than women taking heparin throughout pregnancy ($p < 0.05$). The incidence of stillbirth was also lower in women

taking heparin followed by warfarin than in women treated with Coumadin throughout or heparin throughout ($p < 0.05$). Although the latter report indicated a higher fetal risk with heparin therapy throughout pregnancy, the accuracy of these data could be severely limited by the retrospective nature of the survey, which could have led to incomplete and biased information. This concern is enhanced by other data indicating a high risk with oral anticoagulation. Lee et al[13] followed 151 pregnancies in 88 patients: 31 patients had a mechanical cardiac valve; all received oral anticoagulation medication throughout pregnancy. The rate of fetal loss was significantly greater in patients who were treated with oral anticoagulation than in patients who were not (28 vs. 12%, respectively, $p < 0.05$). No significant difference was found in prematurity (6 vs. 8%) or small-for-date infants (9 vs. 11%). Similarly, a high incidence of spontaneous abortion was reported by Salazar et al (37.5%). These investigators used oral anticoagulants throughout pregnancy except from the 6th week until the end of the 12th week and for the last 2 weeks of gestation, when heparin was used. The incidence of spontaneous abortion was only 14% in the study by Caruso et al,[57] who discontinued oral anticoagulation before conception or soon thereafter and substituted subcutaneous heparin. Another study of the use of heparin in a large number of patients throughout pregnancy (primarily for the treatment of deep vein thrombosis) resulted in normal fetal outcome.[60]

In summary, the use of anticoagulation medications during pregnancy in women with a prosthetic heart valve is associated with increased risk both to the mother and to the fetus. This risk includes maternal bleeding complications, especially during delivery and early postpartum. Anticoagulation has been reported to be associated with increased incidence of fetal loss, prematurity, fetal growth retardation, and birth defect due to Coumadin embryopathy. There is some evidence to suggest that use of Coumadin during the first trimester of pregnancy is associated with increased fetal wastage, although some studies indicate a similar risk with heparin. Vaginal delivery in a patient treated with Coumadin may lead to severe fatal bleeding complications in the fetus and should be avoided.

MANAGEMENT OF A PATIENT WITH PROSTHETIC VALVE DURING PREGNANCY

Prepregnancy Consultation and Evaluation

The following information may help determine the risk of pregnancy in a woman with a prosthetic valve and should be obtained prior to conception: type and position of prosthetic valve(s), cardiac symptoms and functional classification, prosthetic valve function, size and function of the various cardiac chambers (with special emphasis on systolic and diastolic left ventricular function), and presence and severity of native valvular disease.

The exact type and size of the valvular prosthesis can usually be obtained from the patient prosthetic heart valve identification card.[1] This card includes information regarding position of the implant, valve model if applicable, valve size in millimeters, and valve serial number. If the patient cannot provide information about the type of valve implanted, the valve type and location can be determined radiographically (Figs. 6.1–6.6).[1] Prepregnancy evaluation should include a careful history for assessment of the presence and severity of cardiac symptoms and determination of the patient's functional capacity. Exercise testing, including determination of maximum oxygen consumption, is helpful in obtaining objective assessment of functional capacity in women with cardiac symptoms. Physical examination and echo–Doppler study should be performed for evaluation of cardiac function as well as the function of all cardiac valves. In general, since clinical deterioration is likely during pregnancy, patients with impaired functional classification (NYHA class III and IV) or patients with marked impairment in left ventricular function or valvular function should be advised against pregnancy. Patients with lower functional class (I and II) should be advised of the possibility of symptomatic worsening during pregnancy. The patient and her family should be informed of the potential complications to both the mother and the fetus (hemodynamic and symptomatic deterioration, increased risk of thromboembolism, potential harm to the fetus due to anticoagulation and other cardiac drugs, increased incidence of fetal loss, prematurity and fetal growth retardation, and accelerated deterioration of tissue valves during pregnancy).

Management of Complications During Pregnancy

Heart Failure   The assessment of the presence and severity of heart failure during pregnancy is somewhat difficult and often misleading. There may be confusion, for example, resulting from signs and symptoms commonly seen in normal pregnancy (Chapter 2), such as decreased exercise capacity, shortness of breath, palpitations, dizziness, and leg edema, in addition to the physiological presence of a systolic murmur, right and left ventricular heave, and palpable closure of the pulmonic valve. To obtain an accurate hemodynamic assessment, therefore, it is necessary at times to acquire hemodynamic information by either noninvasive (echo–Doppler) or invasive (bedside right heart catheterization) methods. The treatment of heart failure depends on its mechanism. In general, the following drugs are relatively safe: digoxin, diuretics, nitrates, hydralazine, and β-adrenergic blockers (for patients with heart failure due to mitral stenosis). Angiotensin-converting enzyme inhibitors are contraindicated during pregnancy (Chapter 32), and sodium nitroprusside should also be avoided (Chapter 31).

Valve Thrombosis   The clinical presentation of prosthetic valve thrombosis can be subacute with progressive fatigue or shortness of breath, but it can also present acutely with pulmonary edema, stroke, arterial embolization, cardiogenic shock, and even death.[61] Physical examination may reveal decreased intensity of one or both metallic clicks or the presence of a new murmur. Normal auscultatory characteristics of the various prosthetic valves in the aortic and mitral positions and description of abnormal findings are shown in Figure 6.8. The diagnosis of valve thrombosis can be confirmed by either echocardiography or cinefluoroscopy. Since transthoracic echocardiography may not provide the diagnosis,[62] transesophageal technique is preferred. Cinefluoroscopy is useful in demonstrating restriction of leaflet motion[63,64] and provides instantaneous conformation of prosthetic valve thrombosis.[61]

When the thrombus is less than 5 mm in diameter on echocardiography and is not obstructive, the patient can be treated with anticoagulation alone.[65] In the presence of a thrombus 5 mm or larger in diameter, more aggressive therapy is warranted.[66] Thrombolytic therapy has emerged in recent years as a treatment of choice for valve thrombosis.[62–64,67] This form of treatment has a success rate of 70% and a mortality rate of 9–10%. It is more effective for patients with aortic valve thrombosis and for those who have exhibited symptoms for less than 2 weeks.[66] Mortality associated with surgery is approximately 15%[66] and may be substantially higher for emergency operation in cases with hemodynamic instability. Because of high risk of embolization associated with thrombolytic therapy, it has been recently recommended to use this form of therapy for critically ill patients in whom operative risk is high, and consider valve replacement for hemodynamically stable patients who can have surgery with relatively low risk.[66] Thrombolytic therapy has been used in several pregnant women for various indications, including prosthetic valve thrombosis.[68] Although thrombolytic therapy was given without complications in some pregnant patients,[14,15,67,69] uterine hemorrhage requiring transfusion, emergency cesarean section, and even death have been reported.[68]

Anticoagulation

Oral anticoagulant agents have been considered contraindicated in pregnancy because of their reported teratogenic effect and increased fetal bleeding complications[58] (Chapter 33). In contrast, the large heparin molecule does not cross the placenta, and recent experience[58,60] in a large number of patients who received heparin during pregnancy showed normal fetal and neonatal outcomes without increase in maternal bleeding complications.[58,60] It is, therefore, not surprising that earlier recommendations favored the use of heparin when possible throughout pregnancy.

Recently published studies,[14,15,55] however, have reported an increased incidence of valve thrombosis in women treated with subcutaneous heparin. These data are limited by

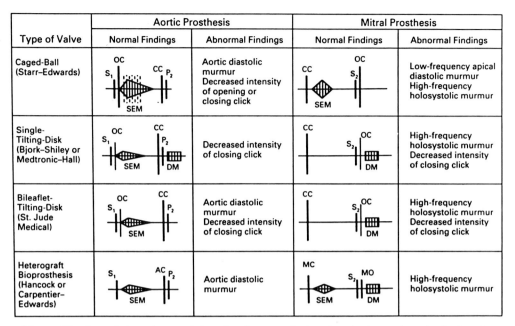

Type of Valve	Aortic Prosthesis		Mitral Prosthesis	
	Normal Findings	Abnormal Findings	Normal Findings	Abnormal Findings
Caged-Ball (Starr–Edwards)		Aortic diastolic murmur Decreased intensity of opening or closing click		Low-frequency apical diastolic murmur High-frequency holosystolic murmur
Single-Tilting-Disk (Bjork–Shiley or Medtronic–Hall)		Decreased intensity of closing click		High-frequency holosystolic murmur Decreased intensity of closing click
Bileaflet-Tilting-Disk (St. Jude Medical)		Aortic diastolic murmur Decreased intensity of closing click		High-frequency holosystolic murmur Decreased intensity of closing click
Heterograft Bioprosthesis (Hancock or Carpentier–Edwards)		Aortic diastolic murmur		High-frequency holosystolic murmur

Figure 6.8   Auscultatory characteristics of various prosthetic valves in the aortic and mitral positions, with schematic diagrams of normal findings and descriptions of abnormal findings. (From Vongpatanasin et al, *N Engl J Med* 1996;335:407, with permission.)
The caged ball aortic prosthesis produces a loud opening click (OC) after the first heart sound (S_1) and a less prominent closing click (CC); an early- to-mid peaking systolic ejection murmur (SEM) is audible, along with multiple systolic clicks (broken lines) of the bouncing poppet within the cage. P_2 denotes the pulmonic component of the second heart sound. The caged ball mitral prosthesis produces a loud opening click after the second heart sound (S_2). An early- to-midsystolic ejection murmur, usually loudest at the left sternal border, is caused by turbulent flow in the left ventricular outflow tract. The aortic single tilting disk valve has a louder closing click than opening click. An early- to-mid peaking systolic ejection murmur is usually best heard at the base and often radiates to the carotid arteries. A soft diastolic murmur (DM) may be noted in an occasional patient. The mitral single tilting disk valve has a louder closing click than opening click. A low frequency diastolic rumbling murmur, which represents turbulent flow across the open valve, is usually audible. The aortic bileaflet tilting disk prosthetic valve produces a loud closing click. An early- to-midpeaking systolic ejection murmur is best heard at the base and often radiates to the carotid arteries. A diastolic murmur is not audible. The mitral bileaflet tilting disk valve has auscultatory characteristics similar to those of the mitral single tilting disk valve. The aortic heterograft bioprosthesis has a closing sound (AC) similar to that of a normal valve. An early- to-midpeaking systolic ejection murmur is audible and often radiates to the carotid arteries. The mitral heterograft bioprosthesis has a closing sound (MC) that may be indistinguishable from a normal first heart sound; an opening sound (MO) is usually audible after the second heart sound, as is an early- to-mid systolic ejection murmur, representing turbulent flow in the left ventricular outflow tract. A low frequency diastolic rumbling murmur may also be audible at the apex.

the small number of patients in some of the studies, by the retrospective design and possible selective and incomplete reporting in other studies, and by lack of information regarding the quality of anticoagulation monitoring. No definitive recommendations can be made at present, given the lack of large, randomized trials. Because of the strong suggestion for potential risk of valve thrombosis, however, women with older generation prosthetic valves in the mitral position should be presented with the available information and the option to use Coumadin throughout gestation with heparin

before delivery.[70] In high risk women who choose not to take Coumadin during the first trimester,[71] in-hospital, continuous intravenous heparin treatment seems justified. If outpatient heparin therapy is provided, very close monitoring of activated partial thromboplastin time (APTT) and frequent physical examinations for early detection of valve thrombosis are recommended.

In patients with older generation prosthetic valves in the aortic position and those with newer generation mechanical valves in any position, subcutaneous heparin may be used during the first trimester and in the last part of gestation. The dose of heparin should be adjusted to prolong the midinterval APTT two to three times control value (Chapter 33), and adequacy of anticoagulation should be monitored at least once every 1–2 weeks. Administration of heparin by subcutaneous infusion with a programmable pump has been demonstrated to achieve a more even control with fewer complications than intermittent subcutaneous injection technique[72] and should be considered in patients with prosthetic valves. Low molecular weight heparin may be an attractive drug for use during pregnancy. Like standard unfractionated heparin, it does not cross the placenta. At the same time, it may provide additional benefits, including reduced incidence of heparin-induced thrombocytopenia, osteoporosis, and bleeding complications; and no blood test is required to monitor its safety.[78] The drug has been used effectively and safely to treat deep vein thrombosis during pregnancy, but data in patients with prosthetic valves are not available.

What is the adequate intensity of oral anticoagulation during pregnancy? For lack of controlled studies, the answer to this question is also not available.

The dose of Coumadin needs to be high enough to prevent thromboembolism mediated by the hypercoagulability associated with pregnancy, but at the same time, it should be kept low enough to prevent maternal bleeding and possible fetal bleeding complications and embryopathy. Table 6.7 shows guidelines for intensity of anticoagulation in the nonpregnant population with prosthetic heart valve as recommended by recent publications. A recent report by Cannegieter et al[74] demonstrated an optimal intensity of anticoagulant therapy

in nonpregnant patients with prosthetic heart valve to be at an international normalized rate (INR) between 2.5 and 4.9. The frequency of thromboemboli seems to be higher in patients with first-generation prosthetic valves (e.g., Starr–Edwards, Bjork–Shiley), prosthetic valves in the mitral position, more than one prosthesis, atrial fibrillation, and history of systemic embolism.[75]

Our recommendations for anticoagulation for patients with mechanical prosthetic valve during pregnancy are summarized in Figure 6.9. Our suggested approach differentiates between patients with higher and lower risk for thromboembolic events. Patients with first-generation prosthetic valves in the mitral position should be informed of the potential resistance to moderate doses of heparin during pregnancy and offered the option of Coumadin therapy throughout pregnancy with intravenous heparin therapy, preferably in-hospital, after the 36th gestational week. An alternative therapy for women who may elect to avoid Coumadin in the first trimester would be intravenous or subcutaneous heparin for the first trimester (APTT 2.5–3.5 of normal), followed by Coumadin between 13 and 36 weeks, and then intravenous heparin. INR in higher risk patients treated with Coumadin needs to be between 3.0 and 4.5. In patients with lower risk for thromboembolic events, including those with a second-generation (e.g., St. Jude Medical, Medtronic–Hall) and those with mechanical prosthesis in the aortic position, the use of subcutaneous heparin (APTT 2.0–3.0) during the first trimester and the last 4 weeks of gestation and Coumadin until the 36th week of gestation seems to be reasonable; an alternative is heparin throughout pregnancy with close follow-

TABLE 6.7   Recommendation of Intensity of Oral Anticoagulation in the Nonpregnant Patient Population

Type of Valve	European Society of Cardiology[70] (1993)	Stein et al[75] (1995)	Vongpatanasin et al[66] (1996)
MECHANICAL VALVES			
Caged ball valves			
Starr–Edwards	3.0–4.5	>2.5–3.5	4.0–4.9
Single tilting disk valves			
Bjork–Shiley	3.0–4.5	2.5–3.5	NA
Medtronic–Hall	2.5–3.0	2.5–3.5	3.0–3.9
Bileaflet tilting disk valves			
St. Jude Medical	2.5–3.0	2.5–3.5	2.5–2.9
> 1 MECHANICAL PROSTHESIS			4.0–4.9
Bioprosthetic valves			
Heterografts			
Mitral, NSR	Oral AC for 3–6 months	2.0–3.0 for 3 months	2.0–3.0 for 3 months
Atrial fibrillation	3.0–4.6	2.0–3.0	2.0–3.0
Aortic, NSR	Oral AC for 3–6 months	Optional AC for 3 months	2.0–3.0 for 3 months
Atrial fibrillation	3.0–4.6	2.0–3.0	2.0–3.0
Homografts			
NSR	NA	NA	No AC
Atrial fibrillation	NA	NA	2.0–3.0

Abbreviations: AC, anticoagulants; NA, not available; NSR, normal sinus rhythm.

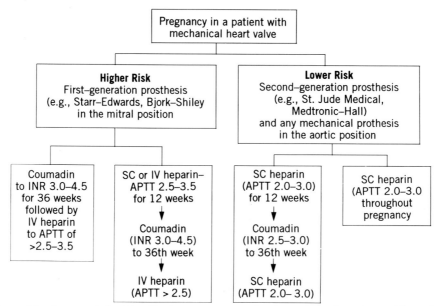

Figure 6.9   Suggested algorithm for the management of anticoagulation in patients with mechanical prosthetic heart valves during pregnancy.

up of APTT. Higher level of anticoagulation seems justified in patients with mechanical prosthesis in the mitral versus the aortic position, in patients with more than one mechanical prosthesis, and in patients with atrial fibrillation and a history of systemic embolization. The intensity of oral anticoagulation should be frequently monitored and immediately corrected if a therapeutic INR is not achieved. A recent study[77] showed a substantial reduction in the incidence of systemic embolization or death with a combination of low dose aspirin (100 mg daily) and warfarin (target INR, 3.0–4.5), compared to warfarin alone, in patients with mechanical valves or tissue valves plus atrial fibrillation or history of thromboembolism. Since a small dose of aspirin is safe during pregnancy,[75] it may be used in addition to anticoagulation to maximize the antithrombotic effect. The concomitant use of dipyridamole has been shown to provide an additional benefit in some reports in nonpregnant patients[75] but is not recommended during pregnancy because of high fetal loss demonstrated in one study.[7]

In the nonpregnant patients with bioprosthetic heart valves in the mitral position, treatment with oral anticoagulants at an INR of 2.0–3.0 is recommended for the first 3 months after valve surgery. Anticoagulation in patients with bioprosthetic aortic valves who are in sinus rhythm during the first 3 months is optional but seems reasonable, since increased incidence of thromboemboli has been reported.[76] Long-term anticoagulation is not recommended in patients with bioprosthetic heart valves except in the presence of atrial fibrillation or evidence of a left atrial thrombus at surgery. The recommended INR for these patients is 2.0–3.0. When

patients with bioprosthetic valve have a history of systemic embolism, the recommendations are to treat with oral anticoagulants for 3–12 months, with doses sufficient to prolong the INR to 2.0–3.0.[75] Intensity of anticoagulation in patients with bioprosthetic valve who require anticoagulation during pregnancy should be comparable to that used in patients with mechanical prosthesis with lower risk for thromboembolic events (Fig. 6.9).

Premature labor frequently occurs in women with prosthetic heart valves. In the study by Salazar et al,[55] 36% of the neonates were born before the 37th week of gestation, and one neonate died of cerebral hemorrhage due to Coumadin treatment that occurred during labor. These data suggest the need to substitute Coumadin with a therapeutic dose of heparin no later than 35 or 36 weeks of gestation to avoid the onset of labor during Coumadin therapy. The switch from Coumadin to heparin and the determination of adequate heparin dose should be performed in the hospital. In patients with older generation mitral prostheses, hospitalization for intravenous heparin therapy and close monitoring of APTT until term may be advisable to minimize the risk of valve thrombosis. Because of the risk of fetal cerebral hemorrhage during vaginal delivery, patients who go into labor during treatment with oral anticoagulation should be scheduled for delivery by cesarean section.

Bacterial Endocarditis Prevention

Endocarditis occurs at some time in 3–6% of patients with prosthetic valves.[66] The risk of valve endocarditis is similar for mechanical and for bioprosthetic valves.[66,79] The mortality associated with the late form (> 60 days following valve replacement) may be as high as 20–40%.[80] Endocarditis prophylaxis was not recommended by the American Heart Association for either uncomplicated vaginal delivery, therapeutic abortion, or cesarean section. The recommendation states, however, that in patients with prosthetic valves, physicians may choose to administer antibiotic prophylaxis even for low risk procedures that involve the genitourinary tract. Because of the potential devastating effect of endocarditis, we strongly recommend antibiotic prophylaxis for vaginal as well as abdominal delivery. For recommended drug regimens for prophylaxis of infective endocarditis, see Chapter 16.

OUTCOME OF WOMEN IN THE CHILDBEARING AGE WITH PROSTHETIC HEART VALVES

Only limited information has been obtained on women in the childbearing age who have prosthetic heart valves. In addition, prognosis of individual patients may not be easily predictable based on group data. Jamieson et al[56] evaluated the outcome of 237 female patients 35 years of age or less who received 255 biological prostheses. The late mortality was 2.26%/patient-year. There were a total of 143 valve-related complications, the majority (43%) of which occurred at a rate of 6.0%/patient-year and included prosthetic valve endocarditis (5.9%) and thromboembolism (5.5%). Valve-related reoperation occurred in 42% of the cases, 8.3 ± 3.2 years after the original surgery, with an overall operative mortality of 6%. The freedom from valve-related mortality at 15 years was approximately 90%. In a recent report on late phase events after valve replacement with the St. Jude Medical prosthesis, Fernandez et al[81] reviewed the outcome of 1200 patients, 585 of whom were women, after valve replacement. The actuarial freedom from all valve-related events and valve-related death at 5 years was 74 and 94%, respectively. Causes of valve-related death included valve thrombosis, peripheral embolization, anticoagulation-related hemorrhage, prosthetic valve endocarditis, paravalvular leak; and sudden death. The outcome in young patients of childbearing age should be better than that reported by Fernandez et al, since higher age was a significant risk factor for late death. Other risk factors included lower preoperative ejection fraction, longer aortic cross-clamp and cardiopulmonary bypass time, previous cardiac operation, and higher preoperative functional class.

In an analysis of risk factors for primary tissue failure in 217 patients with porcine bioprostheses, a valve in the mitral position was found to be a significant predisposing factor.[82] Yamak et al[83] studied the late results of mitral valve replacement with the Carpentier–Edwards high profile bioprosthesis in young adults (mean age 36 ± 11 years); 102 (62.5%) were females. Freedom from structural deterioration was 92% for 5 years and 44% for 12 years. Actuarial survival rate was 87% for 5 years and 76% for 12 years. Scully and Armstrong[84] examined the results of tricuspid valve replacement in 60 patients who underwent 28 bioprosthetic and 32 mechanical tricuspid valve replacements between 1978 and 1993; 68% of the patients were female, and the mean age was 50 ± 15 years. Actuarial survival for hospital survivors was 50% at 15 years, and 10% of the patients required reoperation because of prosthetic failure. Long-term follow-up in young patients (mean age 18 years) following aortic valve replacement with mechanical valves (59%) or bioprostheses showed a survival of 84% at 10 years and repeat valve replacement in 18%.[85]

In summary, therefore, although information on long-term outcome specific for women with prosthetic valves in the childbearing age is not available, there is strong evidence for increased morbidity and mortality in patients with prosthetic valves in general in comparison to the normal population. The available data clearly indicate that women with prosthetic heart valves continue to be subject to an increased incidence of morbidity and decreased longevity even after delivery, a fact that may have an important effect on their ability to fulfill the tasks of motherhood.

REFERENCES

1. Dellsperger KC, Harrison EC. The patient with a prosthetic heart valve. In: Herr RD, Cydulka RK, eds. *Emergency Care of the Compromised Patient.* Philadelphia: JB Lippincott; 1994; 272–285.

2. Ben-Ismail M, Abid F, Trabelsi S, Taktak M, Fekih M. Cardiac valve prostheses, anticoagulation and pregnancy. *Br Heart J* 1986;55:101–105.

3. Iturbe-Alessio I, Del Carmen Fonseca M, Mutchinik O, Santos MA, Zajarias A, Salazar E. Risks of anticoagulant therapy in pregnant women with artificial heart valves. *N Engl J Med* 1986;315:1390–1393.

4. Lee PK, Wang RYC, Chow JSF, Cheung KL, Wong VCW, Chan TK. Combined use of warfarin and adjusted subcutaneous heparin during pregnancy in patients with an artificial heart valve. *J Am College Cardiol* 1986;8:221–224.

5. Pavankumar P, Venugopal P, Kaul U, Iyer KS, Das B, Sampathkumar A, Airon B, Rao IM, Sharma ML, Bhatia ML, et al. Pregnancy in patients with prosthetic cardiac valve. A 10-year experience. *Scand J Thorac Cardiovasc Surg* 1988;22:19–22.

6. Kadri T, Franken RA, Rivetti LA, Tedesco JJ, Suelotto RR, Santos RG. The porcine valve prosthesis and pregnancy. *Arq Bras Cardiol* 1989;52:327–331.

7. Sareli P, England MJ, Berk MR, Marcus RH, Epstein M, Driscoll J, Meyer T, McIntyre J, van Gelderen C. Maternal and fetal sequelae of anticoagulation during pregnancy in patients with mechanical heart valve prostheses. *Am J Cardiol* 1989;63: 1462–1465.

8. Badduke BR, Jamieson WR, Miyagishima RT, Munro AI, Gerein AN, MacNab J, Tyers GF. Pregnancy and childbearing

in a population with biologic valvular prostheses. *J Thorac Cardiovasc Surg* 1991;102:179–186.

9. Ayhan A, Yapar EG, Yuce K, Kisnisci HA, Nazli N, Ozmen F. Pregnancy and its complications after cardiac valve replacement. *Int J Gynaecol Obstet* 1991;35:117–122.

10. Cotrufo M, de Luca TS, Calabro R, Mastrogiovanni G, Lama D. Coumadin anticoagulation during pregnancy in patients with mechanical valve prostheses. *Eur J Cardiothorac Surg* 1991;5:300–304.

11. Born D, Martinez EE, Almeida PA, Santos DV, Carvalho AC, Moron AF, Miyasaki CH, Moraes SD, Ambrose JA. Pregnancy in patients with prosthetic heart valves: the effect of anticoagulation on mother, fetus and neonate. *Am Heart J* 1992;124:413–417.

12. Lecuru F, Taurelle R, Desnos M. Anticoagulant treatment and pregnancy. À propos of 47 cases. *Ann Cardiol Angiol* 1993;42:465–470.

13. Lee CN, Wu CC, Lin PY, Hsieh FJ, Chen HY. Pregnancy following cardiac prosthetic valve replacement. *Obstet Gynecol* 1994;83:353–356.

14. Sbarouni E, Oakley CM. Outcome of pregnancy in women with valve prostheses. *Br Heart J* 1993;71:196–201.

15. Hanania G, Thomas D, Michel PL, Garbarz E, Age C, Millaire J, Acar A. Grossesses chez les porteuses de prothèses valvulaires: étude coopérative retrospective française (155 cas). *Arch Mal Coeur* 1994;87:429–437.

16. Thomas D, Boubrit K, Darbois Y, Seebacher J, Seirafi D, Hanania G. Pregnancy in patients with heart valve prosthesis. Retrospective study à propos of 40 pregnancies. *Ann Cardiol Angiol* 1994;43:313–321.

17. Ross D. Replacement of the aortic valve with a pulmonary autograft: the "switch" operation. *Ann Thorac Surg* 1991;52:1246–1250.

18. Kouchoukos NT, Davila-Roman VG, Spray TL, Murphy SF, Perrillo JB. Replacement of the aortic root with a pulmonary autograft in children and young adults with aortic valve disease. *N Engl J Med* 1994;330:1–6.

19. Magilligan DJ. Advantages and disadvantages of tissue valves. In: Starek PJK, ed. *Heart Valve Replacement and Reconstruction.* Los Angeles: Year Book Medical Publishers; 1987; 237–245.

20. Starek PJK. Advantages and disadvantages of mechanical valves. In: Starek PJK, ed. *Heart Valve Replacement and Reconstruction.* Los Angeles: Year Book Medical Publishers; 1987;221–235.

21. Starr A, Grunkemeier GL. Selection of a prosthesis for aortic valve replacement. *Eur Heart J* 1988;9(suppl E):129–137.

22. Grunkemeier GL, Starr A, Rahimtoola SH. Prosthetic heart valve performance: long term follow-up. *Curr Probl Cardiol* 1992;17:331–406.

23. Khan S, Chaux A, Matloff J, Blanche C, DeRobertis M, Kass R, Tsai TP, Trento A, Nessim S, Gray R, Czer L. The St. Jude Medical valve: experience with 1,000 cases. *J Thorac Cardiovasc Surg* 1994;108:1010–1020.

24. Miller DC, Oyer PE, Stinson EB, Mitchell RS, Baldwin JC, Jamieson W, Shumway NE. Ten year clinical experience in 1651 patients with one type of tissue valve. In: Starek PJK, ed. *Heart Valve Replacement and Reconstruction.* Los Angeles: Year Book Medical Publishers; 1987;175–189.

25. Teoh KH, Ivanov J, Weisel RD, Darcel IC, Rakowski H. Survival and bioprosthetic valve failure: ten-year follow up. *Circulation* 1989;80:18–15.

26. Craver JM, Jones EI, McKeown P, Bone DK, Hatcher CR Jr, Kandrach M. Porcine cardiac xenograft valves: analysis of survival, valve failure and explanation. *Ann Thor Surg* 1982;34:16–21.

27. Jamieson WRE, Rosado LJ, Munro AI, Gerein AN, Burr LH, Miyagishima RT, Janusz MT, Tyers GF. Carpentier–Edwards standard porcine bioprosthesis: primary tissue failure (structural valve deterioration) by age groups. *Ann Thorac Surg* 1988;46:155–162.

28. Yacoub M, Ramsi NR, Sundt TM, Land O, Boyland E, Radley-Smith R, Khaghani A, Mitchell A. Fourteen-year experience with homovital homografts for aortic valve replacement. *J Thorac Cardiovasc Surg* 1995;110:186–193.

29. Cobanoglu A, Jamieson WRE, Miller DC, McKinley C, Grunkemeier GL, Floteu HS, Miyagishima RT, Tyers GF, Shumway NE, Starr A. A tri-institutional comparison of tissue and mechanical valves using a patient-oriented definition of "treatment failure." *Ann Thorac Surg* 1987;43:245–253.

30. Piehler J, Blackstone E, Bailey K, Bailey KR, Sullivan ME, Pluth JR, Weiss NS, Brookmeyer RS, Chandler JG. Reoperation on prosthetic heart valves: patient-specific estimates of in-hospital events. *J Thorac Cardiovasc Surg* 1995;109:30–48.

31. Casale PN, Devereux RB, Milner M, Zullo G, Harshfield GA, Pickering TG, Laragh JH. Value of echocardiographic measurement of left ventricular mass in predicting cardiovascular morbid events in hypertensive men. *Ann Intern Med* 1986;105:173–178.

32. Levy D, Garrison RJ, Savage DD, Kannel WB, Castelli WP. Prognostic implications of echocardiographically determined left ventricular mass in the Framingham heart study. *N Engl J Med* 1990;322:1561–1566.

33. Ghali JK, Liao Y, Simmons B, Castaner A, Cao G, Cooper RS. The prognostic role of left ventricular hypertrophy in patients with or without coronary artery disease. *Ann Intern Med* 1992;117:831–883.

34. Chaitman BR, Bonan R, Lepage G, Tubau JF, David PR, Dyrda IH, Grondin CM. Hemodynamic evaluation of the Carpentier–Edwards porcine xenograft. *Circulation* 1979;60:1170–1182.

35. Yoganathan AP, Chaux A, Gray RJ, Gray RJ, Woo YR, DeRobertis M, Williams FP, Matloff JM. Bileaflet, tilting disc and porcine aortic valve substitutes: in vitro hydrodynamic characteristics. *J Am College Cardiol* 1984;3:313–320.

36. Tindale WB, Black MM, Martin TRP. In vitro evaluation of prosthetic heart valves: anomalies and limitations. *Clin Phys Physiol Meas* 1982;3:115–130.

37. Gabbay S, McQueen DM, Yellin EL, Frater RWM. In vitro hydrodynamic comparison of mitral valve prostheses at high flow rates. *J Thorac Cardiovasc Surg* 1978;76:771–787.

38. Woo Y, Williams FP, Yoganathan AP. Steady and pulsatile flow

studies on a trileaflet heart valve prosthesis. *Scand J Thorac Cardiovasc Surg* 1983;17:227–236.

39. Khan S, Mitchell RS, Derby GC, Oyer PE, Miller DC. Differences in aortic Hancock and Carpentier–Edwards hemodynamics: effect of valve size. *Circulation* 1989;80:II-560. Abstract.

40. Craver JM, Spencer BK, Douglas JS, Franch RH, Jones, EL, Morris DC, Kopchak J, Hatcher, CR Jr. Hancock modified orifice aortic bioprosthesis. *Circulation* 1979;60:II93–97.

41. Jones EL, Craver JM, Morris DC, King SB, Douglas JS, Franch RH, Hatcher CR, Morgan EA. Hemodynamic and clinical evaluation of the Hancock xenograft bioprosthesis for aortic valve replacement (with emphasis on management of the small aortic root). *J Thorac Cardiovasc Surg* 1978;75:300–308.

42. Horstkotte D, Loogen F, Bircks W. Is the late outcome of heart valve replacement influenced by the hemodynamics of the heart valve substitute? In: Horstkotte D, Dieter F, eds. *Update in Heart Valve Replacement: Proceedings of the Second European Symposium on St. Jude Medical Heart Valves.* New York: Springer-Verlag; 1986.

43. Worthan DC, Tri TB, Bowen TE. Hemodynamic evaluation of the St. Jude Medical valve prosthesis in the small aortic annulus. *J Thorac Cardiovasc Surg* 1981;81:615–620.

44. Bove EL, Marvasti MA, Potts JL, Reger MJ, Zamara JL, Eich RH, Parker FB Jr. Rest and exercise hemodynamics following aortic valve replacement. *J Thorac Cardiovasc Surg* 1985;90:750–755.

45. Donaldson RM, Ross DM. Homograft aortic root replacement for complicated prosthetic valve endocarditis. *Circulation* 1984;70:I178–181.

46. Yoganathan AP, Woo YR, Sung HW, Williams FP, Franch RH, Jones M. In vitro hemodynamic characteristics of tissue bioprostheses in the aortic position. *J Thorac Cardiovasc Surg* 1986;92:198–209.

47. Gabbay S, Frater RWM. In vitro comparison of the newer heart valve bioprostheses in the mitral and aortic positions. In: Cohn LH, Gullucci V, eds. *Cardiac Bioprostheses.* New York: Yorke Medical Books; 1982;456–468.

48. Cosgrove DM, Lytle BW, Gill CC, Golding LR, Stewart RW, Taylor PC, Loop FD. In vivo hemodynamic comparison of porcine and pericardial valves. *J Thorac Cardiovasc Surg* 1985;89:358–368.

49. Cohn LH, Allred EN, DiSesa VJ, Cohu LA, Austin JC, Sabik J, Shemin RJ, Collins JJ Jr. Early and late risk of aortic valve replacement: a 12-year concomitant comparison of the porcine bioprosthetic and tilting disc prosthetic aortic valves. *J Thorac Cardiovasc Surg* 1984;88:695–705.

50. Hammermeister KE, Henderson WG, Burchfiel CM, Sethi GK, Souchek J, Oprian C, Cantor AB, Folland E, Khuri S, Rahimtoola S. Comparison of outcome after valve replacement with a bioprosthesis versus a mechanical prosthesis: initial 5 year results of a randomized trial. *J Am College Cardiol* 1987;10: 719–732.

51. Bloomfield P, Kitchin AH, Wheatley DJ, Walbaum PR, Lutz W, Miller HC. A prospective evaluation of the Bjork–Shiley, Hancock and Carpentier–Edwards heart valve prostheses. *Circulation* 1986;73:1213–1222.

52. Cannegieter SC, Rosendaal FR, Briet E. Thromboembolic and bleeding complications in patients with mechanical heart valve prostheses. *Circulation* 1994;89:635–641.

53. Landefeld CS, Rosenblatt MW, Goldman L. Bleeding in outpatients treated with warfarin: relation to the prothrombin time and important remediable lesions. *Am J Med* 1989;87:153–159.

54. Landefeld CS, Goldman L. Major bleeding in outpatients treated with warfarin: incidence and prediction by factors known at the start of outpatient therapy. *Am J Med* 1989;87:144–152.

55. Salazar E, Izaguirre R, Verdejo J, Mutchinick O. Failure of adjusted doses of subcutaneous heparin to prevent thromboembolic phenomena in pregnant patients with mechanical cardiac valve prostheses. *J Am College Cardiol* 1996;27:1698–1703.

56. Jamieson WRE, Miller DC, Akins CW, Munro AI, Glower DD, Moore KA, Henderson C. Pregnancy and bioprostheses: influence on structural valve deterioration. *Ann Thorac Surg* 1995;60:S282–287.

57. Caruso A, deCarolis S, Ferrazzani S, Paradisi G, Pomini F, Pompei A. Pregnancy outcome in women with cardiac valve prosthesis. *Eur J Obstet Gynecol Reprod Biol* 1994;54:7–11.

58. Barbour LA, Pickard J. Controversies in thromboembolic disease during pregnancy: a critical review. *Obstet Gynecol* 1995;86:621–633.

59. Wong V, Cheng CH, Chan KC. Fetal and neonatal outcome of exposure to anticoagulants during pregnancy. *Am J Med Genet* 1993;45:17–21.

60. Ginsberg JS, Kowalchuk G, Hirsh J, Brill-Edwards P, Burrows R. Heparin therapy during pregnancy. *Arch Intern Med* 1989;149:2233–2236.

61. Kontos GJ, Schaff HV, Orszulak TA, Puga FJ, Pluth JR Danielson GK. Thrombotic obstruction of disc valves: clinical recognition and surgical management. *Ann Thorac Surg* 1989;48:60–65.

62. Ledain LD, Ohayon JP, Colle JP, Lorient-Roudaut FM, Foudaut RP, Besse PM. Acute thrombotic obstruction with disc valve prostheses: diagnostic considerations and fibrinolytic treatment. *J Am College Cardiol* 1986;7:743–751.

63. Czer LS, Weiss M, Bateman TM, Plaff JM, DeRobertis M, Eigler N, Vas R, Matloff JM, Gray RJ. Fibrinolytic therapy of St. Jude valve thrombosis under guidance of digital cineflouroscopy. *J Am College Cardiol* 1985;5:1244–1249.

64. Silber H, Khan SS, Matloff JM, Chaux A, DeRobertis M, Gray R. The St. Jude valve: thrombolysis as the first line of therapy for cardiac valve thrombosis. *Circulation* 1993;87:30–37.

65. Gueret P, Vignon P, Fournier P, Chabernaud JM, Gomez M, LaCroix P, Bensaid J. Transesophageal echocardiography for the diagnosis and management of nonobstructive thrombosis of mechanical mitral valve prosthesis. *Circulation* 1995;91: 103–110.

66. Vongpatanasin W, Hills LD, Lange RA. Prosthetic heart valves. *N Engl J Med* 1996;335:407–416.

67. Vasan R, Kaul U, Sanghvi S, Kamlakar T, Negi PC, Shrivastava S, Rajani M, Venugopal P, Wasir HS. Thrombolytic therapy for prosthetic valve thrombosis: a study based on serial Doppler echocardiographic evaluation. *Am Heart J* 1992;123:1575–1580.

68. Turrentine MA, Braems G, Ramirez MM. Use of thrombolytics for the treatment of thromboembolic disease during pregnancy. *Obstet Gynecol Survey* 1995;50:534–541.

69. Ramamurthy S, Talwar KK, Saxena A, Juneja R, Takkar D. Prosthetic mitral valve thrombosis in pregnancy successfully treated with streptokinase. *Am Heart J* 1994;127:446–448.

70. Ad Hoc Committee of the Working Group on Valvular Heart Disease, European Society of Cardiology. Guidelines for prevention of thromboembolic events in valvular heart disease. *J Heart Valve Dis* 1993;2:398–410.

71. Elkayam U. Anticoagulation in pregnant women with prosthetic heart valve: a double jeopardy. *J Am College Cardiol* 1996;27:1704–1706.

72. Ginsberg JS, Barron WM. Pregnancy and prosthetic heart valves. *Lancet* 1994;334:1170–1172.

73. Floyd RC, Gookin KS, Hess LW, Martin RW, Rawlinson KF, Moenning RK, Morrison JC. Administration of heparin by subcutaneous infusion with a programmable pump. *Am J Obstet Gynecol* 1991;165:931–933.

74. Cannegieter SC, Rosendaal FR, Wintzen AR, Van der Meer FJ, Vandenbroucke JP, Briet E. Optimal oral anticoagulant therapy in patients with mechanical heart valves. *N Engl J Med* 1995;333:11–17.

75. Stein PD, Alpert JS, Copeland J, Dalen JE, Goldman S, Turpie AGG. Antithrombotic therapy in patients with mechanical and biological prosthetic heart valves. *Chest* 1995;108:371S–379S.

76. Heras M, Chesebro JH, Fuster V, Penny WJ, Grill DE, Bailey KR, Danielson GK, Orszulak TA, Pluth JR, Puga RJ, Schaff HV, Larsonkeller JJ. High risk of early thromboemboli after bioprosthetic cardiac valve replacement. *J Am College Cardiol* 1995;25:1111–1119.

77. Ginsberg JS, Hirsh J. Use of antithrombotic agents during pregnancy. *Chest* 1995;108:305S–311S.

77. Turpie AG, Gent M, Laupacis A, Latour Y, Gunstenesen J, Basile F, Klimex M, Hirsh J. A comparison of aspirin with placebo in patients treated with warfarin after heart-valve replacement. *N Engl J Med* 1993;329:524–529.

78. Nelson-Piercy C. Low molecular weight heparin for obstetric thromboprophylaxis. *Br J Obstet Gynaecol* 1994;101:6–8.

79. Grover FL, Cohen DJ, Opian C, Henderson WG, Sethi G, Hammermeister KE. Determinations of the occurrence of and survival from prosthetic valve endocarditis: experience of the Veterans Affairs Cooperative Study on valvular heart disease. *J Thorac Cardiovasc Surg* 1994;108:207–214.

80. Thomas P, Sanz E, Permanyer-Miralda G, Almirante B, Planes AM, Soler-Soler J. Late prosthetic valve endocarditis: immediate and long-term prognosis. *Chest* 1992;101:37–41.

81. Fernandez J, Laub GW, Adkins MS, Anderson WA, Chen C, Bailey BM, Nealon LM, McGrath LB. Early and late-phase events after valve replacement with the St. Jude Medical prosthesis in 1200 patients. *J Thorac Cardiovasc Surg* 1994;107: 394–406.

82. Pansini S, Ottino G, Caimmi F, Del Ponte S, Morea M. Risk factors of primary tissue failure within the 11th postoperative year in 217 patients with porcine bioprostheses. *J Card Surg* 1991;6:644–648.

83. Yamak B, Sener E, Kiziltepe U, Mavitas B, Tasdemir O, Bayazit K. Late results of mitral valve replacement with Carpentier–Edwards high profile bioprosthesis in young adults. *Eur J Cardiothorac Surg* 1995;9:335–341.

84. Scully HE, Armstrong CS. Tricuspid valve replacement: fifteen years of experience with mechanical prostheses and bioprostheses. *J Thorac Cardiovasc Surg* 1995;109:1035–1041.

85. Moodie DS, Hanhan U, Sterba R, Murphy DJ Jr, Rosenkranz ER, Kovasc AM. Aortic valve replacement in young patients: long-term follow-up. *Cleveland Clin J Med* 1992;59:473–478.

7

MYOCARDITIS AND PREGNANCY

Avraham Shotan, md, Syed W. H. Bokhari, md, and Uri Elkayam, md

INTRODUCTION

Myocarditis is a focal or diffuse inflammatory process involving the heart muscle. It may be caused by virtually any bacterial, viral, rickettsial, mycotic, or parasitic organism and can also result from several noninfectious processes.[1,2] Viral infection appears to be the most common cause of myocarditis in North America and Europe, with Coxsackie B accounting for nearly 50 percent of all cases[3] and Coxsackie A and echo and polio viruses accounting for most of the remainder. Influenza A and B, rubella, mumps, cytomegalic, rabies, herpes simplex, herpes zoster, varicella, Epstein–Barr, yellow fever, and adenovirus may also cause the disease.[1,2] In animals, there is an initial phase of active viral replication in the heart and direct myocardial damage modified by the humoral immune system. The virus is then cleared by the monocyte–macrophase system followed by a T-cell-mediated cytotoxic reaction, probably in response to antigenic alterations in the myocardium.[4,5] Recent reports have demonstrated the association of myocarditis with acquired immune deficiency syndrome (AIDS) due to opportunistic infections by a variety of organisms, metastatic involvement by Kaposi's sarcoma, or the human immunodeficiency virus (HIV) itself.[6,7] Bacterial myocarditis is uncommon and is usually a complication of bacterial endocarditis.[1] In certain regions of Central America and South America, Chagas' disease, which is caused by *Trypanosoma cruzi,* is the most common cause of acute or chronic myocarditis.[8]

Although any of the above-mentioned causes may produce myocardial inflammation during pregnancy, only a few cases of myocarditis have been reported to occur in pregnancy. In an early review by Sainani et al[9] 4 patients out of 22 patients with viral myocarditis had it in the postpartum period. Grimes and Cates[10] noted a unique myocarditis associated with abortion in four cases; all of them ended fatally within several days of the procedure, and there was autopsy evidence of myocardial inflammation. Gehrke et al[11] reported a case of a 28-year-old asthmatic female who developed acute heart failure accompanied by diarrhea, fever, and hypereosinophilia in the blood in the postpartum period. During steroid treatment, cytomegalovirus-associated myocarditis developed. Chen et al[12] reported a patient with a history of repeated episodes of acute myocarditis who developed congestive heart failure at the 36th week of gestation with rapid deterioration and death.

Several reports have demonstrated a relatively high incidence of histological evidence for myocarditis in patients with peripartum cardiomyopathy.[13–19] These findings have led to the suggestion that myocarditis may be an important etiological factor in patients with peripartum cardiomyopathy.[19] The incidence of active myocardial inflammation in this patient population, however, has varied significantly among different reports. Although some investigators[15,19] reported finding myocarditis in the majority of patients with peripartum cardiomyopathy, other investigators failed to find myocarditis in most of their cases. In the most recent report, Rizeq et al[17] from Stanford University reported a low incidence (9%) of myocarditis in 34 patients with peripartum cardiomyopathy. This incidence was comparable to that found in age- and sex-matched control population undergoing transplantation for idiopathic dilated cardiomyopathy. These results, therefore, do not support the etiological role of myocarditis in patients with peripartum cardiomyopathy. Because of the inconsistent reports, additional data, collected in

Cardiac Problems in Pregnancy, Third Edition
Edited by Uri Elkayam, MD, and Norbert Gleicher, MD
Copyright © 1998 by Wiley-Liss, Inc. ISBN 0-471-16358-9

a systematic, prospective fashion, are needed to further investigate the relationship between acute myocarditis and peripartum cardiomyopathy.

CLINICAL FEATURES

In spite of the variety of the etiological factors in most of the cases, the clinical manifestations of myocarditis are not specific. They may vary with the extent and location of the inflammatory process in the myocardium and the associated systemic illness. Myocarditis may be clinically silent and has been reported as an incidental finding in 0.11–7% of autopsies.[2,20] Sometimes electrocardiographic or chest film abnormalities are detected during a routine evaluation in an infectious disease. The disease often presents initially as a systemic illness with viral symptomatology, such as fever, sore throat, cough, arthralgia, myalgia, abdominal pain, nausea, vomiting, diarrhea, and skin rash. Cardiac manifestations usually become apparent only a few days to a few weeks later and are usually manifested as fatigue, decreased exercise tolerance, dyspnea, palpitations, and, occasionally, precordial discomfort. Pleuropericardial chest pain may occur as a result of associated pericarditis. Focal myocarditis may present with localized electrocardiographic changes and wall motion abnormalities and can mimic acute myocardial infarction.[21] Hemodynamic instability and even circulatory collapse may result secondary to severe left and/or right ventricular dysfunction, a high degree atrioventricular block, ventricular arrhythmias, or associated cardiac tamponade. Myocarditis may result in unexpected sudden death, presumably due to fatal tachyarrhythmia or complete atrioventricular block. Systemic and pulmonary emboli have been reported in myocarditis and may be the presenting feature.[3]

Changes in physical examination will depend on the severity of the disease, and while no abnormal findings can be found in mild cases, persistent fever and excessive tachycardia, both at rest and during exercise, are common. Tachycardia is often disproportionate to the degree of fever. Hypotension is not infrequent, with a narrow pulse pressure. Clinical findings of congestive heart failure with mitral and tricuspid regurgitation may occur in the more severe cases. A pericardial friction rub may be audible in patients with associated pericarditis. In patients with severe cardiac involvement, dilatation of cardiac chambers will result in a diffuse and displaced point of maximal impulse and right ventricular heave. A muffled first heart sound, a third heart sound, and murmurs due to mitral and tricuspid regurgitation can be heard. Neck veins may be distended in patients with heart failure, pericardial effusion, or both. Auscultation of the lungs can reveal bilateral rales. Hepatomegaly and peripheral edema are common in patients with congestive heart failure.

LABORATORY TESTS

Electrocardiogram

In the acute stage, the electrocardiogram is always abnormal, demonstrating ST-segment elevation with inversion or flattening of the T wave.[2,3,21] The Q-T interval may be prolonged. The ST-segment changes usually return to baseline in a few days, while the T-wave changes may persist for several weeks or months. Abnormal Q waves that sometimes develop may mimic acute myocardial infarction. These changes can be diffuse or segmental. Ventricular premature beats are commonly seen, and atrial and ventricular tachyarrhythmias are present in about one-third of the patients. Atrioventricular conduction disturbances of varying degrees and bundle branch block are quite common and usually transient, although permanent complete atrioventricular block has been reported.

Chest X-Ray

Chest roentgenogram may show cardiac enlargement due to chamber dilatation, pericardial effusion, or both. Additional findings may include pulmonary venous congestion, interstitial and even alveolar edema, mild atrial enlargement, prominence of superior vena cava or azygous vein, patchy pulmonary infiltrates, and pleural effusion.

Laboratory Data

The erythrocyte sedimentation rate is elevated in about 70% of the cases and not infrequently exceeds 80 mm/h. White blood cell count may be slightly to moderately elevated, with a neutrophil response in about half of the patients. Eosinophilia may indicate an underlying parasitic etiology. Myocardial necrosis usually results in an increase in cardiac enzymes: creatine phosphokinase (CPK) and its MB isoenzyme, lactic dehydrogenase (LDH), and glutamic oxaloacetic transaminase (GOT).[2,22]

Virus isolation from stool, pharyngeal washings, or other body fluids is usually possible during the first few days of the illness.[2] Recent viral infection may be diagnosed in the acute and convalescent (2–6 weeks after illness) phases of the illness by a fourfold or greater rise in virus antibody titers. Antibodies are usually not found until about 1 week after the onset of the illness. The immunoglobulin class may help in determining the duration of the disease process, since IgM antibody levels peak in 2–3 weeks and are later undetectable, and IgG antibody levels peak later and may remain elevated for months or years. Newer radioimmunoassay and enzyme-linked immunosorbent assay (ELISA) techniques are useful in rapid identification, and polyvalent reagents can be used. Recombinant DNA technology, particularly the polymerase chain reaction method of gene amplification, has allowed characterization of the viral genome and the development of techniques to identify its presence in the myocardial tissue.[23,24]

Echocardiography

An echocardiogram helps in evaluating chamber size, as well as global and regional function, which may vary from normal to substantial enlargement with focal or diffused hypokinesia.[21,23,24] Transient asymmetric septal hypertrophy and transient wall thickening may result, presumably from inhomogeneous edematous inflammation. Mural thrombi are not infrequently found.[23,24] Use of the Doppler technique enables the detection and assessment of the severity of the mitral and tricuspid valves' regurgitation. Pinamonti et al,[25] who studied echocardiographically 41 patients with histologically proven myocarditis, found asynergic ventricular areas in 64%, reversible left ventricular hypertrophy in 20%, ventricular thrombi in 15%, and right ventricular dysfunction in 23% of patients. Tissue characterization showed increased contrast and brightness, with 84% sensitivity and 87% specificity.[26]

Nuclear Imaging

Radionuclide ventriculography may reveal biventricular global dysfunction and enlargement, or regional hypokinesis or dyskinesis, especially at the apex.[11] Myocardial imaging with technetium-99 pyrophosphate,[27] gallium-67 citrate,[28] or indium-111-labeled leukocytes[29] scans may show uptake as evidence of diffuse or focal myocardial inflammation or necrosis. The clinical usage of these procedures in pregnancy is limited due to expected radiation to the fetus (see Chapter 3).

Endomyocardial Biopsy

During the last decade, endomyocardial biopsy has become the "gold standard" for the diagnosis of myocarditis. The established Dallas criteria[30] for the histological diagnosis of myocarditis include findings of inflammatory infiltrate associated with adjacent myocyte necrosis or degeneration (Fig. 7.1). It should be noted that although positive results have diagnostic value, negative results do not rule out myocarditis. In severe cases in which a definite diagnosis has therapeutic implications, a repeat endomyocardial biopsy may be indicated.[31,32]

The ability to perform endomyocardial biopsy during pregnancy is somewhat limited by the need to use fluoroscopy and, therefore, ionizing radiation. In such cases, the procedure can be done by trained individuals under echocardiographic guidance (Fig. 7.2).[33]

Using immunofluorescent methods or viral isolation from a culture of biopsy specimens may be complementary to histopathology in the diagnosis of myocarditis.[34,35] However, the yield of these techniques is relatively low. Because there is a significant homology among enteroviruses, the use of cDNA viral probes has been effective in detecting the presence of the virus in myocardial tissue.[36] Gene amplification by the polymerase chain reaction, which enables the accurate

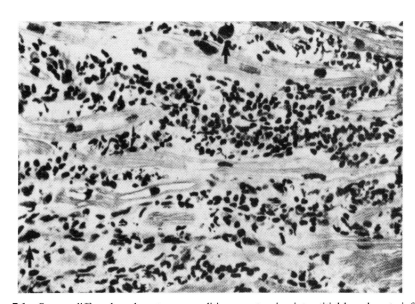

Figure 7.1 Severe diffuse lymphocyte myocarditis: an extensive interstitial lymphocyte infiltrate and myocyte necrosis (arrow) is readily seen; no fibrosis is present. (Stain, Hematoxylin and eosin; magnification, × 350.) (Reproduced from Aretz et al,[30] with permission.)

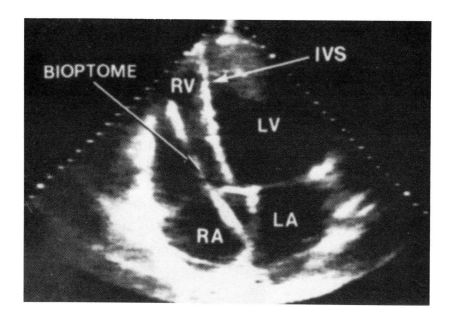

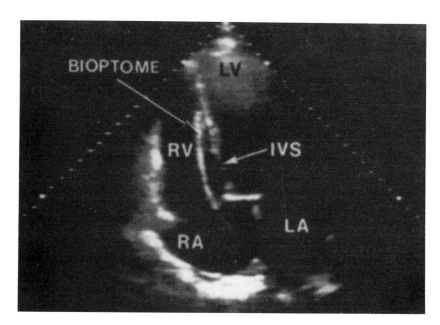

Figure 7.2 Echocardiogram showing the apical four-chamber view of the heart and demonstrating the guidance of the bioptome (black and white arrow) with samples being obtained at (a) the right ventricular (RV) free wall and (b) the interventricular septum (IVS). (From Miller et al,[33] with permission.)

reproduction of large quantities of DNA, has markedly increased our ability to detect viral genome in myocardial biopsy samples from patients with myocarditis.[23,37,38]

TREATMENT

All pregnant women with suspected myocarditis should be hospitalized. Patients with hemodynamic instability, heart failure, significant pericardial effusion at risk of tamponade, and serious arrhythmias should be adequately monitored in an intensive cardiac care unit. Therapy is often mainly supportive and includes rest and adequate oxygenation. Strenuous activity may be deleterious and should be prohibited until the electrocardiogram returns to normal. Congestive heart failure should be treated with diuretics, digoxin, and other vasodilators. Early administration of angiotensin-converting enzyme (ACE) inhibitors produced striking improvements in histologic end points and survival in murine models of myocarditis. Captopril administered 1 or 4 days after infection had consistently and significantly improved myocardial inflammation and necrosis, as well as reduction of heart-to-body weight ratio. When captopril was given 10 days postinoculation, the histologic benefit was undetectable, but the reduction in the ratio of heart to body weight was still apparent[39,40] because of potential severe side effects to the fetus the use of ACE inhibitors in pregnancy is contraindicated (Chapter 32). Patients in cardiogenic shock are treated with intravenous inotropic agents and intraaortic counterpulsation. Temporary circulatory support and cardiac transplantation may be used for end-stage heart failure. Important arrhythmias should be treated with lidocaine, quinidine, or procainamide, which are relatively safe in gestation (see Chapter 30).[41] Temporary pacing should be used for high degree atrioventricular block. This conduction disturbance is transient in the majority of patients with myocarditis, and permanent pacemaker is usually not indicated. Anticoagulation may be added, to reduce the risk of emboli, especially for patients with severe left ventricular dysfunction.

The administration of corticosteroids with or without immunosuppressive drugs is controversial. During the acute tissue invasive stage, immunosuppressive agents may provoke viral replication. Animal studies have shown that corticosteroid administration prolonged viremia, caused persistence of virus in different organs, and aggravated the severity of myocarditis. However, the majority of patients with myocarditis present at the postinvasive stage, when inflammation is due to immune response toward the altered myocardial antigenicity.[2] Although several reports have demonstrated marked improvement following immunosuppression and relapses after discontinuation of the therapy and the resemblance of the inflammatory process to transplant rejection,[41,42] comprehensive review of the literature reveals conflicting reports and insufficient evidence for the role of immunosuppression in patients with myocarditis.[43–52] An overview of 15 uncontrolled small populations (4–34 patients) with a total of 183 patients showed that overall efficacy of corticosteroids was 64% (0–100%).[43–45] In addition to corticosteroids, patients with histologic evidence of myocarditis were treated with a wide range of immunosuppressive agents, including azathioprine, cyclosporin, γ-globulin, antithymocyte globulin, and the anti-CD3 monoclonal antibody OKT3.[46–48] The average rate of improvement was 54%.[49] However, several small groups of patients treated without immunosuppression showed a comparable clinical spontaneous improvement of 48%.[50] The recently published Myocarditis Treatment Trial[51] randomized 111 patients with left ventricular dysfunction and biopsy-proven myocarditis to receive either conventional therapy (47 patients) or an additional immunosuppressive therapy (64 patients): azathioprine and prednisone (18 patients) or cyclosporin and prednisone (46 patients). The immunosuppressive treatment was

administered for 6 months. Mean ejection fraction at one year and actuarial survival curves did not differ significantly between the two groups. Ejection fraction (EF) increased by more than 5% in 76% of the immunosuppressive group versus 53% of the control group. The authors conclude that the sample size may be too small to exclude a survival benefit of immunosuppressive therapy.[51,52]

The mechanisms of immune-mediated myocardial injury vary depending on the genetic makeup of the individual and the strain of the inducing virus, and therefore the response to different immunosuppressive agents varies. Currently, the therapy of myocarditis is mainly supportive, and immunosuppressive therapy is not indicated in most patients.

REFERENCES

1. Wynne J, Braunwald E. The cardiomyopathies and myocarditis. In: Braunwald E, editor, Heart Disease, 5th edition Philadelphia: W. B. Saunders; 1997; 1404.

2. Ensley RD, Renlund DG, Mason JW. Myocarditis. In: Willerson JT, Cohn JN, eds. *Cardiovascular Medicine.* 1st ed. New York: Churchill Livingstone; 1995;894.

3. Reyes MP, Lerner AM. Coxsackievirus myocarditis—with special reference to acute and chronic effects. *Prog Cardiovasc Dis* 1985;27:373–394.

4. Woodruff JF. Viral myocarditis: a review. *Am J Pathol* 1980; 101:425–484.

5. Maze SS, Adolf RJ. Myocarditis: unresolved issues in diagnosis and treatment. *Clin Cardiol* 1990;13:69–79.

6. Cohen IS, Anderson DW, Virmani R, Reen BM, Macher AM, Sennesh J, Di Lorenzo P, Redfield RR. Congestive cardiomyopathy in association with the acquired immunodeficiency syndrome. *N Engl J Med* 1986;35:628–630.

7. Baroldi G, Corallo S, Moroni M, Repossini A, Mutinelli MR, Lazzarin A, Antonacci CM, Cristina S, Negri C. Focal lymphocytic myocarditis in acquired immunodeficiency syndrome (AIDS): a correlative morphologic and clinical study in 26 consecutive fatal cases. *J Am College Cardiol* 1988;12:463–469.

8. Acosta AM, Santos-Buch CA. Autoimmune myocarditis induced by *Trypanosoma cruzi. Circulation* 1985;71:1255–1261.

9. Sainani G, Krompotic E, Slodki S. Adult heart disease due to coxsackievirus B infection. *Medicine* 1968;47:133–147.

10. Grimes DA, Cates W Jr. Fatal myocarditis associated with abortion in early pregnancy. *South Med J* 1980;73:236–238.

11. Gehrke D, Herzum M, Schonian U, Klein HH, Drude L, Mennel HD, Maisch B. Eosinophilic endomyocarditis postpartum or pregnancy related cardiomyopathy. *Herz* 1994;19:176–181.

12. Chen HF, Lee CN, Huang GD, Hsieh FJ, Huang SC, Chen HY. Delayed maternal death after perimortem cesarean section. *Acta Obstet Gynecol Scand* 1994;73:839–841.

13. Melvin KR, Richardson PJ, Olsen EGJ, Daly K, Jackson G. Peripartum cardiomyopathy due to myocarditis. *N Engl J Med* 1982;307:731–734.

14. O'Connell JB, Costanzo-Nordin MR, Subramanian R, Robinson JA, Wallis DE, Scanlon PJ, Gunnar RM. Peripartum car-

diomyopathy: clinical, hemodynamic, histologic and prognostic characteristics. *J Am College Cardiol* 1986;8:52–56.

15. Costanzo-Nordin MR, O'Connell JB. Peripartum cardiomyopathy in the 1980's: etiologic and prognostic considerations and review of the literature. *Prog Cardiol* 1989;212:225.

16. Hershkowitz A, Campbell S, Decker S, Kasper EK, Boehmer J, Hadian D, Neumann DA, Baughman KL. Demographic features and prevalence of idiopathic myocarditis in patients undergoing endomyocardial biopsy. *Am J Cardiol* 1993;71:982–986.

17. Rizeq MN, Rickenbacher PR, Fowler MB, Billingham ME. Incidence of myocarditis in peripartum cardiomyopathy. *Am J Cardiol* 1994;74:474.

18. Carvalho A, Brandao, Martinez EE, Alexopolous D, Lima VC, Andrade JL, Ambrose JA. Prognosis in peripartum cardiomyopathy. *Am J Cardiol* 1989;64:540–542.

19. Midei MG, DeMent SH, Feldman AM, Hutchins GM, Baughman KL. Peripartum myocarditis and cardiomyopathy. *Circulation* 1990;81:992–998.

20. Okada R, Wakafuji S. Myocarditis in autopsy. In Sekiguchi M, Olsen EGJ, Goodwin JF, eds. Myocarditis and related disorders. Berlin: Springer-Verlag; 1985;1:23–29.

21. Chandraratna PAN, Nimalsuriya A, Reid CL, Cohn S, Rahimtoola SH. Left ventricular asynergy in acute myocarditis. *JAMA* 1983;250:1428–1430.

22. Myocarditis Treatment Trial (MTT) investigators. Incidence and clinical characteristics of myocarditis. *Circulation* 1991;84(suppl II):II-2:0007.

23. Nieminen MS, Heikkila J, Karjalainen J. Echocardiography in acute infectious myocarditis: relation to clinical and electrocardiographic findings. *Am J Cardiol* 1984;53:1331–1337.

24. Weinhouse E, Wanderman KL, Sofer S, Gussarsky Y, Gueron M. Viral myocarditis simulating dilated cardiomyopathy in early childhood: evaluation by serial echocardiography. *Br Heart J* 1986;56:94–97.

25. Pinamonti B, Alberti E, Cigalotto A, Dreas L, Salvi A, Silvestri F, Camerini F. Echocardiographic findings in myocarditis. *Am J Cardiol* 1988;62:285–291.

26. Lieback E, Meyer R, Nawrock M, Hetzer R. The clinical value of ultrasonic tissue characterization in the diagnosis of myocarditis. *Circulation* 1991:84(suppl II):II-372.

27. Mitsutake A, Nakamura M, Inou T, Kikuchi Y, Takeshita A, Fujini S. Intense, persistent myocardial avid technetium-99 pyrophosphate scintigraphy in acute myocarditis. *Am Heart J* 1981;101:683–684.

28. O'Connell JB, Henkin RE, Robinson JA, Subramanian R, Scanlon PJ, Gunnar RM. Gallium-67 imaging in patients with dilated cardiomyopathy and biopsy-proven myocarditis. *Circulation* 1984;70:58–62.

29. Yasuda T, Palacios IF, Dec GW, Fallon JT, Gold HK, Leinbach RC, Strauss HW, Khaw BA, Haber E. Indium-111 monoclonal antimyosin antibody imaging in the diagnosis of acute myocarditis. *Circulation* 1987;76:306–311.

30. Aretz HT, Billingham ME, Edwards WE, Factor SM, Fallon JT, Olsen EG, Fenoglio JJ Jr, Schoen FJ. Myocarditis: a histopatho-

logic definition and classification. *Am J Cardiovasc Pathol* 1987;1:3–14.

31. Dec GW, Fallon JT, Southern JF, Palacios I. "Borderline" myocarditis: an indication for repeat endomyocardial biopsy. *J Am College Cardiol* 1990;15:283–289.

32. Factor SM. Borderline myocarditis on initial endomyocardial biopsy: no man's land no more? *J Am College Cardiol* 1990;15:290–291.

33. Miller LW, Labovitz AJ, McBride LA, Pennington DG, Kanter K. Echocardiographic-guided endomyocardial biopsy. A 5-year experience. *Circulation* 1988;78(suppl III):99–102.

34. Hammond EH, Menlove RL, Anderson JL. Predictive value of immunofluorescence and electron microscopic evaluation of endomyocardial biopsies in the diagnosis and prognosis of myocarditis and idiopathic dilated cardiomyopathy. *Am Heart J* 1987;114:1055–1065.

35. Daly K, Richardson PJ, Olsen EG, Morgan Capner P, McSorley C, Jackson G, Jewitt DE. Acute myocarditis: role of histological and virological examination in the diagnosis and assessment of immunosuppressive treatment. *Br Heart J* 1984;51:30–35.

36. Kandolf R, Ameis D, Kirschner P, Cann A, Hofschneider PH. In situ detection of enteroviral genomes in myocardial cells by nucleic acid hybridization: an approach to the diagnosis of viral heart disease. *Proc Natl Acad Sci USA* 1987;84:6272–6276.

37. Jin O, Sole MJ, Butany JW, Chia WK, McLaughlin PR, Lui P, Liew CC. Detection of enterovirus RNA in myocardial biopsies from patients with myocarditis and cardiomyopathy using gene amplification by polymerase chain reaction. *Circulation* 1990;82:8–16.

38. Elstein E, Sole MJ. Frontiers in the diagnosis of viral myocarditis. *Heart Failure* 1992;8:16–23.

39. Rezkalla S, Kloner RA, Khatib G, Khatib R. Beneficial effects of captopril in acute coxsackievirus B_3 murine myocarditis. *Circulation* 1990;81:1039–1046.

40. Suziki H, Matsumori A. Myocardial injury due to viral myocarditis improved by captopril in mice. *Circulation* 1990;82(suppl III):III-674.

41. Mason JW, Billingham ME, Ricci DR. Treatment of acute inflammatory myocarditis assisted by endomyocardial biopsy. *Am J Cardiol* 1980;45:1037–1044.

42. Garrison RF, Swisher RC. Myocarditis of unknown etiology (Fiedler's) treated with ACTH. *J Pediatr* 1953;42:591–599.

43. Mason JW, O'Connell JB. A model of myocarditis in humans. *Circulation* 1990;81:1154–1156.

44. Liu P, McLaughlin PR, Sole MJ. Treatment of myocarditis: current recommendations and future approaches. *Heart Failure* 1992;8:33–40.

45. O'Connell JB, Mason JW. Diagnosing and treating active myocarditis. *West J Med* 1989;150:431–435.

46. Drucker NA, Colan SD, Lewis AB, Beiser AS, Wessel DL, Takahashi M, Baker AL, Perez-Atayde AR, Newburger JW. γ-Globulin treatment of acute myocarditis in the pediatric population. *Circulation* 1994;89:252–257.

47. Salvi A, Di Lenarda A, Silvestri F, Camerini F, Dreas L. Im-

munosuppressive treatment in myocarditis. *Int J Cardiol* 1989;22:329–338.

48. Chan KY, Iwahara M, Benson LN, Wilson GJ, Freedom RM. Immunosuppressive therapy in the management of acute myocarditis in children: a clinical trial. *J Am College Cardiol* 1991;17:458–460.

49. O'Connell JB, Mason JW. Immunosuppressive therapy in experimental and clinical myocarditis. *Pathol Immunopathol Res* 1988;7:292–304.

50. McManus BM, Kandolf R. Evolving concepts of cause, consequence and control of myocarditis. *Curr Opinion Cardiol* 1991;6:418.

51. Mason JW, O'Connell JB, Herskowitz A, Rose NR, McManus BM, Billingham ME, Moon TE. A clinical trial of immunosuppressive therapy for myocarditis. *N Engl J Med* 1995;333: 269–275.

52. McKenna WJ, Davies MJ. Immunosuppression for myocarditis. *N Engl J Med* 1995;333:312–313.

8

PERIPARTAL CARDIOMYOPATHY

ROBERTO M. LANG, MD, MARK B. LAMPERT, MD, ATHENA POPPAS, MD,
AFSHAN HAMEED, MD, AND URI ELKAYAM, MD

INTRODUCTION

Peripartum cardiomyopathy (PPCM) is a rare form of cardiomyopathy of unclear cause that can have life-threatening consequences. This condition is sufficiently uncommon that the practicing cardiologist may see only a few cases during his or her career. At the same time, the consequences of this disorder are potentially devastating. Thus the clinician should be aware of the cumulative experience of the past 20–30 years, to be able to provide optimal treatment to these patients.

DEFINITION

Heart failure associated with pregnancy was recognized as early as in 1849,[1] but it was not until the 1930s that it was fully described as a distinctive entity.[2] In 1971 Demakis et al[3] established diagnostic criteria for PPCM, which included development of cardiac failure in the last month of pregnancy or within 5 months after delivery, absence of a determinable cause, and absence of demonstrable heart disease before the last month of pregnancy. Although these criteria have been widely used, additional information made available over the last three decades suggests that these guidelines may require revision to increase their accuracy. Although the majority of patients with PPCM are diagnosed during the last antepartal or first postpartal month (Fig. 8.1), diagnosis of PPCM has been reported as early as in the third gestational month,[4] and many cases have been diagnosed during the second[5] and third gestational trimester[6–10] (Table 8.1). These data therefore indicate that the diagnosis of PPCM should be considered in patients with heart failure due to systolic left

ventricular dysfunction at any time during pregnancy. Deterioration of left ventricular systolic function typical to PPCM has been described in a number of cases with additional demonstrable heart disease. Oakley[11] described reversible cardiomyopathy diagnosed postpartum in a patient with coincidental Eisenmenger syndrome due to ventricular septal defect. Devlin et al[12] described a patient with a small ventricular septal defect in whom peripartum cardiomyopathy was diagnosed in the 33rd gestational week. Landzberg[13] recently reported a transient but marked decrease in left ventricular systolic function during the peripartum period in a patient with a history of a Fontan operation, and Purcell and Williams[14] described a patient with aortic stenosis who developed peripartum cardiomyopathy 4 weeks after delivery.

The foregoing data indicate that the diagnosis of PPCM should not be excluded in a patient with coincidental heart disease. At the same time, however, other causes of cardiac dysfunction and congestive heart failure, such as infectious, toxic, or metabolic disorders, ischemic or valvular heart disorders, or vascular disease (aortic coarctation or dissection) should be carefully ruled out before the diagnosis of PPCM is made. Also to be ruled out are complications of late pregnancy, including toxemia and amniotic or pulmonary embolism, which may mimic heart failure. In the past, authors reporting cases of PPCM based the diagnosis solely on symptoms and signs of heart failure and radiographic features. With the advent of echocardiographic techniques, it can be clearly demonstrated that pregnant patients exhibiting normal ventricular size and function may at times have clinical features mimicking heart failure. For these reasons, demonstrable impairment in left ventricular systolic function should be added as a criterion for the diagnosis of PPCM (Table 8.2).

Cardiac Problems in Pregnancy, Third Edition
Edited by Uri Elkayam, MD, and Norbert Gleicher, MD
Copyright © 1998 by Wiley-Liss, Inc. ISBN 0-471-16358-9

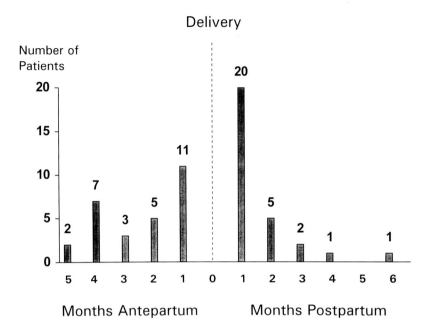

INCIDENCE

The occurrence of PPCM is, in general, rare, but it varies clearly among geographic regions. Recent estimates of incidence range from 1:15,000 in the United States,[15] 1:6000 in Japan,[5] and 1:1000 in South Africa.[16] In Nigeria, estimates as high as 1% have been reported.[17] The majority of the Nigerian cases, however, are likely to be the result of pure volume overload caused by the Hausa tradition of ingesting kanwa, a dried lake salt, while lying on heated mud beds twice daily for 40 days postpartum.

RISK FACTORS

Although early series of patients with PPCM suggested that the syndrome was more prevalent in women over 30 years old, this syndrome has been reported in patients of a wide range of ages.[2,3,6–12,16] The incidence of this disease has been shown repeatedly to be higher in women with multiple pregnancies,[6,8,18–23] but PPCM has also been documented in primiparous women,[4,7,9,11,24–26] Although cases of PPCM have been reported in white, Chinese, Korean, and Japanese women, the majority of affected American patients are of African descent and reside more in tropical climates.[18] Poor nutrition was initially thought to be associated with the development of PPCM;[2] however, numerous cases have since been documented among well-nourished women.[19] Patients with twin pregnancies (7–10% of published cases) appear to

be at higher risk of developing PPCM.[27,28] Other previously described risk factors include a history of toxemia of pregnancy and postpartum hypertension.[2,3,22] Case reports also have suggested an association with maternal cocaine abuse,[18] enterovirus infection,[29] selenium deficiency,[30] and Guillian–Barré neuropathy.[20] Lampert et al have recently reported a link between long-term (> 4 weeks) oral tocolytic therapy and subsequent development of peripartum cardiomyopathy.[31]

The publications that originally outlined these risk factors are relatively old and have not undergone epidemiologic confirmation. Given the possibility that many of the patients in the past harbored diseases that would not meet the modern diagnostic criteria for PPCM, the validity of these early reports must be seriously reconsidered. Further epidemiologic characterization of this patient population may be useful in verifying these and other possible risk factors.

ETIOLOGY

The cause of PPCM is unknown.[18,19,32] In fact, some investigators questioned whether PPCM is indeed a distinct entity.[32] The occurrence of this disease in young women in whom idiopathic cardiomyopathy is rare and the clustering in the peripartum period suggest either that this is a highly vulnerable period for the development of cardiomyopathy or that the condition is truly a separate disease. Whereas patients with underlying cardiac disease (i.e., valvular, ischemic, or idiopathic heart disease) usually have symptoms and signs of heart failure during the second and third trimester of gestation, coinciding with the maximal hemodynamic burden imposed by pregnancy (Chapter 1), the onset of PPCM can occur well after delivery, when the hemodynamic stress associated with pregnancy is resolving. Support for the unique nature of this disease comes from the higher incidence of complete recovery of left ventricular function in patients with PPCM compared to patients with other forms of dilated cardiomyopathy, the propensity to recur with subsequent pregnancies, and the rapid deterioration and early death seen in some patients.[6–9,12,23,25,28,33]

Early suggestions that nutritional disorders may be associated with PPCM[34] have been refuted by many cases of well-nourished patients in whom this disorder has subsequently developed.[18] Although estrogen,[35,36] progesterone,[35] and prolactin[37] have been shown to have profound effects on the cardiovascular system, no distinct hormonal disorder has been identified in PPCM. Small-vessel abnormalities leading to PPCM have been implicated; in cases in which coronary angiography has been performed,[22] however, epicardial coronary arteries have been normal.[19] Pathologic specimens appear to negate the possibility of chronic or intermittent coronary spasm.[37]

It may be tempting to invoke an immunologic mechanism in response to an infection, drugs, or the fetus itself to explain the origin of PPCM. This route has been suggested to explain the increased incidence of the disease in multiparous women and in the mothers of twins.[38] To date, characterization of maternal or fetal immune responses in patients with PPCM has been inadequate. Nevertheless, one study suggested the absence of humoral autoimmunity in these patients.[39]

In 1982 Melvin et al[38] proposed myocarditis as the cause of PPCM. These investigators reported the presence of a dense lymphocytic infiltrate with variable amounts of myocyte edema, necrosis, and fibrosis in right ventricular biopsy specimens obtained from patients with PPCM. Although this study lacked a control group, it was provocative in noting that treatment with prednisone and azathioprine resulted in clinical improvement that coincided with a loss of an inflammatory infiltrate on repeated biopsy in the three patients studied. Subsequently, Sanderson et al[40] performed endomyocardial biopsies in African women with PPCM and found that 5 of 11 patients had histologic specimens consistent with "healing myocarditis." Of interest, among patients with PPCM who subsequently had biopsy specimens showing persistent myocarditis, 3 of 4 went on to have chronic symptoms of heart failure, whereas 4 of 5 of those who had negative results on repeated biopsies clinically improved. More recently, Midei et al[41] also suggested an association between myocarditis and the development of peripartum heart failure. These authors reported that 14 (78%) of 18 patients with newly diagnosed PPCM demonstrated evidence of my-

ocarditis on endomyocardial biopsy. Again, resolution of myocarditis was associated with significant improvement in left ventricular function. Similarly, O'Connell et al[42] studied 14 consecutive patients with PPCM and found a higher incidence (29%) of biopsy-proven myocarditis in these patients compared with patients with idiopathic dilated cardiomyopathy (9%). In contrast to the above-mentioned reports, a recent retrospective review of endomyocardial biopsy specimens from 34 patients diagnosed to have PPCM at Stanford University[10] indicated a low incidence (8.4%) of myocarditis, which was comparable to that of age- and sex-matched patients with idiopathic dilated cardiomyopathy.

The presence of a viral trigger for the development of myocarditis or pericarditis has been recognized for some time. Cenac et al[29] studied the association of a viral cause with the development of PPCM in 38 women. In this report, patients with PPCM and control subjects matched for age, parity, ethnic background, and socioeconomic status underwent blood testing to detect complement fixation to enteroviruses. The results failed to demonstrate a difference in the prevalence of coxsackievirus and echovirus among the two groups. A family history of PPCM has been reported in some cases[4,21,23] and may point toward a possibility of familial predisposition.

In summary, the literature is wealthy with studies attempting to propose etiologies for peripartum heart failure; to date, however, no study has clearly identified a distinct cause of this disease.

PATHOLOGIC FEATURES

Pathologic specimens from patients with PPCM usually demonstrate dilation of the heart and paleness of the myocardium. Although ventricular thrombi are often seen, the heart usually is without obvious structural defects. Endocardial thickening and pericardial fluid have been noted occasionally.[2,43–45] Antemortem biopsy specimens (Fig. 8.2) have demonstrated nonspecific evidence of myofiber hypertrophy, myofiber degeneration, fibrosis, interstitial edema, and, occasionally, lymphocytic infiltration.[3,46–48]

Performing an endomyocardial biopsy on patients with idiopathic dilated cardiomyopathy has fallen out of favor in recent years because of the failure of this procedure to yield diagnostically[49] and clinically[50] relevant information and the paucity of data regarding the benefit of immunosuppressive therapy.[51] Previous reports recommended endocardial biopsies early in the course of PPCM to establish the diagnosis of myocarditis.[38] Until the causes of PPCM have been firmly established, the collection of biopsy data cannot be discouraged. However, based on recent data,[10] it seems that endocardial biopsies are currently of minor diagnostic and therapeutic benefit in patients with PPCM.

TABLE 8.1 Selected Reported Cases of Peripartum Cardiomyopathy

Ref: First Author	Age (years) and Time at Diagnosis	Obstetric History	Symptoms and Signs	ECG/Chest X-Ray Findings	Echocardiogram Findingss
Hovsepian[27] (1989)	20W; 4 days PP	NA	Mild CHF at 4 days PP; pulm edema, tachycardia, $\downarrow$ BP, S_3, S_4, RV and LV heaves	Sinus tach, pulmonary congestion, cardiomegaly	4-chamber enlargement, diffuse LV hypokinesis, 2 + MR
Hoffman[26] (1991)	35; 2 days PP	NA	Dyspnea, tach, tachypnea, S_3, lung crackles, BP 150/100 hypoxemia, hypocapnia	Sinus tach, LVH, borderline cardiac enlargement, interstitial edema, bilateral pleural effusion	LV dilatation, global hypokinesia, FS = 18%, LAE
Klugger[24] (1991)	29; 38 wks	G_1	Dyspnea, orthopnea, chest pain, malaise, tach, tachypnea cyanosis	Sinus tach, bilateral infiltrates	Biventricular hypokinesis
Hagley[20] (1991)	26; 3 wks PP	$G_5 P_5$	Fatigue, dyspnea, orthopnea, PND, cough, pink frothy sputum, pedal edema, tach, tachypnea, inspiratory rales, diffuse PMI displaced laterally MR murmur, S_3	Sinus tach, LAE, LVH, cardiomegaly, pulm congestion	4-chamber dilatation, diffuse LV hypokinesis, severe MR, EF 20% (MUGA)
Brown[6] (1992)	30; 33 wks	$G_3 P_2 Ab_0$	Dyspnea, orthopnea, S_3 systolic murmur, pulm crepitations, mild elevation of LFTs	Sinus tach, interstitial edema	Dilated, diffusely hypokinetic LV, FS = 7%
Bailey[25] (1992)	16; 5 days PP	G_1	CHF (not specified)	Bilateral pleural effusion	Dilated heart with poor function, MR, TR
Leonard[19] (1992)	35; 4 days PP	$G_4 P_4$	Dyspnea, BP 170/90 tach, tachypnea, diaphoresis, diffuse lung crackles, hypoxia, acidosis, S_3, S_4, 4 + pretibial edema	Sinus tach, nonspecific ST-T wave changes, interstitial edema	Markedly dilated LV with global hypokinesis
Mendelson[23] (1992)	30; 1 mo PP	$G_1 P_1$	Orthopnea, dyspnea, tach, JVD, pulm rales, S3, TR murmur, hepatomegaly and tenderness, pitting leg edema	Atrial fibrillation, rapid ventricular response	Ventricular dilatation, EF 19% (MUGA)
Mendelson[23] (1992)	33; 1 mo PP		Dyspnea, orthopnea, PND, tachypnea, bibasilar pulm rales, S_3	NSR, diffusely inverted T waves, cardiomegaly, congestion of pulm vasculature	Marked LV enlargement, hypokinesia
Oakley[11] (1992)	31; 3 mo PP	G_1	Dyspnea, cyanosis, swelling of hands, JVD, S_3, holosystolic murmur	RAD, RVH, cardiomegaly	Global impairment of RV and LV

Ref: First Author	Biopsy Findings	Mode and Time of Delivery	Fetal outcome	Maternal Outcome	Comments
Hovsepian[27] (1989)	Nonspecific changes on biopsy	Uncomplicated vaginal delivery; time NA	NA	Continued deterioration PP, at 3 wks PP LVAD as bridge to transplantation 48 h later. D/C 21 days PS.	
Brown[6] (1992)	NA	Elective C-section under general anesthesia at 34 wks	Female, 2115 g; Apgar 2/6/10 at 1, 5, & 10 min	Pulm edema PP, required mechanical ventilation and inotropic support. D/C from ICU on day 5.	Misdiagnosed as having asthma
Hoffman[26] (1991)	NA	Elective C-section due to preclampsia at 32 wks	Twin girls; 2800 & 2530 g; Apgar 9/9/10 and 5/8/10	Clinical improvement PP, EF at 27 days PP = 43% at 1 yr = 60%.	
Klugger[24] (1991)	NA	Spontaneous vaginal at 39 wks	Newborn required ventilation & inotropic support, died 48 hr PP	Cardiogenic shock with hypoxemia, metabolic acidosis, SVT, renal and hepatic failure. D/C from hospital 3 wks later with EF = 25%.	Misdiagnosed as having anxiety and influenza
Hagley[20] (1991)	NA	Uncomplicated vaginal delivery; time NA	NA	Progressive improvement, 22 wks after diagnosis, nl echo, EF 52%.	
Bailey[25] (1992)	NA	NA	NA	Cardiogenic shock with pulm & renal failure → heart transplantation.	
Leonard[19]	No evidence of myocarditis	C-section for preeclampsia; time NA	NA	Severe symptomatic CHF 5 mo PP.	CHF symptoms during pregnancy attributed to preeclampsia
Mendelson[23] (1992)	NA	Vaginal delivery at term	NA	Clinically improved with tx, EF at 4 mo = 21% at 14 mo 44%, with normal LV size.	Echocardiogram at 38 wks showed FS of 30%
Mendelson[23] (1992)	NA	Vaginal delivery; time NA	NA	Uncomplicated pregnancy 2 yrs pp. Echo-nl LV dimensions and contractility.	
Oakley[11] (1992)	No evidence of myocarditis	Elective C-section at 37 wks	NA	Retinal vein thrombosis 1 mo after dx of PPCM; improvement starting 1 yr after dx with returning RV and LV size and function to former state at 2 yrs.	

(continued

TABLE 8.1 *(Continued)*

Ref: First Author	Age (years) and Time at Diagnosis	Obstetric History	Symptoms and Signs	ECG/Chest X-Ray Findings	Echocardiogram Findingss
Beards[32] (1993)	20; 2 mo PP	NA	Leg, abdominal chest wall, upper limbs, and facial swelling. Coughing, tachypnea, tach, S_3, crepitations	Low voltage QRS complexes, inverted T waves in lateral leads, cardiomegaly, pulm edema	Dilated LV, TR, MR, EF < 20%
Massad[4] (1993)	16; 4 mo after evacuation of molar pregnancy	G_1	Leg edema, cough, hemoptysis, tach, tachypnea, JVD, MR murmurs, S_3, hepatomegaly	LAE, diffuse T-wave inversions, interstitial infiltrates, cardiomegaly	4-chamber enlargement, MR, TR
Abou-Awdi[7] (1994)	34; 33 wks	G_1	Dyspnea, peripheral edema	NA; cardiomegaly, pulm edema	NA
Forssell[8] (1994)	33; NA	G_5P_4	Dyspnea, fatigue, tach, tachypnea, ↓ BP, JVD, enlarged & tender liver, pulm rales, TR murmur, hypoxia, metabolic acidosis	NA	General cardiac dilation with reduced biventricular contraction, TR
Forssell[8] (1994)	37; few wks PP	G_3P_3	Dyspnea, tiredness, JVD, tender liver	NA	Moderate biventricular enlargement
Forssell[8] (1994)	24; during pregnancy	G_3P_3	NA	NA	NA
Yahagi[9] (1994)	26; 32 wks	G_1	Dyspnea, malaise, tach (200 bpm)	Low voltage QRS complex, atrial tach, cardiomegaly	Diffuse biventricular hypokinesis
Devlin[12] (1994)	23; 33 wks	NA	Dyspnea, chest discomfort, tach, hypotension, parasystolic murmur, pulm crepitations	NA	4-chamber enlargement, mural thrombus in LV, small VSD
Pearl[21] (1995)	24; shortly after delivery	G_3P_3	NA	NA	NA

Ref: First Author	Biopsy Findings	Mode and Time of Delivery	Fetal outcome	Maternal Outcome	Comments
Beards[32] (1993)		NA	NA	Resistant to tx with diuretics, inotropes, captopril and vasodilators. Responded to veno-venous hemofiltration, lost > 17 L. D/C 14 days later.	
Massad[4] (1993)	Fibrosis, myocyte hypertrophy, no evidence of myocarditis	Evacuation of molar pregnancy at 3 mo	—	Marked improvement of biventricular function with LVEF of 51%.	Initial symptoms misdiagnosed as respiratory tract infection
Abou-Awdi[7] (1994)	NA	C-section at 34 wks	Normal	Cardiogenic shock on evening of delivery, VT, IABP, and inotropic support. R heart bypass. Hemopump inserted to abdominal aorta; heart transplantation 2 wks later.	Initial symptoms assumed by patient to be "just a part of being pregnant"
Forssell[8] (1994)	NA	NA	NA	No evidence of cardiac disease during 8 yrs F/U	
Forssell[8] (1994)	NA	NA	NA	Gradual improvement PP. Sudden death at 2 mo	
Forssell[8] (1994)	NA	Spontaneous vaginal delivery at 26 wks	Weight 810 g, conventional prematurity tx with satisfactory outcome	Rapid deterioration, intractable CHF 4 mo PP.	
Yahagi[9] (1994)	NA	Emergency C-section at 34 wks	Death during CPR	VT and cardiac arrest at 34 wks, successfully resuscitated. After delivery, multiple organ failure, AT, treated with IABP, hemofiltration, VAD. Patient died 2 mo PP.	
Devlin[12] (1994)	NA	C-section for undetectable fetal heart rate under general anesthesia; time NA	Stillborn	Pulm edema, tach, and ↓ BP during anesthesia, postsurgical course complicated by anuria, ↓ BP, hypoxemia, tachyarrhythmias and pulm edema. Patient died on day 21.	Initial symptoms misdiagnosed as part of normal pregnancy
Pearl[21] (1995)	NA	NA	NA	Patient died 17 days PP in ventricular fibrillation.	Postmortem examination. 520 g heart, biventricular dilatation. Normal coronaries, no evidence of myocarditis.

(continued

TABLE 8.1 *(Continued)*

Ref: First Author	Age (years) and Time at Diagnosis	Obstetric History	Symptoms and Signs	ECG/Chest X-Ray Findings	Echocardiogram Findingss
McIndoe[22] (1995)	32; NA	G$_3$	Hypoxemia, sinus tach, prominent left apical impulse, gallop rhythm	Slight left axis deviation, unremarkable except for borderline cardiomegaly, approximately 12 h later pulm edema	Dilated and poorly contractile LV

Abbreviations: A, abortion; AT, atrial tachycardia; BP, blood pressure; CD, cardioversion, defibrillation; CHF, congestive heart failure; C-section, cesarean section; D/C, discharged; dx, diagnosis; EF, ejection fraction; FS, fractional shortening; F/U, follow-up; G, gravida; IABP, intraaortic balloon pump; ICU, intensive care unit; JVD, jugular venous distension; LAE, left atrial enlargement; LFTs, liver function tests; LV, left ventricle; LVAD, left ventricular assist device; LVH, left ventricular hypertrophy; mo, month; MR, mitral regurgitation; MUGA, nuclear ventriculography; NA, not applicable; nl, normal; NSR, normal sinus rhythm; P, para; PA, pulmonary artery; PMI, point of maximum

CLINICAL PRESENTATION

Physiologic Features and Onset

Pregnancy is normally associated with blood volume expansion, an increase in metabolic demands, relative anemia, and alterations in vascular resistance that are accompanied by mild ventricular dilatation and increases in cardiac output (Chapter 1). These physiologic changes, which are progressive during pregnancy, may lead to hemodynamic and symptomatic decompensation during the second or final gestation trimester in patients with preexisting, subclinical valvular, ischemic, or myopathic heart disease. Because many of the symptoms and signs of normal pregnancy are similar to those of early congestive heart failure (Chapter 2: Table 2.3), and because of the low level of suspicion due to the rarity of PPCM, this condition is often missed in pregnant patients.[4,6,7,20,25] For these reasons, PPCM is most commonly (Fig. 8.1) diagnosed at the end of pregnancy when symptoms become severe or during the first 6 months postpartum when the clinical symptoms continue to exist. Thus, whenever a patient has persistent or worsening heart failure symptoms during pregnancy or in the early puerperium, the diagnosis of PPCM should be seriously considered.

Signs and Symptoms

Commonly described signs and symptoms of patients presenting with peripartum cardiomyopathy are listed in Table

TABLE 8.2 Modified Criteria for Diagnosis of Peripartum Cardiomyopathy

Development of cardiac failure during pregnancy or within 6 months of delivery
Absence of a determinable cause for cardiac failure
Demonstrable impairment in left ventricular systolic function

8.3; for examples of their distribution in reported cases, see Table 8.1. Dyspnea is nearly a universal finding. In addition, cough, orthopnea, hemoptysis, and edema are frequently encountered. Hemoptysis may be the presenting feature of pulmonary embolus, to which these patients are particularly predisposed.[3] Nonspecific fatigue, palpitations, chest pain, and abdominal pain are common and usually tend to confuse the initial clinical evaluation. The New York Heart Association functional classification is confounded by the simultaneously occurring signs and symptoms of normal pregnancy, and therefore categorizations based on this system may not accurately reflect the severity of the underlying cardiac dysfunction.[45]

The physical examination frequently reveals an increased blood pressure,[20,27] although it may be normal or decreased.[8,11,25,28] Typical signs of congestive heart failure (Table 8.3) including cardiomegaly, tachycardia, and third heart sound are noted in more than 85% of patients with PPCM. In addition, increased jugular venous pressure, mitral and tricuspid regurgitation, pulmonary rales, and peripheral edema are commonly found (Table 8.1).

Laboratory Evaluation

Ancillary studies that should be performed routinely in cases of possible PPCM include an electrocardiogram (ECG), chest radiogram, and M-mode and two-dimensional Doppler echocardiographic studies. The ECG usually demonstrates sinus tachycardia. The QRS voltage may be low,[33] or normal or high[27]; nonspecific ST- and T-wave abnormalities may be present,[4,20,24] and occasionally Q waves are seen in the anteroseptal precordial leads. The PR and QRS intervals may be prolonged, suggesting that intraventricular conduction defects and occasionally bundle branch blocks are present.[33] The chest radiogram (Fig. 8.3) invariably shows cardiomegaly. In addition, pulmonary venous congestion, bibasilar infiltrates, and small bilateral pleural effusions are

Ref: First Author	Biopsy Findings	Mode and Time of Delivery	Fetal outcome	Maternal Outcome	Comments
McIndoe[22] (1995)		Emergency C-section due to fetal distress. General anesthesia. Delivery during external cardiac massage; time NA.	3, 92 kg male; Apgar 9/9 at 1, 5 min	Asystole after induction of anesthesia. External cardiac message, emergency C-section, PP-tachyarrhythmias, ↓ BP, pulm edema. D/C home 10 days later.	

impulse (apex beat); PND, paroxysmal nocturnal dyspnea; PP, postpartum; PS, postsurgery; pulm, pulmonary; R, right; RA, right atrium; RAD, right axis deviation; RVH, right ventricular hypertrophy; SVT, supraventricular tachycardia; tach, tachycardia; TR, tricuspid regurgitation; tx, therapy; VAD, ventricular assist device; VF, ventricular fibrillation; VSD, ventricular septal defect; VT, ventricular tachycardia; wks, weeks; yr, years

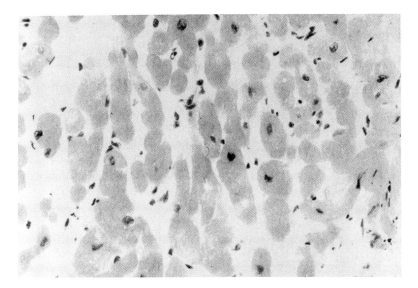

Figure 8.2 Hematoxylin and eosin-stained specimen from right ventricular biopsy obtained from patient with peripartum cardiomyopathy. Myocyte hypertrophy is apparent, with mixed cellular infiltrate and fibrosis. (From Lampert and Lang, *Am Heart J* 1995;130:860–870, with permission.)

TABLE 8.3 Symptoms and Signs of Peripartum Cardiomyopathy

Symptoms	Signs
Dyspnea	Normal or increased blood pressure
	Increased jugular venous pressure
Cough	Cardiomegaly
Orthopnea	Third heart sound
Paroxysmal nocturnal dyspnea	Loud pulmonic valve component of second heart sound
Fatigue	Mitral and/or tricuspid regurgitation
Palpitations	Pulmonary rales
Hemoptysis	Peripheral edema
Chest pain	Ascites
Abdominal pain	Arrhythmias
	Embolic phenomena
	Hepatomegaly

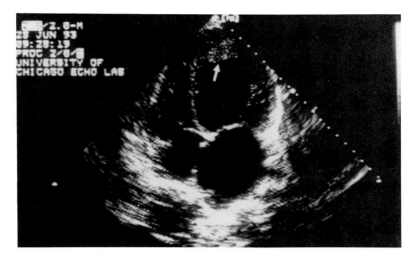

Figure 8.3 Echocardiogram from patient with persistent left ventricular dilatation and dysfunction in whom apical thrombus (arrow) developed. (From Lampert and Lang, *Am Heart J* 1995;130:860–870, with permission.)

commonly seen. The echocardiogram usually shows a dilated left ventricle with marked impairment of overall systolic performance. Right ventricular and biatrial enlargement as well as mitral and tricuspid regurgitation are often found.

To perform a complete hemodynamic assessment and to optimize the treatment of a patient in whom PPCM has been diagnosed, right-side heart catheterization should be considered. If the onset of symptoms occurs prepartum, it is crucial to provide careful hemodynamic management through delivery and the immediate postpartum period. When the initial diagnosis is postpartum, right-side heart catheterization can often be avoided if the patient responds to standard medical therapy. Although the yield of coronary angiography in PPCM patients is low, risk factor analysis should guide the clinician in requesting this study, which poses a small additional risk. Patients with PPCM usually present with tachycardia, have increased right- and left ventricular filing pressures and decreased cardiac output (Table 8.1). Rapid hemodynamic deterioration with cardiogenic shock and multiorgan failure have been described in some cases.[24,25,27]

THERAPY

Medical therapy for PPCM is similar to that for other forms of congestive heart failure.[52] Thus, sodium restriction and the use of digoxin, diuretics, and afterload-reducing agents are the mainstays of medical therapy.[32,45] Digoxin is beneficial for its effects on ventricular inotropy and rate control in cases of atrial fibrillation. In general, digoxin is believed to be safe in pregnancy despite anecdotal reports of adverse effects (Chapter 34). The drug is secreted in breast milk; the infant,

however, ingests a very small percentage of the dose, and no adverse effects have been reported in newborns.

Diuresis is also fundamental in the treatment of heart failure and results in symptomatic relief of exertional and paroxysmal nocturnal dyspnea. Diuretics are also FDA class C agents and are indicated in pregnant women with heart failure when sodium restriction alone has been therapeutically unsuccessful (Chapter 28). Maternal complications of diuretic therapy include pancreatitis, volume contraction, alkalosis, decreased carbohydrate tolerance, hypokalemia, hyponatremia, and hyperuricemia. Bleeding diathesis and hyponatremia have also been reported in neonates of patients who have taken diuretic agents during pregnancy.

Vasodilator therapy can be used to foster a decrease in systemic vascular resistance, an improvement in cardiac output, and a reduction in right and left ventricular end diastolic pressures. A large body of data now supports the use of angiotensin-converting enzyme (ACE) inhibitors to prolong life in nonpregnant patients with heart failure.[52] These drugs, however, have been associated with high incidence of fetal complications (Chapter 32). Reports of severe adverse neonatal renal effects, anuric renal failure, and neonatal death among mothers who ingested ACE inhibitors prepartum have led to the contraindication of these drugs during pregnancy. In the majority of patients, however, the onset of PPCM occurs in the early postpartum months, when the issue of fetal toxicity is no longer a concern. Whenever vasodilator therapy is required prepartum, hydralazine is the agent of choice. This drug has been used parenterally and orally for decades in the treatment of severe hypertension in pregnancy and appears to be safe for the mother and the fetus[53] (Chapter 31).

Thromboembolic phenomena have been commonly reported in cases of PPCM.[54] The use of anticoagulation should therefore be seriously considered. Pregnant patients are at increased risk of thromboembolic complications because of the hypercoagulable state of late pregnancy, which is associated with increased concentrations of coagulation factors II, VII, VIII, and X, and plasma fibrinogen, and with augmented platelet adhesiveness.[55] These changes may persist for as long as 4–6 weeks postpartum.[56,57] In addition, blood stasis in cardiac chambers due to decreased systolic function and decreased stroke volume may predispose the patient to formation of ventricular thrombosis (Fig. 8.3) as well as systemic and pulmonary thromboemboli. In fact, cerebral embolism has been reported as the presenting feature of PPCM.[58] Finally, prolonged bed rest, previously advocated in the treatment of PPCM, may predispose patients to the development of deep venous thrombosis with subsequent pulmonary embolism. This predisposition could partially explain the high incidence of thromboembolism and high mortality rates reported in earlier studies. Currently, bed rest is not recommended and, if possible, should not be prescribed for patients with PPCM.

Oral anticoagulants such as warfarin are FDA class D agents (absolutely contraindicated in pregnancy): they cross the placenta and are associated with fetal teratogenic effects. Before delivery, heparin is the anticoagulant of choice (Chapter 33). Given its short half-life, the drug can be discontinued before delivery to prevent maternal hemorrhage. Although heparin can cause depletion of antithrombin III, thrombocytopenia, and premature maternal osteoporosis, these adverse effects are infrequently seen, especially in patients with PPCM who, because of the onset of their disease in late pregnancy and its transient nature usually require short-term therapy. Neither heparin nor warfarin is secreted into breast milk, and therefore neither drug results in an anticoagulant effect in the breast-fed infant.

Immunosuppressive therapy has been attempted in patients with PPCM and biopsy-proven myocarditis.[38] It is not clear whether reported clinical improvement was related to this therapy. A large prospective, randomized trial of immunosuppression in patients with myocarditis failed to demonstrate a clear benefit. Furthermore, most reported cases had nonspecific biopsy findings, which do not justify the use of these agents. Therefore, until a link between immunosuppressive treatment and resolution of myocarditis can be established in this setting, there is no compelling reason to recommend the use of immunosuppression in patients with PPCM.

Since PPCM may be reversible, the temporary use of an intraaortic balloon pump may help to stabilize patients until improvement occurs.[60] The use of a left ventricular assist device has been reported as a bridge to cardiac transplantation in patients who demonstrated continued deterioration in spite of medical therapy.[27]

Cardiac Transplantation

Cardiac transplantation has been performed successfully in patients with PPCM.[28,61–63] The favorable outcomes are likely attributable to the young age of the recipients and to the recent onset of heart failure and the consequently minimal amount of end-organ damage. Given the successful outcome of cardiac transplantation in these young, otherwise healthy patients, aggressive measures such as temporary life support in the form of cardiopulmonary bypass[61] or a ventricular assist device[28] have been successfully used as a bridge to the arrival of a donor heart. Given that the majority of patients with PPCM recover spontaneously, only those who continue to deteriorate or show no improvement of severe symptoms over a few months should be considered for cardiac catheterization. Two reports[64,65] comparing the results of cardiac transplantation in age-matched females who underwent the operation for PPCM and idiopathic cardiomyopathy demonstrated favorable and comparable long-term survival in both groups. (Two-year survival was 88% in PPCM and 86% in idiopathic cardiomyopathy in the study by Keogh et al[64] and 5-year survival of 60 and 78%, respectively, in the study by Peter and Rickenbacher[65]).

Prognosis

In the United States, mortality from peripartum cardiomyopathy was reported to be 48% by Demakis and Rahimtoola in 1971,[66] and 43% by O'Connell et al[42] in 1986. In contrast, Midei et al[41] in 1990 reported death in only one patient and heart transplantation in two patients out of their group of 18 patients with PPCM. Nearly half of these deaths occured within the first 3 months postpartum, and death was usually caused by chronic progressive congestive heart failure, arrhythmia, or thromboembolic complications. Few data on fetal outcome are available. Reported cases suggest that as in other forms of heart failure, the prognosis is related to left ventricular size,[67,68] severity of left ventricular dysfunction at the time of presentation,[33,69] pulmonary artery and wedge pressures, older age and high parity,[64] and time of diagnosis. Approximately 50% of patients have marked improvement in left ventricular function and clinical symptoms. Recovery usually occurs within 6 months from the time of initial diagnosis.[4] Patients in whom left ventricular function recovers have significantly improved survival.[6,48,69] In a retrospective evaluation of 97 patients with PPCM in South Africa,[16] late presentation of the disease (later than 1 month postpartum) was associated with prognosis worse than that for patients diagnosed earlier.

Effect of Subsequent Pregnancy

Most authors agree that patients with peripartum cardiomyopathy and persistent left ventricular dysfunction are at high

TABLE 8.4   Maternal and Fetal Outcome in 67 Subsequent Pregnancies in 60 Patients with a History of PPCM

Group[a]	Maternal Outcome			Fetal Outcome		
	Normal (%)	LV Dysfunction (%)	Death (%)	Live Birth (%)	Abortions (%)	Stillbirth (%)
A	74	23	2	93	5	2
B	37	54	8	83	17	0

[a]Group A: 43 pregnancies in 40 patients with history of PPCM who had recovery of left ventricular function. Group B: 24 pregnancies in 23 patients with history of PPCM and persistent left ventricular dysfunction.

risk for complications and death, should they become pregnant again. In contrast, the issue of whether patients with peripartum cardiomyopathy and recovered left ventricular function can safely undergo subsequent pregnancy remains controversial. Early data suggest an increased incidence of recurrence of PPCM in patients with recovered left ventricular function who become pregnant again.[4,13] More recent investigators, however, have claimed that when left ventricular function is recovered, patients may safely undergo pregnancy.[70] A recent survey by Ostrzega and Elkayam[71] obtained information on 63 patients post PPCM who had 67 subsequent pregnancies (Table 8.4). Forty patients had recovery of left ventricular function post-PPCM and had 43 subsequent pregnancies (group A) while 23 patients who had 24 subsequent pregnancies had persistent left ventricular dysfunction (group B). Normal maternal outcome was reported in 74% of pregnancies in group A and 37% in group B. Left ventricular dysfunction was reported in 54% of group B patients and 23% of group A patients. Mortality was reported in 2% of group A patients and 8% of group B patients. Incidence of abortions was higher in group B patients (17 vs. 5%) and stillbirth was seen in 2% of group A patients and in none of group B patients. Although these data may be limited by the retrospective and possible biased nature of the study, they may help to guide physicians and patients regarding risk of subsequent pregnancy in a patient with a history of PPCM. More data, however, collected in a prospective fashion, will be needed to confirm the results of this survey.

A recent study by Lampert et al[72] assessed left ventricular contractile reserve in patients with recovered ventricular function by using a dobutamine challenge test. Seven patients who recovered from peripartum cardiomyopathy were compared with control subjects matched for age, race, and parity. The data suggest that contractile reserve is significantly impaired in most patients recovered from peripartum cardiomyopathy. Although impairment in contractile reserve and the safety of subsequent pregnancy cannot be directly linked, these data suggest that the left ventricle of patients who are "recovered" from peripartum cardiomyopathy and who have an abnormal response to dobutamine challenge may respond suboptimally on exposure to hemodynamic stress. On the basis of the above-mentioned data,[71,72] we currently recommend caution to patients with peripartum cardiomyopathy who are considering future pregnancy. Clearly, in patients who show signs of persistent left ventricular dysfunction, subsequent pregnancy should be discouraged. In addition, even patients with a history of PPCM and recovery of left ventricular function cannot be guaranteed an event-free pregnancy, and recurrence of the disease is possible. The risk of mortality, however, seems to be small.

REFERENCES

1. Richie C. Clinical contribution to the pathology, diagnosis and treatment of certain chronic diseases of the heart. *Edinburgh Med Surg J* 1849;2:333.

2. Hull E, Hafkesbring E. Toxic postpartal heart disease. *New Orleans Med Surg J* 1937;89:550–557.

3. Demakis JG, Rahimtoola SH, Sutton GC, Meadows R, Szanto PB, Tobin JR, Gunnar RM. Natural course of peripartum cardiomyopathy. *Circulation* 1971;44:1053–1061.

4. Massad LS, Reiss, CK, Mutch DG, Haskel EJ. Familial peripartum cardiomyopathy after molar pregnancy. *Obstetrics and Gynecology* 1993;81:886–888.

5. Hsieh CC, Chiang CW, Hsieh TT, Soong YK. Peripartum cardiomyopathy. *Jpn Heart J* 1992;33;3:349.

6. Brown G, O'Leary M, Douglas I, Herkes R. Perioperative management of a case of severe peripartum cardiomyopathy. *Anaesth Intensive Care* 1992;20:80–83.

7. Abou Awdi N, Joseph K. Hemopump left ventricular support in the peripartum cardiomyopathy patient. *J Cardiovasc Nurs* 1994;8(2):36–44.

8. Forssell G, Laska J, Olofsson C, Olsson M, Mogensen L. Peripartum cardiomyopathy—three cases. *Journal of Internal Medicine* 1994;235:493–496.

9. Yahagi N, Kumon K, Nakatani T, Ishikawa T, Tanigami H, Eishi K, Takahashi S. Peripartum cardiomyopathy and tachycardia followed by multiple organ failure. *Anesth Analg* 1994;79:581–582.

10. Rizeq MN, Rickenbacher PR, Fowler MB, Billingham ME. Incidence of myocarditis in peripartum cardiomyopathy. *Am J Cardiol* 1994;74:474–477.

11. Oakley CM, Nihoyannopoulos P. Peripartum cardiomyopathy with recovery in a patient with coincidental Eisenmenger ventricular septal defect. *Br Heart J* 1992;67:190–192.

12. Devlin EG, Lavery GG, Lewis MA. Peripartum cardiomyopathy in a patient with a ventricular septal defect. *Eur J Anesth* 1994;11:241–244.

13. Landzberg MJ, Somerville J. Operative and late results following the Fontan procedure in patients older than 15 years. *ACCEL* 1996;28(8).

14. Purcell IF, Williams DO. Peripartum cardiomyopathy complicating severe aortic stenosis. *Int J Cardiol* 1995;52:163–165.

15. Cunningham FG, Pritchard JA, Hankins GD, Anderson PL, Lucas MJ, Armstrong KF. Peripartum heart failure: idiopathic cardiomyopathy or compounding cardiovascular events? *Obstet Gynecol* 1986;67:157–168.

16. Desai D, Moodley J, Naidoo D. Peripartum cardiomyopathy: experience at King Edward VIII Hospital, Durban, South Africa and review of the literature. *Trop Doctor* 1995;25:118–123.

17. Sanderson JE, Adesanya CO, Anjorin FI, Parry EO. Postpartum cardiac failure: heart failure due to volume overload. *Am Heart J* 1979;97:613–621.

18. Veille JC. Peripartum cardiomyopathies: a review. *Am J Obstet Gynecol* 1984;148:805–818.

19. Homans DC. Peripartum cardiomyopathy. *N Engl J Med* 1985;312:1432–1437.

20. Leonard RB, Schwartz E, Allen D, Alson R. Peripartum cardiomyopathy: a case report. *Obstet Gynecol* 1992:157–162.

21. Hagley MT, Mankad SV. Peripartum cardiomyopathy. *JAMA* 1991;46;5:160–163.

22. Pearl W. Familial occurrence of peripartum cardiomyopathy. *Am Heart J* 1995;129:421–422.

23. McIndoe AK, Hammond EJ, Babington PC. Peripartum cardiomyopathy presenting as a cardiac arrest at induction of anaesthesia for emergency Caesarean section. *Br J Anaesth* 1995;75:97–101.

24. Mendelson MA, Chandler J. Postpartum cardiomyopathy associated with maternal cocaine abuse. *Am J Cardiol* 1992;70:1092–1094.

25. Klugger MT, Bersten AD. Multi-organ failure in peripartum cardiomyopathy. *Anaesthes Intensive Care* 1991;19:450–453.

26. Bailey D, Wood MLB, Liban JB. Peripartum cardiomyopathy. *Anaesthes Intensive Care* 1992;20:397–398.

27. Hoffman AC, Masouye P, Rifat K, Suter PM. Peripartum cardiomyopathy: a case report. *Acta Anesthesiol Scand* 1991;35:784–785.

28. Hovsepian P, Ganzel B, Sohi G, Kupersmith J, Gray L. Peripartum cardiomyopathy treated with a left ventricular assist device as a bridge to cardiac transplantation. *South Med J* 1989;82;4:527–528.

29. Cenac A, Gaultier Y, Devillechabrolle A, Moulias R. Enterovirus infection in peripartum cardiomyopathy. *Lancet* 1988;2:968–969. Letter.

30. Cenac A, Simonoff M, Moretto P, Djibo A. A low plasma selenium is a risk factor for peripartum cardiomyopathy: a comparative study in Sahelian Africa. *Int J Cardiol* 1992;36:57–59.

31. Lampert MB, Hibbard J, Weinert L, Briller J, Lindheimer M, Lang R. Peripartum heart failure associated with prolonged tocolytic therapy. *Am J Obstet Gynecol* 1993;168:493–495.

32. Elkayam U, Ostrzega EL, Shotan A. Peripartum cardiomyopathy. In: Gleicher N, ed. *Principles and Practice of Medical Therapy in Pregnancy*. Norwalk, CT: Appleton & Lange; 1992;812–814.

33. Beards SC, Freebairn RC, Lipman J. Successful use of continuous veno-venous haemofiltration to treat profound fluid retention in severe peripartum cardiomyopathy. *Anaesthesia* 1993;48:1065–1067.

34. Brockington IF. Postpartum hypertensive heart failure. *Am J Cardiol* 1971;27:650–658.

35. Ueland K, Parer JT. Effects of estrogens on the cardiovascular system of the ewe. *Am J Obstet Gynecol* 1966;96:400–406.

36. Schaible TF, Malhotra A, Ciambrone G, Scheuer J. The effects of gonadectomy on left ventricular function and cardiac contractile proteins in male and female rats. *Circ Res* 1984;54:38–49.

37. Koide T, Saito Y, Sakemoto T, Murao S. Peripartal cardiomyopathy in Japan: a critical reappraisal of the concept. *Jpn Heart J* 1972;13:488–501.

38. Melvin KR, Richardson PJ, Olsen EG, Daly K, Jackson G. Peripartum cardiomyopathy due to myocarditis. *N Engl J Med* 1982;307:731–734.

39. Cenac A, Beaufils H, Soumana I, Vetter JM, Devillechabrolle A, Moulias R. Absence of humoral autoimmunity in peripartum cardiomyopathy: a comparative study in Nigeria. *Int J Cardiol* 1990;26:49–52.

40. Sanderson JE, Olsen EG, Gatei D. Peripartum heart disease: an endomyocardial biopsy study. *Br Heart J* 1986;56:289–291.

41. Midei MG, DeMent SH, Feldman AM, Hutchins GM, Baughman KL. Peripartum myocarditis and cardiomyopathy. *Circulation* 1990;81:922–928.

42. O'Connell JB, Costanzo-Nordin MR, Subramanian R, Robinson JA, Wallis DE, Scanlon PJ, Gunnar RM. Peripartum cardiomyopathy: clinical, hemodynamic, histologic and prognostic characteristics. *J Am College Cardiol* 1986;8:52–56.

43. Gouley BA, McMillan TM, Bellet S. Idiopathic myocardial degeneration associated with pregnancy and especially the puerperium. *Am J Med Sci* 1937;194:185–199.

44. Meadows WR. Idiopathic myocardial failure in the last trimester of pregnancy and the puerperium. *Circulation* 1957;15:903–914.

45. Lee W. Clinical management of gravid women with peripartum cardiomyopathy. *Obstet Gynecol Clin North Am* 1991;18:257–271.

46. Johnson HB, Hussain G, Flores P, Mann M. Idiopathic heart disease associated with pregnancy and the puerperium. *Am Heart J* 1996;72:809–816.

47. Talwaker PG, Nuralla DV, Mistry CJ, Wagholikar UL. Peripartum cardiomyopathy: a clinico-pathological study. *J Assoc Physicians India* 1978;26:793–798.

48. Tomaru A, Goto Y, Miura S, Takikawa K, Kagawa N, Kudo M. Two cases of peripartum cardiomyopathy. *J Cardiol* 1995;25:43–49.

49. Becker AE, Heijmans D, Essed CE. Chronic non-ischaemic congestive heart disease and endomyocardial biopsies: worth the extra? *Eur Heart J* 1991;12:218–223.

50. Figulla HR, Kellerman AB, Stile SM, Hein A, Kreuger H. Clinical investigations: significance of coronary angiography, left heart catheterization, and endomyocardial biopsy for the diagnosis of idiopathic dilated cardiomyopathy. *Am Heart J* 1992;124:1251–1257.

51. Mason JW, O'Connell JB. Clinical merit of endomyocardial biopsy. *Circulation* 1989;79:971–979.

52. Cohn JN. The management of chronic heart failure. *N Engl J Med* 1996;335:490–498.

53. Sibai BM. Treatment of hypertension in pregnant women. *N Engl J Med* 1996;335:257–265.

54. Wulsch JJ, Burch GE. Postpartal heart disease. *Arch Intern Med* 1961;108:817–823.

55. Lefsky E. Hematologic disorders. In: Barron WM, Lindheimer MD, eds. *Medical Disorders During Pregnancy.* St. Louis: Mosby-Year Book; 1991;272–322.

56. Bonnar J. Venous thromboembolism and pregnancy. *Clin Obstet Gynecol* 1981;8:455–473.

57. Rutherford SE, Phelan JP. Thromboembolic disease in pregnancy. *Clin Perinatol* 1986;13:719–739.

58. Hodgman MT, Pessin MS, Homans DC, Panis W, Prager RJ, Lathi ES, Criscitiello MG. Cerebral embolism as the initial manifestation of peripartum cardiomyopathy. *Neurology* 1982;32:668–671.

59. Mason JW, O'Connell JB, Herskowitz A, Rose NR. A clinical trial of immunosuppressive therapy for myocarditis. *N Engl J Med* 1995;333:269–275.

60. Brantigan CO, Grow JB Sr, Schoonmaker FW. Extended use of intraaortic balloon pumping in peripartum cardiomyopathy. *Ann Surg* 1976;183:1.

61. Dhalla N, Fitzgerald M, Khaghani A, Radley-Smith R, Yacoub MH. Heart transplantation for peripartum cardiomyopathy. *Lancet* 1987;2:1024. Letter.

62. Joseph SG. Peripartum cardiomyopathy: successful treatment with cardiac transplantation. *West J Med* 1987;146:230–232.

63. Carvalho AG, Almeida D, Cohen M, Lima V, Moura L, Buffolo E, Martinez EE. Successful pregnancy, delivery and puerperium in a heart transplant patient with previous peripartum cardiomyopathy. *Eur Heart J* 1992;13:1589–1591.

64. Keogh A, McDonald P, Spratt P, Marshman D, Larbalestier R, Kaan A. Outcome in peripartum cardiomyopathy after heart transplantation. *J Heart Lung Transplant* 1994;13:202–207.

65. Peter R, Rickenbacher MD. Long-term outcome after heart transplantation for peripartum cardiomyopathy. *Am Heart J* 1994;127:1318–1323.

66. Demakis JG, Rahimtoola SH. Peripartum cardiomyopathy. *Circulation* 1971;19:964–968.

67. Ravikishore AG, Kaul UA, Sethi KK, Khalilullah M. Peripartum cardiomyopathy: prognostic variables at initial evaluation. *Int J Cardiol* 1991;32:377–380.

68. Carvalho AG, Almeida D, Cohen M, Lima V, Moura L, Buffolo E, Martinez EE. Successful pregnancy, delivery and puerperium in a heart transplant patient with previous peripartum cardiomyopathy. *Eur Heart J* 1992;13:1589–1591.

69. Hadjimiltiades S, Panidis IP, Segal BL, Iskandrian AS. Recovery of left ventricular function in peripartum cardiomyopathy. *Am Heart J* 1986;112:1097–1099.

70. Sutton MS, Cole P, Piappert M, Saltzman D, Goldhaber S. Effects of subsequent pregnancy on left ventricular cardiomyopathy. *Am Heart J* 1991;121:1776–1778.

71. Ostrzega E, Elkayam U. Risk of subsequent pregnancy in women with a history of peripartum cardiomyopathy: results of a survey. *Circulation* 1995;92(suppl I):I-333. Abstract.

72. Lampert MB, Weinert L, Hibbard J, Roberts L, Lindheimer M, Lang R. Contractile reserve in patients with peripartum cardiomyopathy and recovered left ventricular function. *J Am College Cardiol* 1994;23:428A. Abstract.

9

HYPERTROPHIC CARDIOMYOPATHY AND PREGNANCY

URI ELKAYAM, MD, AND RAVI DAVE, MD

INTRODUCTION

Hypertrophic cardiomyopathy (HCM) is a primary myocardial disease characterized by hypertrophy of the left and/or right ventricular myocardium.[1,2] The hypertrophy is usually asymmetrical, is associated with myocardial fiber disarray, and most commonly involves the interventricular septum close to the base of the heart (asymmetric septal hypertrophy). Other less common forms of HCM include the asymmetrical midventricular and apical and the symmetrical (concentric) hypertrophy. Characteristic pathophysiologic alterations in HCM include (1) hyperdynamic left ventricle; (2) dynamic obstruction of left ventricular outflow, causing a measurable gradient either at rest or on provocation with maneuvers or drugs that increase contractility, decrease ventricular volume, or reduce peripheral vascular resistance; (3) mitral regurgitation secondary either to (a) failure of coaptation of the mitral valve due to the systolic anterior motion of the anterior mitral leaflet or other abnormalities of the mitral valve (e.g., anomalous papillary muscle attachment to the anterior leaflet, mitral valve prolapse) or (b) anterior leaflet damage due to repeated contact with the septum; (4) myocardial ischemia, which may be caused by small-vessel disease with decreased vasodilator capacity, compression of septal perforator arteries, myocardial bridging, decreased coronary perfusion pressure, and decreased capillary myocardial fiber ratio.

CLINICAL MANIFESTATIONS

The wide spectrum of clinical presentations extends from no symptoms to severe illness often manifested in poor effort tolerance, heart failure, or sudden death.[1,2] In a general population of young adults (23–35 years), the prevalence of HCM is about 2 per 1000.[3] The disease occurs in all ages and may be diagnosed in the elderly as well as in the newborn. A large proportion of patients with HCM are asymptomatic; however, clinical manifestations and even severe symptoms may occur in patients with severe left ventricular outflow tract obstruction as well as in those without a significant gradient. Dyspnea is the most common presenting symptom and is frequently accompanied by atypical chest pain, angina, dizziness, presyncope, syncope, and palpitations. Typical symptoms of heart failure such as exertional dyspnea, orthopnea, and paroxysmal nocturnal dyspnea may occur, especially in patients with severe LV outflow obstruction, severe systolic and/or diastolic dysfunction, and in the presence of atrial fibrillation. Sudden death may be the first clinical manifestation of the disease, and its annual incidence is higher in younger patients (6%) than in the elderly (1%).[1,2] Most symptoms are worsened on exertion, and poor effort tolerance is a frequent complaint. Because of the dynamic nature of subaortic obstruction, there is not always a good correlation between the presence or magnitude of resting gradient and severity of symptoms during upright exercise.

Physical examination in the patient who does not have left ventricular outflow obstruction may be entirely normal, or it may reveal only subtle features such as rapid upstroke of the carotid upstroke pulse, prominent left ventricular impulse, and a palpable atrial beat. More characteristic physical signs are found in patients with a large gradient and/or marked myocardial hypertrophy. The jugular venous pulsation is usually normal, but prominent A wave may be seen in patients with hypertrophy of the right ventricle as a result of vigorous atrial contraction. The carotid pulse is of normal volume and

Cardiac Problems in Pregnancy, Third Edition
Edited by Uri Elkayam, MD, and Norbert Gleicher, MD

shows a brisk upstroke; in patients with outflow obstruction it may be followed by a short decline at midsystole and a secondary rise (bifid carotid pulse, or "spike and dome"). The apical precordial impulse is forceful, and a prominent presystolic impulse may be palpable. A systolic thrill can often be palpated along the lower left sternal border and the apex. On auscultation, first heart sound is usually normal and the diagnostic hallmark is a diamond-shaped systolic murmur. This murmur is grade 3-4/6 in patients with resting obstruction; it is heard at or just medial to the apex and radiates to the left sternal border. In addition, a mitral regurgitation murmur can be heard. In patients with latent subaortic obstruction, the murmur increases in intensity in the upright position, during the strain phase of the Valsalva maneuver, on amyl nitrite inhalation, and during exercise or tachycardia. On squatting, on isometric hand grip, and during the overshoot phase of the Valsalva maneuver, the murmur decreases in intensity. Because of prolonged left ventricular ejection time, the second heart sound may be single or may even have a reserved (paradoxical) split. In addition, a fourth heart sound is almost always present.

Electrocardiographic features can include left ventricular hypertrophy, ST-segment and T-wave abnormalities, and abnormal Q waves in the inferior or lateral leads. A finding of giant, negative T waves is typical of apical HCM. On ambulatory electrocardiographic monitoring (Holter), ventricular tachyarrhythmias are frequently seen.[4]

Echocardiography is the test used most frequently to make a definitive diagnosis of HCM.[5] M-mode and two-dimensional echo features of the disease include generalized left ventricular thickening, asymmetric septal hypertrophy (ASH) with a ratio of septal to posterior wall thickening exceeding 1.5, and decreased septal motion. Hypertrophy may also be localized to other segments of the ventricle such as the apex. The size of ventricular cavity is usually decreased, and in the presence of left ventricular outflow obstruction there is a systolic anterior motion (SAM) of the mitral valve; a midsystolic closure of the aortic valve may also be seen. Doppler technique may be helpful in assessing the presence of dynamic left ventricular outflow obstruction and the presence of mitral regurgitation. Transesophageal echo/Doppler study may be useful for the definition of mitral valve abnormalities. Stress thallium studies are useful for the detection of myocardial ischemia.[6] Magnetic resonance imaging may be helpful in the determination of severity of hypertrophy, especially in apical HCM.[7]

HYPERTROPHIC CARDIOMYOPATHY AND PREGNANCY

In the second edition of this book, we described the outcome of pregnancy in 82 pregnancies in 35 patients with HCM reported in the English literature between 1967 and 1985. Although such reports are more likely to describe complicated cases, the available information revealed the occurrence of new onset or exacerbation of signs and/or symptoms of congestive heart failure in approximately 20% of the cases. Other reported symptoms included chest pain (6%), palpitations (4%), syncope and dizziness (1 patient each), and ventricular arrhythmias in two patients, resulting in death in the 39th gestational week in one patient who presented with chest pain, dyspnea, palpitations, and dizzy spells. Several new reports published in the world literature in the last decade continue to demonstrate the risks associated with pregnancy in patients with HCM (Table 9.1).[8-18] Hemodynamic and clinical deterioration and pulmonary edema were described in several cases.[9,11-13] Poorly tolerated, resistant supraventricular tachycardia with fetal distress, necessitating a radiofrequency ablation during the fifth month of gestation, was described in one case,[13] and new onset atrial fibrillation leading to clinical and hemodynamic deterioration controlled by DC cardioversion was described by other investigators.[17] A second fatality of a patient with HCM during pregnancy was described by Pelliccia et al,[15] who reported a sudden death in a 27-year-old asymptomatic woman during her 28 weeks' gestation. We have followed a patient with obstructive HCM during two separate pregnancies following implantation of automatic implantable cardioverter defibrillator for an episode of cardiac arrest. The patient who was free of arrhythmias between her pregnancies had a number of defibrillator discharges during both her pregnancies.

The cases described above demonstrate the potential risk associated with pregnancy in women with HCM. Likelihood for hemodynamic worsening seems to be particularly high in patients who are symptomatic prior to pregnancy and in asymptomatic patients with substantial left ventricular diastolic and/or systolic dysfunction. Several reports have demonstrated an increased incidence of arrhythmias during pregnancy in patients both with and without organic heart disease. The available information suggests an increased risk for both supraventricular and ventricular arrhythmias during pregnancy in patients with HCM.[13,15,17,18] Death associated with pregnancy has been reported in only two patients with HCM. Although the relationship between death and gestation could have been coincidental, pregnancy-induced fetal arrhythmias cannot be excluded as a cause of death in these patients.

Fetal outcome does not seem to be influenced by the presence of maternal HCM. Spontaneous abortion has been reported in 16 or 82 pregnancies (20%) and low birth weight was found in eight cases (10%), an incidence comparable to that reported in women without cardiac disorders. Twelve pregnancies (15%) were delivered by cesarean section, and forceps delivery was reported in only five (6%) cases. Six patients (7%) were reported to have premature delivery, and three babies had respiratory problems either at birth or shortly thereafter. Fetal death occurred in only two cases, one of

TABLE 9.1 Clinical Information on Published Cases with HCM and Pregnancy

Ref: First Author	Age (yrs)	Obstetric History	Form of HCM	Prepregnancy History and Risk Factors	Drugs During Pregnancy	Maternal Complications	Week of Labor	Delivery Mode	Anesthesia	Fetal/ Newborn Outcome/ Complications
Boccio et al[9] (1986)	26	G_1		VT on Holter 1 yr prior to pregnancy; two brothers with IHSS who died suddenly in young adulthood	Propranolol, procainamide	Premature labor at 32 wks not responding to tocolysis with $MgSO_4$; Preinduction pulmonary artery pressure, 40 mm Hg. Patient required intubation following delivery because of pulmonary congestion.	32	C-section due to failure to respond to tocolysis and breach presentation; oxytocin used following delivery	General	
Minnich et al[8] (1987)	18	$G_2P_0Ab_1$	Provokable obstruction	Vertigo and syncope during strenuous exercise 3 yrs before pregnancy		Premature labor at 31 wks controlled with $MgSO_4$.	36	Forceps vaginal delivery after oxytocin induction	Epidural + perineal	None
Lette et al[10] (1989)	32	$G_4P_0Ab_0$	Apical hypertrophy	None	NA	Spontaneous coronary artery dissection 2 days postpartum with acute MI.	NA	C-section because of placenta previa	NA	
Van Kasteren et al[11] (1990)	20	G_1	Obstructive	Dyspnea for 2 yrs; sister with HCM had cardiac arrest during laparoscopy		Worsening of dyspnea after 20th wks; admission at 24 wks.	Term	Spontaneous vaginal with forceps	NA	3365 g male, small VSD
	22	G_2P_1	See above	See above		Hospital admission for dyspnea.	NA	NA	NA	NA
Van Kasteren et al[11] (1990)	30	G_1	Obstructive	Palpitations after exercise		None.	NA	Spontaneous vaginal	NA	2850 g female, normal
	32	G_2P_1	See above	See above		None.	NA	NA	NA	3030 g male, normal
Van Kasteren et al[11] (1990)	23	G_1	Nonobstructive	Family history of HCM, sister died in 6th wk gestation		Bleeding and premature contractions starting at 29 wks; premature delivery.	32	Spontaneous vaginal with forceps	NA	Fetal distress during delivery; 1250 g female, normal
Tessler et al[12] (1990)	27	G_3P_2	Obstructive	None; 2 previous uneventful pregnancies		None.	37	Elective C-section due to previous C-section	General	None
Tessler et al[12] (1990)	29	G_1P_0	Obstructive		IV propranolol during delivery	Dyspnea at rest, occasional palpitations, pulmonary edema during labor, possible fluid overload.	39	Spontaneous vaginal with forceps	Epidural	Neonatal hypoglycemia, possibly due to propranolol
Pelliccia et al[15] (1992)	27		Nonobstructive	None		Sudden death at 28 wks.				
Bascou et al[14] (1993)	29	G_1	Obstructive	Syncope during effort, exertional dyspnea and chest pain, moderate MR	Atenolol	Hospitalized at 30 wks for dyspnea.	39	C-section due to fetal distress	General	Postpartum hypoglycemia

(continued)

TABLE 9.1 (Continued)

Ref: First Author	Age (yrs)	Obstetric History	Form of HCM	Prepregnancy History and Risk Factors	Drugs During Pregnancy	Maternal Complications	Week of Labor	Delivery Mode	Anesthesia	Fetal/ Newborn Outcome/ Complications
Gras et al[13] (1992)	23		Obstructive	Paroxysmal atrial fibrillation requiring electrical cardioversion and treatment with multiple antiarrhythmic drugs; because of sinus nodal dysfunction, rate-responsive atrial pacemaker was implanted		Atrial fibrillation at 10 wks requiring electrical cardioversion at 5 months for fetal distress. Resistant SVT, ablation of AV conduction at 5th month gestation; then rate-responsive ventricular pacemaker implantation.	8th month	Vaginal		Fetal distress induced by maternal tachycardia, normal at delivery
Coven et al[17] (1994)						Rapid atrial fibrillation at 30 wks with dyspnea, hypotension, palpitations. Treated successfully with dc cardioversion.	36	C-section; reason NA	General anesthesia	No effect of dc cardioversion on fetal cardiac rhythm or rate
Rowe et al[18] (1994)	33	NA	Obstructive	Dyspnea, palpitations, decreased activity tolerance, one episode of presyncope	Metoprolol, verapamil	Admission at 22 wks for chest heaviness and palpitations, NSVT. Diagnostic cath at 22 wks. DDD pacemaker in wk 24 with improvement of symptoms; no change in NSVT.	NA	NA	NA	None
Goodwin* (1995)	26	$G_3P_0Ab_2$		Renal transplantation, hypertension, history of seizure disorder; heart failure	Prednisone, imuran, verapamil, clonidine, Inderal, Dilantin	Worsening of CHF admitted with pulmonary edema at 31 wks.	32	Elective C-section due to heart failure	General	1331 g female, normal

Abbreviations: AB, abortion; AV, atrioventricular; C, cesarean; cath, catheterization; CHF, congestive heart failure; dc, direct current; DDD, dual chamber; G, gravida; HCM, hypertrophic cardiomyopathy; IHSS, an obstructive hypertrophic cardiomyopathy; MI, myocardial infarction; NA, information not available; P, para; SVT, supraventricular tachycardia; NSVT, nonsustained ventricular tachycardia; VT, ventricular tachycardia; wk, week; yrs, years.
*, case unpublished or personal communication

which was due to maternal mortality secondary to ventricular arrhythmia.[15]

DIAGNOSIS IN PREGNANCY

In the appropriate clinical setting, such as the presence of suggestive clinical features or a family history of the disease, further testing is indicated to establish the diagnosis. Echocardiography is a definitive test for the diagnosis of HCM and can be safely used during pregnancy. Doppler technique can be used to assess the presence of left ventricular outflow obstruction and mitral regurgitation. Since the use of ionizing radiation is hazardous to the fetus (Chapter 3), cardiac catheterization for diagnosing HCM should be avoided during pregnancy.

MANAGEMENT DURING PREGNANCY

Prepregnancy Evaluation

A detailed evaluation prior to conception is needed to determine the potential risks associated with pregnancy and to develop an appropriate therapeutic strategy aimed at minimizing risks to both mother and fetus. A detailed discussion with the patient and her family prior to pregnancy is essential. The following issues should be thoroughly covered: effect of the disease on safety of pregnancy for both mother and fetus; potential fetal risks due to medications that may be required during pregnancy; risk of sudden death to the mother during and after pregnancy; and likelihood of transmission of HCM to the child.

Every patient should undergo a detailed evaluation, including history and physical examination, 12-lead electrocardiogram, echo–Doppler study, a thallium exercise test, Holter monitoring and, if indicated, cardiac catheterization and electrophysiological evaluation.[6] Likelihood of hemodynamic worsening due to increased plasma volume may occur, particularly in patients with stiff, noncompliant left ventricles. Patients in this relatively small subset (about 10%), characterized by predominantly restrictive physiology, often have only mild hypertrophy but may have atrial enlargement and early presentation, with atrial arrhythmias and emboli. In contrast, in patients with left ventricular outflow tract obstruction and predominantly upper septal hypertrophy, pregnancy-mediated increased plasma volume may result in a favorable hemodynamic effect (personal communication WJ McKenna). Since severity of hemodynamic abnormalities and symptoms may increase during pregnancy, patients with moderate or severe symptoms of heart failure should be advised against pregnancy. Such patients should attempt pregnancy only if a significant symptomatic improvement (to New York Heart Association functional class I or II) can be

easily achieved with drugs safe for the fetus, (β-adrenergic blocking agents, calcium channel blockers, disopyramide), dual-chamber pacing, or surgical treatment (myectomy, mitral valve repair).

The following findings have been associated with increased risk of sudden death in patients with HCM: syncopal or presyncopal episodes, family history of premature sudden death, evidence of ventricular arrhythmias on Holter monitoring, left ventricular outflow obstruction, and evidence of myocardial ischemia. The appropriate approach to the high risk patients prior to concentration is not well established, and the value of electrophysiological studies is not proven. However, because of the well-documented arrhythmogenic effect of pregnancy (Chapter 13), the performance of electrophysiological evaluation makes good clinical sense and should be considered in every patient at high risk for sudden death. Sustained ventricular tachycardia (monomorphic or polymorphic) and ventricular fibrillation have been shown to be strong predictors for subsequent cardiac events. The finding of such arrhythmias, either occurring spontaneously or induced, was suggested by the group from the National Institutes of Health (NIH) as an indication for treatment with an automatic implanted cardiac defibrillator (AICD).[19] This approach has not been supported by other groups with large experience of HCM, and high risk nonpregnant patients with obstructive HCM have been treated successfully with dual-chamber pacing[20] or myectomy[21] alone without AICD. However, because of the potential arrhythmogenic effect of pregnancy itself and the risk of electrophysiological studies during pregnancy, we do recommend the use of AICD in such patients who intend to become pregnant.

Likelihood of Transmission of HCM to the Child

HCM is now known to be caused by mutations in several contractile protein genes. In at least half of the patients, the disease is familial and has an autosomal dominant pattern of inheritance. Relatively recent studies by Maron et al[22] and Greaves et al[23] using cross-sectional and M-mode echocardiography, respectively, evaluated 139 and 75 offsprings of patients with HCM. These studies found echocardiographic evidence for HCM in 14 and 8% of offspring, respectively.

MANAGEMENT OF THE PATIENT WITH HCM DURING PREGNANCY

The Asymptomatic Patient

In the asymptomatic patient with mild disease, no prophylactic treatment is necessary, and the outcome of pregnancy is usually good. Close follow-up is mandatory, however, since hemodynamic and clinical worsening may occur at later stages of pregnancy and during labor and delivery.[12] In patients with resting or provokable left ventricular outflow obstruction, an increase in myocardial contractility and a decrease in ventricular size or left ventricular afterload may cause worsening of left ventricular outflow obstruction and should be avoided or corrected. Such changes may be caused by hypovolemia secondary to diuresis or blood loss, vasodilatation due to drugs or anesthesia, cardiostimulation due to digoxin or sympathomimetic agents, and the Valsalva maneuver. It is important to note, however, that the strain of vaginal delivery is usually well tolerated by women with HCM, and cesarean section is not indicated in most patients (Table 9.1).

Treatment of Symptoms

Specific indications for drug therapy include symptoms such as dyspnea, angina, dizziness, syncope, and palpitations and the presence of arrhythmias. Since a patient's response to the available drugs is variable, therapy should be tailored individually to achieve efficacy while using drugs known to be safe to both the mother and the fetus. The approach to treatment of dyspnea should be based on left ventricular systolic function. In most patients with HCM, symptoms of dyspnea are related to elevated pulmonary venous pressures due to impaired left ventricular diastolic function. In such patients, inotropic intervention such as administration of digoxin is unlikely to help and may even worsen symptoms by increasing outflow obstruction. β-Adrenergic receptor or calcium channel blocking agents are often useful,[6] and diuretic agents may be needed to improve symptoms of dyspnea in such patients.[6a] In the minority of patients, congestive heart failure symptoms are due to decrease in systolic function. In these patients the management of heart failure can include digitalis, diuretics, and vasodilator agents. Because of potential severe side effects, the use of angiotensin-converting enzyme inhibitors is contraindicated during pregnancy (Chapter 32).

β-*Adrenergic* blocking agents have been traditionally used in symptomatic HCM patients during pregnancy with reported good results.[24] The mechanism of action of these drugs in HCM is multifactorial and includes enhancement of left ventricular filling (mainly by reducing heart rate and allowing longer diastolic time) and a direct effect on myocardial distensibility. Beta blockers also decrease myocardial oxygen consumption and sympathetically stimulated left ventricular outflow obstruction and may have antiarrhythmic effects. The use of β-adrenergic blocking agents has been shown to be relatively safe during pregnancy (Chapter 29). It is important, however, to note that complications such as intrauterine growth retardation, neonatal hypoglycemia,[14] bradycardia, and apnea have been described in some newborns. For these reasons, routine use of beta blockers is not recommended, and therapy should be reserved only for symptomatic patients who respond to these drugs. Nonselec-

tive β-adrenergic blocking agents may cause premature uterine contractions; for this reason, drugs with selective effect on β_1 receptors may be preferred during pregnancy.

Calcium channel blockade has also been shown to be effective in the management of patients with symptomatic HCM.[2,6] Verapamil, the drug most widely used and investigated, has been reported to improve both outflow tract obstruction and cardiac symptoms. The mechanisms of the effect of this drug include reduction of myocardial oxygen consumption through its negative chronotropic and inotropic effects and hypotensive action, and improvement of left ventricular diastolic properties. The drug has to be used with caution, since its vasodilating properties may unpredictably increase the obstruction and may even lead to death due to hypotension or pulmonary edema.[25] Verapamil has been used sporadically during pregnancy for the acute treatment of maternal and fetal arrhythmias and in the management of preterm labor and severe eclampsia/preeclampsia without apparent deleterious effects (Chapter 31). *Disopyramide,* a type IA antiarrhythmic agent that has negative inotropic properties, decreases the pressure gradient in a majority of patients with HCM.[26] Oral doses up to 600–800 mg/day are effective.[6] The use of this drug is associated with strong anticholinergic side effects, and in many patients the initial effect is attenuated with time. Although no significant fetal side effects have been reported with disopyramide, the overall experience with the use of this drug in pregnancy is limited (Chapter 30).

A number of recent reports have shown the benefits of *dual-chamber pacing* in reducing or abolishing the left ventricular obstruction.[24,27] This therapeutic technique may work by decreasing or creating paradoxical septal motion, which leads to increased size of the left ventricular outflow track and a progressive reduction of gradient with time. Rowe[18] described a symptomatic pregnant patient with HCM despite treatment with calcium channel and beta blockers; the woman received an atrioventricular sequential pacemaker during pregnancy with improvement of symptoms. Although the initiation of pacemaker therapy during pregnancy seems to be an option in a patient with deteriorating symptoms, the use of ionizing radiation needed for pacemaker implantation is a concern. This therapeutic modality should be reserved for the isolated cases of patients with severe symptoms who do not tolerate or do not respond to medications. *Surgical myectomy* has been used successfully for over 30 years now for the treatment of symptomatic obstructive HCM.[2,6] This technique may provide total relief of resting and provokable outflow obstruction and mitral regurgitation, with improvement in symptoms and decreased risk of atrial fibrillation, syncope, or sudden death. There have been no reports of myectomy surgery during pregnancy. This operation, however, should be considered prior to conception in markedly symptomatic patients with obstructive HCM in spite of medical and pacemaker therapy.

Ventricular Arrhythmias

Since pregnancy is associated with increased incidence of arrhythmias and sudden death has been reported in patients with HCM during gestation,[15] an attempt should be made to identify patients who are at increased risk prior to pregnancy (Fig. 9.1). In a pregnant patient who was not evaluated before conception, this assessment should be done during gestation. Ambulatory electrocardiographic monitoring (Holter) is the best means to detect the presence of arrhythmias during pregnancy. The evaluation of new symptoms of impaired consciousness (syncope, presyncope) is difficult during pregnancy because of high incidence of such symptoms in normal pregnancy.[28] Electrophysiologic studies should be performed only in cases in which the potential benefit of the procedure clearly outweighs the risk. If possible, the procedure should be performed under echocardiographic guidance. When fluoroscopy is used, a strong attempt should be made to minimize fetal exposure to radiation by appropriate shielding, the use of the brachial or internal jugular approach, and a conscious use of minimum fluoroscopy possible.

Supraventricular Arrhythmias

Atrial arrhythmias, especially atrial fibrillation, occur in approximately 10% of patients with HCT, especially in patients with enlarged left atrium (usually > 50 mm),[6] which may be caused by obstructive HCM with concomitant mitral regurgitation and by both diastolic and systolic dysfunction. Both the physiological increase in blood volume and the arrhythmogenic effect of pregnancy increase the likelihood of atrial fibrillation during gestation. The development of this arrhythmia increases risk of systemic emboli and may lead to hemodynamic deterioration.[17] Therapy of this condition should include an attempt to restore sinus rhythm by either drug therapy or electrical cardioversion. Amiodarone has been shown to be the most effective drug for the conversion of atrial fibrillation and maintenance of sinus rhythm in patients with HCM.[29] The use of this drug during pregnancy, however, may be associated with fetal growth restriction, prematurity, and hypothyroidism in the newborn (see Chapter 30). The use of sotalol has also been recommended in young patients with HCM and atrial fibrillation.[6] There is only limited information, however, regarding the safety of this drug during pregnancy. Quinidine is safe for use during pregnancy and may be effective for the conversion of atrial fibrillation and maintenance of sinus rhythm. This drug, however, may be associated with proarrhythmic effect to the mother and increased incidence of malignant ventricular arrhythmias.[30] If quinidine is selected, β-adrenergic blocking agents should be administered concomitantly to prevent an increase in ventricular response due to the vagolytic effect of the drug. Myectomy has been used in patients with obstructive HCM and atrial fibrillation, to reduce left atrial size and restore sinus rhythm.[6] This procedure should be considered prior to pregnancy in a symptomatic patient with atrial fibrillation. Electrical cardioversion has been performed safely during pregnancy for several indications and was used by Coven et al[17] in a patient with HCM who presented during her 30th week of gestation with rapid atrial fibrillation, dyspnea, and hypotension. This procedure should be used for immediate restoration of sinus rhythm in cases entailing hemodynamic compromise. In patients with chronic atrial fibrillation in whom cardioversion has not succeeded despite adequate medical therapy, control of ventricular response is the therapeutic goal. Heart rate control can be achieved in pregnancy with digitalis, calcium antagonists (verapamil, diltiazem), and beta blockers. Because of the potential for hemodynamic deterioration with digitalis in obstructive HCM, and given the more limited experience with chronic use of calcium antagonists during pregnancy, beta blockers should be the first drugs of choice. Atrial fibrillation in patients with HCM has been associated with a substantial risk of thromboembolic complications[2,6] and anticoagulant therapy should therefore be given to such patients. For the recommended approach to anticoagulant therapy in the pregnant patient, see Chapter 33.

MODE OF DELIVERY

Vaginal delivery can be accomplished in patients with HCM without increased risk to the mother or the fetus, even in the symptomatic patient (Table 9.1). Forceps delivery may be used to shorten the second stage of labor,[8,11,12] and cesarean section should be reserved in most cases only for obstetric indications.[9,10,12,14]

Clinical deterioration has been described during labor and delivery in asymptomatic patients with HCM.[12] Such a deterioration may be due to an increase in intravascular blood volume during uterine contraction (Chapter 1). Hemodynamic monitoring using a balloon flotation pulmonary catheter is therefore recommended in symptomatic patients with HCM.

Use of prostaglandins to affect uterine contraction pre- or postpartum should be discouraged in patients with obstructive HCM because of the strong vasodilatory effect of these substances.[31] For similar reasons, a potential detrimental effect of oxytocin has been suggested by some investigators[32] who have, therefore, recommended ergonovine as the preferred agent for induction of labor and involution of the uterus in women with HCM. However, a safe use of oxytocin has been reported in patients with HCM,[8,9,32] and thus the drug does not seem to be contraindicated during pregnancy.

Because of a risk of aggravating left ventricular outflow obstruction, hypovolemia should be avoided during delivery, and blood loss should be estimated and replaced. A good venous access should be established prior to labor, and volume, including cross-matched blood, should be available for potential need. In hypovolemia-induced hypotension, blood pressure can be temporarily restored without inotropic effect by means of vasopressor agents such as phenylephrine or methoxamine. However, the prolonged use of such drugs antepartum is not recommended because they tend to decrease uterine blood flow.

Although epidural anesthesia has been used for delivery in some patients with HCM (Table 9.1), it should be avoided or performed with great caution, especially in patients with spontaneous or provocable left ventricular outflow obstruction. In a personal communication, Dr. William J. McKenna has reported two fatalities following epidural anesthesia. Since tocolytic agents with β-adrenergic stimulating activity may also increase left ventricular outflow obstruction, magnesium sulfate is recommended for tocolysis in patients with obstructive HCM.

ANTIBIOTIC PROPHYLAXIS

HCM, particularly of the obstructive form, is associated with increased risk for bacterial endocarditis.[33] Antibiotic prophylaxis prior to uncomplicated vaginal delivery, cesarean section, and therapeutic abortion is not recommended by the American Heart Association. However, because of the potential devastating effects of bacterial endocarditis and the difficulties of predicting the development of bacteremia, we recommend antibiotic prophylaxis prior to delivery in patients with obstructive HCM.

ACKNOWLEDGMENT

The authors thank Professor William J. McKenna of the Department of Cardiological Sciences at St. George's Hospital Medical School, London, England, for his review of the chapter and his useful comments; many of them were incorporated into this chapter.

REFERENCES

1. Wigle ED. Hypertrophic cardiomyopathy: 1987 view point. *Circulation* 1987;75:311–322.

2. Wynne J, Braunwald E. The cardiomyopathies and myocarditis. In: Braunwald E, ed. *Heart Disease,* 4th ed. Philadelphia: WB Saunders; 1992;1394–1451.

3. Maron BJ, Gardin JM, Flack JM, Gidding SS, Kurosaki TT, Bild DE. Prevalence of hypertrophic cardiomyopathy in a general population of young adults. Echocardiographic analysis of 4,111 subjects in the CARDIA study. Coronary artery risk development in (young) adults. *Circulation* 1995;92:785–788.

4. McKenna WJ, Chetty S, Oakley CM, Goodwin JF. Arrhythmia in hypertrophic cardiomyopathy: exercise and 48-hour ambulatory electrocardiographic assessment with and without beta-adrenergic blocking therapy. *Am J Cardiol* 1980;45:1–5.

5. Feigenbaum H. *Diseases of the Myocardium in Echocardiography,* 5th ed. Philadelphia: Lea & Febiger: 1994:511–526.

6. Wigle ED, Rakowski H, Kimball BP, Williams WG. Hypertrophic cardiomyopathy: clinical spectrum and treatment. *Circulation* 1995;92:1680–1692.

6a. Spirito P, Seidman CE, McKenna WJ, Maron BJ. The management of hypertrophic cardiomyopathy *N Engl J Med* 1997; 336:775 –785.

7. Higgins CB, Byrd BF III, Stark D, McNamara M, Lanzer P, Lipton MJ, Schiller NB, Botvinick E, Chatterjee K. Magnetic resonance imaging in hypertrophic cardiomyopathy. *Am J Cardiol* 1985;55:1121–1126.

8. Minnich ME, Quirk JG, Clark RB. Epidural anesthesia for vaginal delivery in a patient with idiopathic hypertrophic subaortic stenosis. *Anesthesiology* 1987;67:590–692.

9. Boccio RV, Chung JH, Harrison DM. Anesthetic management of cesarean section in a patient with idiopathic hypertrophic subaortic stenosis. *Anesthesiology* 1986;65:663–665.

10. Lette J, Gagnon A, Cerino M, Prenovault J. Apical hypertrophic cardiomyopathy with spontaneous post partum coronary artery dissection. *Can J Cardiol* 1989;5:311–314.

11. Van Kasteren YM, Kleinhout J, Smit MA, von Vugt JMG, van Geijn HP. Hypertrophic cardiomyopathy and pregnancy: a report of three cases. *Eur J Obstet Gynecol Rep Biol* 1990; 38:63–67.

12. Tessler MJ, Hudson R, Naugler MA, Biel DR. Pulmonary edema in two parturients with hypertrophic obstructive cardiomyopathy (HOCM). *Can J Anaesth* 1990;37:469–473.

13. Gras D, Mabo P, Kermarrec A, Bazin P, Varin C, Daubert C. Radiofrequency ablation of atrioventricular conduction during the 5th month of pregnancy. *Arch Mal Coeur Vaiss* 1992;85: 1873–1877.

14. Bascou V, Ferrandis J, Bauer V, Bouret JM, de Meeus JB, Magnin G. Obstructive myocardiopathy and pregnancy. *J Gynecol Obstet Biol Reprod* 1993;22:309–311.

15. Pelliccia F, Cianfrocca L, Gaudio C, Reale A. Sudden death during pregnancy in hypertrophic cardiomyopathy. *Eur Heart J* 1992;13:421–423.

16. Garcia Leon JF, Von der Meden-Alarcon W, Buganza del Castillo A, Ibarrola-Buenabad E, Kably-Ambe A. Hypertrophic cardiomyopathy and pregnancy. Presentation of a case and review of the literature. *Ginecol Obstet Mex* 1993;61:160–162.

17. Coven G, Zizzi S, Cimino F, Demartini L, Noli S, Giordano A, Mapelli A. Electric cardioversion in pregnant patients with obstructive hypertrophic cardiomyopathy. A clinical case. *Minerva Anestesiol.* 1994;60:725–728.

18. Rowe GT. Hypertrophic cardiomyopathy in pregnancy: a case study. *J Cardiovasc Nurs* 1994;8:69–73.

19. Fananapazir L, Chang AC, Epstein SE, McAreavy D. Prognostic determinants in hypertrophic cardiomyopathy: prospective evaluation of a therapeutic strategy based on clinical, Holter, hemodynamic and electrophysiological findings. *Circulation* 1992;86:730–740.

20. McAreavey D, Fananapazir L. DDD pacing may obviate the need for investigation of symptoms of impaired consciousness in hypertrophic cardiomyopathy. *Circulation* 1994;90(suppl II):II–443. Abstract.

21. Borggrete M, Schwammenthal B, Block M, Schalte HD. Pre and postoperative electrophysiologic findings in survivors of cardiac arrest and hypertrophic obstructive cardiomyopathy undergoing myectomy. *Circulation* 1993;88(suppl I):I–210. Abstract.

22. Maron BJ, Nichols PF, Pickle LW, Wesley YE, Mulvihill JJ. Patterns of inheritance in hypertrophic cardiomyopathy: assessment by M-mode and two dimensional echocardiography. *Am J Cardiol* 1984;53:1087–1094.

23. Greaves SC, Roche AHG, Neutze JM, Whitlock RL, Veale AMO. Inheritance of hypertrophic-cardiomyopathy: a cross sectional and M-mode echocardiographic study of 50 families. *Br Heart J* 1987;58:259–266.

24. Fananapazir L, Cannon RO, Triipodi D, Panza JA. Impact of dual-chamber permanent pacing in patients with obstructive hypertrophic cardiomyopathy with symptoms refractory to verapamil and β-adrenergic blocker therapy. *Circulation* 1992; 85:2149–2161.

25. Epstein SE, Rosing DR. Verapamil: its potential for causing serious complication in patients with hypertrophic cardiomyopathy. *Circulation* 1981;64:437–441.

26. Kimball BP, Bui S, Wigle ED. Acute dose–response effects of intravenous disopyramide in hypertrophic obstructive cardiomyopathy. *Am Heart J* 1993;125:1691–1697.

27. Jeanrenaud X, Goy JJ, Kappenberger L. Effects of dual-chamber pacing in hypertrophic obstructive cardiomyopathy. *Lancet* 1992;339:1318–1323.

28. Shotan A, Ostrzega E, Mehra A, Johnson J, Elkayam U. Incidence of arrhythmias in normal pregnancy and relation to palpitations, dizziness and syncope. *Am J Cardiol* 1997;79: 1061–1064.

29. McKenna WJ, Harris L, Rowland E, Kleinebenne A, Krikler DM, Oakley CM, Goodwin JF. Amiodarone for long-term management of patients with hypertrophic cardiomyopathy. *Am J Cardiol* 1984;54:802–810.

30. Coplen SE, Antman EM, Berlin JA, Hewitt P, Chalmers TC. Efficacy and safety of quinidine therapy for maintenance of sinus rhythm after cardioversion. A meta analysis of randomized control trials. *Circulation* 1990;82:1106–1116.

31. Douglas WW. Polypeptides—angiotensin, plasma kinins and other vasoactive agents; prostaglandins. In Gilman AG, Goodman LS, Rall TW, Murad F, eds. *The Pharmacological Basis of Therapeutics,* 7th ed. New York: Macmillan; 1985;639–659.

32. Shah DM, Sunderji SG. Hypertrophic cardiomyopathy and pregnancy: report of a maternal mortality and review of literature. *Obstet Gynecol Survey* 1985;40:444–448.

33. LeJemtel THS, Factor SM, Koenigsberg M, O'Reilly M, Frater R, Sonnenblick EH. Mural vegetations at the site of endocardial trauma in infective endocarditis complicating idiopathic hypertrophic subaortic stenosis. *Am J Cardiol* 1979;44: 569–574.

10

PERICARDIAL DISORDERS AND PREGNANCY

Marla A. Mendelson, MD, and Uri Elkayam, MD

INTRODUCTION

The pericardium, composed of a membranous visceral layer and a fibrous parietal layer, serves to encase and protect the heart.[1] Pericardial fluid is an ultrafiltrate of plasma, and normally there may be 15–50 mL in the pericardial space.[1] The pericardium may become involved in numerous primary and secondary disease processes: the inflammatory response of pericarditis, pericardial effusion, or fibrosis resulting in pericardial constriction. Pericardial inflammation has been found in 2–6% of autopsy studies, (but is clinically recognized only in 0.1% of hospital admissions).[1]

The pericardium may exert a restraining effect on cardiac dilatation, which may explain why the woman with subclinical pericardial disease may first become symptomatic during pregnancy as the heart dilates to accommodate the increased cardiac output. An altered immune response during pregnancy may make a woman of childbearing age more susceptible to infection or inflammation, which in turn may result in pericarditis, the most common form of pericardial disease in the woman of childbearing age. She may also have concomitant illnesses that predispose her to pericardial disease. It is important to consider these historical factors, since the diagnosis of pericardial disease during pregnancy may be difficult and will require a higher index of suspicion if a "risk factor" is present.

ACUTE PERICARDITIS

Probably no serious disease is so frequently overlooked by the practitioner.[2]

—William Osler

Pericarditis is most often a self-limited, mild condition. The severity of disease and hemodynamic consequences vary with the etiology. Often, pericarditis will occur with myocarditis and in conjunction with the already increased blood volume of pregnancy, heart failure may develop. Pericarditis can be detected during pregnancy by the usual diagnostic modalities. Depending on the severity of the presentation, hemodynamic assessment and intervention may be required during pregnancy, but even the most complicated case may be brought safely to term.[3] The incidence is probably similar to the nonpregnant state and the condition can be treated similarly. Therefore there have been a paucity of reported cases.

Etiology

The potential etiologies of acute pericarditis in a woman of childbearing age are summarized in Table 10.1.[1] The pericardium may be involved as a primary process or secondary to another medical illness. Idiopathic pericarditis is probably the most common form of acute pericarditis. The second important category to be considered is trauma, accidental or surgical. Prior chest trauma could include hemopericardium following thoracic surgery, pacemaker insertion, valve replacement, or coronary artery bypass grafting.

Infectious pericarditis may be caused by a variety of viral or bacterial agents. The reported incidence of infectious pericarditis during pregnancy is low. The causative agents discussed would be those most likely to affect a specific population. Viral pericarditis is the most common and may be due to Coxsackie A or B viruses, echovirus, endovirus, mumps, infectious mononucleosis, varicella, hepatitis B, and human immunovirus-1.[1] A case of rubella myopericarditis has been documented during pregnancy.[4] Often there is a nonspecific

Cardiac Problems in Pregnancy, Third Edition
Edited by Uri Elkayam, MD, and Norbert Gleicher, MD
Copyright © 1998 by Wiley-Liss, Inc. ISBN 0-471-16358-9

TABLE 10.1   Etiology of Acute Pericarditis in the Woman of Childbearing Age

Idiopathic
Trauma
Infection
    Viral
    Bacterial
    Fungal
    Tuberculosis
    Other infections: rickettsia, amebiasis, mycoplasma
Radiation
Amyloid
Neoplasm (primary or metastatic)
Sarcoid
Collagen vascular disease
    Rheumatic fever
    Systemic lupus erythematosus
    Rheumatoid arthritis
    Vasculitis
    Scleroderma
    Dermatomyositis
Anticoagulation
Postmyocardial Infarction
Idiopathic thrombocytopenic purpura
Metabolic disorders: uremia, myxedema
Pharmacologic
Dissecting aneurysm
Endocarditis
Thymic cyst

Source: Lorell et al.[1]

viral prodrome with chest pain, lymphadenopathy, or myocarditis. Viral syndromes usually result in fatigue and malaise that may persist for weeks after the chest pain and acute symptoms have abated.

Bacterial pericarditis is often a complication of a bacterial infection elsewhere in the body. The bacterial agents classically involved include pneumococci, staphylococci, streptococci, gram-negative septicemia, *Neisseria,* and *Legionella.*[1] Often, there is a concomitant pneumonia or empyema. The immune-compromised host is susceptible to gram-negative organisms and fungal infections such as histoplasmosis, coccidioidomycosis, *Candida,* and blastomycoses. Other causes of infection are toxoplasmosis, amebiasis, mycoplasma, and *Listeria.*[5]

Tuberculosis should be considered when the patient who has a positive skin test presents with classic signs of weight loss, night sweats, anorexia, arthralgias, and fever. There often are associated large, sanguinous effusions.[6]

It is becoming more common for patients who have had childhood malignancy such as lymphoma or Hodgkin's disease to reach adulthood; therefore, a woman of childbearing age may have undergone prior chest or mediastinal irradiation.[1] This certainly would put her at risk for the development

of pericarditis, pericardial effusion and constrictive pericarditis.

Acute pericarditis may be secondary to another medical illness such as amyloidosis or sarcoidosis.[1] It can be seen in metabolic diseases such as uremia or myxedema. Neoplastic disease also may secondarily involve the pericardium, as seen in lung pathologies including lung cancer, as well as breast cancer, leukemia, Hodgkin's disease, and lymphoma.[1]

Collagen vascular disease often involves the pericardium, specifically in systemic lupus erythematosus, rheumatoid arthritis, and scleroderma. Systemic lupus erythematosus may involve the pericardium in 17–50% of patients, although clinical evidence may only occur in 5% (Table 10.1).[7] There may be exacerbation of lupus during the last trimester of pregnancy and several months postpartum. Treatment with steroids may prevent constriction and tamponade. Pericardial disease is less common in rheumatoid arthritis, and steroid therapy may not be as effective.[8] Other collagen vascular diseases to consider include acute rheumatic fever, Wegener's granulomatosis, and dermatomyositis.[1]

Anticoagulation resulting in hemopericardium is a rare cause of pericarditis. The woman at risk would be taking anticoagulated chronically for atrial fibrillation, pulmonary embolus, or a mechanical prosthetic valve. Either overanticoagulation in the setting of subclinical pericarditis or superimposed trauma with therapeutic anticoagulation could result in a hemopericardium. This patient would have had thoracic surgery or some other disease process present.

As the population of women of childbearing age becomes older, obstetrical patients with a history of coronary artery disease or myocardial infarction may be encountered. Pericarditis has been described after myocardial infarction and as a result of a pericardiotomy and may be the cause, though this is less likely in the woman of childbearing age.

As women with medical illnesses become pregnant, they may be taking medications known to cause pericardial inflammation (e.g., hydralazine, procainamide, diphenylhydantoin, isoniazide, penicillin, methotrexate).[1,9] Though dissecting aneurysm, vascular rupture, a chylopericardium, endocarditis, and thymic cyst are rare clinical events, these conditions have the potential to cause pericardial inflammation, or effusion as well.[1]

Clinical Presentation

Symptoms   Chest pain is the most common complaint in the patient with pericarditis. It is usually sharp and stabbing and may radiate to the back, neck, left shoulder, or upper arm. It may vary in quality and location. Classically, the pain is relieved by leaning forward and is exacerbated by lying supine, swallowing, breathing deeply, or coughing. The differential diagnosis may include acute abdomen, myocardial infarction, esophageal spasm, or pulmonary embolus. Dyspnea is also a common presentation, especially when a moderately large pericardial effusion is present. This occurs with impaired filling of the ventricle due to an effusion and/or mechanical compression of the lung parenchyma (Ewart's sign) and bronchi.[1] Mechanical compression may also cause hoarseness, coughing, and dysphasia. Dyspnea during the latter half of pregnancy may be misconstrued as hyperventilation of pregnancy.

Signs   A pericardial friction rub is a pathognomonic finding in pericarditis described as a "leathery" or grating sound best heard over the second and fourth left intercostal space in the midclavicular line or at the left sternal border. It is best heard with diaphragm on the stethoscope while the patient is leaning forward and deeply inspiring. The rub may be evanescent. It is often of three components corresponding to presystole, systole, and early diastolic filling. It may also have only two components. A third heart sound may also be present. The pericardial friction rub remains constant throughout the respiratory cycle, does not radiate as would a heart murmur, often is loudest in the left sternal border rather than in a specific valve area, and may change in quality at different times of examination.[1] Tachycardia has been noted frequently.

On examination of the chest, lungs are often clear to auscultation. Ewart's sign is dullness below the left scapula if there is lung compression caused by a large pericardial effusion. Neck veins are distended in the presence of large effusion or pericardial constriction due to elevated right ventricular diastolic pressure, causing an elevation in right atrial pressure.

Generalized symptoms, especially in viral pericarditis, may include upper respiratory symptoms preceding the onset of chest pain, a low grade fever, lymphadenopathy, myalgias, or a rash. In a viral illness, symptoms of fatigue and malaise may persist for weeks after the chest pain has subsided. Pericarditis secondary to systemic illnesses may have clinical features to suggest the underlying etiology such as fever, cough, cachexia, edema, or ascites.

Diagnostic Evaluation

Blood tests may suggest the underlying cause of pericarditis: for example, leukocytosis, lymphocytosis, an elevated level of antinuclear antibodies, a positive tuberculin test, positive blood cultures, elevated cardiac enzymes or infections, or specific antibody titers. Diagnostic testing aids in assessing the severity of pericarditis and sequelae of the disease.

Electrocardiogram

Electrocardiographic changes have been reported in up to 80% of patients with acute pericarditis. Initially, there is ST-segment elevation in multiple leads. This elevation often has a characteristic upward concavity with upright T waves. These changes may occur within the first hour after chest pain or fever. Most commonly, the elevations are seen in leads I, II, V_5, and V_6 and persist for hours to days. These phase I changes may also be accompanied with PR-segment depression. The second phase consists of a return of the ST segment to the isoelectric baseline. The T waves remain upright, and the PR segment may be isoelectric or depressed. Late in this phase, T waves begin to flatten and invert. Phase III is characterized by isoelectric ST segments with diffuse T-wave inversion. The PR segment is isoelectric at this time.[1] The fourth phase is characterized by isoelectric ST segments and the return of upright T waves within weeks to months.[10]

Sinus tachycardia is probably the most common cardiac rhythm, and there may be transient atrial fibrillation or atrial flutter. Rarely, sinus bradycardia is seen.[1]

Chest X-Ray

In the pregnant woman, a chest X-ray is indicated only when pneumonia is suspected. If a chest X-ray is obtained for another reason, pericarditis or pericardial effusion may be the explanation for an enlarged cardiac silhouette. A chest X-ray may be helpful for any underlying lung process, such as neoplasm or tuberculosis. In idiopathic pericarditis, pulmonary infiltrates and pleural effusion are not uncommon. The cardiac shadow will not be enlarged until 250–300 mL of pericardial fluid has accumulated.[1]

Echocardiogram

Echocardiography is a very important noninvasive modality in the study of pericarditis. It may reveal thickening of the pericardium, size of pericardial effusion, and most importantly, evidence of cardiac tamponade.[11] Echocardiography also provides information about valvular and myocardial function, which may help to determine the etiology of the pericardial process. In patients with concomitant myocarditis, there may be left ventricular systolic dysfunction. If an effusion has impaired diastolic filling, the diastolic dimension of the left ventricle will be normal or small, with good systolic contraction of left ventricle. Echocardiography permits assessment of course of pericarditis, to determine whether a pericardial effusion is increasing.

In a study of 21 pregnant women without heart disease during the third trimester, 43% had pericardial effusions.[12] The patients were asymptomatic of mild, moderate, or even large pericardial effusions. There was no sign of infection (leukocytosis) or serum protein abnormality.

Ultrafast computed tomography can assess the thickness of the pericardium, but of course carries the risk of radiation during pregnancy. This technique may establish the diagnosis of constriction. Magnetic resonance imaging has also been used in pregnancy and may have value as an aid in determining the etiology of the pericardial effusion and the thickness of the pericardium.

Management

Initially, bed rest and hospitalization for observation may be indicated in the pregnant patient with acute pericarditis, while evaluation ensues to rule out any of the other causes of pericarditis that may be present. In the nonpregnant state, pericarditis is usually self-limited, with the inflammation lasting 2–6 weeks.[13] It is not uncommon for pericarditis to recur in 20–28% of patients.[14] In idiopathic pericarditis associated with a pericardial effusion, 9% may develop mild pericardial constriction.[14] Tamponade has been reported in up to 15% of patients with pericarditis.[13]

Complications of pericarditis may include arrhythmias, which are usually treated as in the nonpregnant state. Sinus tachycardia does not need to be treated but may be an indication of progression to tamponade or constriction. Atrial fibrillation may occur, possibly resulting in heart failure. Especially at risk would be the pregnant woman who has significantly increased blood volume. With hemodynamic compromise and the loss of an atrial "kick," congestive heart failure may ensue. In the setting of atrial fibrillation, the rate can be slowed by a variety of agents, including digoxin and β-adrenergic blocking agents. Quinidine and procainamide can be used to convert the sinus rhythm, although this is rarely necessary because the arrhythmias are transient. Direct current cardioversion should be reserved for situations of hemodynamic compromise.[15]

The pain of pericarditis often responds to nonsteroidal anti-inflammatory agents such as aspirin (325–650 mg) orally every 3–4 hours.[1] Nonsteroidal anti-inflammatory agents, including indomethocin (25–50 mg orally), also can be effective. For severe persistent pain, over 48 hours, corticosteroids could be used. Prednisone may be given in amounts of 60–80 mg per day in divided doses. When the patient is asymptomatic, the steroids may be tapered. Steroids should not be used if tuberculosis is suspected. Exacerbation of symptoms may occur once steroids have been withdrawn. Antibiotics should be used only in cases of documented bacterial or tuberculous pericarditis. The agents and doses used are as in the nonpregnant state.

Pericardiocentesis and/or biopsy may be performed in the pregnant person by the subxyphoid approach. This also may be required for purposes of diagnosis, especially in the case of bacterial pericarditis. Pericardiectomy may be indicated for relapsing pericarditis that is refractory to medical management and can increase the yield of diagnosing tuberculosis during pregnancy. Specific diagnosis of inflammatory or neoplastic pericardial disease can be made by epicardial and pericardial biopsy and by cytologic analysis of the pericardial fluid.[16]

Acute Pericarditis During Pregnancy

Few cases of acute, idiopathic pericarditis during pregnancy responding to conventional therapy and associated with uncomplicated term delivery have been reported.[17–21] The incidence may be the same as in the general population, given the rarity of reports in the literature. Chest pain was the most common initial presentation.[3,17,18] Hagley, Simpson et al described a case of acute idiopathic pericarditis resulting in pulmonary edema complicated by cardiac tamponade.[19,20] Pajuelo-Gallego et al described a case of pericarditis with involvement of the myocardium (myopericarditis) in the third trimester of an uncomplicated pregnancy.[21] Treatment was most often aspirin and/or steroids.[3]

There have been reports of infectious pericarditis during pregnancy caused by staphylococci,[22] meningococci,[23] *Hemophilus influenza*,[24] rubella,[4] and *Listeria*,[5] and secondary to a pleural empyema.[25] The course of pregnancy in these women was complicated by fetal death,[4,23] maternal heart failure,[4] and pericardiectomy.[22,24]

Pericarditis associated with systemic lupus erythematosus has also been reported.[26,27] Both patients developed cardiac tamponade in the postpartum period. It has been suggested that exacerbation of systemic lupus erythematosus may occur during pregnancy.[28] Duclos et al reported on a woman with Takayasu's disease who initially presented with acute pericarditis and tamponade in the fifth month of pregnancy. In addition, there is one reported case of chylopericardium,[30] a rare disorder associated with mechanical obstruction of the thoracic duct or impedance of drainage occurring as a postoperative or posttraumatic complication or due to neoplasm or tuberculosis. The patient had an uneventful delivery but required pericardiocentesis during the postpartum period.

Viral or idiopathic pericarditis usually has a benign course during pregnancy and should not alter the course of the pregnancy.[3] The pain usually responds to aspirin therapy but steroids may be required.

The differential diagnosis in the woman of childbearing age would include pulmonary embolism, myocardial infarction, or aortic dissection. Pulmonary embolism, which may manifest as pleuritic chest pain, may be associated with dyspnea, tachycardia, and hemoptysis. Myocardial infarction is less likely unless associated risk factors are present. The quality of pain is different, since there is often a nonpleuritic exertional component described as a constant, retrosternal chest pressure. It is relieved by nitroglycerin and does not change with position. Even during pregnancy, angina in the nondiabetic female should be readily identifiable. Pericarditis may develop 24–72 hours after the onset of pain. Aortic dissection is described as a sharp, tearing pain, radiating to the back. It is often associated with decreasing loss of distal pulses, aortic insufficiency, hypotension, and possibly hemodynamic compromise.

PERICARDIAL EFFUSION, CARDIAC TAMPONADE, AND PERICARDIAL CONSTRICTION

General Considerations

Pericardial effusion, cardiac tamponade, and pericardial constriction are extremely rare during pregnancy but may occur as sequelae of pericarditis as described above. Small pericardial effusions have been documented by echocardiography in the course of normal pregnancy, regardless of trimester or any etiologic factor.[12,31] In abnormal conditions, the size of the effusion and the rapidity of accumulation of the fluid will determine the effect on diastolic filling and the development of cardiac tamponade. Pericardial effusion may be generalized or regional and can ultimately lead to right atrial and right ventricular collapse with hemodynamic compromise.[1] Initially this occurs during early diastole but later extends throughout the diastole so that ventricular filling becomes impaired. The inability of the right ventricle to expand during end diastole causes a rapid rise of right ventricular end diastolic pressure, followed by an increase in the right atrial pressure. In addition to restriction to right ventricular diastolic filling, a decrease in stroke volume and blood pressure occurs with compensatory tachycardia. The increase in right atrial pressure results in retrograde elevation of the venous pressure clinically manifested by distention of the neck veins. A paradoxical pulse in which the systolic blood pressure decrease is greater than 15–20 mmHg on quiet inspiration is caused by increased venous return and filling of the right ventricle and inspiration. The normal value used for this disparity should be less than 10 mmHg. The right ventricle then encroaches on the left ventricle, causing a decrease in stroke volume and a decrease in cardiac output and systolic blood pressure.

Pericardial constriction occurs when there is fibrosis of the pericardium, often due to a prior process, and this limits the diastolic filling of one or both ventricle. During pregnancy, both ventricles distend to accommodate the increased blood volume. Therefore, it is possible that with the normal hemodynamic changes of pregnancy, the woman with subclinical constriction may become symptomatic during the latter half of pregnancy.

Etiology

The etiologies of the pericardial effusion in a woman of childbearing age are summarized in Table 10.2. The most

TABLE 10.2 The Etiology of a Percardial Effusion During Pregnancy

Acute pericarditis (see Table 10.1)
Neoplastic
Postirradiation
Posttraumatic
Pharmacologic
Collagen vascular disease
Postpericardiotomy (Dressler's) syndrome
AIDS
Chronic myxedema
Idiopathic

common cause in pregnancy is idiopathic or viral pericarditis.[19–21] Other reported causes of pericardial effusion in pregnancy include Takayasu's disease.[29]

The potential acute and subacute etiologies of cardiac tamponade during pregnancy are summarized in Table 10.3. Reported cases have described tamponade secondary to hemopericardium due to rupture of a dissecting aneurysm of the pulmonary artery in a 27-year-old pregnant woman who had uncorrected patent ductus arteriosus and severe pulmonary hypertension.[32] Subacute tamponade has been reported in the setting of idiopathic or viral pericarditis.[19,20]

Pericardial constriction during pregnancy is rare, but potential etiologies in the woman of childbearing age are summarized in Table 10.4. Reported cases during pregnancy described constrictive pericarditis secondary to irradiation[33,34] (which resulted in maternal death in one case[33]), recurrent pericarditis secondary to juvenile rheumatoid arthritis,[35] and unknown cause.[34,36]

Clinical Findings

The presenting symptoms may help distinguish between the clinical entities under discussion. Patients with pericardial effusions may complain of weakness, malaise, dyspnea or or-

TABLE 10.3 The Etiology of Cardiac Tamponade During Pregnancy

ACUTE
Trauma
Cardiovascular rupture
SUBACUTE
Subacute pericarditis
Neoplasm
Uremia
Tuberculosis
Anticoagulation

TABLE 10.4   The Etiology of Pericardial Constriction During Pregnancy

Idiopathic
Pericarditis
Prior cardiothoracic surgery
Neoplasm
Postirradition (mediastinal)
Tuberculosis
Collagen vascular disease

thopnea and, at times, a dull chest pain or pressure. There may be a cough, dysphagia, or hiccups due to mechanical compression of the lungs, esophagus, or phrenic nerve. Compression of the laryngeal nerve may cause hoarseness. The absence of paroxysmal nocturnal dyspnea will help distinguish cardiac tamponade from heart failure. Edema may be present, and hepatomegaly may result in right upper quadrant discomfort and tenderness. Cardiac tamponade is associated with dyspnea, agitation, or stupor. Pericardial constriction is associated with dyspnea, cough, orthopnea, ascites, and edema.

Signs

Neck vein distention and clear lungs are found in both constriction and tamponade. Differentiation between these two diagnoses may be difficult, Table 10.5; compares the clinical presentations of pericardial constriction and cardiac tamponade. In both entities, tachycardia, hypotension, and narrow pulse pressure (<30 mmHg) may be present. Ascites and hepatomegaly may occur in the later stages during pregnancy. In the setting of cardiac tamponade a pericardial friction rub may be heard. Neck veins are distended and demonstrate an X but no Y descent. Systemic arterial pressure decreases. Kussmaul's sign, which is a distention of neck veins increasing with inspiration is pathognomonic for pericardial constriction; neck veins are distended and demonstrate prominent X and Y descents. In addition, the setting of constriction, a prominent diastolic pericardial knock can be heard and can even be palpable.

Diagnostic Evaluation

Chest X-Ray   A large pericardial effusion may increase the cardiac silhouette on chest X-ray, resulting in the so-called water-bottle configuration. Pericardial constriction, however, is associated with a normal or small heart shadow. Calcification of the pericardium may be present on the chest X-ray.[36] Most often lung fields are clear. Pleural effusions may be present.[1]

Electrocardiogram   In the setting of pericardial effusion or constriction, there may be decreased QRS voltage and flattening of the T waves. Electrical alternans is observed, with large effusions or cardiac tamponade. This effect is due to swinging of the heart within the pericardial space.[1] Atrial fibrillation can occur with constrictive pericarditis.

Echocardiogram   An echo-free space between the pericardium and the epicardium is seen in pericardial effusion or tamponade. Echocardiogram permits identification of the location, amount, and extent of the effusion. It is important to document whether there is a diastolic compression of the right atrium and possibly the right ventricle from cardiac tamponade. Posterior motion of the interventricular septum occurs, with the increase in right ventricular end diastolic volume, and a decrease in the left ventricular end diastolic volume during inspiration is seen early in tamponade.[11]

In pericardial constriction, the echocardiogram may demonstrate a thickened visceral pericardium (epicardium) and bright parietal pericardium. An effusion may be absent. Thickening of the pericardium may be better detected on a transesophageal echocardiogram, or by means of magnetic resonance imaging and ultrafast computed tomography. Both in pericardial tamponade and constriction, early mitral flow as recorded by the Doppler technique is reduced with the onset of inspiration and returns to normal with expiration. In contrast, tricuspid flow is diminished with the onset of expiration.[11]

Hemodynamic Evaluation

Right heart catheterization with a pulmonary artery balloon flotation catheter establishes the diagnosis of pericardial tam-

TABLE 10.5   The Clinical Manifestations: Pericardial Constriction Versus Cardiac Tamponade

	Pericardial Constriction	Cardiac Tamponade
Timing of symptoms	Weeks to years	Hours/days
Chest pain history	Remote	Common
Pulsus paradoxus	Often present	Marked
Kussmaul's sign	Present	Absent
Pericardial calcification	Present	Absent
Pericardial effusion	May be absent	Present
Atrial fibrillation	Often present	Absent

ponade at the bedside or in the catheterization laboratory. There is equalization of the mean right atrial pressure, right ventricular diastolic pressure, pulmonary artery diastolic pressure, and mean pulmonary artery wedge pressure (within 5 mmHg). Pericardial constriction would also demonstrate equalization of pressure. However, there would be early diastolic dip-and-plateau ("square root sign") pattern that is often seen in constriction. The right atrial tracing in constriction demonstrates a prominent X and Y descent. The right ventricle also has the dip-and-plateau contour of the pressure tracing.[1]

Treatment and Prognosis

In the pregnant patient with dyspnea or circulatory failure,[34] neck vein distension, and chest pain, a careful search for historical features suggestive of pericardial effusion, constriction, or tamponade should be sought. It is the high index of clinical suspicion that helps establish early diagnosis and intervention. Fortunately, echocardiography can be done at bedside to help establish the diagnosis. Women who are dyspneic and hypotensive, with neck vein distension, may deteriorate clinically in the setting of diuresis, although their symptoms may be mistaken for congestive heart failure. Diuresis further drops the right ventricular filling pressures, stroke volume, cardiac output, and blood pressure. These patients require increased fluids to maintain the ventricular filling.

Pericardiocentesis to remove the pericardial fluid is the treatment for pericardial tamponade. This is often followed by continued drainage of fluid with a temporary indwelling catheter. This can be performed on an emergency basis at the bedside or in the cardiac catheterization laboratory with electrocardiographic monitoring and fluoroscopic guidance. Echocardiography can also be used during the procedure.[37] The subxiphoid approach is most often used. Fluid should be evaluated to detect underlying etiology. While preparations for the procedure are under way, the blood pressure and cardiac filling must be maintained with intravenous fluids or, if appropriate, blood. This volume expansion helps prevent hemodynamic compromise by delaying right ventricular collapse.[32]

Once they become symptomatic, patients with pericardial constriction will often require surgical pericardiectomy. The patient can remain asymptomatic for many years, in which case she can be followed clinically. It is possible for women with subclinical constriction to become symptomatic at the time of pregnancy, due to hemodynamic changes which may necessitate a right heart catheterization during pregnancy. At the time of labor and delivery, monitoring of right heart pressures may be indicated to help maintain adequate filling of the right ventricle.

Pericardial Effusion and Tamponade in Pregnancy

Asymptomatic pericardial effusion is commonly found in women without evidence of cardiac disease.[12,31,38] Such an effusion is noted during all three trimesters but is most commonly found in the third trimester, with resolution postpartum. It has been more often observed in primigravidas with significant weight gain (>12 kg). Two studies of asymptomatic, idiopathic effusion during pregnancy demonstrated a prevalence of up to 40%.[12,31] However, these studies were small and there may have been inherent selection bias.

Pericardial effusion during pregnancy as a result of pericarditis has been reported.[19] The patient presented in the 21st week of gestation with profound dyspnea and orthopnea but no previous history. She was treated initially with digoxin and furosemide and ultimately underwent a surgical pericardiectomy with drainage. After the procedure she went on to a normal term delivery. Methotrexate-related pericarditis complicated by pericardial effusion was described in a patient who was receiving methotrexate for a molar pregnancy.[9] A case of cardiac tamponade during pregnancy was described in 1989 by Simpson et al.[20] The patient presented at 32 weeks' gestation with symptoms of pleuritic chest pain. Examination revealed jugular venous distension, and pulmonary edema was noted on the chest X-ray. The electrocardiogram was remarkable for electrical alternans. An echocardiogram documented a large pericardial effusion. Right heart catheterization revealed equalization of pressures, and the patient underwent pericardiocentesis with drainage. The fluid did not reveal evidence of infection or malignancy. Preterm labor commenced after the procedure. Duclos et al[29] described tamponade in a 21-year-old woman with Takayasu's disease which followed a miscarriage.

Pericardial Constriction During Pregnancy

Review of the medical literature reveals infrequent reports of constrictive pericarditis during pregnancy. Table 10.6 summarizes cases of pericardial constriction during pregnancy reported since 1966.[33,34,39–43] The reported etiologies include postirradiation, postpericarditis, prior thoracic surgery, and juvenile rheumatoid arthritis.

Most often symptoms were manifested during the latter half of pregnancy, when blood volume approaches maximal levels. However, women presented as early as 13 weeks[39] or during the postpartum period.[36] Symptoms were often severe dyspnea, marked edema, and ascites. Hepatomegaly and distended neck veins were observed.[36] Diagnosis was established by right heart catheterization in two reports.[39,40]

Medical therapy consisted of diuretics[39,42] and steroids.[41] Pericardiectomy was required during pregnancy[40,41] or in some cases postpartum.[36,39] Adverse obstetric outcomes included preterm delivery[36,39,41] and infant death.[42]

Successful pregnancies following pericardiectomy for constrictive pericarditis have been reported. In 1966 Mendelson reviewed six patients who had pericardiectomies with 10 subsequent pregnancies among them.[44] One miscarriage occurred, and two pregnancies were terminated for reasons un-

TABLE 10.6 Pericardial Constriction During Pregnancy: Summary of Reported Cases

Ref: First Author	Etiology	Onset of Symptoms (gestational week)	Treatment	Comments
Mendelson[44] (1966)		24	Medical	Viable preterm infant
Szekely[45] (1974)	Calcific		None	Postpartum pericardiectomy
Richardson[40] (1970)		24	Surgical[a]	Mild symptoms during three pregnancies
Watson[41] (1980)	I/P	32		Premature delivery after pregnancies
Szekely[45] (1974)		12	Surgical[a]	Premature delivery
Blake[48] (1984)	S	34	Diuretics	Pericardiectomy 3 months postpartum
Blake[48] (1984)	S	13	Diuretics	Pericardiectomy 3 months postpartum
Sachs[35] (1986)	JRA	32	None	Recurrent pericarditis
Lessing[36] (1987)	Calcific	Postpartum	None	Pericardiectomy
Bakri[42] (1992)	I	20	Diuretics	Preterm labor, nonviable fetus

[a]Pericardiectomy.

Abbreviations: I, postirradiation; JRA, juvenile rheumatoid arthritis; P, pericarditis; S, prior thoracic surgery.

related to the cardiac status. No heart failure or maternal deaths were reported. Jaluvka[43] reported on a woman with two normal pregnancies following pericardiectomy for tuberculous constrictive pericarditis, and Szekely and Snaith briefly reported on one patient who had a normal pregnancy 2 years following pericardiectomy.[45]

The surgical literature reports an estimated mortality of 4–6% for pericardiectomy in nonpregnant patients.[1] Maternal mortality during pericardiectomy was estimated to be similar.[46] Fetal mortality rates from pericardiectomy have not been reported. Richardson et al[40] have suggested that fetal mortality rates associated with pericardiectomy may be comparable to that associated with closed mitral valvulotomy, which is approximately 7–9%.[47] Therefore, the estimated maternal mortality from pericardiectomy is approximately 4% and the associated fetal mortality may be 9%.

In summary, constrictive pericarditis during pregnancy should be managed medically if symptoms and hemodynamic abnormalities are not severe. In symptomatic patients, hemodynamic monitoring during labor, delivery, and the puerperium is helpful in maintaining optimal cardiac output.[35,39,41,48] If constriction appears severe, pericardiectomy can be performed with a reasonable maternal and fetal risk. The clinical response to pericardiectomy is usually very good, and subsequent pregnancies are usually well tolerated.

ABSENCE OF THE LEFT PERICARDIUM

Congenital absence of the pericardium is a rare occurrence, identified at autopsy in 3 of 27,000 patients.[49,50] This congenital anomaly most often involves the left pericardium and usually presents with chest pain, dizziness, syncope, and peripheral emboli. Total absence of the pericardium is not associated with symptoms.[1] As with most congenital anomalies, there may be associated congenital cardiac disorders such as atrial septal defect or bicuspid aortic valve.[1] Death can occur as a result of strangulation of a herniated left atrial appendage.[51] Savage and Nolan reported on a pregnancy in a 22-year-old Malaysian woman with partial absence of the left pericardium, documented by a prominent left atrial appendage on the chest X-ray.[52] The patient presented at 28 weeks of gestation with chest wall pain and had an uncomplicated vaginal delivery under local anesthesia at 41 weeks of gestation.

PERICARDIAL CYSTS

Pericardial cysts are rare congenital anomalies usually found at the right costophrenic angle. There may be chest pain due to enlargement or torsion.[1] Pregnancy complicated by this developmental abnormality has not been reported.

REFERENCES

1. Lorell BH, Braunwald E. Pericardial disease. In: Braunwald E, ed. *Heart Disease,* 4th ed. Philadelphia: WB Saunders; 1992;1465–1516.

2. Osler W. *The Principles and Practice of Medicine.* New York: D Appleton; 1972:1892.

3. Krausz Y, Naparstek E, Eliakim M. Idiopathic pericarditis and pregnancy. *Aust N Z J Obstet Gynaecol* 1978;18:86–89.

4. Fujimoto T, Katoh C, Hayakawa H Yokota M, Kimura E. Two cases of rubella infection with cardiac involvement. *Jpn Heart J* 1979;20: 227–235.

5. Revathi G, Suneja A, Talwar V, Aggarwal N. Fatal pericarditis due to *Listeria monocytogenes. Eur J Clin Microbiol Infect Dis* 1995;14(3):254–255. Letter.

6. Fowler NO, Manitsas GT. Infectious pericarditis. *Prog Cardiovasc Dis* 1973;16:323–336.

7. Elkayam U, Weiss S, Laniado S. Pericardial effusion and mitral valve involvement in systemic lupus erythematosus. *Ann Rheum Dis* 1977;36:349–353.

8. Kirk J, Cosh J. The pericarditis of rheumatoid arthritis. *Q J Med* 1969;38:397–423.

9. Forbat LN, Hancock BW, Gershlick AH. Methotrexate-induced pericarditis and pericardial effusion; first reported case. Postgraduate Medical Journal 1995;71:244–245.

10. Soffer A. Electrocardiographic abnormalities in acute, convalescent and recurrent stages of idiopathic pericarditis. *Am Heart J* 1960;60:729–738.

11. Feigenbaum H. *Echocardiography,* 5th ed. Philadelphia: Lea & Febiger; 1994;556–588.

12. Enein M, Abou Zina AA, Kassem M,el-Tabbakh G. Echocardiography of the pericardium in pregnancy. *Obstet Gynecol* 1987;69: 851–853.

13. Permanyer-Miralda G, Sagrista-Sauleda J, Soler-Soler J. Primary acute pericardial disease: a prospective series of 231 consecutive patients. *Am J Cardiol* 1985;56:623.

14. Sagrista-Sauleda J, Permanyer-Miralda G, Candell-Riera J, Angel J, Soler-Soler J. Transient cardiac constriction: an unrecognized pattern of evoluation in effusive acute idiopathic pericarditis. *Am J Cardiol* 1987;59:961.

15. Schroeder JS, Harrison DC. Repeated cardioversion during pregnancy. *Am J Cardiol* 1971;27:445–446.

16. Maisch B. Pericardial diseases, with a focus on etiology, pathogenesis, diagnostic imaging methods and treatment. *Curr Opin Cardiol* 1994;9:379–388.

17. Adams CW. Postviral myopericarditis associated with the influenza virus. *Am J Cardiol* 1959;4:56–67.

18. Probst R, Mier T. Acute pericarditis complicating pregnancy. *Obstet Gynecol* 1963;22:393–395.

19. Hagley MT, Shaub TF. Acute pericarditis with a symptomatic pericardial effusion complicating pregnancy. *J Reprod Med* 1993;38:813–814.

20. Simpson WG, DePriest PD, Conover WB. Acute pericarditis complicated by cardiac tamponade during pregnancy. *Am J Obstet Gynecol* 1989;160:415–416.

21. Pajuelo-Gallego A, Polo-Velasco A, Ontanilla-Lopez A, Jimenez-Delgado P, Scapini Leon JLI, Herrera-Gonzalez A, Martinez Calderon F, Murillo-Garcia H. Myopericarditis in the third pregnancy trimester. à propos of a case: *Rev Fr Gynecol Obstet* 1988;83:727–729.

22. Valenzuela GJ, Koos BJ, Mejias A. An unusual presentation of a case of staphyloccal pericarditis during pregnancy. *Am J Obstet Gynecol* 1985;151:752–753.

23. Braester A, Nusem D, Horn Y. Primary meningococcal pericarditis in a pregnant woman. *Int J Cardiol* 1986;11:355–358.

24. Weingarten S, Weinberg H, Fang M, Meyer RD. *Hemophilus influenzae* pericarditis in two adults. *West J Med* 1986;145:690–694.

25. Chrobok H, Ogorzal L, Zajiczek J. Suppurative pericarditis during pregnancy as a complication of pleural emphyema. *Przegl Lek* 1966;22:417–419.

26. Quismorio FP. Immune complexes in pericardial fluid in systemic lupus erythematosus. *Arch Intern Med* 1980;140:112–114.

27. Averbuch M, Bojko A, Levo Y. Cardiac tamponade in the early postpartum period as the presenting and predominant manifestation of systemic lupus erythematosus. *J Rheumatol* 1986;13:444–445.

28. Petri M. Systemic lupus erythematosus and pregnancy. *Rheum Dis Clin North Am* 1994;20:87–118.

29. Duclos F, Benchimol D, Lauribe P, Benchimol H, Bonnet J, Bricaud H. Cardiac lesions in Takayasu's disease. A case with initial pericarditis and tamponade. *Presse Med* 1991;20:847–850.

30. Lee CY, DiLoreto PC, Kim S. Isolated primary chylopericardium in pregnancy. *Obstet Gynecol* 1974;43:586–591.

31. Abduljabbar HSO, Marzouki KMH, Zawawi TH, Kahn S. Pericardial effusion in normal pregnant women. *Acta Obstet Gynecol Scand* 1991;70:291–294.

32. Green NJ, Rollason TP. Pulmonary artery rupture in pregnancy complicating patient ductus arteriosus. *Br Heart J* 1992;68:616–618.

33. Gray SF, Muers MF, Scott JS. Maternal death from constrictive pericarditis 15 years after radiotherapy. Case report. *Br J Obstet Gynaecol* 1988;95:518–520.

34. Wojtarowicz A, Cwajda H, Szczygielski A. Constrictive pericarditis as a cause of circulatory failure in a pregnant woman. *Wiad Lek* 1989;42:826–831.

35. Sachs BP, Lorell BH, Mehrez M, Damien N. Constrictive pericarditis and pregnancy. *Am J Obstet Gynecol* 1986;154:156–157.

36. Lessing JB, Landan E, Cohen HS, Baram A, Miller HI, Liron M, Peyser MR. Calcific constrictive pericarditis in pregnancy. *J Reprod Med* 1987;32:551–552.

37. Callahan JA, Seward JB, Nishimura RA. Two-dimensional echocardiography guided pericardiocentesis: experience in 117 consecutive patients. *Am J Cardiol* 1985;55:476.

38. Haiat R, Halphen C, Clement F, Michelon B. Silent pericardial effusion in late pregnancy. *Chest* 1981;79:717.

39. Blake S, Bonar F, McDonald D, et al. Pregnancy with constrictive pericarditis: case reports. *Br J Obstet Gynaecol* 1984;91:404–406.

40. Richardson PM, LeRoux BT, Rogers MA, et al. Pericardiectomy in pregnancy. *Thorax* 1970;25:627–630.

41. Watson PJ, Havelda CJ, Sorosky J, Kochenour NK, Sohi GS, Gray L. Jr. Irradiation-induced constrictive pericarditis requiring pericardiectomy during pregnancy. *J Reprod Med* 1980;24:127–130.

42. Bakri YN, Martan A, Amri A, Amri M. Pregnancy complicating irradiation-induced constrictive pericarditis. *Acta Obstet Gynecol Scand* 1992;71:143–144.

43. Jaluvka V. On the problem of pregnancy following surgical treated constricted pericarditis. *Geburtshilfe Frauenheilkd* 1969;29:260–267.

44. Mendelson CL. *Cardiac Disease in Pregnancy.* Philadelphia: FA Davis; 1966;297–301.

45. Szekely P, Snaith L. *Heart Disease and Pregnancy.* London: Churchill Livingstone; 1974;195–198.

46. Veland K. Cardiac surgery and pregnancy. *Am J Obstet Gynecol* 1965;92:148–162.

47. Becker RM. Intracardiac surgery in pregnant women. *Ann Thorac Surg* 1983;36:453–458.

48. Blake S, Bonar F, McCarthy C, McDonald D. The effect of posture on cardiac output in late pregnancy complicated by pericardial constriction. *Am J Obstet Gynecol* 1984;146:865–867.

49. Morgan J, Rogers A, Forker A. Congenital absence of the left pericardium. *Ann Intern Med* 1971;74:370–376.

50. Nasser W. Congenital absence of the left pericardium. *Am J Cardiol* 1970;26:466–470.

51. Jones J, McManns B. Fetal cardiac strangulation by congenital partial pericardial defect. *Am Heart J* 1984;107:183–185.

52. Savage RW, Nolan TE. Pregnancy in a woman with partial absence of the left pericardium: a case report. *J Reprod Med* 1988;33:385–386.

11

CORONARY ARTERY DISEASE IN THE CHILDBEARING AGE

JOHN D. RUTHERFORD, MB, CHB, FRACP, FACC

INTRODUCTION

Coronary artery disease is the most common cause of death in women and is the leading cause of death in women in the United States.[1] With aging of the post–World War II "baby boomers," there has been a redistribution of the heaviest concentration of childbearing women from ages in the early 20s to ages in the early 30s.[2] In addition the fertility rate for women ages 30–34 years increased by more than a third from a post–baby boom low of 52 births per thousand women in 1975 to 74 births per thousand women in 1988. In 1987, 54% of the births occurred in women ages 30–44 years.[2] Therefore, with increased age and fertility of mothers, and with more than half of the total births occurring in women ages 30–44 years, coronary artery disease during pregnancy is likely to be encountered more frequently.

PRESENTATION OF CORONARY ARTERY DISEASE

Angina pectoris (rather than acute myocardial infarction or sudden death) is the most common symptom of initial presentation of coronary artery disease in women.[3] In pregnancy, coronary disease has presented as angina with smoking as the only obvious risk factor,[4] as vasospastic angina,[5] or in association with preeclampsia,[6] homozygous familial hypercholesterolemia,[7] or diabetes mellitus.[8] Angina has been provoked by terbutaline used for premature labor[9] and a synthetic PGE2 derivative[10] used for pregnancy termination. Acute myocardial infarction presenting during pregnancy is

a rare (incidence 0.01%) but potentially lethal event for both the mother and fetus.[11] Almost all women who have a myocardial infarction before the age of 40 have either insulin-requiring diabetes mellitus,[12] hypertension, hyperlipidemia, or a strong family history of premature coronary artery disease; in the absence of these indices, cocaine abuse should be considered. Spontaneous coronary artery dissection is a rare entity, usually reported in women, which occurs one-third of the time during pregnancy or the puerperium and presents as sudden death or an unstable coronary syndrome. The left anterior descending coronary artery is usually involved. If the initial event is survived, long-term survival is possible.[13] Rarely patients with congenital coronary artery anomalies have also presented during pregnancy[14–16] with coronary syndromes.

RISK FACTORS

In 1993 the U.S. National Cholesterol Education program redefined major coronary heart disease risk factors[17] (Table 11.1).

Cigarette Smoking

The Nurses Health Study provided a direct estimate of the effect of cigarette smoking on the number of cases of coronary heart disease in women. The incidence of coronary artery disease was prospectively examined in a cohort of 119,404 female nurses who were 30–55 years old in 1976 and were free of diagnosed coronary disease.[18] During 6 years of follow-

Cardiac Problems in Pregnancy, Third Edition
Edited by Uri Elkayam, MD, and Norbert Gleicher, MD
Copyright © 1998 by Wiley-Liss, Inc. ISBN 0-471-16358-9

TABLE 11.1   Major Coronary Heart Disease Risk Factors as Determined in 1993 by the U.S. National Cholesterol Education Program

LDL cholesterol ≥ 160 mg/dL
HDL cholesterol < 35 mg/dL
Hypertension
Cigarette smoking
Diabetes
Family history of myocardial infarction or sudden death in parent
    or sibling before 55 years (male) or 65 years (female)
Male ≥ 45 years
Female ≥ 55 years
Subtract one risk factor if HDL ≥ 60 mg/dL

Source: NIH/NHLBI.[17]

up, 65 of the women died of coronary heart disease and 242 had a nonfatal myocardial infarction. In this cohort approximately 30% of the women were current smokers (a fraction similar to that in the general U.S. female population of women of comparable age).[19] There appeared to be no safe level of smoking, and risk increased with heavier smoking (Fig. 11.1, Table 11.2). Risks seemed even higher if the nurses were older, overweight, had a parent with a history of myocardial infarction, or had hypertension, diabetes, or hypercholesterolemia. It was felt that approximately half of the total coronary heart disease in this cohort was attributable to cigarette use. The rates of coronary heart disease were very low in women who had never smoked and did not have other risk factors. These data confirmed a strong, independent

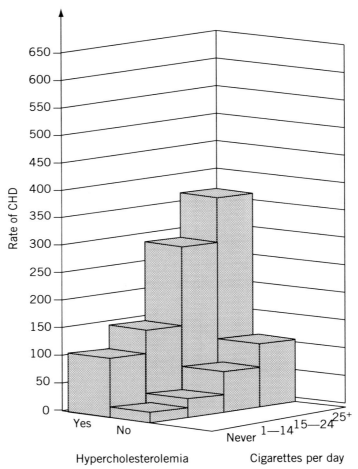

Figure 11.1   Age-standardized rates of coronary heart disease (CHD) per 100,000 person-years (vertical axis) among women according to cigarette use and history of hypercholesterolemia: The rates increase progressively across four categories of increasingly higher cigarette consumption. There appears to be no safe level of smoking, even among women consuming 1–4 cigarettes daily. The risks among women who were smokers and in addition had a history of hypercholesterolemia were even greater. The absolute effect of smoking is particularly strong among women already at risk because of hypercholesterolemia (obesity, hypertension, diabetes, a parental history of coronary disease). (Reproduced from Willett et al., *N Engl J Med* 1987;317;1303–1309, with permission.)

TABLE 11.2   Relative Risk^a of Smoking and Heart Disease in Women

End Point	Nonsmokers	Former Smokers	Smokers (number of cigarettes/day)		
			1–14	15–24	≥25
Fatal coronary heart disease	1.0	1.2	1.9	4.3	5.4
Nonfatal myocardial infarction	1.0	1.5	2.5	4.7	6.3
Angina pectoris	1.0	1.6	1.8	1.5	2.3

^aRisks even higher if patient is older, has parent with myocardial infarction, or is overweight, and hypertension, diabetes, or hypercholesterolemia is present.

Source: The Nurses Health Study: 119,404 female nurses aged 30–55 in 1976, followed for 6 years. In: Willett et al, *N Engl J Med* 1987;317:1303–1309.

positive association between cigarette smoking in women and coronary heart disease.

Alcohol

Women appear to be more susceptible to alcoholic liver disease than men,[20] and those with moderate alcohol consumption also appear to have an increased risk of breast cancer.[21] The Nurses Health Study also provides information concerning alcohol consumption and cardiovascular disease risk.[22] For women under 40 years of age, all levels of alcohol consumption (compared with abstinence) were associated with increased risk of death (probably in large part because of increased risk of accidents); but in women over the age of 50 years, light to moderate drinkers (0.1–29.9 g/day) had a reduced risk of death (largely owing to a decreased risk of fatal cardiovascular disease), and this was especially seen in older women with one or two risk factors. Heavier drinking was found to be associated with increased mortality, especially from noncardiovascular disease (including breast cancer).

Hypertension

Hypertension at any age contributes to the development of coronary artery disease, whether it is systolic hypertension, diastolic hypertension, or labile hypertension. In both women and men, a systolic blood pressure greater than 160 mmHg, or a diastolic pressure of 85 mmHg or higher, increases the risk of coronary heart disease two- to threefold.[23] Hypertension is a powerful independent risk factor for both coronary artery disease and stroke in women (especially black women).[24]

Menopause and Coronary Risk Factors

Three important coronary risk factors affect the time of occurrence of menopause: age, cigarette smoking, and obesity. Cigarette smoking is associated with an earlier menopause

and obesity is associated with a later menopause. Ovarian function begins to decline well before menopause and continues to decline thereafter, and it seems likely that estrogen deficiency contributes to increasing risk of coronary artery disease at this time of a woman's life.[25] Many studies over the last 25 years have suggested that women who take postmenopausal estrogens (noncontraceptive) have a lower risk for coronary heart disease.[26] The approximate dose used in these studies was equivalent to 0.625–1.25 mg of oral conjugated estrogen daily. Estrogen therapy reduces low density lipoprotein (LDL) cholesterol and increases high density lipoprotein (HDL) cholesterol in a dose-dependent fashion. A dose of oral conjugated estrogen of 0.625 mg daily will increase LDL about 10–15% and increase HDL 10–15%.[27]

Oral Contraceptives

Major coronary events are rare in women who use oral contraceptives, and when they occur they are usually related to the combined effects of other risk factors including smoking, diabetes, hypertension, and increasing age.[28,29] While the estrogen and progestin doses in oral contraceptives have decreased over the last 20 years, surveys still suggest that young women who use oral contraceptives are at increased risk for the development of coronary heart disease.[30] Smokers are particularly at hazard, and blood pressure monitoring needs to continue while women take oral contraceptives.

Hyperlipidemia

At all ages, HDL levels are 5–10 mg/dL higher in women than in men. When the ratio of total cholesterol to HDL cholesterol exceeds 7.5, the risk for coronary artery disease in women is similar to that for men. (Optimal ratios are 3.5 or lower). In the presence of a low HDL, elevated serum triglycerides do increase women's risk for coronary heart disease.[31] Long-term use of high estrogen content oral contraceptives is associated with increases in both HDL cholesterol and triglyceride levels. Increases in HDL cholesterol and decreases in LDL cholesterol have been observed in post-menopausal women who receive estrogen replacement.[32] Progestins moderately decrease both HDL cholesterol and triglycerides.

Diabetes Mellitus

Both asymptomatic hyperglycemia and clinically diagnosed diabetes mellitus are risk factors for coronary heart disease in women. Diabetic women have the same risk for coronary artery disease as nondiabetic men of the same age, and diabetes mellitus appears to be a greater risk factor for myocardial infarction in women than in men (exceeding that of cigarette smoking).[33,34] Non-insulin-dependent diabetic women tend to have a larger number of risk factors than insulin-dependent diabetics or nondiabetics. HDL cholesterol levels are consistently lower in diabetics than in nondiabetics,[35] and elevated triglyceride levels are more common in non-insulin-dependent diabetics.

Obesity

The Nurses Health Study reported a strong positive association between obesity and risk of coronary artery disease over an 8-year follow-up[36] (Figure 11.2). Higher levels of body

weight within the "normal range," as well as modest weight gains after the age of 18, appear to increase the risk of coronary heart disease in middle-aged women.[37] The magnitude of the excessive risk with obesity is less than the risk associated with cigarette smoking.

Family History

Women with a parental history of myocardial infarction before age 60 have an age-adjusted relative risk of nonfatal myocardial infarction of 2.8 compared with women with no family history.[38] Furthermore, the relative risk for developing angina was 3.4 for women with a parental history of myocardial infarction before 60 and 2.6 for parental history of angina after age 60.

DIAGNOSTIC TESTING

The accuracy of exercise electrocardiography in diagnosing coronary artery disease is lower in women than in men. Because there is a relatively low prevalence of coronary heart disease in women (under the age of 50 years) Bayes's theorem indicates that the diagnostic value of tests for coronary heart disease will be reduced and the likelihood of "false pos-

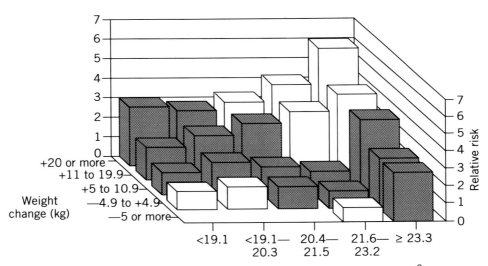

Figure 11.2 The relative risk of coronary heart disease by level of body mass index (BMI) at 18 years of age and weight gain between 18 years of age and 1976 at the commencement of 14 years of follow-up in 115,818 women, ages 30–55 years, without a history of coronary heart disease. Plus signs indicate weight gain; minus signs indicate weight loss. The reference patients were women with a BMI of less than 19.1 kg/m^2 at 18 years of age and with stable weight. The darker shaded categories include the current range of recommended BMI values for adults older than 35 years. Higher levels of body weight within the "normal" range, as well as modest gains after 18 years of age, appear to increase risk of coronary heart disease in middle-aged women. (Reproduced from Willett et al., *JAMA* 1995;273:461–465, with permission.)

itive" test results increased. The diagnostic value of perfusion imaging appears to be greatest in patients with a moderate pretest likelihood (30–60%) of having clinical coronary artery disease; among symptomatic patients, this may include middle-aged women with angina and patients with abnormal baseline electrocardiograms, which preclude accurate interpretation of exercise electrocardiography.[39]

Exercise myocardial perfusion imaging should not be used routinely in patients with either a very low or a very high likelihood of disease. It may be appropriate for women with a very high pretest likelihood of coronary artery disease to proceed to cardiac catheterization for imaging rather than radionuclide testing. Information on the predictive accuracy of stress echocardiography in women is limited, but in populations with a coronary artery disease prevalence from 26 to 67%, the sensitivity was 71–88% and specificity was approximately 65–97%.[40] Information concerning ventricular function derived by two-dimensional echocardiography has obviated the need for nuclear imaging and cardiac catheterization in many patients. During pregnancy, diagnostic testing for coronary artery disease is associated with increased risk to the fetus. Fetal bradycardia has been reported during maximal exercise in normal women,[41] and obviously radionuclide imaging will expose the fetus to radiation and should be recommended only when the value of the derived information outweighs any potential fetal risk. Cardiac catheterization involving fluoroscopy and cineangiography also carries risks for the fetus but has been performed in many pregnant women for important clinical indications. Appropriate "shielding" of the fetus from radiation is important.

ANGIOGRAPHY

The Cleveland Clinic performed an observational study on 1000 women under the age of 50 years who underwent cardiac catheterization for suspected coronary disease from 1961 to 1968.[42] These subjects represented 6.8% of all patients catheterized by that institution during that time period. Significant obstructive coronary artery disease was found in 58% of 222 patients with typical angina, in 27% of 149 patients with atypical angina, and in only 1 of 80 patients not thought to have coronary disease. The Registry of the Coronary Artery Surgery Study (CASS) has also provided information on the angiographic prevalence of high risk coronary artery disease in both men and women with typical angina, probable angina, and nonspecific chest pain.[43] In young women with probable angina, the prevalence of coronary disease was 20% in the age group 30–39 years and 29% in the age group 40–49 years. The prevalence of coronary artery disease in patients with nonspecific chest pain was 10%, and none of the patients under 30 years of age with nonspecific chest pain had obstructive coronary artery disease.[43] In all patients with definite angina (and men with probable angi-

na), there was a high prevalence of coronary artery disease and multivessel disease. In men and women with nonspecific chest pain there appeared to be a low prevalence of severe coronary artery disease, and women with probable angina had an intermediate prevalence.

MEDICAL THERAPY

In general, each of the major classes of therapeutic agents (nitrates, β-adrenergic blocking agents, calcium antagonists) reduced symptoms and improved exercise performance in patients with angina. There is no substantive evidence that any of these therapies mentioned reduces mortality in patients with chronic stable angina. There is evidence that aspirin and effective lipid-lowering regimens will reduce both morbidity and mortality (Table 11.3).

Aspirin

It is likely that aspirin therapy is beneficial in all patients with symptomatic coronary artery disease (including chronic stable angina).[44,45] The efficacy of aspirin in reducing fatal and morbid events is established for patients with acute myocardial infarction.[46] Similarly, three major randomized, placebo-controlled, double-blind studies have shown that in patients with unstable angina or non-Q-wave infarction, aspirin therapy reduces the risk of myocardial infarction or death.[47–49] Aspirin is also beneficial in patients with chronic stable angina. In 2035 male and female patients with a history of angina for more than one month, but no history of prior myocardial infarction, aspirin therapy (75 mg/day) resulted in a 34% risk reduction of the incidence of myocardial infarction and sudden death during a follow-up period of 50 months.[50] It is also possible that women (Nurses Health Study of women free of heart disease, stroke, and cancer aged 34–65 years, who were followed for 475,265 person-years) who regularly

TABLE 11.3 Pharmacology of Chronic Stable Angina

Drug	Benefits		
	Reduces Mortality	Prevents Acute Myocardial Infarction	Reduces Angina or Improves Exercise
Aspirin	+	+	
Lipid lowering	+	+	
Nitrates			+ +
β-Adrenergic blocking agents			+ +
Calcium channel blockers			+ +

use aspirin (1–6/week) have a reduced risk of first acute myocardial infarction and thus derive primary prevention benefits from aspirin.[51]

Aspirin consumption during pregnancy may produce adverse effects in the mother, including hemorrhage, prolonged gestation and labor, and anemia.[52] High doses of aspirin use have been associated with increased perinatal mortality and intrauterine growth retardation, and premature closure of the ductus arteriosis may occur in the latter part of pregnancy. Although aspirin has been used as a tocolytic agent, serious bleeding complications may occur in the newborn. Low doses of aspirin (40–150 mg/day) have been used successfully in mothers with systemic lupus erythematosus with antiphospholipid antibodies, in pregnancies at risk for the development of hypertension and preeclampsia, and in fetuses with intrauterine growth retardation. Aspirin and other salicylates are excreted into breast milk in low concentrations, although adverse affects on platelet function in nursing infants exposed to aspirin through milk have not been reported.

The American Academy of Pediatrics recommends that aspirin be used cautiously by the mother during lactation because of potential adverse effects on the nursing infant. Since the benefits of aspirin in patients with known coronary artery disease are substantial, they have to be weighed against any potential risks in a pregnant mother with symptomatic coronary disease. Certainly, low dose aspirin therapy would provide quite adequate protection for adverse cardiovascular events and minimize the risks to fetus.

Lipid Lowering

Analyses of secondary prevention trials suggest that cholesterol-lowering therapy reduces both recurrent coronary events and mortality.[53,54] Even in myocardial infarct survivors with "average" lipid levels, there is a substantial reduction in coronary events with effective LDL lowering.[54] All patients who have established coronary heart disease or other evidence of clinical atherosclerotic disease should have a lipoprotein analysis for LDL cholesterol determination after an overnight fast, on two occasions, 1–8 weeks apart. In patients who have distinct elevations of LDL cholesterol, the second report of the expert panel on detection, evaluation, and treatment of high blood cholesterol in adults suggested that prompt initiation of drug therapy is acceptable.[17] The target goal for LDL cholesterol reduction should be 100 mg/dL or lower. When it becomes apparent that dietary therapy will not allow this target to be reached, drug therapy should be considered. A number of patients with coronary heart disease have an "isolated" low HDL cholesterol.[55] In this situation cigarette smokers should be encouraged to stop smoking, an effort should be made to control weight optimally and to promote exercise, and careful treatment of any hypertension and diabetes mellitus should be continued. In patients with isolated low HDL cholesterol levels who do not have associated high LDL levels or other risk factors (e.g., a positive family history of premature coronary disease), the use of HDL-raising drugs for primary prevention of coronary disease is not currently recommended.

Other Therapies

Sublingual nitroglycerin remains the treatment of choice for acute anginal episodes, and the prophylactic use of sublingual nitroglycerin (prior to stressful situations or increased physical activity known to produce angina) is encouraged. Long-acting nitrate therapy as an adjunct to this is useful. Organic nitrates dilate both normal and stenotic epicardial coronary arteries, prevent exercise-induced constriction of stenotic arteries,[56] and also attenuate exercise-induced abnormalities in left ventricular function. Careful dosing regimens need to be formulated to provide a 10- or 12-hour nitrate free interval within any 24-hour period. During such a nitrate-free interval, use of sublingual nitroglycerin, either acutely or prophylactically, is important. One of the major determinants of myocardial oxygen demand is heart rate, and therapeutic options for the control of heart rate at rest and during exercise include β-adrenergic blocking agents, diltiazem and verapamil. It has been pointed out that the optimal use of these agents as monotherapy may be as effective in reducing angina and improving exercise performance as combination therapy.[57,58] Nevertheless, it is clear that in patients who continue to have angina despite optimal β-adrenergic blockade, the addition of a calcium antagonist is likely to reduce symptoms and improve exercise performance.[59] Conversely, it is not clear that the addition of a beta blocker to therapy with diltiazem or verapamil improves antianginal efficacy,[57] although combination of a beta blocker and nifedipine does. In patients with chronic stable angina, other conditions such as hypertension, heart failure, atrial fibrillation, diabetes mellitus, and conduction system disease are all going to play a major role in the choice of appropriate therapy. With care, angina frequency can be diminished and exercise performance can both be improved.

The management of the pregnant woman with coronary artery disease is similar to that for the nonpregnant patient except that careful planning among the obstetrician, the anesthesiologist, and the cardiologist is required. The choice of therapeutic agents needs to be discussed, including the use of aspirin, nitrates, beta blockers, and calcium channel blockers (chapters 29 and 31). Beta blockers, which have been used extensively in pregnant patients, form the cornerstone of anti-ischemic therapy of women with coronary disease in pregnancy, since there is less certainty of the safety of long-term therapy with organic nitrates and calcium antagonists in this situation (Table 11.4). Careful hemodynamic monitoring is required throughout labor and delivery and the postpartum

TABLE 11.4 Summary of Anti-Ischemic Therapies for Pregnant Women with Coronary Disease

Drug	Placental Transfer	Risk Factor[a,b]	Fetal Effects	Breast Feed
Aspirin	Yes	C, low dose; D, full dose, 3rd trimester	Increased hemorrhage, increased perinatal mortality, growth retardation, premature closure of ductus arteriosus	Yes
Atenolol	Yes	CM	Low birth weight	Yes
Diltiazem	Yes	CM	No adequate human studies	Yes
Lovastatin	?	XM	Teratogenic in rats but not rabbits; no adequate human studies	No
				No human data
Metoprolol	Yes	BM	No obvious risk—no long-term data	Yes
Nifedipine	Yes	CM	No adequate human studies; use with care	Yes
Nitroglycerin	?	CM	No adequate human studies	No data
Propranolol	Yes	CM	Growth retardation, prematurity, hypoglycemia, bradycardia, respiratory depression	Yes
Verapamil	Yes	CM	No adequate human studies	Yes

[a]*Category B:* Either animal reproduction studies have not demonstrated a fetal risk but there are no controlled studies in pregnant women, or animal reproduction studies have shown an adverse effect (other than a decrease in fertility) that was not confirmed in controlled studies in women in the first trimester (and there is no evidence of a risk in later trimesters). *Category C:* Either studies in animals have revealed adverse effects on the fetus and there are no controlled studies in pregnant women, or studies in women and animals are not available. Drugs should only be given if the potential benefit justifies the potential risk to the fetus. *Category D:* There is positive evidence of human fetal risk, but the benefits from use in pregnant women may be acceptable despite the risk (e.g., if the drug is needed in a life-threatening situation for a serious disease for which safer drugs cannot be used or are ineffective). *Category X:* The drug is contraindicated in women who are or may become pregnant.

[b]Subscript M indicates that the manufacturer has rated the risk of the drug in the professional literature.

Source: Data mainly from Briggs et al.[52]

period, and a normal vaginal delivery is aimed for. When pharmacologic therapy is used during labor, it is important to try to minimize increases in heart rate, and hypotension must be avoided at the time of delivery.

MEDICAL VERSUS REVASCULARIZATION THERAPY

Angina is a diagnosis made by taking a careful history. Two key pieces of information are required to plan overall management strategy. The first is knowledge of the patient's ventricular function. The second is the response of the patient to some form of stress testing. Medical therapy relieves angina in many patients regardless of the severity of disease, and its influence on survival is similar to that of revascularization in patients with single-vessel coronary artery disease or multivessel coronary artery disease and normal systolic function without involvement of the left anterior descending coronary artery.[60] For patients with single-vessel disease, or multivessel disease not involving the proximal left anterior descending coronary artery and normal ventricular systolic function, the choice of medical therapy, angioplasty, or bypass grafting can be individualized.[61] Patients taking appro-

priate medical therapy who have symptomatic limitations in their work or recreational activities should be considered for revascularization. Considerations of revascularization procedures in women appear to indicate increased risks compared with men.

The NHLBI 1985–1986 Coronary Angioplasty Registry[62] reported in 1993 that while there was comparable clinical and angiographic success of percutaneous transluminal coronary angioplasty (PTCA) in men and women, the initial complications were higher in women and the procedural mortality was higher (2.6% in women vs. 0.3% in men, $p < 0.001$). Similarly, women appear to have a higher mortality associated with coronary artery bypass graft surgery. The CASS investigators suggested that women's smaller size (associated with smaller cardiac and coronary artery size) was the reason for the difference, although others have thought that increased age and worse functional status account for the differences.[63] These issues must be considered as the choices between medical therapy and revascularization procedures are weighed. Both PTCA and coronary artery bypass grafting (CABG) have been successfully performed during pregnancy,[64–66] but invasive treatments are used only if medical therapy is failing and the mother's health is thought to be seriously compromised without revascularization.

REVASCULARIZATION

In patients with angina, significant coronary artery disease, and moderately or severely impaired left ventricular function, there is substantial evidence that if significant three-vessel coronary artery disease or two-vessel coronary artery disease with involvement of the proximal left anterior descending coronary artery exists, revascularization should be considered as a means of prolonging survival.[67–69] Patients with significant left main coronary artery stenoses should be revascularized for survival reasons if they are deemed appropriate candidates. In patients with multivessel coronary disease considered good candidates for either PTCA or CABG, the rates of procedure related mortality are similar.[70,71] Patients undergoing bypass grafting are more likely to have procedure-related Q-wave myocardial infarction, but most of these events are well tolerated.[60] Subsequently, patients who undergo bypass grafting appear to have less angina and less requirement for antianginal medication; they also are less likely to need another revascularization procedure[60] than those treated by angioplasty.

SUMMARY

Coronary artery disease, the leading cause of death in women, is encountered during pregnancy with increasing frequency because of increasing maternal age (and fertility). Smoking is probably the major risk factor for coronary artery disease in women of childbearing age, although there are obvious positive associations with a family history of coronary artery disease, obesity, diabetes mellitus, hypertension, and the hyperlipidemias. The most common mode of presentation of women with coronary disease is angina pectoris, and those patients with probable and definite angina should be risk-stratified with stress testing. Some assessment of ventricular function should be made when appropriate, since this is an important determinant of survival and choice of therapy in patients with multivessel coronary artery disease. Both aspirin and effective lipid-lowering therapies have been shown to improve mortality in patients with chronic stable angina, and beta blockers, nitrates, and calcium channel antagonists have been all shown to reduce symptoms and improve exercise performance. All revascularization procedures in women carry increased hazard (compared with men), but symptomatic, angiographic, and mortality outcomes are all favorable in appropriately selected patients.

During the treatment of a pregnant woman with symptomatic coronary disease, the benefits and risks of each of the therapeutic choices must be weighed with respect to the mother's health and any hazard to the fetus. Adequate β-adrenergic blockade is the cornerstone of medical therapy during pregnancy, since the long-term effects of nitrates and calcium channel blockers on the fetus are less well known.

Careful planning and coordination between obstetrician, anesthesiologist, cardiologist, and patient is required.

REFERENCES

1. *Vital Statistics of the United States 1986.* Vol. II, *Mortality,* Part A. Hyattsville, MD: U.S. Department of Health and Human Services; Public Health Service, Centers for Disease Control, National Center for Health Statistics; 1988.

2. Taeuber C. *Statistical Handbook on Women in America.* Phoenix: Oryx Press; 1991.

3. Beard CM, Foster V, Annegers JF. Reproductive history in women with coronary disease. *Am J Epidemiol* 1984;120: 108–114.

4. Shalev Y, Ben-Hur H, Hagay Z, Blickstein I, Epstein M, Ayzenberg O, Gelven A, Caspi A. Successful delivery following myocardial ischemia during the second trimester of pregnancy. *Clin Cardiol* 1993;16:754–56.

5. Maekawa K, Ohnishi H, Hirase T, Yamada T, Matsuo T. Acute myocardial infarction during pregnancy caused by coronary artery spasm. *J. Intern Med* 1994;235:383–385.

6. Dawson PJ, Ross AW. Pre-eclampsia in a parturient with a history of myocardial infarction. A case report and literature review. *Anaesthesia* 1988;43:659–63.

7. Kroon AA, Swinkels DW, van Dongen PW, Stalenhoef AF. Pregnancy in a patient with homozygous familial hypercholesterolemia treated with long-term low-density lipoprotein apheresis. *Metabol: Clin Exp* 1994;43:1164–1170.

8. Pombar X, Straussner HT, Fenner PC. Pregnancy in a woman with class H diabetes mellitus and previous coronary artery bypass graft: a case report and review of the literature. *Obstet Gynecol* 1995;85:825–829.

9. Tye KH, Desser KB, Benchimol A. Angina pectoris associated with use of terbutaline for premature labor. *JAMA* 1980;244: 692–693.

10. Bagni E, Bompani B, Magnavacchi P, Pedrazzini F. Prolonged angina after the administration of a synthetic PGE2 derivative. *G Ital Cardiol* 1993;23:719–721.

11. Hands M, Johnson MD, Saltzman DH, Rutherford J. The cardiac, obstetric, and anesthetic management of pregnancy complicated by myocardial infarction. *J Clin Anesth* 1990;2: 258–268.

12. Gordon MC, Landon MB, Boyle J, Stewart KS, Gabbe SG. Coronary artery disease in insulin-dependent diabetes mellitus of pregnancy (class H): a review of the literature. *Obstet Gynecol Survey* 1996;51:437–444.

13. Bac DJ, Lotgering FK, Verkaaik APK, Deckers JW. Spontaneous coronary artery dissection during pregnancy and post partum. *Eur Heart J* 1995;16:136–138.

14. Chestnut DH, Roberts SL, Laube DW, Martins JB. Pregnancy in a woman with aneurysms of the right coronary artery and an atrioventricular fistula. *J Reprod Med* 1986;31:528–530.

15. Goldberg N, Zisbrod Z, Kipperman R, Krasnow N, Gordon D, Shapir Y, Stein R. Congenital aneurysm of the left coronary sinus and left main coronary artery with fistulous communication

to the right atrium in pregnancy. *J Am Soc Echocardiogr* 1990;3;125–130.

16. Ruszkiewicz A, Opeskin K. Sudden death in pregnancy from congenital malformation of the coronary arteries. *Pathology* 1993;25:236–239.

17. National Institutes of Health/National Heart, Lung, and Blood Institute. Second Report of the Expert Panel on Detection, Evaluation, and Treatment of High Blood Cholesterol in Adults; Washington, DC: NIH/NHLBI; 1993.

18. Willett WC, Green A, Stampfer MJ, Speizer FE, Colditz GA, Rosner B, Monson RR, Stason W, Hennekens CH. Relative and absolute excess risks of coronary heart disease among women who smoke cigarettes. *N Engl J Med* 1987;317;1303–1309.

19. *Smoking and health: a report of the Surgeon General.* Washington, DC: Government Printing office; 1979; U.S. Department of Health, Education, and Welfare publication no. 79-50066.

20. Norton R, Batey R, Dwyer T, MacMahon S. Alcohol consumption and the risk of alcohol cirrhosis in women. *Br Med J* 1987;295:80–82.

21. Longnecker MP. Alcoholic beverage consumption in relation to risk of breast cancer: meta-analysis and review. *Cancer Causes Control* 1994;5:73–82.

22. Fuchs CS, Stampfer MJ, Colditz GA, Giovannucci EL, Manson JE, Kawachi I, Hunter DJ, Hankinson SE, Hennekens CH, Rosner B. Alcohol consumption and mortality among women. *N Engl J Med* 1995;332:1245–1250.

23. The Working Group on Risk and High Blood Pressure. An epidemiological approach to describing risk associated with high blood pressure levels. *Hypertension* 1985;7:641–651.

24. Johnson J, Heineman E, Heiss G, Hames CG, Tyroler HA. Cardiovascular disease risk factors and mortality among black women and white women aged 40–64 years in Evans County, Georgia. *Am J Epidemiol* 1986;123:209–220.

25. Stampfer MJ, Colditz GA, Willett WC. Menopause and heart disease. A review. *Ann NY Acad Sci.* 1990;590:193–203.

26. Grady D, Rubin SM, Petitti DB, Fox CS, Black D, Ettinger B, Ernster VL, Cummings SR. Hormone therapy to prevent disease and prolong life in postmenopausal women. *Ann Intern Med* 1992;117:1016–1037.

27. Cauley JA, La Porte RE, Kuller LH, Bates M, Sandler RB. Menopausal estrogen use, high density lipoprotein cholesterol subfractions and liver function. *Atherosclerosis* 1983;49; 31–39.

28. Hennekens CH, Evans D, Peto R. Oral contraceptive use, cigarette smoking, and myocardial infarction. *Br J Fam Plann* 1979;5:66–67.

29. Rosenberg L, Kaufman DW, Helmrich SP, Miller DR, Stolley PD, Shapiro S. Myocardial infarction and cigarette smoking in women younger than 50 years of age. *JAMA* 1985;253: 2965–2969.

30. Russel-Briefel R, Ezzati T, Fulwood R, Perlman JA, Murphy RS. Cardiovascular risk status and oral contraceptive use: United States, 1976–1980. *Prev Med* 1986;15:352–362.

31. Castelli WP. The triglyceride issue: A view from Framingham. *Am Heart J* 1986;112;432–437.

32. Kaplan NM. Estrogen replacement therapy: effect on blood pressure and other cardiovascular risk factors. *J Reprod Med* 1985;30(suppl 10):802–804.

33. Kannel WB. Lipids, diabetes and coronary heart disease: Insights from the Framingham study. *Am Heart J* 1985;110; 1100–1106.

34. Kannel WB, McGee D. Diabetes and cardiovascular disease: the Framingham study. *JAMA* 1979;241:2035–2038.

35. Nikkila EA. High-density lipoproteins in diabetes. *Diabetes* 1981;30(suppl 2):82–87.

36. Manson JE, Colditz G, Stampfer MJ, Willett WC, Rosner B, Monson RR, Speizer FE, Hennekens CH. A prospective study of obesity and risk of coronary heart disease in women. *N Engl J Med* 1990;322:882–889.

37. Willett WC, Manson JE, Stampfer MJ, Coltitz GA, Rosner B, Speizer FE, Hennekens CH. Weight, weight change, and coronary heart disease in women. Risk within the "normal" weight range. *JAMA* 1995;273:461–465.

38. Colditz GA, Stampfer MJ, Willett WC, Rosner B, Speizer FE, Hennekens CH. A prospective study of parental history of myocardial infarction and CHD in women. *Am J Epidemiol* 1986;123:48–58.

39. American College of Cardiologists/American Heart Association Task Force Report. Guidelines for clinical use of radionuclide imaging. *J Am College Cardiol* 1995;25:521–547.

40. Roger VL. Stress testing for the diagnosis of coronary artery disease in women. *ACC Curr J Rev* (May/June);1995:31–33.

41. Carpenter MW, Sady SP, Hoegsberg B, Sady MA, Haydon B, Cullinane EM, Coustan DR, Thompson PD. Fetal heart rate response to maternal exertion. *JAMA* 1988;259–306.

42. Proudfit WL, Welch CC, Siqueira C, Morcerf FP, Sheldon WC. Prognosis of 1000 young women studied by coronary angiography. *Circulation* 1981;64:1185–1190.

43. Chaitman BR, Bourassa MG, Davis K, Rogers WJ, Tyras DH, Berger R, Kennedy JW, Fisher L, Judkins MP, Mock MB, Killip T. Angiographic prevalence of high-risk coronary disease in patient subsets (CASS). *Circulation* 1981;64:360–367.

44. Fuster V, Dyken ML, Vokonas PS, Hennekens C. Aspirin as a therapeutic agent in cardiovascular disease. AHA Medical/Scientific Statement. *Circulation* 1993;87:659–675.

45. Hirsh J, Dalen J, Fuster V, Harker LB, Salzman EW. Aspirin and other platelet active drugs: the relationship between dose, effectiveness, and side effects. *Chest* 1992;102(suppl):327S–336S.

46. Randomised trial of intravenous streptokinase, oral aspirin, both, or neither among 17,187 cases of suspected acute myocardial infarction: ISIS-2. *Lancet* 1988:(2):349–360.

47. Cairns JA, Gent M, Singer J, Myers MG, Melendez LJ, Finnie KJ, Froggatt GM, Holder DA, Jablonsky G, Kostuk WJ. Aspirin, sulfinpyrazone, or both in unstable angina. Results of a Canadian multicenter trial. *N Engl J Med* 1985;313: 1369–1375.

48. Lewis HD, Davis JW, Archibald GD, Steinke WE, Smitherman TC, Doherty JE 3d, Schnaper HW, LeWinter MM, Linares E, Pouget JM, Sabharwal SC, Chesler E, Demots H. Protective effects of aspirin against acute myocardial infarction and death in men with unstable angina. *N Engl J Med* 1983;309:396–403.

49. Risk of myocardial infarction and death during treatment with low dose aspirin and intravenous heparin in men with unstable coronary artery disease. *Lancet* 1990;340:1421–1425.

50. Juul-Moller S, Edvardsson N, Jahnmatz B, Rosen A, Sorensen S, Omneus R. For the Sweden Angina Pectoris Aspirin Trial (SAPAT) group. Double-blind trial of aspirin in primary prevention of myocardial infarction in patients with stable chronic angina pectoris. *Lancet* 1992;340:1421–1425.

51. Manson JE, Stampfer MJ, Colditz GA, Willett WC, Rosner B, Speizer FE, Hennekens CH. A prospective study of aspirin use and primary prevention of cardiovascular disease in women. *JAMA* 1991;266:521–527.

52. Briggs GG, Freeman RK, Yaffe SJ. *Drugs in Pregnancy and Lactation. A Reference Guide to Fetal and Neonatal Risk.* 4th ed. Baltimore: Williams & Wilkins; 1994.

53. Roussouw JE, Lewis B, Rifkind BM. The value of lowering cholesterol after myocardial infarction. *N Engl J Med* 1990;323;1112–1119.

54. Sacks FM, Pfeffer MA, Moye LA, Rouleau JL, Rutherford JD, Cole TG, Brown L, Warnica JW, Arnold JM, Wunn CC, Davis BR, Braunwald E. The effect of pravastatin on coronary events after myocardial infarction in patients with average cholesterol levels. *N Engl J Med* 1996;335:1001–1009.

55. Miller M, Kwiterovich PO. Isolated low HDL-cholesterol as an important risk factor for coronary heart disease. *Eur Heart J* 1990;11(suppl H):9–14.

56. Gage JE, Hess OM, Murakami T, Ritter M, Grimm J, Krayenbuehl HP. Vasoconstriction of stenotic coronary arteries during dynamic exercise in patients with classic angina pectoris: reversibility by nitroglycerin. *Circulation* 1986;73:865–876.

57. Packer M. Combined beta-adrenergic and calcium entry blockade in angina pectoris. *N Engl J Med* 1989:320:709–718.

58. Strauss WE, Parisi AF. Combined use of calcium-channel and beta-adrenergic blockers for the treatment of chronic stable angina. Rationale, efficacy and adverse effects. *Ann Intern Med* 1988;109:570–581.

59. Nesto RW, White HD, Wynne J, Holman BL, Antman EM. Comparison of nifedipine and isosorbide dinitrate when added to maximal propranolol therapy in stable angina pectoris. *Am J Cardiol* 1987;60:256.

50. Hillis LD, Rutherford JD. Coronary angioplasty compared with bypass grafting. *N Engl J Med* 1994;331:1086–1087. Editorial.

61. Mark DB, Nelson CL, Califf RM, Harrell FE Jr, Lee KL, Jones RH, Fortin DF, Stack RS, Glower DD, Smith LR, Delong ER, Smith PK, Reves JG, Jollis JG, Tcheng JE, Muhlbaier LH, Lowe JE, Phillips HR, Pryor DB. Continuing evolution of therapy for coronary artery disease. Initial results from the era of coronary angioplasty. *Circulation* 1994;89: 2015–2025.

62. Kelsey SF, James M, Holubkov R, Cowley MJ, Detre KM, and investigators from the NHLBI Percutaneous Coronary Angioplasty Registry. Results of Percutaneous Coronary Angioplasty in Women, 1985–1986 National Heart, Lung, and Blood Institute's Coronary Angioplasty Registry. *Circulation* 1993;87: 720–727.

63. Khan SS, Nessim S, Gray R, Czer LS, Chaux A, Matloff J. Increased mortality of women in coronary artery bypass surgery: evidence for referral bias. *Ann Intern Med* 1990;112:561–567.

64. Cowan NC, de Belder MA, Rothman MT. Coronary angioplasty in pregnancy. *Br Heart J* 1988;59:588.

65. Mardini AH, Chapman MK, Gaines TE, Acker JJ. The expanded role of coronary angioplasty during pregnancy. *J Tennessee Med Assoc* 1995;88:423–424.

66. Madjan JF, Walinsky P, Cowchuck JF, Wapner RJ, Plzak L Jr. Coronary bypass surgery during pregnancy. *Am J Cardiol* 1983;52:1145.

67. Varnauskas E, and the European Coronary Surgery Study Group. Twelve-year follow-up of survival in the randomized European Coronary Surgery Study. *N Engl J Med* 1988;319: 332–337.

68. Yusuf S, Zucker D, Peduzzi P, Fisher LD, Takaro T, Kennedy JW, Davis K, Killip T, Passamani E, Morris C, Mathur V, Varnauskas Ed, Chalmers TC, Norris R. Effect of coronary artery bypass graft surgery on survival: overview of 10-year results from randomised trials by the Coronary Artery Bypass Graft Surgery Trialists Collaboration. *Lancet* 1994;344:563–570.

69. Rutherford JD, Braunwald E. Chronic ischemic heart disease. In: Braunwald E, ed. *Heart Disease. A textbook of cardiovascular medicine.* 4th ed. Philadelphia: WB Saunders; 1992; chap. 40.

70. King SB, Lembo NJ, Weintraub WS, Kosinski AS, Barnhart HX, Kutner MH, Alazaraki NP, Guyton RA, Zhao XQ. A randomized trial comparing coronary angioplasty with coronary bypass surgery. *N Engl J Med* 1994;331:1044–1150.

71. Hamm CW, Reimers J, Ischinger T, Rupprecht HJ, Berger J, Bleifeld W. A randomized study of coronary angioplasty compared with bypass surgery in patients with symptomatic multivessel coronary disease. *N Engl J Med* 1994;331: 1037–1043.

12

ACUTE MYOCARDIAL INFARCTION AND PREGNANCY

Arie Roth, MD, and Uri Elkayam, MD

INTRODUCTION

Acute myocardial infarction is a rare event in the childbearing age and has been estimated to occur in only 1 in 10,000 women during pregnancy.[1,2] Since the first report in 1922,[3] many additional cases have been published in the literature,[4–109] indicating the unique features of this condition which can significantly impact on both maternal and fetal outcome (Table 12.1). With the current trend of childbearing at an older age, in addition to the continuing effects of cigarette smoking, stress, and cocaine usage, the occurrence of acute myocardial infarction during pregnancy can be expected to increase. This chapter reviews the clinical aspects of gestational and early postpartal acute myocardial infarction based on 125 well-documented cases and attempts to establish recommendations for the management of this condition.

METHODS

Epidemiology

Although acute myocardial infarction has been reported at any stage of pregnancy and at ages between 16 and 45 years, the highest incidence seems to occur in the third trimester and in women older than 33 years (Table 12.2). Maternal age in patients with postpartum (24 h to 3 months postdelivery) acute myocardial infarction was substantially lower than that of women with antepartal (up to 24 h before labor) or peripartal (within 24 h before and after labor and delivery) acute myocardial infarction (21 ± 6 vs. 33 ± 6 and 34 ± 5 years, respectively). In addition, acute myocardial infarction has been noted to occur more commonly in multigravidas, and its

location during pregnancy is more commonly in the anterior wall. Most maternal deaths occurred either at the time of infarction (usually resulting in an undelivered child) or within two weeks,[1] usually in relation to labor and delivery. No association could be found, however, between maternal mortality and mode of delivery (Table 12.3). The majority of fetal deaths have been associated with maternal mortality, while maternal survival was usually accompanied by normal fetal outcome. The cumulative reported maternal mortality was 21%, with a higher rate found peripartum or postpartum than antepartum. Fetal death was lower (13% overall) than maternal mortality and usually occurred simultaneously with maternal death (10/14, 71%). The remaining cases resulted from abortion or unexplained stillbirth.

When coronary artery morphology had been studied (either by angiography or at autopsy) during pregnancy or shortly thereafter (54% of reported patients), coronary atherosclerosis with or without an intracoronary thrombus was found in 43% (29/68); definite or probable coronary thrombus without evidence of atherosclerotic disease was present in 21% (14/68). Atherosclerotic disease was found more commonly in women with antepartum acute myocardial infarction (58%) than in those with peripartum (12%) or postpartum acute myocardial infarction (29%). Coronary dissection was found in 16% (11/68), being the primary cause of infarction in the post-partum period (33%). Normal coronary arteries were reported in 29% (20/68) of all cases and 75% of those with peripartum acute myocardial infarction.

Etiology

Risk factors for myocardial infarction in young women in general include a family history of coronary artery disease,

Cardiac Problems in Pregnancy, Third Edition
Edited by Uri Elkayam, MD, and Norbert Gleicher, MD

TABLE 12.1 Selected Epidemiological, Clinical, and Pathological Data in 125 Cases of Myocardial Infarction Associated with Pregnancy

Case No.	Year, f/u	Ref: First Author	Age (yr)	Gestational Age	Medical History	Location of MI	Complications	Survival Maternal	Survival Fetal	Mode of Delivery	Anesthesia	Coronary Anatomy
							Antepartum					
1	1935	Reis[63]	45	34 wk	G_6, P_4	?	CHF	+	+	Spontaneous vaginal 48 h P/MI, forceps	Narcotic	?
2	1937, 2 mo f/u	White[59]	22	8 wk	G_1, P_0	Lateral		+	+	Spontaneous vaginal at 40 wk, forceps	Narcotic	?
3	1950, 1 wk f/u	Nolan[18]	37	12 wk	G_5, P_4	Anterior	CHF	+	+	Spontaneous vaginal at 30 wk	?	?
4	1953	Mendelson[62]	42	5 mo	G_2, P_1 PPE AP	Inferior	HTN	+	+	Elective cs at 39 wk	Local	?
5	1952	Mendelson[62]	42	30 wk	G_8, P_7 HTN	Anterior	CHF	Died on day 2 of cardio shock				?
6	1953, 1 wk f/u	Brock[55]	34	8 wk	G_4, P_3 HTN DM	Anterior		+	+	Spontaneous vaginal at 40 wk, forceps	Spinal	?
7	1956, 5 mo f/u	Siegler[74]	38	6w	G_5, P_2 HTN DM	Inferior		+	Stillborn	Spontaneous vaginal at 37 wk		?
8	1957, 1 yr f/u	Myers[61]	39	6 wk	$G_?, P_1$	Inferior		+	+	Spontaneous vaginal at 37 wk		?
9	1957	Forssell[70]	38	2 mo	G_3, P_0 HTN	Anterior		+	+	Elective cs at 2 wk preterm (obst)	?	?
10	1957	Forssell[70]	44	21 wk	G, P: >1	Anterior	CHF	+	–	Spontaneous vaginal at 25 wk	?	?
11	1960	Brown[44]	24	24 wk	G_4, P_3	Anterior	Sudden death at 24 h P/MI	–	–			LAD sten and throm on PM
12	1960, 2.5 yr f/u	Watson[50]	22	38 wk	$G_2, P_?$	Anterior		+	+	Elective cs at 2 wk P/MI		?
13	1961, 1 yr f/u	Shapira[54]	33	28 wk	G_3, P_0 HPLP Fam hx	Inferior		+	+	Spontaneous vaginal at 39 wks, forceps		?
14	1961, 6 mo f/u	Naden[69]	39	3 mo	G_4, P_2	Anterior		+	+	Elective cs at term (obst)		?
15	1961, 1.5 yr f/u	Jacobs[98]	34	5 mo	G_5, P_3	Inferior		+	–	Macerated fetus at 7 mo		?
16	1962, 7 yr f/u	Etienne[100]	26	?	$G_?, P_?$	Anterior		+	+	Spontaneous vaginal	?	?

No.	Year / Notes	Author	Age	Time	G/P	Location	Complication			Delivery	Anesthesia	Outcome
17	1964	Pfaffenschlager[86]	21	7 mo	$G_?, P_?$	Anterior	Hypotension	+	+	Spontaneous vaginal	?	?
18	1964	Bielak[104]	36	29 wk	G_7, P_6 s/p Rec anterior MI PPE	Inferior		+	+	Spontaneous vaginal at term	Pudendal block	?
19	1967, 7 yr f/u	Fletcher[60]	38	29 wk	$G_4, P_?$	Anterior		+	+	Spontaneous vaginal at 38 wk	?	?
20	1967, Sudden death at 2.25 yr of re-MI	Fletcher[60]	36	30 wk	$G_7, P_?$ PPE	Anterior		+	+	Elective cs at 40 wk	?	?
21	1967, 2 yr f/u	Fletcher[60]	36	32 wk	$G_4, P_?$	Inferior		+	+	Spontaneous vaginal at 40 wk	?	?
22	1967	Fletcher[60]	38	30 wk	$G_2, P_?$	Inferior		+	+	Spontaneous vaginal at 38 wk	?	?
23	1967, 14 wk f/u	Fletcher[60]	41	13 wk	$G_2, P_?$ PPE AP	Anterior		+	+	Intrauterine death at 33 wk due to severe preeclampsia	?	?
24	1968	Pantev[87]	26	8 mo	G_2, P_1	Anterior	Cardio shock	−	−	Spontaneous vaginal < 24 h from admission	?	?
25	1968, 8 wk f/u	Adler[81]	40	6 mo	G_4, P_2 Smok	Inferior posterior		+	+	Spontaneous vaginal at term	Pudendal	?
26	1969	Bedford[105]	38	4 mo	G_2	Anterior		+	+	Spontaneous vaginal at term	?	?
27	1970, died 4 yr later of re-MI	Ginz[53]	35	34 wk	G_5, P_2	Inferior		+	+	Spontaneous vaginal at 37 wk	?	?
28	1970	Curry[34]	29	24 wk	G_5, P_2 postinferior AP PPE	Inferior	VF + dc at 300 did not affect fetus	+	−			?
29	1970	Curry[34]		40 wk		Re-inferior	Sudden death	−	−			Diffuse atherosclerosis, 100% throm of CX on PM
30	1971, 1.5 yr f/u	Bruschke[64]	33	36 wk	$G_?, P_2$	Anterior	CHF	+	+	Spontaneous vaginal at 39 wk	?	Prox aneu of LAD at 4 mo P/MI
31	1971, sudden death at 3 mo PP	Husaini[47]	40	12 wk	G_3, P_2 HTN	Interior		+	+	Semielective cs at 35 wk due to CHF	?	3 VD, 100% prox RCA at 1 yr P/MI
32	1971, 2 yr f/u	Husaini[47]	32	33 wk	G_4, P_1	Inferior		+	+	Spontaneous vaginal at 35 wk	?	?
33	1972	Asuncion[52]	39	3 trim	G_4, P_3	Anterior	Sudden death 30 min P/MI	−	+	Emergency cs at 2 min of CPR	?	Diss of LMCA on PM

(continued)

133

TABLE 12.1 (Continued)

Case No.	Year, f/u	Ref: First Author	Age (yr)	Gestational Age	Medical History	Location of MI	Complications	Survival Maternal	Survival Fetal	Mode of Delivery	Anesthesia	Coronary Anatomy
65	1990	Nolan[18]	26	38 wk	G_2, P_1	Anterior	EF = 64%	+	+	Spontaneous vaginal 28 h P/MI	Epidural	Prox and mid LAD and RCA aneu post-MI
66	1991, 10 mo f/u	Frenkel[22]	28	34 wk	G_2, P_1	Anterior	EF = 45%	+	+	Elective cs 40 wk (obst)	Epidural	NCA at 4 mo P/MI
67	1991, 4 mo f/u	Pardo[107]	42	31 wk	G_2, P_3	Anterior		+	+	Semielective cs at 33 wk due to fetal distress	?	Prox LAD, catheter-induced spasm postlabor
68	1992	Perucca[108]	35	38 wk	$G_?$, $P_?$	Lateral	Sudden death 16 days P/MI	−	+	Elective cs at 40 wk	?	?
69	1993	Ottman[23]	25	26 wk	G_6, P_3 AVR	Inferior	Post-MI AP	+	+	Spontaneous vaginal at 35 wk	Narcotic	?
70	1993, 5 mo f/u	Taylor[26]	39	38 wk	G_2, P_1	Anterior	EF = 52%	+	+	Spontaneous vaginal at 40 wk, forceps, SG	Cond	50% prox LAD and 99% IInd Diag at 3 wk P/MI
71	1993	Sheikh[66]	32	16 wk	G_3, P_2 DM HTN Smok	Anterior	EF = 50%	+	+	Elective induced vaginal at 35 wk	Epidural	90% prox LAD sten during MI
72	1993, 6 wk f/u	Sheikh[66]	27	28 wk	G_5, P_2 Smok	Inferior	EF = 65%	+	+ Triplet, CS for severe preecla at 33 wk	Semielective	Epidural	NCA during MI
73	1993, 6 mo f/u	Verkaaik[71]	35	40 wk	G_1 Smok	Anterior	Re-MI infer on day 3	+	+	Semielective cs for fetal distress at 1 + 3 day P/MI	Epidural	3VCA at 1 day P/MI
74	1993, 3 mo f/u	Jessurun[93]	30	33 wk	G_2, P_1 HTN Pheo	Anterior	EF = 50%	+	+	Elective cs at 36 wk (obst)	?	NCA 3 wk P/MI
75	1993	Emori[97]	27	37 wk	G_1	Anterior	Proph pace VF on day 12	+	+	Emergency cs due to fetal distress post-CPR	?	Mid RCA and CX narrowing and diss at 4 wk
76	1994	Sanchez-Ramos[42]	29	26 wk	G_2, P_1 HPLP Fam hx	Inferior		+	+	Elective cs at 39 wk (obst)	Spinal	90% prox RCA at 2 wk P/MI, IC, UK and PTCA
77	1994	Jensen[94]	29	15 wk	G_3, P_2 Fam Hx HTN Smok	Anterior	P/MI, AP	+	+	Induced vaginal at 40 wk	?	Prox LAD sten at 10 wk P/MI and PTCA

Case	Year, f/u	Reference	Age	Timing	G/P	MI Location	Presentation	Maternal	Fetal	Delivery	Anesthesia	Confirmation
78	1994	MHO[99]	35	3 mo	G?, P?	Inferior	EF = 58%	+	+	?	?	NCA at 6 wk P/MI
Peripartum												
1	1955, 2 wk f/u	Antonius[58]	36	28 wk	G2, P1	Anterior	CHF	+	+	Spontaneous vaginal at <1 day P/MI, forceps	Local	?
2	1956, 3 wk f/u	Lewis[84]	37	1 h P/P	G2, P1	Anterior	VF P/MI AP	+	+	Spontaneous vaginal, P/term	?	?
3	1957	Jewett[45]	41	39 wk	G4, P2 Preeclampsia HTN	Anterior	Sudden death before labor	-	+	Delivery by emergency cs 5 min PM		LAD occlusion on PM
4	1958	NA[99]	35	1.5 h P/P	G?, P6 Toxemia Ergot	?	Sudden death (pres)	-	+	Spontaneous vaginal at term	?	
5	1961	Magner[89]	29	39 wk	G3, P1 HTN	Anterior	Cardio shock and death during labor	-	-	Induced vaginal attempted	?	Prox LAD occlusion with throm on PM
6	1963, wk f/u	Bechtel[82]	35	7 mo	G10, P7	Anterior		+	+ twins	Elective cs at term	?	?
7	1965	Dementova[102]	23	?	G1, P0	Anterior	Sudden death in stage II	-	+	Spontaneous with vaginal emergency, Forceps	?	Probably NCA on PM
8	1965	Dementova[102]	27	12 min P/P	G1	Inferior	Sudden death	-	+	Spontaneous vaginal	?	Probably NCA on PM
9	1966	Listo[77]	29	39 wk	G2, P1	Anterior	CHF, shock	+	Stillborn	Cs following severe CHF during vaginal attempt at term	?	?
10	1969	Canning[46]	44	10 min P/P	G7, P5	Anterior	AP	+	+	Spontaneous vaginal at 40 wk	?	
11	1979	Beary[10]	35	At labor	G2, P2 Preeclampsia	Anterior	CH p1713X	+	+	Spontaneous vaginal at term?	?	?
12	1988, 6 mo f/u	Trouton[10]	39	41 wk	G8, P6 Smok	Anterior	VT 14 days P/P, EF = 23%	+	+	Spontaneous vaginal 1 h postadmission	?	NCA at 9 wk P/MI
13	1991, 8 days f/u	Menegakis[80]	37	39 wk	G1 Smok	Anterior		+	+	Spontaneous vaginal at 39 wk	Epidural	NCA at 5 days P/MI
14	1991	Liao[21]	34	12 wk	G3, P2 Smok	Anterior	EF = 32%, spontaneous abortion post-ergot	+	-		?	NCA at 1 h P/MI
15	1992	Liu[24]	33	36 wk	G2, P1 Coca HTN	Anterior	CHF HTN	+	+	Induced vaginal due to fetal distress at 36 wk, forceps, SG	General	?

(continued)

TABLE 12.1 (*Continued*)

Case No.	Year, f/u	Ref: First Author	Age (yr)	Gestational Age	Medical History	Location of MI	Complications	Survival Maternal	Survival Fetal	Mode of Delivery	Anesthesia	Coronary Anatomy
16	1992	Sala[39]	38	39 wk	G_3, P_1 HTN	Anterior	VF on admission CHF, coma	− (26 days P/MI)	+	Emergency cs during CPR		No CAD on PM
17	1992	Van Enk[65]	33	35 wk	P_4 Sickle cell anemia	RVMI	Cardio shock	+	+	Cs on emergency basis		
							Postpartum					
1	1956, 3 yr f/u	Freedom[67]	28	17 days P/P	$G_?, P_1$ Ergot for Migraine	Anterior	P/MI AP	+	+	Spontaneous vaginal 1 wk post-term, forceps	?	?
2	1959	Vasicka[68]	21	4 days P/P	G_2, P_1	Anterior	Sudden death on day 4 P/P; sore throat	−	Stillborn	Spontaneous vaginal at 40 wk, forceps	Local pudendal	Severe LAD sten on PM
3	1959	Urdan[73]	31	4 days P/P	G_6, P_6 HTN	Anterior	Toxemia on HTN, sudden death on day 4 P/P	−	+	Spontaneous vaginal at term	Saddle block	3VCAD and LAD throm on PM
4	1960, 10 mo f/u	Brown[44]	23	3 days P/P	$G_?, P_?$ Preeclampsia	Anterior	—, P/P	+	+	Induced vaginal at term		?
5	1960, 4 mo f/u	Watson[50]	17	3 days P/P	G_1, P_1	Inferior		+	+	Spontaneous vaginal 3 wk preterm		?
6	1960	Wells[90]	42	6 wk P/P	$G_?, P_?$ AP	Anterior	Sudden death at 3 h P/MI	−	+	Spontaneous vaginal at term	?	Prox LAD diss on PM
7	1963	Lewis[84]	28	2 wk P/P	G_3, P_3 HTN in G_3	Anterior	Death from cardi. cardio & # free wall on day 16	−	+	Spontaneous vaginal at term, forceps	?	Throm of the entire LAD on PM
8	1969	Palomino[91]	31	2 wk P/P	$G_?, P_8$	Anterior	Sudden death post chest pain	+	−	Vaginal at ? wk	?	Diss of LAD + CX on PM
9	1970, 6 wk f/u	Ginz[53]	25	11 days P/P	G_1, P_1	?		+	+	Spontaneous vaginal at 36 wk	?	?
10	1970	Ginz[53]	27	8 days P/P	G_2, P_2	Anterior	Sudden death (pres)	−	+	Cs at ? wk	?	?
11	1971	Di Maio[92]	27	2 wk P/P	G_3, P_3	Anterior	Sudden death (pres)	−	+	Vaginal	?	Diss of LAD on PM
12	1971	Glancy[75]	36	11 days P/P	$G_?, P_3$ Smok	Anterior	Sudden death post chest pain	+	+	Spontaneous vaginal		NCA at 57 mo P/MI
13	1972	Asuncion[52]	26	2 wk P/P	G_4, P_4	Anterior	Sudden death at 4 h post-admission	−	+	Spontaneous vaginal at term	Single dose Demerol	Diss of prox LAD on PM
14	1978	Shaver[31]	28	3 wk P/P	G_2, P_2	Anterior		+	+	Cs at term	?	LAD aneurysm at 4 mo P/MI
15	1979, 5 mo f/u	Beary[29]	29	14 days P/P	$G_2, P_?$	Anterior	Sudden death (pres) EF = 36%	+	+	Spontaneous vaginal at term	?	NCA at 20 days P/MI
16	1980	Chant[72]	25	9 wk P/P	G_2, P_2	Anterior		+	+	Spontaneous vaginal at term		NCA at 3 mo P/MI

138

No.	Author	Year, f/u	Age	Timing	G/P, risk	MI location	Complications			Delivery		Angiographic findings
17	Henion[79]	1982, 3 mo f/u	34	4 days P/P	G? P3 Ergot	Anterior	CHF EF = 46%	+	+	Spontaneous vaginal at term	?	NCA at 3 mo P/MI
18	Bornstein[37]	1984	36	1 wk P/P	G? P4	Anterior	CHF VT	+	+	Spontaneous vaginal at term	?	NCA at 17 days P/MI
19	Iffy[7]	1986	36	10 days P/P	G2 P? BrCr Ergot	Anterior	CHF	+	+	Spontaneous vaginal at term	?	?
20	Iffy[7]	1986	22	5 days P/P	G2 P2 BrCr	Anterior	Sudden death (pres)	–	+	Cs due to fetal distress at term	?	Throm of LAD on PM
21	Ruch[14]	1989	27	10 days P/P	G2 P2 PPE BrCr	Anterior	VF Brain damage	+	+	Spontaneous vaginal at term	?	65% sten of mid-LAD at 2 mo P/MI
22	Movesesian[15]	1989, 6 mo f/u	29	3 wk P/P	G? P?	Anterior	CHF	+	+	Vaginal at term	+	Diss of prox LAD at 6 days P/MI
23	Giudici[17]	1989	41	11 days P/P	G? P? BrCr	Anterior	LAD diss post-2nd PTCA	+	+	Vaginal at term	+	Mid-LAD occlusion PTCA and re-PTCA after 24 h
24	Samra[35]	1989, 22 mo f/u	22	14 days P/P	G1 P1	Inferior		+	+	Spontaneous vaginal at term	?	?
25	Wittry[38]	1989	34	12 h P/P	G>1 P>1 Smok	Anterior	Ongoing pain	+	+	Spontaneous vaginal at term	?	Severe sten of LAD during MI
26	McHuge[95]	1990	39	10 days P/P	G? P1 HTN	Anterior		+	+	Elective cs (obst) at term	?	60% LAD tubular narrowing during MI
27	Capro Marzani[106]	1990	38	11 days P/P	G? P? Smok Fam hx	Anterior	CHF VT-DC post-MI AP	+	+	Semielective cs at 39 wk (obst)	?	Diss of LMCA 25 days P/MI
28	Saxena[25]	1992, 6 wk f/u	23	3 days P/P	G2 P2 DM HTN CRF Smok	Inferior	Post-MI AP	+	+	Cs at 37 wk (obst)	?	Occlusion of circumflex marg and PTCA during MI
29	Parry[41]	1992	27	12 wk P/P	G2 P2 HTN	Inferior		+	+	Spontaneous vaginal at term	?	Throm in prox LAD at 9 days P/MI
30	Effstration[96]	1994, 1 yr f/u	27	4 wk P/P	G2 P2 HPLP Smok	Anterior	Pulm embolism	+	+	Elective cs at 8 mo (obst)	?	Prox LAD diss at 3 days P/MI

Abbreviations: Alco, alcohol; Analg, analgesia; Aneu, aneurysm; APA, antiphospholipid antibodies; AVR, aortic valve replacement; BrCr, bromocriptine; Cardio, cardiogenic; CHF, Cognitive Hearty Failure; Coca, cocaine; Cond, conduction anesthesia; CMPT, cardiomyopathy; CPR, cardiopulmonary resuscitation; CRF, chronic renal failure; cs, cesarean section; CX, circumflex coronary artery; Diag, diagonal; Diss, dissection; DM, diabetes; EF, ejection fraction; Ergot, ergotamine derivatives; Fam hx, family history; G_n, gravida; HTN, hypertension; HPLP, hyperlipidemia; IC, intracoronary; IM, intramuscular; IABP, intraaortic balloon counterpulsation; IDDM, insulin-dependent diabetes mellitus; LMCA, left main coronary artery; LAD, Left anterior descending artery; Marg, marginal; NCA, normal coronary arteries; (obst), obstetrical indication; P, post; P_n, para; Pheo, pheochromocytoma; PP, postpartum; P/MI, postmyocardial infarction; PM, post mortem; PPE, previous preeclampsia; Pres, presentation; Prop-pace, prophylactic pacing; Prox, Proximal; PTCA, percutaneous transluminal coronary angioplasty; Pulm, pulmonary; RCA, right coronary artery; Rec, recurring; RVMI, right ventricular infarction; SG, Swan–Ganz catheter in place; Smok, smoking; Sten, stenosis; Throm, thrombus; Trim, trimester; $nVCAD$, 1, 2, 3. . . . vessel coronary artery disease; UK, urokinase.

TABLE 12.2   Comparison of Selected Epidemiological Clinical and Anatomopathological Data in 123 Pregnancies Complicated by 125 Myocardial Infarctions

Parameter	Antepartum: $n = 78$	Peripartum: $n = 17$	Postpartum: $n = 30$	Entire Group: $n = 125$
Age (y)	33 ± 6	34 ± 5	29 ± 6	32 ± 6
Range	16–45	23–44	17–42	16–45
MI location anterior[a]	50/77 (65%)	14/16 (87%)	25/29 (86%)	89/122 (73%)
Multiparous[a]	64/73 (88%)	13/16 (81%)	16/22 (73%)	93/111 (84%)
History (%)				
Hypertension	21	24	17	19
Diabetes mellitus	6	0	3	5
Ischemic heart disease	10	0	3	7
Smoking	32	12	20	26
Family history	12	0	3	8
Hyperlipidemia	1	0	3	2
Preeclampsia	10	18	10	11
Cesarian section (%)				
Elective	15	6	17	14
Semielective or emergency	14	12	7	12
Congestive heart failure post-MI	12 (15%)	7 (41%)	6 (20%)	25 (19%)
Coronary anatomy available in:	36 (46%)	8 (47%)	24 (80%)	68 (54%)
Stenosis	21 (58%)[b]	1 (12%)	7 (29%)[c]	29 (43%)
Thrombus	8 (22%)	1 (12%)	5 (21%)	14 (21%)
Dissection	3 (8%)	0	8 (33%)	11 (16%)
Aneurysm	2 (6%)	0	1 (4%)	3 (4%)
Spasm	1 (3%)	0	0	1 (1%)
Normal	9 (25%)	6 (75%)	5 (21%)	20 (29%)
Mortality				
Mothers	11 (14%)	6 (35%)	9 (30%)	26 (21%)
Infants	12 (15%)	3 (18%)	1 (3%)	16 (13%)
Death of infant associated with mother's death	8/12	1/3	1/1	10/14 (71%)

[a]The antepartum group includes all myocardial infarctions that occurred up to 24 h before labor. The peripartum group includes all myocardial infarctions that occurred within ±24 h from labor. All infarctions that occurred from 24 h to the end of the third postpartal month are included in the postpartum group. The number in the denominator represents the relevant *n* available.
[b]Associated thrombus in 7 cases.
[c]Associated thrombus in 1 case.

familial hyperlipoproteinemia, low levels of high density lipoproteins and/or high levels of low density lipoproteins, diabetes mellitus, cigarette smoking, and previous use of oral contraceptives.[110] Although atherosclerotic disease seems to be the primary cause of acute myocardial infarction during pregnancy, it was found in less than half of patients in whom coronary anatomy was investigated (Table 12.2). Other potential etiologies include thrombosis, coronary artery spasm (either spontaneous[37] or induced by bromocriptine[7,17]), coronary artery dissection,[15,31,71] collagen vascular disease,[16,41] Kawasaki disease,[18] cocaine use,[24] aortic valvular stenosis, aortic prosthetic valve thrombosis,[23] sickle cell chronic lung disease,[65] pheochromocytoma,[93] and fibrosis of a coronary ostium secondary to repeated trauma by a papillary fibroelastoma with a long stalk, which was found to be strategically located in front of the ostium.[100] In spite of the multiplicity of potential etiologies, their rarity during child-bearing age may explain low rate of pregnancy-related acute myocardial infarction.

Twenty-nine percent of cases with defined coronary artery anatomy had normal coronary arteries (Table 12.2). Since thrombus without atherosclerotic disease was found in 21% of the patients, a transient coronary spasm resulting in acute coronary thrombosis as a result of the hypercoagulable state of pregnancy is a possible explanation. Failure to identify similar thrombosis in other cases may be related to late performance of angiography. Since acute myocardial infarction has been related to pregnancy-induced hypertension and preeclampsia, enhanced vascular reactivity to angiotensin II[111] and norepinephrine[112] and endothelial dysfunction[113] reported in these conditions may also promote coronary constriction. Decreased uterine perfusion in the supine position leading to renin release, and angiotensin production,[32] and ergot derivatives which are used to control postpartum[33] or

TABLE 12.3   Comparison of Selected Epidemiological and Clinical Data on Survivors and Nonsurvivors Among Pregnant Women Who Sustained a Myocardial Infarction During Pregnancy and the Puerperium

Parameter	Survivors: $n = 99$	Nonsurvivors: $n = 26$
Age (yr)	32 ± 6	31 ± 7
MI location (%), anterior	70	84
Multiparous[a]	75/89 (84%)	16/22 (73%)
History (%)		
Hypertension	19	24
Diabetes mellitus	5	4
Ischemic heart disease	7	8
Smoking	32	4
Family history	10	0
Hyperlipidemia	3	0
Preeclampsia	10	16
Cesarean section		
Elective	27 (27%)	6 (23%)
semielective or emergency	11/27 (41%)	4 (67%)

[a] See note a, Table 12.2.

postabortion[21] hemorrhage or to suppress lactation,[7,13,14] were also suggested as potential causes of coronary spasm.

Profound alterations in the coagulation and fibrinolytic system occur during pregnancy and increase the risk of thrombosis. These changes include decreased releasable tissue plasminogen activator (tPA),[114–116] increased fast-acting tPA inhibitor,[116,117] change in the level of coagulation factors,[115,118] and reduction in functional protein S levels.[26,119,120] Cigarette smoking during pregnancy further increases risk of thrombosis due to enhanced platelet aggregability.[121] Hypercoagulation is further augmented at the time of separation of the placenta, which is a major source of plasminogen activator inhibitor.[119]

Pregnancy-related coronary arterial dissections have been reported to occur antepartum and postpartum, but the overwhelming majority of cases seem to occur in the immediate postpartum period (Table 12.2, Figure 12.1).[122,123] It has been suggested[15] that angiographically normal coronary arteries seen in many patients with peripartum acute myocardial infarction may represent a healed or spontaneously re-

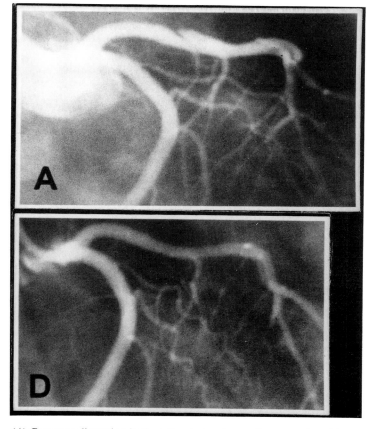

Figure 12.1   (A) Coronary dissection in the left anterior descending artery in a 44-year-old woman who presented with acute anterior myocardial infarction in the early postpartum period. (D) Angiogram 6 months after insertion of a coronary stent at the proximal part of the dissection. (Courtesy of Y Almagor, MD and S. Goldberg, MD; part (A) reproduced with permission from Braunwald, ed., *Heart Disease,* 5th ed, 1996;1854.)

paired coronary dissection. The cause for dissection may be hormonally mediated biochemical and histological changes reported to occur in arterial walls during gestation (e.g., loss of normal corrugation in elastic fibers, fragmentation of reticular fibers, decrease in the content of acid mucopolysaccharide).[124,125]

Marked increase in blood volume, stroke volume, and heart rate usually seen in pregnancy[126] can increase myocardial oxygen demand. At the same time, the physiological anemia and decreased diastolic blood pressure during gestation may reduce myocardial oxygen supply and contribute to the development of myocardial ischemia when coronary blood supply is compromised. These conditions may be further augmented during labor and delivery as a result of anxiety, pain, and uterine contraction, and they may be associated with up to a threefold increase in oxygen consumption. In the puerperium, increased hemodynamic load may be further increased because of enhanced venous return to the heart with relief of caval compression and shift of blood from the contracting emptied uterus into the systemic circulation. The hemodynamic changes normally occurring during late pregnancy and during labor, delivery, and the puerperium[126] may contribute to poor outcome reported in women who suffer an acute myocardial infarction in the peripartum period.

Diagnosis and Clinical Considerations

Early diagnosis of acute myocardial infarction during pregnancy is often hindered by mistaken attributions of its signs and symptoms to normal manifestations of pregnancy[127] and by a low level of suspicion. As in the nonpregnant state, the diagnosis is confirmed primarily by electrocardiographic and enzymatic changes. It is, therefore, important to note that electrocardiographic changes mimicking myocardial ischemia have been reported in up to 37% of parturients undergoing elective cesarean section.[128,129] Echocardiography can be performed safely during pregnancy to confirm the presence of ischemia by demonstrating wall motion abnormalities corresponding to electrocardiographic changes. Although myocardial ischemia is often associated with cardiac arrhythmias,[8] this finding is less helpful in pregnancy when various arrhythmias, especially multiple atrial and ventricular premature beats, but also supraventricular and ventricular tachycardia, may occur in women with normal hearts.[130,131]

In general, use of radiation in pregnancy should be limited as much as possible. The amount of radiation to the fetus from chest radiography is extremely small and probably should be considered safe enough to use when appropriate.[132] Radionuclide ventriculography using technetium-99m and myocardial perfusion scanning using thallium-201 or technetium-99m sestamibi would be expected to yield less than one rad to the conceptus and should be used during pregnancy only when absolutely necessary. Cardiac catheterization and interventional procedures may result in fetal exposure of less than one rad. However, difficult procedures requiring longer fluoroscopy time and multiple cineangiographic views could easily yield a fetal radiation of 5–10 rads. Termination of pregnancy generally is not recommended for fetal doses less than 5 rads, but this measure may be considered when the radiation dose exceeds this amount.

Treatment

Although the management of acute myocardial infarction and its complications should follow usual principles of care, fetal consideration may affect choice of therapy. A close consultation among attending obstetrician, cardiologist, and anesthesiologist is essential to optimize maternal as well as fetal well-being. Ideally, the patient should be treated in an intensive care unit capable of providing maternal and fetal monitoring along with a comprehensive obstetric service. A well-laid plan for prompt rescue of a potentially viable fetus in the event of sudden maternal deterioration should be established.

Drug Therapy: Morphine Sulfate This drug is not known to cause congenital defects. Since it crosses the placenta, however, it may cause neonatal respiratory depression when given shortly before delivery.[133] Morphine enters breast milk in trace amounts only and is considered compatible with breast feeding.[134]

Thrombolytic Therapy Thrombolytic therapy is a first-line treatment in acute myocardial infarction; its use during pregnancy, however, has been limited.[135–148] In fact, pregnancy constitutes a contraindication for thrombolytic treatment.[66,94] The basis for such prohibition, however, is strictly theoretical and probably was adopted from research protocols in which pregnancy traditionally constituted an exclusion criterion. Neither tissue plasminogen activator (TPA) nor streptokinase crosses the placenta in animals. No information, however, is available on passage of streptokinase in the human placenta during early pregnancy, and there are some indications that streptokinase does not cross the placental barrier in late pregnancy and has only a minimal placental passage during labor.[135,139] On the other hand, streptokinase antibodies were detected in the neonatal cord blood of women who received streptokinase several weeks prior to delivery.[137] Urokinase was studied and found not to be teratogenic in rats or mice.[149] Clinical experience with use of thrombolytic therapy during pregnancy has been mostly with streptokinase, being reported primarily in patients with massive and hemodynamically significant pulmonary embolism[136,142,145,146] or deep venous[137] or prosthetic valve thrombosis.[138,143,144,148,150] Because of the pivotal role of thrombolytic therapy in the modern treatment of acute myocardial infarction, published experience with this therapy during pregnancy is shown in Table 12.4. Available

TABLE 12.4 Reported Cases of Thrombolytic Therapy During Pregnancy

Ref: First Author	No. Cases	Therapy	Pregnancy	Dose	Results Maternal	Results Fetal	Disease
Ludwig[137] (1981)	122	SK	9–38 wk	250,000–750,000 IU followed by 200,000 IU/h for 8 h, then 100,000 IU/h. Longest duration, 5 days.	Two uterine hemorrhages leading to emergency CS.	One abruptio placenta with fetal death; one preterm delivery.	DVT
Hall[141] (1972)	1	SK	32 wk	600,000 IU followed by 100,000 IU/h for 41 h throughout delivery.	+ (persistent vaginal bleeding, required transfusion).	+, Preterm delivery.	PE
Fagher[142] (1990)	1	SK	28 wk	100,000 IU/h for 10.5 h, D/C with initiation of labor, episiotomy, and delivery 75 min later. SK reintroduced 8 h after delivery.	NA	+, Preterm delivery.	PE
Ramamurthy[143] (1994)	1	SK	28 wk	250,000 IU/30 min followed by 200,000 IU/24 hr	NA	+, Preterm delivery.	PVT
Sbarouni[144] (1994)	4	SK	NA	NA	NA	NA	PVT
Witchitz[148] (1980)		SK	8 mo	500,000 IU/30 min followed by 100,000 IU/h for 12 hr.	+, Uterine hemorrhage with rupture of membranes leading to cs.	+, Preterm delivery.	PVT
McTaggart[150] (1977)	1	SK	34 wk	250,000 IU followed by 100,000 IU/h for 4 h then 200,000 IU/h for 6 hr, and 2nd dose of 250,000 IU/30 min.	+, Minor bleeding at puncture sites.	−, Fetal death 8 h after initiation of SK.	PE
Flossdorf[145] (1990)	1	TPA	31 wk	10 mg/h for 4 h followed by 2 mg/h for 90 min.	+, Puncture site bleeding, uncomplicated delivery 48 h after TPA.	+, Preterm delivery.	PE
Baudo[146] (1990)	1	TPA	35 wk	100 mg/3 hr	+, Uneventful elective CS 20 h after TPA.	−, Newborn with RDS died on 14th day. Autopsy showed intracranial bleeding.	PE
Barclay[147] (1990)	1	TPA	32 wk	2 mg/h for 48 h.	+, Uneventful delivery 2 days after T PA.	+, Preterm delivery.	PE
Sanchez-Ramos[42] (1994)	1	UK	28 wk	NA	NA	NA	CT
Delclos[136] (1986)	1	UK	28 wk	4400 U/kg over 10 min followed by 4400 U/h.	NA	NA	PE

Abbreviations: +, alive; −, dead; CS, cesarean section; CT, coronary thrombosis; D/C, discontinued; DVT, deep vein thrombosis; NA, not available; PE, pulmonary embolism; PVT, prosthetic valve thrombosis; RDS, Respiratory distress syndrome; SK, streptokinase; TPA, tissue plasminogen activator; TA, thrombolytic agent; UK, urokinase.

reports describe the use of therapeutic dose of streptokinase,[137,141–144] tissue plasminogen activator,[145–147] and urokinase[42,136,138,145] between gestational weeks 9 and 38.[147] Delivery occurred during thrombolytic therapy or 1–2 days after cessation of therapy in many cases.[141,142,145–147] Although maternal and fetal outcome was uneventful in many cases, complications have been reported, including maternal hemorrhage, preterm delivery, and fetal loss.[135,137,141,142] Hemorrhagic complications included spontaneous abortion, minor vaginal bleeding requiring no intervention,[135,138] spontaneous hematoma in the inguinal and axillary region requiring blood transfusion,[135] fatal abruptio placenta with fetal death,[137] uterine bleeding necessitating emergency cesarean section,[137,148] and postpartum hemorrhage that necessitated transfusion.[141,142] Risk of hemorrhagic complication seems to be increased when thrombolytic therapy is given at the time of delivery. Fetal hemorrhage or teratogenic effects have not been reported, and fetal outcome has been favorable in the majority of reported cases. Therapy was used during the first trimester in seven cases[135] with fetal loss in only one case. Most reported cases of fetal loss in patients treated with thrombolytic therapy do not seem to be related to treatment. In one case of fetal death due to abruptio placenta occurring during therapy,[137] however, and in another case in which fetal heart tones disappeared during thrombolytic therapy, such a relationship could not be ruled out.[150] In addition, intracranial hemorrhages were reported in a newborn who died from acute distress syndrome 14 days after delivery[146] by a woman who had received TPA during pregnancy.

In summary, therefore, available reports on the use of thrombolytic therapy during pregnancy do not support teratogenic effect. Although the majority of reported cases resulted in favorable maternal and fetal outcome, therapy is associated with risk of maternal hemorrhage, especially when given at time of delivery. Occasional fetal losses were reported but did not seem to be related to therapy in most cases; such a relationship could not always be ruled out, however. More information will be needed, therefore, before the fetal safety of thrombolytic therapy will be established.

Anticoagulation (See also Chapter 33) Heparin is the anticoagulant of choice during pregnancy because its large molecular size prevents it from crossing the placenta and therefore excludes this agent as a possible teratogen.[151] Since its effect may persist for up to 28 hours, discontinuation of therapy 24 hours before elective induction of labor is desirable.[151] Heparin should be discontinued with onset of spontaneous labor, and judicious use of protamine sulfate may be needed to reduce risk of bleeding and allow safe pudendal and epidural anesthesia.[151,152] Hemostatic stitches should be used to avoid bleeding due to episiotomy, and uterine contraction should be stimulated after delivery by massage and pitocin or ergot derivatives to stop bleeding. Heparin can be resumed after delivery once hemostasis seems adequate. Heparin is not excreted into breast milk because of its high molecular weight.[134]

Aspirin Safety of high dose aspirin during pregnancy is debatable, especially in the third trimester, since large amounts of this drug may lead to increased maternal and fetal hemorrhage, congenital abnormalities, and premature closure of the ductus arteriosus.[153,153] On the other hand, low dose aspirin ($\leq$150 mg/day) proved effective in inhibiting thromboxane synthesis[155] and has been shown to be safe during the second and third trimester in a large number of hypertensive pregnant women.[156] The safety of aspirin during the first trimester is still unclear.[151] Aspirin is excreted into breast milk in low concentrations, and cautious use by lactating women has been recommended, but adverse effects have not been reported.[134]

Organic Nitrates Intravenous as well as oral nitrates have been used in pregnancy for the treatment of hypertension,[157] myocardial ischemia,[66] and infarction,[158] and to arrest preterm labor.[159] There are no known adverse effects of nitrate therapy during pregnancy; careful titration is recommended, however, to avoid maternal hypotension, which can lead to fetal distress.[157] No data are available regarding breast feeding in women treated with these drugs.

β-Adrenergic Blocking Agents (See also Chapter 29) Substantial experience with the use of propranolol, atenolol, labetolol, and metoprolol in pregnancy suggests their safety for gestational use,[160] although anecdotal reports indicate that side effects such as fetal growth retardation, bradycardia, hypoglycemia, hyperbilirubinemia, and apnea at birth should be anticipated. Since nonselective beta blockers may facilitate an increase in uterine activity, use of β_1-selective agents may be preferable. All beta blockers are weak bases and accumulate in breast milk in concentrations higher than in the plasma. Nursing infants should, therefore, be monitored for adverse effects.[160]

Calcium Antagonists Increasing experience with gestational use of nifedipine for treatment of hypertension, preeclampsia, myocardial ischemia, and tocolysis has demonstrated the safety of this drug.[161] Information regarding the use of verapamil and diltiazem during pregnancy is more limited.[162] A recent surveillance study raised the possibility of diltiazem-induced teratogenic effect.[163] All three calcium antagonists mentioned are considered compatible with breast feeding.[134]

Magnesium Although the routine use of magnesium in patients with acute myocardial infarction is still debated, early administration of the drug to high risk patients, especially those who do not receive thrombolytic therapy, has been shown to be useful.[164] Magnesium sulfate is commonly used in pregnancy as a tocolytic agent and as an anticonvulsant for toxemia. Large clinical experience with this drug during pregnancy indicated lack of teratogenic effect or other form of toxicity.[134,165] It should be noted, however, that magnesium sulfate has been rarely used during the first trimester. Newborns of mothers treated with magnesium close to delivery should be observed for signs of respiratory depression, muscle weakness, and loss of reflexes, since these effects were reported in a hypertensive woman treated with 11 g of magnesium sulfate within 3.5 hours of delivery.[166] Maternal hypothermia with maternal and fetal bradycardia due to intravenous magnesium sulfate have been described. In addition, hypotension and pronounced muscle weakness have been reported when the drug was used in combination with nifedipine.[165] Magnesium sulfate is considered compatible with breast feeding.[134]

COMPLICATIONS

Congestive Heart Failure (CHF)

Diuretics should be used cautiously to prevent overdiuresis and hypovolemia and thus reduction in uteroplacental blood flow[167] (see also Chapter 28). *Nitrates* are effective, but careful dose titration is recommended to avoid reduction in blood pressure. *Sodium nitroprusside* has been used in a limited number of patients during pregnancy; its safety is unknown.[167] A large dose of this drug resulted in fetal death in animals, demonstrating a potential for fetotoxicity. There is only limited experience with the use of dopamine in humans during pregnancy. Animal studies have shown both an increase and a decrease in uterine blood flow.[168,169] The drug has been used to increase renal blood flow in oliguric, eclamptic patients and to treat spinal hypotension during cesarean section without apparent adverse effect to the fetuses or newborns.[168–170] Information regarding use of dobutamine during pregnancy is similarly limited. Short-term use of this drug in one patient with myocardial infarction at 18 weeks gestation and in a patient with pulmonary hypertension prior to delivery were not associated with adverse effects.[6,171]

Angiotensin-converting enzyme (ACE) inhibitors are contraindicated during pregnancy because of increased incidence of fetal morbidity and mortality[172] (see also Chapter 32). Reported complications include oligohydramnios, intrauterine growth retardation, premature labor, fetal and neonatal renal failure, bony malformations, limb contractures, persistent patent ductus arteriosus, pulmonary hypoplasia, respiratory distress syndrome, prolonged hypotension, and neonatal death. If heart failure persists or the

patient's clinical condition deteriorates, more aggressive approaches should be sought and undertaken. In one case of severe hemodynamic instability, successful treatment with intraaortic balloon counterpulsation was applied, allowing postponement of delivery until hemodynamic stability had been achieved.[20] Cardiogenic shock accompanying acute myocardial infarction was reported to improve dramatically when cesarean section was undertaken.[11]

Arrhythmias

Drug Therapy Based on substantial clinical experience, the gestational use of digoxin and quinidine is considered to be safe to the fetus.[162] Procainamide and disopyramide have been used successfully to treat maternal and fetal arrhythmias, but experience with these drugs is still limited. Lidocaine has been used safely during pregnancy mainly for epidural or local anesthesia but also, as long as blood levels are closely monitored, as an antiarrhythmic agent. Elevated levels can cause infant central nervous system effect with apnea, hypotonia, dilated pupils, seizures, and bradycardia.[162] A relatively small number of pregnant women have reportedly been treated with newer antiarrhythmic agents such as mexiletine,[173] flecainide,[174] propafenone, and sotalol.[175] Owing to very limited information, these drugs' safety is unknown. The use of amiodarone during pregnancy has been associated with significant side effects, including hypothyroidism and congenital malformations in the newborn.[176] This drug should, therefore, be used only in refractory cases of maternal tachyarrhythmias. A recent survey identified 34 women who received adenosine intravenously during pregnancy for the treatment of maternal supraventricular arrhythmia[177] and showed the efficacy and safety of adenosine for the use during pregnancy.

Cardiac Pacing Indications for cardiac pacing in pregnant patients with acute myocardial infarction are similar to those used in the nonpregnant patient. No problems are anticipated with the use of temporary pacemakers based on reported experience in numerous pregnant patients.[178] These devices, however, should be inserted without fluoroscopy when possible. The availability of external transcutaneous pacing[179] provides the clinician with an ideal alternative for use during pregnancy.

Direct Current (DC) Cardioversion The use of DC cardioversion is recommended for treatment of maternal tachyarrhythmias that are associated with systemic hypotension or heart failure. Several investigators have documented the safety and efficacy of cardioversion and defibrillation in the setting of myocardial infarction during pregnancy.[1,4–6,8,34] Monitoring of fetal heart rate seems advisable, if possible, whenever maternal cardioversion is performed.

Postinfarction Angina

In a case of postinfarction angina pectoris poorly controlled with maximal medical therapy in the early part of pregnancy (up to 20 weeks), consideration should be given to termination of the pregnancy. The approach to this condition after week 20 should be similar to that of the nonpregnant patient. Cardiac catheterization and angiography, if indicated, should be done with fetal shielding, using the brachial or radial approach to reduce scattered radiation to the fetus. Although experience with percutaneous transluminal coronary angioplasty or coronary artery bypass grafting is still limited, these procedures have been performed successfully during pregnancy or the early postpartum period.[12,17,25,180] These forms of therapy, however, should be avoided, if possible, in pregnancy, especially during the first trimester, because of the potential deleterious effects on the fetus of both radiation and cardiopulmonary bypass.[181]

Cardiopulmonary Resuscitation (See also Chapter 25)

Before the onset of fetal viability, about the 24th gestational week, the objectives of cardiopulmonary resuscitation (CPR) can be guided almost exclusively by maternal considerations; later, consideration should also be given to fetal safety. Success of CPR in pregnancy may be hampered by a number of factors:

- The thorax is less compressible to external pressure because of the cephalad displacement of the abdominal contents.
- Chest compressions in the supine position may fail to produce sufficient cardiac output owing to both reduced venous return and increased obstruction to arterial forward flow.
- The elevated diaphragm results in increases of resistance to airflow during artificial respiration and to thoracic compressions, making resuscitation efforts even more difficult.[182]

Because of increased oxygen consumption and increased carbon dioxide and hydrogen ion production by fetoplacental metabolism, any delays in establishing effective ventilation magnify the circulatory compromise of the uteroplacental unit and may accelerate the rate at which the mother and the fetus become unresuscitable despite adequate chest compression.[183] To minimize the effects of the gravid uterus on venous return and cardiac output, a wedge (e.g., a pillow) should be placed under the flank of the right abdomen and hip to displace the uterus to the left side. If having the mother in the left lateral decubitus position makes resuscitative efforts clumsy and ineffective, continuous manual displacement to the left or positioning the back of the resuscitated patient on the thighs of a person kneeling on the floor sitting on the heels ("human wedge" maneuver)[184] may be used as alternative methods.

To date, there have been no studies comparing closed- and open-chest cardiac massage on the hemodynamics of the human uterus and placenta. The uteroplacental circulation, however, offers minimal vascular resistance as long as oxygenation and acid–base balance are not profoundly distorted. Favorable outcomes reported in some cases[185] suggest that the pressure gradients generated even by standard CPR may be adequate to sustain fetal life and should be attempted. At the same time, early evacuation of the uterus by bedside cesarean section resulted in recovery of blood pressure in a patient when generation of adequate blood pressure had failed despite vigorous resuscitative measures. Lee et al[186] recommended thoracotomy and open-chest cardiac massage between the 24th and 32nd weeks of gestation. Cesarean section after the 32nd week should be considered if standard cardiopulmonary resuscitation is ineffective.

Survival of the infant has been directly proportional to the time interval between the death of the mother and delivery.[187] Delivery taking place more than 15 minutes after maternal death rarely produces a viable infant; and virtually all surviving infants had some neurologic sequelae. On the other hand, all surviving infants delivered within 5 minutes after maternal death were healthy. Successful rescue and long-term maintenance of "brain dead" and comatose mothers have been accomplished, allowing for delivery at times more beneficial for the fetus.[187,188] To maximize the chances of both maternal and infant survival,[183–190] rapid cesarean section (within 4–5 min of the arrest) has been recommended.

Several points concerning use of drugs commonly administered during resuscitation should be addressed. Routine administration of bicarbonate has been discouraged in the nonpregnant patient during resuscitation because combined respiratory and metabolic alkalosis caused by vigorous ventilation and bicarbonate administration may be deleterious. During resuscitation of the pregnant woman, however, there is an increased rate of acid metabolite production. Since acidosis increases the α-adrenergic reactivity of the uteroplacental vasculature, use of bicarbonate during the resuscitation of a pregnant patient seems logical. While β- or combined β- and α-adrenergic agonists do not cause any hemodynamic derangement in the uteroplacental blood flow during normal pregnancy, hypoxemia or hypotension enhances sensitivity to the vasoconstrictor action of epinephrine and norepinephrine[191] and may, therefore, further impair uteroplacental flow. For this reason, reduced uteroplacental blood flow due to hypotension may not improve with vasopressors.

LABOR

To allow adequate healing of the infarct, delivery should be postponed, if possible, 2–3 weeks following acute myocardial infarction. Because of the increased hemodynamic requirements during both labor and uterine contractions,[126] myocardial ischemia and cardiac decompensation may occur. In addition, reduced oncotic pressure may predispose the development of pulmonary edema.

Mode of delivery in a pregnant patient with gestational myocardial infarction should be determined by obstetrical reasons and the clinical status of the mother. Both vaginal and cesarean deliveries have their advantages and disadvantages. The outcomes of all 125 patients reviewed for the purpose of this report supports the conclusion reached previously by Cohen et al,[4] who found no convincing support for one mode of delivery versus the other and suggests an individualized approach. Advantages of elective cesarean section include control of the time of delivery and avoidance of long and/or stressful labor. Vaginal delivery, on the other hand, eliminates the risks associated with anesthesia and the major surgical procedure and avoids potential postoperative morbidity (hemodynamic fluctuations, blood loss, pain, infections, respiratory complications, etc.).[2,30] With measures aimed to reduce cardiac workload and oxygen demands, vaginal delivery can be accomplished relatively safely.[5,6,10,40,192] Instrumental delivery is recommended to avoid excessive maternal efforts, and the patient should receive supplemental oxygen. For optimization of cardiac output, left lateral position is preferred. Hemodynamic parameters, as well as oxygen saturation, electrocardiogram, and fetal heart rate, should be monitored continuously. During labor and delivery, it is essential to minimize and control patient pain, fear, and apprehension, all of which can increase myocardial oxygen demand. Tachycardia and hypertension should be prevented and, if they occur, promptly corrected. In view of the possibility of coronary spasm, it may be wise to avoid oxytocin infusion during labor and ergonovine postpartum. Ischemia, which develops during labor and delivery, can be treated by intravenous nitroglycerin, beta blockers, and calcium antagonists. Nitroglycerin, as well as calcium antagonists such as diltiazem and verapamil, have demonstrated some tocolytic effect and may result in prolongation of labor.[159,167]

In summary, selection of delivery mode in patients who have had a myocardial infarction while pregnant should be made on an individual basis. Most patients with coronary artery disease can tolerate and therefore should have a vaginal delivery. Cesarean section is indicated only for obstetrical purposes and in cases of unstable ischemic or hemodynamic condition.

DISCHARGE

The timing of hospital discharge following acute myocardial infarction needs to be individualized. If the pregnancy is well advanced into the third trimester, continued hospitalization with restricted exertional activities until elective delivery may be appropriate in some cases.

Low risk patients and those whose time to delivery is remote may be discharged if their clinical condition is stable. Left ventricular function and the presence of residual myocardial ischemia can be assessed by means of stress echocardiographic study. Such an evaluation was reported 9 days after infarction at 27 weeks of gestation.[42] Because of potential fetal distress during exercise,[12] submaximal exercise protocol and fetal monitoring during exercise are recommended.[193] When high quality echocardiographic evaluation is not possible for technical reasons, thallium exercise test should be considered.

Since myocardial oxygen consumption will progressively increase with the progression of pregnancy, close post discharge follow-up of the pregnant patient after acute myocardial infarction is recommended. Assessment of fetal maturity and reassessment of cardiac status after the 32nd week are important for determination of management plan and feasibility of early delivery, if indicated.

SUBSEQUENT PREGNANCIES

Data on maternal and fetal outcome of pregnancy in patients with a history of prior myocardial infarction are extremely limited.[194] Available cases of pregnancy following myocardial infarction have not been associated with mortality, but there have been reports of increased short- and long-term morbidity.[1,4,20] These data must be interpreted with caution, since the patient number is small; full obstetric and cardiovascular details were not always presented; and the period between the infarction and pregnancy varied substantially (from 6 months to 7 years). As with other infarct survivors, the risks associated with subsequent pregnancy probably depend on many factors, including the cumulative amount of myocardial damage sustained, residual left ventricular function, underlying coronary anatomy, and ongoing myocardial ischemia.

ACKNOWLEDGMENT

This chapter was reproduced with modifications from Roth A, Elkayam U: Acute myocardial infarction associated with pregnancy. *Ann int med* 1996;125:751–762 with permission.

REFERENCES

1. Hankins GDV, Wendel GD Jr., Leveno KJ, Stoneham J. Myocardial infarction during pregnancy: a review. *Obstet Gynecol* 1985;65(1):139–146.
2. Sullivan JM, Ramanathan KB. Management of medical problems in the pregnancy—severe cardiac disease. *N Engl J Med* 1985;313:304–309.

3. Katz H. About sudden natural death in pregnancy: during delivery and the puerperium. *Arch Gynaekol* 1922;115:283–312.

4. Cohen WR, Steinman T, Pastner B, Snyder D, Satwicz P, Monroy P. Myocardial infarction in a pregnant woman at term. *JAMA* 1983;250:2179–2181.

5. Cortis BS, Lee SS, Bacalla M. Acute myocardial infarction and ventricular fibrillation during pregnancy. *Illinois Med J* 1981;160:170–174.

6. Stokes IM, Evans J, Stone M. Myocardial infarction and cardiac arrest in the second trimester followed by assisted vaginal delivery under epidural analgesia at 38 weeks gestation. Case report. *Br J Obstet Gynaecol* 1984;91:197–198.

7. Iffy L, TenHove W, Frisoli G. Acute myocardial infarction in the puerperium in patients receiving bromocriptine. *Am J Obstet Gynecol* 1986;155:371–373.

8. O'Donnell M, Meecham J, Tosson S, Ward S. Ventricular fibrillation and reinfarction in pregnancy. *Postgrad Med J* 1987;63:1095–1096.

9. Dawson PJ, Ross AW. Preeclampsia in a parturient with a history of myocardial infarction. *Anaesthesia* 1988;4:659–663.

10. Trouton TG, Sidhu H, Adgey AA. Myocardial infarction in pregnancy. *Int J Cardiol* 1988;18:35–39.

11. Mabie WC, Anderson GD, Addington MB, Reed CM, Peeden PZ, Sibai BM. The benefit of cesarean section in acute myocardial infarction complicated by premature labor. *Obstet Gynecol* 1988;71:503–506.

12. Cowan NC, de Belder MA, Rothman MT. Coronary angioplasty in pregnancy. *Br Heart J* 1988;59:588–592.

13. Sonel A, Erol C, Oral D, Omulu K, Akyol T, Kaymakcalan. Acute myocardial infarction and normal coronary arteries in a pregnant woman. *Cardiology* 1988;75:218–20.

14. Ruch A, Duhring JL. Postpartum myocardial infarction in a patient receiving bromocriptine. *Obstet Gynecol* 1989;74:448–451.

15. Movesesian MA, Wray RB. Postpartum myocardial infarction. *Br Heart J* 1989;62:154–156.

16. Rallings P, Exner T, Abraham R. Coronary artery vasculitis and myocardial infarction associated with antiphospholipid antibodies in a pregnant woman. *Aust N Z J Med* 1989;19:347–350.

17. Giudici MC, Artis AK, Webel RR, Alpert MA. Postpartum myocardial infarction treated with balloon coronary angioplasty. *Am Heart J* 1989;118:614–616.

18. Nolan TE, Savage RW. Peripartum myocardial infarction from presumed Kawasaki's disease. *South Med J* 1990;83(11):1360–1361.

19. Hands ME, Johnson MD, Saltzman DH, Rutherford JD: The cardiac, obstetric, and anesthetic management of pregnancy complicated by acute myocardial infarction. *J Clin Anesth* 1990;2:258–268.

20. Allen JN, Wewers MD. Acute myocardial infarction with cardiogenic shock during pregnancy: treatment with intraaortic balloon counterpulsation. *Crit Car Med* 1990;18:888–889.

21. Liao JK, Cockrill BA, Yurchak PM. Acute myocardial infarction after ergonovine administration for uterine bleeding. *Am J Cardiol* 1991;68:823–824.

22. Frenkel Y, Etchin A, Barkai G, Reisin L, Mashiach S, Batler A. Myocardial infarction during pregnancy: a case report. *Cardiology* 1991;78:363–368.

23. Ottman EH, Gall SA. Myocardial infarction in the third trimester of pregnancy secondary to an aortic valve thrombus. *Obstet Gynecol* 1993;81:804–805.

24. Liu SS, Forrester RM, Murphy GS, Chen K, Glassenberg R. Anaesthetic management of a parturient with myocardial infarction related to cocaine use. *Can J Anaesth* 1992;39(8):858–861.

25. Saxena R, Nolan TE, von Dohlen T, Houghton JL. Postpartum myocardial infarction treated by balloon coronary angioplasty. *Obstet Gynecol* 1992;79:810–812.

26. Taylor GW, Moliterno DJ, Hillis D. Peripartum myocardial infarction. *Am Heart J* 1993;126:1462–1463.

27. Clark SL. Cardiac disease in pregnancy. *Obstet Gynecol* 1987;18:237–253.

28. Nolan TE, Hankins GDV. Myocardial infarction in pregnancy. *Clin Obstet Gynecol* 1989;32:68–75.

29. Beary JF, Summer WR, Bulkley BH. Postpartum acute myocardial infarction: a rare occurrence of uncertain etiology. *Am J Cardiol* 1979;43:158–161.

30. Aglio LS, Johnson MD. Anaesthetic management of myocardial infarction in a parturient. *Br J Anaesth* 1990;65:258–261.

31. Shaver P, Carrig T, Baker W. Postpartum coronary artery dissection. *Br Heart J* 1978;40:83–86.

32. Sasse L, Wagner R, Murray FE. Transmural myocardial infarction during pregnancy. *Am J Cardiol* 1975;35:448–452.

33. Taylor GJ, Cohen B. Ergonovine-induced artery spasm and myocardial infarction after normal delivery. *Obstet Gynecol* 1985;66:821 822.

34. Curry JJ, Quintana FJ. Myocardial infarction with ventricular fibrillation during pregnancy treated by direct current defibrillation with fetal survival. *Chest* 1970;58:82–84.

35. Samra D, Samra Y, Hertz M, Maier M. Acute myocardial infarction in pregnancy and puerperium. *Cardiology* 1989;76:455–460.

36. Yla-Outinen A, Lyrenas S, Lantz P, Langhoff-Ross J. Myocardial infarction in pregnancy: a case report and review of the literature. *Uppsala J Med Sci* 1989;94:287–290.

37. Bornstein A, Dalal P, Tischler J, Novak S, Michaelson S. Acute myocardial infarction in a thirty-six year old postpartum female. *Angiology* 1984;35:591–594.

38. Wittry MD, Zimmerman TJ, Janosik D, Williams GA. Postpartum myocardial infarction in a patient with intermittent ventricular preexcitation. *Am Heart J* 1989;117:191–194.

39. Sala DJ. Myocardial infarction. *Nurses Assoc Amer Coll Obstet Gynecols* 1992;3:443–453.

40. Bembridge M, Lyons G. Myocardial infarction in the third trimester of pregnancy. *Anaesthesia* 1988;43(3):202–204.

41. Parry G, Goudevenos J, Williams DO. Coronary thrombosis postpartum in a young woman with Still's disease. *Clin Cardiol* 1992;15:305–307.

42. Sanchez-Ramos L, Chami YG, Bass TA, DelValle GO, Adair D. Myocardial infarction during pregnancy: management with

transluminal coronary angioplasty and metallic intracoronary stents. *Am J Obstet Gynecol* 1994;171:1392–1393.

43. Hutchinson SJ, Holden RJ, Lorimer AR. Myocardial infarction in pregnancy. *Scott Med J* 1985;30:116–118.

44. Brown A. Myocardial infarction associated with pregnancy. *N Engl J Med* 1960;23:1163–1165.

45. Jewett JF. Committee on Maternal Welfare. Cholecystitis, cholelithiasis and coronary occlusion. *N Engl J Med* 1957;256;574–575.

46. Canning B St. J, Green AT, Mulcahy R. Coronary heart disease in the puerperium. *J Obstet Gynecol Br Commonw* 1969;76;1018–1020.

47. Husaini MH. Myocardial infarction during pregnancy. Report of two cases with a review of the literature. *Postgrad Med J* 1971;47;660–665.

48. Hughes TBJ. Myocardial infarction and rheumatic heart disease in pregnancy. Case Report. *Br J Obstet Gynaecol* 1975;82;505–507.

49. Sperry KL. Myocardial infarction in pregnancy. *J Forensic Sci* 1987;32:1464–1470.

50. Watson H, Emslie-Smith D, Herring J. Myocardial infarction during pregnancy and puerperium. *Lancet* 1960;ii:523–524.

51. McKeon VA, Perrin KO. The pregnant woman with a myocardial infarction: nursing diagnosis. *Dimensions Crit Care Nurs* 1989;8:92–100.

52. Asuncion CM, Hyun J. Dissecting intramural hematoma of the coronary artery in pregnancy and the puerperium. *Obstet Gynecol* 1972;40:202–210.

53. Ginz B. Myocardial infarction in pregnancy. *J. Obstet Gynaecol Br Commonw* 1970;77:610–615.

54. Shapira E, Rosen RJ, Lederman B, Carey RJ. Myocardial infarction in the third trimester of pregnancy. *JAMA* 1961; 79: 966–977.

55. Brock HJ, Russell NG, Randall CR. Myocardial infarction in pregnancy. Report of a case with normal spontaneous delivery seven months later. *JAMA* 1953;152:1030–1031.

56. Goldberger E, Pokress MJ. Spontaneous delivery in a woman with myocardial infarction. *New York State J Med* 1950;50: 95–96.

57. Stokes M, Evans J, Stone M. Myocardial infarction and cardiac arrest in the second trimester followed by assisted vaginal delivery under epidural analgesia at 38 weeks gestation. Case report. *Br J Obstet & Gynaecol* 1984;91:197–198.

58. Antonius NA, Izzo PA, Hayes GW, Walsh CR, Newark NJ. Myocardial infarction in pregnancy. *Am Heart J* 1955;49; 83–88.

59. White PD, Glendy E, Gustapson P. Myocardial infarction complicating pregnancy in a young woman. *JAMA* 1937;109:863–864.

60. Fletcher E, Knox EW, Morton P. Acute myocardial infarction in pregnancy. *Br Med J* 1967;3:586–588.

61. Myers RF, Sharpe VJH. Acute myocardial infarction occurring during pregnancy. *Can Med Assoc J* 1957;76:754–758.

62. Mendelson CL. Coronary artery disease in pregnancy. *Am J Obstet Gynecol* 1952;63:381–391.

63. Reis RA, Frankenthal Jr LE. Labor in the cardiac patient. *Am J Obstet Gynecol* 1935;29:44–52.

64. Bruschke AVG, Bruyneel KJJ, Bloch A, van Herpen G. Acute myocardial infarction without obstructive coronary artery disease demonstrated by selective cinearteriography. *Br Heart J* 1971;33:585–594.

65. Van Enk A, Visschers G, Jansen W, Van Eps Satius LW. Maternal death due to sickle cell chronic lung disease. *Br J Obstet Gynaecol* 1992;99:162–163.

66. Sheikh AU, Harper MA. Myocardial infarction during pregnancy: management and outcome of two pregnancies. *Am J Obstet Gynecol* 1993;169:279–284.

67. Freedman JR. Coronary occlusion with myocardial infarction in a puerperal patient. *Am J Obstet Gynecol* 1956;71: 1106–1110.

68. Vasicka AI, Lin TJ. Fatal coronary artery disease during the early postpartum period. *Am J Obstet Gynecol* 1959;77: 899–904.

69. Naden RS, Johnson HF, Murray EN. Myocardial infarction during pregnancy. *JAMA* 1961;178:659–661.

70. Forssell J, Brunila T. Cardiac infarction in pregnancy. *Acta Med Scand* 1957;157:387–397.

71. Verkaaik APK, Visser W, Deckers JW, Lotgering FK. Multiple coronary artery dissections in a woman at term. *Br J Anesth* 1993;71:301–302.

72. Chant GN. Coronary anatomy in post partum acute myocardial infarction. *Am J Cardiol* 19890;45:912.

73. Urdan BE, Madden WJ. Pregnancy complicated by myocardial infarction. *Obstet Gynecol* 1959;14:378–380.

74. Siegler AM, Hoffman J, Bloom O. Myocardial infarction complicating pregnancy. *Obstet Gynecol* 1956;7:306–311.

75. Glancy D, Marcus ML, Epstein SE. Myocardial infarction in young women with normal coronary arteriograms. *Circulation* 1971;64:495–501.

76. Lamb MA. Myocardial infarction during pregnancy. A team challenge. *Heart Lung* 1987;16:658–661.

77. Listo M, Bjorkenheim G. Myocardial infarction during delivery. *Acta Obstet Gynecol Scand* 1966;45:268–279.

78. Duke M. Pregnancy, myocardial infarction and normal coronary arteries. *Connecticut Med* 1982;46:626–628.

79. Henion WA, Hilal A, Matthew PK, Lazarus AR, Cohen J. Postpartum myocardial infarction. Associated with normal coronary arteries. *New York State J Med* 1982;1:57–61.

80. Menegakis NE, Amstey MS. Case report of myocardial infarction in labor. *Am J Obstet Gynecol* 1991;165:1383–1384.

81. Adler JJ, Barrash MJ, Lash SR. Myocardial infarction during pregnancy. *Illinois Med J* 1968;134:143–146.

82. Bechtel JT, Lanford WS, Mangone EK. Myocardial infarction associated with twin pregnancy. Report of a case and review of literature. *J Fla Med Assoc* 1963;49:658–661.

83. Levine EL, Lanning RJ. Myocardial infarction immediately following delivery. *Missouri Med* 1956;53:967.

84. Lewis JF. Myocardial infarction during pregnancy: with associated myocardial bacteroides abscess. *South Med J* 1973; 66(3):379–381.

85. Roberts ADG, Low RAL, Hillis WS. Left ventricular aneurysm complicating acute myocardial infarction occurring during pregnancy. Case report. *Br J Obstet Gynaecol* 1983;90:969–970.

86. Pfaffenschlager F. Myokardinfarkt und Schwangerschaft. *Wien Klin Wochenschr* 1964;76:297–299.

87. Pantev I, Piperkov T. On myocardial infarction in pregnant women. *Akush Ginekol (Sofia)* 1968;7:158–161.

88. Ahronheim JH. Isolated coronary periarteritis: report of a case of unexpected death in a young pregnant woman. *Am J Cardiol* 1977;40:287–290.

89. Magner D. Coronary occlusion in labour. *J Obstet Gynaecol Br Commonw* 1961;68:128–129.

90. Wells AL. Dissecting aneurysm of coronary artery in the puerperium. *J Pathol Bacteriol* 1960;79:404–405.

91. Palomino SJ. Dissecting intramural hematoma of left coronary artery in the puerperium. *J Clin Pathol* 1969;51:119–125.

92. Di Maio VJM, Di Maio DJ. Postpartum dissecting coronary aneurysm. *New York State J Med* 1971;767–769.

93. Jessurun CR, Karlina A, Moise KJ, Wilansky S. Pheochromocytoma-induced myocardial infarction in pregnancy. *Texas Heart Institute J* 1993;20:120–122.

94. Jensen SE, Simonsen EE, Thayssen P. Acute myocardial infarction during early pregnancy. *J Intern Med* 1994;235:487–488.

95. McHuge MJ, Taubman MR. Postpartum myocardial infarction: a rehabilitation challenge. *J Cardiovasc Nurs* 1990;4;57–63.

96. Efstratiou A, Singh B. Combined spontaneous postpartum coronary artery dissection and pulmonary embolism with survival. *Cathet Cardiovasc Diagn* 1994;31:29–33.

97. Emori T, Goto Y, Maeda T, Chiba Y, Haze K. Multiple coronary artery dissections diagnosed in vivo in a pregnant woman. *Chest* 1993;104;289–290.

98. Jacobs M, Moress EJ. Myocardial infarction complicating pregnancy. *J Newark Beth Israel Hosp* 1961;12:216–221.

99. Maternal Health in Ohio. Topic this month: maternal deaths involving cardiac disease. *Ohio State Med J* 1958;54:187–188.

100. Etienne Y, Jobic Y, Houel JF, Barra JA, Boschat J, Meunier M, Penther P. Papillary fibroelastoma of the aortic valve with myocardial infarction: echocardiographic diagnosis and surgical excision. *Am Heart J* 1994;127:443–445.

101. Phillips E. Myocardial infarction in pregnancy. *JAMA* 1962;181:63.

102. Dementova MP, Liachov HT, Timosheck EK, Maiden RP. A case of myocardial infarction in a pregnant woman. *Klin Med (Mosc)* 1975;53:141–143.

103. Krawczuk A, Jakowiki J. Two cases of myocardial infarction in the course of labour. *Ginekol Pol* 1965;36:1183–1184.

104. Bielak J, Krystosik J. Myocardial infarction in a 24-year-old pregnant woman. *Wiad Lek* 1973;26:951–954.

105. Bedford JRD. Myocardial infarction in pregnancy. *Obstet Gynecol* 1964;71:459–460.

106. Capra Marzani P, Navazzotti. The myocardial in pregnancy. Description of a case. *Minerva Med* 1969;60:1407–1411.

107. Pardo JG, Gonzalez BR, Novoa OC, Pumarino RD, Oppliger EP, Godoy DI: Acute postpartum infarct of the myocardium secondary to a spontaneous dissection of the coronary artery. *Rev Med Chile* 1990;118:300–305.

108. Perucca E, Cazenave H, Zarate H, Gutierrez I, Barrera C, Fuenzalida JP. Infarto del miocardio y embarazo. *Rev Chil Obstet Ginecol* 1991;53:210–212.

109. Rekosz J, Buczek J, Puchalska-Krotki H, Kapitan-Malinowska B. Cardiac rupture and tamponade in a pregnant woman with acute myocardial infarction. *Kardiol Pol* 1992;36: 224–246.

110. Reece EA, Assimakopoulos A. Coronary artery disease. In: Gleicher N, Gall SA, Sibai BM, Elkayam U, Galbraith RM, Sarto GE, eds. *Principles and Practice of Medical Therapy in Pregnancy.* 2nd ed. Norwalk, CT: Appleton & Lange; 1992;817–822.

111. Gant NF, Daley GL, Chand S, Whalley PJ, MacDonald PC. A study of angiotensin II pressor response throughout primagravid pregnancy. *J Clin Invest* 1973;52:2682–2689.

112. Nisell H, Hjemdahl P, Linde B. Cardiovascular responses to circulating catecholamines in normal pregnancy and in pregnancy-induced hypertension. Clin Physiol 1985;5:479–493.

113. Roberts JM, Taylor RN, Musci TJ, Rodgers GM, Hubel CA, McLaughlin MK. Preeclampsia: an endothelial cell disorder. *Am J Obstet Gynecol* 1989;161:1200–1204.

114. Koh CL, Viegas OA, Yuen R, Chua SE, Ng BL, Ratnam SS. Plasminogen activators and inhibitors in normal late pregnancy, postpartum and in the postnatal period. *Int J Gynaecol Obstet* 1992;38:9–18.

115. Fletcher AP, Alkjaersig NK, Burstein R. The influence of pregnancy upon blood coagulation and plasma fibrinolytic enzyme function. *Am J Obstet Gynecol* 1979;134:743–751.

116. Gore M, Eldon S, Trofatter KF, Soong SJ, Pizzo SV. Pregnancy-induced changes in the fibrinolytic balance: evidence for defective release of tissue plasminogen activator and increased levels of the fast-acting tissue plasminogen activator inhibitor. *Am J Obstet Gynecol* 1987;156:674–680.

117. Mackinnon S, Walker ID, Davidson JF, Walker JJ. Plasma fibrinolysis during and after normal childbirth. *Br J Haematol* 1987;65:339–342.

118. McGehee W. Anticoagulation in pregnancy. In: Elkayam U, Gleicher N, eds. *Cardiac Problems in Pregnancy.* 2nd ed. New York: Alan R. Liss; 1990;397.

119. Yoshimura T, Ito M, Nakamura T, Okamura H. The influence of labor on thrombotic and fibrinolytic systems. *Eur J Obstet Gynecol Reprod Biol* 1992;44:195–199.

120. Comp PC, Thurnau GR, Welsh J, Esmon CT. Functional and immunologic protein S levels are decreased during pregnancy. *Blood* 1986;68:881–885.

121. Davis RB, Leuschen MP, Boyd D, Goodlin RC. Evaluation of platelet function in pregnancy: comparative studies in nonsmokers and smokers. *Thromb Res* 1987;46:175–186.

122. Elkayam U, Rose J, Jamison M. Vascular aneurysms and dissections during pregnancy. In: Elkayam U, Gleicher N, eds.

Cardiac Problems in Pregnancy. 2nd ed. New York: Alan R. Liss; 1990;215.

123. Smith JC. Dissecting aneurysm of coronary arteries. *Arch Pathol Lab Med* 1975;99:117–121.

124. Menalo-Estrella P, Barker AE. Histopathologic findings in human aortic media associated with pregnancy. *Arch Pathol Lab Med* 1967;83:336–341.

125. Bonnet J, Aumailley M, Thomas D, Grosgogeat Y, Broustet JP, Bricaud H. Spontaneous coronary artery dissection: case report and evidence for a defect in collagen metabolism. *Eur Heart J* 1986;7:904–909.

126. Elkayam U, Gleicher N. Hemodynamics and cardiac function during normal pregnancy and the puerperium. In: Elkayam U, Gleicher N, eds. *Cardiac Problems in Pregnancy.* 2nd ed. New York: Alan R. Liss; 1990;5–24.

127. Elkayam U, Gleicher N. Changes in cardiac findings during normal pregnancy. In Elkayam U, Gleicher N, eds. *Cardiac Problems in Pregnancy.* 2nd ed. New York: Alan R. Liss; 1990;31–38.

128. Palmer CM, Norris MC, Giudici MC, Leighton BL, De Simone CA. Incidence of electrocardiographic changes during cesarean delivery under regional anesthesia. *Anesth Analg* 1990;70:36–43.

129. McLintic AJ, Pringle SD, Lilley S, Houston AB, Thorburn J. Electrocardiographic changes during cesarean section under regional anesthesia. *Anesth Analg* 1992;74:51–56.

130. Elkayam U. Pregnancy and cardiovascular disease. In: Braunwald E, ed. *Heart Disease.* 4th ed. Philadelphia: WB Saunders; 1992;1790–1809.

131. Page RL. Treatment of arrhythmias during pregnancy. *Am Heart J* 1995;130:871–876.

132. Brent RL. The effect of embryonic and fetal exposure to X-ray, microwaves and ultrasound: counseling the pregnant and nonpregnant patient about these risks. *Semin Oncol* 1989;16:347–368.

133. Heinonen OP, Slone D, Shapiro S. *Birth Defects and Drugs in Pregnancy.* Littleton, MA: Publishing Sciences Group; 1977;434.

134. American Academy of Pediatrics Committee on Drugs. The transfer of drugs and other chemicals into human milk. *Pediatrics* 1994;93:137–150.

135. Turrentine MA, Braems G, Ramirez MM. Use of thrombolytics for the treatment of thromboembolic disease during pregnancy. *Obstet Gynecol Survey* 1995;50:534–541.

136. Delclos GL, Davila F. Thrombolytic therapy for pulmonary embolism in pregnancy: a case report. *Am J Obstet Gynecol* 1986;155(2):375–376.

137. Ludwig H, Genz HJ. Thrombolytic treatment during pregnancy. *Thromb Haemostasis* 1981;46:438. Abstract.

138. Tissot H, Vergnes C, Rougier P, Bricaud H, Dallay D. Fibrinolytic treatment with urokinase and streptokinase for recurrent thrombosis in two valve prostheses for the aortic and mitral valves during pregnancy. *J Gynecol Obstet Biol Reprod* 1991;20:1093–1096.

139. Pfeifer GW. The use of thrombolytic therapy in obstetrics and gynaecology. *Australasian Annals of Medicine* 1970;19 (suppl 1):28–31.

140. Amas AG. Streptokinase, cerebrovascular disease—and triplets. *Br Med J* 1977;5:1414–1415.

141. Hall RJC, Young C, Sutton GC, Campbell S. Treatment of acute massive pulmonary embolism by streptokinase during labor and delivery. *Br Med J* 1972;4:647–649.

142. Fagher B, Ahlgren M, Astedt B. Acute massive pulmonary embolism treated with streptokinase during labor and the early puerperium. *Acta Obstet Gynecol Scand* 1990;69;659–661.

143. Ramamurthy S, Talwar KK, Saxena A, Juneja R, Takkar D. Prosthetic mitral valve thrombosis in pregnancy successfully treated with streptokinase. *Am Heart J* 1994;127:446–448.

144. Sbarouni E, Oakley CM. Outcome of pregnancy in women with valve prostheses. *Br Heart J* 1994;71:196–201.

145. Flossdorf TH, Breulmann M, Hopf HB. Successful treatment of massive pulmonary embolism with recombinant tissue type plasminogen activator (rt-PA) in a pregnant woman with intact gravidity and preterm labour. *Intensive Care Med* 1990;16:454–456.

146. Baudo F, Caimi TM, Redaelli R, Nosari AM, Mauri M, Leonardi G, deCataldo F. Emergency treatment with recombinant tissue plasminogen activator of pulmonary embolism in a pregnant woman with antithrombin III deficiency. *Am J Obstet Gynecol* 1990;163(4):1274–1275.

147. Barclay GR, Allen K, Pennington CR. Tissue plasminogen activator in the treatment of superior vena caval thrombosis associated with parenteral nutrition. *Postgrad Med J* 1990;66: 398–400.

148. Witchitz S, Veyrat C, Moisson P, Scheinman N, Rozenstain L. Fibrinolytic treatment of thrombus on prosthetic heart valves. *Br Heart J* 1980;44:545–554.

149. Shepard TH. *Catalog of Teratogenic Agents.* 6th ed. Baltimore: Johns Hopkins University Press; 1989;655.

150. McTiggart DR, Ingran TG. Massive pulmonary embolism during pregnancy treated with streptokinase. *Med J Aust* 1977;1:18–20.

151. Ginsberg JS, Hirsh J. Use of antithrombotic agents during pregnancy. *Chest* 1995;108:3055–3115.

152. Anderson DR, Ginsberg JS, Burrows R, Brill-Edwards P. Subcutaneous heparin therapy during pregnancy: a need for concern at the time of delivery. *Thromb Haemostasis* 1991;65: 248–250.

153. Stuart MJ, Gross SJ, Elrad H, Graeber JE: Effects of acetylsalicylic-acid ingestion on maternal and neonatal hemostasis. *N Engl J Med* 1982;307:909–912.

154. Zierler S, Rothman KJ. Congenital heart disease in relation to maternal use of Bendectin and other drugs in early pregnancy. *N Engl J Med* 1985;313:347–352.

155. Viinikka L, Hartikainen-Sorri AL, Lumme R, Hiilesmaa V, Ylikorkala O. Low dose aspirin in hypertensive pregnant women: effect on pregnancy outcome and prostacyclin–thromboxane balance in mother and newborn. *Br J Obstet Gynaecol* 1993;100:809–815.

156. CLASP. A randomised trial of low dose aspirin for the prevention and treatment of preeclampsia among 9364 pregnant women. *Lancet* 1994;343;619–629.

157. Cotton DB, Longmire S, Jones MM, Dorman KF, Tessem J, Joyce TH III. Cardiovascular alterations in severe pregnancy-induced hypertension: effects of intravenous nitroglycerin coupled with blood volume expansion. *Am J Obst Gynecol* 1986;154:1053–1059.

158. Shalev Y, Ben-Hur H, Hagay Z, Blickstein I, Epstein M, Ayzenberg O, Gelven A, Caspi A. Successful delivery following myocardial ischemia during the second trimester of pregnancy. *Clin Cardiol* 1993;16:754–756.

159. Lees C, Campbell S, Jauniaux E, Brown R, Ramsay B, Gibb D, Moncada S, Martin JF. Arrest of preterm labour and prolongation of gestation with glyceryl trinitrate, a nitric oxide donor. *Lancet* 1994;343:1325–1326.

160. Frishman W, Chesner M. Use of beta-adrenergic blocking agents in pregnancy. In: Elkayam U, Gleicher N, eds. *Cardiac Problems in Pregnancy.* 2nd ed. New York: Alan R. Liss; 1990;351–359.

161. Childress CH, Katz VL. Nifedipine and its indications in obstetrics and gynecology. *Obstet Gynecol* 1994;83:616–624.

162. Widerhorn J, Shotan A, Widerhorn ALM, Elkayam U. Antiarrhythmic. In: Lee RV, Garner PR, Barron WM, Coustan DR, eds. *Curr Obstet Med* 1995;3:95–116.

163. Briggs GG, Freeman RK, Yaffe SJ, eds. Diltiazem. *Drugs in Pregnancy and Lactation.* 4th ed. Baltimore: Williams & Wilkins; 1994;287–288.

164. Shechter M, Hod H, Chouraqui P, Kaplinsky E, Rabinowitz B. Magnesium therapy in acute myocardial infarction when patients are not candidates for thrombolytic therapy. *Am J Cardiol* 1995;75:321–323.

165. Briggs GG, Freeman RK, Yaffe SJ, eds. Magnesium sulfate. *Drugs in Pregnancy and Lactation.* 4th ed. Baltimore: Williams & Wilkins; 1994;513–518.

166. Brady JP, Williams HC. Magnesium intoxication in a premature infant. *Pediatrics* 1967;40:100–103.

167. Widerhorn J, Widerhorn ALM, Elkayam U. Cardiovascular pharmacotherapy in pregnancy and lactation. In: Gleicher N, Gall SA, Sibai BM, Elkayam U, Galbraith RM, Sarko GE, eds. *Principles and Practice of Medical Therapy in Pregnancy.* Norwalk, CT: Appleton & Lange; 1992;/767–783.

168. Clark RB, Brunner JA III. Dopamine for the treatment of spinal hypotension during cesarean section. *Anesthesiology* 1980;53:514–517.

169. Fishburne JI Jr, Dormer KJ, Payne GG, Gill PS, Ashrafzadeh AR, Rossavik IK. Effects of amrinone and dopamine on uterine blood flow and vascular responses in the gravid baboon. *Am J Obstet Gynecol* 1988;158:829–837.

170. Kirshon B, Lee W, Mauer MB, Cotton DB. Effects of low dose dopamine therapy in the oliguric patient with preeclampsia. *Am J Obstet Gynecol* 1988;159:604–607.

171. Waring PH, Shaw DB, Brumfield CG. Anesthetic management of a parturient with Osler–Weber–Rendu syndrome and rheumatic heart disease. *Anesth Analg* 1990;71:96–99.

172. Shotan A, Widerhorn J, Hurst A, Elkayam U. Risks of angiotensin-converting enzyme inhibition during pregnancy: experimental and clinical evidence, potential mechanisms, and recommendations for use. *Am J Med* 1994;96:451–456.

173. Gregg AR, Tomich PG. Mexilitene use in pregnancy. *Journal of Perinatology* 1988;8:33–35.

174. Perry JC, Ayres NA, Carpenter RJ Jr. Fetal supraventricular tachycardia treated with flecainide acetate. *J Pediatr* 1991;118:303–305.

175. Wagner X, Jouglard J, Moulin M, Miller AM, Petitjean J, Pisapia A. Coadministration of flecainide acetate and sotalol during pregnancy: lack of teratogenic effects, passage across the placenta and excretion in human breast milk. *Am Heart J* 1990;119:700–702.

176. Widerhorn J, Bhandari AK, Bughi S, Rahimtoola SH, Elkayam U. Fetal and neonatal adverse effects profile of amiodarone treatment during pregnancy. *Am Heart J* 1991;122:1162–1166.

177. Elkayam U, Goodwin TM. Adenosine therapy for supraventricular tachycardia during pregnancy. *Am J Cardiol* 1995;75:521–523.

178. Jaffe R, Gruber A, Fejgin M, Altaras M, Ben-Aderet N. Pregnancy with an artificial pacemaker. *Obstet Gynecol Survey* 1987;42:137–139.

179. Zoll PM, Zoll RH, Falk RH, Clinton JE, Eitel DR, Antman EM. External noninvasive temporary cardiac pacing: clinical trials. *Circulation* 1985;71:937–944.

180. Majdan JF, Walinsky P, Cowchock SF, Wapner RJ, Plzak L Jr. Coronary artery bypass surgery during pregnancy. *Am J Cardiol* 1983;52(8):1145–1146.

181. Gazzaniga AB. Cardiac surgery during pregnancy. In: Elkayam U, Gleicher N, eds. *Cardiac Problems in Pregnancy.* 2nd ed. New York: Alan R. Liss; 1990;264.

182. Troiano NH. Cardiopulmonary resuscitation of the pregnant woman. *J Perinatal Neonatal Nurs* 1989;3:1–13.

183. Marx GF. Cardiopulmonary resuscitation of late-pregnant women. *Anesthesiology* 1982;56:156. Letter.

184. Goodwin APL. The human wedge. *Anesthesia* 1992;47:433–444.

185. DePace NL, Betesh JS, Kotler MN. "Postmortem" cesarean section with recovery of both mother and offspring. *JAMA* 1982;248:971–973.

186. Lee RV, Rodgers BD, White LM, Harvey RC. Cardiopulmonary resuscitation of pregnant women. *Am J Med* 1986;81(2):311–318.

187. Katz VL, Dotters DJ, Droegemueller W. Perimortem cesarean delivery. *Obstet Gynecol* 1986;68:571–576.

188. Dillon WP, Lee RV, Tronolone MJ, Buckwald S, Foote RJ. Life support and maternal death during pregnancy. *JAMA* 1982;248:1089–1091.

189. Hill LM, Parker D, O'Neill BP. Management of maternal vegetative state during pregnancy. *Mayo Clinic Proc* 1985;60:469–472.

190. Strong TH Jr., Lowe RA. Perimortem cesarean section. *Am J Emergency Med* 1989;7:489–494.

191. Karlsson K. The influence of hypoxia on uterine and maternal placental blood flow, and the effect of alpha-adrenergic blockade. *J Perinatal Med* 1974;2:176–184.

192. Chestnut DH, Zlatnik FJ, Pitkin RM, Varner MW. Pregnancy in a patient with a history of myocardial infarction and coronary artery bypass grafting. *Am J Obstet Gynecol* 1986;155: 372–373.

193. Carpenter MW, Sady SP, Hoegsberg B, Sady MA, Haydon B, Cullilnane EM, Coustan DR, Thompson PD. Fetal heart rate response to maternal exertion. *JAMA* 1988;259;3006–3009.

194. Frenkel Y, Barkai G, Reisin L, Rath S, Mashiach S, Battler A. Pregnancy after myocardial infarction: are we playing safe? *Obstet Gynecol* 1991;77:822–825.

TABLE 13.1 Prevalence of Arrhythmia in Young Nonpregnant Healthy Females of Childbearing Age

Cardiac Rhythm	Number of Subjects	% of Total
Normal sinus rhythm	50	100
Sinus tachycardia (>100 bpm)	50	100
Sinus bradycardia (<60 bpm)	50	100
Sinus arrhythmia	50	100
Atrial arrhythmia: atrial premature beats, isolated	32	64
Ventricular arrhythmias		
Ventricular premature beats, isolated	27	54
Ventricular premature beats, multifocal	5	10
Ventricular tachycardia	1	2
Atrioventricular junctional arrhythmias		
AV junctional escape beats	2	4
Accelerated AV junctional rhythm	1	2
Atrioventricular block		
First degree	6	12
Second degree	2	4

Source: Adapted from Sobotka et al,[2] with permission of CV Mosby Co.

served out of 92,315 pregnancies over a 23-year period in the New York Lying-In Hospital (Table 13.2).[4] In that evaluation, arrhythmias occurred significantly more often in patients with organic heart disease such as rheumatic valvular disease or congenital heart disease.

Some authors have suggested that paroxysmal SVT occurs with increased frequency in pregnant women.[5–11] Some of the patients experienced their first attack during pregnancy. Others, with a history of prepregnancy arrhythmia, had an increase in the frequency, duration, and severity of the arrhythmia.

The apparent increase in incidence of cardiac arrhythmia is not limited to SVT. Brodsky et al reported seven patients who developed their initial manifestation of VT during pregnancy.[12] There have been other reports of VT during pregnancy.[12] These reports of both SVT and VT taken together suggest that significant symptomatic cardiac tachyarrhythmia directly related to pregnancy is relatively uncommon. A consistent theme in these publications is the previously stable and healthy asymptomatic woman who develops significant symptomatic arrhythmias during pregnancy. The majority of these patients had no apparent structural heart disease. Such patients may have an increase in arrhythmia or greater sensitivity to their usual symptoms.

Relationship of Structural Heart Disease to Cardiac Arrhythmia

SVT typically occurs in otherwise healthy individuals without significant structural heart disease. Other specific arrhythmias have been described in patients with structural heart diseases. For example, atrial fibrillation, atrial flutter, and atrial tachycardia are most often observed in patients with disease in the atrium resulting from rheumatic mitral valve disease or septal defects. Chronic atrial fibrillation is most often seen in patients with rheumatic mitral stenosis or

TABLE 13.2 Prevalence of Cardiac Arrhythmias Observed During Pregnancy

Arrhythmias	Prevalence Among Patients with Organic Heart Disease (N = 3252)	Prevalence Among All Pregnancies (N = 92,315)
Paroxysmal supraventricular tachycardia	0.5	0.03
Chronic atrial fibrillation	0.7	0.02
Atrioventricular block		
First degree	0.5	0.02
Second or third degree	0.2	<0.02
Intraventricular conduction delay[a]	0.1	<0.002

[a]Left bundle branch block, right bundle branch block.
Source: Adapted from Mendelsohn.[4]

regurgitation. VT seems to occur in pregnant patients without obvious structural heart disease.[12] In contrast, VT in nonpregnant individuals usually occurs in patients with significant heart disease. AV block of a benign type such as first-degree and second-degree type I, occurs commonly in patients without disease. More serious types of AV block occur in patients with significant heart disease, such as rheumatic or congenital heart disease.

The Physiological and Psychological Influence on Cardiac Arrhythmia During Pregnancy

Theoretically, the physiological and psychological effects that occur during pregnancy could provoke complex cardiovascular problems.

Physiological Changes Intravascular volume increases during pregnancy, augmenting the preload on the ventricles, hence enhancing contractility (Chapter 1).[3] This increase in preload may lead to an increase in myocardial irritability, or it may uncover an arrhythmogenic focus in atrial or ventricular tissue. During pregnancy, there is also typically an increase in the heart rate that may promote cardiac arrhythmia by modifying the effective refractory period, velocity of conduction, and spatial dispersion of refractoriness.[13] Hormonal influence due to elevation of estrogen, progesterone, or other pregnancy-related hormones and electrolytes shifts that occur with volume changes during pregnancy could be factors in generating cardiac arrhythmias.

Autonomic Changes Alteration in adrenergic responsiveness has been implicated in abnormal cardiovascular events during pregnancy.[14–17] In general, during pregnancy catecholamine levels do not change from prepregnancy values. In addition, most women have a decreased responsiveness to catecholamines during pregnancy. Some investigators have suggested that pregnancy-associated hypertension can occur because of a continuation of prepregnancy sensitivity to catecholamines. This relative overresponsiveness may be due to changes in the amount or function of adrenoreceptors or catecholamine binding. Cardiac arrhythmias could also result from changes of these types or an increase in catecholamine level or both. A variety of situations will increase the catecholamine level during pregnancy, including stretching of the uterus and physical or emotional stress.

Stress Pregnancy in general has been described as a psychologically stressful experience.[18,19] Stress, anxiety, and fear activate the pituitary–adrenal axis and stimulate the sympathetic nervous system, with potential arrhythmogenic effects.[13] As a result, pregnant women may be prone to catecholamine-sensitive arrhythmia. It is unclear whether pregnancy is the sole cause of these arrhythmias or just exacerbates or brings out the underlying arrhythmia (known substrate). The debate continues as to whether pregnancy can predispose otherwise healthy women to cardiac arrhythmias. There is no universal agreement on whether pregnancy per se can cause arrhythmias in an otherwise healthy woman.

Approach to Pregnant Patient with Arrhythmia

There are more similarities than differences in the clinician's approach to the pregnant versus nonpregnant patient with cardiac arrhythmias. In considering whether the symptoms are referable to cardiac arrhythmias, one should start with a detailed history and physical examination, with emphasis on the cardiovascular system. Patients with symptoms suggestive of cardiac arrhythmia may present with a variety of complaints, including palpitations, dizziness, presyncope, syncope, chest discomfort, symptoms of congestive heart failure, or even nonspecific symptoms described as generalized tiredness. Awareness of an irregular rhythm varies greatly. While some patients can be very symptomatic with just premature beats, others can be relatively asymptomatic even with VT. Sometimes, a woman may complain of palpitations even when the rhythm is entirely normal. It is necessary to document carefully the nature, frequency, and severity of the symptoms; the presence of precipitants such as excessive alcohol, caffeine, or drug use (legal or illegal); and details relating to exercise and psychosocial stress.[19] History of a previously documented cardiac disorder such as rheumatic heart disease, the results of diagnostic testing, and response to any drug treatment should be solicited. Physical examination is also an important part of the workup. Frequently, since most of the patients are relatively healthy females, no cardiac abnormalities are detected. Nevertheless, emphasis should be focused on physical evidence of congenital and rheumatic heart disease, since arrhythmia may be the initial manifestation of these disorders.

Laboratory workup should include blood tests for electrolytes and thyroid function, at a minimum. Noninvasive cardiac testing is particularly helpful in pregnant patients, since invasive testing is relatively contraindicated. A 12-lead ECG, which can provide for direct evidence of the arrhythmia in question, should be standard as part of the workup. Often, a static ECG may be unrevealing, but a dynamic ECG, including ambulatory (Holter) monitoring or transtelephonic monitoring, will be particularly helpful.

A complete echocardiogram is extremely useful from a diagnostic and prognostic standpoint. It can provide structural information in rheumatic valvular disease and congenital heart disease. It can also measure left ventricular function, potentially yielding important prognostic information in patients with cardiomyopathy.

Pregnancy itself is a stress test, but exercise testing may be carried out during pregnancy to help establish the diagnosis of ischemic heart disease and to assess functional capacity and cardiac reserve. It is especially useful in a patient with exercise-induced symptoms and can form a basis for determining whether the arrhythmia is catecholamine sensitive.[12]

However, the safety of stress testing in pregnancy has not been fully established. Fetal bradycardia has been reported with maximal but not with submaximal exercise.[20] A low level exercise protocol with fetal monitoring is recommended when stress testing is indicated (Chapter 3).

The risk/benefit ratio of therapy for arrhythmia in pregnant women changes traditional concepts of management in these patients. In considering therapy for cardiac arrhythmia, it is important to recognize that any treatment that affects maternal arrhythmias will probably directly or indirectly affect the fetus (Chapter 30). Most therapies have not been thoroughly tested in pregnancy and therefore are unlikely to be definitely safe. Therefore the general approach should be to avoid all but the absolutely safe or necessary therapies.[21] In addition, invasive testings are usually excluded, hence reducing the physician's ability to make a definitive diagnosis. The physician must therefore rely more on an empiric approach, including a more exhaustive noninvasive workup and use of mild therapies to reduce symptoms. It is also important to realize that in otherwise healthy pregnant women, symptoms of palpitation are often due to premature beats such as APDs or VPDs.[22,23] These premature beats are often of no clinical importance, and only a simple reassurance to the patient is necessary. Often, the avoidance of stimulating agents such as caffeine, alcohol, and illegal drugs may relieve patients from further symptoms. In general, immediate medical attention is indicated for arrhythmias such as SVT, VT, or severe bradyarrhythmias that affect the mother and result in hemodynamic compromise that jeopardizes not only the patient but also the fetus (by decreasing the uterine blood flow). In these situations, antiarrhythmic therapy must be initiated as soon as possible after the appropriate diagnosis has been made.

Since virtually all drugs can cross the placenta, selection of a pharmacologic agent should be based on both its therapeutic efficacy and its proven safety during pregnancy.[21] Since no antiarrhythmic drug is completely safe, selected medications should be used in the smallest effective dose, with periodic drug level monitoring. With this in mind, management of cardiac arrhythmia in pregnancy differs from what is done in a nonobstetrical practice only in that drug choices are more restricted.

MECHANISM, CLINICAL FEATURES, DIAGNOSIS, AND MANAGEMENT OF CARDIAC ARRHYTHMIAS DURING PREGNANCY

Commonly Benign Arrhythmias

Sinus Arrhythmia   Sinus arrhythmia is commonly seen in healthy young women; in general it has no clinical significance and therefore requires no medical therapy. Electrocardiographically, the P wave is upright in leads II, III, and aVF, but irregular. If the maximum P-P cycle length exceeds the minimum P-P cycle length by more than 10%, sinus arrhythmia is considered to be present. Vara and Halminen noted sinus arrhythmia in half of the 60 normal pregnant patients.[23] Sinus arrhythmia commonly occurs in young people, especially those with a slower heart rate or following enhanced vagal tone, such as after the administration of digitalis. It also decreases with age or with autonomic dysfunction such as diabetic neuropathy. Sinus arrhythmia appears in two forms. In the respiratory form, the P-P interval cyclically shortens during inspiration (a result of reflex inhibitions of the vagal tone) and widens during expiration. Nonrespiratory sinus arrhythmia is characterized by a phasic variation in P-P intervals unrelated to the respiratory cycle and may be the result of digoxin intoxication.

Sinus Tachycardia   Sinus tachycardia is defined as a sinus rhythm at a rate greater than 100 beats per minute. The P waves appear upright in leads I, II, III, and aVF as in normal sinus rhythm, and there is a 1:1 association of P waves to each QRS complex. The rate of sinus tachycardia at rest rarely exceeds 180 beats per minute in the adult and except under certain circumstances such as thyrotoxicosis, can the rate reach 200 beats per minute. The onset is gradual, and the response to vagal maneuvers is gradual slowing with prompt resumption of the tachycardia. Reviewing a long rhythm strip and instituting vagal maneuvers are particularly helpful measures in differentiating sinus tachycardia from other types of supraventricular arrhythmia. In pregnant women, for physiological reasons, the heart rate increases on an average of 15 beats per minute (or approximately 20% above baseline) and peaks between 32 weeks and the end of gestation.[24,25] It is not unusual to see a transient increase in heart rate above 100 beats per minute. In addition, the heart rate tends to fluctuate during labor and delivery in association with uterine contraction.[24,25] Therefore, transient sinus tachycardia is commonly seen in pregnancy. However, a persistent increase in heart rate may be a manifestation of an underlying pathological state. Causes and conditions associated with persistent sinus tachycardia include fever, infection, thyrotoxicosis, congestive heart failure, myocarditis, pulmonary embolism, amniotic embolism, and stimulating agents. Eliminating the underlying cause may be sufficient to relieve the symptoms.

Sinus Bradycardia   Sinus bradycardia, heart rate less than 60 beats per minute, commonly occurs in young healthy females.[2] It is not commonly seen during pregnancy.[4] Sinus bradycardia, as low as 35–45 beats per minute, is usually seen during sleep or in highly trained athletes in excellent aerobic condition. It is usually caused by an excess of vagal tone or a decrease in sympathetic tone or a combination of the two. It is often associated with sinus arrhythmia. It may also be a manifestation of underlying diseases such as hypothyroidism, sick sinus syndrome, carotid hypersensitivity, or drug toxicities. Mild sinus bradycardia, 45–60 beats per minute, may occur transiently after normal delivery and may persist for a few days in the postpartum period.[4] The mechanism of this condition is unclear. It may represent a return to normal from an elevated heart rate of pregnancy, and it appears to be of no clinical significance in the absence of heart block or markedly prolonged pauses (>3 s). Treatment of sinus bradyarrhythmia per se is usually not necessary. In the absence of structural heart disease or any pathological conditions, sinus bradycardia is seldom associated with symptoms and requires no intervention.

Atrial Premature Depolarizations APDs are caused by an electrical impulse originating within the atrium but outside the sinus node. The impulse is premature, producing atrial depolarization and a P wave that differs in morphology from the P wave of sinus node origin. The exact etiology is unknown but may be associated with use of stimulating agents or anxiety, infection, inflammation, pericarditis, or sympathomimetic drugs such as theophylline. APDs may be a sign of organic heart disease and may trigger atrial tachycardia or atrial fibrillation or flutter in patients with rheumatic heart disease or cardiomyopathy. However, APDs are usually not associated with heart disease and are rarely of clinical significance. APDs are commonly observed during pregnancy.[22] Upshaw noted the occurrence of APDs in 4 of 13 patients undergoing ECG monitoring during labor and delivery.[26]

APDs are common among young healthy females, and therefore no therapy is necessary in asymptomatic patients. Symptomatic patients may improve with reassurance and elimination of the precipitating factors. If antiarrhythmic therapy is deemed necessary for treatment of intolerable symptoms, the risk and benefit of the treatment must be clearly explained to the mother and digoxin or a β-adrenergic blocking agent should be tried initially.

Ventricular Premature Depolarizations VPDs are common among young healthy females.[2] In a study of 50 young nonpregnant women without evidence of heart disease, isolated VPDs occurred in 54% of the subjects, but only 5 (10%) had 10 or more VPDs during a 24-hour Holter recording. Therefore, isolated VPDs are fairly common among young healthy females but frequent VPDs are rare.

The clinical significance of VPDs is intimately related to the presence and severity of underlying heart disease.[27] The mere presence of VPDs does not appear to increase the risk of sudden death in patients without identifiable heart disease. In patients with structural heart disease, VPDs occur with increased frequency, commonly more than 10 per hour. In these patients, ventricular arrhythmia has been shown to be an independent risk factor for sudden death. The risk is further increased when VPDs are repetitive and complex in morphology and occur in association with left ventricular dys-

function. VPDs occur in association with a variety of toxins and complex medical conditions such as myocardial ischemia and hypercatecholamine state. The mechanism of VPDs is believed to entail a ventricular focus with enhanced automaticity; or it may represent a form of reentry within the bundle of His, or ventricular myocardial system. Both mechanisms may be operative under different circumstances.

Mendelsohn reported that VPDs were increased as a result of pregnancy.[4] VPDs by themselves without accompanying structural heart disease do not have any clinical significance. It is not clear whether pregnancy increases just the number of VPDs (isolated) or the complexity of the arrhythmia.

Shotan et al,[22,28] who performed Holter monitoring in 86 consecutive pregnant women, referred mostly for symptoms of palpitations, found multiple VPDs, APDs, or both in 18% of the patients. The presence of multiple ectopic beats was not associated with any adverse effect on mother or fetus, and there was a significant reduction in the number of premature beats postpartum.

The approach to pregnant women with VPDs depends on the underlying heart disease and the frequency and severity of the symptoms. The arrhythmia could be investigated by a combination of noninvasive tests, such as 24-hour Holter monitoring and echocardiogram. Common precipitating factors such as alcohol, caffeine, and smoking should be avoided, and electrolyte abnormality or hypoxia should be corrected. Treatment of asymptomatic VPDs in patient with or without structural heart disease is not necessary. In symptomatic patients with no structural heart disease, treatment is undesirable because all antiarrhythmic drugs have potential side effects to both the mother and fetus, and none of the drugs are particularly effective. Indeed, satisfactory results may be obtained by eliminating the precipitating factors and reassuring the patient. If the patient is severely symptomatic, however, the use of a beta blocker such as metoprolol or, under extreme circumstances, quinidine or procainamide, has demonstrated relative safety and efficacy in pregnancy. After initiation of antiarrhythmic therapy, repeat 24-hour Holter monitoring is recommended to assess the degree of efficacy and any evidence of proarrhythmia.

First-Degree Atrioventricular Block First-degree block is usually due to a delay in conduction time of the atrial impulse through the AV junction. In general, the etiology of first-degree AV block consists of an increase in parasympathetic tone, drugs that prolong AV conduction (digoxin, beta blockers, calcium channel blockers), conduction system diseases (fibrosis, inflammation with myocarditis), or acute ischemia. First-degree AV block has been noted occasionally during labor, but pregnancy itself does not appear to be a cause.[4] Transient first-degree AV block is common in young healthy females, especially during sleep.[2] Whether there is an increased incidence of first-degree AV block during pregnancy is unclear. Mendelsohn reported 17 cases of first-degree AV block (PR > 0.2 s) among 92,315 consecutive pregnancies (0.02%).[4] The incidence would have been 0.5% if only patients with organic heart disease had been taken into account. First-degree AV block in pregnancy appeared to be associated with rheumatic heart disease, inasmuch as 16 of 17 (93%) had that disorder. Prognosis of these patients was good and was related to the underlying heart function. All 17 patients described by Mendelsohn survived, and fetal losses were due to the associated serious cardiac abnormality, rather than being directly related to the delay in conduction time.

Unless accompanied by severe sinus bradycardia, first-degree AV block usually does not cause any symptoms. Therefore it does not require treatment. Emphasis should be placed on identifying and eliminating the underlying causes.

Arrhythmias of Clinical Significance

Many episodes of SVT and VT are benign, since they may be of short duration (>3 beats; < 10) and usually are not associated with any symptoms.[12,28] Treatment of the arrhythmia may be more harmful than the arrhythmia itself. Some episodes of tachycardia are associated with severe or even life-threatening symptoms, all of which will be discussed.

Ventricular Fibrillation   The incidence of ventricular fibrillation in pregnant women is unknown. Numerous sudden cardiac deaths presumably due to ventricular fibrillation have been reported in the literature. Etiologies of maternal death have been described as associated with a history of coronary artery diseases, proarrhythmic effects of antiarrhythmic drugs, complex congenital heart disease, hypertrophic cardiomyopathy, prosthetic valves, pulmonary hypertension, prolonged QT syndrome, and abuse of drugs such as cocaine.[28-36] Acute treatment of ventricular fibrillation should follow the cardiopulmonary resuscitation guidelines recommended by the American Heart Association.[37] If sudden death is aborted, careful evaluation by a cardiologist and electrophysiologist is important in finding out the etiology of the event and in future management. Evaluation and treatment of these patients should be extensive and often includes invasive techniques. Termination of the pregnancy may be necessary.

Ventricular Tachycardia   VT can occur in a structurally normal heart; in the general population, however, it is more commonly associated with structural heart disease (e.g., coronary artery disease, cardiomyopathy, right ventricular dysplasia, mitral valve prolapse). In the study by Sobotka et al[2] of 50 healthy women who underwent 24-hour ECG monitoring, only one episode of an asymptomatic 3-beat VT was recorded. VT is probably an unusual event in pregnancy. Although the exact incidence is unknown, most of the cases of

symptomatic VT reported during pregnancy were paroxysmal and occurred in young women with structurally normal hearts, as documented by noninvasive and invasive techniques.[12,38] However cases of VT with associated coronary artery disease, rheumatic heart disease, mitral valve prolapse, long QT, hypertension, and hypomagnesemia in pregnancy have been reported (Table 13.3).[12,39-42]

VT is typically defined by at least three consecutive ventricular beats at a rate between 100 and 250 beats per minute. Because the sequence of ventricular depolarization and repolarization is abnormal, the QRS complex during VT is wide, usually greater than 0.12 second. The duration of VT can be classified into two types. Nonsustained VT terminates spontaneously in less than 30 seconds and causes no hemodynamic compromise. Sustained VT lasts more than 30 seconds and frequently causes hemodynamic compromise. The basic sinus rhythm is usually intact and antegrade atrial depolarization persists, leading to AV dissociation. On occasion, if the AV node and the ventricular myocardium are not refractory, the sinus or atrial impulse may capture the ventricle, producing fusion beats. Therefore AV dissociation, capture, and fusion beats are not necessary for the diagnosis of VT but are helpful if found. Sometimes, slow VT may represent an idioventricular escape rhythm, VT with 2:1 exit block from the site of tachycardia or antiarrhythmic effects on the tachycardia. On occasion, VT may appear to be have a narrow complex on a single monitoring lead; therefore, multiple or 12-lead ECG should be obtained to better clarify the diagnosis.

The mechanism of VT in patients with structural heart disease is typically reentry, involving a disparity in conduction between normal and diseased myocardium. However, the most common mechanism of VT in pregnancy may be explained by catecholamine sensitivity. In a review of 26 cases of VT during pregnancy, Brodsky et al[12] reported that a variety of factors were related to VT in those patients (Table 13.3). These investigators found that 21 of 26 cases of VT reported in the literature were not associated with structural heart disease. In fact, most of the arrhythmias were related to physical exertion or emotional stress. In addition, in the evaluation of 7 patients, the frequency of these arrhythmias appears to decrease during sleep and, consistent with the hypothesis of catecholamine sensitivity, responded to treatment with β-adrenergic blockers.[12]

In the general population, the prognostic significance of VT depends on the severity of associated heart disease and the type of presenting arrhythmia.[43] In patients with structural heart disease, several studies have documented an association between VT and subsequent mortality from sudden death. The risk of sudden death is further increased when concomitant left ventricular dysfunction is present. Of the 26 patients reported by Brodsky et al, 21 were without structural heart disease.[12] Of the 5 patients with structural heart dis-

TABLE 13.3   Ventricular Tachycardia During Pregnancy

Year of Report	Number of Patients (Pregnancies)	Heart Disease	Other Factors	Therapy	Maternal Outcome	Fetal Outcome
1931	1	None	ex, psy	dig, quin	OK	Unknown
1946	1	None	ex, psy	None	OK	Unknown
1962	1	None	ex	quin	OK	OK
1962	1 (1,2)	None	ex, psy	quin	OK	Unknown
	2 (1–4)	None	ex, psy	quin	OK	Unknown
	3 (1)	None	ex, psy	quin	OK	Unknown
1962	1	None	ex	pca	Death	Death
1965	1	None	psy	quin, pca, ph	OK	OK
1967	1	None	ex	quin, prop	Unknown	Unknown
1969	1	None	QT	prop	OK	OK
1969	1 (1)	None	ex, psy	quin, pca, dig	OK	OK
	1 (2)	None	ex, psy	quin, lido, ph	OK	OK
1970	1	RHD	an/lab	None	OK	OK
1970	1	CAD	AMI	defib	Death	Death
1974	1	None	psy	lido, pca, ph, prop	OK	*a*
1979	1	Unknown	None	diso	OK	OK
1979	1	Unknown	None	quin	OK	OK
1980	1	None	None	mex, prop	OK	brady
1982	1	None	ex	None	Unknown	Unknown
1982	1 (1)	None	ex, psy, QT	prop	OK	Death
	1 (2)	None	ex, psy, QT	prop, ph	OK	Apnea
	1 (3)	None	ex, psy, QT	prop, ph	OK	OK
1984	1	None	hypok	lido	OK	OK
1986	1 (1)	None	psy	met	OK	OK
	2 (1)	None	ex	met	OK	OK
1987	1	MVP	None	mex, aten	OK	OK
1987	1	*b*	None	amio, prop	OK	OK
1987	1	None	Unknown	prop	OK	OK
1987	1	CAD	AMI	defib	OK	OK

a Intrauterine growth retardation, apnea, bradycardia, first-degree atrioventricular block, hypoglycemia.
b Myocardial fibrosis.

Abbreviations: AMI, acute myocardial infarction; amio, amiodarone; an/lab, anesthesia during labor; aten, atenolol; brady, bradycardia, CAD, coronary artery disease; defib, defibrillation; dig, digoxin; diso, disopyramide; ex, exercise; HD, heart disease; hypok, hypokalemia; lido, lidocaine; met, metoprolol; mex, mexiletine; MVP, mitral valve prolapse; pca, procainamide; ph, phenytoin; prop, propanolol; psy, emotional/psychological in complaints; quin, quinidine; QT, QT interval prolongation; RHD, rheumatic heart disease.

Source: Adapted from Brodsky et al.[12]

ease, there was one maternal death due to myocardial infarction and ventricular fibrillation.

General Approach to VT Treatment   A number of clinical factors influence the management of VT in patients during their pregnancy. The duration of the VT (sustained vs. nonsustained) and severity of symptoms would influence the speed of initiating treatment. The etiology of the VTs (catecholamine sensitive vs. noncatecholamine sensitive) will influence the use of various antiarrhythmic agents. In general, in patients who have nonsustained VT, comprehensive evaluation (Holter and echocardiography) and correction of precipitating factors must be performed before the type of ther-

apy is decided. The possible proarrhythmic as well as teratogenic effects of antiarrhythmic agents must be considered with caution before initiation of drug therapy.

VT Without Structural Heart Disease   In patients with no apparent heart disease, whether symptomatic or asymptomatic, the presence of nonsustained runs of VT may be so disturbing to the physician that treatment is favored. There is little evidence to support the use of antiarrhythmic agents, however, since these patients overall have a good prognosis.[38] Nevertheless, the patients should be followed closely because the arrhythmias may increase in complexity and duration over time. Medical therapy in this patient population should probably be withheld unless the patient is very symptomatic. In patients without structural heart disease, the etiology of VT is likely to be mediated by catecholamine.[12] If those patients have risk factors for catecholamine-sensitive VT (exercise, stress) most of these tachycardias will respond to beta blockers such as metoprolol.

VT with Structural Heart Disease   No definitive pharmacology studies show that treating patients with asymptomatic VT improves their survival, nor are there studies to show improved maternal or fetal morbidity or mortality with drug treatments. Therapy is usually indicated, however, in patients with significant structural heart disease and symptomatic VT. Quinidine and procainamide have shown to be safe in treating VT during pregnancy.[45] Isolated cases of use of acebutolol,[43] bretylium,[44] and flecainide[39] have been reported. Amiodarone, a type III antiarrhythmic agent, has been used successfully in the management of recurrent, life-threatening supraventricular and ventricular arrhythmias in pregnant women.[46–51] Other agents such as flecainide,[39,52] propafenone,[53] bretylium,[44] and acebutolol[43] are reportedly useful in the treatment of recurrent or refractory VT, although their relative safety has not yet been established.[45]

Acute Treatment of Sustained VT   The general approach to the acute treatment of sustained VT is similar to the recommendation in the guidelines for cardiopulmonary resuscitation and critical cardiac care.[38] In hemodynamically well-tolerated VT, intravenous lidocaine or procainamide should be the treatment of choice. Bretylium or magnesium should be reserved for VT that is refractory to lidocaine and procainamide. Intravenous amiodarone is available for treatment of sustained VT, although the safety to the fetus of this therapy is not well established. Direct current synchronized cardioversion could be used if the VT is hemodynamically unstable or if it does not respond to antiarrhythmic therapy (see section of dc cardioversion). In VT secondary to digoxin toxicity, synchronized cardioversion is relatively contraindicated. Instead, the use of lidocaine or beta blocker is the treatment of choice.

Atypical Ventricular Tachycardia/Torsades de Pointes   This arrhythmia can be secondary to a number of different etiologies including congenital QT prolongation, drug-induced QT prolongation, and electrolyte abnormality. In a hemodynamically stable patient, precipitating factors should be corrected if possible and intravenous magnesium ($>$ 2 g) should be the initial treatment of choice.[54] If this regimen is ineffective, overdrive pacing should be used while infusion of isoproterenol is being started.[55]

Differentials of Tachyarrhythmias   Since the therapy can differ very greatly for SVT and VT, it is important to make an accurate diagnosis of the rhythm in patients who present with acute, sustained, and symptomatic arrhythmias.[56] A brief summary of a number of common arrhythmias will be presented (Table 13.4), and an approach to the differential diagnosis of each arrhythmia will be discussed. In managing patients with sustained or acute tachyarrhythmia, it is important to differentiate tachyarrhythmias supraventricular versus ventricular in origin. The width of the QRS, the regularity of the rhythm, and atrial activity are the key factors in the differential diagnosis of tachyarrhythmia. Other helpful factors include clinical information such as ischemic heart disease manifest as previous myocardial infarction.

Tachyarrhythmias can be generally classified into four categories depending on regularity of the rhythm and QRS width. The major differential diagnosis of a wide complex and regular tachycardia includes VT, SVT (including atrial flutter and atrial tachycardia) with aberrancy, or antidromic tachycardia with antegrade conduction through a bypass tract. Wide complex but irregular tachycardia usually suggests atrial fibrillation or multifocal tachycardia with a fixed or rate-related aberrancy or antegrade conduction through a bypass tract or erratic VT. Narrow, complex, and regular tachycardias include sinus tachycardia, sinoatrial reentry tachycardia, atrial tachycardia (reentry or automatic), junctional tachycardia, AV nodal reentry tachycardia, AV reciprocating tachycardia, and atrial flutter with fixed AV conduction. Irregular, narrow, complex tachycardias include atrial fibrillation and multifocal tachycardia.

TABLE 13.4   Classification of Tachyarrhythmias: QRS Complex

Wide ($\geq$0.12 s)		Narrow ($<$0.12 s)	
Regular	Irregular	Regular	Irregular
VT	AFIB with aberrancy or BBB	ST	AFIB
SVT with aberrancy	AAT with aberrancy or BBB	SVT	AAT
(AVNRT, SNART, IART		NJPT	
AVRT (antidromic)		AFLUT	
		AVRT (orthodromic)	

Abbreviations: AAT, automatic atrial tachycardia; AFIB, atrial fibrillation; AFLUT, atrial flutter; AVNRT, atrioventricular nodal reentry tachycardia; AVRT, atrioventricular reciprocating tachycardia; BBB, bundle branch block; IRAT, intraatrial reentry tachycardia; NJPT, nonparoxysmal junctional tachycardia; SNRT, sinus nodal reentry tachycardia; ST, sinus tachycardia; SVT, supraventricular tachycardia; VT, ventricular tachycardia.

Supraventricular Tachycardia

Paroxysmal Supraventricular Tachycardia Paroxysmal SVT includes a number of different types of tachycardia with distinctive features and clinical mechanisms (Table 13.5). The mechanisms of SVTs may be reentry or automatic. Electrophysiologic studies have demonstrated that reentry is the most common mechanism of standard paroxysmal SVT (>90% of cases) and that abnormal automatically accounts for a small minority of the cases (< 10%).[1]

AV Nodal Reentry Tachycardia and AV Reciprocating Tachycardia AV nodal reentry, the most common narrow, complex, regular tachycardia, is responsible for about two-thirds of the cases of paroxysmal SVT. The mechanism of this arrhythmia is reentry within the region of the AV node. The ventricular rate is usually between 160 and 250 beats per minute. The tachycardia is usually initiated by either an atrial or a ventricular premature beat. The PR interval of the initiating atrial extra beat is longer than the PR interval of the regular sinus beat. During tachycardia, abnormal atrial depolarization occurs as the impulse travels from the AV node and proceeds superiorly and leftward. It is recognized by "inverted" P waves in the inferior ECG lead. In most cases, atrial depolarization occurs during inscription of the QRS complex and a retrograde P wave is not seen.[56] If P waves are seen, they occur in a 1:1 relationship with the QRS, provided there is no VA block. Approximately 30% of the time, an inverted retrograde P wave will be seen to closely follow each QRS complex. The RP interval is usually less than 100 ms.

In about 20% of patients, the reentry may involve a concealed accessory pathway where the impulse usually travels in antegrade manner over the AV node and His–Purkinje system and in retrograde manner to the atrium over a concealed accessory pathway. If this extra nodal conduction pathway (bypass tract) conducts in an antegrade direction, then overt preexcitation is present and the patient has Wolff–Parkinson–White syndrome. If the extra nodal tract conducts in only a retrograde fashion, then a concealed bypass tract exists. In orthodromic AV reciprocating tachycardia, the impulse travels in an antegrade fashion through the AV node and up in a retrograde fashion through the bypass tract. Electrical alternans described in AV reciprocating tachycardia occurs when QRS complexes vary in amplitude from beat to beat. The ventricular rate is usually slightly faster than tachycardia from AV nodal reentry. The sequence of atrial depolarization is abnormal and the P waves are usually seen after the QRS complexes. The RP interval usually exceeds 100 ms.

AV nodal reentry and AV reciprocating tachycardia are usually very well tolerated, especially in patients with no structural heart disease. In general, short runs of these arrhythmias require no specific pharmacological therapy.

TABLE 13.5 Mechanisms of Clinical Features of Common Arrhythmias During Pregnancy

Arrhythmias	Common Mechanisms	Associated Conditions	Treatment
SNRT	Reentry	Usually none	Vagal maneuvers, digoxin, beta blockers
IART	Reentry	Usually none	Vagal maneuvers, digoin, beta blockers
AAT	Automatic	Digoxin toxicity	Reverse underlying causes; magnesium, verapamil, or withdrawal of digoxin
MAT	Automatic	Pulmonary disease	Reverse underlying causes; magnesium, verapamil, or withdrawal of digoxin
AVNRT	Reentry	Usually none	Adenosine, verapamil, digoxin
AVRT	Reentry	Usually none	Quinidine, procainamide, ± beta blockers, ± digoxin
AFIB	Reentry	Mitral valve disease, hypertensive heart disease cardiomyopathies, pericarditis, thyrotoxicosis, alcohol	Digoxin, beta blockers for rate control; type IA antiarrhythmics (quinidine, procainamide) for conversion
AFLUT	Reentry	Mitral valve disease, hypertensive heart disease cardiomyopathies, pericarditis, thyrotoxicosis, alcohol	Digoxin, beta blockers for rate control; type IA antiarrhythmics (quinidine, procainamide) for conversion
VT	Reentry	Commonly none	Depending on underlying heart disease (see text); if none, consider beta blockers
VF	Reentry, automatic	Ischemia, proarrhythmia, complex congenital heart, HCM, pulmonary hypertension, prolonged QT, cocaine, prosthetic valve	Underlying disease, implantable defibrillator amiodarone

Abbreviations: AAT, automatic atrial tachycardia; AFIB, atrial fibrillation; AFLUT, atrial flutter; AVRT, atrioventricular reciprocating tachycardia; BBB, bundle branch block; HCM, hypertensive cardiomyopathy; IART, intraatrial reentry tachycardia; MAT, multifocal atrial tachycardia; NJPT, nonparoxysmal junctional tachycardia; PSVT, paroxysmal supraventricular tachycardia; SNRT, sinus nodal reentry tachycardia; ST, sinus tachycardia; SVNRT, atrioventricular nodal reentry tachycardia; SVT, supraventricular tachycardia; VF, ventricular fibrillation; VT, ventricular tachycardia.

However, prolonged episodes producing hemodynamic deterioration may require medical therapy or even cardioversion. The general approach would include the use of vagal maneuvers or intravenous adenosine to terminate the arrhythmias.[57] Adenosine (6–12 mg) has been shown to terminate more than 90% of supraventricular tachycardias involving the AV node as part of the reentry circuit. Such termination is both prompt—about 15 seconds following peripheral intravenous injection—and safe. In addition, adenosine has been shown to be safe and effective in pregnancy.[58,59] If adenosine is unsuccessful, intravenous verapamil may be used effectively to terminate these arrhythmias.[45,60] Intravenous verapamil is usually given at 5–10 mg (0.075–0.15 mg/kg) over a period of 1–3 minutes and can be repeated in 30 minutes. The safety of verapamil during pregnancy is less well known than that of adenosine. Intravenous digoxin should be considered as an alternative for acute termination, although it may not have an effect until 30 minutes after administration. In patients with AV reciprocating tachycardia, agents such as type IA drugs (quinidine or procainamide) that slow the conduction of the bypass tract can also terminate the arrhythmia. The long-term therapy of these patients will depend on the frequency and severity of the symptoms. Any long-term use of an antiarrhythmic agent should be considered cautiously because of the potential transfer of drug to the fetus. If attacks are infrequent, antiarrhythmic prophylaxis is not indicated. However, for patients with severe symptomatic attacks, a combination of digoxin and other therapy such as quinidine or a beta blocker appear to be safe and effective for use during pregnancy.[45]

In patients with AV nodal reentry tachycardia, digoxin is the drug of first choice, followed by the addition of beta blockers. For patients with a concealed bypass tract, digoxin is still one of the drugs of choice, along with type IA antiarrhythmic agents. For severely symptomatic patients who become refractory to medications, radiofrequency ablation of the bypass tract or slow pathway has been successfully performed during pregnancy.[61]

Sinoatrial node and Intraatrial Reentry Tachycardias Reentry involving supraventricular areas such as the atrium or sinus node produce tachycardias such as intraatrial or sinoatrial reentry tachycardias. The mechanism of sinoatrial reentry tachycardia results from reentry around the region of the sinus node. SVT is typically initiated by an atrial premature depolarization, but subsequent P waves are morphologically similar to sinus P waves. The atrial rate is usually regular (160–260 beats per minute). AV conduction may be 1:1, or variable AV block may occur. The RP interval is usually greater than half the RR interval. Vagal maneuvers or adenosine may terminate the tachycardia. This rhythm may mimic sinus tachycardia.

The mechanism of intraatrial reentry tachycardia entails reentry within the atrium. It is usually initiated by an atrial premature depolarization. The onset is usually sudden, and the rate is typically between 130 and 180 beats per minute.[62] The RP interval is influenced by the rate. Adenosine may terminate the tachycardia or produce AV block. Vagal maneuvers rarely terminate the arrhythmias.

Sinus nodal reentry and atrial tachycardia due to reentry account for less than 10% of cases of SVT and can be managed by either AV nodal blockers or antiarrhythmic agents that prevent recurrent reentry. AV block can occur without affecting the tachycardia, and vagal maneuvers can slow and then abruptly terminate the tachycardia. Of all the potent AV blocking drugs, digoxin is the safest and most effective. Beta blockers should be considered as a second-line therapy, with metoprolol being the best tolerated. Type IA antiarrhythmic agents can be used to prevent reentry but often are ineffective. Recently, flecainide was reported to be effective in terminating atrial tachycardia in pregnancy.[63]

Atrial Flutter Paroxysmal atrial flutter usually occurs in patients without structural heart disease, while chronic (persistent) atrial flutter is usually associated with underlying heart disease such as rheumatic mitral or ischemic heart disease, or cardiomyopathies.[64] Atrial flutter often occurs in association with other SVT, particularly atrial fibrillation. It may occur as a result of atrial dilatation from septal defects, pulmonary emboli, mitral or tricuspid stenosis, or regurgitation or chronic ventricular failure. It may also be associated with toxic and metabolic conditions that affect the heart, such as acute alcohol ingestion, thyrotoxicosis, or constrictive pericarditis. Atrial flutter is uncommon during pregnancy. Its incidence is unknown.

Paroxysmal atrial flutter tends to be unstable, reverting to sinus rhythm or degenerating into atrial fibrillation. In atrial flutter, the atria contract, a fact which may in part account for the presence of fewer systemic emboli than are seen in atrial fibrillation. In patients with associated overt preexcitation, the ventricular response rate can be very fast, with rates over 300 beats per minute secondary to 1:1 AV conduction. (In that situation, the patient may become hemodynamically unstable.) The mechanism of atrial flutter often entails atrial macro reentry or, rarely, focal ectopic origin due to enhanced automaticity.[64] Atrial flutter is typically characterized by an atrial rate between 280 and 320 beats per minute. In typical flutter, the atrial depolarization is usually seen as negative deflections in the inferior leads (II, III, aVF), although the flutter waves can be seen as positive deflections in atypical flutter. The ventricular rate depends on the refractory period of the AV node. Usually 2:1 AV block occurs, resulting in a regular ventricular rate of 140–160 beats per minute. If variable block occurs, the ventricular rate may become irregular. If higher degree AV block occurs, the flutter waves may become more obvious, appearing in a sawtooth pattern in the inferior leads. Indeed, any regular, narrow, complex tachycardia at 150 beats per minute should be considered to be atrial flutter until proven otherwise. Vagal maneuvers will usually not terminate the arrhythmia but will increase the AV block, making the sawtooth waves more apparent, especially in the inferior leads. Therapy such as type IA antiarrhythmic drugs will reduce the flutter rate from the typical 300–250 beats per minute or less. If the flutter rate is sufficiently slowed, it is possible to have 1:1 conduction. Therefore, in some patients, administration of class IA drugs without concomitant use of drugs to block the AV junction may result in acceleration of heart rate.

The approach to atrial flutter depends on the hemodynamic status of the pregnant patient. The underlying cause must be sought and eliminated. For the hemodynamically stable patient, ventricular response rate should be controlled first with intravenous digoxin. If this is ineffective, calcium channel blockers or beta blockers can be used to bring the ventricular rate down to 100 beats per minute. After the desired ventricular rate has been achieved, class I antiarrhythmic agents such as procainamide or quinidine can be used to convert atrial flutter to sinus rhythm. In patients who are hemodynamically compromised, urgent synchronized cardioversion should be applied. Drugs for sedation may be necessary in conscious patients. Whether the patients will require continuous antiarrhythmic agents for sinus rhythm maintenance, as is necessary for other SVTs, will depend on the severity and frequency of the symptoms.

Narrow Complex Irregular Tachycardia

ATRIAL FIBRILLATION   While atrial fibrillation occurs in approximately 5% of the population greater than 65 years old, its incidence in women of childbearing age is rare (<0.1%).[4] Most affected younger people have underlying heart disease, including valvular disease, cardiomyopathy, hypertensive heart disease, and heart failure. Other causes include thyrotoxicosis, pulmonary embolism, and alcohol ingestion. Atrial fibrillation can be paroxysmal or chronic. The exact incidence of atrial fibrillation during pregnancy is not known. Pregnancy does not appear to predispose otherwise healthy hearts to atrial fibrillation. In patients with heart disease, however, pregnancy may cause an increased incidence of paroxysms of atrial fibrillation.[4] Mendelsohn reported a total of 31 cases of atrial fibrillation (10 paroxysmal and 21 chronic) over 92,315 consecutive pregnancies.[4] All the patients with chronic atrial fibrillation and 80% of patients with paroxysmal atrial fibrillation had rheumatic mitral diseases. The remaining 2 patients with paroxysmal atrial fibrillation had thyrotoxicosis. In 13 of 21 patients with chronic atrial fibrillation, heart failure developed during the course of the pregnancy. Of these, 4 of 21 of the mothers and 11 of 21 of the fetuses died. Therefore, Mendelsohn concluded that atrial fibrillation by itself (without any structural heart disease) was rare in pregnancy, whereas chronic atrial fibrillation in pregnancy was usually associated with structural heart dis-

ease and carried a high maternal and fetal morbidity and mortality. The increased morbidity and mortality in patients with atrial fibrillation and rheumatic mitral valve diseases can be explained by the impaired hemodynamic changes and thromboembolic complications.

Hemodynamically, atrial fibrillation is poorly tolerated in mitral stenosis. The left atrial emptying is severely impaired because of the shortened diastolic filling time during atrial fibrillation with fast ventricular response rate. This results in a rise in left atrial pressure and pulmonary venous hypertension, as well as pulmonary edema and decrease in cardiac output.

The risk of systemic embolization in atrial fibrillation is probably due to circulatory stasis in the left atrial appendage with subsequent thrombus formation and chance of detachment causing embolic events. The risk of stroke in patients with atrial fibrillation in the setting of valvular heart disease is 17 times that of the control population without atrial fibrillation.[65] The risk of nonvalvular atrial fibrillation is about five times that of the control population without atrial fibrillation. Certain patients with atrial fibrillation and other risk factors appear to have a higher risk of embolization. These conditions include advanced age, hypertension, diabetes mellitus, congestive heart failure, and history of embolization. The exact incidence of systemic embolism in pregnancy is not known, but the condition appears to depend on the presence of underlying heart disease (mitral stenosis, mitral valve prolapse, congestive heart failure) and the chronicity of atrial fibrillation. Mendelsohn reported an occurrence of systemic embolic events in 5 of 31 (16%) pregnant patients with rheumatic mitral stenosis and atrial fibrillation.[4] In contrast, the risk of embolism is relatively low in patients with "lone" atrial fibrillation.[66] Results from the Framingham heart study indicated an increased risk of stroke in these patients, while another study, from the Mayo Clinic did not.[67]

The etiology of atrial fibrillation is associated with atrial tissue injury or damage and increased atrial pressure. The risk of developing atrial fibrillation has been related to left atrial dimension as determined by echocardiography.[68] The most common cardiac condition associated with the development of this arrhythmia during pregnancy is mitral stenosis. Electrophysiologically, atrial fibrillation is due to simultaneous discharge of multiple atrial foci, resulting in an atrial rate between 400 and 700 beats per minute with variable conduction through the AV node, producing an irregular ventricular rhythm. There are no P waves, and there is no effective atrial contraction. The fibrillatory waves are best seen in V_1 and the inferior leads. The ventricular rate depends on the AV node refractoriness. The average ventricular response rate is between 140 and 180 beats per minute. The ventricular rate is typically irregular because of the random conduction through the AV node. Patients who present with a ventricular rate between 60 and 100 beats per minute and are not on any AV nodal slowing agents should be evaluated for intrinsic AV nodal disease.

The initial approach to the management of atrial fibrillation is similar to that of atrial flutter. The underlying cause of atrial fibrillation should be investigated (thyrotoxicosis, rheumatic valvular disease, cardiomyopathy). In a hemodynamically stable patient, the ventricular response rate should be controlled with digoxin, beta blockers, or calcium channel blockers alone or in combination. Frequently, sinus rhythm may return spontaneously while the rate is being controlled. After the rate has been controlled, drugs such as quinidine or procainamide are useful in the conversion to sinus rhythm by chemical means. Synchronized cardioversion can be utilized to convert atrial fibrillation to sinus rhythm on an emergency basis (in a patient with compromised hemodynamics). In an elective situation, quinidine or procainamide should be started and therapeutic level achieved before cardioversion is instituted to prevent relapse. Because of the significant risk of systemic embolization in patients with atrial fibrillation for more than 2 days, 3 weeks of anticoagulation both before and after attempted reversion to sinus rhythm is recommended. One study suggested that electrical cardioversion can be safely performed without the need for 3 weeks of anticoagulation therapy beforehand if transesophageal echocardiography reveals no left atrial thrombus, as long as anticoagulation is maintained for 3 weeks afterward.[69] Earlier literature suggested that if the left atrial size were greater than 4.5 cm by echocardiography, it was unlikely that sinus rhythm would be maintained for more than a brief period (weeks to months). Recent literature suggested that sinus rhythm can be maintained in patients with left atrial size greater than 4.5 cm, provided class IC or III antiarrhythmic drugs are used.[70]

Cardioversion to sinus is likely to be successful and atrial fibrillation is unlikely to recur in patients who have no heart disease if left atrial size is less than 5 cm and atrial fibrillation is of short duration (< 6 months).[71,72] Whether pregnant patients with chronic nonvalvular atrial fibrillation should be anticoagulated is controversial, since the use of warafin during pregnancy is associated with a substantial teratogenic risk. Heparin, which does not cross the placenta, is the drug of choice. It is recommended that systemic anticoagulation be used in pregnant patients with atrial fibrillation associated with mitral valve disease and history of embolic events.[73] Lone atrial fibrillation (atrial fibrillation in the absence of underlying organic heart disease) in patients under the age of 60 is associated with a very low risk of clinical embolic event. It is unclear whether pregnancy will increase the risk of systemic embolism in patients with lone atrial fibrillation and whether anticoagulation would decrease this hypothetical risk.

AUTOMATIC ATRIAL TACHYCARDIA Automatic atrial tachycardias including multifocal atrial rhythms are uncommon SVTs, seen in the setting of a variety of physiologic and metabolic derangements.[75] These arrhythmias commonly occur in the elderly and are associated with chronic obstructive airway disease, disease of the atrium, and hypoxia. Their occurrence in young healthy pregnant females is extremely rare. Few cases of persistent automatic atrial tachycardia during pregnancy have been reported.[74,75] Electrophysiologically, the condition results from an automatic ectopic focus within the atrium. It may be initiated by an atrial extra beat, but the P-wave vector is usually similar to sinus (inferior and leftward). The P-wave morphology usually changes and there may be three or more different P-waves morphologies. The ventricular rate is usually less than 200 beats per minute and irregular. It is often confused with atrial fibrillation.

The most important first step in managing this arrhythmia is to minimize obviously reversible conditions such as hypoxia or electrolyte imbalance. Because this rhythm does not involve a reentry "loop," vagal maneuvers, such as carotid sinus massage, the Valsalva maneuver, or the use of pharmacological agents that alter AV conduction, will not terminate the arrhythmias but may transiently increase the AV block.[74] In general, short runs of this tachycardia are usually well tolerated, and no specific therapy is required. The current treatment of choice is to use intravenous magnesium,[76] beta blockers, or calcium channel blockers (diltiazem or verapamil),[77] which may convert the tachycardia to sinus rhythm. In case the tachycardia is due to digitalis toxicity, withholding digitalis and repletion of the serum potassium to normal level will usually suffice. In two recent cases of atrial tachycardia reported to have accelerated during pregnancy, the patients returned to normal sinus rhythm postpartum.[74,75]

Preexcitation and Associated Tachycardias Preexcitation syndromes refer to a variety of conditions with accessory electrical conduction pathways between the atrium and the ventricle. The most common type of preexcitation, Wolff–Parkinson–White syndrome, is defined by a short PR interval, wide QRS, delta wave, and tachyarrhythmias. The incidence of preexcitation varies from 0.1 to 3.7 per thousand patients.[78] It is found in all age groups, from the fetal and neonatal period to the elderly. The prevalence is higher in males and decreases with age, apparently because of spontaneous loss of preexcitation. The majority of adults with preexcitation have normal hearts, although preexcitation can be associated with Ebstein's anomaly, mitral valve prolapse, septal defects, and hypertrophic cardiomyopathy. The anomalous complexes caused by the accessory pathways can mask or mimic myocardial infarction, bundle branch block, or ventricular hypertrophy. The exact incidence of preexcitation during pregnancy is not known, but several reports have indicated that pregnancy may facilitate the onset of tachyarrhythmias or increase their incidence.[8,10,46,57,79,80]

The mechanism of the tachycardia is related to the accessory pathways between the atrium and the ventricle. The bypass tract is usually capable of bidirectional conduction. Many patients are capable of having more than one type of tachycardia. Approximately 80% of patients with tachycardia have orthodromic AV reciprocating tachycardia, where the QRS is narrow and tachycardia impulse travels down the AV node–His axis, returning to the atrium over the accessory pathway. Approximately 15% of the patients have antidromic tachycardia where the impulse pattern is reversed, creating a wide complex tachycardia that is regular and can mimic VT. In patients with atrial flutter or atrial fibrillation (approximately 20% of total), the accessory pathway is not a requisite part of the mechanism responsible for tachycardia, and the flutter or fibrillation occurs in the atrium unrelated to the accessory pathway. Atrial fibrillation presents a potentially serious risk because of the possibility for very rapid conduction over the accessory pathway, permitting an extremely rapid ventricular response that can lead to ventricular fibrillation. The prognosis is excellent in a patient without tachycardia or an associated cardiac anomaly. The prognosis is good for most patients with recurrent tachycardia, but, rarely, sudden death occurs. In one study, sudden death occurred in 1 of 151 patients followed 1–11 years.[56]

No diagnostic or therapeutic intervention is suggested in patients with asymptomatic preexcitation. Patients with preexcitation can have symptomatic paroxysmal SVT, including atrioventricular reciprocating tachycardia (antidromic or orthodromic). Treatment of atrioventricular reciprocating tachycardias was described in an earlier section. A small percentage of these patients can have paroxysmal atrial fibrillation, a potentially life-threatening condition. Accessory pathways lack the normal decremental properties of the AV node and may therefore permit transmission of an extremely fast number of atrial impulses (350–600 per minute) to the ventricle, leading to ventricular fibrillation. The use of digoxin and verapamil is contraindicated, since both may increase transmission of impulses through the accessory pathway to the ventricle and thus facilitate degeneration of atrial fibrillation to ventricular fibrillation. For a hemodynamically stable patient, management of atrial fibrillation should begin with intravenous procainamide (10–15 mg/kg at an infusion rate of 50 mg/min) followed by a maintenance infusion of 1–4 mg/min. Synchronized cardioversion is the treatment of choice if mother or fetus becomes hemodynamically compromised. Consideration of the chronic use of antiarrhythmic therapy in a patient with preexcitation depends on the frequency and severity of the patient's symptoms. Obviously, if the attacks are rare and of short duration and well tolerated hemodynamically, no therapy is recommended. Atrioventricular reciprocating tachycardia in very symptomatic patients can be managed with a combination of a beta blocker and either quinidine, disopyramide, or procainamide. For atrial fibrillation, multiple regimens have been described as effective, including disopyramide, quinidine, procainamide, flecainide, amiodarone, and esmolol.[46–49,81] After pregnancy, electrophysiological study is recommended in patients with symptomatic tachycardias.

Wide Complex Regular Tachycardia

SUPRAVENTRICULAR TACHYCARDIA WITH ABERRANCY Any type of SVT conducted with a functional or persistent bundle branch block or antidromic AV reciprocating tachycardia with antegrade conduction through a bypass tract can mimic VT. The QRS duration during this type of SVT is wide but usually less than 0.14 second. Right bundle branch block pattern is more commonly seen with aberrant conduction, although it is nonspecific. The relationship of one P wave to each QRS complex can help differentiate SVT from VT. Carotid sinus massage, vagal maneuvers, or intravenous adenosine can terminate SVT if the mechanism of the tachycardia is reentry involving the AV node. These interventions may also terminate VT, although less frequently. Carotid sinus massage can also slow the AV node conduction, making the flutter waves more noticeable if the SVT is atrial flutter. Certain physical findings can help differentiate SVT from VT. In SVT, the heart sounds S_1 and S_2 do not vary in intensity, but this is not so in VT. Cannon *a* waves indicate VT because of AV dissociation. Major features in differentiating SVT with aberrancy and VT are summarized in Table 13.6.

WIDE COMPLEX IRREGULAR TACHYCARDIA In patients with an underlying intraventricular conduction disorder or rate-related conduction disturbance or preexcitation syndrome, acute onset of automatic atrial tachycardia or atrial fibrillation with very rapid ventricular response rate may create a rhythm that is irregular, with wide QRS complex. Sometimes, the rate is so fast that it appears to be regular, and the rhythm can be confused with VT. However, careful examination of the cycle length and use of vagal maneuvers or adenosine can help in differentiation. Treatment is similar to that of automatic atrial tachycardia, atrial fibrillation, or the preexcitation-related tachycardias described earlier.

Electrical Therapy: Synchronized Cardioversion and Defibrillation

Electrical therapy will effectively terminate most tachycardias whether supraventricular (e.g., atrial fibrillation, AV nodal reentry) or ventricular (e.g., ventricular tachycardia, ventricular fibrillation). The electric shock, by depolarizing all excitable myocardium and possibly by prolonging refractoriness, interrupts reentry circuits, discharges foci, and establishes electrical homogeneity that terminates reentry. Synchronized electrical cardioversion may be necessary in patients with tachyarrhythmias unresponsive to drug therapy or when hemodynamic decompensation develops. This procedure reportedly has been performed safely during all stages of pregnancy in over a dozen cases.[57,74,75,82–88]

In general, any tachycardia that produces hypotension, pulmonary edema, or unstable angina and does not respond promptly to medical management should be terminated elec-

TABLE 13.6   Diferential Diagnosis of Regular Wide Complex Tachycardia

	VT	SVT with Aberration
AV dissociation	$+++$	$-$
Fusion beats	$+++$	$-$
QRS width	> 140 ms	< 140 ms
R/S ratio in V_6	< 1.0	> 1.0
QRS Morphology V_1		
Triphasic (rSR′)	$-$	$+++$
Triphasic (RSr′)	$+++$	$-$
Biphasic	$++$	$+$
Monophasic	$+++$	$-$
Onset	VPB	APB with wide QRS
CSM or vagal maneuvers or adenosine	No effect or very rarely termination.	May terminate tachycardia or create AV blocks
Frontal plane axis	< -30 or LAD	Normal or rightward

Abbreviations and symbols: AV, atrioventricular; APB, atrial premature beat; CSM, carotid sinus massage; LAD, left-axis deviation; SVT, supraventricular tachycardia; VPB, ventricular premature beat; VT, ventricular tachycardia; $+++$, strongly favors; $++$, helpful; $+$, does not help; $-$, goes against.

trically. Atrial fibrillation with rapid ventricular response rate in patients with preexcitation is often best treated with electrical cardioversion. In general, the patient's hemodynamic status improves immediately after cardioversion. If after the first shock, reversion to sinus rhythm does not occur, a higher energy level should be tried. The recommended energy varies for arrhythmias (see Table 13.7).

Reported fetal complications from electrical therapy include the occurrence of transient fetal bradycardia that resolved spontaneously or immediately after birth. Occasionally, maternal complications from electrical therapy can occur, including arrhythmias induced by inadequate synchronization, with the shock occurring during the T wave and possibly precipitating ventricular fibrillation. Embolic episodes have been reported in patients converted from atrial fibrillation to sinus rhythm. If atrial fibrillation does not create any hemodynamic compromise, drug treatment should be considered first. Elective cardioversion can be performed after an adequate trial of antiarrhythmic therapy. Because of the risk of systemic embolization, anticoagulation should be performed at least 3 weeks prior to elective cardioversion for atrial fibrillation and should continue for several more weeks after successful cardioversion. Elevation of cardiac enzymes after electrical cardioversion have been reported, although it is not very common.

Radiofrequency Ablation

Both electrophysiological (EP) evaluation and radiofrequency ablation require the use of ionizing radiation and therefore are usually avoided during pregnancy. Lee et al[40] reported four cases of echo-guided placement of EP catheters during pregnancy for the evaluation of presyncope, syncope, or ventricular tachycardia. Gras et al[61] reported radiofrequency ablation of atrioventricular conduction in a patient with hypertrophic cardiomyopathy; the procedure was performed during the fifth month of pregnancy to treat a poorly controlled SVT, which had led to fetal distress.

TABLE 13.7   Recommended Energy (joules) for Cardioversion

Arrhythmia	Initial Energy (J)	Mode
AFIB	50–100	Synchronized
AFLUT	25–50	Synchronized
VT, unstable	200	Synchronized
VT, stable	25–50	Synchronized
SVT, stable	100–200	Synchronized
VFIB	200–360	Asynchronized
SVT, unstable WPW with AFIB	200–360	Synchronized

Abbreviations: AFIB, atrial fibrillation; AFLUT, atrial flutter; SVT, supraventricular tachycardia including atrial flutter; VFIB, ventricular fibrillation; VT, ventricular tachycardia; WPW, Preexcitation (Wolff–Parkinson–White).

Automatic Implantable Cardioverter Defibrillator (AICD)

Although the insertion of AICD during pregnancy has not been reported, pregnancies in women who had had these devices implanted before pregnancy have been shown to be uneventful.[89,90]

Bradyarrhythmia of Clinical Significance

Approach to Bradyarrhythmia Many types of bradyarrhythmia and conduction abnormality are not clinically significant. Patients with bradyarrhythmias can have a variety of symptoms or, frequently, none. The frequency of attacks and associated symptoms may resemble those of patients with tachyarrhythmia, from mild dizziness to syncope. It is important to correlate the symptoms with actual electrocardiographic abnormalities. Static and dynamic ECG monitoring are the most useful modalities for documentation. It is also important to distinguish normal variant (vagal) and pharmacologically induced bradyarrhythmias from those of pathologic origin. Pharmacological agents such as digoxin, beta blockers, calcium channel blockers, and/or type I and III antiarrhythmic agents can produce profound bradycardia or conduction abnormality. Pathologic conditions, such as myocardial ischemia, hypothermia, myxedema, subarachnoid hemorrhage, should also be investigated. Bradyarrhythmias usually include disease of the sinoatrial node and AV node and the conduction pathways.

Sinus Node Disease or Dysfunction Some degree of sinus nodal dysfunction may manifest as sinus bradycardia, prolonged sinus pause or sinus arrest greater than 3 seconds, and/or chronotropic incompetence. This condition is occasionally associated with paroxysmal supraventricular tachyarrhythmias. However, marked sinus bradycardia (heart rate < 40 beats per minute) or long pauses (> 2 seconds) may be seen in young healthy females without any symptoms.[2] The manifestation of sinus node dysfunction includes various degrees of sinoatrial block, usually a disorder of impulse transmission from the sinus node to the atrial tissue. This may appear as intermittent sinus pauses or a prolonged sinus pause interrupted by an escape beat. The incidence of sinus node dysfunction occurring during pregnancy is unknown. Other conditions that may be associated with sinus bradycardia, although rare in pregnant women, include myocarditis, cardiomyopathy, hypothyroidism, carotid hypersensitivity, hypothermia, acute inferior myocardial infarction, drugs or intoxication. (Beta blockers, calcium channel blockers, organophosphate, lithium, clonidine, digoxin, and class I or III antiarrhythmic drugs). Usually, diagnosis of sinus node disease can be made based on the history, physical examination, and static or dynamic ECG. In some cases, provocative tests such as atropine or isoproterenol infusions, or tests to measure the sinus nodal recovery time, may be necessary to establish the diagnosis. As a rule, however, it is not advisable to perform these tests on pregnant patients.

For management (Table 13.8), emphasis should be placed on eliminating the underlying causes. If symptoms occur, they usually respond to intravenous atropine (1 mg). In very extreme or rare occasions, when bradycardia produces symptoms of severe hemodynamic compromise and does not respond to atropine, isoproterenol hydrochloride in a form of continuous infusion (2–4 μg/min) may be used. Intravenous calcium chloride (100–500 mg of 10% CaCl) can be used in cases of calcium channel blocker toxicity. Glucagon (2–4 mg IV) is the drug of choice in beta-blocker overdose. A pacemaker (temporary or permanent) may be necessary if persistent symptomatic bradycardia occurs, such as in sick sinus syndrome.[91,92] In women of childbearing age, atrial or dual-chamber pacing is usually preferable to ventricular pacing, to preserve sequential atrioventricular contraction.[93]

Second- and Third-Degree Atrioventricular Block Although pregnancy does not appear to predispose patients to the development of second- or third-degree heart block,[96–104] several cases of pregnancy in women with heart block have been reported. If the condition is first noted at pregnancy, it was usually present before the pregnancy. Common cardiac conditions associated with high degree AV block are con-

TABLE 13.8 Management of Bradyarrhythmias and Conduction Disturbances in Pregnancy

Arrhythmia	Treatment
Sinus bradycardia (SB), symptomatic	Atropine, repeat if necessary; isoproteronol, calcium chloride, glucagon, temporary pacing
Persistent SB (sick sinus syndrome)	Theophylline, dual-chamber permanent pacing
Atrioventricular block	
First degree	No treatment
Second degree, type I	No treatment necessary
Second degree, type II symptomatic	Permanent pacing
Third degree, congenital	± Permanent pacing
Third degree, acquired	Permanent pacing
Bi- or trifascicular blocks	Pacing only if symptoms are associated with bradyarrhythmias

genital heart disease (especially ventricular septal defect) and rheumatic valvular disease.[4] The prognosis and the need for pacemaker are usually related to the underlying escape rhythm and the cardiac disease.[4,94–102] In patients with high grade AV block, Mendelsohn reported that maternal and fetal mortality usually can be attributed to the underlying heart diseases, not the conduction defect.

Second-degree AV block is characterized by a partial transmission of the atrial impulses to the ventricle. It is classified into two types. In type I, the block in conduction usually occurs at the AV node. Type I second-degree AV block is characterized by progressive prolongation of the PR interval, indicating progressive decrease in conduction velocity and a decreasing RR interval before a P wave is completely blocked. In a nonpathological state, type I block is usually seen in young adults with excessive parasympathetic tone, such as highly conditioned athletes. In a pathological state, it can be associated with an acute inferior myocardial infarction because the right coronary artery supplies the inferior wall as well as the AV nodal branch 90% of the time. It is generally transient and requires no treatment in the majority of patients. In type II, the block occurs below the level of the AV node and is usually the result of disease in the His bundle or bundle branch system, (the QRS complexes are generally wide due to the presence of concomitant bundle branch block). The PR is usually fixed, and the conduction ratio is 2:1 or less. This is usually an unstable condition and usually antedates the development of Adams–Stokes syncope and is progressive to complete AV block. In third-degree AV block, there is a complete dissociation between atrial and ventricular activity. If the block is at the AV node, the QRS is narrow and the escape rhythm is usually stable ($>$ 40 beats per minute) and may respond to autonomic maneuvers. If the block is at the level of the His bundle or lower, the escape rhythm usually originates from the ventricle and the rate is slower ($<$ 40 beats per minute). This is an unstable rhythm and is associated with an increased incidence of syncope and sudden death.

Second-degree AV block type I in general does not produce any symptoms until the ventricular rate has fallen at least below 40 beats per minute. Treatment is similar to symptomatic sinus bradycardia. Should it produce hemodynamic instability, use of atropine or isoproterenol is usually enough to increase the ventricular rate. However temporary pacing may be necessary. Second-degree AV block type II, when it is not associated with fast atrial rate, is usually not a transient event. The ventricular rate may become slow enough to produce hemodynamic symptoms. It tends to be persistent and recurrent and may progress to complete heart block, especially the infranodal type. It has a more serious prognosis, since it is occasionally associated with extensive organic damage to the conduction system. Artificial pacing will be required in most instances, and atropine is unlikely to be successful.

It is debatable when a patient with congenital complete heart block would require a permanent pacemaker.[101] Pacemaker therapy instituted to correct slow escape rate and related symptoms has been reported during pregnancy.[100] In contrast, Holdright and Sutton[98] reported normalization of AV conduction in a woman with complete heart block during two consecutive pregnancies and return to complete AV block immediately postpartum. Usually, if there is no associated heart disease and a reasonable junctional escape mechanism, a pacemaker is not necessary. However, if the heart block is acquired and associated with structural heart disease, permanent pacemaker implantation is indicated.

Intraventricular Conduction Block Bundle branch block is rare among the adult population, with an estimated incidence of 1–2%.[96,97] Most of the individuals affected are over 40 years old and have associated structural heart disease. The presence of bundle branch block in the young adult population is rare, especially in the pregnant women. No claims of pregnancy itself causing bundle branch block have been reported, but a pregnant patient may present with fascicular blocks, isolated or in combination with bundle branch block. Rheumatic valvular disease was reported to be responsible for bundle branch block during pregnancy.[4]

Bundle branch block, especially left, is usually associated with structural heart disease (e.g., rheumatic, congenital), although it can be functional in origin. Fascicular blocks, left anterior/superior hemiblock, and left posterior/inferior hemiblock are due to individual conduction delay in respective fascicles. Fascicular blocks are associated with conditions causing bundle branch blocks and may occur alone or in association with AV block. In asymptomatic patients without structural heart disease, the incidence of progression to complete heart block from bi- or trifasicular disease is quite low ($<$ 1.2%). Bundle branch block per se does not alter the outcome of pregnancy and has no special implication regarding type of delivery. In Mendelsohn's review of bundle branch block, most instances of maternal death or cardiac failure were due to advanced heart disease.[4]

Pregnant patients may present with fascicular blocks,[101] isolated or in combination with bundle branch block. In asymptomatic patients without structural heart disease, the incidence of progression to complete heart block is quite low ($<$ 1.2% per year). In patients with symptoms of dizziness or syncope, the cause of symptoms should be established by appropriate clinical investigations. Permanent pacing is indicated only if the symptom is proven to be associated with bradyarrhythmia.

In managing a pregnant patient with asymptomatic heart block, continuous ECG monitoring during labor and puerperium should be instituted. A temporary pacemaker should be available, to be used in the event of excessive slowing of the rate or syncope. When the block is accompanied by underlying heart disease, pacemaker insertion at the onset of labor should be seriously considered, and provision should be made to prevent fluid overload and to treat heart failure. Patients with block from acquired heart disease are usually exposed to greater risk than those with congenital disease. Digoxin is contraindicated in heart block because of its vagal action, which may induce further rate slowing. Digoxin can be administered effectively once a pacemaker has been inserted.

Uncomplicated implantation of pacemaker during pregnancy has been reported in a few cases.[61,99,100,103] Similarly, uncomplicated pregnancies have been reported in women with permanent pacemaker.[104,105] To reduce the amount of ionizing radiation used, pacemaker implantation can be guided electrocardiographically.[99,100]

Summary

Serious cardiac arrhythmias, including tachyarrhythmias and bradyarrhythmias, are rare during pregnancy. While most of these arrhythmias are of unknown etiology, they sometimes are associated with organic heart disease and other metabolic derangements. Detailed history and physical examinations and noninvasive diagnostic tests should be obtained to provide an accurate diagnosis. Treatments of rhythm disorders in general are no different for pregnant and nonpregnant females. While withdrawal of causative agents may suffice to eliminate the underlying arrhythmias, a conservative approach is usually preferred: antiarrhythmic agents given cautiously, or electrical cardioversion. Even cardiac pacing may be necessary in life-threatening symptomatic arrhythmias.

REFERENCES

1. Zipes DP. Specific arrhythmias: diagnosis and treatment. In Braunwald E, ed. *Heart Disease* 5th ed. Philadelphia: WB Saunders; 1992;97:640–704.

2. Sobotka PA, Mayer JH, Bauernfeind RA, Kanakis C Jr, Rosen KM. Arrhythmias documented by 24-hour continuous ambulatory electrocardiographic monitoring in young women without apparent heart disease. *Am Heart J* 1981;101:573–759.

3. Brodsky M, Wu D, Denes P, Kanikisc C, Rosen KM. Arrhythmias documented by 24 hour continuous electrocardiographic monitoring in 50 male medical students without apparent heart disease. *Am J Cardiol* 1977;39:390–395.

4. Mendelsohn CL. Disorders of the heartbeat during pregnancy. *Am J Obstet Gynecol* 1956;72:1268–1301.

5. Szekely P, Snaith L. Paroxysmal tachycardia in pregnancy. *Br Heart J* 1953;15:195–198.

6. Panja M, Mitra K, Kar AK, Chhetri M, Panja S, Mitra J, Lahiri D. A clinical profile of heart disease in pregnancy. *Indian Heart J* 1986;38:392–396.

7. Hubbard WH, Jenkins BAG, Ward DE. Persistent atrial tachycardia in pregnancy. *Br Med J* 1983;287:327.

8. Widerhorn J, Widerhorn AL, Rahimtoola SH, Elkayam U. WPW syndrome during pregnancy: increased incidence of supraventricular arrhythmias. *Am Heart J* 1992;123:796–798.

9. Kounis NG, Zavras GM, Papadaki PJ, Soufras GD, Kitrou MP, Poulos EA. Pregnancy-induced increase of supraventricular arrhythmias in Wolff–Parkinson–White syndrome. *Clin Cardiol* 1995;18;137–140.

10. Tawam M, Levine J, Mendelson M, Goldberger, J, Dyer A, Kadish A. Effect of pregnancy on paroxysmal supraventricular tachycardia. *Am J Cardiol* 1993;72:838–840.

11. Lee SH, Chen SA, Wu TJ, Chiang CE, Cheng CC, Tai CT, Chiou CW, Ueng KC, Chang MS. Effects of pregnancy on first onset and symptoms of paroxysmal supraventricular tachycardia. *Am J Cardiol* 1995;76:675–678.

12. Brodsky M, Doria R, Allen B, Sato D, Thomas G, Sada M. New-onset ventricular tachycardia during pregnancy. *Am Heart J* 1992;123:933–941.

13. Schwartz PJ, Priori SG. Sympathetic nervous system and cardiac arrhythmias. In: Zipes PD, Jalife J, eds. *Cardiac Electrophysiology: From Cell to Bedside*. Philadelphia: WB Saunders; 1990:330–343.

14. Zuspan FP. Catecholamines: their role in pregnancy and the development of pregnancy-induced hypertension. *J Reprod Med* 1979;23:143–150.

15. Natrajan PG, McGarrigle HH, Lawrence DM, Lachelin GC. Plasma noradrenaline and adrenaline levels in normal pregnancy and in pregnancy-induced hypertension. *Br J Obstet Gynaecol* 1982;89:1041–1045.

16. Whittaker PG, Gerrard J, Lind T. Catecholamine responses to changes in posture during human pregnancy. *Br J Obstet Gynaecol* 1985;92:586–592.

17. Barron WM, Mujais SK, Zinaman M, Bravo EL, Lindheimer MD. Plasma catecholamine responses to physiologic stimuli in normal human pregnancy. *Am J Obstet Gynecol* 1986;154:80–84.

18. Bibring GL, Dwyer TF, Huntington DS, Valenstein AF. A study of the psychological processes in pregnancy and of the earliest mother–child relationship. *Psychoanal Study Child* 1961;16:9–72.

19. Hensleigh PA, Brown EL. Psychosocial stress and pregnancy. In: Gleicher N, ed. *Principles of Medical Therapy in Pregnancy*. New York: Plenum Medical Book Co; 1985:885–888.

20. Carpenter MW, Sady SP, Hoegsberg B, Sady MA, Hagdon B, Cullinane EM, Coustan DR, Thomson PD. Fetal heart rate response to maternal exertion. *JAMA* 1988;259:3006–3009.

21. Page RL. Treatment of arrhythmias during pregnancy. *Am Heart J* 1995;130;871–876.

22. Shotan A, Ostrzega E, Mehra A, Johnson JV, Elkayam U. Incidence of arrhythmias in normal pregnancy and relation to palpitations, dizziness, and syncope. *Am J Cardiol* 1997;79:1061–1064.

23. Vara P, Halminen E. Electrocardiographic examinations during pregnancy and labor. *Acta Obstet Gynecol Scand* 1946;26:402–412.

24. Burch GE. Heart disease and pregnancy. *Am Heart J* 1977;93:104–116.

25. Metcalfe J, McAnulty JH, Ueland K. Cardiovascular physiology. *Clin Obstet Gynecol* 1981;24:693–710.

26. Upshaw C. A study of maternal electrocardiograms recorded during labor and delivery. *Am J Obstet Gynecol* 1970;107:17–27.

27. Moss AJ. Clinical significance of ventricular arrhythmias in patients with and without coronary artery disease. *Prog Cardiovasc Dis* 1980;23:33–52.

28. Elkayam U: Pregnancy and cardiovascular disease. In: Braunwald E, ed. *Heart Disease* 5th ed. Philadelphia: WB Saunders; 1997:1843–1864.

29. O'Donnell M, Meecham J, Tosson SR, Ward S. Ventricular fibrillation and reinfarction in pregnancy. *Postgrad Med J* 1987;63:1095–1096.

30. Rally CR, Walters MB. Paroxysmal ventricular tachycardia without evident heart disease. *Can Med Assoc J* 1962;86: 268–273.

31. Ruszkiewicz A, Opeskin K. Sudden death in pregnancy from congenital malformation of the coronary arteries. *Pathology* 1993;25:236–239.

32. Pelliccia F, Cianfrocca C, Gadio C, Reale A. Sudden death during pregnancy in hypertrophic cardiomyopathy. *Eur Heart J* 1992;13:421–423.

33. Robinson DE, Leicht CH: Epidural analgesia with low-dose bupivacaine and tontange for labor and delivery in a parturient with severe pulmonary hypertension. *Anesthesiology* 1988; 68:285–288.

34. McCurdy CM, Rutherford SE, Coddington CC. Syncope and sudden arrhythmic death complicating pregnancy. A case report of Romano–Ward syndrome. *J Reprod Med* 1993;38: 233–234.

35. Fox CH. Cocaine use in pregnancy. *J Am Board Fam Fract* 1994;7:225–228.

36. Hanania G, Thomas D, Michel PL, Garbarz E, Age C, Millaire A, Acar J. Pregnancy and prosthetic heart valves: a French cooperative retrospective study of 155 cases. *Eur Heart J* 1994;15:1651–1681.

37. Guidelines for CPR and Emergency Cardiac Care. Emergency Cardiac Care Committee and Subcommittee. American Heart Association. Part III. Adult advance cardiac life support. IV. Special resuscitation situations. *JAMA* 1992;268:2199–2242, 2242–2250.

38. Chandra NC, Gates EA, Thamer M. Conservative treatment of paroxysmal ventricular tachycardia during pregnancy. *Clin Cardiol* 1991;14:347–350.

39. Field LM, Barton FL. The management of anesthesia for caesarean section in a patient with paroxysmal ventricular tachycardia. *Anaesthesia* 1993;48:593–595.

40. Lee MS, Evans SJ, Blumberg S, Bodenheimer MM, Roth SL. Echocardiographically guided electrophysiologic testing in pregnancy. *J Am Soc Echocardiogr* 1994;7:182–186.

41. Nadioo DP, Bhorat I, Moodley J, Nadioo JK, Mitha AS. Continuous electrocardiographic monitoring hypertensive crises in pregnancy. *Am J Obstet Gynecol* 1991;164;530–533.

42. Varon ME, Sherer DM, Abramovicz JS, Akiyama T. Maternal ventricular tachycardia associated with hypomagnesemia. *Am J Obstet Gynecol* 1992;167:1352–1355.

43. Akhtar M. Management of ventricular tachyarrhythmias. *JAMA* 1982;247:671–674.

44. Gutgesell M, Overholt E, Boyle R. Oral bretylium tosylate use during pregnancy and subsequent breastfeeding: a case report. *Am J Perinatol* 1990;7:144–145.

45. Cox IL, Gardner MJ. Treatment of cardiac arrhythmias during pregnancy. *Prog Cardiovasc Dis* 1993;36:137–178.

46. McKenna WJ, Harris L, Rowland E, Whitelaw A, Storey G, Holt D. Amiodarone therapy during pregnancy. *Am J Cardiol* 1983;51:1231–1233.

47. Rey E, Bachrach LK, Burrow GN. Effects of amiodarone during pregnancy. *Can Med Assoc J* 1987;136:959–960.

48. Robson DJ, Jeeva Raj MV, Storey GC, Holt DW. Use of amiodarone during pregnancy. *Postgrad Med J* 1985;61:75–77.

49. Widerhorn J, Bhandari AK, Bughi S, Rahimtoola SH, Elkayam U. Fetal and neonatal adverse effect profile of amiodarone treatment during pregnancy. *Am Heart J* 1991;122: 1162–1166.

50. Strunge P, Frandsen J, Andreasen F. Amiodarone during pregnancy. *Eur Heart J* 1988;9:106–109.

51. Penn IM, Barrett PA, Pannikote V, Barnaby PF, Campbell JB, Lyons NR. Amiodarone in pregnancy. *Am J Cardiol* 1985;56:196–197.

52. Wagner X, Jouglard J, Moulin M, Miller AM, Petitjean J, Pisapia A. Coadministration of flecainide acetate and sotalol during pregnancy: lack of teratogenic effects, passage across the placenta, and excretion in human breast milk. *Am Heart J* 1990;119:700–702.

53. Brunozzi LT, Meniconi L, Chiocchi P, Liberati R, Zuanetti G, Latini R. Propafenone in the treatment of chronic ventricular arrhythmias in a pregnant patient. *Br J Clin Pharmacol* 1988;26:489–490.

54. Tzivoni D, Banai S, Schugar C, Schuger C, Benhorin J, Kerena A, Gottlieb S, Stern S. Treatment of torsade de pointes with magnesium sulfate. *Circulation* 1988;77: 392–397.

55. Jackman WM, Friday KJ, Clark M, Anderson JL, Aliot EM, Clark M, Lazzara R. The long QT syndromes: a critical review, new clinical observations and unifying hypothesis. *Prog Cardiovasc Dis* 1988;31;115–172.

56. Wellens HJJ. Supraventricular tachycardias in Willerson JT, Cohn JN (editors): Cardiovascular medicine. New York Churchill Livingstone 1995;1327–1342.

57. DiMarco JP, Miles W, Akhtar M, Milstein S, Sharma AD, Platia E, McGovern B, Scheinman MM, Govier WC. Adenosine for paroxysmal supraventricular tachycardia: dose ranging and comparison with verapamil assessment in placebo-controlled, multicenter, trials. *Ann Intern Med* 1990;113:104–110.

58. Harrison JK, Greenfield RA, Wharton JM. Acute termination of supraventricular tachycardia by adenosine during pregnancy. *Am Heart J* 1992;123:1386–1388.

59. Elkayam U, Goodwin TM. Adenosine therapy for supraventricular tachycardia during pregnancy. *Am J Cardiol* 1995;75: 521–523.

60. Klein V, Repke JT. Supraventricular tachycardia in pregnancy: cardioversion with verapamil. *Obstet Gynecol* 1984;63: 16S–18S.

61. Gras D, Mabop, Kermarrec A, Bazin P, Varin C, Daubert C. Interruption de la conduction auriculo-ventriculaire par radiofréquence au 5e mois d'une grossesse. Arch Mal Coeur Vaiss 1992;85:1873–1877.

62. Haines DE, DiMarco JP. Sustained intra-atrial re-entrant tachycardia. Clinical, electrocardiographic and electrophysiologic characteristics and long-term follow-up. J Am College Cardiol 1990;15:1345–1354.

63. Ahmed K. Issawi I, Peddireddy R. Use of flecainide for refractory atrial tachycardia of pregnancy. Am J Crit Care 1996;5:306–308.

64. Waldo AL, Henthorn RW, Plumb VJ: Atrial flutter—recent observations in man. In: Josephson ME, Wellens HJJ, eds. Tachycardia: Mechanisms, Diagnosis, and Treatment. Philadelphia: Lea & Febiger; 1984;113.

65. Wolf PA, Dawber TR, Thomas HE, Kannel WB. Epidemiologic assessment of chronic atrial fibrillation and risk of stroke: the Framingham study. Neurology 1978;28:973–977.

66. Brand FN, Abbott RD, Kanell WB, Wolff PA. Characteristics and prognosis of lone atrial fibrillation. JAMA 1985;254:3449–3453.

67. Kopecky SL, Gersh BJ, McGoon MD, Whisnant JP, Holmes DR Jr, Ilstrup DM, Frye RL. The natural history of lone atrial fibrillation. A population-based study over three decades. N Engl J Med 1987;317;669–674.

68. Henry WL, Morganroth J, Pearlman AS, Clark CE, Redwood DR, Itscoitz SB, Epstein SE. Relations between echocardiographically determined left atrial size and atrial fibrillation. Circulation 1976;53:273–279.

69. Manning WU, Silverman DI, Gordon SP, Krumholz HM, Douglas PS. Cardioversion from atrial fibrillation prolonged anticoagulation with use of transesophageal echocardiography to exclude the presence of atrial thrombi. N Engl J Med 1993;328:750–775. (See Comments.)

70. Brodsky MA, Allen BJ, Capparelli EV, Luckett CR, Morton R, Henry WL. Factors determining maintenance of sinus rhythm after chronic atrial fibrillation with left atrial dilatation. Am J Cardiol 1989;63:1065–1068.

71. Byrene-Quinn E, Wing AJ. Maintenance of sinus rhythm after DC reversion of atrial fibrillation. A double-blind controlled trial of long acting quinidine bisulfate. Br Heart J 1970;32:370–376.

72. Dittrich HC, Erickson JS, Schneiderman T, Blacky AR, Savides T, Nicod PH. Echocardiographic and clinical predictors for outcome of elective cardioversion of atrial fibrillation. Am J Cardiol 1989;63:193–197.

73. Hirsh J, Fuster V. Guide to anticoagulant therapy: 2. Oral antigoagulants. Circulation 1994;89:1469–1480.

74. Doig JC, McComb JM, Reid DC. Incessant atrial tachycardia accelerated by pregnancy. Br Heart J 1992;67:266.

75. Murphy JJ, Hutchon DJ. Incessant atrial tachycardia accelerated by pregnancy. Br Heart J 1992;68:342. Letter.

76. Iseri LT, Fairshter RD, Hardemann JL, Brodsky MA. Magnesium and potassium therapy in multifocal atrial tachycardia. Am Heart J 1985;110:789–794.

77. Levine JH, Michael JR, Guarnieri T. Treatment of multifocal arterial tachycardia with verapamil. N Engl J Med 1985;313;21–25.

78. Wellens HJ. Wolff–Parkinson–White syndrome: diagnosis, arrhythmias and identification of the high risk patient. Modern Concepts Cardiovasc Dis 1983;52:53–59.

79. Munger TM, Hammill SC, Packer DL, Feldman BJ, Bailey KR, Ballard DJ, Holmes DR Jr, Gersh BJ. A population study of the natural history of Wolff–Parkinson–White syndrome in Olmsted County, Minnesota 1953–1989. Circulation 1993;87:866–873.

80. Gleicher N, Meller J, Sandler R, Sullum S. Wolff–Parkinson–White syndrome in pregnancy. Obstet Gynecol 1981;58:748–752.

81. Plomp TA, Vulsma T, de Vijlder JJ. Use of amiodarone during pregnancy. Eur J Obstet Gynecol Reprod Biol 1992;43:201–207.

82. Curry JJ, Quintana FJ. Myocardial infarction with ventricular fibrillation during pregnancy treated by direct current defibrillation with fetal survival. Chest 1970;58:82–84.

83. Grand A, Bernard J. Cardioversion et grossesse: conséquences foetales. Nouv Presse Med 1973;2:2327–2329.

84. Robards GJ, Saunders PM, Donnelly GL. Refractory supraventricular tachycardia complicating pregnancy. Med J Aust 1973;2:278–280.

85. Schroeder JS, Harrison DC. Repeated cardioversion during pregnancy: treatment of refractory paroxysmal atrial tachycardia during three successive pregnancies. Am J Cardiol 1971;27:445–446.

86. Sussman HI, Duque D, Lesser ME. Atrial flutter with 1:1 conduction: report of a case in a pregnant woman successfully treated with dc countershock. Dis Chest 1966;49:99–103.

87. Swartjes JM, Schutte MF, Bleker OP. Management of eclampsia: cardiopulmonary arrest resulting from magnesium sulfate overdose. Eur J Obstet Gynecol Reprod 1992;47:73–75.

88. Treakie K, Kostic B, Hulkowers. Supraventricular tachycardia resistant to treatment in a pregnant woman. J Fam Pract 1992;35:581–584.

89. Isaacs JD, Mulholland DH, Hess LW, Allbert JR, Martin RW. Pregnancy in a woman with an automatic implantable cardioverter–defibrillator: a case report. J Reprod Med 1993;38:487–488.

90. Gerger MJ, Newby KH, Natale A. Impact of implantable defibrillators on the outcome of pregnancy. Circulation 1995;92(suppl I):I-783. Abstract.

91. Schatz JW, Fischer JA, Lee RF, Lampe RM. Pacemaker therapy in pregnancy for management of sinus bradycardia–junctional tachycardia syndrome. Chest 1974;65:461–463.

92. Abramovici H, Faktor JH, Gonen Y, Brandes JM, Amikan S. Maternal permanent bradycardia: pregnancy and delivery. Obstet Gynecol 1984;63:381–383.

93. Rosenqvist M, Brandt J, Schuller H. Long-term pacing in sinus node disease: effects of stimulation mode on cardiovascular morbidity and mortality. Am Heart J 1988;116:16–22.

94. Epstein JR, Altman HE. Heart block in pregnancy. Med Ann DC 20:660–663.

95. Schonbrum M, Rowland W, Quiroz AC. Complete heart block in pregnancy. *Am J Obstet Gynecol* 1966;27:243–246.

96. Eddy W, Frankenfeld R. Congenital complete heart block in pregnancy. *Am J Obstet Gynecol* 1977;128:223–225.

97. Ginns HM, Holliurake K. Complete heart block in pregnancy treated with an internal pacemaker. *Br J Obstet Gynaecol* 1970;77:710–712.

98. Holdright DR, Suttton GC. Restoration of sinus rhythm during two consecutive pregnancies in a woman with congenital complete heart block. *Br Heart J* 1990;64:338–339.

99. Jordaens LJ, Vandenbogaerde JF, Van De Bruaene P, De buyzere M. Transesophageal echocardiography for insertion of a physiological pacemaker in early pregnancy. *PACE* 1990;13:955–957.

100. Lau CP, Lee CP, Wong CK, Cheng CH, Leung WH. Rate responsive pacing with a minute ventilation sensing pacemaker during pregnancy and delivery. *PACE* 1990;13:158–163.

101. Dalvi BV, Chaudhuri A, Kulkarni HL, Kale PA. Therapeutic guidelines for congenital complete heart block presenting in pregnancy. *Obstet Gynecol* 1992;79:802–804.

102. Ramsewak S, Persad P, Perkins S, Narayansingh G. Twin pregnancy in a patient with complete heart block. *Clin Exp Obstet Gynecol* 1992;19:166–167.

103. Rosen A, Klein M, Ambros O, Pfemeter G. Implantation eines Herzschrittmachers in der 25.SSW bei erworbenem AV Block III. Grades. Geburtshilfe *Frauenheilkd* 1991;51: 239–240.

104. Terhaar M, Schakenbach L. Care of the pregnant patient with a pacemaker. *J Perinatal Neonatal Nurs* 1991;5:1–12.

105. Walsh T, Savage R, Hess DB. Successful pregnancy in a patient with a double inlet left ventricle treated with a septation procedure. *South Med J* 1990;83:358–359.

14

MITRAL VALVE PROLAPSE AND PREGNANCY

William F. Rayburn, MD

INTRODUCTION

Mitral valve prolapse (MVP), one of the most common cardiac abnormalities, results from a variety of congenital and acquired mechanisms. The exact prevalence of MVP is unknown, but its reported incidence in the general population is about 3% of adults.[1] Diagnosis of MVP should be based on history, physical examination, and echocardiography. Most patients are asymptomatic, and the condition is often discovered incidentally during a routine physical examination. Women predominate in most studies, and the diagnosis is frequently made in young women of childbearing age.

BACKGROUND

Natural History

The major anatomic abnormality of MVP is an enlargement of one or both mitral leaflets, most frequently the posterior leaflet. Histologic examination of an affected mitral valve reveals a wide spectrum of findings. The valve leaflets may be normal, or they may demonstrate various degrees of myxomatous degeneration (especially the posterior leaflet in cases seen at autopsy or surgery). Redundancy of mitral leaflets may produce either a localized protrusion or a generalized ballooning of leaflet tissue into the left atrium. The chordae tendineae may also appear normal or be elongated. Mitral annular dilation may be moderate or marked.

Two theories prevail about the causes of MVP.[2] The first postulates that a primary inheritable abnormality of the connective tissues allows for weakness and stretching of the mitral leaflets, chordae tendineae, and annulus, resulting in prolapse. The second, a "response to injury" hypothesis, proposes that minor congenital variations in the mitral valve allow the leaflets and chordae tendineae to be injured with prolonged systolic stress. Repair and reinjury then set the stage for progressive weakening and collagen disruption.

MVP may be associated with conditions such as rheumatic heart disease, congestive cardiomyopathy, Marfan's syndrome, Ehlers–Danlos syndrome, pseudo–xanthoma elasticum, osteogenesis imperfecta, coronary heart disease, and ostium secundum atrial septal defect. Infective endocarditis and severe mitral regurgitation are rare conditions. Significant coronary artery disease has been found in about 5% of patients with MPV who have undergone coronary arteriography for evaluation of chest pain.[3] This finding is age related, however, and the condition would be less common in young women of reproductive age.

The long-term outlook for MVP in children and women of reproductive age is generally excellent. Most remain asymptomatic for many years without change in clinical or laboratory findings. Heart failure from MVP is highly unlikely. Progressive mitral regurgitation occurs in about 15% of patients over a 10- to 15-year period, especially if there is a murmur along with a click.[4] Infective endocarditis and rupture of chordae tendineae are usually responsible for intensification of mitral regurgitation. Valve replacement may be necessary when regurgitation becomes severe.

Cerebral emboli may result from an accompanying paroxysmal arrhythmia, loss of endothelial continuity, or tearing of the endocardium overlying any myxomatous valve. These events may lead to platelet aggregation and the formation of mural platelet–fibrin complexes. In young people with undetected cerebral vascular disease, cerebral embolization secondary to MVP may be present as unexplained strokes, oth-

Cardiac Problems in Pregnancy, Third Edition
Edited by Uri Elkayam, MD, and Norbert Gleicher, MD
Copyright © 1998 by Wiley-Liss, Inc. ISBN 0-471-16358-9

er cerebral and retinal complications, and mild cardiac infarctions.

Signs and Symptoms

Most nonpregnant patients are asymptomatic and do well. Symptoms of palpitations, anxiety, fatigue, lightheadedness, and chest pain are not often associated with objective findings. One or more midsystolic clicks, with or without a late systolic murmur, are the auscultatory hallmarks of MVP. The "snapping" click usually occurs during maximal valve prolapse and may be absent, single, or multiple at any time.[1]

The typical mid- or late systolic murmur begins with or just follows the click and is usually crescendo in quality. Any maneuver that reduces left ventricular volume will lead to an earlier occurrence and accentuation of MVP. Therefore, a click and murmur will occur earlier while sitting, standing, or performing the Valsalva maneuver. The intensity of the murmur may decrease unless the mitral regurgitation is severe. Prompt squatting and isometric exercises will increase left ventricular volume and may therefore move the click toward the second heart sound and delay the onset of the louder murmur.

A classification of patients with mitral valve prolapse has been proposed: anatomic MVP (or "floppy mitral valve") and MVP syndrome.[5] The category of anatomic mitral valve prolapse includes a wide spectrum of mitral valve abnormalities.

Symptoms and physical findings in these patients directly relate to mitral dysfunction and progressive regurgitation. Mitral valve prolapse syndrome refers to the occurrence of symptoms such as palpitations, chest pain, fatigue, exercise intolerance, dyspnea, and syncope that cannot be explained on the basis of a mitral valve abnormality alone. The pathogenesis of these symptoms may relate to metabolic neuroendocrine dysfunction. The theory of autonomic nervous dysfunction is intriguing, but specific delineation of the problem is unclear at this time.

Laboratory Evaluation

Echocardiographic findings are becoming standard criteria for confirming the diagnosis and for following patients with MVP. Use of this test would seem to be especially important during pregnancy because of the characteristic late- or pansystolic murmur found in healthy pregnant women without MVP. A standard M-mode and two-dimensional echocardiographic machine with a 2.25 MHz transducer is commonly used, although two-dimensional echocardiography should provide a yield superior to that from M mode alone. M-mode echocardiographic evidence for MVP is typically defined as a systolic hammocking greater than 2 mm posterior to C–D point or midsystolic buckling.[6] MVP is defined by two-dimensional echocardiography as superior motion and bowing of either or both mitral valve leaflets above the level of the

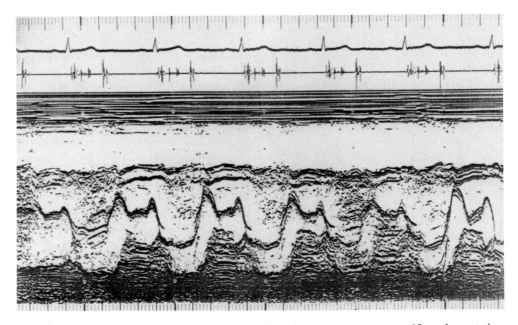

Figure 14.1   Echocardiogram of mitral valve prolapse in a pregnant woman at 18 weeks gestation reveals a pansystolic prolapse of the posterior leaflet at the level of the mitral valve. The phonocardiogram demonstrates a midsystolic click and a systolic murmur. A normal sinus rhythm is seen on the electrocardiogram.

valve ring during systole, with the leaflet coaptation point at or superior to the ring.[7]

Late systolic prolapse of one or both leaflets can be directly visualized by echocardiography as posterior movement interrupting normal anterior motion (Fig. 14.1). Other echocardiographic abnormalities suggestive of, but not specific for, MVP include exaggerated mitral leaflet mobility, producing diastolic contact with the interventricular septum; minimal systolic sagging, diminishing normal anterior motion of the mitral leaflets; and a multiplicity of parallel mitral leaflet echoes. Hemodynamic measurements and left ventricular function are usually normal in patients with uncomplicated MVP.[3,8] Echocardiograms or right ventricular cineangiograms may demonstrate tricuspid prolapse. Care must be taken not to overdiagnose mitral prolapse angiographically in the presence of normal radiographic variants.

Electrocardiographic (ECG) abnormalities occur in up to two-thirds of patients with MVP.[3,8] The most typical abnormality consists of a flattened or inverted T wave in leads II, III, and aVF. Less common ECG changes include prolongation of the QT interval, premature ventricular contractions, atrial fibrillation, and first-degree atrioventricular block. Ambulatory ECG monitoring is the most sensitive method for detecting arrhythmias. Except for the effect of any thoracic bony abnormalities, chest X-ray films are normal in patients with uncomplicated mitral prolapse.[9]

Management

Endocarditis may occur in individuals with isolated clicks and in those with late systolic murmurs. The value of antibiotic prophylaxis against infective endocarditis is unknown but doubtful in patients with echocardiographic prolapse that is unaccompanied by auscultatory signs of regurgitation.[1] Spontaneous rupture of the delicate, attenuated chordae tendineae may suddenly augment mitral regurgitation, causing the murmur to be louder and holosystolic.

People in whom the diagnosis is made accidentally on routine physical examination are usually asymptomatic and require no therapy. Reassurance that symptoms, if present, do not signal cardiac compromise or impending danger is usually sufficient. Prevention of endocarditis is the major consideration in these patients. In general, patients with a systolic murmur should receive antibiotic prophylaxis for any diagnostic and therapeutic procedures that may induce bacteremia.

Patients with anatomic MVP should be evaluated periodically for mitral regurgitation and preventing endocarditis. Progressive regurgitation is accompanied with left atrial enlargement and failure. Medical therapy is directed toward atrial fibrillation (control of ventricular rate) and treatment of congestive failure associated with mitral regurgitation (va-sodilators and diuretic therapy). If very limited or no benefit is gained, surgery should be considered.

Ventricular arrhythmias require individual assessment and identification of precipitating factors. Caffeine or other stimulants such as alcohol, tobacco, and sympathomimetic drugs should be avoided, especially among those with tachyarrhythmias. β-Adrenergic-blocking agents such as propranolol may control arrhythmias (premature ventricular contractions, supraventricular tachycardia) and limit symptoms of chest pain and palpitations. Use of these drugs may increase left ventricular volume and decrease contractility and thus may decrease valve prolapse and tension on the chordae and adjacent myocardium. Quinidine has been used in combination with propranolol; however, digitalis, procainamide, or quinidine alone is less effective (see Chapter 29).[9]

Patients with MVP syndrome do not progress to develop mitral regurgitation. It is important to educate and reassure them about the relatively benign course. Drugs with increased adrenergic receptor sensitivity (e.g., thyroxine) and catecholamines or other cyclic adenosine monophosphate stimulants should be avoided.

EFFECTS OF PREGNANCY ON MVP

Approximately 1.2% of pregnant women were suspected of having MVP during pregnancy.[10] On close evaluation, only half of these women may have a previously suspicious or positive echocardiogram. In most obstetric studies, the diagnosis of MVP may not have been made by an echocardiogram. Clinically evident hemodynamic abnormalities are uncommon during pregnancy in women with MVP.

Clicks, murmurs, and possibly symptoms are less obvious during pregnancy, probably because the intravascular volume is expanded and peripheral vascular resistance reduced (see Chapter 2). The increased blood volume may realign the mitral valve complex by increasing left ventricular and end diastolic volume and by lengthening the long axis of the left ventricle.[10] For example, Haas[11] found on two of three pregnant patients with MVP that both the click and late systolic murmur disappeared, while in the third, only the click remained by the third trimester. In all the patients, the characteristic click and murmur had returned by 3 months postpartum. Auscultatory findings of MVP diminish with advancing gestation.

Any hospitalization for cardiac complications is rare. Propranolol is commonly taken before conception but is often discontinued during early gestation with no apparent adverse effect. Other illnesses (asthma, seizure disorder, drug addiction) are uncommon and do not usually influence the heart condition. Castillo et al [12] reported a case of acute mitral insufficiency secondary to bacterial endocarditis and ruptured chordal tendineae at 30 weeks of gestation in a 29-year old woman with echocardiographic demonstration of MVP. Induced uterine contractions were generally well tolerated, and the delivery and postpartum courses were uncomplicated.

EFFECTS OF MVP ON PREGNANCY

Only a few investigations have reported on pregnancy outcomes in patients with MVP. Most patients deliver vaginally at term after an uncomplicated antepartum course. In our experience of 96 cases, the incidence of spontaneous abortion or premature delivery in women with MVP is no higher than in women without an apparent cardiac disorder.[10,13] The frequency of intrapartum complications is also not significantly greater among patients with MVP compared to those with no cardiac disorder (Table 14.1). All but 11 of the 91 patients received prophylactic antibiotics during labor. Local anesthesia was commonly used, but epidural or spinal anesthesia was given in 7 patients without signs of hypotension or congestive heart failure. Twenty cesarean sections (21% of total deliveries) were performed because of failure of labor to progress, breech presentation, repeat cesarean section, or a nonreassuring fetal heart rate pattern. All tolerated pregnancy well, and most infants were appropriately sized and delivered without low Apgar scores (Table 14.1). Prolonged neonatal hospitalization was unnecessary for reasons other than prematurity or congenital anomalies.

Another study by Tang et al[14] in Hong Kong confirmed these impressions. The obstetrical performances and outcomes of 37 women with MVP were reviewed. Thirteen patients were diagnosed as having had the cardiac defect before pregnancy, while 24 patients were detected initially during prenatal examinations. Thirty-four of the 37 women underwent uneventful vaginal deliveries at term, while three ended in cesarean sections as a result of obstetrical complications. No maternal mortality or cardiac complications occurred. Although one infant was hydropic from a hemoglobinopathy, the remaining 36 babies were born without apparent difficulties.

The safety of labor and delivery of women with MVP was investigated by Shapiro and colleagues[15] in Baltimore. Twenty-three patients with auscultatory and echocardiographic evidence for MVP were compared with a similar group of women without such findings. A maximum rate of cervical dilation (3.3 cm/h) was found in both groups. Durations of the first and second stages of labor were not different, and birth weights and Apgar scores of newborn infants were similar. No clinically significant advantage in the speed of labor and delivery was found for patients with MVP over the general population. Thus, the laxity of joints and connective tissue that can be associated with MVP may not necessarily facilitate childbirth or quicken delivery.

Two recent reports confirm that MVP, despite comprising a large proportion of obstetric cardiac problems, is well tolerated. Chia et al[16] from Singapore reported about 28 patients with echocardiographic proven nonmyxomatous MVP. Progress during the antepartum and intrapartum periods and use of analgesia did not differ significantly from patterns seen in noncardiac patients. The numbers in this study were too small to permit a valid comparison of the higher cesarean section rate in the MVP group to the department average. Jana et al[17] from Chandigarsh, India, reported on 34 pregnancies

TABLE 14.1   Pregnancy Outcomes of Patients With or Without Mitral Valve Prolapse (MVP)

Outcome	With MVP ($n = 96$)	Without MVP ($n = 235$)	Statistical Significance[a]
ANTEPARTUM			
Hospitalization	0	11 (5%)	NS
Other Medical illnesses	15 (16%)	24 (10%)	NS
INTRAPARTUM			
Premature delivery	9 (10%)	29 (12%)	NS
Meconium	16 (15%)	38 (16%)	NS
Cesarean section	20 (21%)	42 (18%)	NS
NEONATAL			
Spontaneous abortion	14 (15%)	24 (10%)	NS
Low birth weight (< 2500 g)	9 (9%)	45 (19%)	
5-minute Apgar score ≤ 6	6 (6%)	8 (3%)	NS
Major anomaly	2 (2%)	5 (2%)	NS
Perinatal mortality	1 (1%)	4 (2%)	NS

[a]As determined by Rayburn et al.[10,13]

in 15 women with MVP, all of whom remained well throughout pregnancy and labor. The frequencies of preterm deliveries and congenital abnormalities were not higher than those in the reference group of patients.

Despite this reassurance, case reports do document that rare but dreaded complications of MVP can occur during pregnancy. Artal et al[18] describe the course of a 32-year-old patient (gravida 4, para 1, spontaneous abortion 2), whose diagnosis of MVP was confirmed by echocardiography at 14 weeks after an episode of palpitations. At 37.5 weeks, the patient experienced a 4-minute syncopal episode, which resulted in a left hemiparesis. Transient thromboembolic ischemia was diagnosed, and it was believed to be secondary to the MVP. A repeat cesarean section was performed after the onset of spontaneous labor. The hemiparesis resolved by the first day postpartum. The patient was treated with low dose aspirin in a subsequent pregnancy without complication. In another case, Bergh et al[19] described a 26-year-old patient (gravida 2, para 1), who had a history of asymptomatic MVP and presented with a sudden, painless loss of vision in her right eye at 10 weeks of gestation. Ophthalmologic evaluation demonstrated branch retinal artery occlusion with near complete loss of vision. Echocardiographic findings were consistent with MVP and a bicuspid aortic valve. Therapy throughout gestation consisted of aspirin 50 mg twice daily and dipyridamole 50 mg three times daily. The pregnancy progressed without complications. Examination 6 months after the vaginal delivery revealed no change in the patient's status. Relatively recently, a case of postpartum group B streptococcal endocarditis was reported following uncomplicated spontaneous vaginal delivery.[12] Echocardiography showed moderate to severe MVP, and vegetation on the atrial surfaces of both leaflets.

SPECIAL CONSIDERATIONS DURING PREGNANCY

Prenatal Genetic Counseling

There is no clear genetic pattern of inheritance, and an autosomal dominant inheritance with variable expressivity has been suggested.[1,20] Inheritance may be underestimated because of asymptomatic prolapse. Familial occurrence has been uncommon in most large series.[1,8] Questioning about or examining family members is recommended. Otherwise, genetic counseling for MVP alone is not recommended routinely before or during pregnancy.

Maternal MVP was suggested as a risk factor for congenital heart disease in the offspring.[21] A higher prevalence of MVP was found in mothers of infants with congenital heart disease compared to mothers of a control group of normal infants. The presence of multiple malformation in several of

the infants is consistent with Pickering's hypothesis of biosynthetic defect.[22]

Propranolol Medication

Despite its widespread use in human pregnancies, propranolol has been mentioned in few reports describing abnormal births. In three prospective studies, women with chronic hypertension experienced an increase in fetal and neonatal survival when propranolol treatment was used to control hypertension in pregnancy.[23–25]

Propranolol exposure in late pregnancy has been associated with neonatal apnea, respiratory distress, bradycardia, and hypoglycemia.[23–20] All these effects are consistent with the known pharmacologic effects of propranolol and are likely to be residual influences of the maternally administered agent (see Chapter 29).

Echocardiographic Changes

Echocardiographic observations by Lutas et al[31] indicate that mitral valve prolapse is most likely overdiagnosed before pregnancy or that the prolapse disappears during pregnancy in more than half of a population of women whose echocardiograms performed elsewhere had been suspicious or positive for MVP.[10] We later applied the described standard echocardiographic criteria, and found no evidence of MVP either throughout pregnancy or after delivery. These findings also suggest that pregnancy is associated with either no change, an improvement, or a disappearance of a previously documented mitral prolapse.

We followed 21 women with echocardiographic evidence for MVP throughout pregnancy.[10] No evidence for MVP at midgestation, later in pregnancy, and postpartum was present in 62% (13/21) of the study pregnancies. A prolapsed valve was present in the remaining 38% (8/21) women at midgestation. The prolapse disappeared late in pregnancy in five cases and persisted in three cases (Fig. 14.2). Any MVP observed in late gestation persisted on the postpartum examination.

Any decrease or disappearance in mitral prolapse may relate to increases in left atrial and ventricular volumes during pregnancy (Chapter 1). Sufficient increases may eliminate or decrease evidence for MVP during pregnancy and explain its reappearance after the reequilibration of intravascular volume in the postpartum period. Furthermore, pregnancy is thought to ameliorate rather than adversely affect hemodynamics in women with mild or moderate insufficiency.[31] The decrease in peripheral vascular resistance results in better forward flow and reduced valvular stress and regurgitation. A repeat echocardiogram is recommended postpartum to determine whether the MVP exists, since an absence of MVP during pregnancy does not exclude the

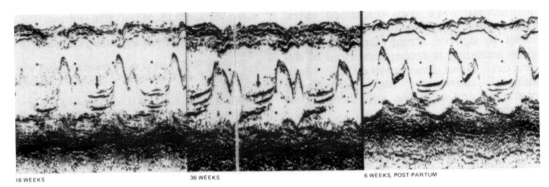

16 WEEKS   36 WEEKS   6 WEEKS, POST PARTUM

Figure 14.2   Echocardiographic changes in a woman in whom mitral valve prolapse appeared at 16 weeks gestation, disappeared by 36 weeks, and reappeared by 6 weeks postpartum.

diagnosis once the intra- and cardiovascular volumes have decreased to normal.

Antibiotic Prophylaxis

The relative risk of infective endocarditis among nonpregnant patients with MVP is five times that of the general population.[1,8] When MVP is accompanied by diffusely thickened, redundant leaflets (myxomatous change), patients are more prone to deformity, degeneration, and infection than patients with MVP but without thickened leaflets (no myxomatous change). Whether patients with cardiac disease and an uncomplicated vaginal delivery benefit from antibiotic prophylaxis has been examined in a series of 2165 women, none of whom received prophylactic antibiotics.[2,32] Asymptomatic puerperal bacteremia was found in only 1% of blood cultures taken at placental separation and at 5, 10, and 30 minutes after delivery.

The issue of antibiotic prophylaxis during delivery for patients with MVP remains unsettled.[32,33] Any person with MVP and mitral regurgitation or a redundant valve (thickened leaflets) is at increased risk of developing infective endocarditis, and therefore prophylactic antibiotics should be prescribed before procedures associated with bacteremia are undertaken. It is generally accepted that prophylaxis should be given for any complicated delivery; however, the necessity of antibiotic prophylaxis for an uncomplicated vaginal delivery has not been firmly established. A report by Sugrue et al[34] concluded that antibiotic prophylaxis was not needed for routine vaginal delivery in patients with heart disease. Since the development of complications and bacteremia during normal delivery cannot always be predicted, however, it is reasonable to administer prophylaxis prior to any vaginal delivery of women with MVP.

The issue is complicated by the difficulties in diagnosing MVP during pregnancy due to the almost inevitable presence of a parasternal systolic ejection murmur during normal pregnancy and the variability of the murmur, depending on the left ventricular volume and contractility in the presence of MVP. Recommendations for antibiotic prophylaxis should likely be based on the diagnosis made at any point in a patient's life. The risk of bacterial endocarditis is not likely to decline in a patient with clear-cut evidence for prolapse before pregnancy who if, because of volume changes, shows no prolapse on echocardiography before labor. The risk for endocarditis has more to do with histologic abnormalities of the valve, and improvement of echocardiographic and auscultatory findings during pregnancy may mask the extent of the valve's abnormality.

For the foregoing reasons, we suggest antibiotic prophylaxis for all women with documented MVP with a thickened mitral valve or mitral insufficiency who are about to deliver. Antibiotics should be given according to recommendations of the American Heart Association[35] (see Chapter 16), although controversy regarding efficacy continues and revisions will likely occur.

Analgesia and Anesthesia

Anesthetic goals include the prevention of increased myocardial contractility and heart rate, maintenance of normal circulatory blood volume, and avoidance of elevation in airway pressure (see Chapter 24).[32] Regional analgesia should be used with caution in patients with MVP because the concomitant sympathetic denervation increases venous capacity and decreases peripheral resistance.[36] The reduced ventricular volume may increase the degree of prolapse and regurgitation.

Alcantara et al[37] reported a case in which epidural analgesia was chosen despite a history of MVP because of the presence of pneumonia and bronchial asthma. The obstetricians repaired the uterus without exteriorization, so that a sensory level to T-6 sufficed and the local anesthetic was administered in incremental doses to permit development of compensatory mechanisms. If these preventive measures are used, with frequent monitoring of arterial pressure, volume status, and denervation level, epidural analgesia should be safe and effective.

SUMMARY

Mitral valve prolapse is the most common heart lesion encountered during pregnancy, and the diagnosis is frequently made in young women of childbearing age. Patients with no connective tissue, skeletal, or other cardiovascular disorders tolerate pregnancy well and are unlikely to develop any remarkable cardiac complications. Clicks, murmurs, and possibly symptoms remain the same or become less evident during gestation. The incidences of antepartum and intrapartum complications and signs of fetal compromise are not more frequent than they are in pregnant patients with no known cardiac disorders. No special precautions during pregnancy seem to be necessary in women with MVP alone, except for the select use of antibiotics prior to dental work, surgical procedures, and delivery, and monitoring of arrhythmias. Rare complications associated with MVP while nonpregnant may also occur during gestation.

REFERENCES

1. Savage D, Garrison R, Devereaux R, Castelli W, Anderson S, Levy D, McNamara P, Stokes J, Kannel W, Feinliet M. Mitral valve prolapse in the general population. I. Epidemiologic features: the Framingham study. *Am Heart J* 1983;106:571–576.

2. Cowles T, Gonik B. Mitral valve prolapse in pregnancy. *Semin Perinatol* 1990;14:34–41.

3. Scampardonis G, Yang SS, Maranhao V, Goldbert H, Gooch AS. Left ventricular abnormalities in prolapsed mitral leaflet syndrome. Review of 87 cases. *Circulation* 1973;48:287–297.

4. Braunwald E. The mitral valve prolapse syndrome. In: Braunwald E, ed. *Heart Disease.* (4th ed.) Philadelphia: WB Saunders; 1992;1029–1035.

5. Jacquet-Davis, P. Mitral valve prolapse. *Prim Care Update Ob/Gyn* 1995;2:1–5.

6. Nishimura R, McGoon M, Shub C, Miller FA Jr, Ilstrup DM, Tajik AJ. Echocardiographically documented mitral valve prolapse: long-term follow-up of 237 patients. *N Engl J Med* 1985;313:1305–1309.

7. Fergenbaum H: Mitral valve prolapse. In: Fergenbaum H, ed. *Echocardiography* Philadelphia: Lea & Febiger; 1994; 262–269.

8. Jeresaty RM. Mitral valve prolapse: an update. *Trans-Am Acad Insur Med* 1993;76:24–33.

9. Zuppiwli A, Mori F, Favilli S, Barchielli A, Corti G, Montereggi A, Dolara A. Arrhythmias in mitral valve prolapse, relation to anterior mitral leaflet thickening clinical variables, and color Dop-pler echocardiography parameters *Am Heart J* 1994;128:919–927.

10. Rayburn WF, LeMire MS, Bird JL, Buda A. Mitral valve prolapse: echocardiographic changes during pregnancy. *J Reprod Med* 1987;32:185–187.

11. Haas JH. The effect of pregnancy on the middiastolic click and murmur of the prolapsing posterior leaflet of the mitral valve. *Am Heart J* 1976;92:407–408.

12. Castillo RA, Llado I, Adamsonns K. Ruptured chordae tendineae complicating pregnancy: a case report. *Reprod Med* 1987;32:137–139.

13. Rayburn WF, Fontana ME. Mitral valve prolapse and pregnancy. *Am J Obstet Gynecol* 1981;141:9–11.

14. Tang L, Chang S, Wong, V, Ma H. Pregnancy in patients with mitral valve prolapse. *Int J Gynaecol Obstet* 1985;23:217–221.

15. Shapiro E, Trimble E, Robinson J, Estruch M, Gottlieb S. Safety of labor and delivery in women with mitral valve prolapse. *Am J Cardiol* 1985;56:806–807.

16. Chia Y, Yeoh S, Lim M, Viegas O, Ratnam S. Pregnancy outcome and mitral valve prolapse. *Asia-Oceania J Obstet Gynecol* 1994;20:383–388.

17. Jana N, Vasishta K, Khunnu B, Dhall GI, Grover A. Pregnancy in association with mitral valve prolapse. *Asia-Oceania J Obstet Gynecol* 1993;19:61–65.

18. Artal R, Greenspoon JS, Rutherford S. Transient ischemic attack: a complication of mitral valve prolapse in pregnancy. *Obstet Gynecol* 1988;71:1028–1030.

19. Bergh PA, Hollander D, Gregori C, Breen J. Mitral valve prolapse and thromboembolic disease in pregnancy: a case report. *Int J Gynecol Obstet* 1988;27:133–137.

20. Pyeritz RE: Genetics andCardiovascular Disease in Braunwald E (editor): Heart Disease 5th edition. Philadelphia: W.B. Saunders; 1997, pp 1650–1686.

21. Ferencz C, Rubin JD, McCarter RJ, Brenner JI, Neill CA, Perry W, Hepner SI, Downing JW. Maternal mitral valve prolapse and congenital heart disease in the offspring. *Am Heart J* 1985;110:899.

22. Pickering NJ, Bordy JI, Barret MJ. Von Willebrand syndromes and mitral valve prolapse. Linked mesenchymal dyspasias. *N Engl J Med* 1981;305:131.

23. Eliahou HE, Silverberg DS, Reisin E, Romem I, Mashiach S, Serr DM. Propranolol for the treatment of hypertension in pregnancy. *Br J Obstet Gynaecol* 1978;85:431–436.

24. Tcherdakoff PH, Colliard M, Berrard E, Kreft C, Dupay A, Bernaille JM. Propranolol in hypertension during pregnancy. *Br Med J* 1978;2:670.

25. Bott-Kanner G, Schweitzer A, Reisner SH, Joel-Cohen SJ, Rosenfeld JB. Propranolol and hydralazine in the management of essential hypertension in pregnancy. *Br J Obstet Gynaecol* 1980;87:110–114.

26. Cottrill CM McAllister RG, Gettes L Jr, Noonan JA. Propranolol therapy during pregnancy, labor and delivery: evidence for transplacental drug transfer and impaired neonatal drug disposition. *J Pediatr* 1977;91:812–814.

27. Turnstall MI. The effect of propranolol on the onset of breathing at birth. *Br J Anaesth* 1969;41:792.

28. Campbell JW. A possible teratogenic effect of propranolol. *N Engl J Med* 1985;313:158–162.

29. Mitrani A Oettinger M, Abinader EG, Sharf M, Klein A. Use of propranolol in dysfunctional labour. *Br J Obstet Gynaecol* 1975;82:651–655.

30. Pruyn SC, Phelan J, Buchanan G. Long-term propranolol therapy in pregnancy: maternal and fetal outcome. *Am J Obstet Gynecol* 1979;135:485–489.

31. Lutas E, Devereux R, Kramer-Fax R, Spitzer M. Disappearance of mitral valve prolapse during pregnancy. *J Cardiovasc Ultrasonogr* 1984;3:183–186.

32. Bor DH, Himmelstein DU. Endocarditis prophylaxis for patients with mitral valve prolapse. A quantitative analysis. *Am J Med* 1984;76:711–717.

33. Devereux RB, Frary CJ, Kramer-Fox R, Roberts RB. Cost effectiveness of injective endocarditis prophylaxis for mitral valve prolapse with or without a mitral regurgitant murmur. *Am J Cardiol* 1994;74:1024–1029.

34. Sugrue D, Blake S, Troy P, MacDonald D. Antibiotic prophylaxis against infective endocarditis after normal delivery: is it necessary? *Br Heart J* 1980;44:499–502.

35. Dajani AS, Taubert KA, Wilson W, Bolger AF, Bayer A, Ferrieri P, Gewitz MH, Shulman ST, Nouri S, Newburger JW, Hutto C, Pallasch TJ, Gage TW, Levison ME, Peter G, Zuccaro G Jr. Prevention of bacterial endocarditis. Recommendations by the American Heart Association. JAMA 1997;277:1794–1801.

36. Thiagarajah S, Frost EAM. Anesthetic consideration in patients with mitral valve prolapse. *Anaesthesia* 1983;38:560.

37. Alcantara LG, Marx GF. Cesarean section under epidural analgesia in a parturient with mitral valve prolapse. *Anesth Analg* 1987;68L902.

15

PRIMARY PULMONARY HYPERTENSION AND PREGNANCY

Uri Elkayam, md, Ravi Dave, md, and Syed W. H. Bokhari, md

INTRODUCTION

Primary pulmonary hypertension (PPH) is an uncommon form of pulmonary hypertension without a demonstrable cause.[1,2] Diagnostic criteria as used in the National Institutes of Health (NIH) Registry[3] include a mean pulmonary artery pressure of more than 25 mmHg at rest, or more than 30 mmHg during exercise, without left-sided valvular disease, myocardial disease, congenital heart disease, or respiratory, connective tissue, or chronic thromboembolic disease.[1] The incidence of PPH ranges from one to two cases per million population.[1] It is therefore not surprising that this condition has been only rarely described in association with pregnancy. A grave prognosis, however, has been associated with pregnancy in many patients with PPH, and early recognition of this clinical syndrome is important, since prevention of pregnancy or early therapeutic abortion must be strongly considered.

ETIOLOGY

Although the cause of PPH is still unknown, a number of potential mechanisms have been proposed. These include loss of endothelial cell integrity[4], stimulation of the pulmonary arterial system by catecholamines,[2] enhanced secretion of endothelin,[5] enhanced growth factor release leading to intimal proliferation,[6] and occult thrombosis in situ of small pulmonary arteritis,[7] possibly caused by coagulation abnormalities found to exist in patients with PPH.[7] A recent case-control study demonstrated an increased risk of PPH as-

sociated with the use of any appetite suppressant, especially if the drugs were used for more than 3 months.[8] In addition, familial PPH inherited as an autosomal dominant trait, was reported in 6% of cases in the NIH Registry.[3]

CLINICAL PRESENTATIONS

PPH is a progressive disease that occurs most frequently in the young and predominantly in women[9] (63% of patients represented in the NIH Registry were females, and the mean age was 36 ± 15 years).[3] Patients usually come to medical attention relatively late in the course of the disease, and death usually occurs a few months to several years after onset of symptoms.[1,2,9,10] The most common presenting symptoms are dyspnea, fatigue, chest pain, palpitations, syncope or near syncope (particularly with exertion), and Raynaud's phenomenon.[1,2] In the late phase of the disease, dyspnea at rest, cough, and hemoptysis occasionally develop. A compression of the recurrent nerve by the dilated pulmonary artery may result in hoarseness.

Physical Examination

The characteristic physical findings are a consequence of a marked pressure increase in the pulmonary circulation and the resulting right ventricular hypertrophy and failure. Cyanosis, although not commonly seen in the early stages of the disease, can be present later on. The factors contributing to this finding are an increased tissue O_2 extraction due to low cardiac output, ventilation perfusion mismatches in the

Cardiac Problems in Pregnancy, Third Edition
Edited by Uri Elkayam, MD, and Norbert Gleicher, MD
Copyright © 1998 by Wiley-Liss, Inc. ISBN 0-471-16358-9

lungs, and right-to-left shunting via vascular anastomoses in the lungs or, at times, via a patent foramen ovale.[2]

The jugular venous pulse shows an exaggerated A wave, reflecting poor compliance of the right ventricle. The common development of tricuspid insufficiency due to right ventricular dilation is usually accompanied by a jugular V wave. The carotid arterial pulses have normal rates of rise but low volume, owing to a decreased stroke volume. Palpation of the chest usually reveals a right ventricular heave due to hypertrophy and a palpable P_2 reflecting dilation of the pulmonary artery.

Auscultation of the heart reveals a normal first heart sound (S_1), which often is followed by an ejection sound (click) and a systolic ejection murmur caused by the ejection of blood into a dilated pulmonary artery. Both the click and the murmur are heard maximally over the pulmonic auscultatory area, and the ejection sound usually decreases during inspiration. When tricuspid insufficiency has developed, a holosystolic murmur can be heard maximally at the left lower sternal border or at the apex when this area is being taken over by the enlarged right ventricle. The characteristic inspiratory accentuation of the murmur is lost with the onset of right ventricular failure. The second heart sound (S_2) is characterized by a loud pulmonic component (P_2). The splitting of S_2 is initially normal or prolonged. Failure of the right ventricle in later stages results in an earlier P_2 and loss of the characteristic respiratory variation of the second heart sound. The development of pulmonic valve incompetence due to dilation of the valvular apparatus is identified by a high-pitched, early diastolic decrescendo murmur (Graham–Steel murmur), heard loudest at the left sternal border. A right-sided S_4 is usually heard along the lower left sternal border and increases with inspiration. It is the result of a hypertrophied, poorly compliant right ventricle. Right ventricular failure is characterized by the development of S_3 along the lower left sternal border, as well as peripheral signs, including hepatomegaly, peripheral edema, and ascites.

LABORATORY FINDINGS

Hematological and Chemical Studies

Hematological abnormalities in patients with PPH can include polycythemia, a hypercoagulable state, abnormal platelet function, and defects in fibrinolysis.[1] In patients with right ventricular failure, liver functions test may also be abnormal.

Pulmonary Function

Pulmonary functions are often normal; however, mild reduction in total lung capacity and forced vital capacity can be found in many patients with PPH.[3] In addition, diffusion capacity for carbon monoxide is often reduced. This effect is probably due to an increase in capillary to alveolar distance secondary to hypertrophy of vascular endothelial cells.

Electrocardiogram

The electrocardiogram commonly reveals normal sinus rhythm or slight sinus tachycardia with right axis deviation, right atrial enlargement, and right ventricular hypertrophy.[11]

Radiology

Chest X-ray films usually demonstrate enlargement of the heart with right ventricular and right atrial prominence, and dilatation of the pulmonary trunk and its major divisions. The peripheral pulmonary vasculature is usually decreased.[12]

Echocardiogram

The echocardiogram often reveals an enlarged, hypertrophied right ventricle with a normal or small left ventricle. The E-F slope of the anterior leaflet of the mitral valve is decreased as a result of decreased flow. In addition, an increased incidence of mitral valve prolapse[13] and thickened ventricular septum with an abnormal motion[14] have been shown in patients with PPH.[13] Bidimensional echocardiography allows visualization of the right atrium, which is enlarged in patients with PPH. Doppler examination usually shows tricuspid regurgitation and, less frequently, pulmonary regurgitation.

Lung Ventilation–Perfusion Scan

Ventilation–perfusion scans of the lungs either are within normal limits or demonstrate diffuse patchy patterns with low probability of pulmonary embolisms.[15] It has been suggested that the performance of lung scans in the late stage of the disease can be hazardous because the luminal area of the pulmonary circulation is further reduced by macroaggregation of albumin used for scanning. A recent prospective study, however, reported no such adverse reactions in any of 163 patients with PPH who underwent lung perfusion scans.[15]

Exercise Testing

Cardiopulmonary exercise usually demonstrates reduced maximal oxygen consumption, high minute ventilation, a low aerobic threshold, reduced maximal oxygen pulse, and an increased alveolar–arterial oxygen gradient. The distance walked during the six-minute walk test correlates with the severity of pulmonary hypertension.[1]

Cardiac Catheterization

The hemodynamic profile is fairly typical. A marked increase in pulmonary resistance results in pulmonary hypertension and decreased cardiac output. Pulmonary capillary wedge pressure is either low or normal but tends to increase somewhat in the late stage of the disease because left ventricular compliance is impaired secondary to increased right ventricular pressure.[14,16] The pulmonary capillary wedge pressure is usually normal also in veno-occlusive disease, owing to the patency of the larger pulmonary veins and the patchy nature of the disease in the veins, but it may be elevated in several sites.[1] Right ventricular end diastolic pressure increases initially secondary to myocardial hypertrophy and decreased compliance and later as a result of systolic dysfunction. Right atrial pressure is elevated and demonstrates an increased A wave and, in the presence of tricuspid valve regurgitation, a tall V wave. Cardiac catheterization is usually indicated in patients with pulmonary hypertension, to exclude correctable causes for increased pulmonary pressures. The procedure should be performed cautiously and by experienced operators, since isolated cases of deaths have been reported.[6]

PPH AND PREGNANCY

In the earlier edition of this text (1990), we described the outcome of pregnancy in 35 patients with PPH. Fourteen of these patients (40%) died during pregnancy or in the early postpartum period. Although the information was limited by its anecdotal and retrospective nature, it reemphasized the high risk to women with PPH who become pregnant. Since our last report, an additional 16 patients have been identified in the literature[17–29] and we were involved in the care of another whose case was not published. Out of the 17 new cases, seven died[16–20,22,23,29] early postpartum, and one patient had a therapeutic abortion at 8 weeks of gestation.[28] Death occurred between a few hours to several days postpartum in the majority of cases and was usually due to sudden cardiovascular collapse or to progressive right ventricular failure and clinical deterioration.[14,18–21,29] New onset of clinical symptoms[16–18,29,30] or worsening of clinical status has been common during pregnancy, occurring mostly during the second or third gestational trimester. Most common symptoms were dyspnea on exertion, and fatigue. Other signs and symptoms included peripheral edema, chest pain, palpitations, syncope, nonproductive cough, and hemoptysis. One patient developed hoarseness because her left recurrent laryngeal nerve became completely paralyzed secondary to dilated left pulmonary artery.[19] Worsening of symptoms during pregnancy required early hospitalization in many cases. The duration of symptoms prior to pregnancy did not seem to affect the outcome of pregnancy. Similarly, the severity of pulmonary hypertension or level of pulmonary vascular resistance failed to provide a predictor for high risk of mortality. Right ventricular filling pressure, however, was elevated in most patients who died, suggesting that right ventricular failure may increase the likelihood of death in pregnant patients with PPH.

Vaginal delivery has been reported in the majority of cases with PPH[16,19,25,31,32] and seems to be safe in the stable patient (Table 15.1). Hemodynamic monitoring during labor usually shows either no significant change or some increase in pulmonary artery pressure.[20,21,32] Cesarean section was performed in several reported cases for obstetrical reasons,[22] because of failure of labor to progress[22,30] and for right ventricular failure,[26] or in cases of early delivery, because of worsening maternal clinical status.[18,22,23,26,29] Abrupt increase in pulmonary pressure in the early puerperium has been described.[19] Epidural anesthesia for delivery has been used in the majority of reported cases with PPH[16,19,20,22,25,27] and has produced good analgesia with very little hemodynamic effect. The use of general anesthesia for cesarean section has been described and was associated with hemodynamic stability.[22,29]

FETAL OUTCOME IN PATIENTS WITH PPH

Live-born infants have been reported in the majority of recently published cases (Table 15.1). One, however, was stillborn,[22] and one newborn who was delivered by cesarean section in the 26th week of gestation because of deterioration of maternal clinical status died of pulmonary insufficiency.[23] In addition, increased incidences of fetal growth retardation[18,19,25,26,32] and low birth weight for gestational age have been reported. Impairment of fetal growth may be secondary to low and fixed cardiac output in women with PPH and inadequate blood supply to the uterus.[28]

MANAGEMENT OF THE PREGNANT WOMAN WITH PPH

Pregnancy seems to be contraindicated in patients with PPH for the following reasons: (1) high incidence of maternal morbidity and mortality; (2) inability to predict the course and outcome of pregnancy, even in asymptomatic or only mildly symptomatic women with PPH; and (3) high incidence of fetal growth retardation, with increased morbidity and mortality. In addition, the patient and/or her family should be informed about the expected grave prognosis and limited life span in patients with PPH even if they survive their pregnancy.[1] Available information regarding survival and natural history suggests a median period of survival of 2.5 years after diagnosis. High pulmonary artery pressure and functional classification, decreased exercise tolerance (6-minute walk test), and poor response of pulmonary pressure to vasodilators are predictors of worse prognosis.[1] Lung or heart–lung transplantations have been performed in patients with PPH. The results of these procedures are equally limited, with the one-year survival rate ranging between 65 and 70%.[33]

Patients have to be adequately informed about the means to prevent unwanted pregnancies (Chapter 37). Selection of

TABLE 15.1 Maternal and Fetal Outcome in Recently Published Cases with PPH

Ref: First Author	Signs and Symptoms During Gestation	Mode of Delivery	Anesthesia	Outcome Maternal	Outcome Fetal
Takeuchi[19] (1988)	Exertional dyspnea, hoarseness	Oxytocin-induced vaginal delivery with vacuum extraction at 39 weeks	Epidural	Sudden collapse and death 7 days postpartum	Small for gestational age
Robinson[20] (1988)	Progressive exertional dyspnea, syncope, pitting edema to knees	Oxytocin-induced vaginal delivery with forceps at 35 weeks	Epidural	Sudden collapse and death 5 days postpartum	
Scomka[21] (1988)	Exertional dyspnea	Vaginal delivery induced at 38 weeks	Epidural	Favorable	Favorable
Roberts[22] (1990)	Increasing shortness of breath	Spontaneous labor at 36 weeks; C-section due to failure of labor to progress	Epidural	Death immediately post C-section	Stillborn
Roberts[22] (1990)	Increasing exertional dyspnea, palpitations	Spontaneous labor at 34 weeks; C-section due to failure of labor to progress and mother's deteriorating condition	General	Favorable	Transient tachypnea after delivery
Pfisteter[23] (1991)	Dyspnea on exertion	Elective C-section at 26 weeks due to mother's deteriorating condition	NA	Died on second day post-delivery	Died of pulmonary insufficiency
Nootens[25] (1993)	Progressive exertional dyspnea	Oxytocin-induced vaginal delivery at 36 weeks due to oligohydramnios	Epidural	Favorable	Favorable
Torres[26] (1994)	Dyspnea, fatigue, syncope, preeclampsia	Elective C-section at 35 weeks due to preeclampsia and fetal growth retardation	NA	Favorable	Small for gestational age
Smedstad[27] (1994)	Cough, fatigue, palpitations, weight gain, orthopnea, chest pain	Vaginal delivery induced at 34 weeks with prostaglandin gel	Epidural	Clinical deterioration post-partum; heart–lung transplantation 18 months postpartum	Favorable
Martinez[29] (1994)	Fatigue, resting dyspnea, cough, chest pain	Elective C-section due to worsening of maternal condition	General	Sudden collapse and death 6 h after delivery	Favorable
Martinez[29] (1994)	Fatigue, dyspnea, chest pain, syncope, systemic hypertension	Elective C-section at 35 weeks	Epidural	Death 48 h after delivery	Favorable
Kiss[30] (1995)	Progressive exertional dyspnea	Induced at 34th week with prostaglandin gel; C-section due to failure of labor to progress and right ventricular failure	Epidural	Favorable	Favorable

the most adequate means of birth control for a patient with PPH may not be easy. Although the role of oral contraceptives as an etiological factor in PPH has not been proven, several reports in the literature suggest an etiological link between pulmonary hypertension and oral contraceptive use.[34] Moreover, the development of internal vascular lesions in both veins and arteries, including the pulmonary arteries, has been reported in women using oral contraceptives.[35] The effect of oral contraceptives on the evolution of the disease in women with PPH is unknown. It has been suggested that the development of pulmonary hypertension with oral contraceptive usage may be enhanced in women with predisposing causes such as collagen vascular disease, family history of pulmonary hypertension, and congenital disease. Tubal ligation can be considered for asymptomatic or mildly symptomatic patients but may be hazardous in sicker patients.[9] The procedure should be performed under local or epidural anesthesia with adequate monitoring of systemic and pulmonary pressures and the electrocardiogram.[31] The safe use of general anesthesia for laparoscopic sterilization and termination of pregnancy in a patient with PPH was described in 1994.[28] Intrauterine devices, which are not recommended in patients with valvular heart disease because of the increased susceptibility to infection and valvular bacterial endocarditis, can be used in patients with PPH. Other means of birth control should not be recommended because of their lower efficacy in preventing pregnancy (Chapter 37).

If pregnancy occurs, abortion is indicated as early as possible.[28] This procedure should be performed with hemodynamic and electrocardiographic monitoring so that stability can be maintained and complications prevented. Patients who decide not to terminate pregnancy should be followed closely. Physical activity, especially involving isometric exercise, should be minimized to avoid a further increase in the circulatory burden. To assure restriction of activity and to optimize monitoring, symptomatic patients should be hospitalized when there are signs of progression of symptoms or clinical deterioration.

A recommended algorithm for the management of the nonpregnant patients with PPH is shown in Figure 15.1. Because of the hypercoagulable state of pregnancy and the recently demonstrated prognostic importance of anticoagulation therapy in nonpregnant PPH patients,[1,9] We recommend anticoagulation therapy during pregnancy and the puerperium in all patients with PPH. Guidelines for anticoagulation during pregnancy are detailed in Chapter 33.

A successful use of vasodilators has been well documented in patients with PPH.[36–39] Although individual effect is unpredictable, initial response to vasodilator challenge can predict patients who are likely to respond to long-term therapy.[37] Recent studies have demonstrated a sustained improvement in 25–30% of patients with large doses of nifedipine and diltiazem[36] (Table 15.2). The use of vasodilator therapy to lower pulmonary artery pressures in patients with PPH during pregnancy, has also been described. Increasing data suggest that nifedipine may be safe for the use during pregnancy (Chapter 31). One report[27] showed a 27% decrease in mean pulmonary artery pressure and a 47% reduction in pulmonary vascular resistance after acute testing of nifedipine given at a dose of 20 mg/h for 3 hours in a symptomatic patient with PPH in her 33rd week of pregnancy. Additional experience with the use of a calcium antagonists in

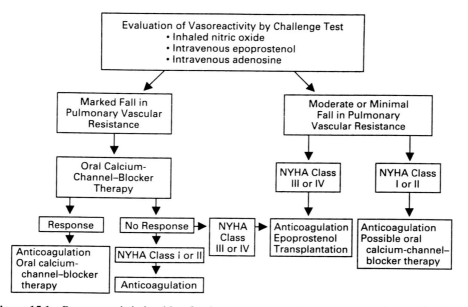

Figure 15.1 Recommended algorithm for the management of nonpregnant patients with primary pulmonary hypertension. (From Rubin, *N Engl J Med* 1997;336:111–117 with permission.)

TABLE 15.2 Dose Ranges and Routes of Administration of the Most Frequently Used Vasodilators in Patients with Primary Pulmonary Hypertension[a]

Drug	Route	Dose Range
Epoprostenol[b]	Intravenous	2–20 ng/kg of body weight/min
Adenosine	Intravenous	50–200 μg/kg of body weight/min
Nitric oxide	Inhaled	5–80 ppm
Nifedipine	Oral	30–240 mg/day
Diltiazem	Oral	120–900 mg/day

[a]As recommended for the nonpregnant patient. Efficacy and safety of these drug regimens in pregnancy are not known.
[b]The dose range shown is for a short-term infusion; the dose range for long-term infusions often exceeds 100–150 ng/k/min.
Source: Modified from Rubin, *N Engl J Med* 1997;336:111–117.

pregnancy was published by Slomka et al,[21] who used intravenous diltiazem (200 mg/h) in a patient with PPH prior to her induction in the 38th week. The drug resulted in a significant reduction in pulmonary vascular resistance and pulmonary artery pressures and increased cardiac output. No information, however, is available regarding the safety in pregnancy of a very high dose of calcium antagonists, which would seem to be required for the treatment of PPH (Table 15.2). Side effects of long-term vasodilator therapy include systemic hypotension, edema, and hypoxemia.[1]

The use of continuous infusion of prostaglandins has shown to improve hemodynamic characteristics, exercise tolerance, quality of life, and survival in symptomatic patients with PPH.[38,39] Prostaglandin E_1[22] and prostacyclin[28] have been used in pregnancy for a short period to lower pulmonary pressures. In addition, use of prostacyclin has been reported in the treatment of hypertension in pregnancy.[40,41] Infusion of the drug for a few hours to several days seemed to be effective and safe. In a comparison of prostacyclin and dihydralazine in patients with acute hypertensive crises of pregnancy, both drugs caused similar reduction in blood pressure and resulted in a comparable obstetric and neonatal outcome. No reports however are available regarding chronic use of prostacycline during pregnancy. The efficacy and safety of such therapy is therefore not known. The main adverse effects of long-term treatment with prostacyclin reported in the nonpregnant population have been related to their complex delivery system. Side effects included pump malfunction, catheter-related infections, and thrombosis.[38,39] Drug-induced side effects are common and include jaw pain, cutaneous erythema, diarrhea, and arthralgias.[1]

Other intravenous vasodilators may be of value in the short-term prevention or treatment of increased pulmonary artery pressure during labor and delivery and in the early puerperium. The following drugs have been used for this purpose during pregnancy: nitroprusside,[22,31] nitroglycerin,[20,22]

adenosine,[25] diltiazem,[21] isoproterenol,[21,28] and hydralazine.[26] In general, however, the use of vasodilators in patients with PPH is limited by the concomitant effect of these drugs on systemic blood pressure.[22,27] For this reason, it is preferable to use drugs with short half-life (e.g., adenosine, prostacyclin, nitroglycerin, nitroprusside), to allow careful titration and rapid discontinuation in case of adverse effects. Adenosine may also be used to evaluate pulmonary vasodilator reserve prior to initiation of chronic vasodilator therapy. The acute response to this drug has been predictive of the subsequent effects of intravenous prostacyclin and oral calcium channel blockers.[42,43]

Nitric oxide (NO) is another agent that may be useful for lowering of pulmonary artery pressure in patients with PPH. Since this drug binds to hemoglobin and is thereby inactivated, inhalation of NO gas leads to selective vasodilatory effect on the pulmonary vascular bed without a systemic effect. Inhalation of NO by patients with PPH resulted in an effect similar to that seen after intravenous administration of adenosine.[44] We have recently used the drug successfully to lower pulmonary artery pressure during delivery in a patient with pulmonary hypertension secondary to Eisenmenger's syndrome. A recent communication reported the use of NO in a young woman with end stage PPH.[45] During and after 9 hours of NO administration, the patient developed systemic hypotension and myocardial ischemia, which led to hemodynamic collapse and death. More information is obviously needed before the use of NO in PPH can be established.

Because of the stress and hemodynamic changes associated with labor, delivery, and the early postpartum period, hemodynamic and electrocardiographic monitoring is advisable during these times in all patients with PPH. Pulmonary artery pressure, systemic blood pressure, and cardiac output should be measured regularly during labor and delivery.[17,23,25–27] The placement of the pulmonary catheter may be difficult in patients with PPH because of dilation of the right atrium and ventricle and the presence of tricuspid regurgitation. The procedure should, therefore, be performed as soon as labor starts, using a specially designed guidewire catheter. Every effort should be made to minimize blood loss during delivery, and significant loss should be replaced promptly.

Blood gases should be measured repeatedly during labor, delivery, and the puerperium, to assure adequate oxygenation. Hypoxemia should be prevented by oxygen administration.[20,27,30]

Mode of delivery should be determined by obstetric indications and the clinical status of the mother during labor and delivery. Delivery should be carefully planned by all specialties involved in the care of the patient, including cardiology, obstetrics, anesthesia, neonatology, critical care, and nursing.[46] Planned delivery is preferred, to allow for presence and coordination of all services involved in the care of the patient. It is important to provide effective analgesia for labor and delivery. Epidural anaesthesia has been used in the majority of reported cases and has provided excellent analgesia with minimal hemodynamic changes. Abboud et al[32] reported that the use of intrathecal morphine also produced effective analgesia with no significant hemodynamic effect. Epidural anesthesia has been used successfully for cesarean deliveries in patients with PPH.[22,30] This form of anesthesia was associated with good analgesia, but one patient experienced significant hypotension that required fluid loading and intravenous ephedrine and was associated with fetal tachycardia and occasional type-2 dips, which resolved with improvement of systemic blood pressure. General anesthesia for cesarean delivery was reported in two cases.[22,29] In patients with PPH, however, the use of general anesthesia may be associated with some risks, which include increased pulmonary artery pressure mediated by intubation, and the negative inotropic effects of the anesthetic agents. These adverse effects can be minimized by the use of narcotic-based induction and maintenance techniques as well as by avoiding any anesthetics with known negative inotropic effect[46] (Chapter 24).

Since the supine position can result in further decline in cardiac output due to diminution of venous return, the patient should be kept in the left lateral position during labor and delivery. As the incidence of premature delivery is high in women with PPH, premature labor should be anticipated. Postpartum patients should continue to be monitored hemodynamically and electrocardiographically for 24–28 hours to prevent potential deterioration due to postpartum increase in venous return to the heart. Prolonged postpartum hospitalization of 7–10 days is recommended to ensure stability prior to discharge.

REFERENCES

1. Rubin LJ. Primary pulmonary hypertension. *N Engl J Med* 1997;336:11–117.

2. Rich S, Braunwald E, Grossman W. Pulmonary hypertension. IN: Braunwald E, ed. *Heart Disease.* 5th ed. Philadelphia: WB Saunders; 1997;780–806.

3. Rich S, Dantzker DR, Ayres SM, Bergofsky EH, Brundage BH, Detre KM, Fishman AP, Goldring RM, Groves BM, Koerner SK, Levy PC, Reid LM, Vreim CE, Williams GW. Primary pulmonary hypertension: a national prospective study. *Ann Intern Med* 1987;107:216–223.

4. Vane JR, Anggard EE, Botting RM. Regulatory functions of the vascular endothelin. *N Engl J Med* 1990;323:27–36.

5. Stewart DJ, Levy RD, Cernacek P, Langleben D. Increased plasma endothelin-1 in pulmonary hypertension: marker or mediator of disease? *Ann Intern Med* 1991;111:464–469.

6. Botney MD, Bahadori L, Gold LI. Vascular remodeling in primary pulmonary hypertension, potential role for transforming growth factor-beta. *Am J Pathol* 1994;144:286–295.

7. Rich S, Brundage BH. Pulmonary hypertension: a cellular basis for understanding the pathophysiology and treatment. *J Am College Cardiol* 1989;14:545–550.

8. Abenhaim L, Moride Y, Brenot F, Rich S, Benichou J, Kurz X, Higgenbottam T, Oakley C, Wouters E, Aubier M, Simmoneau G. Appetite suppressant drug and the risk of primary pulmonary hypertension. International Primary Pulmonary Hypertension Study Group. *N Engl J Med* 1996;325:609–616.

9. Fuster V, Steele PM, Edwards WD, Gersh BJ, McGoon MD, Frye RL. Primary pulmonary hypertension: natural history and the importance of thrombosis. *Circulation* 1984;70:580–587.

10. D'Alonzo GE, Barst RG, levy PS P-T-O, et al. Survival in patients with primary pulmonary hypertension: results of a national prospective registry. *Ann Intern Med* 1991;115:343–349.

11. Kanemoto N. Electrocardiographic and hemodynamic correlations in primary pulmonary hypertension. *Angiology* 1988;39:781–787.

12. Kanemoto N, Furuya H, Etoh T, Sasamoto H, Matsuyama S. Chest roentgenograms in primary pulmonary hypertension. *Chest* 1978;76:45.

13. Goodman DJ, Harrison DC, Poppl RL. Echocardiographic features of primary pulmonary hypertension. *Am J Cardiol* 1974;33:438.

14. Louie EK, Rich S, Brundage BH. Doppler echocardiographic assessment of impaired left ventricular filling with right ventricular pressure overload due to primary pulmonary hypertension. *J Am College Cardiol* 1986;8:1298–1306.

15. Rich S, Pietra GG, Kieras K, Hart K, Brundage BH. Primary pulmonary hypertension: radiographic and scintigraphic patterns of histologic subtypes. *Ann Intern Med* 1986;105:499–502.

16. Rozkovec A, Montanes P, Oakley CM. Factors that influence the outcome of primary pulmonary hypertension. *Br Heart J* 1986;55:449–458.

17. Srensen MB, Korshin JD, Fernandes A, Secher O. The use of epidural analgesia for delivery in a patient with pulmonary hypertension. *Acta Anaesth Scand* 1982;26:180–182.

18. Feijen HWH, Hein PR, Van Lakwijk-Vondrovicova EC, Nijhuis GM. Primary pulmonary hypertension and pregnancy. *Eur J Obstet Gynecol Reprod Biol* 1983;15:159–164.

19. Takeuchi T, Nishii O, Okamura T, Yaginuma T. Primary pulmonary hypertension in pregnancy. *Int J Gynecol Obstet* 1988;26:145–150.

20. Robinson DE, Leicht CH. Epidural analgesia with low-dose bupivacaine and fontange for labor and delivery in a parturient with severe pulmonary hypertension. *Anesthesiology* 1988;68:285–288.

21. Slomka F, Salmeron S, Zetlaoui P, Cohen H, Simoneau G, Samii K. Primary pulmonary hypertension and pregnancy: anesthetic management for delivery. *Anesthesiology* 1988;69:959–961.

22. Roberts NV, Keast PJ. Pulmonary hypertension and pregnancy—a lethal combination. *Anaesth Intensive Care* 1990;18:366–374.

23. Pfisterer J, Runge HM, Kommoss F, Herbst EW, Hillemanns HG. Primare pulmonale Hypertonie und Schwangerschaft. *Geburtshilfe Frauenheilkd* 1991;51:236–238.

24. Kuroiwa M, Meno H, Higashi H, Hamanaka N, Takita J. A case report of primary pulmonary hypertension: congestive heart failure induced by pregnancy and delivery. *Kokyu To Junkan* 1992;40:691–694.

25. Nootens M, Rich S. Successful management of labor and delivery in primary pulmonary hypertension. *Am J Cardiol* 1993;71:1124–1125.

26. Torres PJ, Gratacos E, Magrina J, Martinez-Crespo JM, Cardach V. Primary pulmonary hypertension and pre-eclampsia: a successful pregnancy. *Br J Obstet Gynaecol* 1994;101:163–165.

27. Smedstad KG, Cramb R, Morison DH. Pulmonary hypertension and pregnancy: a series of eight cases. *Can J Anaesth* 1994;41:502–512.

28. Myles PS. Anaesthetic management of laparoscopic sterilization and termination of pregnancy in a patient with severe primary pulmonary hypertension. *Anaesth Intensive Care* 1994; 22:465–469.

29. Martinez JM, Comas C, Sala X, Gratacos E, Torres PJ, Fortung A. Maternal primary pulmonary hypertension associated with pregnancy. *Am J Obstet Gynecol Reprod Biol* 1994;54:143–147.

30. Kiss H, Egarter C, Asseryanis E, Putz D, Kneussl M. Primary pulmonary hypertension in pregnancy: a case report. *Am J Obstet Gynecol* 1995;172:1052–1054.

31. Nelson DM, Main E, Crafford W, Ahumada GG. Peripartum heart failure due to primary pulmonary hypertension. *Obstet Gynecol* 1983;62:595–635.

32. Abboud TK, Raya J, Noueihed R, Daniel J. Intrathecal morphine for relief of labor pain in a parturient with severe pulmonary hypertension. *Anesthesiology* 1983;59:477–479.

33. Hosenpud JD, Novick RJ, Bennet LE, Keck BM, Fiol B, Daily OP. The Registry of the International Society for Heart and Lung Transplantation: Thirteenth Official Report—1996. *J Heart Lung Transplant* 1996;15:655–674.

34. Kleiger RE, Boxer M, Ingham RE, Harrison DC. Pulmonary hypertension in patients using oral contraceptives: a report of six cases. *Chest* 1976;69:143–147.

35. Irey NS, Norris HJ. Intimal vascular lesions associated with female reproductive steroids. *Arch Pathol* 1973;96:227–234.

36. Weiz WK, Rubin LJ, Ayres SM, Bergofsky EH, Brundage BH, Detre KM, Elliot CG, Fishman AP, Goldring AM, Groves BM.

The acute administration of vasodilators in primary pulmonary hypertension: experiences from the National Institutes of Health Registry on Primary Hypertension. *Am Rev Respir Dis* 1989;140:1623–1630.

37. Rich S, Kaufmann E, Levy PS. The effect of high doses of calcium-channel blockers on survival in primary pulmonary hypertension. *N Engl J Med* 1992;327:76–81.

38. Barst RJ, Rubin LJ, McGoon MD, Caldwell EJ, Long WA, Levy PS. Survival in primary pulmonary hypertension with long-term continuous intravenous prostacycline. *Ann Intern Med* 1994;121:409–415.

39. Barst RJ, Rubin LJ, Long WA, McGoon MD, Rich S, Badesch DB, Groves BM, Japson VF, Bourge RC, Brundage BH, Koerner SK, Langleben D, Keller CA, Wretsky, Clayton ML, Jobsis MM, Blackburn SD Jr, Shortimo D, Crow JW. A comparison of continuous intravenous Eprostenol (prostacyclin) with conventional therapy for primary pulmonary hypertension. *N Engl J Med* 1996;334:296–302.

40. Belch JJF, Inorburn J, Greer IA, Saafo S, Prentice CRM. Intravenous prostacyclin in the management of pregnancies complicated by severe hypertension. *Thrombosis Haemostasis J* 1983;50:460 (Abstract).

41. Moodley J, Gouws E. A comparative study of the use of epoprostenol and dihydralazine in severe hypertension in pregnancy. *Br J Obstet Gynaecol* 1992;99:727–730.

42. Schrader B, Inbar S, Kaufman L, Vestal RE, Rich S. Comparison of the effects of adenosine and nifedipine in pulmonary hypertension. *J Am College Cardiol* 1992;19:1060–1064.

43. Nootens M, Schrader B, Kaufman E, Vestal R, Long W, Rich S. Comparative acute effects of adenosine and prostacyclin in primary pulmonary hypertension. *Chest* 1995;107:54–57.

44. Pepke-Zaba J, Higenbottam TW, Dinh-Xuan AT, Stone D, Wallwork J. Inhaled nitric oxide as a cause of selective pulmonary vasodilatation in pulmonary hypertension. *Lancet* 1991;338:1173–1174.

45. Partanen J. Death in a young woman suffering from primary pulmonary hypertension during inhaled nitric oxide therapy. *Arch Intern Med* 1995;155:875–876.

46. Weeks SU, Smith B. Obstetric anaesthesia in patients with primary pulmonary hypertension. *Can J Anaesth* 1991;38:814–816.

16

INFECTIVE ENDOCARDITIS

Ramin Ebrahimi, MD, Cyril Y. Leung, MD, Uri Elkayam, MD, and Cheryl L. Reid, MD

INTRODUCTION

Infective endocarditis is a rare occurrence during pregnancy.[1–7] However, more than 50 cases of infective endocarditis during pregnancy or the early peripartum period have been reported in the last decade, some of them with devastating consequences for the mothers and/or fetuses.[8–39] Early diagnosis of this disease in pregnancy is, therefore, critical. The management of a pregnant woman with infective endocarditis involves general principles similar to those applied to the nonpregnant patient. At the same time, however, in order to reduce the risk to the fetus, special considerations should be made in the diagnostic and therapeutic approach to this disease when it occurs during gestation.

PREDISPOSING FACTORS

Rheumatic heart disease, although declining in incidence, still accounts for the majority of the cases. Correction of many congenital heart abnormalities allows more women who are at risk of developing infective endocarditis to reach childbearing age.[31] Mitral valve prolapse, an abnormality with a female to male predominance of 2:1,[39] is another predisposing factor for endocarditis in pregnancy [8,11,23,34,40] as well as intravenous drug abuse.[16] Although preexisting valvular abnormalities are common in patients with infective endocarditis, infection occurring on functionally normal cardiac valves has been reported.[20,21]

A variety of diagnostic and therapeutic procedures may result in bacteremia and can lead to infective endocarditis during pregnancy. These include dental as well as genitourinary and gastrointestinal procedures.[41] Obstetric and gyne-

cologic procedures have been reported to be the cause in 26% of cases with infective endocarditis in females.[5,42] Pregnancy-related bacteremia may occur following abortion, vaginal delivery with manual removal of the placenta, curettage, implantation of infected intrauterine contraception devices, development of pelvic infections,[42] and cesarean section.[42–44]

MICROBIOLOGY

Streptococcal infection is the most common cause for infective endocarditis during pregnancy.[8,13,17,18,21,22] Infection with *Streptococcus viridans* is often subacute with symptoms present for several months before diagnosis. The patient may present with an acute fulminant picture, however, because of a complication of the disease such as valvular rupture and the occurrence of congestive heart failure.[9] When symptoms are present for only a few weeks, however, acute bacterial endocarditis is often due to *Staphylococcus aureus, Streptococcus pneumoniae,* and *Streptococcus pyogenes.*[45] Isolated case reports have described a variety of organisms causing infective endocarditis, including *Pseudomonas aeruginosa, Listeria monocytogenes,*[46] *Chlamydia trachomatis,*[47] *Salmonella,*[48] *Mycobacterium tortuitum, Neisseria gonorrhea,*[25,49] and *Clostridium perfringens.*[29] In patients with a history of intravenous drug usage, *Staphylococcus aureus* is the predominant organism, although polymicrobial infections may also occur. Many of the organisms reported to cause infective endocarditis during pregnancy have also been cultured from the normal vagina and postpartum uterus.[50–52] McCormack et al in 1975[53] showed a 5% incidence of positive blood cultures in women studied less than an hour following delivery with mostly streptococci, including anaerobic, microaerophilic,

Cardiac Problems in Pregnancy, Third Edition
Edited by Uri Elkayam, MD, and Norbert Gleicher, MD
Copyright © 1998 by Wiley-Liss, Inc. ISBN 0-471-16358-9

and hemolytic streptococci. Blanco et al[54] found bacteremia in 10% of obstetrical patients who develop complications including endoparametritis and pyelonephritis. Organisms predominantly isolated in these patients included group B streptococci and *Escherichia coli*. More recently, Tiossi et al[43] collected blood cultures from 100 women 45 minutes after delivery and found positive cultures in seven: six for staphylococcus and one for candida, penicillium, clandosporum, and aspergillus that were found in association. Four of the patients had premature amniorrhexis longer than six hours before delivery and six of the patients had labor more than six hours after admission. In another recent study, Boggess et al[44] found bacteremia in 14% of 93 women undergoing a cesarean delivery after a minimum of four hours labor or ruptured membranes, compared to zero of 26 women not in labor.

CLINICAL FEATURES

The clinical features are related to the infectious process itself, the cardiovascular complications, and the noncardiac complications.[55,56] The onset of the disease may be acute or subacute. The classic triad of fever, murmur, and anemia should certainly raise the suspicion of infective endocarditis. Fever is present in almost 100% of patients, but it may be absent in patients taking antipyretics or steroids, or in those who have had recent antibiotic therapy. Headaches, malaise, fatigue, and musculoskeletal pain are common. The acute form of the disease may be associated with chills, sweats, nausea, vomiting, chest pain, peripheral emboli, or dyspnea.

A finding of a new cardiac murmur or a change in character or intensity of a preexisting murmur has been considered to be an important characteristic of the disease. However, neither the presence of, nor a change in character of, a murmur is found invariably. The common development of murmurs or change in intensity of existing murmurs are common in pregnancy and can make the diagnosis of endocarditis difficult (Chapter 2).

Peripheral Manifestations

Cutaneous Manifestations Four lesions involving the skin have been described in patients with infective endocarditis: petechiae, subungual hemorrhages, Osler nodes, and Janeway lesions. Petechiae (most commonly involving the conjunctival or oral mucosa) are the most frequent finding and are reported to occur in 26% of patients.[56] Subungual splinter hemorrhages are most often the result of trauma and, therefore, have less diagnostic value. Osler nodes are tender, erythematous lesions noted on the palms and terminal phalanges of the hand or soles of the feet, and are considered to be due to a hypersensitivity reaction. Janeway lesions are small nontender macular nodular hemorrhagic spots that are present on the palms and soles. Both Osler nodes and Janeway lesions are uncommon today.

Renal Manifestations There are three types of renal abnormalities that may occur in infective endocarditis: renal infarctions (renal infarction due to usually sterile emboli occurs in approximately 60% of patients with left-sided infective endocarditis[56]), local embolic glomerulonephritis, and diffuse, proliferative glomerulonephritis. Two types of glomerulonephritis are due to immune-complex glomerular injury. Renal insufficiency may result from either of these lesions, although control of the infection frequently reverses the serologic abnormalities and thus the azotemia.

Because many of the drugs used to treat infective endocarditis are excreted by the kidneys and may cause nephrotoxicity, appropriate reductions in dosages must be made in cases with renal insufficiency. Differentiation between renal failure due to immune-complex injury and nephrotoxicity secondary to drug therapy can be difficult. Recovery from drug-related nephrotoxicity usually occurs following discontinuation of the antibiotics. If renal abnormalities persist, renal biopsy may become necessary to diagnose immune-complex injury.

Neurologic Manifestations Neurologic or psychiatric symptoms due to embolization, rupture of mycotic aneurysms, and meningitis or meningocerebritis occur in approximately one-third of patients with infective endocarditis.[56] Aphasia, ataxia, cortical sensory loss, and homonymous hemianopsia can be caused by emboli or rupture of a mycotic aneurysm. Embolic cerebral infarction is the most common neurologic complication of infective endocarditis, occurring in approximately 20% of patients, and usually within the first two weeks of therapy.[56a] Roth spots (oval, retinal hemorrhages with a clear pale center) are seen in less than 5% of patients. Meningitis is most often aseptic; cerebrospinal fluid cultures may be positive in acute bacterial endocarditis, particularly when it is due to *Staphylococcus aureus*.[57] A variety of neurologic manifestations may occur, including headaches, seizures, or mental aberrancy.

Cardiac and Noncardiac Complications

The most common cause of death (60%) in patients with infective endocarditis is congestive heart failure,[56] which is usually a result of valvular regurgitation (Table 16.1), particularly of the aortic valve. Valve disruption from the infection may result from erosion of valve edges, total destruction of the valves by highly invasive organisms, perforation or prolapse of a leaflet, or rupture of chordae tendineae. Stenosis of a valve may cause valvular stenosis. The valve most frequently involved in infective endocarditis is the aortic valve (55%), followed by the mitral valve (28%).

Extension of the infection into the myocardium can lead to sinus of Valsalva aneurysm rupture and septal perforation with the development of a ventricular septal defect, aortopulmonary fistula, and ventriculoatrial fistula. Congestive heart failure due to the left-to-right shunt can result from these defects.

Systemic emboli occur in one-third of cases of infective endocarditis. Hemiplegia, aphasia, and sensory loss are the usual clinical manifestations of this complication. Pulmonary emboli are commonly seen with infections of the tricuspid valve. Other sites of emboli include the coronary arteries (may result in a myocardial infarction), spleen, and kidney. Myocardial abscesses have been noted at autopsy in 20% of patients,[56] and can result from direct extension of the infection or from bacteremia. Myocardial abscesses should be suspected when conduction abnormalities or arrhythmias occur, and can lead to intracardiac fistula, which may precipitate congestive heart failure and antibiotic failure. Extension into the pericardial space may result in suppurative pericarditis. Pericardial effusions occur in greater than 50% of patients but are generally associated with a benign clinical course.[58]

Mycotic aneurysms may develop as a result of direct invasion of bacteria into the arterial wall, embolic occlusion of the vasa vasorum, or deposition of immune complexes. Such can be found in the brain, the abdominal aorta, the superior mesenteric, splenic, coronary, and pulmonary arteries, the sinus of Valsalva, and the ligated ductus arteriosus. Mycotic aneurysms that have not ruptured may be associated with few or no symptoms, but can cause persistent sepsis, fever, pain, and neurologic symptoms. Diagnosis is difficult, but is best made by angiography. Since rupture and hemorrhage can occur at any time during or after therapy, surgery is recommended if the aneurysm is recognized and is in a surgically accessible site.

DIAGNOSIS

The most useful clinical findings suggestive of infective endocarditis are fever, cardiac murmur or history of preexisting cardiac disease, and positive blood cultures. The Duke criteria, a new diagnostic schema, use clinical, microbiologic, and echocardiographic data to increase the number of definite diagnoses of infective endocarditis (Tables 16.2 and 16.3).[59]

Bacteremia associated with infective endocarditis is continuous. Blood cultures are positive in over 80% of cases. In approximately 16% of patients with infective endocarditis, blood cultures will be negative.[56] Negative blood cultures are usually found in patients who have received antibiotic therapy, or in whom the causative agent cannot be easily cultured with standard techniques. In patients who have received antibiotic therapy within two weeks, the antibiotics should be discontinued if possible, and cultures redrawn beginning 24–48 hours later. Blood cultures should be repeated twice during a seven-day interval, and if they remain negative, a diagnosis other than infective endocarditis should be considered (e.g. collagen vascular disease, atrial myxoma, or

TABLE 16.1   Cardiovascular Complications of Endocarditis

Valve destruction with resultant regurgitation
Localized suppuration
    Perivalvular or myocardial abscesses
    Creation of left-to-right shunts (sinus of Valsalva rupture, ventricular septal defects, aortopulmonary fistula, ventriculoatrial fistula)
Emboli
    Systemic
    Coronary artery with myocardial infarction
Mycotic aneurysms
Conduction abnormalities; rhythm disturbances
Pericarditis

marantic endocarditis). Blood for serologic studies for Q fever, psittacosis, and tularemia should also be obtained in patients with negative blood cultures.

Elevated erythrocyte sedimentation rate, although nonspecific, is found in over 90% of patients with infective endocarditis. Anemia is common but may also be related to the pregnancy. White blood cell count is frequently elevated and a leftward shift is common in patients with infective endocarditis. Presence of an active sediment in the urine suggests renal involvement such as glomerulonephritis or renal infarction.

Chest X-ray is helpful in the diagnosis of pulmonary complications such as embolization and congestion. Echocardiography is useful to detect vegetations of the cardiac valves and intracardiac complications. Two-dimensional and transesophageal echocardiography demonstrate vegetations in over 80% of patients with infective endocarditis.[51,52] Because of its superior imaging capabilities, transesophageal echocardiography is particularly helpful in defining small vegetations and intracardiac complications. During pregnancy, transesophageal echocardiography can be performed safely either without conscious sedation or, if necessary, with judicious use of medications accompanied by fetal monitoring. Contrast two-dimensional echocardiography can be used to detect complications of infective endocarditis such as tricuspid insufficiency or intracardiac shunts. Doppler echocardiography is useful in the assessment of the severity of valvular stenosis, pressure gradients, and valvular regurgitation. Color Doppler echocardiography may also provide a clinically useful estimate of the presence and severity of valvular regurgitation.

MANAGEMENT OF INFECTIVE ENDOCARDITIS

Antibiotic Therapy of Infective Endocarditis

The choice of antibiotics for infective endocarditis depends on proper microbiological identification of isolated organisms or blood cultures and susceptibility testing. In pregnan-

TABLE 16.2   Proposed New Criteria for Diagnosis of Infective Endocarditis

DEFINITE INFECTIVE ENDOCARDITIS

Pathologic criteria
  Microorganisms: demonstrated by culture or histology in a vegetation, *or* in a vegetation that has embolized, *or* in an intracardiac abscess, *or*
  Pathologic lesions: Vegetation or intracardiac abscess present, confirmed by histology showing active endocarditis
Clinical criteria
  Two major criteria, *or*
  One major and three minor criteria, *or*
  Five minor criteria

POSSIBLE INFECTIVE ENDOCARDITIS

Findings consistent with infective endocarditis that fall short of "definite", but not "rejected"

REJECTED

Firm alternate diagnosis for manifestations of endocarditis, *or*
Resolution of manifestations of endocarditis, with antibiotic therapy for 4 days or less, *or*
No pathologic evidence of infective endocarditis at surgery or autopsy, after antibiotic therapy for 4 days or less

Source: Durack et al,[59] with permission.

TABLE 16.3   Terminology Used in the Proposed New Criteria

Major criteria

POSITIVE BLOOD CULTURES FOR INFECTIVE ENDOCARDITIS

Typical microorganism for infective endocarditis from two separate blood cultures *viridans* streptococci,[a] *Streptococcus bovis,* HACEK[b] group, or community-acquired *Straphyloccus aureus* or enterococci, in the absence of a primary focus, *or*
Persistently positive blood culture, defined as recovery of a microorganism consistent with infective endocarditis from:
  Blood cultures drawn more than 12 hours apart, *or*
  All of three or a majority of four or more separate blood cultures, with first and last drawn at least one hour apart

EVIDENCE OF ENDOCARDIAL INVOLVEMENT

Positive echocardiogram for infective endocarditis
  Oscillating intracardiac mass, on valve or supporting structures, *or* in the path of regurgitant jets, *or* on implanted material, in the absence of an alternative anatomic explanation, *or*
  Abscess, *or*
  New partial dehiscence of prosthetic valve, *or*
New valvular regurgitation (increase or change in preexisting murmur not sufficient)

Minor Criteria

Predisposition: predisposing heart condition or intravenous drug use
Fever: ≥ 38.0°C (100.4°F)
Vascular phenomena: major arterial emboli, septic pulmonary infarcts, mycotic aneurysm, intracranial hemorrhage, conjunctival hemorrhages, Janeway lesions
Immunologic phenomena: glomerulonephritis, Osler's nodes, Roth spots, rheumatoid factor
Microbiologic evidence: positive blood culture but not meeting major criterion as noted above,[c] *or* serologic evidence of active infection with organism consistent with infective endocarditis
Echocardiogram: consistent with infective endocarditis but not meeting major criterion

[a] Including nutritional variant strains.
[b] Comprising *Haemophilus* spp, *Actinobacillus actinomycetemomitans, Cardiobacterium hominis, Eikenella* spp, and *Kingella kingae.*
[c] Excluding single positive cultures for coagulase-negative staphylococci and organisms that do not cause endocarditis.

Source: Durack et al,[59] with permission.

cy, the choice of antibiotics must also be based on consideration of the possible adverse effects on the fetus.[60]

Proper microbiologic identification and susceptibility testing are important because of the increasing incidence of infective endocarditis caused by uncommon organisms, including gram-negative organisms and fungi, and of antibiotic resistance. Usually, in subacute infective endocarditis, treatment does not need to be instituted before the two to three days required for microbiologic testing. In contrast, acute infective endocarditis is often caused by highly destructive organisms requiring antibiotic therapy with no delay. In such patients, the etiology of infective endocarditis can be suspected on the basis of the clinical setting, including infected skin lesions, urinary tract infection, or intravenous drug abuse and antibiotic therapy initiated against the most likely causative organism. Initial therapy should consist of a penicillin, a penicillinase-resistant penicillin, and an aminoglycoside. If the results of microbiologic isolation dictate a different antibiotic therapy, substitution can be made at that time. Antibiotic therapy is given intravenously in intermittent doses at four- to six-hour intervals in patients with normal renal function, or by continuous infusion. The optimum duration of antibiotic therapy is still debated; however, it is generally accepted that therapy should be continued for at least four and preferably six weeks.

In patients with culture-negative infective endocarditis, acute illnesses should be handled as discussed earlier. When there is a favorable clinical response, the antibiotics should be continued. In cases with subacute endocarditis, it is rea-

sonable to start therapy with penicillin, a penicillinase-resistant penicillin, and an aminoglycoside. If there is a clinical response, antibiotics should be continued; if not, they should be stopped and the patient reevaluated.

Early prosthetic valve endocarditis (within two months of surgery) is usually due to contamination of the implant site, often by staphylococci or gram-negative organisms. Late prosthetic infections are caused by the same organisms as those found in native valve endocarditis. About half the patients can be treated successfully with antibiotics alone, while the rest require surgical treatment for cure of infection,

TABLE 16.4   Indications for Surgery in the Treatment of Infective Endocarditis

Congestive heart failure
Infections
    Uncontrolled by antibiotic therapy
    Fungal, usually with staphylococcal infections of aortic and mitral valves, *Serratia,* and gram-negative bacillary infections
Recurrent systemic emboli despite adequate antibiotic therapy
Acquired heart block
Other
    Acquired intraventricular conduction defects
    Pericarditis, suppurative
    Mycotic aneurysm of coronary artery
    Mycotic aneurysm of sinus of Valsalva
    Rupture of sinus of Valsalva, rupture of ventricular or atrial septa, or others (e.g., development of arteriovenous and ventriculoatrial shunts)

Source: Reid et al,[62] with permission.

heart failure, or both. The antibiotics chosen for the treatment of endocarditis should be bactericidal.[61] Effectiveness of therapy should be monitored with serial blood cultures at 48 hours and frequently throughout the course of therapy, even in cases with defervescence and clinical improvement.[62,63]

Congestive Heart Failure

Congestive heart failure is the most common cause of death in patients with infective endocarditis and every effort should be made for diagnosis and treatment.[62] Treatment of heart failure during pregnancy should, in general, be similar to the treatment of nonpregnant patients. Drugs such as digoxin, di-

TABLE 16.5   Chemoprophylaxis of Infective Endocarditis

CARDIAC ABNORMALITIES REQUIRING PROPHYLAXIS

Prosthetic heart valves
Congestive heart disease
Rheumatic or other acquired valvular heart disease
Hypertrophic cardiomyopathy
Mitral valve prolapse syndrome with mitral insufficiency
Previous episode of infective endocarditis

PROPHYLAXIS NOT REQUIRED

Uncomplicated scundum atrial septal defect
Previous coronary artery bypass surgery
Six months after cardiac surgery for uncomplicated secundum atrial septal defect; ventricular septal defect or patent ductus arteriosus
Mitral valve prolapse without valvular regurgitation
Physiologic, functional, or innocent heart murmurs
Cardiac pacemakers and implanted defibrillators
Previous rheumatic fever without valvular dysfunction

Source: Adapted from the recommendations of the American Heart Association.[65]

TABLE 16.6   Procedures for Which Prophylaxis Is Recommended

Respiratory Tract
    Tonsillectomy and/or adenoidectomy
    Surgical operations that involve respiratory mucosa
    Broncoscopy with rigid bronchoscope
    Broncoscopy with a flexible bronchoscope, with or without biopsy[†]
Gastrointestinal Tract*
    Sclerotherapy for esophageal varices
    Esophageal structure dilation
    Endoscopic retrograde cholangiography with biliary obstruction
    Biliary tract surgery
    Surgical operations that involve intestinal mucosa
    Transesophageal echocardiography[†]
    Endoscopy with or without gastrointestinal biopsy[†]
Genitourinary Tract
    Cystoscopy
    Urethral dilatation
    Vaginal hysterectomy[†]
    Vaginal delivery[†]

Source: Adapted from the recommendations of the American Heart Association.[65]

*Prophylaxis is recommended for high-risk patients; it is optional for medium-risk patients.
[†]Prophylaxis is optional for high-risk patients.

uretics, organic nitrates, and hydralazine can be used safely during gestation (Chapters 28, 31, and 34). In contrast, nitroprusside is not recommended due to a potential risk of cyanide toxicity, and angiotensin-converting enzyme inhibitors are contraindicated because of fetal toxicities (Chapters 31 and 32).

Surgical Therapy

Surgical intervention, especially valve replacement, has had a dramatic impact on the mortality of patients with moderate-to-severe congestive heart failure (Table 16.4).[64] Successful cardiac surgery during pregnancy has been reported,[19,20,22,26,30,32] and patients with infective endocarditis in whom medical therapy fails, should receive surgical intervention. Fetal loss associated with open heart surgery has been reported to be approximately 30% (Chapter 23). Cardiac surgery is theoretically best performed after the 24th to 28th week, when organogenesis is complete. Good perfusion of the placenta must be maintained during cardiopulmonary bypass and, therefore, invasive hemodynamic monitoring of the mother seems indicated during surgery. Indications for surgical intervention include: uncontrolled infection despite appropriate antibiotic therapy, congestive heart failure, and, in most cases of fungal endocarditis and recurrent systemic emboli. The development of a sinus of Valsalva aneurysm with rupture into a cardiac chamber, as well as ventricular septal defects and other structural abnormalities, are indica-

TABLE 16.7   Prophylactic Regimens for Dental, Oral, Respiratory Tract, or Esophageal Procedures

Situation	Agent	Regimen
Standard general prophylaxis	Amoxicillin	2.0 g orally 1 h before procedure
Unable to take oral medications	Ampicillin	2.0 g IM or IV within 30 min before procedure
Allergic to penicillin	Clindamycin **or**	600 mg orally 1 h before procedure
	Cephalexin[†] or cefadroxil[†] **or**	2.0 g orally 1 h before procedure
	Azithromycin or clarithromycin	500 mg orally 1 h before procedure
Allergic to penicillin and unable to	Clindamycin **or**	600 mg IV within 30 min before procedure
take oral medications	Cefazolin[†]	1.0 g IM or IV within 30 min before procedure

IM indicates intramuscularly, and IV, intravenously.

[†]Cephalosporins should not be used in individuals with immediate-type hypersensitivity reaction (urticaria, angioedema, or anaphylaxis) to penicillins.

Source: Adopted from the recommendations of the American Heart Association.[65]

PREVENTION

Chemoprophylaxis is appropriate whenever patients with increased susceptibility to the development of infective endocarditis undergo manipulation or surgical procedures likely to result in bacteremia (Table 16.5). The severe consequences of the disease emphasize the importance of this preventive measure. Prophylaxis is appropriate when these patients undergo manipulations or surgical procedures likely to be associated with bacteremia. These include most dental and upper respiratory tract procedures; lower gastrointestinal, gallbladder, and genitourinary surgery; and instrumentation (Table 16.6). Chemoprophylaxis for surgical procedures involving instrumentation of the genitourinary or gastrointestinal tract should be directed against the enterococcus (Table 16.8). Cardiac abnormalities likely to be encountered during pregnancy that should be covered with prophylactic antibiotics are listed

tions for surgery, since these conditions are usually associated with congestive heart failure and uncontrolled infection.

in Table 16.5. Procedures likely to result in significant bacteremia are shown in Table 16.6. Recommendations for antibiotic prophylaxis made by the American Heart Association (Tables 16.7 and 16.8) include the following indications:[65] presence of prosthetic valves, a history of endocarditis, or surgically constructed systemic pulmonary shunts or conduits. In addition, endocarditis prophylaxis is recommended for vaginal deliveries in the presence of infection in patients at risk for cardiac complications (Table 16.5). The use of antibiotic prophylaxis is not recommended in cases of uncomplicated vaginal or abdominal delivery based on early studies indicating a low likelihood for bacteremia associated with these procedures.[3] Recent studies, however, have provided information suggesting that bacteremia is common after labor and delivery, and should be considered as high risk for patients susceptible to endocarditis.[43,44] Because of this documented risk of bacteremia even after uncomplicated vaginal and cesarean delivery, the relatively low risk and cost of therapy, and the potentially devastating effect of endocarditis, prophylactic antibiotic treatment is given routinely in our medical center to all patients who are susceptible to bacterial endocarditis.

TABLE 16.8   Prophylactic Regimens For Genitourinary/Gastrointestinal (Excluding Esophageal) Procedures

Situation	Agents	Regimen[†]
High-risk patients	Ampicillin plus gentamicin	Ampicillin 2.0 g IM or IV plus gentamicin 1.5 mg/kg (not to exceed 120 mg) within 30 min of starting procedure; 6 h later, ampicillin 1 g IM/IV or amoxicillin 1 g orally
High-risk patients allergic to ampicillin/amoxicillin	Vancomycin plus gentamicin	Vancomycin 1.0 g IV over 1–2 h plus gentamicin 1.5 mg/kg IV/IM (not to exceed 120 mg); complete injection/infusion within 30 min of starting procedure
Moderate-risk patients	Amoxicillin or ampicillin	Amoxicillin 2.0 g orally 1 h before procedure, or ampicillin 2.0 g IM/IV within 30 min of starting procedure
Moderate-risk patients allergic to ampicillin/amoxicillin	Vancomycin	Vancomycin 1.0 g IV over 1–2 h complete infusion within 30 min of starting procedure

IM indicates intramuscular, and IV, intravenously.

[†]No second dose of vancomycin or gentamicin is recommended.

Source: Adopted from the recommendations of the American Heart Association.[65]

REFERENCES

1. McFaul PB, Dornan JC, Lamki H, Boyle D. Pregnancy complicated by maternal heart disease: review of 519 women. *Br J Obstet Gynaecol* 1988;95:861–867.

2. Payne DG, Fishburne JI, Rufty AJ, Johnston FR. Bacterial endocarditis in pregnancy. *Obstet Gynecol* 1982;60:247–250.

3. Sugrue D, Blake S, Troy P, McDonald D. Antibiotic prophylaxis against infective endocarditis after normal delivery—is it necessary? *Br Heart J* 1980;44:499–502.

4. Sugrue D, Blake S, MacDonald D. Pregnancy complicated by maternal heart disease at the National Maternity Hospital, Dublin, Ireland. *Am J Obstet Gynecol* 1981;139:1–6.

5. Seaworth BJ, Durack DT. Infective endocarditis in obstetric and gynecologic practice. *Am J Obstet Gynecol* 1986;154:180–188.

6. Szekely P, Turner R, Snaith L. Pregnancy and the changing pattern of rheumatic heart disease. *Br Heart J* 1973;35:1293–1303.

7. Conradsson T, Werko L. Management of heart disease in pregnancy. *Prog Cardiac Dis* 1974;16:407–419.

8. Strasberg GD. Postpartum group B streptococcal endocarditis associated with mitral valve prolapse. *Obstet Gynecol* 1987; 70:485–487.

9. Castillo RA, Llado I, Adamsons K. Ruptured chordae tendineae complicating pregnancy. A case report. *J Reprod Med* 1987;32:137–139.

10. Cox SM, Hankins GD, Leveno KJ, Cunningham FG. Bacterial endocarditis. A serious pregnancy complication. *J Reprod Med* 1988;33:671–674.

11. Carpenter V, Jansson G, Magnusson K, Savela M, Carlsson H, Hogberg U. Enterococcal endocarditis following legal abortion. *Lakartidningen* 1988;85:2657–2658.

12. Dommisse J. Infective endocarditis in pregnancy. A report of 3 cases. *S Afr Med J* 1988;73:186–187.

13. Hughes LO, McFadyen IR, Raftery EB. Acute bacterial endocarditis on a normal aortic valve following vaginal delivery. *Int J Cardiol* 1988;18:261–262.

14. Mooij PN, de Jong PA, Bavinck JH, Korsten HH, Bonnier JJ, Berendes JN. Aortic valve replacement in the second trimester of pregnancy: a case report. *Eur J Obstet Gynecol Reprod Biol* 1988;29:347–352.

15. Korsten HH, Van Zundert AA, Mooij PN, De Jong PA, Bavinck JH. Emergency aortic valve replacement in the 24th week of pregnancy. *Acta Anaesthesiol Belg* 1989;40:201–205.

16. Cox SM, Leveno KJ. Pregnancy complicated by bacterial endocarditis. *Clin Obstet Gynecol* 1989;32:48–53.

17. Pimentel M, Barbas CS, de Carvalho CR, Takagaki TY, Mansur AJ, Grinberg M, Barbas Filho JV. Septic pulmonary embolism and endocarditis caused by *Staphylococcus aureus* in the tricuspid valve after infectious abortion. Report of 2 cases. *Arq Bras Cardiol* 1989;52:337–340.

18. Zamprogno R., Neri G, Alitto F, Moro E, Sandri R. Bacterial endocarditis in pregnancy. Description of 2 cases and review of the literature. *Minerva Cardioangiol* 1990;38:85–88.

19. Shevchenko IuL, Guriev AV, Shikhverdiev NN, Tsvetkova TV, Gridasov VF, Zhuravlev VP, Ashinov NA, Airiian SG. Successful surgical treatment of infectious endocarditis in a pregnant woman. *Vestn Khir Im I I Grek* 1990;144:42–44.

20. Avila WS, Grinberg M, Tarasoutchi F, Pomerantzeff P, Bellotti G, Jatene A, Pileggi F. Cerebral malformation of the conceptus associated with maternal bacterial endocarditis and with aortic valve replacement during pregnancy. *Arq Bras Cardiol* 1990;55:201–204.

21. Atri ML, Cohen DH. Group B streptococcus endocarditis following second trimester abortion. *Arch Intern Med* 1990; 150:2579–2580.

22. Souma T, Yokosawa T, Iwamatsu T, Irisawa T. Successful mitral valve replacement for infective endocarditis in pregnancy. *Nippon Kyobu Geka Gakkai Zasshi* 1990;38:1035–1038.

23. Pereira M de B, Timerman S, Timerman A, Negrisoli AL, Bub RF, Smith MR, Akamine N, Aun R, Knobel E. *Staphylococcus aureus* endocarditis in a puerperal woman with mitral and tricuspid valve prolapse. *Arq Bras Cardiol* 1990;55:385–388.

24. Jeyamalar R, Sivanesaratnam V. Management of infective endocarditis in pregnancy. *Aust N Z J Obstet Gynaecol* 1991;31:123–124.

25. Bataskov KL, Hariharan S, Horowitz MD, Neibart RM, Cox MM. Gonococcal endocarditis complicating pregnancy: a case report and literature review. *Obstet Gynecol* 1991;78:494–496.

26. Westaby S, Parry AJ, Forfar JC. Reoperation for prosthetic valve endocarditis in the third trimester of pregnancy. *Ann Thorac Surg* 1992;53:263–265.

27. Deger R, Ludmir J. *Neisseria sicca* endocarditis complicating pregnancy. A case report. *J Reprod Med* 1992;37:473–475.

28. Nkoua JL,Kimbally Kaky G, Ekoba J, Gombet T, Onkani AH, Oumba C, Bouramoue C. Infectious endocarditis of gyneco-obstetric origin. Apropos of 15 cases. *J Gynecol Obstet Biol Reprod* 1993;22:425–428.

29. Janion M, Kurzawski J, Konstantynowicz H, Wozakowska Kaplon B, Tracz W. Myocardial infarction in pregnancy. *Kardiol Pol* 1993;38:351–353.

30. Matsumoto H, Shimokawa S, Umebayashi Y, Watanabe S, Taira A. Simultaneous cesarean section and mitral valve replacement for infective endocarditis during pregnancy–a case report. *Nippon Kyobu Geka Gakkai Zasshi* 1993;41:329–331.

31. Presbitero P, Somerville J, Stone S, Aruta E, Spiegelhalter D, Rabajoli F. Pregnancy in cyanotic congenital heart disease. Outcome of mother and fetus. *Circulation* 1994;89:2673–2676.

32. Ishibashi Y, Sasamura Y, Ohe K, Ishizaka M, Kiyota M, Kataoka K, Ohta S. A case report of mitral valve replacement for infective endocarditis in pregnancy. *Kyobu Geka* 1994;47: 474–476.

33. Felice PV, Salom IL, Levine R. Bivalvular endocarditis complicating pregnancy. A case report and literature review. *Angiology* 1995;46:441–444.

34. Hagay ZJ, Weissman A, Geva D, Snir E, Caspi A. Labor and delivery complicated by acute mitral regurgitation due to ruptured chordae tendineae. *Am J Perinatol* 1995;12:111–112.

35. Jorge S do C, Mejia BI, Zamorano MM, de Andrade J, Arnoni AS, Sousa JE. Infective endocarditis associated with pregnancy. *Arq Bras Cardiol* 1995;64:319–322.

36. Raumanns J, Kaufhold A, Behrendt W, Peters G. Lethal, non-menstrual toxic shock syndrome associated with *Staphylococcus aureus* sepsis. *Anaesthesist* 1995;44:869–874.

37. Garini A, Astorri E, Cimolato B, Bonifazi C, Bianchi C, Ferrari O. Bacterial endocarditis in pregnancy. Report of a clinical case diagnosed postpartum. *Minerva Cardioangiol* 1995;43:443–447.

38. Caraballo V. Fatal myocardial infarction resulting from coronary artery septic embolism after abortion: unusual cause and complication of endocarditis. *Ann Emerg Med* 1997;29:175–177.

39. Levy D, Savage D. Prevalence and clinical features of mitral valve prolapse. *Am Heart J* 1987;113:1281–1290.

40. MacMahon SW, Roberts JK, Kramer-Fix R, Zucker DM, Roberts RB, Devereux RB. Mitral valve prolapse and infective endocarditis. *Am Heart J* 1987;113:1291–1298.

41. Everett ED, Hirschmann JV. Transient bacteremia and endocarditis prophylaxis. Review. *Medicine* (Baltimore) 1977;56:61–77.

42. Levin JN, Stander RW. Subacute bacterial endocarditis following obstetric and gynecologic procedures: report of eight cases. *Obstet Gynecol* 1959;13:568–573.

43. Tiossi CL, Rodrigues FO, Santos AR, Franken RA, Mimica L, Todesco JJ. Bacteremia induced by labor. Is prophylaxis for infective endocarditis necessary? *Arq Bras Cardiol* 1994;62:91–94.

44. Boggess KA, Watts DH, Hillier SL, Krohn MA, Benedetti TJ, Eschenbach DA. Bacteremia shortly after placental separation during cesarean delivery. *Obstet Gynecol* 1996;87:779–784.

45. Holt S, Hicks DA, Charles RG, Coulshed N. Acute staphylococcal endocarditis in pregnancy. *Practitioner* 1978;220:619–622.

46. Holshouser CA, Ansbacher R, McNitt T, Steele R. Bacterial endocarditis due to *Listeria monocytogenes* in a pregnant diabetic. *Obstet Gynecol* 1978;51:9S–10S.

47. Bel-Kahn MJ, Watanakunakorn C, Menefee MG, Long H, et al. *Chlamydia trachomatis* endocarditis. *Am Heart J* 1978;95:627–636.

48. Gill GV. Endocarditis caused by *Salmonella* enteritis. *Br Heart J* 1979;42:353–356.

49. Alvarez-Elcordo S, Mateos-Mora M, Zajarias A. *Mycobacterium tortuitum* endocarditis after mitral valve replacement with a bovine prosthesis. *South Med J* 1985;78:865–866.

50. Hunter CA, Long KR. A study of the microbiological flora of the vagina. *Am J Obstet Gynecol* 1958;75:865–871.

51. Hesseltine HC, Hite KE. Bacteriology of the gynecologic and involuting puerperal uterus. *Am J Obstet Gynecol* 1949;57:143–153.

52. Rabe LK, Winterscheid KK, Hillier SL. Association of viridans group streptococci from pregnant women with bacterial vaginosis and upper genital tract infection. *J Clin Micro* 1988;26:1156–1160.

53. McCormack WM, Rosner B, Lee YH, Rankin JS, Lin JS. Isolation of genital mycoplasmas from blood obtained shortly after vaginal delivery. *Lancet* 1975;1:596–601.

54. Blanco JD, Gibbs RS, Castaneda YS. Bacteremia in obstetrics: clinical course. *Obstet Gynecol* 1981;58:621–625.

55. Karchmer AW. Infective endocarditis. In Braunwald E (editor), *Heart Disease,* 5th Edition. W.B. Saunders Co. Philadelphia, 1997:1077–1104.

56. Pruitt AA, Rubin RH, Karchner AW, Dunchan GW. Neurologic complications of bacterial endocarditis medicine. *Medicine* (Baltimore) 1978;57:329–343.

57. McComb JM, McNamee PT, Sinnamon DG, Adgey AAJ. Staphylococcal endocarditis presenting as meningitis in pregnancy. *Int J Cardiol* 1982;1:325–327.

58. Reid CL, Rahimtoola SH, Chandraratna PAN. Frequency and significance of pericardial effusion detected by two-dimensional echocardiography in infective endocarditis. *Am J Cardiol* 1987;60:394–395.

59. Durack DT, Lukes AS, Bright DK. New criteria for diagnosis of infective endocarditis: utilization of specific echocardiographic findings. *Am J Med* 1994;96:200–209.

60. Garland SM, O'Reilly MA. The risks and benefits of antimicrobial therapy in pregnancy. *Drug Saf* 1995;13:188–205.

61. Wilson WR, Guiliani ER, Danielson GK, Geraci JE. General considerations in the diagnosis and treatment of infective endocarditis. *Mayo Clin Proc* 1982;57:81–85.

62. Reid CL, Leedom JM, Rahimtoola SH. Infective endocarditis. In: Cohn HF, ed. *Current Therapy.* 28th ed. Philadelphia: WB Saunders, 1983;190–197.

63. Richardson JV, Karp RB, Kirklin JW, Dismukes WE. Treatment of infective endocarditis: 10-year comparative analysis. *Circulation* 1978;58:589–597.

64. Hubbell G, Cheitlen MD, Rapaport E. Presentation, management, and follow-up evaluation of infective endocarditis in drug addicts. *Am Heart J* 1981;102:85– .

65. Dajani AS, Taubert KA, Wilson W, Bolger AF, Bayer A, Ferrieri P, Gewitz MH, Shulman ST, Nouri S, Newburger JW, Hutto C, Pallasch TJ, Gage TW, Levison ME, Peter G, Zuccaro G. Prevention of bacterial endocarditis. Recommendations by the American Heart Association. *JAMA* 1997;277:1794–1801.

PART IV

VASCULAR DISEASE IN PREGNANCY

17

VASCULAR DISSECTIONS AND ANEURYSMS DURING PREGNANCY

URI ELKAYAM, MD, AND AFSHAN HAMEED, MD

AORTIC DISSECTION

Aortic dissection is an uncommon but potentially catastrophic illness that is initiated by a tear in the aortic intima. Driven by the pressure in the aorta, the blood entering through the tear separates the media in a course parallel to the blood flow in the aortic lumen, with propagation of the dissection to variable distances.[1] The dissection channel is usually in the outer part of the aortic media, and its containment is nearly adventitial, explaining the high frequency of extravasation of blood outside the aorta. Any branch arising from the aorta may be involved in the dissection process; the manifestations of the disease are therefore related to the specific anatomic structures involved.

Etiology

The etiology of aortic intimal tear and its propensity for medial dissection is unknown. Pregnancy is one of several clinical settings that have been described in association with an increased incidence of aortic dissection.[2] In nontraumatic cases, the intimal disruption may represent an aberration of a more or less continuous process of vascular endothelial injury and repair. This process may be compromised by the pregnant state. Other conditions that may affect this process include congenital abnormalities of collagen, such as the Marfan and Ehlers–Danlos syndromes, or abnormal morphological development, such as coarctation of the aorta or bicuspid aortic valve.[3] Other conditions that have been associated with nontraumatic aortic dissection include Noonan and Turner syndromes and cocaine abuse.[1] The most common denominator noted in nearly three-fourths of general adult patients with aortic dissection including women under the age of 40 is hypertension.[1,4,5] In the reported cases occurring in coincidence with pregnancy, there is however no evidence to associate preeclampsia/eclampsia and aortic dissection.

Pathogenesis

Although dissection of the aorta is uncommon in young people, a relationship has been demonstrated between this vascular event and pregnancy. Older literature reported that up to 50% of dissections in patients of less than 40 years of age occurred during a or shortly after pregnancy.[4] In contrast, a recent review of 1253 patients with acute aortic dissection published in the literature found no instance of associated pregnancy,[5] indicating the rare occurrence of aortic dissection during pregnancy.

Physiological increase in blood volume and cardiac output have been suggested as a potential cause for aortic dissection during pregnancy. Since, however, dissections occur infrequently during labor and often develop in the early postpartum period, the stress of labor can be dismissed as a relevant factor.[2] Alterations in the structure of the vascular wall have been demonstrated during pregnancy.[6–9] They are similar to changes described in cystic medial necrosis and increase in their severity toward term.[6] Although these changes may predispose patients to the development of aortic dissection in pregnancy, normal aortas have been found at necropsy in pregnant women[10] and even in those with aortic dissection.[11] Some hormonal influence on connective tissue has been shown in experimental animals and in humans and may be related to the development of arterial dissection during pregnancy; however, the exact role of this factor is unclear. Estrogens have been shown to inhibit collagen and elastin deposition in the aorta and progestogens to minimally accelerate the deposition of aortic noncollagenous proteins in the rat model.[12–15] Pregnancy-related changes in the microscopic appearance of arteries in rabbits are also inducible by the administration of norethynodrel and ethynyl estradiol. In addition, intimal hyperplasia, which is seen in pregnancy or hypertensive women, has been found in women treated with oral contraceptives.[14]

Pathology

In most cases, a continuous intimal tear is identified in addition to disruption of the aortic media.[1] This tear, which marks the beginning of the dissection, occurs about 2 cm above the aortic valve cusps in 70% of patients and at the descending thoracic aorta, just beyond the origin of the left subclavian artery, in 20% of patients. Uncommonly, it is located in the aortic arch or below the diaphragm. The entrance tear is accompanied by a reentry tear in about 10% of patients, producing the so-called double-barrel aorta. Although dissection is a longitudinal separation of the media, the percentage of aortic circumference involved by the dissection at any particular level is variable. Usually half of the aortic circumference is dissected; the other half stays intact.[3] Dissections beginning in the ascending aorta generally involve the right lateral wall and course downstream along the greater curvature of the ascending, transverse, and descending thoracic aortas. Because of their location, involvement of the right coronary, innominate, left common carotid, and left subclavian arteries is common. The progression of the dissection is usually limited by extensive atherosclerotic plaquing, aortic isthmus, coarctation, or inflammatory fibrosis, all of which are uncommon in women of childbearing age.

Classification

Three classification systems are most commonly used to define the location and extent of aortic dissection.

1. DeBakey classification type I, which begins at the ascending aorta and extends to the descending aorta, type II, which begins at the ascending aorta and does not extend beyond, and type III, which involves the descending thoracic aorta only. Type III dissection is subdivided into type IIIA, in which the dissection is limited to the thoracic aorta, and type IIIB, where the dissection extends below the diaphragm.
2. The Stanford classification divides all aortic dissections into two types: type A—proximal dissections and distal dissections with extension into the aortic arch and ascending aorta, and type B—distal dissections.

3. More recently, a simplified descriptive classification has been widely accepted; it differentiates between proximal dissection (DeBakey types I and II or Stanford type A) and distal dissection (DeBakey type III or Stanford type B).[1]

Epidemiology

Aortic dissection occurs two to three times more frequently in males than in females at any age, including the childbearing age.[5] No more than 200 cases of pregnancy-related aortic dissections have been reported. However, a predisposition to this condition during pregnancy has been suggested by many.[15–25] McGeachy and Paullin[23] reported in 1937 that 6 of 24 cases of dissecting aneurysm in females of childbearing age occurred in association with pregnancy. Schnitker and Bayer[24] noted that 24 of 49 dissecting aneurysms in females below the age of 40 occurred in association with pregnancy. Twenty of the cases were diagnosed antepartum, two during labor, and two postpartum. In 1954 Mandel et al[25] reviewed 70 cases of aortic dissection in females of childbearing age and found that 36 of them occurred in association with pregnancy. In the nonpregnant population, increasing age, male sex, hypertension, aortic coarctation, bicuspid aortic valve, and the Marfan syndrome all seem to indicate an increased risk for aortic dissection.[1,4] In pregnancy, it is much more difficult to weigh risk factors. Konishi et al[26] showed that 60% of 52 cases of aortic dissection during pregnancy and the puerperium were over age 30 and 77% occurred in multiparous women; 20% had coarctation of the aorta, and a few were marfanoid. Others have not demonstrated increasing maternal parity as an important predisposing factor toward aortic dissection in pregnancy.

Pregnancy-related aortic dissection occurs most frequently in the third trimester. Pedowitz and Perell[27] described 48 patients with aortic dissection during pregnancy. One patient presented in the first trimester, 8 in the second, 23 in the third trimester, 6 during labor or the first 24 hours postpartum, and 10 two days or more after delivery.[27] Two recently published cases have described aortic dissection in pregnant patients with congenital bicuspid aortic valve (Table 17.1).[6,16]

DIAGNOSIS

Clinical Manifestations

Most dissections are associated with severe pain, typically in the chest, which may radiate to the back, shoulders, and abdomen (Table 17.2).[1,4] Other symptoms are related to complications of the dissection. The most catastrophic complication is due to rupture of the aorta with extravasation of blood into the pericardial space,[6,9] pleural space, mediastinum, retroperitoneum, wall of the pulmonary artery, interatrial or interventricular septum (involvement of the atrioventricular

TABLE 17.1 Selected Published Cases of Aortic Dissection During Pregnancy

Ref: First Author (year)	Age (years)	Aortic Wall Histology	Risk Factors for Dissection	Gestational Week	Site of Dissection	Clinical Presentation	Treatment	Outcome Maternal	Outcome Fetal
Pumphrey[16] (1986)	19	Normal	Bicuspid aortic valve	37	Intimal tear 3 cm above a bicuspid aortic valve; large dissecting hematoma without exit point	Chest vibration and new cardiac murmurs mild chest discomfort. Aortic insufficiency.	Delivery by C-section, sodium nitroprusside for 48 h, then replacement of ascending aorta by a Dacron prosthesis containing a Bjork–Shiley valve.	Postsurgical atrioventricular dissociation requiring permanent pacemaker.	Favorable
Anderson[6] (1994)	25	Accumulation of acid mucopolysaccharides within the media with focal degeneration of elastic fibers and loss of cell nuclei	Bicuspid aortic valve	38	Ascending aorta rupturing into pericardial cavity	Sudden onset of retrosternal burning and pain. Worse on inspiration.	Erroneously diagnosed initially as tracheitis and treated with analgesia.	Cardiac arrest and death in spite of pericardiocentesis and thoracotomy in an attempt to relieve cardiac tamponade.	Fetus delivered by C-section during resuscitation of the mother; died shortly after delivery
Wahlers[19] (1994)	31	Mucoid degeneration of the media		39	A tear 2 cm distal to noncoronary cusp; dissection continued into the supraaortic branches. Minor hemorrhage, pericardial effusion.	Acute severe breast pain, 3+ aortic regurgitation, flap in the ascending aorta. Small pericardial effusion. Impaired pulses in left leg.	Hypertension controlled with IV nitroglycerin, C-section followed by repair of the aortic arch with a vascular prosthesis.	Good postoperative recovery except atelectasis of left lower lobe requiring repeated bronchoscopic treatment.	Favorable
Jayram[20] (1995)	33	NA		26	Started distal to left subclavian artery with patent false lumen reentering true lumen at level of midabdominal aorta.	Acute abdominal pain; abdominal aortic dissection extending into the left iliac artery by ultrasound.	Initial control of blood pressure with IV nitroglycerin followed by oral hydralazine, nifedipine, and labetalol until 36 weeks, when C-section performed with extradural anesthesia after confirmation of fetal maturity.	Abdominal dissection repaired 6 months later because of progression of dissection in spite of medical therapy. Favorable outcome.	Favorable
Khalil[21] (1995)	26	Perivascular infiltration of vasa vasorum by lymphocytes, fragmentation of the media with microcalcification. Intima-unremarkable.	Gestational hypertension	2 weeks postpartum	Infrarenal abdominal dissection with secondary aneurysm formation.	Abdominal and low back pain; pulsating midline, supraumbilical, abdominal mass.	Aortobilateral iliac artery bypass.	Smooth postoperative recovery.	Live twins delivered vaginally at full term
Nolte[8] (1995)	25	Minute areas of dissection and loss of fragmentation of the internal elastic lamina and elastic tissue of the media. Focal increase in ground substance.		3 days after delivery	Right iliac artery, left external iliac artery.	Acute onset of right lower quadrant pain followed by cardiogenic shock.	Laparotomy and hemostasis.	Hemorrhagic shock, death on 8th postoperative day of massive pulmonary embolism	—
Nolte (1995)	25	Blood and fibrin between media and external elastic lamina. Marked decrease in medial smooth muscles; loss of elastic fibers; increase in micropolysaccharides in the ground substance.		2 days following elective cesarean section	Beginning beyond the left subclavian artery origin, extending into infrarenal abdominal aorta.	Sudden onset of left parascapular back pain. Worse with inspiration.	Medical therapy with IV nitroprusside, labetalol, and oral enalapril and metoprolol for blood pressure control.	Nine months later, surgery due to extension of dissection	—

TABLE 17.2 Diagnostic Modalities for the Evaluation of Suspected Aortic Dissection

Characteristics	Aortography	CT	MRI	TEE
Sensitivity	+ +	+ +/+ + +	+ + +	+ + +
Specificity	+ + +	+ +/+ + +	+ + +	+ +/+ + +
Demonstration of intimal tear	+ +	+	+ + +	+ +
Thrombus	+ + +	+ +	+ + +	+
Aortic insufficiency	+ + +	−	+	+ + +
Percardial effusion	−	+ +	+ + +	+ + +
Branch vessel involvement	+ + +	+	+ +	+
Coronary artery involvement	+ +	−	−	+ +
Rapid performance	Fair	Fair	Fair	Very
Ability to perform at bedside	No	No	No	Yes
Noninvasive	No	Yes	Yes	Yes
IV contrast	Yes	Yes	No	No
Risk during pregnancy	Radiation	Radiation	Probably safe	Safe

Abbreviations: CT, computerized tomography; IV, intravenous; MRI, magnetic resonance imaging; TEE, transesophageal echocardiography.

conduction system), lung, or esophagus. In addition, partial or complete obstruction of any artery arising from the aorta by the medial hematoma can occur.[19,20] Arteries affected may include the coronaries (sudden death or myocardial infarction), innominate or common carotid (syncope, confusion, stroke, or coma), innominate or subclavian (upper limb ischemia or paralysis), intercostal or lumbar (spinal cord ischemia), celiac, renal, mesenteric, or common iliac arteries. Acute and severe aortic regurgitation can result from dilatation of the aorta or extension of the dissection to the level of the valve,[16,19] and may produce pulmonary edema. Obstruction of the aorta or pulmonary artery may produce circulatory collapse. The physical findings most commonly found in patients with aortic dissection include pulse deficits,[19] murmur of aortic regurgitation, and neurological manifestations (cerebrovascular accident, altered consciousness, and, in distal dissections, paraparesis or paraplegia due to ischemic spinal cord damage).[1]

Laboratory Findings

The most common abnormal finding on chest X-ray is a temporal widening of the mediastinum.[29] Pleural effusion may be present (mostly on the left side in patients with distal dissection). It should be noted that chest X-ray findings in aortic dissection are nonspecific, and absence of abnormal finding should not exclude the possibility of a dissection. Aortography has been the gold standard diagnostic modality for the diagnosis of aortic dissection. However, other diagnostic tests such as contrast-enhanced computerized tomography (CT), magnetic resonance imaging (MRI), ultrasound, and transesophageal echocardiography (TEE) provide the clinician with a choice of diagnostic modalities[30,31] (Table 17.2). Aortography provides the ability to accurately assess the extent of the dissection, including branch vessel involvement.[1] In addition, it allows the assessment of the presence

and severity of aortic regurgitation and the status of the coronary arteries. The limitations of this procedure include its inherent risks related to its invasive nature and the use of ionizing radiation and contrast material. Contrast-enhanced CT scanning has a sensitivity of 80% to 90% and a specificity of 87% to 100% in the detection or exclusion of aortic dissection.[1,30] Unlike aortography, CT scanning is noninvasive but is also associated with the use of radiation and contrast material. This technique is somewhat less sensitive for the detection of aortic dissection than other available modalities and cannot reliably diagnose aortic regurgitation or involvement of branch vessels.[1] In a recent evaluation, MRI has demonstrated a sensitivity of 98% to 100% and a specificity of 94% to 98% for aortic dissections (Table 17.2).[1,30,31] MRI is especially useful to distinguish aortic dissection from other aortic abnormalities such as thoracic aortic aneurysm or prior aortic graft repair.[1] In addition, this modality is effective in diagnosing the presence of a thrombus, the site of an intimal tear, pericardial effusion, and aortic regurgitation. Magnetic resonance imaging, however, has a number of limitations, which include limited view of branch vessels and inability to use it for unstable patients and for patients with pacemakers and old types of metallic heart valve.

Transthoracic echocardiography provides only limited diagnostic information in patients with aortic dissection. The yield of Doppler echocardiography is high in the diagnosis of aortic dissection–related complications such as bleeding into the pericardial sac and aortic regurgitation. Transesophageal echocardiography overcomes the limitations of transthoracic echocardiography and has a sensitivity of 98–100% for aortic dissection, as well as high specificity. (94%)[1,30,31] The procedure, which is relatively noninvasive, can be performed at the bedside and has been shown to be safe during pregnancy (Chapter 2). Transesophageal echocardiography, however, cannot be used in patients with esophageal disease: It is not tolerated by some patients, and it provides only a limited visibility of the proximal aortic arch.

The electrocardiogram is of little value in the diagnosis of aortic dissection, but it may be useful in revealing an acute myocardial infarction, which usually indicates involvement of the coronary arteries. In addition, the electrocardiogram may demonstrate pericarditis in patients with bleeding into the pericardial sac, and left ventricular hypertrophy in patients with long-standing hypertension or aortic coarctation, which may predispose to dissection.

If subdiaphragmatic dissection is suspected, abdominal ultrasonography may be of considerable value. Abdominal roentgenograms, although of some use in the patient who might have atherosclerosis, have no role in the pregnant population, where atherosclerosis is rare and radiation should be avoided.

Differential Diagnosis

The differential diagnosis of aortic dissection is that of other catastrophic illnesses, including acute pulmonary and amniotic fluid embolism, myocardial infarction, aortic regurgitation due to other causes, pneumothorax, cerebrovascular accident, uterine rupture, abruptio placentae, and mesenteric infarction. Given the availability of reasonably sophisticated diagnostic modalities, antemortem diagnosis of aortic dissection should be the rule.

Treatment

Since without treatment aortic dissection is associated with a high incidence of mortality, an urgent and aggressive approach to management is mandatory. The patient should be moved to an intensive care setting, preferably with the capability for hemodynamic monitoring. Invasive measurement of systemic arterial pressures will facilitate optimal care.

Surgery is not always indicated in patients with distal aortic dissection, since no difference in outcome has been demonstrated with either medical or surgical therapy.[1] Medical therapy is recommended for the stable patients with uncomplicated acute distal dissection or chronic aortic dissection and for patients who must be stabilized prior to surgery. Surgical therapy is indicated in patients who fail medical therapy (rupture or impending rupture, dissection progression, inability to control pain or blood pressure).[1] Current practice recommends the use of intravenous β-adrenergic blocking agents such as propranolol, metoprolol, or atenolol to achieve a 20% reduction in heart rate followed by an oral maintenance dose. In the nonpregnant patient, blood pressure should be lowered by nitroprusside infusion[16] to systolic levels of 100–120 mmHg, or to the lowest values that still allow adequate blood flow and perfusion to vital organs. This drug, which has a rapid onset of action and a very short half-life, can be titrated quickly. The use of nitroprusside during pregnancy, however, may produce thiocyanate toxicity to the fetus (see Chapter 31). Maternal toxicity is rare and can occur at large doses, especially in patients with renal impairment. Such toxicity may be manifested by metabolic acidosis, severe hypotension, confusion, coma, absent reflexes, widely dilated pupils, pink color, and shallow breathing. Because experience with the use of nitroprusside during pregnancy is limited, and because of the potential for fetal toxicity of this agent, it should be used only in cases refractory to other drugs. Hydralazine, an arterial dilator, is generally the drug of choice for blood pressure reduction in pregnancy and should be given in combination with beta blockers. This drug has been widely used for blood pressure reduction during pregnancy and its safety has been established (see Chapter 31).

To avoid the stress of labor, delivery in a patient with aortic dissection should be performed by means of cesarean section under epidural anesthesia.[16,19,20] In patients with proximal dissection, corrective surgery should be performed as soon as possible, since this measure is associated with improved outcome.[16,19] Replacement of the aortic valve is not necessary in every case and should be avoided if possible. Cardiac surgery with the use of extracorporeal circulation has been performed during pregnancy without increased risk to the mother but is associated with increased fetal loss.[32,33]

RUPTURE OF SPLENIC ARTERY ANEURYSM

Splenic artery aneurysm is the third most common abdominal aneurysm, following infrarenal and iliac artery aneurysms.[34] The incidence of this vascular abnormality has been determined to be 0.16% in a large autopsy study published in 1958[35] and 0.78% by a later angiographic evaluation.[36]

Despite the observation that other arterial aneurysms are three to five times more common in males, splenic artery aneurysms occur two to three times more frequently in females. Rupture of these aneurysms is twice as common in women, with up to 20% occurring during pregnancy.[37–40] Macfarlane and Thorbjarnarson[40] reviewed the first 61 reported cases of ruptured splenic artery aneurysms in pregnancy and found that 69% occurred in the third trimester, 13% during labor, and 6% in the puerperium. Only 30% were associated with hypertension. The definitive cause of splenic artery aneurysms is unknown, but pregnancy, especially multiparity, seems to be an important etiological factor.[37,41,42] Other associated conditions include atherosclerotic vascular disease, arterial dysplasia, focal arterial inflammatory processes, and portal hypertension with splenomegaly. The role of pregnancy in the pathogenesis of these aneurysms may be related to hormone-induced alterations in elastic tissue and medial ground substance, and repeated gestation may cause irreversible damage. Martinez et al[42] noted significant histological findings in women: subendothelial thickening, internal elastic lamina fragmentation, medial fibrodysplasia, accumulation of acid glycosaminoglycans in both the subintimal and medial layers of the aneurysmatic zone, and disorganization of the medial elastic fibers. It is feasible that some women with splenic artery aneurysm have preexisting splenic vessel pathology, either acquired or congenital. In addition, increased blood volume and intraabdominal pressure, as well as splenomegaly, may also play a role during pregnancy.

Splenic artery aneurysms usually occur in the distal portion of the main trunk of the splenic artery, are mostly asymptomatic prior to rupture, and may be found incidentally during angiography or laparotomy. Common symptoms of rupture include nausea, vomiting, diarrhea, or constipation. Pain is a frequent symptom and may be located in the epigastrium or left flank, with radiation to the left shoulder; it is often associated with diaphoresis, hypotension, tachycardia, and shock.[43] Hypotensive episodes may be associated with deceleration of fetal heart rate manifesting fetal distress due to compromise in placental circulation and hypoxia. Onequarter of all patients develop a two-stage or double rupture, with the initial bleed into the lesser sac followed minutes to weeks later by a second rupture into the peritoneal cavity with shock and, if not appropriately treated, death. Gastrointestinal bleeding may occur, but it is rare in pregnant patients. X-ray film may show a calcified curvilinear shadow in the upper left quadrant. Fluoroscopy occasionally demonstrates a pulsatile filling defect in the posterior wall of the stomach, but definitive diagnosis is established by angiography. All these diagnostic procedures are somewhat limited during pregnancy owing to the risk of radiation to the fetus. Ultrasonography, computerized tomography, and magnetic resonance imaging can also provide important diagnostic and follow-up information. The differential diagnoses of splenic artery aneurysm include a rupture of other arterial aneurysm, abdominal aortic dissection, acute pancreatitis, ischemic bowel, splenic infarction, renal colic, cholecystitis, appendicitis, gastritis, and myocardial infarction.[34] The diagnosis of splenic artery aneurysm rupture is even more difficult during pregnancy, when it may mimic other potential conditions such as uterine rupture and premature separation of the placenta with concealed hemorrhage. The following findings should help in ruling out uterine causes: history of transient severe pain in the upper left quadrant, lack of predisposing factors for uterine rupture or obstruction, relaxed uterus, absence of vaginal bleeding, normal fetal heart sounds, and presence of upper abdominal mass.

Early clinical suspicion is crucial in pregnancy and in cases of suspected rupture, hemodynamic support and emergency laparotomy are necessary to avoid maternal and fetal mortality.[34,44–59] Recent recommendations suggest that asymptomatic aneurysms 1 cm or larger in women of childbearing age should be electively resected or be treated with percutaneous embolization therapy.[60,61] A mortality rate has been associated with rupture of splenic artery aneurysm as high as 25% in the nonpregnant population.[43] Review of the first 99 cases reported in the world literature until 1993[34] demonstrated a 69% maternal and 90% fetal mortality in women with ruptured splenic artery aneurysm during pregnancy and only 10 cases of both maternal and fetal survival. More recent publications however, have reported favorable outcome of mothers and fetuses in several cases with rupture of splenic artery aneurysm during pregnancy.[34,44–58]

RUPTURE OF RENAL ARTERY ANEURYSM

The experience in 123 patients who had surgery for renal artery aneurysm was described in 1995.[62] Sixty percent of the patients were females, and the average age was 43 years. Renal artery aneurysms are usually of fibrodysplastic origin, have a saccular shape with a fibrous neck, and are located at or near an arterial bifurcation. These aneurysms may have a very thin wall and therefore may rupture. A predisposition for rupture of renal artery aneurysm during pregnancy has been suggested.[63] Of the first 24 reported cases, 6 occurred during pregnancy. Most of the reported cases of pregnancy-related rupture of renal artery aneurysms have occurred antepartum. Both fetal and maternal death were common in early reports.[27,64–67] Survival of both mother and fetus has been, however, reported recently in several cases.[68–72] Maternal age and parity are felt to be unrelated to the development of renal artery aneurysms.

Noted cases recently reported have included a rupture of a transplant renal artery aneurysm[69] and a giant, 5.8 cm right renal artery aneurysm diagnosed 8 weeks postpartum and successfully treated surgically with salvage of the kidney.[73] Seven cases of ruptured congenital arteriovenous malformation of the kidney during pregnancy have been reported.[72–79] Saito et al[80] described the most recent case, a woman who presented with gross hematuria and left flank pain at 22 weeks of her second pregnancy. These authors elected to use transcatheter embolization, which was successful, resulting in a delivery of a healthy newborn 4 months later. Since this technique involves the use of ionizing radiation, it has potential risks to the fetus. Therefore, treatment of this condition when associated with pregnancy should probably be surgical.[73,76,77]

RUPTURE OF OVARIAN ARTERY ANEURYSM

Pregnancy-related rupture of ovarian artery aneurysms has been reported in nine cases.[81–85] Similar to rupture of other intraabdominal vessels, this situation also presents with acute abdominal and flank pain and hypovolemic shock. Multiparity seems to predispose patients to rupture of the ovarian artery, and treatment is surgical. Seven of these cases occurred in the postpartum phase,[83,84] while one of the cases occurred during the third trimester close to term[83] and one patient experienced a rupture during the second stage of labor.

UTERO-OVARIAN VEIN RUPTURE

Rupture of a uterine or ovarian vein is another rare event, which may result in maternal and fetal morbidity and mortality. Review of the literature reveals more than 100 cases of utero-ovarian vein rupture associated with pregnancy.[86–91] The cause of spontaneous utero-ovarian vein rupture is unknown. Multiparity may be a predisposing factor.[88] Sudden increase in venous pressure, previous surgery, underlying leiomyomata uteri, and abnormal placental implantation have been suggested as other predisposing factors.[89] Ginsburg et al[86] reviewed 28 cases and reported that 61% of them occurred before the onset of labor and 21% presented postpartum. Similar to rupture of an ovarian artery, utero-ovarian vein rupture may also present as acute abdominal and flank pain, followed by the development of hypovolemic shock and fetal distress. Cases of retroperitoneal bleeding or bleeding confined to the broad ligament may present with rectal and back pain and may demonstrate a palpable mass. Peritoneal signs will be evident in cases with intraperitoneal bleeding.

Treatment is clearly surgical, although in most cases the laparotomy is combined with a delivery by cesarean section. Ginsburg et al[86] reported a successful surgical treatment of a lacerated uterine vein at 26 weeks of gestation with continuation of pregnancy and uneventful vaginal delivery of a normal infant at term.

REFERENCES

1. Williams GM, Gott VL, Brawley RK, et al. Aortic dissection associated with pregnancy. *J Vasc Surg* 1988;8:470–475.

2. Larson EW, Edwards WD. Risk factors for aortic dissection: a necropsy study of 161 patients. *Am J Cardiol* 1984;53: 849–855.

3. Isselbacher EM, Eagle KKA, DeSanctis RW. Disease of the aorta. In: Braunwald E, ed. *Heart Disease.* 5th ed. Philadelphia: WB Saunders; 1997;1546–1581.

4. Spittell PC, Spittell JA Jr, Joyce JW, Tajik AJ, Edwards WD, Schaff HV, Stanson AW. Clinical features and differential diagnosis of aortic dissection: experience with 236 cases (1980 through 1990). *Mayo Clin Proc* 1993;68:642–651.

5. Oskoui R, Lindsay J Jr. Aortic dissection in women < 40 years of age and the unimportance of pregnancy. *Am J Cardiol* 1994;73:821–823.

6. Anderson RA, Fineron FW. Aortic dissection in pregnancy: importance of pregnancy-induced changes in the vessel wall and bicuspid aortic valve in pathogenesis. *Br J Obstet Gynaecol* 1994;101:1085–1088.

7. Manolo-Estrella P, Barker AE. Histopathologic findings in human aortic media associated with pregnancy. *Arch Pathol* 1967;83:336–341.

8. Nolte JE, Rutherford RB, Nawaz S, Rosenberger A, Speers WC, Krupski WC. Arterial dissections associated with pregnancy. *J Vasc Surg* 1995;21:515–520.

9. Cavanzo FJ, Taylor HB. Effect of pregnancy on the human aorta and its relationship to dissecting aneurysms. *Am J Obstet Gynecol* 1969;105:567–568.

10. Cecchi E, Trucano G, Parisi F, Di-Summio M, Triorchero R. Aortic dissection in pregnancy: report of 2 cases. *G Ital Cardiol* 1994;24:441–444.

11. Foidart JM, Rorive G, Nusgens B. Aortic collagen biosynthesis during renal hypertension, pregnancy and hypertension during pregnancy in the rat. *Biomedicine* 1978;28:215–219.

12. Wolinsky H. Effects of estrogen and progestogen treatment on the response of the aorta of male rats to hypertension. *Circ Res* 1972;30:341–349.

13. Danforth DN, Manolo-Estrella P, Buckingham JC. Effect of pregnancy and of Enovid on the rabbit vasculature. *Am J Obstet Gynecol* 1964;88:952–962.

14. Irey NS, Norris HJ. Intimal vascular lesions associated with female reproductive steroids. *Arch Pathol* 1973;96:227–234.

15. Barrett JM, Van Hooydonk JE, Boehm FH. Pregnancy related rupture of arterial aneurysms. *Obstet Gynecol Survey* 1982;37: 557–566.

16. Pumphrey LW, Fay T, Weir I. Aortic dissection during pregnancy. *Br Heart J* 1986;55:106–108.

17. Heid M, Nos S, Cristalli B, Batellier J, Levardon M. Acute aortic dissection during pregnancy. Surgical treatment with maternal and fetal rescue. *J Gynecol Obstet Biol Reprod* 1993;22: 66–67.

18. Oliveira M, Quininha J, Serra J, Ferreira R, Galrinho A, Rosario L, Vitoriano I, Castelao N, Antunes AM. Acute aortic dissection in pregnancy. Report of a clinical case. *Rev Port Cardiol* 1994;13:227–231.

19. Wahlers T, Lass J, Alken A, Borst HG. Repair of acute type A aortic dissection after cesarean section in the thirty-ninth week of pregnancy. *J Thorac Cardiovasc Surg* 1994;107:314–315. Letter.

20. Jayram A, Carp HM, Davis L, Jacobson SL. Pregnancy complicated by aortic dissection: cesarean delivery during extradural anaesthesia. *Br J Anaesth* 1995;75:358–360.

21. Khalil I, Fahl M. Acute infrarenal abdominal aortic dissection with secondary aneurysm formation in pregnancy. *Eur J Vasc Endovasc Surg* 1995;9:481–484.

22. Helms E, Uguen T, Amaranto P, Carton MJ, Ducreux JC, Tempelhoff C. Aortic dissection and pregnancy. À propos of a case. *Arch Mal Coeur Vaiss* 1995;88:397–399.

23. McGeachy TE, Paullin JE. Dissecting aneurysm of aorta. *JAMA* 1937;108:1690–1698.

24. Schnitker MA, Bayer CA. Dissecting aneurysm of the aorta in young individuals, particularly in association with pregnancy. With report of a case. *Ann Intern Med* 1944;20:486–511.

25. Mandel W, Evans EW, Walford RL. Dissecting aortic aneurysm during pregnancy. *N Engl J Med* 1954;251:1001–1059.

26. Konishi Y, Tatsuta N, Kumada K, Minami K, Matsuda K, Yamusato A, Usui N, Muraguchi T, Hirkasa Y, Okamoto E, Watanabe R. Dissecting aneurysms during pregnancy and the puerperium. *Jpn Circ J* 1980;44:726–733.

27. Pedowitz P, Perell A. Aneurysms complicated by pregnancy. I. Aneurysms of the aorta and its major branches. *Am J Obstet Gynecol* 1957;73:720–735.

28. Shalev Y, Ben-Hur H, Hagay Z, Blickstein I, Epstein M. Successful delivery following myocardial ischemia during the second trimester of pregnancy. *Clin Cardiol* 1993;16:754–756.

29. Vu FH, Young N, Soo YS: Imaging of thoracic aortic dissection Australas Radiol 1994;38:170–175.

30. Sommer T, Fehske W, Holzknecht N, Smekal AR, Keller E, Lutterbey G, Kreft B, Kuhl C, Greseke J, Abu-Ramadan D, Schmed H. Aortic dissection: a comparative study of diagnosis with spiral CT, multiplanar transesophageal echocardiography, and MR imaging. Radiology 1996;198:347–352.

31. Sarasin FP, Louis-Simonet M, Gaspoz JM, Junod AF. Detecting acute thoracic aortic dissection in the emergency department: time constraints and choice of the optimal diagnostic test Ann Emerg Med 1996;28:278–288.

32. Thornhill ML, Camann WC. Cardiovascular disease. In: Chestnut DH, ed. *Obstetric Anesthesia*. St. Louis: Mosby-Year Book; 1994;746–779.

33. Khandelwal M, Rasanen J, Ludormirski A, Addonizio P, Reece A. Evaluation of fetal and uterine hemodynamics during maternal cardiopulmonary bypass. *Obstet Gynecol* 1996;88:667–671.

34. Angelakis EJ, Bair WE, Barone JE, Lincer RM. Splenic artery aneurysm rupture during pregnancy. *Obstet Gynecol Survey* 1993;48:145–147.

35. Sheps S, Spittel J, Fairbaim JF II. Proceedings of staff meeting. *Mayo Clinic* 1958;33:381–390.

36. Stanley JC, Fry WJ. Pathogenesis and clinical significance of splenic artery aneurysms. *Surgery* 1974;76:898–909.

37. Macfarlane JR, Thorbjarnarson B. Rupture of splenic artery aneurysm during pregnancy. *Am J Obstet Gynecol* 1966;95:1025–1037.

38. Vassalotti SB, Schaller JA. Spontaneous rupture of splenic artery aneurysm during pregnancy. Report of first known antepartum rupture with maternal and fetal survival. *Obstet Gynecol* 1967;30:264–268.

39. O'Grady JP, Day EJ, Toole AL, Paust JC. Splenic artery aneurysm rupture in pregnancy. A review and case report. *Obstet Gynecol* 1977;50:627–630.

40. Macfarlane JR, Thorbjarnarson B. Rupture of splenic artery aneurysm during pregnancy. *Am J Obstet Gynecol* 1966;95:1025–1037.

41. Trastek VF, Pairolero PC, Joyce JW, Hollier LH, Bernatz PE. Splenic artery aneurysms. *Surgery* 1982;91:694–699.

42. Martinez E, Menendez AR, Ablanedo P. Splenic artery aneurysms. *Int Surg* 1986;71:95–99.

43. deVries JE, Shuttenkerk ME, Malt RA. Complications of splenic artery aneurysm other than intraperitoneal rupture. *Surgery* 1982;91:200–204.

44. Lowry SM, O'Dea T, Gallagher DI, Mozenter R. Splenic artery aneurysm rupture: the seventh instance of maternal and fetal survival. *Obstet Gynecol* 1986;67:291–292.

45. Czekelius P, Deichert L, Gesenhues T, Schulz KD. Rupture of an aneurysm of the splenic artery and pregnancy: a case report. *Eur J Obstet Gynecol* 1990;38:229–232.

46. Dunlop W, Iwanicki S, Akierman A, Pasieka J, Higgin Jr. Spontaneous rupture of splenic artery aneurysm: maternal and fetal survival. *Can J Surg* 1990;33:407–408.

47. Hayde SM, Gillett WR, Thompson IA. Rupture of a spleen artery aneurysm in pregnancy. *Aust N Z J Obstet Gynaecol* 1990;30:132–133.

48. Czekelius P, Deichert L, Genenhues T, Schulz KD. Rupture of an aneurysm of the splenic artery and pregnancy: a case report. *Eur J Obstet Gynecol Reprod Biol* 1991;38:229–232.

49. Hunka D, Csordas T, Domany Z. Rupture of the splenic artery aneurysm during pregnancy. *Acta Chir Hung* 1991;32:77–82.

50. McNeely RG, Anderle LJ, Conklin CR. Splenic artery aneurysm rupture in pregnancy with maternal and fetal survival: a case report. *J Reprod Med* 1992;37:939–942.

51. Tanchev S, Popova M, Slavov I. The splenic emergency syndrome during pregnancy: a report of 2 cases. *Akush Ginekol* 1992;31:32–34.

52. Williams J. Splenic artery aneurysm rupture: an uncommon obstetrical catastrophe. *J Fam Pract* 1988;26:73–74.

53. Veschambre PU, Coppo B, Grosieux P. Rupture of splenic artery aneurysm during the first three months of pregnancy. *Presse Med* 1993;22:1693–1694.

54. Carllouett JC, Merchant FB. Ruptured splenic artery aneurysm in pregnancy. Twelfth reported case with maternal and fetal survival. *Am J Obstet Gynecol* 1993;168:1810–1811.

55. Chen CW, Chen CP, Wang KG. Splenic artery aneurysm rupture in the second trimester. *Int J Gynecol Obstet* 1995;49:199–200.

56. Jotkowitz MW, Polglase AL. Splenic artery aneurysm in pregnancy. *Aust N Z J Obstet Gynaecol* 1995;35:232–233. Letter.

57. Simpson KR. Rupture of splenic artery aneurysm in pregnancy. *Crit Care Nurse* 1995;15:25–29,31–32.

58. Loke SS, Bullard MJ, Liaw SJ, Liao HC. Splenic artery aneurysm rupture in pregnancy: a review and case report. *Chang Keng I Hsueh* 1995;18:166–169.

59. Walker JS, Dire DJ. Vascular abdominal emergencies. *Emergency Med Clin North Am* 1996;14:571–592.

60. McGinnis HD, DeLuca SA. Splenic artery aneurysms. *Am Fam Physician* 1993;47:1199–1202.

61. McDermott VG, Shlansky-Goldberg R, Cope C. Endovascular management of splenic artery aneurysm and psuedoaneurysms. *Cardiovasc Intervent Radiol* 1994;17:179–184.

62. Lacombe M. Aneurysms of the renal artery. *J Mal Vasc* 1995;20:257–263.

63. Harrow BR, Sloane JA. Aneurysm of renal artery: report of five cases. *J Urol* 1959;81:35–41.

64. Burt RL, Johnston FR, Silverthorne RG, Lock FR, Dickerson AJ. Ruptured renal artery aneurysm in pregnancy. Report of a case with survival. *Obstet Gynecol* 1956;7:229–233.

65. Thomas GP, Gillis OS. Spontaneous rupture of a renal artery associated with pregnancy. *Am J Obstet Gynecol* 1970;106: 628–629.

66. Cohen SG, Cashdan A, Burger R. Spontaneous rupture of a renal artery aneurysm during pregnancy. *Obstet Gynecol* 1972;39:897–902.

67. Patterson WM. Maternal death due to undiagnosed left renal artery aneurysm associated with an absent right kidney. *Proc R Soc Med* 1973;66:761–762.

68. Saleh YZ, McLeod FN. Ruptured renal artery aneurysm in pregnancy. Case report. *Br J Obstet Gynaecol* 1977;84: 391–393.

69. Dayton B, Helgerson RB, Sollinger HW, Acher CW. Ruptured renal artery aneurysm in a pregnant uninephric patient: successful ex vivo repair and autotransplatnation. *Surgery* 1990;107:708–711.

70. Richardson AJ, Liddington M, Jaskowski A, Murie JA, Gillmer M, Morris PJ. Pregnancy in a renal transplant recipient complicated by rupture of a transplant renal artery aneurysm. *Br J Surg* 1990;77:228–229.

71. Murakami M. Rupture of renal arterial aneurysm in a pregnant patient. *MASUI* 1993;42:1367–1370.

72. Rijbroek A, Van Dijk HA, Roex AJ. Rupture of renal artery aneurysm during pregnancy. *Eur J Vasc Surg* 1994;8:375–376.

73. Plrskin MJ, Orebner ML, Hassel LH, Gusz JR, Balkin PW, Lerud KS, Larson AW. A giant renal artery aneurysm diagnosed post partum. *J Urol* 1990;144:1459–1461.

74. Waltzer WC. The urinary tract in pregnancy. *J Urol* 1981;125:271–276.

75. Scheifley CH, Daughtery GW, Greene LF, Priestley JT. Arteriovenous fistula of the kidney. New observations and report of three cases. *Circulation* 1959;19:662–671.

76. Boijsen E, Kohler R. Renal arteriovenous fistulae. *Acta Radiol* 1962;57:433–445.

77. Koizumi H, Hirano S, Chikazawa H. Renal arteriovenous fistula in pregnancy: a case reprot. *Nishinihon J Urol* 1984;47: 465.

78. Klimberg I, Wilson J, Davis K, Finlayson B. Hemorrhage from congenital renal arteriovenous malformation in pregnancy. *Urology* 1984;23:381–386.

79. MacMillan RDH, Robinette MA. Congenital arteriovenous malformation of kidney in pregnancy. *Urology* 1985;26: 441–445.

80. Saito S, Iigaya T, Koyama Y. Transcatheter embolization for the rupture of congenital arteriovenous malformation of the kidney in pregnancy. *J Urol* 1987;137:964–965.

81. Caillouette JC, Owen HW. Postpartum spontaneous rupture of an ovarian-artery aneurysm. *Obstet Gynecol* 1963;21:510–511.

82. Burnett RA, Carfrae DC. Spontaneous rupture of ovarian artery aneurysm in the puerperium. Two case reports and a review of the literature. *Br J Obstet Gynaecol* 1976;83:744–750.

83. King WL. Ruptured ovarian artery aneurysm: a case report. *J Vasc Surg* 1990;12:190–193.

84. Jafari K, Saleh I. Postpartum spontaneous rupture of an ovarian artery aneurysm. *Obstet Gynecol* 1977;49:493–494.

85. Barrett JM, Van Hooydonk JE, Bohem FH. Pregnancy-related rupture of arterial aneurysms. *Obstet Gynecol Survey* 1982;37: 557–566.

86. Ginsburg KA, Valdes C, Schnider G. Spontaneous utero-ovarian vessel rupture during pregnancy: three case reports and a review of the literature. *Obstet Gynecol* 1987;69:474–476.

87. Hodgkinson CP, Christensen RC. Hemorrhage from ruptured utero-ovarian veins during pregnancy. *Am J Obstet Gynecol* 1950;59:1112–1172.

88. Belfort MA, Simon T, Kirshon B, Howell JF. Ruptured ovarian artery aneurysm complicating a term vaginal delivery. *South Med J* 1993;86:1073–1074.

89. Johnston CC, Arban AT. Hemorrhage from rupture of utero-ovarian vein. *JAMA* 1960;174:528–530.

90. Weitzman CC, Capalbo JL. Utero-ovarian vein rupture associated with pregnancy. *New York State J Med* 1966;66: 2282–2285.

91. LaRose P, Sehdeva PK. Spontaneous rupture of a uterine vein during labor. *South Med J* 1978;71:1446–1447.

18

MARFAN SYNDROME AND PREGNANCY

Uri Elkayam, md, Enrique Ostrzega, md, Avraham Shotan, md, and Anilkumar Mehra, md

INTRODUCTION

Marfan syndrome is a hereditary disorder of the connective tissue[1-5] with an estimated prevalence of 4–6 per 10,000 persons; prevalence does not differ according to sex, race, or ethnicity.[4] The syndrome is caused by abnormalities in the relation between fibrillin and fibers due to an abnormal gene for fibrillin[1,2] on chromosome 15.[3] A family history of the disease is present in 65–75% of patients and is sporadic in the rest. Cardiovascular involvement, including mitral and tricuspid valve prolapse with or without valvular regurgitation, dilatation of the aorta (primarily of the ascending portion), and aortic regurgitation, is a common feature of the disease.[4-6] Life expectancy is greatly reduced in patients with this syndrome, predominantly because of cardiac complications (aortic dilatation, dissection, and rupture).[7]

CARDIOVASCULAR RISK OF PREGNANCY

Pregnancy in women with the Marfan syndrome poses two problems: a potential catastrophic and often lethal acute aortic dissection and the risk for having a child who inherits the syndrome. In a review of the literature published up to 1980, Pyeritz[8] found reports of 32 women with the Marfan syndrome who had had at least one pregnancy. Acute aortic dissection was diagnosed in 20 of these women, of whom 16 died during or shortly after pregnancy and 4 died later in the postpartum period because of aortic rupture or regurgitation. Most of these patients had had preexisting cardiovascular abnormalities, including aortic dilatation, aortic regurgitation, coarctation of the aorta, hypertension, cardiomegaly, and ductus arteriosus. A review of the literature since 1980

and some of our complicated cases (Table 18.1, Figures 18.1–18.5) reveal additional data of pregnancy in women with the Marfan syndrome.[9-19] Most of these case reports describe cardiovascular complications during pregnancy, including (1) dilatation of the ascending aorta with the development of aortic regurgitation and congestive heart failure, and (2) proximal and distal dissections of the aorta with occasional involvement of the iliac[9,11] and coronary arteries.[13] Most women developed cardiac complications in the second and third trimesters, although aortic dissection occurred in isolated patients a few days after conception,[15] during labor,[9] and 8 days after delivery.[16] Aortic dissections occurring in the 14th, 28th, and 32nd gestational weeks and postpartum resulted in maternal death in each case.[10,14] Live babies were delivered before surgery by cesarean sections at the 32nd week in one patient,[17] the 36th week in two patients,[11,12] and 38th and 42nd weeks in one patient each.[13] In all patients, surgical repair was done successfully up to 8 weeks after delivery. In two other patients, surgery was performed during pregnancy. In one of these patients,[15] aortic arch replacement and triple coronary artery bypass were done a few days after conception, and a normal baby was delivered by cesarean section in the 34th gestational week. In the other patient, who had a sinus of Valsalva aneurysm and aortic regurgitation, the aortic valve was successfully replaced in the 22nd week of pregnancy. The operation, however, was complicated by maternal hypotension that resulted in a decrease in fetal heart rate from 120 to 40 beats per minute. On day 10 after surgery, the patient had cardiac arrest caused by cardiac arrhythmia and was successfully resuscitated. Pregnancy was continued for 6 more weeks, after which the patient delivered a premature baby with the Marfan syndrome and respiratory distress.

Cardiac Problems in Pregnancy, Third Edition
Edited by Uri Elkayam, MD, and Norbert Gleicher, MD
Copyright © 1998 by Wiley-Liss, Inc. ISBN 0-471-16358-9

TABLE 18.1 A Summary of Cases Published Since 1980 Reporting Peripartum Cardiovascular Complications in Women with the Marfan Syndrome

Case	Ref: First Author (year)	Age (years)	Prior Cardiovascular Disease	Complications Maternal	Complications Fetal	Gestational Stage	Procedure	Outcome Maternal	Outcome Fetal	Obstetrical History
1	Ferguson et al[9] (1983)	42	Mild gestational hypertension; cardiac evaluation including M-mode echo 2 years PTA reported normal	Proximal and distal aortic dissection extending to the iliac bifurcation. Aortic insufficiency.	Fetal bradycardia	39 weeks, early labor	Cesarean section followed by surgical repair of aortic dissection with aortic valve and ascending aorta replacement	Discharged on 10th postoperative day	Good	G_2, P_0, Ab_1
2	Baltazar et al[10] (1983)	31	Heart murmur present since age of 2 years	Proximal and distal aortic dissection extending to abdominal aortal below the renal arteries, aortic regurgitation, ventricular tachycardia.		14 weeks	Unsuccessful resuscitation	Death	Death	G_1, P_0, Ab_0
3	Mor-Yosef et al[11] (1988)	35	Aortic aneurysm, aortic and mitral insufficiency diagnosed 2 years PTA	Congestive heart failure starting at 28 weeks gestation.		36 weeks	Cesarean section followed by surgical correction of aortic aneurysm and AVR 6 weeks postpartum	Good	Good	G_4, P_2, Ab_1
4	Mor-Yosef et al[11] (1988)	26	None; normal size aorta by echo prior to and during pregnancy	Distal aortic dissection distal to origin of left subclavian artery to and iliac arteries.		20 weeks	Hysterotomy and delivery of 270 g fetus; medical therapy of aortic aneurysm	Good	Death	G_1, P_0, Ab_0
5	Rosenblum et al[12] (1983)	28	MVP, normal aortic root diameter by echo at 13, 20, and 28 weeks	Distal aortic dissection distal to origin of left subclavian artery.		36 weeks	Cesarean section followed by surgical replacement of distal thoracic aorta on third postpartum day	Discharged on 11th postoperative day	Good	G_2, P_1, Ab_0
6	Shime et al[13] (1987)	Not reported		Aortic dissection with extension to the coronary arteries followed by cardiac arrest.		38 weeks	Successful resuscitation; cesarean section followed by immediate surgical repair of aortic dissection	Admitted 3 months postpartum with dissection of abdominal aorta	Good	G_3, P_2, Ab_0
7	Metcalfe et al[14] (1986)	31	Hypertension	Distal aortic dissection extending the length of the thoracic and abdominal aorta; cardiogenic shock.		28 weeks	Emergency AVR	Death 7 h after beginning of surgery	Not reported	G_2
8	Cola et al[15] (1985)	34	Hypertension	Proximal and distal aortic dissection on the 1–8 days postconception.		1–8 days postconception	Replacement of the aortic valve and arch. Cesarean section at 34 weeks gestation and tubal ligation under epidural anesthesia	Discharged on postoperative day	Good	G_1, P_0, Ab_0
9	Barker et al[16]	40	Severe retrosternal chest pain radiat-	Dissection of the abdominal aorta.		8 days postpartum	Medical therapy	Good	Good	G_3

No.	Author (year)	Age	History	Clinical presentation	Timing	Treatment	Maternal outcome	Fetal outcome	G/P
	(1989)		ing to the back for 10 days during first pregnancy 6 years PTA						Not reported
10	Smith et al[17] (1989)	19	Dilatation of aortic annulus to 5.5 cm 2 years PTA	Sinus Valsalva aneurysm, mild aortic insufficiency, continued severe chest pain.	22 weeks	AVR	Cardiopulmonary arrest 10 days postsurgery; successfully resuscitated	Fetal bradycardia during surgery, premature (29 weeks), respiratory distress, Marfan syndrome	Not reported
11	Maruyama et al[18] (1993)	32		Proximal aortic dissection with acute aortic insufficiency.	32 weeks	Emergency surgery with cesarean section, reconstruction of ascending aorta and aortic arch; AVR and aortocoronary bypass of right coronary artery	Good	Good	
12	Chow[19] (1993)	34	Mitral regurgitation; aortic root dilatation	Dissection of descending aorta one week postpartum.	One week postpartum	Medical therapy	Good	Premature (32 weeks)	G_1P_0
13	Marshall[a] (1995)	34		Progressive pedal edema and DOE during 3rd trimester; 8–9 cm proximal ascending aortic aneurysm and moderate to severe AI diagnosed postpartum.	Fetal distress	Emergency aortic valve and ascending aorta replacement	Good	Good	G_2P_1
14	[b]	34	MVP (Fig. 18.1) slightly dilated aortic root diameter at 42 mm	Sudden death 2 days postpartum due to proximal aortic dissection and pericardial tamponade (Fig. 18.2).	2 days postpartum		Death	Good	$G_6P_2Ab_3$
15	[b]	23	Episodes of sharp chest pain radiating to the back starting 1 year PTA	Increased frequency and severity of chest pain III/VI systolic murmur. Thoracoabdominal aortic aneurysm and descending aortic dissection (Figs. 18.3–18.5).	16 weeks	Elective therapeutic abortion at 19 weeks; medical therapy	Good	Aborted	G_2P_1
16	[b]	25	Severe chest pain at 42 weeks, aortic root dilatation and 2+AI. Ascending aortic dissection 2 months postpartum and severe AI.		42 weeks	Emergency cesarean section at 42 weeks; AVR and ascending aorta replacement 2 months postpartum	Good	Good	G_1P_0

[a]Personal communications, Erik S. Marshall, 1995.

[b]Patient seen at LAC & USC Medical Center, Los Angeles.

Abbreviations: Ab, abortion; AI, Aortic insufficiency; AVR, aortic valve replacement; DOE, dyspnea on exertion; G, gravida; MVP, mitral valve prolapse; P, para; PTA, prior to admission.

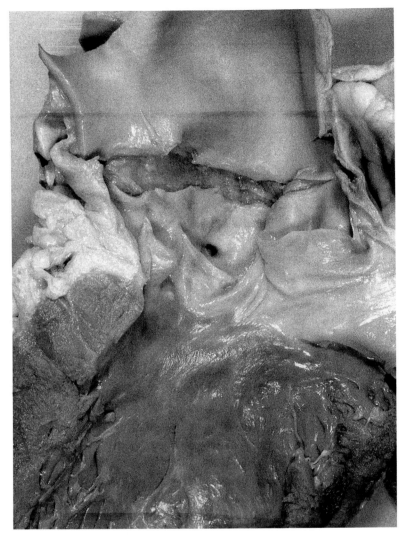

Figure 18.1   Pictured just above the cusps of the aortic valve is a transverse tear across nearly the entire diameter of the ascending aorta (Table 18.1, case 14).

The cause of the increased incidence of aortic dissection during pregnancy is not clear. An association between predisposition to dissection and the hyperdynamic and hypervolemic cardiocirculatory state of pregnancy is possible. In addition, estrogen has been reported to inhibit collagen and elastin deposition in the aorta, and progestogen has been shown to accelerate deposition of noncollagenous proteins in the aortas of rats.[20] Such structural changes in the arterial wall during pregnancy may also contribute to aortic dissection.[21]

Although most reports describe severe complications related to pregnancy in women with the Marfan syndrome, this literature probably overpresents pregnancy-related complications because of a bias toward reporting complicated rather than uncomplicated cases. Such an assumption is supported by Pyeritz,[8] whose retrospective analysis of 105 pregnancies in 26 patients with the Marfan syndrome and prospective follow-up of 10 patients with the syndrome who had minimal or no preexisting cardiovascular disease showed only a low risk for maternal complications and death. The same group published the results of a prospective longitudinal evaluation of the outcome of 45 pregnancies in 21 Marfan syndrome patients seen in the investigators' institution between 1983 and 1992.[22] Aortic dissection or dilatation requiring surgery occurred in three patients who had prior evidence of compromise including aortic regurgitation in two and history of aortic graft replacement and a chronic thoracic dissection in the third case. Serial echocardiograms performed during pregnancy showed little or no change in aortic root diameter in most patients. Cardiac status was not affected by pregnancy,

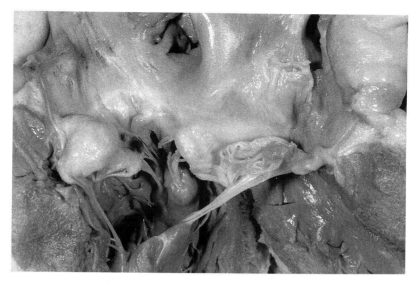

Figure 18.2   The mitral valve displays prolapsed leaflets, which balloon upward toward the left atrium, along with attenuated and elongated chordae tendinea (Table 18.1, case 14).

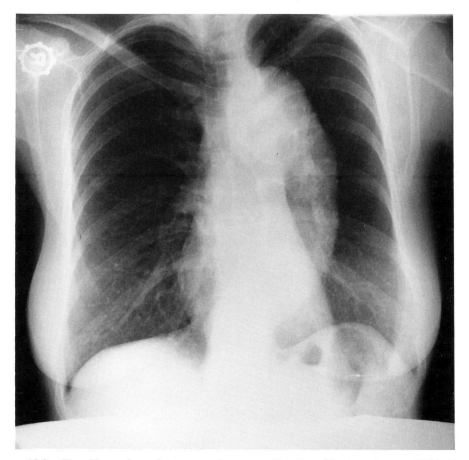

Figure 18.3   Chest X-ray of case 2 demonstrating severe dilatation of the thoracic aorta (Table 18.1, case 15).

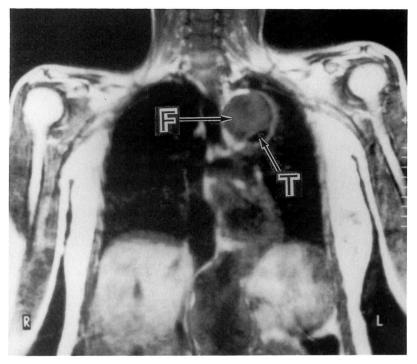

Figure 18.4 Coronal view of spin-echo magnetic resonance image showing dilated aorta with dissection: F, false lumen; T, true lumen (Table 18.1, case 15).

and the incidence of obstetric complications was comparable to the incidence seen in the general population. This report, therefore, showed that in contrast to patients with preexisting cardiac abnormalities,[8] patients without major cardiac involvement tolerate pregnancy well, and in addition, pregnancy does not seem to aggravate aortic root dilatation over time. These data are further supported by two recent reports[23,24] describing successful pregnancies in 3 cases despite mild to moderate aortic root enlargement and mitral valve prolapse in all 3 patients, as well as a moderate degree of left ventricular systolic dysfunction in 1 patient.

In addition to maternal risk associated with pregnancy in the Marfan syndrome, there is a risk for transmitting the disease to the fetus. The Marfan syndrome is inherited as an autosomal dominant disorder,[25] and the fetus has a 50% chance of inheriting the mutant gene.[5]

PRECONCEPTION EVALUATION AND CONSULTATION

Because no large clinical trials of pregnancy in patients with the Marfan syndrome have been reported, our recommendations are based on general principles rather than trial data. Women with the Marfan syndrome should be counseled before conception about potential pregnancy-related complications and about the risk for transmitting the syndrome to the

offspring. Mildly affected patients should be informed about the different presentations of the disease and the possibility of more severe expression in the offspring.[5] It should be noted that because of better understanding of the gene defect of the Marfan syndrome,[2,3,26–29] prenatal diagnosis of this disease may be possible in some patients of informative families (i.e., those in which the disease cosegregates with marker alleles).[5,30,30a,30b] Before conception occurs, physicians should carefully counsel the patient and her family about the expected morbidity of the mother in years to come and the possibility of reduced life expectancy.

Many pregnancy-related complications described in patients with the Marfan syndrome emphasize the great potential for risk associated with gestation, especially in patients with cardiovascular involvement. Such cardiovascular abnormalities should be carefully evaluated before and frequently throughout pregnancy. Dilatation of the ascending aorta before conception seems to be an important predictor of aortic dissection during gestation, and this condition should be excluded before pregnancy. Reports of aortic dissection in the Marfan syndrome in pregnant[12] and nonpregnant patients with normal aortic root diameter[31,31a] show that event-free pregnancy cannot be guaranteed to any patient with this syndrome. Recently, Simpson and colleagues[32] showed that transesophageal echocardiography was superior to transthoracic echocardiography in the assessment of aortic diameter and the diagnosis of aortic dissection and other

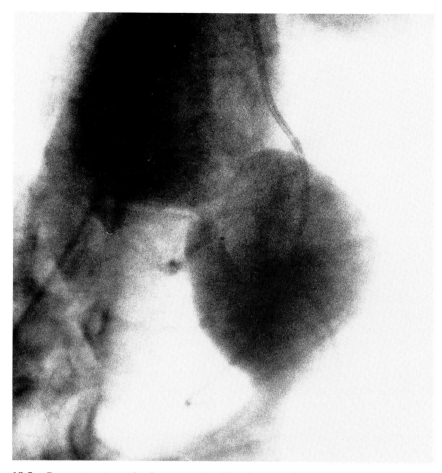

Figure 18.5   Contrast aortography demonstrating dilated aorta and severe aortic regurgitation (Table 18.1, case 15).

cardiovascular manifestations of the Marfan syndrome. The use of transesophageal echocardiography should, therefore, be preferred for preconception risk stratification in women with the Marfan syndrome.

SURGERY DURING PREGNANCY

If a pregnant patient with the Marfan syndrome has substantial dilatation of the aorta, therapeutic abortion or surgical intervention should be considered. Surgery for marked dilatation of the aorta[17] and for aortic dissection[15,15a] has been reported during gestation. Cola and Lavin[15] recently reported successful aortic arch replacement and coronary artery bypass grafting for aortic dissection in a patient with the Marfan syndrome; the surgery was done a few days after conception, with normal fetal outcome. Smith and coworkers[17] reported successful replacement of the aortic valve and the ascending aorta during the 22nd week of gestation; this was

done because of symptomatic dilatation of the aorta from 5.5 cm to 7.7 cm during pregnancy.

Gott and colleagues[33] showed a 5-year survival rate of 85% in 50 patients with the Marfan syndrome after composite graft repair of the ascending aorta. They recommended preventive replacement of the ascending aorta if the aorta reaches or exceeds 60 mm. A recent study by Murgatroyd and colleagues[31] reported aortic root dimension to be 5.1 ± 1.3 cm. On the basis of these data, a recent editorial[34] recommended elective replacement of the aortic root when or before the root reaches 5.5 cm in patients with the Marfan syndrome who show progressive dilatation of the aortic root by serial echocardiographic assessments, in patients with a family history of aortic dissection, and in women who are planning pregnancy.

Successful surgery for aortic dissection during pregnancy has been reported in a few cases.[35–39] It should be noted, however, that cardiac surgery in general has been shown to result in increased fetal loss.[38] For this reason, if fetal maturity can be confirmed, a cesarean section should be done before or concomitantly with thoracic surgery.[8,10,12]

PROPHYLACTIC USE OF β-ADRENERGIC BLOCKING AGENTS

Several preliminary studies[39–42] have suggested that β-adrenegic blocking agents may have a beneficial effect on the rate of aortic root dilatation in children and adolescents. These initial results are strongly supported by a recent report by Shores and colleagues,[43] who did a randomized study of the effect of propranolol (mean dose, 212 ± 68 mg/d) on the progression of aortic dilatation in adolescents and adults with the Marfan syndrome for approximately 10 years. These investigators showed a lower rate of aortic dilatation and a significantly reduced rate of aortic regurgitation, aortic dissection, cardiovascular surgery, congestive heart failure, and death in the patients treated with propranolol. The applicability of these data to pregnant patients needs to be further studied but, on the basis of available information, the prophylactic use of beta-blockers during pregnancy seems to make good clinical sense.

Propranolol has been extensively used during pregnancy to treat various conditions, including hypertension,[44–47] thyrotoxicosis,[48,49] hypertrophic cardiomyopathy,[50,51] and maternal[46,52,53] and fetal supraventricular tachyarrhythmias.[44,53–57] Although the overall experience with this drug in pregnancy has been favorable,[58] potential side effects, including fetal growth retardation,[46] bradycardia, hypoglycemia, hyperbilirubinemia, and apnea at birth in the newborn, have been reported.[59,60] Such side effects should be anticipated by the clinician. Barden and Stander[61] have shown that propranolol given to pregnant women blocks the inhibitory effects of epinephrine on myometrial activity. The nonselective β-adrenergic blocking effect of propanolol may, therefore, facilitate an increase in uterine activity. Although the clinical relevance of these findings is not clear, the use of β_1-adrenergic receptor blocking agents, such as metoprolol and atenolol, may be preferred during pregnancy. Several studies have shown these agents to be safe when used to treat hypertension during pregnancy.[62–64] A few studies, however, have reported lower birth weight in association with exposure to atenolol during gestation.[65] β-Adrenergic blocking agents are excreted in breast milk.[66–68] However, unless hepatic function in the newborn is markedly impaired, breast feeding should not be discouraged.

DIAGNOSIS OF AND MEDICAL THERAPY FOR AORTIC DISSECTION DURING PREGNANCY

Transthoracic echocardiography has traditionally been used to assess the ascending aorta in patients with the Marfan syndrome. The recent introduction of transesophageal echocardiography has provided the clinician with a highly effective tool for the diagnosis of aortic dissection both in nonpregnant and pregnant patients.[69,70] Because aneurysm of the aorta in the patients with the syndrome can occasionally also involve the descending aorta,[71] transesophageal echocardiography seems preferable to transthoracic echocardiography for both preconception assessment and periodic follow-up during pregnancy. This bias is further supported by the report by Simpson and coworkers[32] that this technique was superior to transthoracic echocardiography in the diagnosis of aortic dissection and dilation in patients with the Marfan syndrome.

Magnetic resonance imaging may be equally effective in the stable patient, but the safety of this technique during pregnancy has not been completely established. No evidence suggests that short-term exposure to an electromagnetic field can harm the fetus, but prolonged or high level exposure to electromagnetic radiation has been linked to unfavorable effects on embryogenesis and chromosomal structure.[72,73] Until conclusive information about the effect of magnetic resonance imaging on the fetus is established in many studies with long follow-up periods, echocardiography seems preferable.[72] If contrast aortography is done, an attempt should be made to minimize the use of radiation and to adequately shield the fetus.[74]

Standard medical therapy for aortic dissection includes the use of intravenous nitroprusside and beta-blockers to control blood pressure and decrease left ventricular contractility, thereby reducing ejection velocity and minimizing shear forces.[75] The use of nitroprusside during pregnancy, however, may lead to thiocyanate toxicity in the fetus.[58] Thus, the gestational use of hydralazine to control blood pressure is preferred. Hydralazine has been used extensively to control blood pressure during pregnancy, and its safety has been well established.[58]

LABOR AND DELIVERY

The available literature and our own experience show that patients with the Marfan syndrome who have normal results on cardiovascular examination and no evidence of aortic dilatation can tolerate vaginal delivery[22]. In these patients, cesarean section should be reserved for obstetrical indications.[23,24,76,77] At the same time, however, the stress of labor should be reduced by means of epidural anesthesia, to minimize pain, and forceps or vacuum, to shorten the second stage of labor. Both systolic and diastolic blood pressures increase markedly during uterine contractions.[78] These changes should be anticipated and prevented with beta-blockers or vasodilators. In patients with aortic dilatation, aortic dissection, or other important cardiac abnormalities, cesarean section should be the preferred method of delivery because it minimizes the hemodynamic changes associated with vaginal delivery. A recent report by Irons and Pollard[79] described postpartum hemorrhage of the uterine vasculature 3 days after cesarean section secondary to the Marfan syndrome. Similar postpartum hemorrhage, reported by Pyeritz[8] in 4 of 11 women with the Marfan syndrome, should be anticipated in such patients.

ACKNOWLEDGMENT

This chapter has been modified from Elkayam U et al. *Ann Int Med* 1995;123:117–122, with permission.

REFERENCES

1. Milewcz DM, Pyeritz RE, Crawford ES, Byers PH. Marfan syndrome: defective synthesis, secretion and extracellular matrix formation of fibrillin by cultured dermal fibroblast. *J Clin Invest* 1991;88:79–86.

2. Dietz HC, Cutting GR, Pyeritz RE, Maslen CL, Sakai LY, Corson GM, Puffenberger EG, Hamash A. Marfan syndrome caused by a recurrent de novo missense mutation in the fibrillin gene. *Nature* 1991;352:337–339.

3. Kainulainen K, Sakai LY, Child A, Pope M, Puhakka L, Ryhanen L, Palotie A, Kaitila I, Peltonen L. Two mutations in Marfan syndrome resulting in truncated fibrillin. *Proc Natl Acad Sci USA* 1992;89:5917–5921.

4. Pyeritz RE, McKusick VA. The Marfan syndrome: diagnosis and management. *N Engl J Med* 1979;300:772–777.

5. Rossiter JP, Johnson TRB. Management of genetic disorders during pregnancy. *Obstet Gynecol Clin North Am* 1992;19:801–813.

6. Beighton P, de Paepe A, Danks D, Finidori G, Gedde-Dahl-T, Goodman R, Hall JG, Hollister DH, Horton N, McKusick VA. International nosology of heritable disorders of connective tissue. *Am J Med Genet* 1988;29:581–594.

7. Murdoch JL, Walker BA, Halpern BL, Kuzma JW, McKurick VA. Life expectancy and causes of death in the Marfan syndrome. *N Engl J Med* 1972;286:804–808.

8. Pyeritz RE. Maternal and fetal complications of pregnancy in the Marfan syndrome. *Am J Med* 1981;71:784–790.

9. Ferguson JE II, Ueland K, Stinson EB, Maly RP. Marfan's syndrome: acute aortic dissection during labor, resulting in fetal distress and cesarean section, followed by successful surgical repair. *Am J Obstet Gynecol* 1983;147:759–762.

10. Baltazar RF, Mower MM, Aquino N, Udoff EJ, Friedman R. Acute pulmonary edema in a pregnant patient. *Arch Intern Med* 1983;143:781–783.

11. Mor-Yosef S, Younis J, Granat M, Kedari A, Migalter A, Schenker JG. Marfan's syndrome in pregnancy. *Obstet Gynecol Survey* 1988;43:382–385.

12. Rosenblum NG, Grossman AR, Gabbe SG, Mennuti MT, Cohen AW: Failure of serial echocardiographic studies to predict aortic dissection in a pregnant patient with Marfan's syndrome. *Am J Obstet Gynecol* 1983;146:470–471.

13. Shime J, Mocarski EJM, Hastings D, Webb GD, McLaughlin PR. Congenital heart disease in pregnancy: short- and long-term implications. *Am J Obstet Gynecol* 1987;156:313–322.

14. Metcalfe J, McAnulty JH, Ueland K. Heart disease and pregnancy: physiology and management. Boston: *Little, Brown;* 1986;144–149.

15. Cola LM, Lavin JP. Pregnancy complicated by Marfan's syndrome with aortic arch dissection, subsequent aortic arch replacement and triple coronary artery bypass grafts. *J Reprod Med* 1985;30:685–688.

15a. Trirapepe L, Voci P, Pinto G, Brauneis S, Menichetti A. Anaesthesia for caesarean section in a Marfan patient with recurrent aortic dissection *Can J Anasth* 1996;43:1153–1155..

16. Barker SGE, Burnand KG. Retrograde iliac artery dissection in Marfan's syndrome. *J Cardiovasc Surg* 1989;30:953–954.

17. Smith VC, Eckenbrecht PD, Hankins DV, Leach CL. Marfan's syndrome, pregnancy and the cardiac surgeon. *Mil Med* 1989;154:404–406.

18. Maruyama T, Totsuka N, Akahane K, Yoshioka J, Shinohara M, Kouzu S, Fujii N, Yajima H, Shimotori M. Two cases of Marfan syndrome complicated with aortic dissection during pregnancy. *Kokyu To Junkan* 1993;41:85–88.

19. Chow SL. Acute aortic dissection in a patient with Marfan's syndrome complicated by gestational hypertension. *Med J Aust* 1993;159:760–762.

20. Wolinsky H. Effects of estrogen and progestogen treatment on the response of the aorta of male rats to hypertension. *Circ Res* 1972;30:341–349.

21. Elkayam U, Rose J, Jamison M. Vascular aneurysms and dissections during pregnancy. In: Elkayam U, Gleicher N, eds. *Cardiac Problems in Pregnancy.* 2nd ed. New York: Alan R. Liss; 1990;215–229.

22. Rossiter JP, Repke JT, Morales AJ, Murphy EA, Pyeritz RA. A prospective longitudinal evaluation of pregnancy in the Marfan syndrome. *Am J Obstet Gynecol* 1995;173:1599–1606.

23. Bailey MK, Hwu-Yun R, Baker JD III, Cooke JE, Conroy JM. Marfan syndrome in the parturient. *J Soc Can Med Assoc* 1989;85:327–330.

24. Gordon CF III, Johnson MD. Anesthetic management of the pregnant patient with Marfan syndrome. *J Clin Anesth* 1993;5:248–251.

25. Pyeritz RE. The Marfan syndrome. *Am Fam Physician* 1986;34:83–94.

26. Dietz HC, Pyeritz RE, Hall BD, Cadle RG, Hamosh A, Schwartz J, Meyers DA, Francomano CA. The Marfan syndrome locus: confirmation of assignment to chromosome 15 and identification of tightly linked markers at 15q15q-21.3. *Genomics* 1991;9:355–361.

27. Kainulainen K, Pulkkinen L, Savolainen A, Kaitila I, Peltonea L. Location on chromosome 15 of the gene defect causing Marfan syndrome. *N Engl J Med* 1990;323:935–939.

28. Lee B, Godfrey M, Vitale E, Hori H, Mattei M-G, Sarfarazi M, Tsipouras P, Ramirez F, Hollister DW. Linkage of Marfan syndrome and a phenotypically related disorder to two different fibrillin genes. *Nature* 1991;352:330–334.

29. Maslen CL, Corson GM, Maddox BK, Glanville RW, Sakai LY. Partial sequence of a candidate gene for the Marfan syndrome. *Nature* 1991;352:334–337.

30. Godfrey M, Vandemark N, Wang M, Velinov M, Wargswski D, Tsipouras P, Han J, Becker J, Robertson W, Droste S, Rao VH. Prenatal diagnosis and a donor splice site mutation in fibrillin in a family with Marfan syndrome. *Am J Hum Genet* 1993;53:472–480.

30a. Wang M, Mata J, Price CF, Iversen PL, Godfrey M. Prenatal and presymptomatic diagnosis of the Marfan symdrome using fluorescence PCR and an automated sequencer. *Prenat Diagn* 1995;15:499–507.

30b. Rantamaki T, Raghunath H, Karttunen L, Lonnqvist L, Chico A, Peltonen L. Prenatal diagnosis of Marfan sundrome: identification of a fibrillin-1 mutation in chorionic villus sample. *Prenat Diagn* 1995;15:1176–1181.

31. Murgatroyd F, Child A, Poloniecki J, Treasure T, Pumphrey C. Does routine echocardiographic measurement of the aortic root diameter help predict the risk of aortic dissection in the Marfan syndrome? *Eur Heart J* 1991;12:410. Abstract.

31a. Lipscomb KJ, Smith JC, Clarke B, Donnai P, Harris. Outcome of opregnancy in women with Marfan's sy,mdrome. *Br J Obstet Gynaeco* 1997;104:201–206.

32. Simpson IA, de Belder MA, Treasure T, Camm AJ, Pumphrey CW. Cardiac manifestations of Marfan's syndrome: improved evaluation by transesophageal echocardiography. *Br Heart J* 1993;69:104–108.

33. Gott VL, Pyeritz RE, Magovern GJ Jr, Cameron DE, McKusick VA. Surgical treatment of aneurysms of the ascending aorta in the Marfan syndrome: results of composite graft repair in 50 patients. *N Engl J Med* 1986;311:1070–1074.

34. Treasure T. Elective replacement of the aortic root in Marfan's syndrome. *Br Heart J* 1993;69:101–103. Editorial.

35. Katz NM, Collea JV, Moront MG, MacKenzie RD, Wallace RB. Aortic dissection during pregnancy: treatment by emergency cesarean section immediately followed by operative repair of the aortic dissection. *Am J Cardiol* 1984;54:699–701.

36. Pumphrey CW, Fay T, Weir I. Aortic dissection during pregnancy. *Br Heart J* 1986;55:106–108.

37. Snir E, Levinsky L, Salomon J, Findler M, Levy MJ, Vidne BA. Dissecting aortic aneurysm in pregnant women without Marfan disease. *Surg Gynecol Obstet* 1988;167:463–465.

38. Becker RM. Intracardiac surgery in pregnant women. *Ann Thorac Surg* 1983;36:453–458.

39. Ose L, McKusick VA. Prophylactive use of propranolol in the Marfan syndrome to prevent aortic dissection. *Birth Defects* 1977;13:163–169.

40. Pyeritz RE. Propranolol retards aortic root dilatation in the Marfan syndrome. *Circulation* 1983;68(suppl III):365. Abstract.

41. Zahka KG, Hensley C, Glesby M, Pyeritz RE. The impact of medical and surgical therapy on the cardiovascular prognosis of the Marfan syndrome in early childhood. *J Am College Cardiol* 1989;13:119A. Abstract.

42. Rosen SE, Roman MJ, Pini R, Kramer-Fox R, Devereux RB. The impact of chronic beta-blockade therapy on arterial compliance in the Marfan syndrome. *Am J Med Genet* 1993;47:157. Abstract.

43. Shores J, Berger KR, Murphy EA, Pyeritz RE. Progression of aortic dilatation and the benefit of long-term β-adrenergic blockade in Marfan's syndrome. *N Engl J Med* 1994;330: 1335–1341.

44. Eliahou HE, Silverbeg DS, Reisin E, Romen I, Mashiach S, Serr DM. Propranolol for the treatment of hypertension in pregnancy. *Br J Obstet Gynaecol* 1978;85:431–436.

45. Tcherdakoff PH, Colliard M, Berrard E, Kreft C, Dupay A, Bernaille JM. Propranolol in hypertension during pregnancy. *Br Med J* 1978;2:670.

46. Pruyn SC, Phelan JP, Buchanan GC. Long-term propranolol, therapy in pregnancy: maternal and fetal outcome. *Am J Obstet Gynecol* 1979;135:485–489.

47. Bott-Kanner G, Schweitzer A, Reisher SH, Kreft C, Dupay A, Bernaille JM. Propranolol and hydralazine in the management of essential hypertension in pregnancy. *Br J Obstet Gynaecol* 1980;87:110–114.

48. Bullock JL, Harris RE, Young R. Treatment of thyrotoxicosis during pregnancy and propranolol. *Am J Obstet Gynecol* 1975;121:242–245.

49. Langer A, Hung CT, McA'Nulty JA, et al. Adrenergic blockade: a new approach to hyperthyroidism in pregnancy. *Obstet Gynecol* 1974;44:181–186.

50. Turner GM, Oakley CM, Dixon HG. Management of pregnancy complicated by hypertrophic obstructive cardiomyopathy. *Br Med J* 1968;4:281–284.

51. Oakley GDG, McGarry K. Limb DG, Oakley CM. Management of pregnancy in patients with hypertrophic cardiomyopathy. *Br Med J* 1979;1:1749–1750.

52. Cottrill CM, McAllister RG Jr, Gettes L, Noonan JA. Propranolol therapy during pregnancy, labor and delivery: evidence for transplacental drug transfer and impaired neonatal drug disposition. *J Pediatr* 1977;91:812–814.

53. Schroeder JS, Harrison DC. Repeated cardioversion during pregnancy: treatment of refractory paroxysmal atrial tachycardia during three successive pregnancies. *Am J Cardiol* 1971;27:445–446.

54. Dumesic DA, Silverman NH, Tobias S, Golbus MS. Transplacental cardioversion of fetal supraventricular tachycardia with procainamide. *N Engl J Med* 1982;307:1128–1131.

55. Wladimiroff JW, Stewart PA. Fetal therapy: treatment of fetal cardiac arrhythmias. *Br J Hosp Med* 1985;34:134–140.

56. Kleineman CS, Copel JA, Weinstein EML, Santulli TV Jr, Hobbins JC. Treatment of fetal supraventricular tachyarrhythmias. *J Clin Ultrasound* 1985;13:265–273.

57. Teuscher A, Bossi E, Imhof P, Erb E, Stocker FP, Weber JW. Effect of propranolol on fetal tachycardia in diabetic pregnancy. *Am J Cardiol* 1978;42: 304–307.

58. Widerhorn J, Widerhorn ALM, Elkayam U. Cardiovascular pharmacotherapy in pregnancy. In: Gleicher N, Gall SA, Sibai BM, Elkayam U, Galbraith RM, Santo GE, eds. *Principles and Practice of Medical Therapy in Pregnancy*. 2nd ed. Norwalk, CT: Appleton & Lange, 1992;767–783.

59. O'Connor PC, Jick H, Hunter JR, Sterachis A, Madsen S. Propranolol and pregnancy outcome. *Lancet* 1981;2:1168.

60. Tursntall MB. The effect of propranolol on the onset of breathing at birth. *Br J Anaesthesia* 1969;41:792.

61. Barden TP, Stander RW. Effects of adrenergic blocking agents and catecholamines in human pregnancy. *Am J Obstet Gynecol* 1968;102:226–235.

62. Hogstedt S, Lindeberg S, Axelsson O, Lindmark, G, Rane A, Sandstrom B, Lindberg BS. A prospective controlled trial of metoprolol–hydralazine treatment in hypertension during pregnancy. *Acta Obstet Gynecol Scand* 1985;64: 505–510.

63. Sandstrom B. Adrenergic beta-receptor blockers in hypertension of pregnancy. *Clin Exp Hypertension* 1982;B1:127–141.

64. Liedholm H. Atenolol in the treatment of hypertension of pregnancy. *Drugs* 1983;25:206–211.

65. Lardoux H, Gerard J, Blazquez G, Chouty F, Flouvat B. Hypertension in pregnancy: evaluation of two beta blockers, atenolol and labetolol. *Eur Heart J* 1983;4(suppl G):35–40.

66. Karlberg B, Lundberg D, Aberg H. Excretion of propranolol in human breast milk. *Acta Pharmacol Toxicol* 1974;34:222–224

67. Bauer JH, Pape B, Zajicek J, Groshong T. Propranolol in human plasma and breast milk. *Am J Cardiol* 1979;43:860–862.

68. Liedholm H, Melander A, Bitzeu PO, Helm G, Lonnerholm G, Mattiasson I, Nilsson B, Wahlin-Boll E. Accumulation of atenolol and metoprolol in human breast milk. *Eur J Clin Pharmacol* 1981;20:229–231.

69. Cigarroa JE, Isselbacher EM, DeSanctis RW, Eagle KA. Diagnostic imaging in the evaluation of suspected aortic dissection. *N Engl J Med* 1993;328:35–43.

70. Stoddard MF, Longaker RA, Vuocolo LM, Dawkins PR. Transesophageal echocardiography in the pregnant patient. *Am Heart J* 1992;124:785–787.

71. Pruzinsky MS, Katz NM, Green CE, Salter LF. Isolated descending thoracic aortic aneurysm in Marfan's syndrome. *Am J Cardiol* 1988;61:1159–1160.

72. Elser AD. Does MR imaging have any known effects on the developing fetus? *Am J Roentgenol* 1994;162:1493.

73. Beers GL. Biological effects of weak electromagnetic field from 0 Hz to 200 MHz: A survey of the literature with special emphasis on possible magnetic resonance effect. *Magn Resonance Imaging* 1989;7:309–331.

74. Elkayam U, Gleicher N. Diagnostic approaches to maternal heart disease. In: Elkayam U, Gleicher N, eds. *Cardiac Problems in Pregnancy*. 2nd ed. New York: Alan R. Liss; 1990;41–45.

75. Eagle KA, DeSanctis R. Diseases of the aorta. In: Braunwald E, ed. *Heart Disease*. 4th ed. Philadelphia: WB Saunders; 1992;1528–1557.

76. Donaldson LB, DeAlverez RP. The Marfan syndrome and pregnancy. *Am J Obstet Gynecol* 1965;62:629–641.

77. Elias S, Berkowitz RL. The Marfan syndrome and pregnancy. *Obstet Gynecol* 1976;47:358–361.

78. Elkayam U, Gleicher N. Hemodynamics and cardiac function during normal pregnancy and the puerperium. In Elkayam U, Gleicher N, eds. *Cardiac Problems in Pregnancy*. 2nd ed. New York: Alan R. Liss. 1990;5–24.

79. Irons DW, Pollard KP. Post partum hemorrhage secondary to Marfan's disease of the uterine vasculature. *Br J Obstet Gynaecol* 1993;100:279–281.

19

THROMBOEMBOLIC DISEASE IN PREGNANCY

Karen Rosene-Montella, MD, and Jeffrey Ginsberg, MD

INTRODUCTION

Venous thromboembolism (VTE) during pregnancy remains a leading cause of maternal morbidity and mortality.[1-3] Pregnancy confers a five- to sixfold increase in the risk of venous thrombosis, but the absolute risk in an individual patient is difficult to determine. Diagnosis and management of thromboembolism during pregnancy, although critical, are problematic for several reasons. First, anatomic and physiologic changes that occur during pregnancy and postpartum not only increase the risk of VTE, but also have the potential to cause false-positive tests for deep vein thrombosis (DVT). Second, there is often an understandable reluctance to expose the fetus to the radiation associated with the necessary diagnostic procedures and to teratogens, such as the agents used in maternal oral anticoagulant therapy. Third, there is a paucity of published results from clinical trials establishing valid recommendations for the diagnosis, prevention, and treatment of VTE. Despite these limitations, several key studies have elucidated important information about the epidemiology, diagnosis, and management of pregnant patients with suspected or established venous thromboembolism. In this chapter, we summarize these studies and provide recommendations for diagnostic and management strategies as well as for future clinical trials.

EPIDEMIOLOGY OF VENOUS THROMBOEMBOLISM DURING PREGNANCY

Incidence

The true incidence of VTE during pregnancy and the postpartum period is unknown. There is reasonable evidence that the incidence of thrombosis during pregnancy is increased compared to the nonpregnant state.[4-7] Studies using radiographic documentation place the combined risk of DVT and pulmonary embolism (PE) at 0.5–3.0 per thousand deliveries.[8,9] The subclinical risk may be higher, a 3% incidence of asymptomatic calf DVT postpartum was found in one study using fibrinogen scanning.[10] A personal history of prior thrombosis and/or the presence of an underlying hypercoagulable state may significantly increase the incidence of VTE in given individuals.

Location

There is an overwhelming propensity for DVT during pregnancy to occur in the left leg.[11,12] In a study of 60 consecutive pregnant women presenting with a first episode of DVT, 58 episodes occurred in the left leg and the remaining two were bilateral; there were no cases of isolated right leg DVT.[12] Although the reason for this finding is not known, one plausible explanation is the exaggerated compression by the right iliac artery on the left common iliac vein during pregnancy.[13]

Timing

Although venous stasis in the legs is greatest near term, there is no evidence that the incidence of VTE during pregnancy is highest during the third trimester. Further, there are studies reporting that the incidence of VTE during pregnancy is equally distributed during the three trimesters. In the study cited earlier in which 60 consecutive women with a first episode of DVT were evaluated, 13 (22%) developed DVT during the first trimester, 28 (47%) during the second

Cardiac Problems in Pregnancy, Third Edition
Edited by Uri Elkayam, MD, and Norbert Gleicher, MD
Copyright © 1998 by Wiley-Liss, Inc. ISBN 0-471-16358-9

trimester, and 19 (32%) during the third trimester.[12] A similar distribution has been reported in other studies.[14,15] In the largest series, comprising 170,000 pregnant women with no prior thromboembolic events, 75% of the DVTs occurred antepartum, and half of these occurred by 15 weeks of gestation.[8] The proportion of women presenting with nonthrombotic causes of leg pain and swelling is highest during the third trimester, probably because of the obstruction of venous outflow due to the enlarging gravid uterus.[11] There is evidence from some studies that the risk of VTE in a given patient is higher postpartum than antepartum, particularly after cesarean section.[16–18] In the study of 170,000 pregnancies just referred to, 66% of PEs occurred postpartum, and 80% of these occurred following cesarean section; as noted above, however, the majority (75%) of the DVTs occurred antepartum.[8]

Predisposing Factors

Pregnancy itself may predispose a woman to thrombosis resulting from a combination of factors: stasis, due to both hormonal and mechanical effects, and hypercoagulability, due to increased clotting factors, decreased fibrinolysis, and decreased fibrinolytic proteins (Table 19.1). Other factors predisposing to thrombosis include cesarean section or other operative procedures, obesity, prolonged hospitalization, and advanced age and parity.[4,14,19,20] Similar to the general non-pregnant population, it is likely that women with congenital deficiencies of antithrombin III, protein C, or protein S, resistance to activated protein C, or the persistent presence of antiphospholipid antibodies have an increased risk of thromboembolic disease during pregnancy and the puerperium.[18,21,22] In women of childbearing age who develop thrombosis, strong consideration should be given to testing for coagulation abnormalities.

Women with previous venous thromboembolism probably have an increased risk for recurrent VTE during pregnancy and the puerperium.[23–26] Retrospective studies have reported the incidence of recurrent thrombembolic disease to be as high as 15%.[25,26] The risk of recurrence in a questionnaire study[25] was not affected by the etiology of the initial event. Women whose initial event was associated with oral contraceptive use had the same risk as those whose initial event was unprovoked. Prophylaxis trials aimed at decreasing this recurrence risk are limited. The results of one randomized trial reported that one of 20 untreated patients (5%) with previous thrombosis developed recurrent antepartum VTE,[24] whereas a cohort study (published in letter form) reported that none of 59 pregnant patients with previous VTE developed antepartum recurrence.[23] Conclusions from these studies are limited by the relatively small numbers and lack of description of the inception cohorts. In addition, the majority of prophylactic failures occurred in the presence of underlying hypercoagulable state and may have in part been due

TABLE 19.1   Change in Coagulation During Pregnancy

Factor[a]	Effect of Pregnancy
Platelets	Slow decrease during pregnancy; further decrease after delivery; marked increase 3rd–5th postpartum day; increase in aggregation
Fibrinogen	Marked increase during antepartum period; no change during labor, but prompt decrease after placental delivery: increase to predelivery level by day 3–5 with slow decrease thereafter
Prothrombin	No change
V	Immediate increase after placental delivery; slow decrease to normal by day 7
VII, IX, X	Progressive increase during pregnancy; gradual decrease in puerperium
VIII	Progressive increase during pregnancy; decrease after delivery with secondary increase then gradual decrease
XI, XIII	Decrease during pregnancy; gradual increase to normal in puerperium
Fibrin split products	Increase in labor and immediately postpartum
Fibrinolysis	Decrease after first trimester with prompt increase to normal after delivery
Protein S	Gradual decrease in free levels during pregnancy
Protein C	No change
Antithrombin III	No change or decrease; decrease in preeclampsia and nephrotic syndrome

[a]Clotting factors return to normal by 8 weeks postpartum.

to inadequate heparin dosing. Trials in nonpregnant patients have demonstrated a greater recurrence risk among patients with true idiopathic VTE than in patients with reversible risk factors, suggesting that the former groups be treated differently with respect to prophylaxis for VTE.[27] It is difficult to extrapolate these data to pregnant women because pregnancy itself may represent a reversible risk factor, one that obviously cannot be removed for the period in question. Controlled clinical trials are required to establish the true incidence of recurrent VTE in pregnant women, as well as the safety and efficacy of anticoagulant therapy in preventing recurrent VTE.

Conclusions

Based on the results of the cited studies of the epidemiology of VTE during pregnancy, several clinically useful conclusions can be made:

1. Pregnant women presenting with symptoms in the left leg are far more likely to have DVT than women presenting with symptoms in the right leg. Nevertheless, DVT does occur in the right leg; thus when a woman presents with symptoms in the right leg, investigation with objective tests is necessary.
2. Women presenting with suspected DVT during the first two trimesters are more likely to have DVT than women presenting during the third trimester; the incidence of nonthrombotic causes of leg symptoms is highest during the third trimester.
3. Pregnancy predisposes patients to venous thromboembolism.

DIAGNOSIS OF DVT AND PULMONARY EMBOLISM DURING PREGNANCY

Diagnostic Problems Associated with Pregnancy

Clinical diagnosis of DVT and PE is somewhat unreliable in nonpregnant patients[28,29] and is further complicated during pregnancy. First, nonthrombotic causes of leg swelling and pain are common during pregnancy.[11] In support of this, a recent cohort study reported that the majority of pregnant patients evaluated with objective tests for clinically suspected DVT during pregnancy (leg pain and swelling) did not have DVT.[11] Second, the compressive effects of the gravid uterus can make interpretation of diagnostic studies difficult.[30] In particular, tests such as impedance plethysmography (IPG), which is sensitive to venous outflow obstruction, may give false-positive results during pregnancy.[30] Third, there is a clinical impression that isolated iliac vein thrombosis, which is not detected by routine diagnostic modalities, occurs with increased frequently during pregnancy.[31-36] Special efforts

(see below) should be made to detect iliac vein thrombosis when it is suspected, because tests such as compression ultrasonography (CUS) are insensitive to this condition. Fourth, the mean age of pregnant patients presenting with clinically suspected PE is lower than the mean age of nonpregnant patients presenting with clinically suspected PE. One implication of this difference is that pregnant patients are less likely than nonpregnant patients to have comorbid conditions, such as chronic airflow limitation, that cause lung scan abnormalities. Additionally, pregnant patients may look clinically "well" and be more likely to have a normal alveolar–aterial oxygen gradient. A recent retrospective review of 17 pregnant patients with documented PE demonstrated normal alveolar–arterial gradients in 58%.[36a]

Radiologic Procedures During Pregnancy

There is considerable reluctance on the part of pregnant women and their physicians to expose the fetus to radiation. This reluctance has the potential to lead to suboptimal care, particularly for the management of patients with suspected PE in whom lung scanning may be the pivotal diagnostic test.

The risks to the fetus associated with the radiologic procedures used to make the diagnosis of maternal DVT and PE were estimated in 1989.[37] This study critically reviewed the literature concerning the adverse effects to the fetus with radiation exposure and attempted to arrive at the amounts of radiation absorbed by the fetus with the procedures (Table 19.2). A small increase in the relative risk of childhood cancer is the only adverse experience suggested with low dose (< 5 rads total pregnancy exposure) in utero radiation exposure. Further, with the available procedures, it is possible to recommend to women with suspected DVT or PE diagnostic approaches that are associated with fetal radiation exposure of less than 0.5 rad. The risk of such exposure is small both in relative and absolute terms and strongly supports the judicious use of radiologic procedure when indicated clinically (see below).

Clinical Diagnosis of DVT

Pregnant patients must receive accurate, objective testing to confirm the diagnosis of DVT, to avoid unnecessary use of anticoagulant therapy, to avoid adverse consequences of untreated DVT, and to assess recurrence risk. Although objective tests are mandatory, the assignment of a pretest likelihood is useful when the estimate is interpreted in conjunction with the results of a noninvasive test.[38] This can be done by determining the signs and symptoms at presentation, the presence of risk factors for VTE, and the presence of an alternate diagnosis for the patients presentation. For example, a patient who presents with typical clinical features of DVT, has one or more risk factors for DVT (e.g., cesarean section), and has no alternate explanation for their symptoms

TABLE 19.2 Estimated Fetal Exposure to Radiation from Various Diagnostic Procedures

Procedure	Estimated Fetal Radiation Exposure (rads)
Bilateral venography without abdominal shield	0.628
Unilateral venography without abdominal shield	0.314
Limited venography	<0.050
Pulmonary angiography via femoral route	0.221–0.374
Pulmonary angiography via brachial route	<0.050
Perfusion lung scan using ^{99m}Tc-MAA	
3 mCi	0.018
1–2 mCi	0.006–0.012
Ventilation lung scan	
using ^{133}Xe	0.004–0.019
using ^{99m}Tc-DTPA	0.007–0.035
using ^{99m}Tc SC	0.001–0.005
Radioisotope venography using ^{99m}Tc	0.001–0.005
^{125}I-fibrinogen leg scanning	2.000
Chest X-ray	<0.001

Abbreviations: ^{99m}Tc-MAA, ^{99m}Tc-DTPA, radioisotope in macroaggregated albumin, diethylenetriomine-pentaacetic acid.

^{99m}Tc-MAA: → Technetium labelled macro aggregiated albumin.

^{99m}Tc-DTPA: → Technetium labelled diethylenetriamamine Pentaacetic acid. Technetium Pentate (Generic name)

^{99m}Tc SC: → Technetium labelled sulfur colloid.

^{133}XE → Xenon 133 (Isotope itself) (gas).

(e.g., cellulitis, baker's cyst) would be considered to have a high pretest probability. In a recent study in nonpregnant patients, the combination of a high pretest likelihood and a normal IPG at presentation was associated with a posttest likelihood of DVT of 55% necessitating further investigation with CUS or venography in such patients.

Distribution of Thrombi in Patients with DVT

In nonpregnant patients with DVT, approximately 80% of the thrombi occur in the proximal (popliteal or more proximal) veins, with or without calf DVT, whereas the remaining 20% are isolated in the calf veins.[39] Of the patients with isolated calf vein thrombosis, approximately 30% develop clinically important extension into the proximal veins within 7–14 days of presentation; the remaining 70% will not extend and do not require treatment.[39] An approach that has been validated in large clinical trials of nonpregnant patients is the performance of a test that is sensitive to proximal DVT, such as IPG[39–41] or CUS.[42,43] If the initial test is normal, it should be repeated on a serial basis over 7–14 days. A test that re-

mains normal indicates that the patient had either no DVT or calf DVT that did not extend into the proximal veins, and thus anticoagulant therapy can be withheld safely. Using the IPG, this diagnostic approach has been validated in pregnant patients. However, it is likely that not enough patients with actual calf DVT in this study had treatment withheld to permit the drawing of definite conclusions about the safety of withholding treatment in this instance.[11] Therefore, if calf vein is found during pregnancy, the current recommendation is to fully anticoagulate.

Objective Tests for the Diagnostic of DVT

The three tests that are useful for the diagnosis of DVT during pregnancy are impedance plethysmography (IPG), compression ultrasonography (CUS), and contrast venography. Studies published before 1990 reported that the IPG was highly sensitive to proximal DVT in symptomatic outpatients.[39–41] However, two recent studies from McMaster University have reported sensitivities of IPG for proximal DVT that are much lower than those found in earlier studies.[44,45] It may be that the contemporary studies showed lower sensitivity because the patients with DVT who were referred to McMaster-based hospitals had minimal symptoms. Asymptomatic patients with proximal DVT have a higher likelihood of having small, nonocclusive popliteal vein thrombi that are less likely to cause an abnormal IPG. The safety of withholding anticoagulant therapy if serial IPG remains normal has been demonstrated in several clinical trials, including one trial in 152 pregnant patients tested in the left lateral decubitus posterior.[11,39–41] However, the results of another study, in which a new IPG machine was used, reported an unacceptably high event rate (including deaths) in patients with normal IPG.[46] It is not clear whether the high event rate reported in this study was due to the IPG machine used. Therefore, because of concerns about the sensitivity of IPG for nonocclusive proximal DVT and the high event rate in the one clinical management study of IPG in nonpregnant patients, it seems reasonable to take several precautions. If IPG is used as the initial test and is normal, further testing (with CUS or venography) should be performed in patients with a high pretest probability, whereas strict adherence to the performance of serial IPG should be maintained in patients with a moderate or low pretest probability. Alternatively, until it is clear that anticoagulation can be safely withheld when IPG is used, CUS can be selected as the initial test.

Compression ultrasonography has been developed over the last few years and is highly sensitive to proximal DVT in symptomatic outpatients.[42] The most reliable finding is that of a noncompressible venous segment that has a very high positive predictive value for DVT.[42,43] In nonpregnant patients, the safety of withholding anticoagulant therapy if serial CUS remains normal within 7 days of presentation has been demonstrated in a large clinical trial.[43] Although CUS is highly sensitive and specific for thrombi in the common femoral, superficial femoral, and popliteal veins, it may be insensitive to isolated iliac DVT. Magnetic resonance imaging (MRI) or indirect approaches such as measuring the diameter of the iliac vein or applying pulsed Doppler sampling of the common femoral vein may be useful in detecting iliac vein thrombosis. These methods should be considered when a patient presents with a clinical suspicion of iliac vein thrombosis (severe back or flank pain and/or cramping abdominal pain in conjunction with unilateral leg pain and swelling of the entire extremity).[32–36]

Adequately performed contrast venography is the reference standard for the diagnosis of DVT.[47] In the pregnant patient, a limited venogram can be performed using pelvic and abdominal shielding with a lead-containing apron.[37] The shielding minimizes the amount of radiation absorbed by the fetus but does not allow visualization of the iliac vein. If iliac vein thrombosis is suspected and CUS is nondiagnostic, consideration should be given to magnetic resonance imaging. A recent prospective study that included 54 cases with confirmatory venograms demonstrated 100% sensitivity and 92% specificity of MRI. With ultrasonography of the thigh and computed tomography of the pelvis, as in reference studies involving an additional 79 patients, MRI has a sensitivity of 97% and a specificity of 95%.[48]

A Practical Approach for the Diagnosis of Clinically Suspected DVT During Pregnancy

Either CUS or IPG can be used as the initial diagnostic test in pregnant patients with clinically suspected DVT (Figs. 19.1 and 19.2). If neither test is available, consideration should be given to transferring the patient to a facility that offers one or both. It is the opinion of the authors that compression ultrasonography is the noninvasive test of choice because it is more sensitive and specific for DVT than IPG in nonpregnant patients and is likely to be more sensitive and specific in pregnant patients.[43] However, because CUS has not been evaluated in a large cohort of pregnant patients and IPG has, we believe that the use of either test is reasonable in pregnant patients.

If CUS is positive at any time during pregnancy, DVT can be diagnosed. If the test is normal, calf DVT or isolated iliac DVT may still be the cause of the patient's symptoms. If the latter is clinically suspected (see above), the indirect methods of evaluating the iliac vein by duplex and/or MRI should be considered. Alternatively, IPG, which should be sensitive to iliac DVT, or venography can be performed. If iliac DVT is not a consideration and the initial CUS is normal, serial CUS over 7–14 days or, alternatively, a limited venogram can be performed.

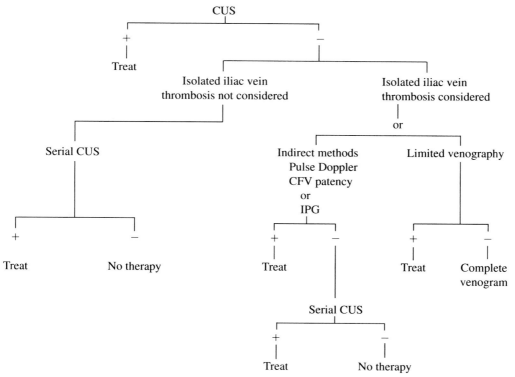

Figure 19.1   Diagnosis by means of CUS of clinically suspected DVT during pregnancy. Abbreviations: CFV, CUS, compression ultrasonography; IPG, impedance plethysmography.

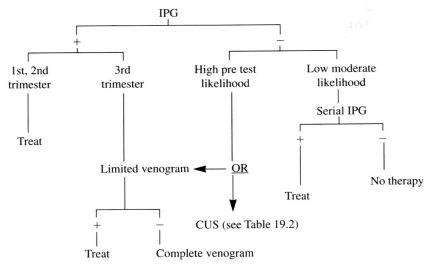

Figure 19.2   Diagnosis by means of impedance plethysmography of clinically suspected deep vein thrombosis during pregnancy. Abbreviation as in Figure 19.1.

If IPG is used and is abnormal during the first two trimesters, DVT can be diagnosed. An abnormal IPG during the third trimester, however, may be falsely positive because of outflow obstruction by the gravid uterus; repeating the test in a lateral position may identify such patients.[30] If the test remains abnormal in spite of this maneuver, further investigation with a limited venogram or CUS should be considered; if these procedures return abnormal results, DVT can be diagnosed. If a limited venogram is normal, a complete venogram should be performed in case the patient has iliac vein thrombosis. If the initial IPG is negative, serial IPG testing should be performed over 7–14 days. If the test becomes abnormal, DVT can be diagnosed, whereas if the test remains normal, clinically important DVT can be excluded. The recent concern about the sensitivity of IPG for proximal DVT prompts consideration to performing venography or CUS in a patient with a high pretest probability of DVT (most pregnant patients) and a normal initial IPG; if CUS is performed, the diagnostic algorithm in Figure 19.1 can be followed.

If neither IPG nor CUS is available, or if there is a strong clinical suspicion of calf DVT, venography should be performed, limited at first and, if normal, complete venography. It is our belief that the risks associated with clinical diagnosis and unnecessary or suboptimal treatment are greater than the risks of performing contrast venography.

Objective Tests for the Diagnosis of Pulmonary Embolism

The tests that are useful in patients with clinically suspected PE include ventilation–perfusion lung scanning, pulmonary angiography, and the tests described above for the diagnosis of DVT. The latter are used because this condition frequent-

ly is present in patients with PE, and the detection of DVT in a patient with clinically suspected PE provides grounds to make a diagnosis of PE and to treat with anticoagulation, without performing further tests.[49]

Although pulmonary angiography is the reference standard for the diagnosis of PE,[49] it is invasive and expensive and, therefore, is reserved for situations in which less invasive tests are not diagnostic. Fetal radiation exposure should be minimized by using the brachial or internal jugular approach when possible; when the femoral approach is used, fluoroscopy over the pelvis should be avoided.

Ventilation–perfusion lung scanning is currently the test of choice in patients with clinically suspected PE. When technetium macroaggregates of human albumin are used for the perfusion scan and radioactive technetium sulfur colloid for the ventilation scan, the amount of radiation absorbed by the fetus is well under 50 mrad.[37] In some centers, a perfusion scan is performed alone as the initial test. The advantage of this approach is that if the perfusion scan is normal, PE can be excluded without the need for a ventilation scan. If the perfusion scan is abnormal, however, the patient must wait 24 hours before the ventilation scan can be performed. In nonpregnant patients, a normal perfusion scan [segmental or large (> 75% of the segment) subsegmental perfusion defect with normal ventilation] has a positive predictive value of approximately 90%.[49,50] Approximately half of nonpregnant patients with suspected PE have neither a normal perfusion scan nor a high probability lung scan; this type of scan result can be referred to as a nondiagnostic, nonhigh, indeterminant, or intermediate probability.[49–51] The prevalence of PE in patients with a nonhigh lung scan pattern is approximately 25%.[49–51] In patients with nonhigh lung scans, therefore, further investigation is indicated.

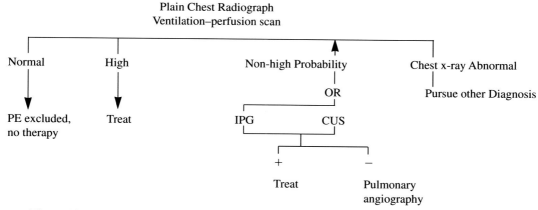

Figure 19.3 Diagnosis of clinically suspected pulmonary embolism (PE) during pregnancy by means of ventilation–perfusion scan/plain chest radiograph. Abbreviations as in Figure 19.1.

A Practical Approach to the Diagnosis of Clinically Suspected Pulmonary Embolism During Pregnancy

An approach to the pregnant patient with clinically suspected PE is summarized in Figure 19.3. A chest radiograph is useful to exclude conditions such as fractured rib, pneumonia, or pneumothorax, which can cause symptoms similar to those seen with PE. Both a ventilation and a perfusion lung scan are recommended. In some centers, it may be easier to perform a noninvasive test of the legs, such as IPG or CUS. These tests are useful only if positive, since it is reasonable to diagnose PE in a patient with suspected PE who has an abnormal IPG or CUS. However, a normal IPG or CUS result does not exclude PE, and further investigation with a lung scan is indicated if a normal result is indeed obtained.

If the results of the perfusion scan are normal, PE can be excluded. If the lung scan is high probability, PE can be diagnosed. In patients with nonhigh lung scans, further investigation is indicated. IPG or CUS can be performed and the patient treated if the results are abnormal. However, if the results are normal, a pulmonary angiogram should be strongly considered. An approach that has been validated in nonpregnant patients with nonhigh scans is the performance of serial IPG over 14 days and, if the results are normal, withholding anticoagulants.[52] This approach has not been evaluated in pregnant patients and, therefore, cannot be recommended.

ANTICOAGULANT THERAPY DURING PREGNANCY

The agents currently available for the prevention and treatment of VTE are heparin-like compounds [unfractionated heparin, low molecular weight (LMW) heparins, and heparinoids] and coumarin derivatives.

Safety of Anticoagulant Therapy During Pregnancy

Fetal Complications of Anticoagulants During Pregnancy
There are two potential fetal complications of maternal anticoagulant therapy: teratogenicity and bleeding (see also Chapter 33). Heparin, which does not cross the placenta, does not have the potential to cause fetal bleeding or teratogenicity, although bleeding at the uteroplacental junction is possible.[53] Two recent studies strongly suggest that heparin therapy is safe for the fetus.[54,55]

In contrast to heparin, coumarin derivatives cross the placenta and have the potential for causing both bleeding in the fetus and teratogenicity.[56,57] Coumarin derivatives can cause an embryopathy, which consists of nasal hypoplasia and/or stippled epiphyses after in utero exposure to oral anticoagulants during the first trimester of pregnancy, as well as central nervous system abnormalities, which can occur after exposure to such drugs during any trimester.[56] It is possible that oral anticoagulants are safe during the first 6 weeks of gestation, but there is a risk of embryopathy if coumarin derivatives are taken between 6 and 12 weeks of gestation.[58] In addition, these oral anticoagulants cause an anticoagulant effect in the fetus that is a concern, particularly at the time of delivery.

Maternal Complications of Anticoagulant Therapy During Pregnancy
In one cohort study, the rate of major bleeding in pregnant patients treated with heparin therapy was 2%,[55] which is consistent with the reported rates of bleeding associated with heparin therapy in nonpregnant patients[59] and with warfarin therapy[60] when used for the treatment of DVT. The risk of bleeding with heparin is dose dependent.[55] Adjusted-dose (therapeutic) subcutaneous heparin can cause a persistent anticoagulant effect at the time of delivery.[61] In a recent cohort study, an anticoagulant effect persisted for up to 28 hours after the last injection of adjusted-dose (30,000–40,000

units/day) subcutaneous heparin, frequently resulting in deliveries that were complicated by a prolonged activated partial thromboplastin time (APTT).[61] Although this prolongation of APTT results was not associated with significant bleeding, most anesthetists felt it to be a contraindication to epidural anesthesia. The mechanism for this is unclear; to avoid an anticoagulant effect during delivery in women receiving adjusted-dose subcutaneous heparin therapy, however, a reasonable approach is to discontinue heparin 12–24 hours prior to elective induction of labor, depending on the heparin dose and degree of prolongation of the APTT. The use of intravenous heparin in high risk patients may be indicated during this interval. If spontaneous labor occurs in women receiving adjusted-dose subcutaneous heparin, careful monitoring of the APTT is required. If the APTT is prolonged near delivery, the use of protamine sulfate will neutralize plasma heparin and may reduce the risk of bleeding without adverse effects on the fetus.

Long-term heparin therapy may be associated with osteoporosis. Four recent studies provide estimates of the risk of heparin-induced osteoporosis with long-term heparin.[62–65] The results of these studies show that although the risk of symptomatic fractures is low (2% or less), a subclinical reduction in bone density, detected radiographically, occurs in up to one-third of women receiving long-term heparin therapy. The radiologic effects of heparin are at least partly reversible. It is unknown whether women with reduced bone density due to heparin are predisposed to future fractures.

The mechanism for heparin-induced osteoporosis is not known. It was initially thought that the risk of osteoporosis might depend on the dose of heparin used and the duration of heparin therapy. At least one prospective study, however, found no correlation between degree of decrease in bone density and dose or duration of heparin therapy, although this conclusion is limited by the small number of patients studied. Since none of the studies has addressed separately patients with prior heparin exposure, it is unclear whether prior exposure is a risk factor for subsequent osteopenia.

Some women report considerable discomfort associated with twice daily self-administered heparin injections. Therefore, the use of an indwelling subcutaneous Teflon catheter, which must be replaced weekly, can be considered in pregnant patients who require long-term heparin and have considerable discomfort with injections.[66]

Use of Anticoagulants in the Nursing Mother   Heparin is not secreted into breast milk and can be administered safely to nursing mothers.[67] There have been two convincing reports that warfarin does not induce an anticoagulant effect in the breast-fed infant when the drug is administrated to a nursing mother.[68,69] Therefore, we recommend the use of warfarin in women who require anticoagulant therapy postpartum; breast feeding may be encouraged in these women.

Low Molecular Weight Heparin and Heparinoids   There is accumulating experience with the use of LMW heparin and heparinoids both in pregnant and nonpregnant patients for the prevention and treatment of DVT.[70–77] Based on the results of large clinical trials in nonpregnant patients, there is good evidence that LMW heparin and heparinoids are at least as good as (and perhaps better than) unfractionated heparin for the treatment of patients with acute proximal DVT[71,72] and for the prevention of DVT in patients who undergo surgery.[49]

There is also evidence that LMW heparin and heparinoids do not cross the placenta.[78–80] These agents have potential advantages over unfractionated heparin during pregnancy because they cause less heparin-induced thrombocytopenia,[81] have the potential for once-daily administration, and may have a lower risk of heparin-induced osteoporosis.[77] However, these agents are more expensive than unfractionated heparin and, therefore, until further comparative clinical trials, comparing their efficacy and safety with unfractionated heparin have been performed, there is insufficient evidence to endorse them for routine clinical use in pregnant patients who require anticoagulant therapy. A recent review of the published experience with LMW heparin in obstetrics and gynecology suggests that they are both safe and effective for thromboprophylaxis and treatment of VTE in pregnancy.[2]

Efficacy of Anticoagulant Therapy During Pregnancy

There is a paucity of data about the efficacy of anticoagulants for the prevention and treatment of VTE during pregnancy. Accordingly, the recommendations about the use of these agents during pregnancy is based largely on extrapolations from data in nonpregnant patients and on case reports and case series of pregnant patients. Based on the safety data, heparin is the drug of choice for the prevention and treatments of VTE during pregnancy.

The results of a large randomized trial in nonpregnant patients have shown that a regimen consisting of full-dose intravenous (IV) heparin, followed by 3 months of 12-hourly subcutaneous (SC) heparin therapy, in doses adjusted to prolong a midinterval APPT into the therapeutic range (adjusted-dose SC heparin), is safe and effective.[59] Therefore, it seems reasonable to extrapolate these results to pregnant patients with DVT and PE and use IV heparin followed by at least 3 months of adjusted-dose SC heparin. A reduction in SC heparin after 3 months to a dose that produces a lesser prolongation of the APTT is worth considering in women with smaller thrombi who present early during pregnancy, to minimize the risks of bleeding and osteoporosis. However, there are no trials comparing efficacy of therapeutic adjusted dose versus prophylactic doses in the prevention of recurrence later in pregnancy.

Pregnant women with previous VTE are probably at increased risk for recurrent VTE, but the magnitude of the risk is unknown.[23,24] It is possible that the risk of recurrence is higher in women with previous idiopathic VTE than in women who developed VTE in association with a transient risk factor.[75,76,82] However, none of the available data in pregnant patients have stratified risk of recurrence according to the circumstance of the prior event. It is not clear whether women who developed VTE in association with a previous pregnancy are at a relatively higher risk of recurrence.

There are two reasonable approaches to pregnant patients with previous VTE: active prophylaxis with heparin, and clinical surveillance with or without regular noninvasive tests such as CUS or IPG. Subcutaneous heparin (5000 U 12-hourly) is effective and safe for the prevention of VTE in high risk nonpregnant patients,[83] and its use has been recommended in pregnant patients.[84] However, there is a concern about the use of the same dose of SC heparin every 12 hours because it does not reliably produce detectable heparin levels during the second and third trimesters.[85] Case reports of prior prophylaxis failures occurred at this dose or in the presence of a hypercoagulable defect. There also exist published data on the use of more intense heparin therapy, in doses that produce plasma heparin levels (measured as antifactor X_a activity) of 0.1–0.2 U/mL, and the recurrence rate is reportedly less that 3%,[55] This approach is more likely to produce a consistent anticoagulant effect throughout pregnancy; the use of heparin (5000 U every 12 hours throughout pregnancy), on the other hand, is likely to result in variable (and, in many patients, undetectable) plasma levels of heparin.

In pregnant women with previous VTE who cannot or refuse to use heparin, an alternative is clinical surveillance with or without regular IPG or CUS.[23] The safety of this approach has never been demonstrated in a large clinical trial and is dependent on detection and treatment of VTE before the development of major PE. Some authors deem this approach to be reasonable in women who developed VTE in association with a previous risk factor (e.g., leg fracture), since the risk of recurrence may be lower in these patients. The uncertainty in approach to pregnant women with previous VTE underlines the urgent need to perform appropriate clinical trials.

SUMMARY AND RECOMMENDATIONS

Diagnosis of VTE

Principles of the Diagnosis of DTE and PE

1. It is mandatory to investigate women who present with symptoms suggestive of DVT or PE.
2. It is reasonable to err on the side of "overinvestigation." It is the strong opinion of the authors that when indicated, the performance of diagnostic procedures that expose the fetus to radiation should be undertaken rather that risk a wrong diagnosis. Prior to the performance of any such procedures, the risks and benefits should be discussed with the patient.
3. Although diagnostic algorithms for nonpregnant patients with suspected DVT or PE have been validated in large clinical trials, there are few such trials in pregnant patients.
4. Special efforts, such as lead shielding the pelvis, performing pulmonary angiography via the brachial or internal jugular route, and reducing the dose of radioisotope used to perform perfusion lung scans, should be made to minimize radiation exposure to the fetus.

Diagnosis of DVT

1. We recommended the use of compression ultrasonography (CUS) as the initial diagnostic test in patients with clinically suspected DVT. The algorithm in Figure 18.1 should be used.
2. Suspicion of isolated iliac DVT indicates further testing with IPG, venography, pulsed Doppler, or MRI, or evaluation of the patency of iliac veins by ultrasound.
3. IPG is a reasonable alternative to CUS as the initial test (Fig. 19.2).
4. If CUS and IPG are not available, the patient should be transferred to a facility offering these tests or contrast venography should be performed.

Diagnosis of PE

1. A lung scan should be performed in pregnant patients with suspected PE (Fig. 19.3).
2. If the lung scan is normal, PE can be excluded, whereas if the lung scan shows a high probability, PE can be diagnosed in the majority of patients. In a patient with a nondiagnostic lung scan, further investigation is indicated, beginning with a test to detect DVT. If testing for DVT is normal, pulmonary angiography should be performed.
3. It is reasonable to perform IPG or duplex before a lung scan, but these tests are helpful only if positive. If the results are normal, PE cannot be excluded, and it is important to perform a lung scan.

Prevention and Treatment of DVT and PE
Prevention of Venous Thromboembolism

1. In pregnant women with a history of VTE, we recommend heparin prophylaxis or surveillance.

2. We recommend adjusted-dose subcutaneous heparin therapy throughout pregnancy for women for whom it has been decided to use long-term oral anticoagulant therapy, such as (a) patients with antiphospholipid antibodies, resistance to activated protein C, or a deficiency of protein C or S or antithrombin III (AT III) and history of VTE, and (b) those with recurrent VTE.

3. In AT III-deficient women who are treated with heparin throughout pregnancy, the use of antithrombin III concentrates around the time of delivery is a reasonable alternative to (or in combination with) heparin.

4. In pregnant women with previous VTE, a workup for thrombophilia (deficiencies of protein C, protein S, or AT III, as well as resistance to activated protein C and antiphospholipid antibodies) should be considered, particularly in women with recurrent VTE and/or a strong family history of VTE. Interpretation of protein S and AT III results can be difficult during pregnancy. Pregnant women without congenital deficiencies have a normal physiologic decrease in free protein S levels.[86,87] Antithrombin III levels are lowered by heparin therapy and in certain conditions such as preeclampsia. If the assays for hypercoagulability are suggestive of thrombophilia, adjusted-dose SC heparin should be administered throughout pregnancy.

5. In pregnant women with previous VTE and no thrombophilia, the need for heparin and the optimum heparin regimen remain to be determined. In a recent debate on this issue, a consensus among experts was not reached. Some authors use unfractionated heparin (5000 U every 12 h SC, throughout pregnancy), whereas other use unfractionated heparin (5000 U every 12 h SC) during the first trimester and higher doses (7500 U 12-hourly or adjusted to produce plasma heparin levels of 0.1–0.2 U/mL) during the second and third trimesters. Until the results of comparative trials are available, either regimen seems reasonable.

6. LMW heparins and heparinoids are likely to be effective and safe as alternatives to unfractionated heparin.

7. Alternatively, clinical surveillance, with or without regular IPG or CUS, can be performed to detect DVT.

8. Controlled clinical trials, to determine the relative efficacy and safely of heparin for the prevention of recurrent VTE, and to clarify the optimal heparin regimen, are needed urgently.

9. To avoid an anticoagulant effect from adjusted-dose subcutaneous heparin at the time of delivery, heparin can be discontinued or substituted with IV heparin near term and, 12–24 hours later, labor can be induced electively. If labor is prolonged, or if there is a major concern about recurrent VTE, an injection of prophylactic SC heparin or dextran can be given.[10] Because of the risk of recurrence is high postpartum, especially for PE or following cesarean section, and oral anticoagulants are not excreted in breast milk, postpartum therapy should include heparin, followed by 4–6 weeks of warfarin [in doses adjusted to prolong the international normalized ratio (INR) to 2.0–3.0]. Heparin should be started only after hemostasis is secure, and the dose and rate of administration of heparin should be individualized. To avoid warfarin-induced skin necrosis, full heparinization is necessary in the presence of protein C or S deficiency until adequate anticoagulation has been achieved on oral anticoagulants.

Treatment of VTE During Pregnancy

1. In patients who develop venous thrombosis during pregnancy, full doses of IV heparin should be given for at least 5 days, followed by adjusted-dose SC heparin for at least 3 months to prolong the PTT into the therapeutic range.

2. One approach to avoiding an anticoagulant effect from subcutaneous heparin at delivery is to discontinue SC heparin near term and, 12–24 hours later, to induce labor electively.

3. Both heparin (full-dose IV or adjusted-dose SC) and warfarin should be started postpartum as soon as hemostasis is achieved; when a therapeutic INR of 2.0–3.0 is achieved, heparin can be discontinued and warfarin administered for at least 4–6 weeks.

Planned Pregnancy During Long-Term Oral Anticoagulant Therapy

1. When pregnancy is planned in patients receiving long-term oral anticoagulant therapy, two options can be considered: Frequent pregnancy tests can be performed and heparin substituted for warfarin when pregnancy is achieved, or warfarin can be replaced with heparin before conception is attempted. Both approaches have limitations. The first assumes that warfarin is safe during the first 6 weeks of gestation, whereas the second increases the duration of exposure to heparin and, therefore, the risk of osteoporosis.

2. It is important to discuss these approaches with women prior to conception.

SUMMARY

It is clear that further prospective trials to elucidate the risk of venous thromboembolism during pregnancy and to arrive at an optimum treatment and prophylaxis regimen are urgently needed. When VTE is suspected during pregnancy, it is imperative that a rigorous diagnostic strategy be employed to ensure that treatment is not withheld unnecessarily. It is important to recognize during the evaluation that isolated iliac vein thrombosis may occur. Moreover, the clinical diagnosis of pulmonary embolism may be even more subtle in the pregnant population, owing to the absence of comorbid conditions. Low molecular weight heparins hold promise for both prophylaxis and treatment of VTE in pregnancy.

REFERENCES

1. Kaunitz AM, Hughes JM, Grimes DA, Smith JC, Rochat RW, Kafrissen ME. Causes of maternal mortality in the U.S. *Obstet Gynecol* 1985;65:605–612.

2. Fejgin MD, Lourwood DL. Low molecular weight heparins and their use in obstetrics and gynecology. *Obstet Gynecol Survey* 1994;46:424–431.

3. Her Majesty's Stationery Office. Report on confidential inquiries into maternal deaths for England and Wales, 1979–1981. London: HMSO; 1986.

4. Bonnar J. Venous thromboembolism and pregnancy. *Clin Obstet Gynecol* 1981;8:455–473.

5. Rothbard MJ, Gluck D, Stone ML. Anticoagulation therapy in antepartum pulmonary embolism. *New York State J Med* 1976;76:582–584.

6. Villasanta U. Thromboembolic disease in pregnancy. *Am J Obstet Gynecol* 1965;93:142–160.

7. Nordstrom M, Lindblad B, Bergqvist D, Kjellstrom T. A prospective study of the incidence of deep vein thrombosis within a defined urban population. *J Intern Med* 1992;232: 155–160.

8. Rutherford S, Montoro M, McGehee W, Strong T. Thormboembolic disease associated with pregnancy: an 11 year review. *Am J Obstet Gynecol* 1991;164:286. Abstract.

9. Dixon JE. Pregnancies complicated by previous thromboembolic disease. *Br J Hosp Med* 1987;37:449–452.

10. Friend JR, Kakkar VV. The diagnosis of deep venous thrombosis in the puerperium. *J Obstet Gynaecol Br Commonw* 1970;77:820–823.

11. Hull RD, Raskob GE, Carter CJ. Serial impedance plethysmography in pregnant patients with clinically suspected deep-vein thrombosis. Clinical validity and negative findings. *Ann Intern Med* 1990;112:663–667.

12. Ginsberg JS, Brill-Edwards P, Burrows RF, Bona R, Prandoni P, Buller HR, Lensing A. Venous Thrombosis during pregnancy: leg and trimester of presentation. *Thromb Haemostasis* 1992;67:519–520.

13. Cockett FB, Thomas ML, Negus D. Iliac vein compression. Its relation to iliofemoral thrombosis and the post-thrombotic syndrome. *Br Med J* 1967;2:14–19.

14. Hellgren M, Nygards EB. Long term therapy with subcutaneous heparin during pregnancy. *Gynecol Obstet Invest* 1982;13:76–89.

15. Bergqvist A, Bergqvist D, Hallbook T. Diagnosis and treatment of patients with deep vein thrombosis during pregnancy. A prospective study. *Acta Obstet Gynecol Scand* 1983;62: 443–448.

16. Bergqvist A, Bergqvist D, Hallbook T. Acute deep vein thrombosis after caesarian section. *Acta Obstet Gynecol Scand* 1979;58:473–476.

17. Laros RK, Alger LS. Thromboembolism and pregnancy. *Clin Obstet Gynecol* 1979;22:871–888.

18. Conard J, Horellou MH, Van Dreden P, Lecompte T, Samama M. Thrombosis and pregnancy in congenital deficiencies in AT III, protein C or protein S: study of 78 women. *Thromb Haemostasis* 1990;63:319–320.

19. de Swiet M. Thromboembolism. *Clin Haematol* 1985;14: 643–661.

20. Moseley P, Kerstein M. Pregnancy and thrombophlebitis. *Surg Gynecol Obstet* 1980;150:593–599.

21. Long AA, Ginsberg JS, Brill Edwards P, Johnston M, Turner C, Denburg JA, Bensen WG, Cividino A, Andrew M, Hirsh J. The relationship of antiphospholipid antibodies to thromboembolic disease in systemic lupus erythematosus: A cross-sectional study. *Thromb Haemostasis* 1991;66:520–524.

22. Svensson PJ, Dahlback B. Resistance to activated protein C as basis for venous thrombosis. *N Engl J Med* 1994;330:517–522.

23. de Swiet M, Floyd E, Letsky E. Low risk of recurrent thromboembolism in pregnancy. *Br J Hosp Med* 1987;38:264.

24. Howell R, Fidler J, Letsky E, de Swiet M. The risk of antenatal subcutaneous heparin prophylaxis: a controlled trial. *Br J Obstet Gynaecol* 1983;90:1124–1128.

25. Badaracco MA, Vessey M. Recurrent venous thromboembolic disease and use of oral contraceptives. *Br Med J* 1994;1: 215–217.

26. Tengborn L, Bergqvist D, Matzsch T, Bergqvist A, Hedner U. Recurrent thromboembolism in pregnancy and puerperium. Is there a need for thromboprophylaxis? *Am J Obstet Gynecol* 1989;160:90–94.

27. Levine MN, Hirsh J, Gent M, Turpie AG, Weitz J, Ginsberg J, Geerths W, LeClerc J, Neemeh J, Powers P, Plovella F. Optimal direction of oral anticoagulant therapy: a randomized trial comparing four weeks with three months of warfarin in patients with proximal deep vein thrombosis *Thromb Haemostasis* 1995;74:606–711.

28. McLachlin J, Richard T, Paterson JC. An evaluation of clinical signs in the diagnosis of venous thrombosis. *Arch Surg* 1962;85:738–743.

29. Haeger K. Problems of acute deep venous thrombosis. I. The interpretation of signs and symptoms. *Angiology* 1969;20: 219–224.

30. Ginsberg JS, Turner C, Brill-Edwards P, Harrison L, Hirsh J. Pseudothrombosis in pregnancy. *Can Med Assoc J* 1988;139: 409–410.

31. Effeney DJ. Ileofemoral venous thrombosis: real-time ultrasound diagnosis, normal criteria, and clinical application. *Radiology* 1983;150:787–792.

32. Gree IA, Barry J, Mackon N, Allan PL. Diagnosis of deep venous thrombosis in pregnancy: a new role for diagnostic ultrasound. *Br J Obstet Gynaecol* 1990;97:53–57.

33. Frede TE, Ruthberg BN. Sonographic demonstration of iliac vein thrombosis in the maternity patient. *J Ultrasound Med* 1988;7:33–37.

34. Polak JF, O'Leary DH. Deep vein thrombosis in pregnancy: noninvasive diagnosis. *Radiology* 1989;166:377–379.

35. Ankri I, Seebacher J, Ancri D. Diagnostic non invasif des thrombses veineuses profondes par echo Doppler. *J Mal Vasc* 1988;11:325–329.

36. Abbitt PL, Thiagarajah S. Venous sonography for pregnancy related thrombosis: case report. *Virginia Med* 1989;116:277–278.

36a. Powrie RO, Larson L, Rosene-Montella K, Abarca M, Barbouri L, Trujillo N. Aveolar-arterial gradient is not useful as a diagnostic test for acute pulmonary embolism associated with pregnancy. *Am J Obstet Gynecol* in press 1997).

37. Ginsberg JS, Hirsh J, Rinabow AJ, Coates G. Risks to the fetus of radiologic procedures used in the diagnosis of maternal venous thromboembolic disease. *Thromb Haemostasis* 1989;61:189–196.

38. Wells PS, Hirsh J, Anderson DR, Foster G, Kearon C, Weitz J, D'Ovidio R, Cogo A, Prandoni P, Girolami, Ginsberg JS. Accuracy of the clinical assessment of deep vein thrombosis: complementary role with noninvasive testing. *Lancet* 1995;345:1326–1330.

39. Hull RD, Hirsh J, Carter CJ, Jay RM, Ockelford PA, Buller HR, Turpie AG, Powers P, Kinch D, Dodd PE, Gill GJ, LeClerc JR, Gent M.. Diagnostic efficacy of impedance plethysmography for clinically suspected deep-vein thrombosis: a randomized trial. *Ann Intern Med* 1985;102:21–28.

40. Huisman MV, Buller HR, ten Cate JW, Vreeken J. Serial impedance plethysmography for suspected deep venous thrombosis in outpatients. *N Engl J Med* 1986;314:823–828.

41. Husiman MV, Buller HR, ten Cate JW, Heijermans HS, Van Der Laan J, Van Maanen DJ. Management of clinically suspected acute venous thrombosis in outpatients with serial impedance plethysmography in a community hospital setting. *Arch Intern Med* 1989;149:511–513.

42. Lensing AWA, Prandoni P, Brandjes D, Huisman PM, Vigo M, Tomasella G, Kiekt J, Wouter Ten Cate J, Huisman MV, Buller HR. Detection of deep-vein thrombosis by real-time B-mode ultrasonography. *N Engl J Med* 1989;320:342–345.

43. Heijboer H, Buller HR, Lensing AWA, Turpie AGG, Colly LP, ten Cate JW. A comparison of real time compression ultrasonography with impedance plethysmography for the diagnosis of deep-vein thrombosis in symptomatic outpatients. *N Engl J Med* 1993;329:1365–1369.

44. Anderson DR, Lensing AW, Wells PS, Levine MN, Weitz JI, Hirsh J. Limitations of impedance plethysmography in the diagnosis of clinically suspected deep-vein thrombosis. *Ann Intern Med* 1993;118:25–30.

45. Ginsberg JS, Wells PS, Hirsh J, Panju AA, Patel A, Malone DE, McGinnis J, Stevens P, Brill-Edwards P. Reevaluation of the sensitivity of impedance plethysmography for the detection of proximal deep vein thrombosis. *Arch Intern Med* 1994;154;1930–1933.

46. Prandoni P, Lensing AWA, Buller HR, Carta M, Vigo M, Cogo A, Cuppini S, ten Cate JW. Failure of computerized impedance plethysmography in the diagnostic management of patients with clinically suspected deep-vein thrombosis. *Thromb Haemostasis* 1991;65:233–236.

47. Rabinov K, Paulin S. Roentgen diagnosis of venous thrombosis in the leg. *Arch Surg* 1972;104:134–144.

48. Spritzer CE, Norconk JJ, Sostman HD, Coleman RE. Detection of deep venous thrombosis by magnetic resonance imaging. *Chest* 1993;104:54–60.

49. Hull RD, Hirsh J, Carter CJ, Jay RM, Dodd PE, Ockelfield PA, Coates G, Grill GJ, Turpie AG, Doyle DJ, Buller HR, Raskob GE. Pulmonary angiography, ventilation lung scanning and venography for clinically suspected pulmonary embolism with abnormal perfusion lung scan. *Ann Intern Med* 1983;98:891–899.

50. Hull RD, Raskob GE, Hirsh J. The diagnosis of clinically suspected pulmonary embolism. Practical approaches. *Chest* 1986;89:417s–424s.

51. PIOPED. Value of the ventilation/perfusion scan in acute pulmonary embolism. Results of the prospective investigation of pulmonary embolism diagnosis (PIOPED). *JAMA* 1990;263:2753–2759.

52. Hull RD, Raskob GE, Ginsberg JS, Panju AA, Brill-Edwards P, Coates G, Pineo GF. A noninvasive strategy for the treatment of patients with suspected pulmonary embolism. *Arch Intern Med* 1994;154:289–297.

53. Flessa HC, Kapstrom AB, Glueck MJ, Will JJ. Placental transport of heparin. *Am J Obstet Gynecol* 1965;93:570–573.

54. Ginsberg JS, Hirsh J, Turner DC, Levine MN, Burrows R. Risks to the fetus of anticoagulant therapy during pregnancy. *Thromb Haemostasis* 1989;61:197–203.

55. Ginsberg JS, Kowalchuck G, Hirsh J, Brill-Edwards P, Burrows R. Heparin therapy during pregnancy: risks to the fetus and mother. *Arch Intern Med* 1989;149:2233–2236.

56. Hall JAG, Paul RM, Wilson KM. Maternal and fetal sequelae of anticoagulation during pregnancy. *Am J Med* 1980;68:122–140.

57. Becker MH, Genvesser NB, Finegold M, Miranda D, Spackman T. Chondrodysplasia punctata: is maternal warfarin a factor? *Am J Dis Child* 1975;129:356–359.

58. Iturbe-Alessio I, Fonseca MC, Mutchinik O, Santos MA, Zajarias A, Salazar E. Risks of anticoagulant therapy in pregnant women with artificial heart valves. *N Engl J Med* 1986;315:1390–1393.

59. Hull R, Delmore T, Carter C, Hirsh J, Genton E, Gent M, Turpie G, McLaughlin D. Adjusted subcutaneous heparin versus warfarin sodium in the long-term treatment of venous thrombosis. *N Engl J Med* 1982;306:189–194.

60. Hull, Hirsh J, Jay R, Carter C, England C, Gent M, Turpie AGG, McLoughlin D, Dodd P, Thomas M, Raskob G, Ockelford P. Different intensities of oral anticoagulant therapy in the treatment of proximal-vein thrombosis. *N Engl J Med* 1982;307:1676–1681.

61. Anderson DR, Ginsberg, Burrows R, Brill-Edwards P. Subcutaneous heparin therapy during pregnancy: a need for concern at the time of delivery. *Thromb Haemostasis* 1991;63:248–250.

62. Ginsberg JS, Kowalchuck G, Hirsh J, Brill-Edwards P, Burrows R, Coates G, Webber C. Heparin effect on bone density. *Thromb Haemostasis* 1990;64:286–289.

63. Dahlman T, Lindvall N, Hellgren M. Osteopenia in pregnancy during long-term heparin treatment: a radiologic study postpartum. *Br J Obstet Gynaecol* 1990;97:221–228.

64. Barbour LA, Kick SD, Steiner JF, LoVerde MF, Heddleston LN, Lear JL, Baron AE, Barton PL. A prospective study of heparin-induced osteoporosis using bone densitometry. *Am J Obstet Gynecol* 1994;170:862–869.

65. Dahlman TC. Osteoporotic fractures and the recurrence of thromboembolism during pregnancy and the puerperium in 184 women undergoing thromboprophylaxis with heparin. *Am J Obstet Gynecol* 1993;168:1265–1278.

66. Anderson DR, Ginsberg JS, Brill-Edwards P, Demers C, Burrows RF, Hirsh J. The use of an indwelling Teflon catheter for subcutaneous heparin administration during pregnancy. *Arch Intern Med* 1993;153:841–844.

67. O'Reilly R. Anticoagulant, antithrombotic and thrombolytic drugs. In: Gilman AG, et al, eds. *The Pharmacologic Basis of Therapeutics.* 6th ed. New York: Macmillan, 1980;347–1366.

68. Orme ML, Lewis PJ, de Swiet M, Serlin MJ, Sibeon R, Baty JD, Breckenridge M. May mothers given warfarin breast-feed their infants? *Br Med J* 1977;1:1564–1565.

69. McKenna R, Cale ER, Vasan U. Is warfarin sodium contraindicated in the lactating mother? *J Pediatr* 1983;103:3225–3227.

70. Gillis S, Shushan A, Eldor A. Use of low molecular weight heparin for prophylaxis and treatment of thromboembolism in pregnancy. *Int J Gynecol Obstet* 1992;39:297–301.

71. Melissari E, Parker CJ, Wilson NV, Monte G, Kanthou C, Pemberton KD, Nicolaides KH, Barrett JJ, Kakkar VV. Use of low molecular weight heparin in pregnancy. *Thromb Haemostasis* 1992;68:652–656.

72. Hull RD, Raskob GE, Pineo GF, Green D, Trowbridge AA, Elliott CG, Lerner RG, Hall J, Sparling T, Brettell R, Norton J, Carter CJ, George R, Merli G, Ward J, Mayo W, Rosenbloom D, Brant R. Subcutaneous low-molecular-weight heparin compared with continuous intravenous heparin in the treatment of proximal-vein thrombosis. *N Engl J Med* 1992;326:975–982.

73. Hull RD, Raskob GE, Coates G, Panju AA. Clinical validity of a normal perfusion lung scan in patients with suspected pulmonary embolism. *Chest* 1990;97:23–26.

74. Hull R, Raskob G, Pineo G, Rosenbloom D, Evans W, Mallory T, Anquist K, Smith F, Hughes G, Green D, Elliott CG, Panju A, Brant R. A comparison of subcutaneous low-molecular-weight heparin with warfarin sodium for prophylaxis against deep-vein thrombosis after hip or knee implantation. *N Engl J Med* 1993;329:1370–1376.

75. Prandoni P, Lensing AWA, Buller HR, Carta M, Cogo A, Vigo M, Casara D, Ruol A, ten Cate JW. Comparison of subcutaneous low-molecular-weight heparin with intravenous standard heparin in proximal deep-vein thrombosis. *Lancet* 1992;339:441–445.

76. Prandoni P, Lensing AWA, Buller HR, Cogo A, Prins MH, Cattelan AM, Cuppini S, Noventa F, ten Cate JW. Deep-vein thrombosis and the incidence of subsequent symptomatic cancer. *N Engl J Med* 1992;327:1128–1133.

77. Monreal M, Lafoz E, Olive A, del Rio L, Vedia C. Comparison of subcutaneous unfractionated heparin with a low molecular weight heparin (Fragmin) in patients with venous thromboembolism and contraindications for coumarin. *Thromb Haemostasis* 1994;71:7–11.

78. Forestier F, Daffos F, Capella-Pavlovsky M. Low molecular weight heparin (PK 10169) does not cross the placenta during the second trimester of pregnancy: study by direct fetal blood sampling under ultrasound. *Thromb Res* 1984;34:557–560.

79. Forestier F, Daffos F, Rainaut M, Toulemonde F. Low molecular weight heparin (CY 216) does not cross the placenta during the third trimester of pregnancy. *Thromb Haemostasis* 1987;57:234.

80. Omri A, Delaloye JF, Andersen H, Bachmann F. Low molecular weight heparin NOVO (LHN-1) does not cross the placenta during the second trimester of pregnancy. *Thromb Haemostasis* 1989;61:55–56.

81. Warkentin TE, Levine MN, Roberts RS, Gent M, Horsewood P, Kelton JG. Heparin-induced thrombocytopenia is more common with unfractionated heparin than with low molecular weight heparin. *Thromb Haemostasis* 1993;89:1336. Abstract.

82. Research Committee of the British Thoracic Society. Optimum duration of anticoagulation for deep-vein thrombosis and pulmonary embolism. *Lancet* 1992;340:873–876.

83. Collins R, Scrimgeour A, Yusof S, Peto. Reduction in fatal pulmonary embolism and venous thrombosis by perioperative administration of subcutaneous heparin. Overview of results of randomized trials in general, orthopedic, and urologic surgery. *N Engl J Med* 1988;318:1162–1173.

84. Ginsberg JS, Hirsh J. Use of antithromboitc agents during pregnancy. *Chest* 1992;102:385s–390s.

85. Dahlman TC, Hellgren MSE, Blomback M. Thrombosis prophylaxis in pregnancy with the use of subcutaneous heparin adjusted by monitoring heparin concentration in plasma. *Am J Obstet Gynecol* 1989;161:420–425.

86. Comp PC, Thurnau GR, Welsh J, Esmon CT. Functional and immunologic protein S levels are decreased during pregnancy. *Blood* 1986;68:881–885.

87. de Boer K, ten Cate JW, Sturk W, Borm JJ, Treffers PE. Enhanced thrombin generation in normal and hypertensive pregnancy. *Am J Obstet Gynecol* 1989;160:95–100.

20

TAKAYASU'S ARTERITIS AND PREGNANCY

URI ELKAYAM, MD, AND AFSHAN HAMEED, MD

INTRODUCTION

Takayasu's arteritis (TA) is a chronic inflammatory arteriopathy of unknown origin involving the aorta and its main branches.[1] The disease is most common in Asian countries; increasing reports from Europe, Africa, the Middle East, and North America, however, indicate the occurrence of TA worldwide.[2] The main clinical features as well as distribution of arterial involvement may vary somewhat in different geographical regions.[1] The incidence of TA in North America is 1.2–2.6 cases per million per year.[2] The disease is found with a high prevalence among women and during the childbearing age in most geographical areas. Ninety-seven percent of 60 patients recently reported in the United States were female, and the median age was 25 years.[3] Similarly, the average age at the time of onset of symptoms in a group of 57 Japanese patients was reported to be 22 years.[4]

The clinical presentation of TA has been described by means of triphasic pattern.[1] The early stage of the disease (phase I) is an inflammatory period involving a granulomatous arteritis of the aorta and its branches. This stage may present with fever, night sweats, arthralgias, fatigue, and loss of appetite. Phase II involves vessel inflammation and is presented symptomatically as vessel tenderness and pain. The chronic phase (phase III) occurs months or years after the acute phase and is related to arteritic changes including intimal proliferation, degeneration of medial elastic fibers, and involvement of the vasa vasorum, eventually leading to narrowings and aneurysms of the aorta, its main branches, and the pulmonary arterial tree (Fig. 20.1). Common physical findings include decreased or absent pulses, unequal limb blood pressure, and bruits. Blood vessels of the neck and upper limbs are more commonly involved than those of the low-er limbs. Frequency of clinical features of TA at presentation and during the course of the disease is shown in Figure 20.2. Symptoms are usually limb claudication and organ ischemia. Since stenoses progress slowly, collateral blood flow develops and patients may be asymptomatic. Secondary complications include hypertension (mainly due to narrowing of the aorta and the renal arteries), aortic regurgitation, abdominal and myocardial ischemia, congestive heart failure, cerebrovascular accidents, and pulmonary hypertension. The most common skin manifestations of TA are erythema nodosum and pyoderma gangrenosum.

It should be noted that TA has a chronic recurrent pattern, and both active inflammatory and fibrotic changes may be present concomitantly. There is no laboratory test that is diagnostic for TA. The erythrocyte sedimentation rate (ESR) has been considered as an excellent marker for the activity of the disease.[5] In a more recent study, however, Kerr et al[3] found an elevated ESR in 72% of patients with active disease and also in 56% of patients in remission, indicating a low specificity for elevated ESR as a marker of disease activity.

Long-term survival in patients with TA is usually high. Ishikawa and Maetani[6] reported an 83% survival in 120 Japanese patients followed for 15 years, Zheng et al[4a] reported 5-year and 10-year survival rates of 93 and 91%, respectively, of 530 Chinese patients followed on the average for 8 years, and Kerr et al reported a 97% survival in 60 patients followed for 5 years.[3] Predictors of poor outcome include the presence of aneurysms, hypertension, cardiac involvement, extensive disease and severe functional disability.[1] Long-term morbidity is not uncommon and is related to the disease itself, its secondary manifestations, and complications of medical as well as surgical treatment. Forty-seven percent of patients reported by Kerr et al[3] were placed on

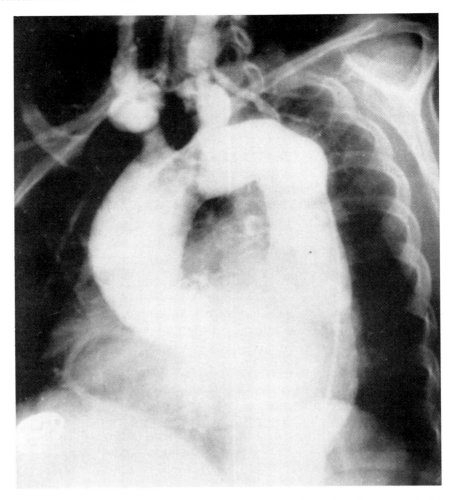

Figure 20.1   Aortogram of a 26-year-old woman with Takayasu's arteritis who presented with massive hemoptysis during her 28th week of pregnancy: areas of stenosis and aneurysmal dilations involving the aorta and both carotid arteries are visible. (From Rocha et al, *Chest* 1994;106:1619–1622 with permission.)

permanent disability because they were unable to consistently perform full daily functions.

TREATMENT

The administration of high dose glucocorticoids is the primary therapy for active, inflammatory TA. Approximately 40% of patients, however, may fail to respond to steroid therapy, and those who do not improve will require additional cytotoxic therapy.[1] Both cyclophosphamide and methotrexate have been used with some success. According to Kerr,[1] methotrexate should receive preferential consideration. Both percutaneous angioplasty and surgery have been applied for correction of vascular complications in patients with TA. Surgery is usually used to correct renovascular hypertension or cerebral ischemia, or to repair aortic or branch aneurysms,

or to treat aortic regurgitation or coronary artery disease. The outcome of surgery is most favorable when disease is quiescent; such treatment should therefore be postponed when possible until active inflammation is subsided. A high degree of success has been reported recently with the use of angioplasty for stenotic lesions of the aorta and renal arteries.[7]

PREGNANCY AND TAKAYASU'S ARTERITIS

A higher prevalence of TA in young women[1–3] indicates the likelihood of pregnancy in patients with this disease. In a review of the literature, we have been able to find reports published in the last decade in pregnancies in over 50 patients with TA.[3,8–32] In an attempt to evaluate the influence of pregnancy on the morbid condition of TA, Matsumura et al[21] followed C-reactive protein (CRP) scores in 20 pregnancies and

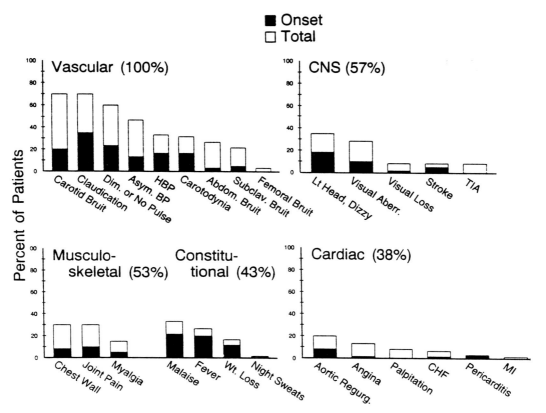

Figure 20.2 Frequency of clinical features of Takayasu's arteritis at presentation and during the course of disease: Abdom, abdominal; Aberr, aberration; Asym, asymmetric; CHF, congestive heart failure; CNS, central nervous system; Dim, diminished; HBP, high blood pressure; Lt, light; MI, myocardial infarction; Regurg, regurgitation; Subclav, subclavian; TIA, transient ischemic attack; Wt, weight. (From Kerr et al, *Ann Intern Med* 1994;120:919–929 with permission.)

evaluated their digital plethysmograms. This study demonstrated favorable change in CRP scores and digital plethysmography during pregnancy, indicating improvement rather than deterioration of TA with pregnancy.

Early experience showed no maternal or fetal complications during 30 pregnancies in 13 Chinese patients with TA.[33] In contrast, Ishikawa and Matsuura[34] found gestation to be more eventful in 27 Japanese patients with a total of 33 pregnancies. Marked increase in systolic blood pressure during uterine contractions was found in 10 pregnant women. In one of these patients, a cerebral hemorrhage occurred just before delivery. The majority of more recently published cases (Table 20.1) have reported favorable maternal outcome. However, increased blood pressure during pregnancy[1,16] and the development of heart failure[13] have been described.

Although fetal growth retardation[9,10,21,31,32] as well as premature labor and delivery[9,13,31] are commonly found, a favorable fetal outcome has been reported in most cases. Neonatal death on the seventh day postpartum was reported in one case of a woman whose pregnancy was complicated

by toxemia; cesarean section had to be performed because of fetal distress at 31 weeks.[19] The mode of delivery applied in the majority of patients was vaginal, and forceps often were used to expedite the second stage of labor.[3,9–32] Cesarean section deliveries have been performed mainly for obstetrical indications or for maternal hypertension and vascular disorders.[9,11,23,25,31] In the great majority of cases, abdominal delivery has been performed under epidural anesthesia with favorable results. Hypotension, nausea, and lightheadedness secondary to this form of anesthesia were reported in one case and required the use of ephedrine.[25]

RECOMMENDATIONS

The management of pregnancy in a patient with TA should be initiated prior to conception by careful evaluation of the disease status with special emphasis on patient's functional capacity, cardiac function, and the presence and severity of systemic hypertension. Patients should be informed of the

TABLE 20.1 Selected Reports of Pregnancy in Cases with Takayasu's Arteritis

Ref: First Author (year)	Age (years)	Obstetrical History	Clinical Presentation	Treatment	Vascular Involvement	Outcome Maternal	Outcome Fetal	Mode of Delivery
Chua[10] (1987)	27		S/p acute myocardial infarction, s/p angioplasty of right renal artery stenosis, diminished right carotid pulse, absent right upper limb pulse. BP 130/90 mmHg.	Propranolol for hypertension	Subtotal occlusion of right renal artery; total occlusion of right coronary artery	Uncomplicated	Live 2420 g female; uncomplicated	Elective C-section at 38 weeks under general anesthesia
Giles[11] (1987)	34	G_7P_2 Ab_4	Diminished femoral pulses, dyspnea. BP 140/90 mmHg	Oxprenolol and hydralazine for hypertension	Bicuspid aortic valve	Uncomplicated	Live 860 g male; d/c without problems	C-section at 26 weeks after spontaneous rupture of membranes
Graca[9] (1987)	27	G_2P_0 Ab_0	Absent upper limb pulses; diminished carotid pulses with bruits bilaterally; systolic murmurs over precordial, carotid, and abdominal areas. BP arms, 125/100 mmHg; legs, 240/140 mmHg.	Diazepam, methyldopa, hydralazine, mepindolol for hypertension	Complete occlusion of left renal artery, narrowing of aorta below the emergence of celiac trunk; total occlusion of both subclavian arteries	Poor control of BP in spite of medications	Live-born 910 g, uncomplicated; growth retardation after 28 weeks	Elective C-section at 30 weeks due to intrauterine growth retardation
Railton[12] (1988) Case 1	30	G_2P_1	Weak right brachial pulse		90% right brachiocephalic artery stenosis; total block of both carotids and left subclavian arteries; suprarenal aortic aneurysm	Uncomplicated	Live 2920 g infant; uncomplicated	Induced vaginal delivery at 38 weeks
Case 2	22	G_1	S/p unsuccessful subclavian bypass operation, AR due to rheumatic valvular disease, left arm claudication.	NA	Total occlusion of left subclavian and carotid arteries; narrowing of thoracic aorta	Uncomplicated	Live 3150 g infant; uncomplicated	Induced vaginal delivery at 39 weeks
Case 3	24	G_4P_0	Impalpable arm pulses, s/p unsuccessful right axillofemoral bypass.	NA	NA	Uncomplicated	Live 3900 g infant; uncomplicated	Vaginal delivery with forceps at term
Case 4	37	G_3P_2	Absent left arm pulses, MR secondary to rheumatic valvular disease. BP 180/80 mmHG.			Uncomplicated	Live 3400 g infant; uncomplicated	Vaginal delivery at term
Winn[13] (1988)	23	G_1	S/p aortorenal artery bypass and left common carotid and vertebral endarterectomy. Bilateral carotid and	Methyldopa, hydralazine, and propranolol for hyperten-	Totally occluded bilateral subclavian arteries; severe stenosis of left common carotid; superior mesenteric and left renal arteries	Pulmonary edema several hours postpartum; in	Live infant; uncomplicated	Premature labor at 33 weeks controlled with terbutaline induction with pito-

(continued)

Reference (year)	Age	Gravida/Para	Clinical presentation	Treatment	Angiographic findings	Maternal outcome	Neonatal outcome	Delivery
			subclavian bruits; nearly impalpable brachial and radial pulses. Brachial BP 150/80 mm Hg; central BP (femoral), 210/120 mm Hg.	sion; hemodynamic monitoring during labor and delivery, diuresis and ACE inhibition postpartum		good condition 5 days after delivery		cin 24 h later due to decelerations of FHR; vaginal delivery with low outlet forceps; discharged
Crofts[16] (1991)	23	G_1	Hypertension and proteinuria after 30 weeks.	Intravenous hydralazine to control hypertension postpartum	Total occlusion of right subclavian and brachial arteries; distal occlusion of left subclavian artery	Increased BP to 200/92 mm Hg during labor	Live 2230 g male; transient, mild respiratory distress	Induced vaginal delivery with forceps under epidural anesthesia at 36 weeks
McKay[22] (1992)	20	G_2P_1	S/p CVA with hemiplegia and expressive aphasia. BP = right arm, 80/60 mm Hg; left thigh, 140/80 mm Hg; right femoral artery, 180/95 mm Hg.		Total right and brachycephalic artery occlusion; subtotal left carotid artery occlusion	Favorable; discharged home 2 days post-delivery	Live 3422 g female; uncomplicated	Induced vaginal delivery with low outlet forceps under epidural anesthesia
Beillin[25] (1993)	24	G_2P_1	Absent pulses in left upper extremity; decreased carotid pulses bilaterally. Asymptomatic throughout pregnancy.		Alternating areas of stenosis and dilatation in aortic arch and left subclavian artery, thoracic aorta, abdominal aorta, and renal arteries	Hypotension, nausea, and lightheadedness during anesthesia corrected with ephedrine	Normal newborn	Elective C-section under epidural anesthesia
Delcorsoc[26] (1993)	25	NA	Patient conceived while on maintenance dose of prednisone (7.5 mg/d for acute TA 2 years ago.)	Prednisone reduced to 5 mg on alternate days	Narrowing abdominal aorta below the renal arteries; stenosis of both renal arteries and subclavian arteries; stenosis of left common carotid artery; aneurysmal dilatation of right internal carotid artery	Favorable	Live 3820 g female; uncomplicated	C-section at 38 weeks because of breech presentation
Buffolo[a] (1994)	28	NA	Back pain radiating to precordium and left shoulder, hemoptysis, dizziness and syncope, systolic murmurs, anemia.	Surgical closure of 2 aneurysmal holes distal to left subclavian artery and at the transition of left carotid and subclavian artery; bypass graft ascending aorta to innominate	Chest X-ray—enlargement of mediastinum. Echocardiogram—aneurysm of transverse aorta, angiogram—subocclusion of innominate artery, aneurysm at posterior wall of transverse aorta and descending aorta and thoraco-abdominal transitional area	Favorable	Loss of fetal heart beat during hypothermic circulatory arrest; 2650 g infant; uncomplicated	Premature labor resolved with terbutaline. C-section at 39 weeks

TABLE 20. (Continued)

Ref = First Author (year)	Age (years)	Obstetrical History	Clinical Presentation	Treatment	Vascular Involvement	Outcome		Mode of Delivery
						Maternal	Fetal	
Rocha[29] (1994)	26		Hematemesis due to Mallory Weiss tear. Pulmonary hypertension; cardiomegaly; diffuse lung infiltrate; diminished pulses in upper extremities; bilateral carotid bruits.	artery. Prednisone (50 mg/d) postsurgery	Paucity of peripheral pulmonary vessels; aneurysmal dilatation of ascending and descending aorta	Carotid surgery; thoracic aortic aneurysm resection after pregnancy; died of postoperative complications	2270 g infant; uncomplicated	Assisted vaginal at 35 weeks with outlet forceps under epidural anesthesia
Bassa[31] (1995) Case 1	21	G_1	Absent pulses in both upper limbs; diminished carotid pulses, popliteal BP 190/100 mm Hg.	Prednisone (50 mg/d) for 2 weeks. Methyldopa for hypertension		Favorable	Birth weight 2000 g; no complications	C-section under epidural anesthesia for fetal distress
Case 2	33	P_6	Hypertension, upper limb ischemia.		Bilateral subclavian artery occlusion; stenosis at origin of right common carotid and abdominal aorta at renal arteries level		Live 3750 g infant; uncomplicated	Uncomplicated vaginal delivery
Case 3	35	G_8P_7	Absent left upper limbs pulses; weakly palpable right upper limb pulse. BP 150/100 mm Hg.				Live 4400 g male; uncomplicated	Emergency C-section under epidural anesthesia for cephalopelvic disproportion
Case 4	33	G_3P_2	Intermittent claudication of both upper limbs. Bilateral carotid and subclavian bruits. Absent right brachial and radial pulses; diminished left brachial and radial pulses.	Patient conceived on prednisone therapy (4 mg/d); drug stopped at 10 weeks	ESR, 88 mm/hr	Favorable	Live 2400 g male; uncomplicated	Emergency C-section at 38 weeks due to fetal distress under epidural anesthesia

[a]Buffolo

Abbreviations: Ab, abortion; ACE, angiotension-converting enzyme; AR, aortic regurgitation; BP, blood pressure; C-section, cesarean section; CVA, cerebral vascular accident; d/c, discharged; ESR, erythrocyte sedimentation rate; FHR, fetal heart rate; G, gravida; MR, mitral regurgitation; NA, not available; P, para; s/p, status post; TA, Takayasu's arteritis.

potential risk of maternal and fetal morbidity during pregnancy, including exacerbation of hypertension, heart failure, high incidence of fetal growth retardation, and increased likelihood for surgical abdominal delivery. The need for vascular surgery or percutaneous angioplasty should be assessed before conception, to avoid such procedures during pregnancy.

Hypertension should be vigorously treated from early pregnancy in an attempt to prevent complications such as congestive heart failure and cerebral hemorrhage. However,

because of marked variations in regional blood flow, excessive reduction in arterial blood pressures may further decrease blood flow to organs with compromised perfusion. Aggressive reduction of blood pressure in patients with thoracic or abdominal aortic narrowing can result in low blood pressure distal to the narrowing (Fig. 20.3) with a potential compromise of placental blood flow and increased likelihood of fetal growth retardation.[9] Considerations for selection of antihypertensive therapy should include fetal safety, and drugs with established safety should be preferred (Chapter

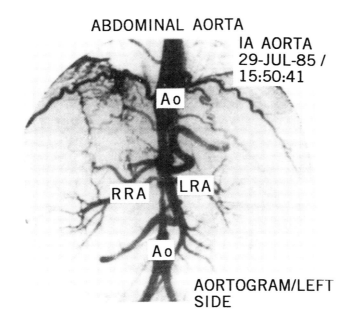

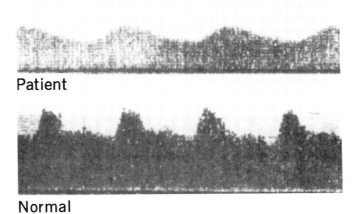

Figure 20.3 Infrarenal stenosis of the abdominal aorta in a pregnant patient with Takayasu's arteritis leading to a marked reduction in uterine artery blood flow velocity.

22). Reported antihypertensive therapy in patients with TA included β-adrenergic blocking agents, hydralazine, and methyldopa (Table 20.1).

Adrenal corticosteroids are the first modality of treatment for active inflammatory TA disease.[1] The use of these drugs has been reported during pregnancy for various indications and in several cases with TA.[10,29,31,34] Available information suggests that both prednisone and prednisolone pose very little risk to the developing fetus.[35] In addition, the American Academy of Pediatrics considers prednisone to be compatible with breast feeding.[36] Since pregnancy does not seem to affect the inflammatory activity of TA, adrenal corticosteroids should not be used prophylactically and can be reserved for patients who become pregnant during the acute phase of the disease. The indication for prednisone therapy should be reassessed in patients who conceive while on therapy.[26,30,31]

A reported 40% of patients with active inflammatory TA fail to respond to glucocorticoids and require additional cytotoxic therapy with either cyclophosphamide or methotrexate.[1] The safety of cyclophosphamide in pregnancy is not entirely clear. Although normal fetal outcome has been reported among patients receiving the drug in pregnancy, other infants were born with birth defects including flattened nasal bridge, palate defect, skin tag, missing toe, hypoplastic middle phalanx fifth finger, single coronary artery, hemangioma, umbilical hernia, imperforate anus, rectovaginal fistula, and growth retardation.[35]

Review of the literature by Griggs et al[35] has identified the use of methotrexate, a folic acid antagonist, in 26 pregnancies. In three cases of the use of this drug during the first trimester, infants were born with the following anomalies: absence of lambdoid and coronial sutures, oxycephaly, absence of frontal bone, low set ears, hypertelorism, dextroposition of the heart, absence of digits on feet, growth retardation, wide posterior fontanel, hypoplastic mandible, multiple anomalous ribs, large anterior fontanel, and long webbed fingers. In addition, newborn myelosuppression has been reported after methotrexate use during pregnancy. Aso et al[23] reported the performance of therapeutic abortion in the first trimester in four women who became pregnant during the active state of the disease. Although there is no evidence for an adverse influence of pregnancy and delivery on TA, patients should be aware of potential risks of the above-mentioned drugs so that the option of therapeutic abortion can be considered in early stages of pregnancy.[23,37]

Prophylactic antibiotics prior to delivery are recommended in patients with aortic regurgitation and narrowing of blood vessels. Since thromboembolic complications have not been reported during pregnancy and because of the potential complication of therapy (Chapter 33), anticoagulation or antiplatelet therapy does not seem to be indicated in the majority of cases. In patients at high risk for the development of heart failure (severe hypertension, evidence for systolic and/or diastolic left ventricular dysfunction, valvular heart disease, coronary artery disease) and in those with clinical signs and/or symptoms of congestive heart failure, hemodynamic monitoring with the aid of a pulmonary artery catheter is recommended during labour and delivery.[13] Accurate blood pressure monitoring may require an arterial line inserted into a nonobstructed artery. Vaginal delivery should be allowed in the majority of women with TA. Forceps (Table 20.1) or vacuum extraction may be used to shorten the second stage of labor if needed. Cesarean section delivery should be performed for obstetrical indications,[26,31] and when there is resistant hypertension or heart failure not responding to medical therapy.[23] Epidural anesthesia has been used for delivery in the majority of reported cases (Table 20.1) and has been shown to be safe. Blood pressure should not be allowed to fall excessively,[25] however, since organs with already compromised perfusion must be protected from damage due to further decreased blood flow. In contrast, rise in blood pressure has been reported to be more common during the first and second stages of labor and should be prevented.[31] Vasoconstrictor drugs should be avoided during labor and delivery, and ergot preparations should not be used during delivery or for suppression of lactation.

REFERENCES

1. Kerr GS. Takayasu's arteritis. *Rheum Dis Clin North Am* 1995;21:1041–1058.

2. Hall S, Buchbinder R. Takayasu's arteritis. *Rheum Dis Clin North Am* 1990;16:411.

3. Kerr GS, Hallahan CW, Giordano J, Leavitt RY, Fauci AS, Rottem M, Hoffman GS. Takayasu arteritis. *Ann Intern Med* 1994;120:919–929.

4. Ishikawa K. Natural history and classification of occlusive thromboaortopathy (Takayasu's disease). *Circulation* 1977;57: 27–35.

4a. Zheng D, Fan D, Liu L. Takayasu arteritis in China: a report of 530 cases *H,V,S.* 1992;7:32–36.

5. Weaver FA, Yellin AE. Surgical treatment of Takayasu's arteritis. *Heart Vessels Suppl* 1992;7:154–158.

6. Ishikawa K, Maetani S. Long-term outcome for 120 Japanese patients with Takayasu's disease. *Circulation* 1994;90:1855.

7. Tyagi S, Singh B, Kaul UA, Sethi KK, Arora R, Khalilullah M. Balloon angioplasty for renovascular hypertension in Takayasu's arteritis. *Am Heart J* 1993;125:1386–1393.

8. Galvez J. Takayasu arteritis with secondary hypertension in pregnancy. *Rev Med Chil* 1987;115:1085–1087.

9. Graca LM, Cardoso MC, Machado FS. Takayasu's arteritis and pregnancy: a case of deleterious association. *Eur J Obstet Gynecol Reprod Biol* 1987;24:347–351.

10. Chua S, Viegas OA, Tan AT, Ratnam SS. Successful outcome of pregnancy in a subfertile patient with severe aortoarteritis (Takayasu's disease). *Eur J Obstet Gynecol Reprod Biol* 1987;25:249–253.

11. Giles WB, Young AA, Howlin KJ, Cook CM, Irudinger BJ. Doppler ultrasound features of stenosis of the aorta in a pregnancy complicated by Takayasu's arteritis: case report. *Br J Obstet Gynaecol* 1987;94:907–909.

12. Railton A, Allen DG. Takayasu's arteritis in pregnancy: a report of 4 cases. *S Afr Med J* 1988;73:123.

13. Winn HN, Setaro JF, Mazor M, Reece EA, Black HR, Hobbins JC. Severe Takayasu's arteritis in pregnancy: the role of central hemodynamic monitoring. *Am J Obstet Gynecol* 1988;159: 1135–1136.

14. Gaida BJ, Gervais HW, Mauer D, Leyser KH, Eberle B, Dick W. Takayasu syndrome. *Med Klin* 1991;86:367–373.

15. Jilek D, Dlowhy P, Svoboda J, Burianova Z, Svejda J. Takayasu's disease. Detection of the early systemic stage of the disease in a pregnant woman. *Cas Lek Cesk* 1991;130:20–23.

16. Crofts SL, Wilson E. Epidural analgesia for labour in Takayasu's arteritis. *Br J Obstet Gynaecol* 1991;98:408–409.

17. Guidozzi F, Louridas G, Grant MG, Koller AB, King P, Naylor S. Takayasu's arteritis in a pregnant woman. *S Afr J Surg* 1991;29:159–160.

18. Duclos F, Benchimol D, Lauribe P, Benchimol H, Bonnet J, Bricaud H. Cardiac lesions in Takayasu's disease. A case with initial pericarditis and tamponade. *Presse Med* 1991;20:847–850.

19. Cristalli B, Morice P, Heid M, Levardon M. Takayasu's disease and pregnancy. *J Gynecol Obstet Biol Reprod* 1992;21:969–970.

20. Ben-Zineb N, Zine S, Bellasfar M, Mesaad MJ, Sfar R. Association of Takayasu arteritis, Crohn disease and pregnancy. *Rev Fr Gynecol Obstet* 1992;87:591–593.

21. Matsumura A, Moriwaki R, Numano F. Pregnancy in Takayasu arteritis from the view of internal medicine. *Heart Vessel Suppl* 1992;7:120–124.

22. McKay RS, Dillard SR. Management of epidural anesthesia in a patient with Takayasu's disease. *Anesth Analg* 1992;74:297–299.

23. Aso T, Abe S, Yaguchi T. Clinical gynecologic features of pregnancy in Takayasu arteritis. *Heart Vessels Suppl* 1992;7:125–132.

24. Rao K. Pregnancy and Takayasu's aorto-arteritis. *J Indian Med Assoc* 1992;90:107.

25. Beilin Y, Bernstein H. Successful epidural anesthesia for a patient with Takayasu's arteritis presenting for cesarean section. *Can J Anaesth* 1993;40:64–66.

26. Del Corso L, De Marco S, Vannini A, Pentimone F. Takayasu's arteritis: low corticosteroid dosage and pregnancy—a case report. *Angiology* 1993;44:827–831.

27. Alavacek K, Janik V, Twma S. Takayasu's arteritis with primary involvement of the pulmonary artery. *Unifr-Lek* 1993;39: 773–777.

28. Coel M, Saito R, Endo PM. Use of magnetic resonance imaging in the diagnosis of Takayasu's arteritis during pregnancy: a case report. *Am J Perinatol* 1993;10:126–129.

29. Rocha MP, Gunterpalli KK, Moise KJ Jr., Lockett LD, Khawli F, Rokey R. Massive hemoptysis in Takayasu's arteritis during pregnancy. *Chest* 1994;106:1619–1622.

30. Bloechle M, Bollmann R, Chaoui R, Birnbaum M, Bartho S. Pregnancy in Takayasu arteritis. *Z Geburtshilfe Neonatol* 1995;199:116–119.

31. Bassa A, Desai DK, Moodley J. Takayasu's disease and pregnancy: three case studies and a review of the literature. *S Afr Med J* 1995;85:107–112.

32. Fignon A, Marret H, Alle C, Jacquet A, Avigdor S, Descamps P, Body G, Lansac J. Association of Takayasu's arteritis, pregnancy and Still's disease. *J Gynecol Obstet Biol Reprod (Paris)* 1995;24:747–750.

33. Wong VCW, Wang RYE, Tse TF. Pregnancy and Takayasu's arteritis. *Am J Med* 1983;75:597–601.

34. Ishikawa K, Matsuura S. Occlusive thromboaortopathy (Takayasu's disease) and pregnancy: clinical course and management of 33 pregnancies and deliveries. *Am J Cardiol* 1982;50:1293–1300.

35. Briggs GG, Freeman RK, Yaffe SJ. *Drugs in Pregnancy and Lactation.* 4th ed. Baltimore: Williams & Wilkins; 1994;713–716.

36. Committee on Drugs, American Academy of Pediatrics. The transfer of drugs and other chemicals into human milk. *Pediatrics* 1994;93:137–150.

37. Hampl KF, Schneider K, Skarvan J, Bitzer J, Graber J. Spinal anesthesia in a patient with Takayasu's disease. *Br J Anaesth* 1994;72:129–132.

21

AMNIOTIC FLUID EMBOLISM

Steven L. Clark, MD

INTRODUCTION

Amniotic fluid embolism (AFE) is an uncommon obstetric disorder with a mortality of 60–70%.[1,2] This condition is classically characterized by hypoxia, hypotension, and coagulopathy. Despite numerous attempts to develop an animal model, AFE remains incompletely understood. Nevertheless, the past decade has seen several significant advances in our understanding of this enigmatic condition.

HISTORICAL CONSIDERATIONS

The earliest description of AFE was by Meyer in 1926.[3] However, the condition was not widely recognized until the report of Steiner and Luschbaugh in 1941.[4] These investigators described autopsy findings in 8 pregnant women with sudden shock and pulmonary edema during labor. In all cases the pulmonary vasculature contained squamous cells or mucin, presumably of fetal origin. In a follow-up report in 1969 by Liban and Raz, fetal debris was also observed in the kidneys, liver, spleen, pancreas, and brain of several patients, in contrast to control patients, who did not produce such findings.[5] However, squamous cells were identified in uterine veins of several patients in this series, a finding confirmed in a report of Thompson and Bud in a patient without AFE.[6]

Since the initial descriptions of AFE, more than 300 case reports have appeared in the literature. Although most cases were reported during labor, sudden death in pregnancy has been attributed to AFE under many widely varying circumstances, including cases of first- and second-trimester abortion.[7–10] In 1948 Eastman, in an editorial review, stated "Let us be careful not to make [the diagnosis of AFE] a waste bas-

ket for cases of unexplained death in labor."[11] Fortunately, increased understanding of the syndrome of AFE makes such errors highly unlikely today.

EXPERIMENTAL MODELS

The first animal model of AFE was that of Steiner and Luschbaugh, who showed that rabbits and dogs could be killed by the intravenous injection of heterologous amniotic fluid and meconium.[4] Several subsequent reports of AFE in experimental animals have yielded conflicting results (Table 21.1).[4,11–27] In most series, experimental injection of amniotic fluid had adverse effects, ranging from transient alterations in systemic and pulmonary artery pressures in dogs, sheep, cats, and calves to sudden death in rabbits. However, only two of these studies involved pregnant animals, and heterologous amniotic fluid was used in most. In several studies the effects of whole or meconium-enriched amniotic fluid were contrasted with those of filtered amniotic fluid. A pathological response was obtained only in particulate-rich amniotic fluid in four such studies, whereas three reports demonstrated physiologic changes with filtered amniotic fluid as well. Data produced with the models involving particulate-enriched amniotic fluid may have little relevance to the human model, since the concentration of particulate matter injected has been many times greater than that present in human amniotic fluid, even in the presence of meconium. In the four studies in which amniotic fluid was injected into both the arterial and venous systems, three showed toxic effects with both arterial and venous injection, implying a pathologic humoral substance or response. In studies in which autopsy was performed, pulmonary findings ranged

Cardiac Problems in Pregnancy, Third Edition
Edited by Uri Elkayam, MD, and Norbert Gleicher, MD
Copyright © 1998 by Wiley-Liss, Inc. ISBN 0-471-16358-9

TABLE 21.1 Animal Models of Amniotic Fluid Embolism

Ref: First Author (year)	Animal	Anesthetized	Pregnant	Filtered AF	Pathology with Whole/Concentrated AF	AF Species	Pathologic Injection Arterial	Pathologic Injection Venous	Hemodynamic Changes	Coagulopathy	Autopsy
Steiner[4] (1941)	Rabbit/dog	No	No	No	Yes	Human	NE	Yes	NE (death)	No	Debris in pulmonary artery
Cron[12] (1952)	Rabbit	No	No	NE	Yes	Human	No	Yes	NE (death)	No	Debris in pulmonary artery
Schneider[13] (1955)	Dog	No	No	NE	Yes	Human	NE	Yes	NE (death)	5 of 8	Debris in pulmonary artery
Jacques[14] (1960)	Dog	Yes	No	NE	Yes	Human/dog	NE	Yes	↑PAP, Nl BP	Fibrinogen 12 of 13	Debris in pulmonary artery
Halmagyi[15] (1962)	Sheep	Yes	No	No	Yes	Human	NE	Yes	↑PAP, Nl SVR, nl CO,	No	NE
Attwood[16] (1965)	Dog	Yes	No	Yes (mild)	Yes	Human	Yes	Yes	↑PAP, ↑PVR, ↓SVR, Nl to ↑LAP, BP	4 of 12	NE
Stolte[17] (1967)	Monkey	Yes	Yes	No	No	Human/monkey	No	No	Nl BP, Nl P	1 of 12	NE
MacMillan[18] (1968)	Rabbit	No	No	No	Yes	Human	Yes	Yes	NE (death)	2 of 12	Minimal debris, hemorrhage

	Species					Species			Hemodynamic findings		Autopsy findings
Reis[19] (1965)	Sheep	Yes	Yes	Yes	Yes	Sheep	Yes	Yes	↑PAP, ↑PVR, ↓SVR ↑BP, Nl LAP, Nl PCWP	No	Normal
Dutta[20] (1970)	Rabbit	Yes	No	NE	Yes	Human	NE	Yes	NE (death)	No	Minimal debris, massive infarction
Adamsons[21] (1971)	Monkey	Yes	Yes	NE	No	Monkey	NE	No	Nl BP, Nl P, Nl RR	No	NE
Kitzmiller[22] (1972)	Cat	Yes	No	No	Yes	Human	NE	Yes	↓BP, ↑P, ↑CVP	No	NE
Spence[23] (1974)	Rabbit	No	Yes	No	No	Rabbit	NE	No	Nl BP, Nl P, Nl RR	No	NE
Reeves[24] (1974)	Calf	No	No	NE	Yes	Calf	NE	Yes	↓BP, ↑PAP, Nl CO Nl PCWP	No	
Azegami[26] (1986)	Rabbit	No	No	No	Yes	Human	NE	Yes	NE (death)	No	Pulmonary edema, debris pulmonary vessels
Richards[25] (1988)	Rat[a]	Yes	No	Yes	NE	Human	NE	Yes	Coronary flow	No	
Hankins[27] (1993)	Goat	Yes	Yes	Yes	Yes	Goat	NE	Yes	↑PVT, ↑SVR ↓CO, ↑PCWP	No	NE

[a]Isolated heart preparation.

Abbreviations: AF, amniotic fluid; BP, blood pressure; CO, cardiac output; CVP, central venous pressure; LAP, left atrial pressure; NE, not examined; Nl, normal; P, pulse; PAP, pulmonary artery pressure; PCWP, pulmonary capillary wedge pressure; PVR, pulmonary vascular resistance; RR, respiratory rate; SVR, systemic vascular resistance.

Source: Modified with permission from SL Clark, GDV Hankins, DB Cotton, JP Phelan, eds., *Critical Care Obstetrics*, 2nd ed. Boston: Blackwell Scientific; 1991.

from massive vascular plugging with fetal debris (after embolization with particulate-enriched amniotic fluid) to normal.

In contrast, three studies (including the only two carried out in primates) showed the intravenous injection of amniotic fluid to be entirely innocuous, without effects on blood pressure, pulse, or respiratory rate. In one study, the volume of amniotic fluid infused would in the human represent 80% of the total amniotic fluid volume. More recently, a carefully controlled study in the goat model using homologous amniotic fluid demonstrated hemodynamic and clinical findings similar to what is seen in humans, including an initial transient rise in pulmonary and systemic vascular resistance and myocardial depression.[27] These findings were especially prominent when the injection included meconium. Importantly, the initial phase of pulmonary hypertension has in all animal models studied been transient and in survivors has resolved within 30 minutes.

HUMAN HEMODYNAMIC DATA

In humans, an initial, transient phase that apparently involves both systemic and pulmonary vasospasm leads to a more often recognized secondary phase involving hypotension and depressed ventricular function.

Figure 21.1 demonstrates in a graphic manner the depression of left ventricular function seen in five patients studied with pulmonary artery catheterization. The mechanism of left ventricular failure is unknown.[28,29] Work in the rat model by Richards and coworkers suggests the presence of possible coronary artery spasm and myocardial ischemia in

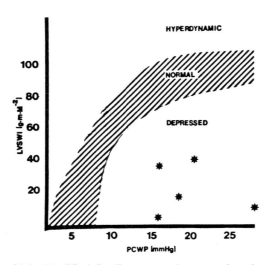

Figure 21.1 Modified Starling curve demonstrating depressed left ventricular function in five patients with amniotic fluid embolism. (Reproduced from SL Clark, Amniotic fluid embolism in critical care obstetrics, SL Clark, JP Phelan, DB Cotton, eds., *Critical Care Obstetrics.* Oradell, NJ: Medical Economics Books; 1987; pp 393–411, with permission of the publisher.)

animal AFE.[25] On the other hand, global hypoxia could certainly account for left ventricular dysfunction. The in vitro observation of decreased myometrial contractility in the presence of amniotic fluid suggests the possibility of a similar effect of amniotic fluid on myocardium.[30]

COAGULOPATHY

Patients surviving the initial hemodynamic insult may succumb to a secondary coagulopathy. The exact incidence of the coagulopathy is unknown. Coagulopathy was an entry criterion for inclusion in the initial analysis of the National AFE Registry; however, several patients whose cases were submitted to the registry clearly had AFE but gave no clinical evidence of coagulopathy.[2] In a similar manner, a number of patients have been observed to develop an acute obstetric coagulopathy alone, in the absence of placental abruptio, and these women suffered fatal exsanguination without any evidence of primary hemodynamic or pulmonary insult.[31]

As with experimental investigations into hemodynamic alterations associated with AFE, investigation of this coagulopathy has yielded contradictory results. From in vitro studies it is seen that amniotic fluid shortens whole-blood clotting time, has a thromboplastin-like effect, induces platelet aggregation and release of platelet factor III, and activates the complement cascade.[32–35] In addition, Courtney and Allington show that amniotic fluid contains a direct factor X activating factor.[36] However, while confirming the factor X activating properties of amniotic fluid, Phillips and Davidson[37] concluded that there is not enough procoagulate in clear amniotic fluid to cause significant intervascular coagulation, a finding disputed by more recent studies of Lockwood and colleagues.[38]

In the experimental animal models discussed earlier, coagulopathy has likewise been an inconsistent finding. Thus, the exact nature of the consumptive coagulopathy demonstrated in humans with AFE has yet to find a satisfactory explanation. The powerful thromboplastin effects of trophoblast are well established. The coagulopathy associated with severe placental abruption and that seen with AFE are probably similar in origin, representing an activation of the coagulation cascade following exposure of the maternal circulation to a variety of fetal antigens with varying thromboplastin-like effects.[2]

PATHOPHYSIOLOGY

In a recent analysis of the National AFE Registry, a marked similarity was noted between the clinical, hemodynamic, and hematologic manifestations of AFE and both septic and anaphylactic shock.[2] Clearly the clinical manifestations of this

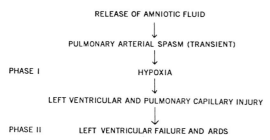

RELEASE OF AMNIOTIC FLUID

↓

PULMONARY ARTERIAL SPASM (TRANSIENT)

↓

PHASE I   HYPOXIA

↓

LEFT VENTRICULAR AND PULMONARY CAPILLARY INJURY

↓

PHASE II   LEFT VENTRICULAR FAILURE AND ARDS

Figure 21.2 Proposed pathophysiologic relationship between amniotic fluid embolism, septic shock, and anaphylactic shock. Each syndrome also has specific and different direct physiologic effects (for example, fever in endotoxin mediated sepsis.) (Reprinted with permission from Clark et al.[2])

condition are not identical; fever is unique to septic shock and cutaneous manifestations are more common in anaphylaxis. Nevertheless the marked similarities of these conditions suggest similar pathophysiologic mechanisms.

A detailed discussion of the pathophysiologic features of anaphylactic and septic shock is beyond the scope of this chapter. However, both these conditions involve the entrance into the circulation of a foreign substance (bacterial endotoxin or specific antigens) that then results in the release of various primary and secondary endogenous mediators (Fig. 21.2). It is the release of these mediators that results in the principal physiologic derangements characterizing these syndromes. These include profound myocardial depression and decreased cardiac output described in both animals and man,[39–41] as well as pulmonary hypertension, demonstrated in lower primate models of anaphylaxis,[2] and disseminated intervascular coagulation in both human anaphylactic reactions and septic shock.[2,39–48] Further, the temporal sequence of hemodynamic decompensation and recovery seen in experimental AFE is virtually identical to that described in canine anaphylaxis.[44] An *anaphylactoid* response is also well described in man and involves the nonimmunologic release of similar mediators.[48]

The ability of arachidonic acid metabolites to cause the same physiologic and hemodynamic changes observed in human AFE has been reported.[49] Further, in the rabbit model of AFE, pretreatment with an inhibitor of leukotriene synthesis has been shown to prevent death.[26] A final intriguing clue to the pathophysiologic origin of AFE is the observation that 41% of patients in the AFE registry gave a history of either drug allergy or atopy on admission to the hospital.[2]

Earlier anecdotal reports suggested a possible relationship between hypertonic uterine contractions or oxytocin use and AFE.[1] Although disputed on statistical grounds by Morgan in 1971, this misconception persisted in some writings until recently.[50] The historic anecdotal association between hypertonic uterine contractions and the onset of symptoms in AFE was made clear by the analysis of the National Registry.[2] The data demonstrated that the hypertonic contrac-

tions commonly seen in association with AFE appear to be a result of the release of catecholamines into the circulation as part of the initial human hemodynamic response to any massive physiologic insult. Under these circumstances norepinephrine, in particular, acts as a potent uterotonic agent.[2,51] Thus, while the association of hypertonic contractions and AFE appears to be valid, it is the response to AFE that causes the hypertonic uterine activity rather than the converse.[2] Indeed, there is a complete cessation of uterine blood flow in the presence of even moderate uterine contractions; thus a tetanic contraction is the least likely time during an entire labor process for any exchange between maternal and fetal compartments.[52] Oxytocin use has no relationship to the occurrence of AFE.[32,50,53]

Thus, the syndrome of AFE appears to be initiated after maternal intervascular exposure to various types of fetal tissue.[2] Such exposure may occur during the course of normal labor and delivery, after potentially minor traumatic events such as intrauterine pressure catheter placement, or during cesarean section. Because fetal-to-maternal tissue transfer is virtually universal during the labor and delivery process, actions by health care providers such as intrauterine manipulation or cesarean delivery may affect the timing of the exposure; no evidence, however, exists to suggest that exposure itself can be avoided by altering clinical management. Whereas much has been written about the importance to the fetus of an immunologic barrier between the mother and the antigenically different products of conception, little attention has been paid to the potential importance of this barrier to maternal well-being. The observations of the National AFE Registry as well as cumulative data for the past several decades suggest that breeches of this barrier may, under certain circumstances, and in susceptible mother/fetus pairs, be of immense significance to the mother as well.[2]

Experimental evidence both in animals and humans unequivocally demonstrates that the intervenous administration of even large amounts of amniotic fluid per se is innocuous.[17,21,54] Further, the clinical findings described in the National Registry are not consistent with an embolic event as commonly understood. Thus the term "amniotic fluid embolism" itself appears to be a misnomer. The authors of the National Registry analysis suggested that the name "amniotic fluid embolism" be discarded and the syndrome of acute peripartum hypoxia hemodynamic collapse and coagulopathy be designated in a more descriptive manner, as *anaphylactoid syndrome of pregnancy.*[2]

CLINICAL PRESENTATION

Clinical signs and symptoms noted in patients with AFE are listed in Table 21.2. In a typical case, a patient who is laboring or has just undergone cesarean delivery, or one who is in the period immediately following vaginal delivery or preg-

TABLE 21.2 Frequency of Signs and Symptoms in Patients with Amniotic Fluid Embolism

Sign or Symptom	No. of Patients	%
Hypotension	43	100
Fetal distress[a]	30	100
Pulmonary edema or adult respiratory distress syndrome[b]	28	93
Cardiopulmonary arrest	40	87
Cyanosis	38	83
Coagulopathy[c]	38	83
Dyspnea[d]	22	49
Seizure	22	48
Atony	11	23
Bronchospasm[e]	7	15
Transient hypertension	5	11
Cough	3	7
Headache	3	7
Chest pain	1	2

[a]$n = 30$. Includes all live fetuses in utero at time of event.

[b]$n = 30$. Eighteen patients did not survive long enough for these diagnosis to be confirmed.

[c]$n = 38$. Eight patients did not survive long enough for this diagnosis to be confirmed.

[d]$n = 45$. One patient was intubated at the time of the event and could not be assessed.

[e]Difficult ventilation was noted during cardiac arrest in 6 patients, and weezes were auscultated in 1 patient.

Source: Reprinted with permission from Clark et al.[2]

TABLE 21.3 Interval Between Cardiac Arrest and Delivery and Neonatal Outcome in Patients with Amniotic Fluid Embolism

Interval (min)	Outcome	
	Number Survived	Number Survived Intact
<5	3/3	2/3 (67%)
5–15	3/3	2/3 (67%)
16–25	2/5	2/5 (40%)
26–35	3/4	1/4 (25%)
36–54	0/1	0/1 (0%)

Source: Reprinted with permission from Clark et al.[2]

nancy termination, suffers the acute onset of profound hypoxia and hypotension followed by cardiopulmonary arrest. The initial episode is often complicated by the development of a consumptive coagulopathy, which may lead to exsanguination even if attempts to restore hemodynamic and respiratory function are successful. However, it must be emphasized that in any individual patient, any of the three principal phases (hypoxia, hypotension, coagulopathy) may either dominate or be entirely absent. Clinical variations in this syndrome appear to be related to variations in antigenics exposure and maternal response.[2]

Maternal outcome is dismal in patients with AFE syndrome. Overall maternal mortality rate appears to be 60–80%.[1,2] Only 15% of patients survive neurologically intact.[2] In a number of cases, following successful hemodynamic resuscitation and reversal of disseminated intravascular coagulation, life support systems were withdrawn because of brain death resulting from the initial profound hypoxia. In patients progressing to cardiac arrest, only 8% survive neurologically intact.[2] In the National Registry, no form of therapy appeared to be associated with improved outcome.[2]

Neonatal outcome is similarly poor. Among fetuses in utero at the time of onset of maternal symptoms, survival rate is approximately 80%. However, only half of these fetuses survive neurologically intact.[2] Fetuses surviving to delivery generally demonstrate profound respiratory acidemia. Although no form of therapy appears at the present time to result in improved maternal outcome, there is a clear relationship between neonatal outcome and event to delivery interval in those women suffering cardiac arrest (Table 21.3).[2]

DIAGNOSIS

In the past, histologic confirmation of the clinical syndrome of AFE was often sought by the detection of cellular debris of presumed fetal origin, either in the distal port of a pulmonary artery catheterization or at autopsy.[1] However, several studies in the past decade suggest that such findings are commonly encountered even in normal pregnant women (Fig. 21.3).[55–57] In the analysis of the National AFE Registry, fetal elements were found in roughly 50% of cases in which pulmonary artery catheter aspirate was analyzed and in roughly 75% of patients who went to autopsy.[2] The frequency with which such findings are encountered varies with the number of histologic sections obtained. In addition, multiple special stains are often required to document such debris.[1] Given the nature of the data at present, it is impossible to make any reliable statement regarding the frequency with which such histologic findings can be said to help confirm the clinical diagnosis of AFE. It is clear, however, that the diagnosis of anaphylactic syndrome of pregnancy remains today a clinical one; histologic findings are neither sensitive nor specific.[1,2]

TREATMENT

Treatment remains disappointing, with the overall mortality rate of 60–80%, noted earlier. In the National Registry we found no difference in survival among patients suffering ini-

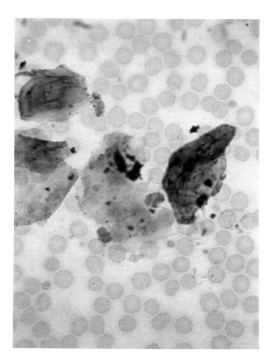

Figure 21.3 Squamous cells recovered from the pulmonary arterial circulation of a pregnant woman with New York Heart Association functional class IV rheumatic mitral stenosis. (Reproduced from SL Clark, Amniotic fluid embolism in critical care obstetrics, SL Clark, JP Phelan, DB Cotton, eds., *Critical Care Obstetrics.* Oradell, NJ: Medical Economics Books; 1987; pp. 393–411, with permission of the publisher.) (See color plates.)

tial cardiac arrest in small rural hospitals attended by family practitioners and those presenting identical clinical signs and symptoms at tertiary level centers, attended by board-certified anesthesiologists, cardiologists, and specialists in maternal/fetal medicine. Nevertheless, several generalizations can be drawn:

1. The initial treatment for AFE is supportive. Cardiopulmonary resuscitation is performed if the patient is suffering from a lethal dysrhythmia, and oxygen should be provided at high concentrations.

2. In the patient who survives the initial cardiopulmonary insult, it should be remembered that left ventricular failure is commonly seen. Thus the most appropriate course seems to be volume expansion to optimize ventricular preload and, if the patient remains significantly hypotensive, the addition of an inotropic agent such as dopamine. In patients who remain unstable following the initial resuscitative efforts, pulmonary artery catheterization (to guide hemodynamic manipulation) may be of benefit.

3. Although no evidence exists to document the benefit of corticosteroids in patients with AFE, the similar

pathophysiologies proposed in the National Registry suggest that the administration of high doses of corticosteroids would be a consideration. However, in the absence of any data to suggest the benefit of this, such steroid treatment is not be mandated by standard of care.

4. In patients suffering AFE with the fetus still in utero, careful attention must be paid to the fetal condition. In a mother who is hemodynamically unstable but has not yet undergone cardiorespiratory arrest, maternal considerations must be carefully weighed against those relating to the fetus. The decision to subject such an unstable mother to a major abdominal operation (cesarean section) is a difficult one. Under these circumstances there is clearly no standard of care; all cases must be individualized. However, it is axiomatic in these situations that when a choice must be made, maternal well-being must take precedence over that of the fetus.

5. In mothers who have progressed to frank cardiac arrest, the situation is different. Under these circumstances maternal survival is extremely unlikely regardless of the therapy rendered. It is highly unlikely that the imposition of cesarean section would significantly alter the outcome for such women. Even properly performed CPR (difficult at best in a pregnant woman) provides only a maximum of 30% of normal cardiac output. Under these circumstances it is fair to assume that the proportion of blood shunted to the uterus and other areas in the splanchnic bed approaches zero. Thus the fetus will be for practical purposes anoxic at all times following maternal cardiac arrest, even during the performance of CPR. Because the interval from maternal arrest to delivery is directly correlated with newborn outcome, perimortem cesarean section should be initiated immediately on the diagnosis of maternal cardiac arrest in patients with AFE, assuming sufficient personnel are available to continue to provide care to the mother and deliver the baby.[2,58] For the pregnant patient, the standard ABCs of cardiopulmonary resuscitation should be modified to include a fourth category, D: delivery.

SUMMARY

Despite many advances in the understanding of the condition, amniotic fluid embolism, or anaphylactoid syndrome of pregnancy, remains enigmatic and in most cases is associated with dismal maternal and fetal outcomes regardless of the quality of care rendered. Thus, AFE remains unpredictable, unpreventable, and, for the most part, untreatable. It is anticipated that the new directions in pathophysiology suggested by the analysis of the recent registry data may allow future advances in the treatment of this condition.

REFERENCES

1. Clark SL. New concepts of amniotic fluid embolism: a review. *Obstet Gynecol Survey* 1990;45:360–368.

2. Clark SL, Hankins GDV, Dudley DA, Dildy GA, Porter TF. Amniotic fluid embolism: analysis of a national registry. *Am J Obstet Gynecol* 1995;172:1158–1169.

3. Meyer JR. *Bras/Med* 1926;2:301–303.

4. Steiner PE, Luschbaugh CC. Maternal pulmonary embolism by amniotic fluid. *JAMA* 1941;117:1245–1253.

5. Liban E, Raz S. A clinicopathologic study of fourteen cases of amniotic fluid embolism. *Am J Clin Pathol* 1969;51:477–481.

6. Thompson WB, Budd JW. Erroneous diagnosis of amniotic fluid embolism. *Am J Obstet Gynecol* 1963;91:606–617.

7. Guidotti RJ, Grimes DA, Cates W. Fatal amniotic fluid embolism during legally induced abortion in the United States, 1972–1978. *Am J Obstet Gynecol* 1981;141:257–348.

8. Meier PR, Bowes WA. Amniotic fluid embolus-like syndrome presenting in the second trimester of pregnancy. *Obstet Gynecol* 1983;61(suppl):31–33.

9. Cromley MG, Taylor PJ, Cummings DC. Probable amniotic fluid embolism after first trimester pregnancy termination. *J Reprod Med.* 1983;28:209–210.

10. Resnik R, Schwartz WH, Plumer MH. Amniotic fluid embolism with survival. *Obstet Gynecol* 1976;47:295–298.

11. Eastman NJ. Obstet Gynecol Surv. 1948;3:35. Editorial comment.

12. Cron RS, Kilkenny GS, Wirthwein C. Amniotic fluid embolism. *Am J Obstet Gynecol* 1952;64:1360.

13. Schneider CL. Coagulation defects in obstetric shock: meconium embolism and defibrination. *Am J Obstet Gynecol* 1955;69:748.

14. Jacques WE, Hampton JW, Bird RM, Bolten KA, Randolph B. Pulmonary hypertension and plasma thromboplastin antecedent deficiency in dogs. *Arch Pathol* 1960; 69:248–255.

15. Halmagyi DFJ, Starzecki B, Shearman RP. Experimental amniotic fluid embolism: mechanism and treatment. *Am J Obstet Gynecol* 1962;84:251.

16. Attwood HD, Downing SE. Experimental amniotic fluid embolism. *Surg Gynecol Obstet* 1965;120:255.

17. Stolte L, van Kessel H, Seelen J, Eskes T, Wagatsuma T. Failure to produce the syndrome of amniotic fluid embolism by infusion of amniotic fluid and meconium into monkeys. *Am J Obstet Gynecol* 1967;98:694.

18. Macmillan D. Experimental amniotic fluid embolism. *J Obstet Gynaecol Br Commonw* 1968;75:8.

19. Reis RL, Pierce WS, Behrendt DM. Hemodynamic effects of amniotic fluid embolism. *Surg Obstet Gynecol* 1965;129:45.

20. Dutta D, Bhargava KC, Chakravarti RN, Dhall SR. Therapeutic studies in experimental amniotic fluid embolism in rabbits. *Am J Obstet Gynecol* 1970;106:1201.

21. Adamsons K, Mueller-Heubach E, Myer RE. The innocuousness of amniotic fluid infusion in the pregnant rhesus monkey. *Am J Obstet Gynecol* 1971;109:977.

22. Kitzmiller JL, Lucas WE. Studies on a model of amniotic fluid embolism. *Obstet Gynecol* 1972;39:626.

23. Spence MR, Mason KG. Experimental amniotic fluid embolism in rabbits. *Am J Obstet Gynecol* 1974;119:1073..

24. Reeves JT, Daoud FS, Estridge M, Stone WH, McGrary D. Pulmonary pressor effects of small amounts of bovine amniotic fluid. *Respir Physiol* 1974;20:231.

25. Richards DS, Carter LS, Corke B, Spielman F, Cefalo RC. The effect of human amniotic fluid on the isolated per fused rat heart. *Am J Obstet Gynecol* 1988;158:210.

26. Azegami M, Mori N. Amniotic fluid embolism and leukotrienes. *Am J Obstet Gynecol* 1986;155:1119–1123.

27. Hankins GDV, Snyder RR, Clark SL, Schwartz L, Patterson WR, Butzin CA. Acute hemodynamic and respiratory effects of amniotic fluid embolism in the pregnant goat model. *Am J Obstet Gynecol* 1993;168(4):1113–1129.

28. Clark SL, Cotton DB, Gonik B, Greenspoon J, Phelan JP. Central hemodynamic alterations in amniotic fluid embolism. *Am J Obstet Gynecol* 1988;158(5):1124–1126.

29. Girard P, Mal H, Laine JF, Petitpretz P, Rain B, Duraux P. Left heart failure in amniotic fluid embolism. *Anesthesiology* 1986;64:262.

30. Courtney LD. Coagulation failure in pregnancy. *Br Med J* 1970;1:691.

31. Porter TF, Clark SL, Dildy GA, Hankins GDV. Isolated disseminated intravascular coagulation and amniotic fluid embolism. Society of Perinatal Obstetricians, 16th Annual Meeting. Poster presentation.

32. Beller FK, Douglas GW, Debrovner CH. The fibrinolytic system in amniotic fluid embolism. *Am J Obstet Gynecol* 1963;87:48.

33. American College of Obstetricians and Gynecologists Prologue. *Obstetrics.* 3rd ed. Washington, DC: ACOG; 1993.

34. Duff P. Defusing the dangers of amniotic fluid embolism. *Contemp Ob/Gyn* August 1984;127–149.

35. Ratnoff OD, Vosbugh GJ. Observations of the clotting defect in amniotic fluid embolism. *N Engl J Med* 1952;247:970.

36. Courtney LD, Allington LM. Effect of amniotic fluid on blood coagulation. *Br J Haematol* 1972;113:911.

37. Phillips LL, Davidson EC. Procoagulant properties of amniotic fluid. *Am J Obstet Gynecol* 1972;113:911.

38. Lockwood CJ, Bach R, Guha A, Zbou X, Miller WA, Nemerson Y. Amniotic fluid contains tissue factor, a potent initiator of coagulation. *Am J Obstet Gynecol* 1991;165:1335–1141.

39. Raper RF, Fisher MM. Profound reversible myocardial depression after anaphylaxis. *Lancet* 1988;1:386–388.

40. Smedegard G, Revenas B, Lundberg C, Arfors KE. Anaphylactic shock in monkeys passively sensitized with human reaginic serum. I. Hemodynamics and cardiac performances. *Acta Physiol Scand* 1981;111:239–247.

41. Parrillo JE. Pathogenic mechanisms of septic shock. *N Engl J Med* 1993;328:1471–1477.

42. Enjeti S, Bleecker ER, Smith PL, Rabson J, Permutt S, Traystman RJ. Hemodynamic mechanisms in anaphylaxis. *Circ Shock* 1983;11:297–307.

43. Smith PL, Kagey-Sobotka A, Bleecker ER, Traystman R, Kaplan AP, Gralnick H, Valentine MD, Permutt S, Lichtenstein LM. Physiologic manifestations of human anaphylaxis. *J Clin Invest* 1980;66: 1072–1080.

44. Kapin MA, Ferguson JL. Hemodynamic and regional circulatory alterations in dog during anaphylactic challenge. *Am J Physiol* 1985;249:H430–H437.

45. Wong S, Dykewicz MS, Patterson R. Idiopathic anaphylaxis—a clinical summary of 175 patients. *Arch Intern Med* 1990;150: 1323–1328.

46. Silverman HJ, Van Hook C, Haponik EF. Hemodynamic changes in human anaphylaxis. *Am J Med* 1984;77:341–344.

47. Lee WP, Clark SL, Cotton DB, Bonik B, Phelan J, Faro S, Giebel R. Septic shock during pregnancy. *Am J Obstet Gynecol* 1988;159(2):410–416.

48. Parker CW. Systemic anaphylaxis. In: Parker CW (ed) *Clinical Immunology*. Philadelphia: WB Saunders;1980:1208–1218.

49. Clark SL. Arachidonic acid metabolites and the pathophysiology of amniotic fluid embolism. *Semin Reprod Endocrinol* 1985;3:253.

50. Morgan M. Amniotic fluid embolism. *Anaesthesia* 1979;34:29.

51. Paul RH, Koh BS, Bernstein SG. Changes in fetal heart rate: uterine contraction patterns associated with eclampsia. *Am J Obstet Gynecol* 1978;130:165–169.

52. Towell ME. Fetal acid–base physiology and intrauterine asphyxia. In: Godowin JW, Godden JO, Chance GW, eds. *Perinatal Medicine*. Baltimore: Williams & Wilkins; 1976;200.

53. American College of Obstetricians and Gynecologists Prologue. Amniotic fluid embolism syndrome. In: *Obstetrics*. 3rd ed. Washington, DC: ACOG; 1993:94–95.

54. Sparr RA, Pritchard JA. Studies to detect the escape of amniotic fluid into the maternal circulation during parturition. *Surg Gynecol Obstet* 1958;107:550–564.

55. Plauche WC. Amniotic fluid embolism. *Am J Obstet Gynecol* 1983;147:982–983.

56. Clark SL, Pavlova Z, Horenstein J, Greenspoon J, Phelan JP. Squamous cells in the maternal pulmonary circulation. *Am J Obstet Gynecol* 1986;154:104–106.

57. Lee W, Ginsburg KA, Cotton DB, Kaufman RH. Squamous and trophoblastic cells in the maternal pulmonary circulation identified by invasive hemodynamic monitoring during the peripartum period. *Am J Obstet Gynecol* 1986;155:999–1001.

58. Katz VJ, Dotters DJ, Droegenmueller W. Perimortem cesarean delivery. *Obstet Gynecol* 1986;68:571–576.

22

HYPERTENSION DURING PREGNANCY: DIAGNOSIS, PATHOPHYSIOLOGY, AND MANAGEMENT

R.S. CHARI, MD, A.Y. FRANGIEH, MD, AND B.M. SIBAI, MD

INTRODUCTION

Hypertensive disorders in pregnancy are a leading cause of maternal and perinatal morbidity and mortality. Overall, hypertension complicates approximately 10% of pregnancies. The incidence is higher in patients with predisposing factors including nulliparity, multifetal gestation, preexisting hypertension or diabetes, a previous pregnancy complicated by preeclampsia/eclampsia, familial history of preeclampsia, hydrops fetalis, and rapidly growing hydatidiform moles.

The maternal complications associated with the hypertensive disorders of pregnancy include abruptio placentae, pulmonary edema, respiratory failure, disseminated intravascular coagulopathy, cerebral hemorrhage, hepatic failure, and acute renal failure. Most of the maternal deaths worldwide are attributed to these complications.

Fetal complications occurring in pregnancies with hypertensive disease include prematurity, intrauterine growth restriction, stillbirth, and neonatal death. The presence of severe hypertension (160/110 mmHg) increases the perinatal mortality by approximately 10- to 20-fold.[1,2]

CLASSIFICATION OF HYPERTENSIVE DISEASES IN PREGNANCY

Currently, there are a number of classification systems for hypertensive disease in pregnancy (see Tables 22.1 and 22.2).[3,4] These different classification systems vary with respect to the level at which high blood pressure is defined, as well as the significance of nonhypertensive features in the definition of gestational hypertension.

In general, hypertension in pregnancy can be defined as a blood pressure greater than 140 systolic and 90 diastolic on at least two occasions 6 hours apart.

To facilitate an approach to the management of hypertension in pregnancy, the classification of hypertensive disorders in pregnancy can be divided into two broad categories: chronic hypertension and gestational hypertension.

CHRONIC HYPERTENSION IN PREGNANCY

Definition and Classification

The prevalence of chronic hypertension in women of reproductive age is not known and likely varies according to population, race, and geographic location. However, it is estimated that chronic hypertension is present in approximately 1–5% of pregnancies.[5] Chronic hypertension in pregnancy is defined as (1) hypertension that precedes pregnancy, (2) hypertension that occurs in pregnancy prior to 20 weeks of gestation, or (3) hypertension that persists beyond the sixth postpartum week.

The presentation of chronic hypertension implies either primary (essential) hypertension or secondary hypertension. Essential hypertension, which is not linked to a single etiology, accounts for 90% of the chronic hypertension seen during pregnancy.[6] Secondary hypertension is due to an underlying abnormality (e.g., renal disease, certain endocrine disorders, collagen vascular disease, pheochromocytoma, renal artery stenosis, aortic coarctation).

Chronic hypertension can be further subclassified as mild or severe, depending on the systolic and diastolic blood pres-

Cardiac Problems in Pregnancy, Third Edition
Edited by Uri Elkayam, MD, and Norbert Gleicher, MD
Copyright © 1998 by Wiley-Liss, Inc. ISBN 0-471-16358-9

TABLE 22.1   Modified Classification of the American College of Obstetricians and Gynecologists

PREGNANCY-INDUCED HYPERTENSION

Hypertension that develops as a consequence of pregnancy and regresses postpartum
   Hypertension: without proteinuria or pathological edema
   Preeclampsia: with proteinuria or pathological edema
      Mild
      Severe
   Eclampsia: with proteinuria or pathological edema

PREGNANCY-AGGRAVATED HYPERTENSION

Underlying hypertension worsened by:
   Superimposed preeclampsia
   Superimposed eclampsia

COINCIDENTAL HYPERTENSION

Chronic hypertension that antecedes pregnancy or persists post partum

Source: Cunningham et al.

sure readings. If the systolic blood pressure is less than 160 mmHg, and the diastolic blood pressure is less than 110 mmHg, the hypertension is defined as mild. Blood pressure readings exceeding 160 mmHg systolic and 110 mmHg diastolic are defined as severe.

Management

The pregnancy outcome in patients who have chronic hypertension and one receiving antihypertensive therapy depends on the severity of the hypertension. Antihypertensive treatment is necessary for the mother with severe hypertension to reduce the acute risk of cerebral hemorrhage or hypertensive encephalopathy. In addition, these patients are at increased risk for superimposed preeclampsia and require frequent antepartum assessment as well as antihypertensive therapy for blood pressure control.[7]

The role of therapy in patients with mild uncomplicated chronic hypertension is uncertain, despite many prospective studies that have examined the pregnancy outcome in the treatment of mild chronic hypertension (Table 22.3).[8–15] Although maximal blood pressure in pregnancy was lowered in mild chronic hypertensive patients on therapy, neither the controlled nor the uncontrolled studies have shown a reduction in the incidence of superimposed preeclampsia or abruptio placentae with the use of antihypertensive medications.[6]

Therefore, to further delineate an approach to therapeutic management in pregnant patients with chronic hypertension, these patients can be classified as low risk or high risk on the basis of patient history and clinical presentation.

Low Risk Chronic Hypertension in Pregnancy   Chronic hypertensive patients considered to be at low risk (mild hypertension without target organ involvement or damage) have a favorable maternal and perinatal prognosis without the use of antihypertensive therapy. This observation was made in a prospective trial by Sibai et al[12] in which 300 mild chronic hypertensive women were randomized at 6–13 weeks of gestation to receive either no medication or an antihypertensive agent (methyldopa or labetalol). There were no differences among the three groups in the incidence of superimposed preeclampsia, abruptio placentae, preterm delivery, and perinatal outcome. As a result, antihypertensive therapy in this low risk group (95% of all pregnant women with chronic hypertension)[6] may not be of added benefit in pregnancy. In fact, the potential association between low birth weight infants and the long-term use of β-adrenergic block-

TABLE 22.2   Classification of the International Society for the Study of Hypertension in Pregnancy

Hypertension in pregnancy is:
   Diastolic blood pressure > 110 mmHg on any one occasion
   Diastolic blood pressure > 90 mmHg on two or more occasions > 4 hours

Proteinuria in pregnancy is:
   Excretion of > 300 mg total protein per 24 hours, two clean-catch midstream specimens of urine
   collected > 4 hours apart with albumin 1 g/L, or 2+ on a reagent strip

These definitions are then used for the clinical classification into:
A. 1. Gestational hypertension (without proteinuria)
     2. Gestational proteinuria (without hypertension)
     3. Gestational proteinuric hypertension (preeclampsia)
B. 1. Chronic hypertension (without proteinuria)
     2. Chronic renal disease (with or without hypertension)
     3. Chronic hypertension with superimposed preeclampsia
C. Unclassified hypertension or proteinuria
D. Eclampsia

Source: Svensson et al.

TABLE 22.3   Pregnancy Outcome in Randomized Controlled Trials of Chronic Hypertension[a]

| Ref: First Author (year) | Groups | Gestational Week | | Birth Weight (g) | IUGR (%) | Preeclampsia (%)[b] | Perinatal Death (%) |
		At Entry	At Delivery				
Leather[8]	Control, n = 24	< 20	36.5	2520	N/A	N/A	8.3[c]
(1968)	Treated, n = 23		38.0	2840			0
Redman[9]	Control, n = 107	20.6 ± 0.5	38.1 ± 0.2	3130 ± 49	N/A	4.7	1.9[c]
(1976)	Treated, n = 101	21.9 ± 0.5	38.1 ± 0.2	3090 ± 60		6.7	1.0
Arias[10]	Control, n = 29	16.4 ± 1.1	38.3 ± 0.4	3011 ± 103	14.2	10.3	3.4
(1979)	Treated, n = 29	14.7 ± 1.0	38.1 ± 0.5	2926 ± 131	14.2	3.4	0
Weitz[11]	Control, n = 12	< 34	37.6 ± 0.5	2820	25	33.3	0
(1987)	Treated, n = 13		39.0 ± 0.4	3140	0	38.4	0
Sibai[12]	Control, n = 90	11.3 ± 0.2	39.0 ± 0.2	3123 ± 69	8.9	15.6	1.1
(1990)	Treated, n = 173	11.2 ± 0.2	38.7 ± 0.2	3060 ± 72	7.5	17.3	1.2
Butters[13]	Control, n = 14	15.9	39.5	3530	0	N/A	0
(1990)	Treated, n = 15	15.8	38.5	2620	66		6
Gallery[14]	Methyldopa, n = 27	32 ± 4.2	37.5 ± 3.1	2654 ± 821	N/A	7.4	7.4
(1979)	Oxprenolol, n = 26	31 ± 9.1	38.0 ± 2.0	3051 ± 663		7.6	0
Fidler[15]	Methyldopa, n = 22	23.9 ± 6.7	37.7 ± 2.3	2992 ± 732	N/A	9.1	4.5
(1983)	Oxprenolol, n = 24	22.5 ± 7.2	37.1 ± 3.4	2715 ± 919		8.3	4.2

[a]Date are presented as mean ± SEM where available.
[b]Preeclampsia = blood pressure plus proteinuria.
[c]Excludes second trimester loss.
Abbreviations: IUGR, intrauterine growth retardation; N/A, not available.

ing agents in pregnancy[13,16,17] raises further questions regarding the use of these agents in treating patients with mild chronic hypertension. Because the trials performed to date do not establish a justification for treating low risk chronic hypertension in pregnancy, antihypertensive therapy should be reserved for patients who have chronic hypertension classified as high risk.

Although patients with low risk hypertension do not require drug therapy, careful antepartum management and antenatal evaluation are still essential. At the initial prenatal visit, the importance and implications of hypertension in pregnancy should be discussed with the patient. The patient should be encouraged to avoid smoking and excess caffeine consumption, and she should be advised about the benefits of proper nutritional intake. The frequency of visits can be adjusted based on clinical findings. Maternal laboratory evaluation should include a 24-hour urine collection for protein and creatinine clearance in the first trimester. Further laboratory testing can follow in the subsequent trimesters depending on the patient's clinical course. For example, further laboratory testing may not be necessary in patients whose blood pressure and clinical condition remain stable, and in whom fetal growth continues to be reassuring. With the advent of clinical symptoms and signs of possible preeclampsia, however, immediate laboratory reevaluation should be undertaken and further management effected accordingly.

Fetal evaluation should include serial ultrasound for fetal growth and antenatal fetal testing starting at 34–36 weeks of gestation. Timing for delivery should be individualized to each particular clinical situation.

In general, however, patients with uncomplicated low risk hypertension can continue the pregnancy until cervical ripening or until the 41st week of gestation. Obvious indications for hospitalization include superimposed preeclampsia and/or a deterioration in fetal growth prior to 37 weeks. If the clinical or laboratory status of the patient continues to worsen, preterm delivery must be considered. Patients greater than 37 weeks of gestation who develop superimposed preeclampsia or abnormal fetal testing or growth should also be considered for delivery.

High Risk Chronic Hypertension in Pregnancy Patients with chronic hypertension should be considered to be at high risk if they have severe hypertension or if mild hypertension is complicated by target organ involvement or damage. The specific characteristics of high risk include blood pressure greater than 160 mmHg systolic or 110 mmHg diastolic prior to 20 weeks of gestation, or the presence of other clinical and laboratory abnormalities that reflect target organ involvement (see Table 22.4). It is important to note that a patient classified as low risk early in pregnancy may eventually qualify for the high risk category. Pregnancies in women considered to be at high risk are associated with increased maternal and perinatal complications, including superimposed preeclampsia, abruptio placentae, and prematurity.[7,18–21]

TABLE 22.4 Chronic Hypertension in Pregnancy: High Risk Characteristics

Blood pressure > 160 mmHg systolic / 110 mmHg diastolic[a]
Maternal age > 40 years
Duration of hypertension > 15 years
Diabetes (class B to F)
Renal disease (all causes)
Cardiomyopathy
Collagen vascular disease
Coarctation of the aorta
Presence of lupus anticoagulant
Previous pregnancy with perinatal loss

[a]At gestational age < 20 weeks.

The initial prenatal visit in patients with high risk hypertension should include counseling measures similar to those outlined for patients with low risk hypertension. Antepartum care should involve outpatient evaluation every 2 weeks in the first two trimesters, and then more frequently if needed. Consideration for hospitalization should be made whenever adequate control of blood pressure cannot be successfully obtained otherwise, or if there is a concern regarding patient compliance. It is not unusual for such a hospitalization to be necessary at the time of the first prenatal assessment, particularly if antihypertensive medication adjustment is required. Laboratory testing should include renal and liver function tests at the initial evaluation, along with a 24-hour urine collection. We recommend further laboratory evaluation at the beginning of each trimester, and more frequent laboratory testing if clinically indicated. Fetal surveillance should begin at 28–30 weeks of gestation.

Indications for hospitalization in patients with high risk chronic hypertension include the complications previously outlined: specifically, superimposed preeclampsia and nonreassuring fetal growth. In preterm patients who develop severe superimposed preeclampsia, we recommend daily measurements of the maternal platelets and hepatic function, along with daily fetal evaluation after 26 weeks. Delivery may be required in patients who have further maternal or fetal deterioration.[22] In pregnant patients with superimposed preeclampsia who stabilize after hospitalization, delivery may be delayed until 34–36 weeks of gestation, or until pulmonary maturity is verified by an amniocentesis. Preterm patients with high risk chronic hypertension complicated by superimposed severe preeclampsia should be allowed to deliver if spontaneous labor ensues and should not receive tocolytics. Finally, pregnancy can continue until 40 weeks of gestation in patients with high risk chronic hypertension who remain otherwise uncomplicated throughout the course of the pregnancy.

The management of antihypertensive therapy in these patients involves consideration of a therapeutic goal as well as patient understanding and compliance. Antihypertensive medications should be adjusted to keep the systolic blood pressure between 140 and 160 mmHg and the diastolic blood pressure between 90 and 105 mmHg. In patients with mild hypertension and target organ damage, antihypertensive therapy is also recommended for short-term maternal benefit.[21,23] Therapy should be adjusted to maintain the diastolic blood pressure at less than 90 mmHg in this patient population.

The preferred approach for starting medical treatment in high risk chronic hypertension is to initiate monotherapy whenever feasible. Methyldopa remains the drug of choice because thus far it is the most extensively studied antihypertensive agent in pregnancy. The dose of methyldopa ranges from 750 to 4000 mg/day, as titrated to blood pressure response. If this dose is ineffective or insufficient, polytherapy can be instituted. Additional medications we currently consider for use in patients with high risk chronic hypertension are nifedipine (40–120 mg/day), followed by labetalol (300–2400 mg/day). Although the risk for low birth weight infants has been associated with the long-term use of beta blockers,[13,16,17] we believe that the benefit of maintaining the diastolic blood pressure below 105 mmHg probably supersedes the risk of a low birth weight infant in this clinical situation. Nevertheless, the associated risk of low birth weight infants in all pregnancies complicated by severe hypertension should not be overlooked. Therefore, close antenatal surveillance is recommended after 32 weeks of gestation in all patients with high risk chronic hypertension.

GESTATIONAL HYPERTENSION

Definition and Classification

Gestational hypertension is defined as hypertension induced by pregnancy beginning after 20 weeks of gestation and resolving by the sixth postpartum week. The number of women who become hypertensive during pregnancy is not certain, and as with chronic hypertension, the incidence may vary with population, race, and geographic location. Estimates range from 13% in indigent populations to as high as 20% in nulliparous women.[24,25]

Within the classification of gestational hypertension are transient hypertension (hypertension without proteinuria) and preeclampsia (hypertension with proteinuria).

Preeclampsia can be further subclassified into mild and severe. This classification is related primarily to the level of hypertension and the absence or presence of specific clinical and laboratory findings. In mild preeclampsia, the blood pressure exceeds 140 mmHg systolic or 90 mmHg diastolic but is less than 160 mmHg systolic or 110 mmHg diastolic. Aside from mild proteinuria (< 5.0 g in 24 h), there are no clinical or laboratory abnormalities. Severe preeclampsia is diagnosed in the presence of blood pressure exceeding 160 mmHg systolic or 110 mmHg diastolic, new onset protein-uria exceeding 5.0 g in 24 hours, platelet count below 100,000/mL, evidence of microangiopathic hemolytic ede-ma, or elevated hepatic liver enzymes. Persistent headache, visual disturbances, pulmonary edema, and epigastric pain are also consistent with severe disease.

PATHOPHYSIOLOGY OF PREECLAMPSIA

In normal pregnancy, there is decreased vascular resistance, leading to decreased blood pressure through the first half of gestation and a gradual rise to prepregnant levels by the be-ginning of the third trimester.

The normal maternal vascular response to placentation consists of transforming the uteroplacental bed into a low re-sistance, low pressure, high flow system. These physiologi-cal changes during normal pregnancy are initiated by an in-vasion of endovascular trophoblastic cells into the walls of the spiral arteries that replace the endothelial cells and digest their subjacent musculoelastic lamina. These changes begin in the decidual portion of the spiral arteries in the first trimester and extend to the radial arteries of the inner one-third of the myometrium later in pregnancy. As a result, the arteries in the uterus are converted from narrow lumen, mus-cular vessels to distended thin-walled vessels.

Despite decades of intensive research, the etiology of preeclampsia/eclampsia remains uncertain. One of the earli-est abnormalities noted in women who later develop preeclampsia is a failure of the second wave of trophoblastic invasion into the maternal spiral arterioles. As a result of this defective invasion by trophoblastic cells, the maternal spiral arterioles are not transformed into the high volume, low re-sistance capacitance vessels capable of supplying the pla-centa with maximal blood flow. It has been hypothesized that as a result of impaired perfusion, the placenta may elaborate one or more substances that are toxic to endothelial cells. Therefore, the placenta has been recognized as an essential component to the disease process. This connection is sup-ported by observations of the disease in hydatidiform mole and abdominal pregnancies, suggesting that neither fetal nor uterine factors contribute to the pathogenesis of this process. Thus, the placenta is hypothesized as an initiator in the patho-genesis of preeclampsia, whereby placental hypoperfusion results in the liberation of cytotoxic factors, leading to dis-ruption of the maternal vascular endothelial cells, resulting in the maternal syndrome.

There is increasing evidence to suggest that endothelial cell injury plays an important role in the pathogenesis of preeclampsia. Shanklin and Sibai found extensive injury from both placental bed and uterine boundary vessels in all specimens from preeclamptic patients, but not in those of normotensive patients.[26] Roberts et al proposed that aberra-tions of endothelial cell function in preeclampsia could ac-count for the activation of the coagulation cascade and loss of vascular integrity that accompany the disorder.[27] These in-vestigators also suggested that reduced placental perfusion might be behind the release of cytotoxic factors. Tsukimori et al demonstrated that a circulating cytotoxic agent to en-dothelial cells is present in women with preeclampsia.[28] The presence of such cytotoxic agents directed against endothe-lial cells validates the vascular histopathological findings suggestive of endothelial cell damage in women with preeclampsia, including deposition of plasma constituents and proliferation of myointimal cells.

Endothelial cells are able to secrete a variety of signaling molecules into the circulation. Specifically, the endothelium can release both dilator (prostacyclin and endothelium-de-rived hyperpolarizing factor) and constrictor (thromboxane A_2, endothelin, superoxide anion/endoperoxidases) sub-stances, which help to control the tone of smooth muscle.

Prostacyclin, a vasodilator, and thromboxane A_2, a vaso-constrictor and platelet aggregator, are produced by the en-dothelial cell. In the urine and serum of preeclamptic women, the ratio of prostacyclin to thromboxane A_2 has been found to be reduced compared to normotensive pregnant women.[29] Many of the clinical features seen in preeclampsia/eclampsia could be explained by the established effects of prostacyclin deficiency and/or thromboxane excess with resultant va-sospasm. These clinical features of vasospasm include hy-pertension and the ultimate, vascular, end organ involvement of maternal disease (eclampsia, liver infarction or rupture, glomerular capillary endotheliosis, fetal growth restriction secondary to placental insufficiency, etc.). This extensive in-volvement of the endothelium was confirmed by Kraayen-brink et al, who demonstrated an increased urinary excretion ratio of thromboxane B_2/6-keto-prostaglandin $F_{1\alpha}$.[30] They speculated that vessel wall and endovascular trophoblast pro-duction of prostacyclin may be a pivotal escape mechanism of the uteroplacental circulation.

Endothelial cells in cell culture have also been shown to release vasoconstrictor peptides, identified as endothelins.[31] Endothelin is one of the most potent endogenous vasocon-strictors known, and it is therefore speculated to be a con-tributor to the pathogenesis of preeclampsia. Taylor et al have demonstrated that endothelin is increased in preeclamptic women.[32] More recent work by Mento et al examined whether endothelin binding is altered in the fetoplacental ar-teries of placentas from high risk pregnancies complicated by pregnancy-induced hypertension.[33] The findings from this study demonstrated a 41% increase in the density of vascu-lar endothelin receptors in placentas affected by pregnancy-induced hypertension. The authors concluded that the combination of increased endothelin concentrations and in-creased number of placental artery endothelin receptors may contribute to decreased placental perfusion in pregnancy in-duced hypertension.

Further evidence of endothelial cell injury or dysfunction

has been demonstrated with the use of markers for endothelial cell injury. Hsu et al demonstrated that thrombomodulin is also increased in preeclamptic women.[34] Thrombomodulin (TM) is an endothelial cell surface glycoprotein. More recent work by the same group has shown significantly higher serum TM levels in patients with preeclampsia[35] than in either patients with gestational hypertension or chronic hypertension, or in normotensive controls. This finding suggests that TM represents a marker for endothelial cell injury or damage, confirming this underlying abnormality in the pathogenesis of preeclampsia. Another possible marker of endothelial cell injury is tumor necrosis factor α. This cytokine is derived from macrophages and lymphocytes and is involved with the biologic function of endothelial cell function. Tumor necrosis factor α (TNF-α) is increased in the plasma and amniotic fluid of patients with preeclampsia.[36] However it is not shown to be causative, and may represent endothelial cell injury after TNF-α-mediated activation of the immune system, resulting in the secretion of vasoactive substances, increased vascular permeability, and intravascular coagulation.

Other contributors to an increased vascular tone include active oxygens, such as superoxide and hydrogen peroxide. These active oxygens have been shown to influence the derived relaxing factor (nitric oxide) and to reduce the vascular tone, either indirectly, by inactivating endothelium release of prostacyclin, or directly by contracting smooth muscles.[37,38] Tsukmori et al explored this area further by examining whether preeclampsia enhances the superoxide generation of neutrophils.[39] The findings of these investigators illustrated that patients with preeclampsia could be characterized by the presence of a neutrophil activator that enhances superoxide production, therefore contributing to the pathogenesis of preeclampsia. Other studies have demonstrated similar findings.[40–44]

Gant and coworkers demonstrated that increased vascular sensitivity to angiotensin II (a potent vasoconstrictor) precedes the onset of preeclampsia.[45] The operative factors in mediating this vascular refractoriness to angiotensin II are not certain. A number of studies have concluded that the blunted pressor response in normotensive women may be mediated by the vascular endothelial synthesis of prostaglandins.[46–48] Work evaluating the identification of women with elevated angiotensin-converting enzyme (ACE) activity in preeclampsia through ACE genotyping was undertaken recently.[49] Further study as to whether the ACE genotypes will be useful in identifying women at risk for preeclampsia is required.

An important vasodilator is endothelium-derived growth factor (EDRF), identified as nitric oxide. Nitric oxide relaxes smooth muscle and inhibits aggregation and adhesion of platelets.[50] In normal human pregnancy, nitrate concentrations (indirect indices of NO synthesis) are maximal at 20 weeks of gestation and correlate inversely with diastolic blood pressure.[51] Pinto et al, using perfused umbilical vessels, demonstrated that EDRF is reduced in umbilical vessels of preeclamptic women compared to controls.[52] The exact role of EDRF in the pathogenesis of preeclampsia is currently an area of active research.

Other theories not related to alterations in vasoconstrictor/vasodilator substances also exist. Arbogast et al proposed that very low density lipoproteins (VLDLs) may be responsible for the endothelial injury seen in preeclampsia.[53] Such damage may be mediated by direct injury to the endothelium and reduced toxicity-preventing activity, which protects against VLDL-induced injury.

Finally, a genetic component to the disorder has been described. The possibility was entertained initially because the incidence of preeclampsia in daughters of preeclamptic women was noted to be eightfold greater than in the normal population.[54] A correlation between the disease and the HLA-DR4 locus has been described.[55,56] Subsequently, Hayward et al constructed an exclusion map using DNA markers on two-generation families with preeclampsia.[57] These authors assumed an autosomal recessive disorder with complete penetrance and homogeneity in the families studied. A positive linkage was not found, but this result does not exclude the possibility of a genetic etiology in preeclampsia through another mode of inheritance. Chelsey et al proposed that fetal genes may also play a role in the development of preeclampsia.[58] Further study and investigation is needed to establish the role of genetics in the development of preeclampsia.

Whatever the underlying pathogenesis of preeclampsia may be (see Fig. 22.1),[59] it is important to recognize that the clinical syndrome, particularly hypertension, is but one late manifestation of this disease, not a feature of pathogenesis. Therefore, the ultimate cure for the disease is delivery. The institution of antihypertensive therapy in this patient population should be approached with caution, since lowering in blood pressure does not necessarily mean an improvement or stabilization of the underlying disease process.

Management of Gestational Hypertension

The management of gestational hypertension is dependent on whether the diagnosis is one of transient hypertension or preeclampsia. From a clinical standpoint, the presence of proteinuria may occur late in the course of preeclampsia/eclampsia. Therefore, the distinction between transient hypertension and preeclampsia can be both difficult and retrospective. When the diagnosis is in question, it is prudent to assume the more serious process (preeclampsia).

Transient Hypertension Generally, transient hypertension presents in the late third trimester. Since there is an absence of other organ involvement in transient hypertension, theoretically there should not be a requirement for intrapartum or

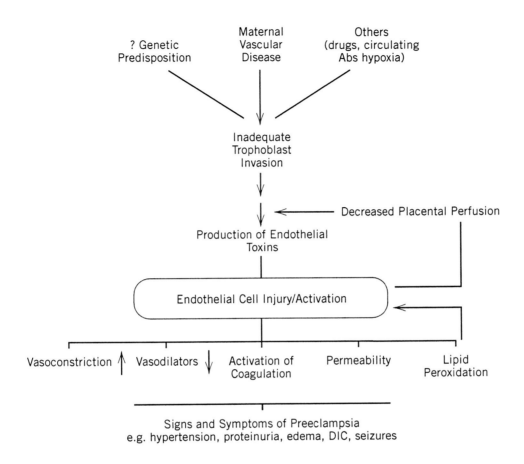

Figure 22.1 Proposed pathology of preeclampsia. (Modified from De Groot et al.[59])

postpartum seizure prophylaxis. As stated earlier, however, it may be clinically difficult to differentiate between this condition and preeclampsia. As well, the lack of proteinuria on a urine dipstick may not reliably indicate the absence of proteinuria, and awaiting the results of a 24-hour urine collection may not be clinically feasible in the face of impending delivery.[60] Therefore, again, in uncertain situations, preeclampsia should be considered and seizure prophylaxis instituted empirically in patients with blood pressures exceeding 160/110 mmHg.

Recent cocaine use should also be considered in the patient presenting with isolated hypertension. This complication is best addressed by a urine drug screen for cocaine at the time of admission.

In patients with idiopathic transient hypertension in pregnancy, the blood pressure returns to normal usually by the tenth postpartum day.[2] The favorable pregnancy outcome in this population was described by Hjertberg et al[61] in a prospective study involving 55 patients with transient hypertension. None of these patients were treated with antihypertensive agents, and they were comparable in pregnancy and perinatal outcome to nonhypertensive women. Long-term follow-up studies indicate that transient hypertension recurs in 80–88% of women in subsequent pregnancies and predicts possible future chronic hypertension.[2]

The use of antihypertensive therapy should be reserved for patients in whom blood pressure exceeds 160 mmHg systolic or 110 mmHg diastolic. Antihypertensive agents that can be considered in this acute situation include parenteral hydralazine, parenteral labetalol, and oral nifedipine. The dosing and administration of these medications is addressed shortly.

Mild Preeclampsia   Patients with stable, mild preeclampsia may be managed conservatively until fetal pulmonary maturity is verified or until after 37 weeks of gestation with cervical ripening.

At our institution, the conservative management of preterm patients (< 37 weeks of gestation) with mild preeclampsia consists of initial hospitalization for observation, bed rest, fetal evaluation, and laboratory investigation. With stabilization of blood pressure, reassuring fetal evaluation, and normal laboratory results, the decision to maintain conservative management as an inpatient or outpatient depends on patient compliance and the degree of proteinuria on the 24-hour urine collection. If the patient is reliable, will maintain bed rest at home, will return for twice weekly fetal nonstress testing (NST) and for fetal growth assessment every 2 to 3 weeks, and if the protein urine excretion is less than 1g/24h, outpatient management can be instituted. If none of the criteria are met, inpatient management with the same frequency of fetal testing and surveillance is indicated. Laboratory investigations, including platelets, liver function tests, and a 24-hour urine collection, should be repeated at intervals of at least 7–10 days.

The use of antihypertensive agents in patients with mild preeclampsia has been addressed in several studies (see Table 22.5).[62–73] These studies have examined the use of α-methyldopa and beta blockers in the treatment of mild preeclampsia before term. The rationale for the utilization of antihypertensive therapy in mild preeclampsia is not to lower the blood pressure readings, but to improve perinatal outcome by prolonging pregnancy safely in patients remote from term. Pickles et al[66] showed that both the maximum blood pressure prior to labor and the incidence of proteinuria were reduced in patients treated with labetalol. However the

TABLE 22.5   Randomized Trials of Antihypertensive Therapy in Mild Preeclampsia[a]

Ref: First Author (year)	Groups	Gestational Week		Admission/ Delivery Interval (days)	IUGR (%)	Perinatal Death (%)
		At Entry	At Delivery			
Sibai[62] (1987)	Bed rest, $n = 94$	32.4 ± 2.4	35.5 ± 3.0	1.3 ± 13	9.3	0
	Labetalol, $n = 92$	32.6 ± 2.4	35.4 ± 3.0	20.1 ± 14	19.1	1.1
Plouin[63] (1988)	Lebetalol, $n = 91$	28.5 ± 7.5	37.8 ± 2.6[b]	N/A	12[b]	1.1
	Methyldopa, $n = 85$	26.2 ± 6.8	37.8 ± 2.6[b]		15[b]	4.7
Pickles[64] (1989)	Placebo, $n = 74$	34.2 ± 2.6	37.5 ± 1.9	N/A	1	0
	Labetalol, $n = 70$	34.0 ± 2.7	37.8 ± 2.2		9	0
Plouin[65] (1990)	Placebo, $n = 78$	28.0	38.4	N/A	11	1.2
	Oxprenolol/ hydralazine, $n = 78$	28.0	38.1		7	2.6
Pickles[66] (1992)	Placebo, $n = 74$	4 ± 2.7	37.8 ± 2.3	9.5	N/A	N/A
	Labetalol, $n = 70$	34 ± 2.6	37.5 ± 2.0	11.5		
Rubin[67] (1983)	Placebo, $n = 39$	33.8 ± 4.3	38.7 ± 1.8	N/A	15	2.2
	Atenolol, $n = 46$	33.8 ± 4.9	39.1 ± 1.5		18	5.1
Wichman[68] (1984)	Metropolol, $n = 26$	33.0	38.0	N/A	N/A	0
	Placebo, $n = 26$	33.0	38.0			4
Cruikshank[69] (1992)	Labetalol, $n = 31$	34.2	37.5	N/A	N/A	0
	No therapy, $n = 45$	35.3	37.4			0
Phippard[70] (1991)	Clonidine, $n = 25$	30.7	N/A	N/A	20	0
	Placebo, $n = 27$	31.6			7	0
Sibai[71] (1992)	Nifedipine, $n = 98$	32.8 ± 2.8	36.1 ± 2.8	N/A	15	0
	No therapy, $n = 99$	33.4 ± 2.7	36.7 ± 2.5		13	0
Blake[72c] (1991)	Atenolol/thiazide/ Aldomet, $n = 17$	N/A	37.0 ± 2.6	N/A	N/A	12
	No therapy, $n = 19$		38.3 ± 1.8			5
Jannet[73] (1994)	Nicardipine, $n = 50$	29.6 ± 6.7	N/A	N/A	N/A	0
	Metoprolol, $n = 50$	28.8 ± 7.2				2

[a]Data are presented as mean ± SEM where available.

[b]Live births.

[c]Hypertension without proteinuria.

Abbreviations: IUGR, intrauterive growth retardation; N/A, not available.

length of gestation was not significantly prolonged and the indices of clinical outcome were not significantly improved in the group receiving labetalol. In a study by Sibai et al,[62] 200 women with mild preeclampsia between 26 and 35 weeks were randomized to treatment with hospitalization alone versus hospitalization with labetalol. This study also showed that treatment in mildly preeclamptic patients did not improve perinatal outcome. In fact, the incidence of infants small for gestational age was significantly higher in the labetalol group. These findings are similar to those of studies cited earlier also involving the long-term use of beta-blocker therapy in pregnancy.[13,16,17] Finally, other authors have argued that the mild hypertension is a physiologic response to a relatively ischemic fetoplacental unit, analogous to the ischemic kidney.[74] Therefore, there is currently little evidence to support the use of antihypertensive therapy in the management of mild preeclampsia remote from term.

Severe Preeclampsia Traditional teaching has advocated delivery in patients with severe preeclampsia remote from term. The rationale behind this management was based on presumed acceleration of pulmonary and neurological development in the preterm fetus of the preeclamptic patient, in the face of maternal disease undisputedly improved by delivery.[3] However, recent studies addressing the issue of fetal pulmonary maturity and neurological development in newborns of preeclamptic women have raised doubts about the accelerated development in utero of these "stressed" fetuses.[75,76] As well, recent prospective studies by Sibai and others,[77–79] have confirmed that the perinatal outcome in patients with severe preeclampsia remote from term and managed expectantly tended to be more favorable than that in those managed aggressively (i.e., delivered within 48 h of admission).

At our institution, we expectantly manage carefully selected patients with severe preeclampsia remote from term. Patients greater than or equal to 34 weeks of gestation are delivered for reasons of maternal disease (Fig. 22.2).

Patients who qualify for expectant management include those who are at 24–34 weeks of gestation and have severe preeclampsia as determined by blood pressure criteria (blood pressure persistently > 160 mmHg systolic, 110 mmHg diastolic). Patients with eclampsia, HELLP (Hemolysis, Elevated Liver enzymes, Low Platelet count) syndrome, or fetal distress at the time of admission are promptly delivered.

Expectant management comprises admission, bed rest, and 24 hours of intravenous magnesium sulfate therapy for seizure prophylaxis. During the period, patients undergo blood pressure stabilization with antihypertensive agents, as well as fetal assessment, including NST, biophysical profile (BPP), and fetal growth assessment by ultrasound. Steroids for the acceleration of pulmonary maturity are initiated at this time. Patients who stabilize on this regimen are transferred to the antepartum floor and undergo daily assessment of maternal platelets and liver enzymes (AST, LDH, and total

bilirubin), as well as daily fetal testing [NST, biophysical profile (BPP), and amniotic fluid index (AFI)].

Indications for delivery include eclampsia, severe hypertension refractory to maximal doses of three antihypertensive agents, completion of 34 weeks of gestation, HELLP syndrome (platelets < 100,000/mL, AST > 72, LDH > 600, and total bilirubin > 1.3), and nonreassuring fetal testing (NST with severe variable or late decelerations, BPP < 4 on two occasions 6 h apart or < 2 on single test; AFI < 5 cm).

In the initial acute setting of severe preeclampsia, antihypertensive therapy should be initiated to protect the patient from the complications of severe hypertension, especially stroke. The goal of antihypertensive therapy in this clinical setting is to maintain the systolic blood pressure between 150 and 160 mmHg, and the diastolic blood pressure between 90 and 100 mmHg. Uncontrolled reduction in blood pressure may be dangerous to both the mother and the fetus and may result in coma, stroke, myocardial infarction, acute renal failure, or fetal distress.

We currently use the following antihypertensive agents in the acute treatment of severe preeclampsia: parenteral hydralazine, parenteral labetalol, and oral nifedipine. The doses are titrated to blood pressure response. Comparative trials of hydralazine, nifedipine, and labetalol have not shown one agent to be superior in the acute management of severe hypertension in pregnancy (see Table 22.6).[80–82]

Hydralazine is given in intravenous boluses of 5–10 mg at intervals of 15–20 minutes, until a satisfactory response has been achieved. Nifedipine is given at 10–20 mg as an initial oral dose. It is then repeated in 30 minutes if required to achieve an adequate reduction in blood pressure. The total dose of nifedipine should not exceed 120 mg over a 24-hour period. Labetalol is administered in repeated bolus intravenous injections. The initial dose of 20 mg is given, and if no improvement in blood pressure is noted, repeated doses of 40 mg and then 80 mg can be given every 10–20 minutes, to a maximum total dose of 300 mg.

In patients with severe preeclampsia, managed expectantly, chronic antihypertensive therapy is often required to maintain blood pressure control. Antihypertensive therapy that we use in this clinical situation includes oral nifedipine and oral labetalol. Nifedipine is started at a dose of 10 mg every 6 hours, increased as necessary to a maximal daily dose of 120 mg. Labetalol is administered at a starting dose of 200 mg every 8 hours, to a maximum dose not exceeding 2400 mg over 24 hours. Again, the goal of antihypertensive therapy in patients with severe preeclampsia managed expectantly is to achieve a systolic pressure between 150 to 160 mmHg, and a diastolic pressure of 90 to 100 mmHg. Adequate blood pressure control will not prevent progress of the nonhypertensive complications of severe preeclampsia, however, and thus careful daily assessment, as described earlier, is warranted.

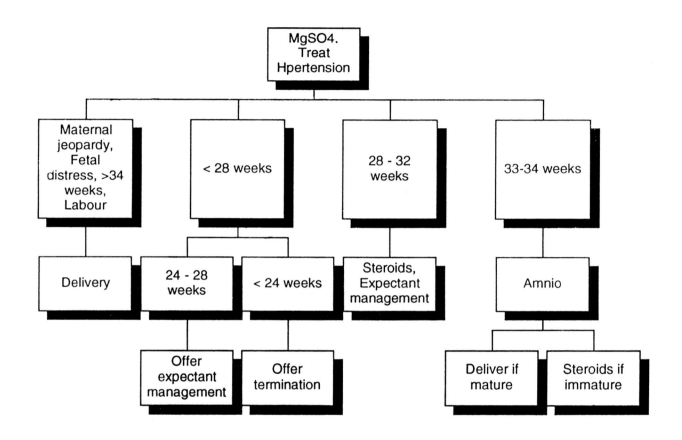

Figure 22.2   Management of severe preeclampsia.

ANTIHYPERTENSIVE DRUGS IN PREGNANCY

Drugs for the Long-Term Treatment of Hypertension in Pregnancy

Therapy options for patients with high risk chronic hypertension (see Table 22.7A) include:

Methyldopa   Methyldopa is the only antihypertensive agent whose long-term safety for both the mother and the fetus has been adequately assessed. Methyldopa is the most commonly prescribed medication for hypertension in pregnancy, and the standard to which all other antihypertensive medications are compared.

Methyldopa reduces central sympathetic outflow by stimulating α_2-adrenoreceptors in the brain stem. In addition, it may act as an α_2-adrenergic peripheral blocking agent via a false neurotransmitter effect. It reduces systemic vascular resistance without causing significant physiological changes in heart rate or cardiac output, while renal blood flow is maintained. The maternal side effects include dry mouth, lethargy, drowsiness, liver function abnormalities, postural hypotension, hemolytic anemia, and a positive Coomb's test. Methyldopa should be avoided in patients who are predisposed to depression, since the condition is sometimes, although uncommonly, a side effect of this medication. The plasma half-life is approximately 2 hours, and peak plasma

TABLE 22.6   Randomized Controlled Trials of Antihypertensive Drugs in the Treatment of Severe Hypertension in Pregnancy[a]

Ref: First Authors (year)	Anihypertensive Drugs	Blood Pressure Treatment Failure (%)	Antenatal Therapy (number)	Gestation Age at Delivery (weeks)	Acute Fetal Distress (%)
Mabie[80]	Labetalol, $n = 40$	10	13	35.5 ± 2.6[b]	0[b]
(1987)	Hydralazine, $n = 20$	0	2	34.5 ± 2.6[b]	33[b]
Fenakel[81]	Nifedipine, $n = 24$	4.2	24	34.6 ± 2.3	4.1
(1991)	Hydralazine, $n = 25$	32	25	33.6 ± 2.4	44
Moodley[82]	Epoprostenolol, $n = 22$	0	22	36	50
(1992)	Hydralazine, $n = 25$	8	25	36	56

[a]Data are presented as mean ± SEM where available.
[b]Patients who received antenatal therapy only.

levels occur within 2 hours after oral administration. However, the fall in arterial pressure is maximal about 4–8 hours following a dose of medication.

Methyldopa crosses the placenta freely so that concentrations in maternal and fetal sera are the same, reflecting the low protein binding of the drug. Methyldopa is excreted in the urine (50–70%) after sulfate conjugation in the liver. The usual dosage in women with severe hypertension is an initial loading dose of 1 g, followed by a maintenance dose of 1–2 g/day given in four divided doses. This dose may be increased to a maximum of 4 g/day as needed. In patients with mild hypertension and target organ damage (high risk chronic hypertension), the usual dose is 250 mg three times daily.

Methyldopa is the only antihypertensive drug for which extensive evaluation of the pediatric outcome[83] is available: There were no differences in developmental tests or intelligence quotients between children aged 7.5 years who were exposed to methyldopa in utero and a control population.

Clonidine   This medication is a potent α_2-adrenoreceptor central stimulant. Its potential side effects include sedation, dry mouth, and rebound hypertension following an abrupt discontinuation. Approximately 40–60% is excreted unaltered in the urine. The usual oral dose in pregnancy is 0.1–0.3 mg/day given in two divided doses. This dosage can be increased up to a maximum of 1.2 mg/day as needed.

The safety and efficacy of clonidine in pregnancy have not been fully studied. Horvath et al[84] reported no significant dif-

TABLE 22.7   Antihypertensive Drugs in Pregnancy

Class	Drug	Starting Dose	Maximum Dose
A. Drugs for the Long-Term Treatment of Hypertension			
Central α_2-agonist	Methyldopa	250 mg tid	4 g/day
	Clonidine	0.1–0.3 mg bid	1.2 mg/day
α_1-Adrenergic blocker	Prazosin	1 mg bid	20 mg/day
Calcium channel blocker	Nifedipine	10 mg qid	120 mg/day
β-Adrenergic blocker	Atenolol	100 mg qd	100 mg/bid
α/β-Adrenergic blocker	Labetalol	100 mg tid	2400 mg/day
Diuretics	Hydrochlorothiazide	25 mg qd	50 mg/day

Class	Drug	Dose	
B. Drugs for the Acute Treatment of Severe Hypertension			
Arterial dilator	Hydralazine	5–10 mg IV q 15–30 min	
	Diazoxide	30–60 mg IV q 10–15 min	
Calcium channel blocker	Nifedipine	10–20 mg PO q 30 min	
α/β-Adrenergic blocker	Labetalol	20–40–80 mg IV q 10–20 min (up to 300 mg)	
Arterial/venous dilator	Sodium nitroprusside	(50 mg/250 mL saline): 0.5–5.0 μg/kg/min	

Abbreviations: bid, twice a day; IV, intravenous; PO, oral; q, every; qid, four times a day; tid, three times a day.

ference in blood pressure control or maternal/fetal outcome in 100 pregnant patients randomized to either clonidine or methyldopa therapy. As a result, these authors concluded that clonidine was a safe and effective antihypertensive agent in pregnancy.

Prazosin Prazosin is a selective postsynaptic α-adrenergic blocking agent. It reduces both the systolic and diastolic blood pressures, while producing less tachycardia and sodium retention than methyldopa. It causes vasodilatation of both the resistance and capacitance vessels, thereby reducing the cardiac preload and afterload without a reduction in the glomerular filtration rate and the renal blood flow. In addition, it produces a decrease in the plasma renin activity and is therefore the drug of choice in pregnancy for the treatment of hypertension characterized by high renin levels. Side effects include fluid retention, orthostatic hypotension, and nasal congestion. The median time to peak concentration in nonpregnant individuals is 2 hours, and the mean elimination half-life is 2–3 hours. The drug is metabolized in the liver and almost completely excreted in the bile. The usual dose of prazosin is 1 mg twice daily; however, the drug has been used in doses as high as 20 mg/day.

The use of this drug in pregnancy has undergone limited evaluation thus far. Lubbe et al,[85] who assessed the pregnancy outcome in 14 women receiving prazosin and oxprenolol, reported no incidence of superimposed preeclampsia. Sibai and Tabb (unpublished data) compared pregnancy outcomes in 80 women with chronic hypertension; half were treated with prazosin and half with methyldopa. Both drugs were effective in controlling hypertension, and the incidence of superimposed preeclampsia was similar in the two groups. There was no difference in perinatal outcome between the two groups; however, patients receiving prazosin had a higher plasma volume at term than those receiving methyldopa.

Calcium Channel Blockers These drugs (dihydropyridines) act by inhibiting transmembrane calcium influx from the extracellular space into the cytoplasm. Therefore, a blocking of the excitation–contraction coupling in smooth muscle fibers results in vasodilatation and reduction in the peripheral vascular resistance. Drugs included in this group are nifedipine, nicardipine, nitrendipine, isradipine, and nimodopine. Nifedipine is the drug that has been used most extensively in pregnant women with chronic hypertension. The main maternal adverse effects are facial flushing, headache, and palpitations. No adverse fetal effect have been reported, and no change has been observed in either uteroplacental flow measured by radioisotopes[86] or placental resistance measured by umbilical Doppler flow velocities in women treated with short-term or long-term nifedipine.[87,88] Nifedipine is rapidly absorbed orally. The two oral preparations that are available are nifedipine capsules and nifedipine slow-re-

lease tablets. The peak activity of each drug occurs at 10–15 minutes and at 40–60 minutes after ingestion, respectively. The maximum dose should not exceed 120 mg/day.

Controlled trials and pediatric follow-up studies involving the long-term use of calcium channel blockers in pregnancy are currently lacking. However, smaller studies have shown that nifedipine slow-release tablets can be used as a second-line antihypertensive agent when combined with methyldopa or a beta blocker.[89,90]

Beta Blockers The drugs in this category have different hemodynamic effects that depend on their receptor selectivity, presence of intrinsic sympathomimetic activity (ISA), and lipid solubility. The basic mode of action of beta blockers is competitive inhibition of catecholamines at the β_1- (heart) and β_2- (peripheral circulation, bronchi, and uterus) adrenoreceptors. Side effects in the nonpregnant patient include bronchial spasm, hypoglycemia, cold extremities, and a disturbance in lipid metabolism. The use of these agents in pregnancy reportedly has been associated with neonatal bradycardia, hypoglycemia, fetal growth retardation, altered adaptation to perinatal asphyxia, and neonatal respiratory depression.[91] However most of these neonatal side effects may be seen as a complication of the severe maternal hypertensive disease itself. The metabolism and route of excretion of the drugs depend on the solubility of each particular beta blocker. The lipid-soluble drugs (e.g., propanolol, oxprenolol, metoprolol) are metabolized in the liver, and the water-soluble drugs (e.g., atenolol) are excreted by the kidney. The lipid-soluble drugs have a short plasma half-life, necessitating more frequent daily dosing (2–4 doses per day). The water-soluble drugs have a much longer plasma half-life and therefore can be given once daily.

Because of the concern for fetal growth restriction, the long-term use of beta blockers in pregnancy should be approached with caution until further data are available to clarify this issue. Their use should be limited to patients with high risk chronic hypertension in whom methyldopa and nifedipine have provided unsatisfactory control of sever hypertension.

Labetalol Labetalol is a combined α- and β-adrenoreceptor blocker. Its theoretical advance over other beta blockers lies in the treatment of hypertension in preeclampsia/eclampsia. The additional property of alpha blockade induces vasodilatation, thereby diminishing the primarily vasospastic process of this disorder. The side effects of this medication include scalp tingling, tremulousness, and headache. A starting dose of 300 mg daily can be increased to a maximum daily dose of 2400 mg/day.

Labetalol appears to be as safe as methyldopa in the short-term use in the third trimester.[63] However, the long-term use in mild preeclampsia was associated with small-for-gestational-age infants in a study by Sibai et al.[62] Therefore, as in the case of other beta blockers, the long-term use of this medication during pregnancy must be approached with caution.

Diuretics   Diuretics lower blood pressure by decreasing the intravascular volume and cardiac output. The most commonly prescribed diuretics in nonpregnant hypertensives are the thiazide diuretics. Side effects of these medications include hypokalemia, hypomagnesemia, hyponatremia, hyperglycemia, hyperuricemia, hyperlipidemia, and hemorrhagic pancreatitis. Reported neonatal adverse effects have included electrolyte imbalance, thrombocytopenia, and small-for-gestational-age newborn. The usual dosage of this medication is 25 mg orally once a day.

A meta-analysis of nine randomized trials of more than 7000 subjects taking diuretics during pregnancy revealed a decrease in the tendency of these women to have edema and hypertension. No increase in the incidence of adverse fetal effects was seen.[92] However, since diuretic therapy causes a fall in blood volume and cardiac output, our policy is to discontinue diuretics in patients at the initial prenatal visit. We have found very few patients who later require reinstitution of chronic diuretic therapy in pregnancy. We restrict diuretic therapy (in the form of Lasix) to patients whose pregnancy is complicated by pulmonary edema or excessive fluid retention, and certain patients with renal disease.

Drugs for the Acute Treatment of Severe Hypertension

Medications used for the urgent/emergent control of blood pressure greater than 160/110 mmgH in pregnancy are listed in Table 22.7B.

Hydralazine   Hydralazine causes a direct relaxation of arterial smooth muscle, which is associated with stimulation of the sympathetic nervous system resulting in increased heart rate and contractility. This drug has been studied in pregnancy for almost 40 years. Maternal adverse effects include headache, flushing, palpitations, nausea, and vomiting. Drug-induced lupus syndrome is generally observed only after long-term oral use of this medication. Uteroplacental flow may decrease following parenteral administration, leading to fetal distress. The drug is inactivated by acetylation prior to being excreted. Individual variations in acetylation, which is genetically determined, do not pose a problem with the short-term use of hydralazine.

The onset of the effect of therapy may be delayed for 20–30 minutes. Hyrdalazine may accumulate after continuous intravenous infusion, resulting in hypotension and, therefore, it should be administered in small intravenous boluses of 5–10 mg at intervals of 15–30 minutes.

Diazoxide   Diazoxide, a nondiuretic thiazide, is a potent arterial vasodilator. There have been reports of precipitous hypotension resulting in maternal cerebral ischemia and fetal distress.[93,94] Hyperglycemia is another side effect. The drug is rapidly protein-bound and inactivated. Intravenous bolus infusion lowers the blood pressure within 30 seconds, with a peak effect seen within 3–5 minutes.

This medication should be administered in bolus intravenous form at a dose of 30–60 mg every 10–15 minutes until an acceptable blood pressure reading is obtained.[95]

Calcium Channel Blockers   Dihydropiridines are potent antihypertensive agents that depress the myogenic tone of precapillary arterioles. The most frequent side effects associated with these drugs are secondary to the acute vasodilatation.

Nifedipine   Large controlled trials using this drug in pregnancy are currently lacking. In a study by Walters and Redman,[96] nifedipine was found to be extremely effective in the acute treatment of severe hypertension in pregnancy. The onset of action occurs within 10 minutes of administration, and the peak action occurs after 30 minutes, with blood pressure control maintained for approximately 4 hours. We give an initial dose of 10–20 mg orally, repeating it every 30 minutes as necessary. The daily maximum dose should not exceed 120 mg/day.

Nicardipine   This drug has been used for treatment of hypertension in nonpregnant patients. In a study by Carbonne et al,[97] nicardipine was given by the oral route for mild hypertension (20 mg, three times a day) and by the intravenous route for severe hypertension (1 μg/kg/min). Long-term therapy (9 ± 2.1 weeks) was well tolerated by the mother with no adverse fetal/neonatal effects noted. Nine of the 20 patients who received intravenous therapy reported headache. Further larger, controlled studies are required before the routine use of this medication can be recommended.

Isradipine   The use of this medication in pregnancy has been reported. Ingemarsson[98] used intravenous isradipine (0.3 mg over 5 mins) and found a normalization of the blood pressure 15–30 minutes after injection. There was no change in Doppler velocimetry of the umbilical or uterine arteries. Further controlled trials to evaluate this drug in pregnancy are required.

Nitrendipine   Allen et al[99] investigated the acute effects of 20 mg of oral nitrendipine in 10 pregnant hypertensive patients. These authors found that a single oral dose induced a decrease in maternal systolic and diastolic blood pressure. The side effects included flushing and headaches. No significant fetal adverse effects were reported. Again, controlled trials are required prior to routine use of this medication in treating severe hypertension in pregnancy.

Nimodipine   One study by Belfort et al[100] examined the effects of Nimodipine in 10 consecutive patients with severe preeclampsia. The results demonstrated that nimodipine is rapidly absorbed after oral administration. Significant maternal and fetal cerebral vasodilator activity was noted. There was a reduction in the pulsatility index in maternal ophthalmic and central retinal arteries, and a reduction in the systolic/diastolic ratio in the fetal middle cerebral arteries. Because nimodipine appears to be associated with a decrease in cerebral vasospasm, its benefit may lie in the treatment of patients with severe preeclampsia/eclampsia. Its use in these patients is currently under investigation.

Labetalol Labetalol has been used in the management of acute hypertensive emergencies in pregnancy.[80] This drug may provide a faster onset of action and a smoother control of blood pressure reduction than hydralazine. However, the dose required to lower the blood pressure acutely may vary considerably, from 20 mg to 300 mg (given in divided doses of 20 mg, 40 mg, and 3 doses of 80 mg every 10–20 mins). The acute administration of this drug results in fewer side effects than are observed with hydralazine.[80,101]

Sodium Nitroprusside This drug is a potential arterial and venous dilator, used extensively in the treatment of malignant hypertension in the nonpregnant population. Sodium nitroprusside is noted for a rapid onset of action with short duration. Because of the potent hypotensive properties of this drug, invasive arterial pressure monitoring is recommended. This drug should be used only in extreme emergencies in pregnancy because of the potential risks of fetal cyanide poisoning and metabolic acidosis.[102,103]

CONCLUSION

Patients presenting with hypertension in pregnancy must undergo thorough examination and laboratory investigation. The decision to begin antihypertensive treatment will ultimately depend on the findings of a complete evaluation. Many drugs are available for treating hypertension in pregnancy. Some have been studied extensively (methyldopa, beta blockers), while others are still currently under investigation (calcium channel blockers, prazosin). As with all medications in pregnancy, the benefit of starting drug therapy must outweigh the expected or presumed complications of withholding therapy. Inherent to this decision-making process is an understanding of the mechanisms of drug action and drug metabolism. Consideration of the potential adverse outcome(s) of drug therapy must be made not only for the mother, but also for the fetus and the neonate.[104–107] Medical treatment should be initiated only when careful clinical assessment supports the suggestion that drug therapy would offer more benefit than harm to the patient and the fetus.

REFERENCES

1. Druzin ML. Pregnancy induced hypertension and preeclampsia: the fetus and the neonate. In: Rubin PC, ed. *Handbook of Hypertension, X, Hypertension in Pregnancy.* New York: Amsterdam Elsevier; 1988; 267–289.

2. National High Blood Pressure Education Program Working Group Report on High Blood pressure in Pregnancy, *Am J Obstet Gynecol* 1990; 163; 1689–1712.

3. Hypertensive Disorders in Pregnancy. Cunningham FG, MacDonald PC, Gant NF, Leveno KJ, Gilstrap LC. Williams 19th Ed., Appleton and Lange, 1993; Chapter 36:pg. 764.

4. Svensson A. Hypertension in pregnancy. *Clin Exp Hypertension* 1993;15 (6):1353–1361.

5. Chelsey LC. *Hypertensive Disorders in Pregnancy.* New York: Appleton-Century-Crofts; 1978.

6. Sibai BM, Usta IM. Chronic hypertension in Pregnancy. In Sciarra JJ, ed. 4th ed.

7. Sibai BM, Anderson GD. Pregnancy outcome of intensive therapy in severe hypertension in first trimester. *Obstet Gynecol* 1986;67:517.

8. Leather HM, Humphreys DM, Baker PB, Chadd MA. A controlled trial of hypotensive agents in hypertension in pregnancy. *Lancet* 1968;1:488–490.

9. Redman CWE, Beilin LJ, Bonnar J. Fetal outcome in a trail of antihypertensive treatment in pregnancy. *Lancet* 1976;1:753–756.

10. Arias F, Zamora J. Antihypertensive treatment and pregnancy outcome in patients with mild chronic hypertension. *Obstet Gynecol* 1979;53:489–494.

11. Weitz C, Khouzami V, Maxwell K, Johnson JWC. Treatment of hypertension in pregnancy with methyldopa: a randomized double-blind study. *Int J Gynecol Obstet* 1987;25:35.

12. Sibai BM, Mabie WC, Shamsa F, Villar MA, Anderson GD. A comparison of no medication versus methyldopa or labetolol in chronic hypertension during pregnancy. *Am J Obstet Gynecol* 1990;162:906–907.

13. Butters L, Kennedy S, Rubin PC. Atenolol in essential hypertension during pregnancy. *Br Med J,* 1990;3.

14. Gallery EDM, Saunders DM, Hunyor DM. Randomized comparison of methyldopa and oxprenolol for treatment of hypertension in pregnancy. *Br Med J Obstet Gynecol* 1979;1:1591.

15. Fidler J, Smith V,Fayers P. Randomized controlled comparative study of methyldopa and oxprenolol in the treatment of hypertension in pregnancy. *Br Med J Obstet Gynecol* 1983; 286:1927.

16. Saotome T, Minoura S, Terashi K, Sato T, Echizen H, Ishizaki T. Labetalol in hypertension during the 3rd trimester of pregnancy: its antihypertensive effect and pharmacokinetic–dynamic analysis. *J Clin Pharmacol* 1993;33:979–988.

17. Kaja R, Hiilesmaa V, Holma K, Jarvenpaa AL. Maternal antihypertensive therapy with beta blockers associated with poor outcome in very low birth weight infants. *Int J Gynecol Obstet* 1992;38:195–199.

18. Mabie WC, Pernoll ML, Biswas NK. Chronic hypertension in pregnancy. *Obstet Gynecol* 1986;67:197–205.

19. Branch DW, Silver RM, Blackwell JL. Outcome of treated pregnancies in women with antiphospholipid syndrome: an update of the UTAH experience. *Obstet Gynecol* 1992;80:614.

20. Abe S, Amagesaki Y, Konishi K, Kato, Sakaguchi H, Iyori S. The influence of antecedent renal disease on pregnancy. *Am J Obstet Gynecol* 1985;153:508–514.

21. Hou SH, Grossman SD, Madias NE. Pregnancy in women with renal disease and moderate renal insufficiency. *Am J Med* 1985;78:185–194.

22. Schiff E, Friedman SA, Sibai BM. Conservative management of severe preeclampsia remote from term. *Obstet Gynecol* 1994;84(4):626–630.

23. Mabie WC, Ratts TE, Ramanathan KB, Sibai BM. Circulatory congestion in obese hypertension: a subset of pulmonary edema in pregnancy. *Obstet Gynecol* 1988;71:553–558.

24. Cunningham FG, Leveno KJ. Management of pregnancy-induced hypertension. In: Rubin PC, ed. *Handbook of Hypertension, X, Hypertension in Pregnancy*. New York: Amsterdam Elsevier; 1988;290–319.

25. MacGillivray I. Some observations on the incidence of preeclampsia. *J Obstet Gynecol BR Emp* 1958;65:536–539.

26. Shanklin DR, Sibai BM. Ultrastructural aspects of preeclampsia. I. Placental bed and uterine boundary vessels. *Am J Obstet Gynecol* 1989;161:735–741.

27. Roberts JM, Taylor RN, Musci TJ, Rogers GM, Hubel CA, McLaughlin MK. Preeclampsia and endothelial cell disorder. *Am J Obstet Gynecol* 1989;161:1200–1204.

28. Tsukimori K, Maeda H, Shinguy M, Koyanagi T, Nobunaga M, Nakano H. The possible role of endothelial cells in hypertensive disorders during pregnancy. *Obstet Gynecol* 1992;80:229–233.

29. Keith JC, Spitz B, Van Assch FA. Thromboxane synthetase inhibition as a new therapy for preeclampsia animal and human studies: minireview. *Prostaglandins* 1993;45:3–13.

30. Kraayenbrink AA, Dekker GA, van Kamp GJ, van Geijn HP. Endothelial vasoactive mediators in preeclampsia. *Am J Obstet Gynecol* 1993;169:160–166.

31. Vanhoutte P. Is endothelin involved in the pathogenesis of hypertension? *Hypertension* 1992;21:747–751.

32. Taylor RN, Varma M, Teng NNH, Roberts JM. Women with preeclampsia have higher plasma endothelin than women with normal pregnancies. *J Clin Endocrin Metab* 1990;71(6):1675–1677.

33. Mento PF, Macica CM, Petrikovsky BM, Wilkes BM. Increased density of endothelin receptors in pregnancy-induced hypertension, *Am J Obstet Gynecol* 1995; 172 (no 1, pt 2). Abstract 420.

34. Hsu CD, Iriye B, Johnson TRB, Witter FR, Honf BF, Chang DW. Elevated circulation of thrombomodulin in severe preeclampsia. *Am J Obstet Gynecol* 1993;169:148–149.

35. Hsu CD, Hong SF, Chan DW. Circulating thrombomodulin is elevated in pregnant women with preeclampsia, but not with gestational hypertension or chronic hypertension. *Am J Obstet Gynecol* 1995;72 (no 1, pt 2). Abstract 433.

36. Kupferminc MJ, Peaceman AM, Wigton JR, Rehnberg KA, Socol ML. Tumor necrosis factorα is elevated in plasma and amniotic fluid in patients with severe preeclampsia. *Am J Obstet Gynecol* 1994;170:1752–1759.

37. Gryglewski RJ, Palmer RMJ, Mancada S. Superoxide anion is involved in the breakdown of endothelium-derived vascular relaxing factor. *Nature* 1986;320:454–456.

38. Whorton R, Montgomery ME, Kent RS. Effect of hydrogen peroxide on prostaglandin production and cellular integrity in cultured porcine endothelial cells. *J Clin Invest* 1985;76:295–306.

39. Tsukimori K, Maeda H, Ishida K, Nagat H, Koyanagi T, Nakano H. The superoxide generation of neutrophils in normal and preeclamptic pregnancies. *Obstet Gynecol* 1993;40:536–540.

40. Warso MA, Lands WEM. Lipid peroxidation in relation to prostaglandin and thromboxane physiology and pathophysiology. *Br Med Bull* 1983;139:277–280.

41. Sacks T, Moldaro CF, Craddock PR, Bowers TK, Jacobs HS. Oxygen radicals mediated endothelial cell damage by complement stimulated granulocytes. An in vitro model of immune vascular damage. *J Clin Invest* 1978;61:1161–1167.

42. Weis SJ, Young J, LoBuglio AF, Slivka A, Nimeh NF. Role of hydrogen peroxide in neutrophil cultured endothelial cells *J Clin Invest* 1981;68:714–721.

43. Hubel CA, Roberts JM, Taylor RN, Musci TJ, Rodgers GM, McLaughlin MK. Lipid peroxidation in pregnancy: new perspectives in preeclampsia. *Am J Obstet Gynecol* 1989;161:1025–1034.

44. Haeger M, Unander M, Norder-Hansson B, Tylman M, Bengston A. Complement, neutrophil, and macrophage activation in women with severe preeclampsia and the syndrome of hemolysis, elevated liver enzymes, and low platelet count. *Obstet Gynecol* 1992;79:19–26.

45. Gant NF, Daley GL, Chand S, Whalley PJ, MacDonald PC. A study of angiotensin II pressor response throughout the primigravid pregnancy. *J Clin Invest* 1973;52:2682–2689.

46. Cunningham FG, Cox K, Kant NF. Further observations on the nature of pressor responsivity to angiotensin II in human pregnancy. *Obstet Gynecol* 1975;146:581.

47. Everett RB, Worley RJ, MacDonald PC, Gant NF. Effect of prostaglandin synthetase inhibitors on pressor response to angiotensin II in human pregnancy. *J Clin Endocrin Metab* 1978;46:1007.

48. Gant NF, Chand S, Whalley PJ, MacDonald PC. The nature of pressor responsiveness to angiotensin II in human pregnancy. *Obstet Gynecol* 1974;43:854–860.

49. Dizon-Towson D, Lempe I, Hasting S, Nelson LM, Verner M, Ward K. A common genetic variant of angiotensin converting enzyme is associated with both preeclampsia and chronic hypertension. *Am J Obstet Gynecol* 1995;172 (no 1, pt 2). Abstract 420.

50. Masaki T, Kimura S, Yanagisawa M, Goto K. Molecular and cellular mechanism of endothelin regulation. Implication of vascular function. *Circulation* 1991;84:1457–1468.

51. Myatt L, Brewer A, Prada J. Nitric oxide production in normotensive pregnancy; measurement of urinary nirtate. *Proc Soc Gynecol Invest* 1992;155. Abstract 193.

52. Pinto A, Sorrentino R, Sorrentino P. Endothelial-derived relaxing factor released by endothelial cells of human umbilical vessels and its impairment in pregnancy induced hypertension. *Am J Obstet Gynecol* 1991;164:507–513.

53. Arbogast BW, Leeper SC, Merrick RD, Olive KE, Taylor RN. Which plasma factors bring about disturbance of endothelial function in preeclampsia? *Lancet* 1994;343:340–341.

54. Zahradnik HP, Schafer W, Wetzka B, Breckwoldt M. Hypertensive disorders in pregnancy. The role of eicosanoids. *Eicosanoids* 1991;4:123–136.

55. Kilpatrick DC, Liston WA, Gibson F, Livingston J. Association between susceptibility to preeclampsia within families and HLA DR4. *Lancet* 1989;2:1063–1065.

56. Zahradnik HP, Schafer W, Wetzka B, Breckwould M. Hypertensive disorders in pregnancy. the role of eicosanoids. *Eicosanoids* 1991;4:123–136.

57. Hayward C, Livingston J, Holloway S, Liston WA. An exclusion map for preeclampsia; assuming autosomal recessive inheritance. *Am J Human Genet* 1992;50:749–757.

58. Chelsey LC, Cooper DW. Genetics of hypertension and pregnancy: possible single gene control of preeclampsia and eclampsia in the descendants of eclamptic women. *Br J Obstet Gynecol* 1986;93:898–908.

59. DeGroot CJM, Taylor RN. New insights into the etiology of preeclampsia. *Am Med J* 1993;25:243–249.

60. Meyer NL, Mercer BM, Friedman SA, Sibai BM. Urinary dipstick protein: poor predictor of absent or severe proteinuria. *Am J Obstet Gynecol* 1994, 170:137–141.

61. Hjertberg R, Belfrage P, Hanson V. Conservative treatment of mild and moderate hypertension in pregnancy. *Acta Obstet Gynecol Scand (Denmark)*, August 1992;71(6) :439–446.

62. Sibai BM, Gonzalez AR, Mabie WC, Moretti M. A comparison of labetalol plus hospitalization versus hospitalization alone in the management of preeclampsia remote from term. *Obstet Gynecol* 1987;70:323.

63. Plouin PF, Breart GL, Maillard F, Papiernik E, Relier JP. Comparison of anithypertensive efficacy and perinatal safety of labetalol and methyldopa in the treatment of hypertension in pregnancy: a randomized controlled trial. *Br J Obstet Gynaecol* 1988;95:868–876.

64. Pickles CJ, Symonds EM, Broughton-Pipkin F. The fetal outcome in a randomized double blind induced hypertension. *Br J Obstet Gynaecol* 1989;96:38–43.

65. Plouin F, Breart G, Llado J, Dalle M, Keller ME, Goujon H, Berchel C. A randomized comparison of early with conservative use of antihypertensive drugs in the management of pregnancy induced hypertension. *Br J Obstet Gynaecol* 1990;97: 134–141. Year 1990, pages 134–141.

66. Pickles CJ, Broughton-Pipkin F, Symonds EM. A randomized placebo-controlled trail of labetalol in the treatment of mild to moderate pregnancy-induced hypertension. *Br J Obstet Gynaecol* 1992;99(12):964–968.

67. Rubin PC, Clark DM, Sumner DJ, Low RA, Butters L, Reynolds B, Steedman D, Reid JL. Placebo-controlled trial of atenolol in the treatment of pregnancy-associated hypertension. *Lancet* 1983;i:431–434. Saturday Feb, 26, 1983/Pg. 431–434.

68. Wichman K, Ryden G, Karlberg BE. A placebo-controlled trial of metoprolol in the treatment of hypertension in pregnancy. *Scand J Clin Lab Invest* 1984;44:90–95.

69. Cruikshank DJ, Robertson AA, Campbell DM, MacGillivray I. Does labetalol influence the development of proteinuria in pregnancy hypertension A randomized controlled study. *Eur J Obstet Gynecol* 1992;45:47–51.

70. Phippard AF, Fischer WE, Horvath JS, Child AG, Korda AR, Henderson-Smart D, Duggin GG, Tiller DJ. Early blood pressure control improves pregancy outcome in primigravid women with mild hypertension. *Med J Aust* 1991;154: 378–382.

71. Sibai BM, Barton JR, Akl S, Sarinoglu C, Mercer BM. A randomized prospective comparison of management of preeclampsia remote from term. *Am J Obstet Gynecol* 1992; 167(4):879–884.

72. Blake S, MacDonald D. The prevention of the maternal manifestations of preeclampsia by intensive antihypertensive treatment. *Br J Obstet Gynaecol* 1991;98:244–248.

73. Jannet D, Carbonne B, Sebban E, Milliez J. Nicardipine versus metoprolol in the treatment of hypertension during pregnancy: a randomized controlled trial. *Obstet Gynecol* 1993;169(5):1096–1101.

74. Broughton-Pipkin F. The renin–angiotensin system in normal pregnancies. In Rubin PC, ed. *Hypertension in Pregnancy.* Amsterdam: Elsevier; 1988;118–151.

75. Schiff E, Friedman SA, Mercer BM, Sibai BM. Fetal lung maturity is not accelerated in preeclamptic pregnancies. *Am J Obstet Gynecol* 1993;169(5):1096–1101.

76. Chari RS, Schiff E, Friedman SA, Sibai BM. Are fetal neurologic and physical development accelerated in preeclampsia? Society of Gynecologic Investigation, Mar 1995. Abstract P-450.

77. Sibai BM, Mercer BM, Schiff E, Friedman SA. Aggressive versus expectant management of severe preeclampsia at 28 to 32 weeks gestation. A randomized controlled trial. *Am J Obstet Gynecol* 1194;171:818–822.

78. Odendaal H, Pattinson R, Bam R, Grove D, Kotze T. Aggressive or expectant management for patients with severe preeclampsia between 28 to 34 weeks gestation: a randomized controlled trial. *Obstet Gynecol* 1990;76:1070–1074.

79. Sibai BM, Akl S, Fairlie F, Moretti M. A protocol for managing sever preeclampsia in the second trimester. *Am J Obstet Gynecol* 1990;163(3):733–738.

80. Mabie WC, Gonzales AR, Sibai BM, Amone A. A comparative trial of labetalol and hydralazine in the acute management of severe hypertension complicating pregnancy. *Obstet Gynecol* 1987;70:328.

81. Fenakel K, Fenakel G, Appleman Z, Lurie S, Katz Z, Shoham Z. Nifedipine in the treatment of severe preeclampsia. *Obstet Gynecol* 1991;77:331.

82. Moodely J, Gouws E. A comparative study of the use of epoprostenol and dihydralazine in severe hypertension in pregnancy. *Br J Obstet Gynaecol* 1992;99:727–730.

83. Cockburn J, Moar VA, Ounsted NM, Redman CWG. Final report of study on hypertension during pregnancy: the effects of specific treatment on the growth and development of the children. *Lancet* 1982;1:647–649.

84. Horvath JS, Phippard A, Korda A. Clonidine hydrochloride: a safe and effective antihypertensive agent in pregnancy. *Obstet Gynecol* 1985;66:634.

85. Lubbe WF, Hodge JV, Kellaway GSM. Antihypertensive treatment and fetal welfare in essential hypertenson in pregnancy. *N Med J* 1982;95:1.

86. Lindow S, Davies N, Davey DA, Smith JA. The effect of sublingual nifedipine on utero-placental blood flow in hypertensive pregnancy. *Br J Obstet Gynaecol* 1988;95:1276–1281.

87. Hanretty KP, Whittle MJ, Howie CA, Rubin PC. Effect of nifedipine on Doppler flow velocity waveforms in severe preeclampsia. Br Med J 1989;299:1205–1206.

88. Moretti MM, Fairlie FM, Akl S, Khaury A. Sibai BM. The effect of nifedipine therapy on fetal and placental Doppler waveforms in preeclampsia remote from term. *Am J Obstet Gynecol* 1990; 163:844–848.

89. Constantine G. Beevers DG, Reynolds AL, Luesley DM. Nifedipine as a second line antihypertensive drug in pregnancy. *Br J Obstet Gynaecol* 1987;94:1136–1142.

90. Rubin PC, Butters L, McCabe RT. Nifedipine and platelets in preeclampsia. *Am J Hypertension* 1988;1:175–177.

91. Van Zweiten PA, Timmermans PBMWM. Differential pharmacological properties of beta adrenonoeceptor blocking drugs. *J Cardiovasc Pharmacol* 1983; 5 (suppl 1): S1–S7.

92. Collins R, Yusuf S, Peto R. Overview of randomized trials of diuretics in pregnancy. *Br Med J* 1985;290;17–23.

93. Henrich WL, Cronin R, Miller PP, Anderson RD. Hypotensive sequelae of diazoxide and hydralazine therapy. *JAMA* 1977; 237:264–265.

94. Neuman J, Weiss B, Rabello Y, Cabal I, Freeman RK. Diazoxide for the acute control of sever hypertension complicating pregnancy: a pilot study. *Obstet Gynecol* 1979;53:50–55.

95. Dudley DKL. Minibolus diazoxide in the management of severe hypertension in pregnancy. *Am J Obstet Gynecol* 1985;151:196–200.

96. Walters BNJ, Redman CWG. Treatment of severe pregnancy-associated hypertension with the calcium antagonist nifedipine. *Br J Obstet Gynaecol* 1984;91:330–336.

97. Carbonne B, Jannet D, Touboul C, Khelifati Y, Milliez J. Nicardipine treatment of hypertension during pregnancy. *Obstet Gynecol* 1993;81:908–914.

98. Ingemarsson I, Wide-Swensson D, Andersson KE, Arulkumaran S. Maternal and fetal cardiovascular changes after intravenous injection of isradipine to pregnant women. *Drugs* 1990;40 (suppl 2):58–59.

99. Allen J, Maigaard S, Forman A, Jacobsen P, Jespersen LT, Hansen KPB, Andersson KE. Acute effects of nitrendipine in pregnancy-induced hypertension. *Br J Obstet Gyncaecol* 1987;94:222–226.

100. Belfort MA, Saade GR, Moise KJ, Cruz A, Adam K, Kramer W, Kirshon B. Nimodipine in the management of preeclampsia: maternal and fetal effects. *Am J Obstet Gynecol* 1994; 171(2):417–424.

101. Jouppila P, Kirkinen P, Koivula A, Ylikorkala O. Labetalol does not alter the placenta and fetal blood flow or maternal prostanoids in preeclampsia. *Br J Obstet Gynaecol* 1986;93: 543–547.

102. Shoemaker CT, Meyers M. Sodium nitroprusside for control of severe hypertensive disease of pregnancy: a case report and discussion of potential toxicity. *Am J Obstet Gynecol* 1981; 139:708–711.

103. Naulty J, Cefalo RC, Lewis PE. Fetal toxicity of nitroprusside in the pregnant ewe. *Am J Obstet Gynecol* 1981;139:708–711.

104. Are ACE inhibitors safe in pregnancy? *Lancet,* 1989; Aug 26:482.

105. Are ACE inhibitors safe in pregnancy? *Lancet,* 1989; Sept 23:750. Letter.

106. Rosa F, Bosco W, Graham CF, Milstein JB, Dreis N, Creamer J. Neonatal anuria with maternal angiotensin-converting enzyme inhibition. 1989;74:371–374. *Obstetric & Gynaecology*

107. Scott AA, Purohit DM. Neonatal renal failure: a complication of maternal antihypertensive therapy. *Am J Obstet Gynecol* 1989,160:1223–24.

23

CARDIAC SURGERY DURING PREGNANCY

Robbin G. Cohen, MD, and Luis J. Castro, MD

INTRODUCTION

A number of hemodynamic changes occur during pregnancy that increase the load on the cardiovascular system. These include increases in intravascular volume, stroke work, heart rate, and a decrease in systemic and pulmonary vascular resistance (Chapter 1). Such changes may not be tolerated in pregnant patients with preexisting cardiac disease (e.g., rheumatic valvular lesions, congenital heart disease, or, less often in this age group coronary artery disease) and may require cardiac surgery during pregnancy. Furthermore, cardiovascular catastrophes such as endocarditis (Chapter 16) or acute dissections of the aorta (Chapter 17) may occur, forcing the cardiac surgeon to operate on the pregnant patient. As techniques in cardiac surgery and cardiopulmonary bypass continue to improve, surgical results in pregnant women have become similar to those of the general population. It is the risk to the fetus that remains high. Finally, in the near future, the advent of "in utero" cardiac surgery may enable surgeons to attempt correction of selected congenital cardiac lesions prior to the birth of the infant. This chapter discusses the many challenges of cardiac surgery and the pregnant patient.

HISTORY

Few cardiac surgeons have much experience operating on the heart or great vessels during pregnancy. As a result, extensive clinical series are few. The first reports of cardiac surgery during pregnancy were published in 1952, prior to the clinical availability of cardiopulmonary bypass. At that time, 90–95% or cardiac lesions occurring in pregnant women

were due to chronic rheumatic valvulitis, of which 75% were felt to be confined to the mitral valve.[1–5] This operative experience in the early 1950s consisted of a total of 11 cases of closed mitral commissurotomies, performed with one maternal death and one premature delivery. One of these reports was by Cooley and Chapman,[3] who described fracturing the mitral valve commissures with a finger placed through the left atrial appendage via a left anterior thoracotomy incision in two patients: one in her fourth month of pregnancy and one at 36 weeks of gestation. Harken and Taylor reviewed the literature in 1961 and included 394 cases of mitral valve surgery in pregnant patients with a maternal mortality rate of 1.8% and a fetal mortality rate of 9%.[6]

In 1957 Daley et al used hypothermia and brief circulatory arrest to perform a pulmonary valvotomy with a good outcome.[7] The first report of an open cardiac procedure performed on cardiopulmonary bypass, which appeared in 1959, described a pulmonary valve commissurotomy and repair of atrial septal defect performed at 6 weeks of gestation.[8] Though the mother survived, the fetus aborted spontaneously 3 months later. With improvements in both surgical and cardiopulmonary bypass techniques, however, results with cardiac surgery on cardiopulmonary bypass have improved. Bernal and Miralles's review of the literature in 1986 revealed 22 cardiac surgical cases performed cardiopulmonary bypass between 1968 and 1983.[9] Of these, 18 patients went on to have normal deliveries of normal infants. One patient required a cesarean delivery during cardiopulmonary bypass, and one infant was stillborn 3 days after the cardiac procedure. There were no maternal deaths. In fact, one patient underwent two cardiac surgical procedures with cardiopulmonary bypass during the same pregnancy; a mitral valve prosthesis was implanted at 2 weeks of gestation, and was re-

Cardiac Problems in Pregnancy, Third Edition
Edited by Uri Elkayam, MD, and Norbert Gleicher, MD
Copyright © 1998 by Wiley-Liss, Inc. ISBN 0-471-16358-9

placed by another prosthetic valve at 35 weeks. Six hours after the second procedure, the patient went into labor and delivered a normal infant.[10] More recent reports continue to confirm the increasing safety of the routine use of cardiopulmonary bypass in pregnant patients requiring cardiac surgical procedures.[11]

INDICATIONS

Despite the improved results now achieved with cardiac surgery during pregnancy, these procedures should be avoided unless it is clear that surgery will yield the best result with acceptable risk. Because of the assumed risk to both mother and fetus, surgery under these circumstances has traditionally been confined to patients with cardiovascular emergencies and those with preexisting cardiac disease that has become refractory to medical management during the pregnancy. For women of child-bearing age with known preexisting cardiac disease, the optimal scenario is patient education, with prevention of conception until the cardiac lesion has been corrected surgically. When faced with a pregnant patient with congestive heart failure early in pregnancy, aggressive evaluation and institution of medical therapy is indicated. Many patients with New York Heart Association functional class I or II symptoms can deliver a term infant with medical therapy alone. Patients with more advanced or worsening symptoms will continue to deteriorate as the pregnancy progresses into the third trimester. Cardiac surgery is indicated in this scenario if a correctable cardiac lesion is present. If the cardiac lesion is not correctable with acceptable risk, termination of the pregnancy should be considered.

Historically, rheumatic valvular lesions have accounted for the majority of cases of significant heart disease during pregnancy. The ratio of rheumatic to congenital heart disease complicating pregnancy, which was 16:1 in 1954, was 3:1 in 1967 and continues to decline as childhood rheumatic fever becomes less common.[12,13] Other important but less common causes of cardiovascular disease requiring surgery during pregnancy are native and prosthetic endocarditis (Chapter 16), and acute aortic dissections in pregnant women with the Marfan syndrome (Chapter 18). These indication for cardiac surgery during pregnancy are discussed in detail in the sections that follow.

Valvular Disease During Pregnancy

The majority of early reports of cardiac surgery during pregnancy involve procedures on the mitral valve, most commonly, closed valvotomies for mitral stenosis. Maternal mortality, as expected, has been no different from mortality for similar operations in nonpregnant patients, and is usually less than 2%. Fetal mortality ranges from 10 to 15%.[14,15] A survey of the Society of Thoracic Surgeons in 1983 included 101

closed mitral commissurotomies performed during pregnancy by 54 surgeons.[16] Most procedures were performed in the second trimester of pregnancy in women with progressive congestive heart failure refractory to medical therapy. This survey indicated no maternal mortality and a low perinatal mortality rate of 3%.[16] However, as pointed out by Chambers and Clark,[17] self-reporting surveys tend to be subject to an underreporting of adverse outcomes, and actual perinatal mortality from closed commissurotomy is probably significantly higher.

Despite acceptable morbidity and mortality with closed mitral commissurotomy, advances in mitral valve surgery have led practically all surgeons to prefer the open approach. Though maternal results have been excellent, loss of the fetus continues to be a serious concern. In the Society of Thoracic Surgeons survey reported by Becker,[16] 68 valve procedures were performed during cardiopulmonary bypass: 23 were open mitral valvotomies and 19 were mitral valve replacements. There was one maternal death due to postoperative hepatitis, and the fetal mortality was 16% ($n = 11$). Most fetal deaths occurred as spontaneous abortions within 4 days of surgery. In addition, two mothers delivered premature infants that survived at 29 and 32 weeks of gestation within 24 hours of cardiac surgery. Three mothers had cesarean sections just prior to cardiac surgery, with deliveries of healthy infants at 35–36 weeks of gestation.[16] Recent review of the literature from 1959 to 1990 summarized 77 valve cases performed during pregnancy.[17] There were 33 open mitral commissurotomies, 29 mitral valve replacements, and 15 aortic valve replacements; 1 maternal death and 13 fetal deaths were reported. In a recent report from Brazil, Born et al[18] described the outcome of surgery in 30 pregnant women with rheumatic valvular disease. In this study, between 1981 and 1992, mitral commissurotomy was performed in 24 patients, double commissurotomy (mitral and aortic) in 1 patient, and valve replacement in 5 patients. Cardiopulmonary bypass was utilized in all procedures. Deaths related to surgery were reported as 13 and 33% for mothers and fetuses, respectively.

Other valvular lesions also occasionally require cardiac surgery during pregnancy. Though fortunately rare, both native and prosthetic forms of endocarditis have been known to occur during this period. Conventional management of native valve endocarditis remains primarily medical, with aggressive institution of intravenous antibiotics (Chapter 16). Given the known natural history of this disease, clinical indications for surgical intervention should remain the same in pregnant patients as in the general population, namely, evidence of persistent sepsis, infection with particularly virulent organisms such as *Staphylococcus aureus* or fungus, progressive heart failure, septic emboli, or the development of heart block. If medical therapy is not successful, prompt operative intervention is warranted.[19]

The goals of operative intervention should include complete excision and debridement of all devitalized/infected tissue, followed by valve replacement. When selecting a valve prosthesis, the surgeon must consider the potential for curing the infection, the durability of the prosthesis, and the risks of postoperative anticoagulation. The patient's age and desire for future pregnancies must also be taken into account. Bioprostheses do not require future anticoagulation in patients in sinus rhythm, therefore minimizing known risks associated with warfarin and heparin during subsequent pregnancies (see Chapter 33). However, degeneration of the bioprosthesis due to accelerated calcification and wear may require reoperation in young patients in as little as 5 years.[20] Durability is clearly superior with mechanical valves. Mechanical valves are the valve of choice in most young women who do not desire future pregnancies or are fearful of reoperation. Mechanical valve prostheses require life-long anticoagulation to prevent thromboembolic events.

Recent success has been reported with the use of both aortic homografts and pulmonary autografts for aortic valve replacement on the setting of endocarditis. These valves offer the advantages of reduced incidence of reinfection and improved durability compared with porcine or bovine bioprostheses. Furthermore, anticoagulation is usually not required, which allows for future pregnancies without the risk of anticoagulation.[21–23] As experience with homograft and pulmonary autografts continues to increase, these may become attractive procedures for valve replacement in the pregnant patients with aortic endocarditis.[24]

A pregnant woman with implanted prosthetic heart valve and clinical evidence of infection with positive blood cultures may harbor prosthetic valve endocarditis (PVE). The incidence of PVE in the general population is low. Agnihotri and associates[25] reviewed 2443 patients who underwent primary or redo aortic valve replacements and found an incidence of prosthetic endocarditis of 3.7%. The results of PVE can be catastrophic, with reported mortality rates ranging from 20 to 50%.[26,27] This high mortality reflects the difficulty of abolishing aortic root or mitral annular infection with myo-cardial extension. The pathologic features of PVE include valve annular abscesses, paravalvular leak, and prosthetic dehiscence. Both bioprosthetic and mechanical valves can be affected; however, the incidence of annular abscesses may be more common with mechanical valves. Infections of tissue valves more commonly involve the valve leaflets, with fewer abscesses observed.[28]

Medical therapy of prosthetic valve endocarditis begins with appropriate intravenous antibiotics specific to the organisms cultured. The historical outcome with antibiotics alone is discouraging, and mortality rates between 56 and 70% are cited in the literature.[27,29,30] Given the rarity of cases of pregnancy complicated by PVE, and the high mortality associated with this disease in the general population, treatment to reduce maternal mortality should be aggressive. Therefore, all patients with systemic infection and new periprosthetic leaks or echocardiographic findings consistent with annular involvement require prompt/early reoperation, which offers the greatest chance for cure. Other indications prompting early operative intervention include heart failure, ongoing sepsis, valve obstruction, valve dehiscence, and fungal PVE.[31] Evidence of vegetations, without annular involvement or embolization, may be approached initially with antibiotic therapy alone.[32] The choice of a valve prosthesis in this setting continues to evolve.[22,33] As with surgery for native endocarditis, recent reports suggest superior results utilizing unstented homograft valves in the setting of PVE.[21,34] The data supporting the superiority of homografts in the setting of native and prosthetic valve endocarditis, along with potential long-term durability profiles and freedom from anticoagulation, suggest better outcomes in the future for both the pregnant patient and the unborn fetus.

As with native valve endocarditis, operative success with the surgical treatment of PVE depends on radical debridement, with removal of all infected tissue, closure of cardiac defects created by the infection, and valve replacement.[32] Depending on the extent of the infection, a large amount of tissue may require debridement, with extensive reconstruction of the heart. Since these operations are associated with considerable morbidity and mortality in nonpregnant patients, pregnant patients with congestive heart failure secondary to prosthetic endocarditis are particularly at risk.

Coronary Artery Disease During Pregnancy

The entire spectrum of cardiovascular disease may affect and complicate pregnancy. Though the incidence of myocardial ischemia infarction during pregnancy has been small, the trend toward childbearing at an older age in western society may influence the incidence of this problem (Chapter 12). Patients with unstable angina and coronary disease refractory to medical therapy or not amenable to percutaneous angioplasty, and those with other critical coronary lesions (e.g., left main disease) may require coronary artery bypass grafting. Other indications for surgical intervention include the complication of myocardial infarction such as rupture of a papillary muscle, acute ventricular septal defect, ventricular rupture, or cardiogenic shock. Fortunately, these life-threatening conditions are extremely rare in the childbearing age group. If they occur, however, surgical efforts should be focused on maternal survival, with consideration given to termination of the pregnancy.

Congenital Heart Disease

Excluding patients with significant pulmonary hypertension, women with many forms of congenital heart disease can proceed with pregnancy with minimal risks to themselves. However, miscarriage, prematurity, low birth weight, and fetal congenital defects are seen with significantly increased incidence. Rarely, worsening heart failure and clinical deterioration mandate early termination of pregnancy or surgical repair. The spectrum of congenital heart disease complicating pregnancy is discussed in Chapter 4.

Acute Aortic Dissections

Hemodynamic alterations associated with pregnancy, along with hormonal changes, may lead to alteration in both intima and media of the aorta and peripheral arteries. As a result, the incidence of acute aortic dissection is believed to be increased with pregnancy. In fact, 50% of acute aortic dissections in women under the age of 40 occur during pregnancy (Chapter 17). Women with Marfan's syndrome are particularly susceptible to aortic dissection during pregnancy and must be carefully followed for evidence of aortic disease (Chapter 18). Prompt diagnosis and institution of therapy are essential, because it is estimated that approximately 50% of patients die within the first 48 hours of the acute event.[35] Thus, in the setting of pregnancy, the risk of death to both mother and fetus is high.

The primary event leading to acute aortic dissection is a tear in the aortic intima permitting blood to penetrate the aortic wall.[35] The direction of dissecting blood usually extends distally from the intimal tear, albeit proximal propagation frequently occurs. The dissection can affect the organ of any aortic branch, producing ischemia by compression of the true lumina of important arterial tributaries. This may result in end organ ischemia or infarction, resulting in any of a number of severe complications (e.g., stroke, myocardial infarction, paraplegia, acute renal failure, infarcted bowel, limb ischemia). In fact, aortic dissection is commonly referred to as "the great clinical masquerader" because of its wide spectrum of clinical presentations. These manifestations are clearly complicated by pregnancy, and the presence of such complexity has the potential to further delay diagnosis.

Many classification schemes have been introduced representing aortic dissection by utilization of general descriptive features.[36] The Stanford classification simplifies aortic dissection based on its location and biologic behavior.[37] Dissections involving the ascending aorta, regardless of the site of primary tear or involvement of the distal aorta, are termed "type A." All other aortic dissections not involving the ascending aorta are described as "type B." Undiagnosed and/or untreated type A aortic dissections are frequently fatal within the first 48 hours, the majority of cases resulting in intrapericardial rupture and tamponade.[38] As a result, control of blood pressure and urgent repair of the ascending aorta is indicated to save the life of the pregnant mother. Blood pressure control should be accomplished with hydralazine or β-adrenergic blocking agents, since nitroprusside poses a potential for fetal toxicity (Chapter 22). Operative goals are to replace the ascending aorta, resect the primary intimal tear if possible, preserve the native aortic valve when possible, and reconstitute distal flow into the true aortic lumen.

Conventional management of patients with type B dissections (no involvement of ascending aorta) is focused on blood pressure control and close observation. Operative intervention is reserved for patients developing major complications (e.g., rupture, acute expansion, vital end organ ischemia).[39] Though consideration for elective/early termination of pregnancy may be prudent and should be discussed with the patient, cases of favorable outcome to both mother and fetus have been reported.[40]

Acute aortic catastrophes in "normal" pregnant women cannot be foreseen. Pregnancy counseling/education has a definite place in the management of patients with the Marfan syndrome, however. In these patients, close medical observation throughout pregnancy is mandated. Pregnancy should not be recommended in Marfan patients with known cardiovascular involvement or significant aortic dilatation (> 4 cm). Early termination of pregnancy has been advocated by some to reduce the maternal mortality associated with aortic complications (Chapter 18).

CARDIOPULMONARY BYPASS AND PREGNANCY

Because of the many hemodynamic and physiologic changes that occur during pregnancy, surgical procedures using cardiopulmonary bypass during this period pose a significant challenge to the cardiac surgeon, the anesthesiologist, and the perfusionist alike. Though maternal mortality for cardiac surgical procedures in pregnant women now is similar to that for nonpregnant women, fetal mortality is reported as approximately 14%.[41] Many have suggested that the safest time during pregnancy for cardiac surgical intervention is early in the second trimester, when organogenesis of the first trimester is complete. Also, maximum maternal hemodynamic changes of pregnancy, which might further compromise the myocardium, have not yet occurred.[42,43] Though successful pregnancies have been reported after surgical correction of cardiac disease using cardiopulmonary bypass during the first trimester, others have shown that congenital malformations were more common when these procedures occurred during this period. Therefore, cardiac surgery during early pregnancy is to be discouraged.[42,44] As gestation progresses beyond early second trimester, the potential for induction of premature labor increases. As a result, waiting until later in pregnancy will increase the chances of neonatal survival.

Perfusion Techniques for Cardiopulmonary Bypass During Pregnancy

Cardiopulmonary bypass (CPB) in the pregnant patient is complicated by the accompanying maternal hemodynamic and physiologic alterations, as well as by the need to protect the fetus. The technical aspects of CPB in the pregnant patient, which were nicely detailed by Josephs and Hindman,[45] are summarized.

Positioning, Monitoring, and Cannulation

To avoid aortocaval compression by the gravid uterus, the pregnant patient should be placed with the right hip elevated 15 degrees. This position rotates the uterus away from the inferior vena cava and enhances venous return to the venous cannula during cardiopulmonary bypass.[46] Decompressing the posterior circulation in this manner may also increase placental perfusion.[43,47]

Standard cannulation should be performed, using the aorta for the arterial cannulation, and the right atrium or vena cava for venous drainage. Cannulation of the femoral artery and vein should be avoided. Femoral arterial cannulation has the potential to result in hypoperfusion of the uterine blood vessels. Venous return through femoral venous cannulas may be compromised by obstruction of the inferior vena cava by the fetal and uterine position.[45]

Aggressive monitoring of both mother and fetus is essential for cardiac surgery to affect cardiopulmonary bypass during pregnancy. The mother should have a radial arterial catheter, Swan–Ganz catheter, continuous ECG, and continuous O_2 saturation monitor placed at the beginning of the procedure. Many centers also routinely use intraoperative transesophageal echocardiography (TEE). TEE provides important information regarding volume status, ventricular filling and function, segmental wall motion, and valvular function, and such results are used to evaluate the heart prior to initiating bypass. TEE monitoring can assist in weaning from CPB and is valuable in assessing the postoperative result of surgery for valvular disease, congenital heart disease, and coronary artery disease.

An abdominal Doppler for detecting the fetal heart rate should be positioned on the patient's abdomen and continuously monitored by experienced personnel from the labor and delivery unit. Some centers prefer bilateral abdominal Doppler probes, so that fetal heart tones will not be lost if fetal movement occurs.

Anticoagulation

Because of its large molecular weight (MW = 20,000), heparin does not cross the placental barrier. As a result, the anticoagulation required for cardiopulmonary bypass does not increase the risk of intraabdominal or intracranial hemorrhage in the fetus. However, maternal heparinization can cause uterine hemorrhage and placental disruption, necessitating close monitoring of the patient's level of anticoagulation (Chapter 33).

Fetal Heart Rate

It is essential that the fetal heart rate be monitored throughout the procedure, and especially during cardiopulmonary bypass. The normal fetal heart rate is between 120 and 160 beats per minute. Insufficient fetal blood flow and hypoxia result from inadequate uterine blood flow,

insufficient umbilical blood flow, or a decrease in maternal arterial oxygen content. Low blood flow rates during cardiopulmonary bypass result in decrease blood flow to the fetus, which in turn results in fetal bradycardia. Restoration of normal blood flow to the fetus usually restores the fetal heart rate to normal.[48] Prolonged periods of fetal distress cause the fetus to autoregulate available blood flow to the brain, heart, and adrenal glands, and to decrease the volume of oxygen by 50%. Fetal survival becomes unlikely after 10 minutes of oxygen deprivation. Lesser periods of hypoxemia are associated with an increased incidence of cerebral palsy or other neurological sequelae.[49]

Fetal bradycardia will frequently respond to increases in flow rates on CPB. Other measures that have been noted to reduce fetal distress on CPB are adjustments in maternal position (to relieve umbilical cord compression), correction of maternal acid–base deficits, maintenance of normal maternal glucose levels, minimization of the use of vasopressors, increasing maternal oxygen saturation, and maintaining volume status and oxygen-carrying capacity by replacing blood loss with packed red blood cells.[49]

Uterine contractions can also be monitored during surgery. Werch et al noted that uterine contractions increase in frequency before and during cardiopulmonary bypass but can be suppressed with medication.[49]

Priming Volume and Flow Rates

The pregnant patient's blood volume is significantly expanded. As a result, a short circuit with decreased pump prime volume is recommended. Since the resting cardiac output of the pregnant patient is increased by as much as 45% (with a coexisting decrease in peripheral vascular resistance), high flow rates are necessary to achieve adequate mean arterial pressure.[45] Pump flow rates to maintain a cardiac index of between 2.6 and 3.0 L/min/m² should be used. One method for estimating adequate pump flow is to calculate a cardiac index of 2.4 L/min/m² based on prepregnant body surface area measurements, and then add 30–50% to the calculated flow, depending on the stage of pregnancy.[50] It should be noted that there is a direct correlation between blood flow and fetal heart rate. Because fetal arterial oxygen saturation varies between 52 and 65%, oxygen supply to the fetus is flow dependent.

Temperature Management

Whenever possible, normothermic or mildly hypothermic conditions should be maintained when cardiopulmonary bypass becomes necessary in pregnant patients. Fetal cardiac arrhythmias including ventricular fibrillation may occur in response to moderate or deep hypothermia. Furthermore, rewarming can result in decreased fetal heart rate and uterine contractions with premature labor.[50] A recent study by Pomini et al reported a fetal mortality of 24% when hypothermia was used in heart surgery during pregnancy[51] compared to 0% while operating in normothermia. During cardiopulmonary bypass, maternal core temperature should start near normothermic levels and be allowed to drift slowly to 34°C. Maternal blood temperature should not be permitted to fall below 30°C.[50]

Myocardial Protection Potassium ions traverse the placental barrier with ease and may induce depression of fetal cardiac activity or cardiac arrest.[45] As a result, the use of high potassium cardioplegia solutions should be confined to the first cardioplegic dose, with normothermic solutions for subsequent doses. An attempt should be made to recover the high potassium solution from the right atrium in the case of antegrade cardioplegia (by use of bicaval cannulation and opening the right atrium), and from the aorta when retrograde cardioplegia is used with the used of an aortic vent. The maternal serum potassium level should be closely monitored and, if it rises significantly above normal levels, steps to promote normalization should be taken. Ultrafiltration during and after the cardiopulmonary bypass run can help to control maternal potassium levels.

Cardiovascular Medications During Surgery Josephs and Hindman[45] emphasize that pregnant patients have unique responses to medications that alter their hemodynamic status. They stress that a number of factors must be taken into account when medications of these types are selected during cardiac surgical procedures. These include the effect on uteroplacental blood flow, the effect on uterine muscle tone and labor, direct and indirect effects on the fetus, and undesirable maternal and fetal side effects. In general, α-adrenergic agonists are contraindicated during pregnancy because the uterine vasculature is controlled by α-adrenoreceptors. Low dose-epinephrine is the vasopressor of choice because at low doses, epinephrine is primarily a β-adrenergic agonist. Sodium nitroprusside is contraindicated during pregnancy because of the risk of cyanide toxicity to mother and fetus. Any medication that lowers blood pressure must be used with care because of its effects on uterine blood flow. Hydralazine is useful for treating hypertension during cardiopulmonary bypass because it decreases blood pressure in the mother while increasing renal and uterine blood flow.

FUTURE CONSIDERATIONS

In Utero Cardiac Surgery for Congenital Heart Defects

The widespread use of prenatal ultrasound examination has made possible the early identification of many congenital anomalies. The pioneering efforts of Adzick and Harrison[52] have allowed "fetal surgery" to emerge as a rapidly developing branch of pediatric surgery, with many as yet unexplored applications for the future. Although most correctable lesions diagnosed in utero are more safely managed after planned delivery, certain life-threatening fetal malformations are being recognized as best managed by the "in utero" approach. One example is the treatment of congenital diaphragmatic hernia, which has been repaired in a select group of patients at the University of California, San Francisco.

It remains to be seen whether the in utero approach will find application and prove feasible and beneficial for the fetus with correctable cardiac anomalies. Currently, animal models in which the fetus is subjected to cardiopulmonary bypass are providing valuable insight into the many obstacles remaining before such technology can be applied clinically.[53,54]

REFERENCES

1. Shaffer CF, Chapan DW. *Correlative Cardiology.* Philadelphia: WB Saunders; 1952.

2. Brock RC. Valvulotomy in pregnancy. *Proc R Soc Med* 1952;45:538–542.

3. Cooley DA, Chapman DW. Mitral commissurotomy during pregnancy. *JAMA* 1952;150:1113–1116.

4. Logan A, Turner RWD. Mitral valvulotomy during pregnancy. *Lancet* 1952;1:1286–1289.

5. Mason J, Stable FE, Szekely PJ. Cardiac disease in pregnancy. *J Obstet Gynaecol Br Emp* 1952;59:569–575.

6. Harken DE, Taylor WJ. Cardiac surgery during pregnancy. *Clin Obstet Gynecol* 1961;4:697–709.

7. Daley, R, Harrison GK, McMillan IK. Direct-vision pulmonary valvotomy during pregnancy. *Lancet* 1957;2:875–876.

8. Dubourg G, Broustet H, Bricaud H. Correction complete d'une triade de Fallot, en circulation extra-corporelle, chez une femme enceinte. *Arch Mal Coeur Vaiss* 1959;52:1389–1393.

9. Bernal JM, Miralles PJ. Cardiac surgery with cardiopulmonary bypass during pregnancy. *Obstet Gynecol Survey* 1986;41:1–6.

10. Miller M, Buchanan N, Cane RD, Kinsley R. Two mitral valve replacements during the course of a single pregnancy. *Intensive Care Med* 1978;4:41.

11. Rossouw GJ, Knott-Craig CJ, Barnard PM, Macgregor LA, Van Zyl WP. Intracardiac operation in seven pregnant women. *Ann Thorac Surg* 1993;55:1172–1174.

12. Niswander KR, Berendes H, Dentschberger J, Lipko N, Westphal MC. Fetal morbidity following potential anoxygenic obstetric conditions. V. Organic heart disease. *Am J Obstet Gynecol* 1967;98:871–876.

13. Szekely P, Turner R, Snaith L. Pregnancy and the changing pattern of rheumatic heart disease. *Br Heart J* 1973;35:1293–1299.

14. Vosloo S, Reichart B. The feasibility of closed mitral valvotomy in pregnancy. *J Thorac Cardiovasc Surg* 1987;93:675–679.

15. Knapp RXC, Ardin Ll. Closed mitral valvulotomy in pregnancy. *Clin Obstet Gynecol* 1968;11:978–991.

16. Becker RM. Intracardiac surgery in pregnant women. *Ann Thorac Surg* 1983;36:453.

17. Chambers CE, Clark SL. Cardiac surgery during pregnancy. *Clin Obstet Gynecol* 1994;37:316–323.

18. Born D, Massonetto JC, de Almeida PA, Moron AF, Buffolo E, Gomes WJ, Martinez-Filho EE. Heart surgery with extracorporeal circulation in pregnant women. Analysis of materno-fetal outcome. *Arq Bras Cardiol* 1995;64:207–211.

19. Westaby S, Parry AJ, Forfar JC. Reoperation for prosthetic valve endocarditis in the third trimester of pregnancy. *Ann Thorac Surg* 1992;53:263–265.

20. Sbarouni E, Oakley CM. Outcome of pregnancy in women with valve prostheses. *Br Heart J* 71:196–201.

21. McGiffin DC, Galbraith AJ, McLachlan GG, Stower RE, Wong ML, Stafford EG, Gardner MA, Pohlner PG, O'Brian MF. Aortic valve infarction: risk factors for death and recurrent endocarditis after valve replacement. *J Thorac Cardiovasc Surg* 1992;104:511–520.

22. Tuna IC, Orzulak TA, Schaff HV, Danielson GK. Results of homograft aortic valve replacement for active endocarditis. *Ann Thorac Surg* 1990;49:619–624.

23. Ross DN. Replacement of the aortic and mitral valves with a pulmonary autograft. *Lancet* 1967;2:956–958.

24. Joyce F, Tingleff J, Aagaard J, Pettersson G. The Ross operation in the treatment of native and prosthetic valve endocarditis. *J Heart Valve Disease* 1994;3:371–376.

25. Agnihotri AK, McGiffin DC, Galbraith AJ, O'Brient MF. The prevalence of endocarditis after aortic valve replacement. *J Thorac Cardiovasc Surg* 1995;110:1708–1724.

26. Nunez L, del la Llana R, Aguado MG, Iglesias A, Larrea JL, Celemin D. Bioprosthetic valve endocarditis: indications for surgical intervention. *Ann Thorac Surg* 1983;35:262–270.

27. Miller DC. Predictors of outcome in patients with prosthetic valve endocarditis and potential advantages of homograft aortic root replacement for prosthetic ascending valve-graft infections. *J Cardiac Surg* 1990;5:53–62.

28. Mandell GL, Bennett JE, Dolin R. *Principles and Practices of Infectious Disease.* 4th ed. New York: Churchill Livingstone; 1995;783–791.

29. Fang G, Keys TF, Gentry LO, Harris AA, Rivera L, Getz K, Fuchs PC, Gustafson M, Wong ES, Goetz A, Wagener MM, Yu VL. Prosthetic valve endocarditis resulting from nosocomial bacteremia: a prospective multicenter study. *Ann Intern Med* 193;119:560–567.

30. Ivert TS, Dismukes WE, Cobbs CG, Blackstone EH, Kirklin JW, Bergdahl LA. Prosthetic valve endocarditis. *Circulation* 1984;69:223–232.

31. Kirklin JW, Barret-Boyes BG. *Cardiac Surgery.* 2nd ed. New York: Churchill Livingstone; 1993.

32. Lytle B. Surgical treatment of prosthetic valve endocarditis. *Semin Thorac Cardiovasc Surg* 1995;7:13–19.

33. Kirklin JW, Kirklin JW, Pacifico AD. Aortic valve endocarditis with aortic root abscess cavity: surgical treatment with aortic valve homograft. *Ann Thorac Surg* 1988;45:674–677.

34. Haycock D, Barret-Boyes BG, Macedo T, Kirklin JW, Blackstone E. Aortic valve replacement for active infectious endocarditis in 108 patients: a comparison of free allograft valves with mechanical prostheses and bioprostheses. *J Thorac Cardiovasc Surg* 1992;103:130–139.

35. Anagnostopoulos E. *Acute Aortic Dissections.* Baltimore: University Press; 1975.

36. Deakey ME, Henly WS, Cooley DA, Morris GC, Crawford ES, Beall AC. Surgical management of dissecting aneurysms of the aorta. *J Thorac Cardiovasc Surg* 1965;49:130–149.

37. Daily P, Trueblood W, Stinson E, Wuerflein R, Shumway NE. Management of aortic dissections. *Ann Thorac Surg* 1970;10:237–247.

38. Hirst A, Johns V, Kime S. Dissecting aneurysm of the aorta: a review of 505 cases. *Medicine* 1958;37:217–279.

39. Glower D, Fann AJ, Speir M, Morrison L, White W, Smith R, Rankin S, Miller DC, Wolfe W. Comparison of medical and surgical therapy for uncomplicated descending aortic dissection. *Circulation* 1990;82(suppl IV)IV39–IV46.

40. Elkayam U, Ostrzega E, Shotan A, Mehra A. Cardiovascular problems in pregnant women with the Marfan syndrome. *Ann Intern Med* 1995;123:117–122.

41. Parry AJ, Westaby S. Cardiopulmonary bypass during pregnancy. *Perfusion Rev* 1994;3:8–18.

42. Zitnik RS, Brandenberg RO, Sheldon R, Wallace RB. Pregnancy and open heart surgery. *Circulation* 1969;39:257–262.

43. Meffert WG, Stansel HC. Open heart surgery during pregnancy. *Am J Obstet Gynecol* 1968;102:1116–1120.

44. Lapiedra OJ, Bernal JM, Ninot S, Gonzalez I, Pastor E, Pedro PJ. Open heart surgery for mitral prosthetic thrombosis during pregnancy. Fetal hydrocephalus. *J Thorac Cardiovasc Surg* 1986;27:217.

45. Josephs J, Hindman R. Cardiopulmonary bypass and the pregnant patient: a review. *J Extracorporeal Technol* 1993;25:61–66.

46. Sutton RG. Cardiopulmonary bypass and related issues involving the pregnant patient. Mechanics of Cardiopulmonary Bypass VI; Lake Buena Vista, FL; 1990.

47. Lalone B, Snow S. *Cardiopulmonary Bypass Methods.* Indianapolis, IN: Extracorporeal Technology; 1990;41–42.

48. Levy DL, Warriner RA, Burgess GE. Fetal response to cardiopulmonary bypass. *Obstet Gynecol* 1980;56:112–115.

49. Werch A, Lambert HM, Cooley D, Reed CC. Fetal monitoring and maternal open heart surgery. *South Med J* 1977;70:1024.

50. Sutton RG. Cardiopulmonary bypass and related issues involving the pregnant patient. Mechanics of Cardiopulmonary Bypass VI; Lake Buena Vista, FL; 1990.

51. Pomini F, Mercogliano D, Cavalletti C, Caruso A, Pomini P. Cardiopulmonary bypass in pregnancy. *Ann Thorac Surg* 1996;61:259–268.

52. Adzick NS, Harrison MR. The unborn surgical patient. *Curr Probl Surg* 1994;31:176.

53. Fenton KN, Zinn HE, Heinemann MK, Liddicoat JR, Hanley FL. Long-term survivors of fetal cardiac bypass in lambs. *J Thorac Cardiovasc Surg* 1994;107:1423–1427.

54. Hanley FL. Fetal cardiac surgery. *Adv Cardiac Surg* 1994;5:47–74.

24

ANALGESIA AND ANESTHESIA DURING PREGNANCY

JAYA RAMANATHAN, MD, JOHN G. D'ALESSIO, MD, ERAN GELLER, MD, VALERY RUDICK, MD, AND DAVID NIV, MD

INTRODUCTION

Much progress has been made since Simpson's first attempt to administer ether to a woman in labor in 1847. Today, thanks to the development of modern obstetric anesthesia, parturients can look forward to a relatively painless, safe, and stress-free labor and delivery, and often even enjoy participating in the birth of their children.

The parturient with complex cardiac disease offers a special challenge, even to the most experienced anesthesiologist, for various reasons. For instance, there have been no large-scale, controlled, prospective or retrospective studies on anesthetic management of pregnant women with cardiac diseases. Therefore, data regarding the safety or superiority of any anesthetic agent or technique for a given patient with a specific cardiac lesion are not clearly defined. Thus, to choose the most appropriate anesthetic for these patients, the obstetric anesthesiologist has no choice other than deriving information from isolated case reports and relying on personal experience.

When planning a safe anesthetic for a pregnant woman with a serious cardiac problem, the obstetric anesthesiologist is often in the unenviable position of having to play many different roles—as a critical care specialist, a pulmonologist, and even a cardiologist. Anesthesiologists are often involved in the placement of invasive monitoring lines; in the intensive care unit, they are often called on to interpret the hemodynamic data and electrocardiographic findings and to initiate appropriate therapeutic interventions as well as to participate in the management of patients on ventilators. To achieve this formidable complex of tasks, obstetric anesthe-

siologists should be familiar with and able to integrate their knowledge of the following:

the anesthetic significance of normal cardiovascular changes of pregnancy, labor, and delivery

the pathophysiology of the preexisting cardiac disease and the current cardiac status

the direct effects of anesthetic agents on the heart as well as the indirect effects mediated through the autonomic nervous system by regional blockade

The opinion expressed by Lunn and Mushin,[1] that the "quality of the anesthetist is more important in terms of outcome than the drugs or techniques he chooses to use" assumes special significance in the context of anesthetic considerations in the cardiac parturient.

LABOR PAIN AND ANALGESIC CONSIDERATIONS

Pain of parturition arises as soon as the uterus begins to contract. During the first stage of labor, distension, stretching and tearing of the cervix, as well as contraction and distension of the uterus, are considered to be the major stimuli causing pain.[2] No direct relationship exists between the intensity of pain during the first stage of labor and the degree of cervical dilatation, but the commonly accepted dictum is that pain tends to be augmented toward the end of the first stage of labor. These painful stimuli can be effectively interrupted two ways: peripherally, by blocking the paracervical nerves, and centrally, by performing paravertebral, epidural, or sub-

Cardiac Problems in Pregnancy, Third Edition
Edited by Uri Elkayam, MD, and Norbert Gleicher, MD
Copyright © 1998 by Wiley-Liss, Inc. ISBN 0-471-16358-9

arachnoid blocks on T10–L1 nerve roots before their entrance into the spinal cord.

A sharp perineal pain dominates the second stage of labor. This pain can be effectively relieved by peripheral blockade of the pudendal nerves, which originate from the perineal structures, or by using caudal, low epidural, and low subarachnoid blocks. The latter blocks interrupt nociceptive stimuli traveling via the S2–S4 nerves into the spinal cord.

IMPACT OF PREGNANCY-INDUCED CHANGES ON ANESTHESIA

The impact of the physiologic changes of pregnancy on the conduct of anesthesia must be taken into account and is summarized briefly herein.

Anesthetic Significance of Cardiovascular Changes in Pregnancy

For a detailed review of cardiac function during pregnancy, consult Chapter 1. A brief description of pregnancy-related changes in cardiac output, heart rate, preload, afterload, and myocardial contractility is appropriate.[3,4]

Cardiac output begins to increase from the 5th week of pregnancy and reaches the maximum of 45% above the preconception values around the 24th week of gestation. The increases in heart rate and stroke volume contribute toward the increase in cardiac output. The heart rate begins to rise by the 5th week of gestation and continues well into the third trimester. Stroke volume starts to rise by about the 8th week and continues until the 20–24th week of gestation. During labor, cardiac output increases further, and at full dilatation of the cervix it reaches the maximum of 34% above prelabor values. Again, both heart rate and stroke volume increase, contributing to this effect. After delivery, the cardiac output remains high because of the additional, dramatic increase in the stroke volume due partly to the augmented venous return from the relief of venacaval compression.

Preload increases during pregnancy because of expanded blood volume and increased venous return. On the other hand, *afterload* decreases significantly (by about 34%) by 20 weeks of pregnancy as a result of progressive decrease in systemic vascular resistance. Myocardial *contractility* increases slightly but not to a significant degree in healthy pregnant women.[5] The central venous and pulmonary arterial pressures remain essentially unchanged.

All the foregoing changes are important in terms of anesthetic management of pregnant women with cardiac diseases as described below.

- Increased heart rates of pregnancy pose additional stress on the diseased myocardium. Some of the commonly used anesthetic agents and drugs (ephedrine, ketamine,

enflurane, etc.) can cause additional rise in heart rate, thus compounding the problem.

- Similarly, many anesthetic gents—specifically, inhalation agents and intravenous induction agents—depress myocardial contractility and therefore are to be avoided.
- The fall in peripheral vascular resistance of pregnancy may worsen (right-to-left shunts) or improve (aortic incompetence) the clinical status. The sympathetic blockade resulting from regional anesthesia further decreases the systemic vascular resistance; therefore in a given patient, depending on the clinical situation, epidural anesthesia can improve or worsen forward flow, alter intracardiac shunt fraction, and even change the direction of shunt flow. These factors are discussed in detail later.
- The pregnant cardiac patient is more likely to have cardiac failure during the second stage or immediate postpartum period. All anesthetic interventions should be undertaken with extreme caution to prevent further compromise of the cardiac status. Appropriate choice of anesthetic drugs and inotropes is important, as is judicious fluid management, preferably with invasive hemodynamic monitoring.

Anesthetic Significance of Respiratory System Changes

- Water retention and increased vascularity tend to cause swelling of the upper respiratory tract, with production of copious amounts of secretions. Therefore, direct laryngoscopy and visualization of larynx can be difficult and endotracheal intubation traumatic.[6]
- The decrease in oxygen reserve due to reduced functional residual capacity and increased oxygen consumption causes rapid desaturation and hypoxia, especially during difficult tracheal intubation or upper airway obstruction caused by deep sedation.[7]
- Increased minute ventilation and decreased functional residual capacity can cause rapid uptake of inhalation agents. Therefore, the parturient can quickly lose her upper airway reflexes and become unconscious at far lower concentrations of inhalation anesthetics when these agents are used to provide analgesia for labor.

In parturients with cardiac diseases, continuous administration of oxygen during labor and delivery, and adequate oxygenation before the induction of general anesthesia, are mandatory.[8–10]

Anesthetic Implications of Gastrointestinal System Changes

Interference with gastric emptying occurs when the enlarging uterus causes a shift in the position of the stomach, thus changing the angle of the gastroesophageal junction. Intragastric pressure increases and gastric motility decreases in pregnancy. Several investigators have studied gastric motility in pregnant women with conflicting results.[11,12] While some authors found decreased gastric motility early in the first trimester, others reported that the gastric emptying time remained unchanged until the 34th week of pregnancy or even until the onset of labor.[11,12] With the onset of labor, other factors such as fear, labor pain, and opioid drugs inhibit gastric motility. Finally, the lithotomy position, as well as muscle fasciculations caused by succinylcholine, can cause further rise in intragastric pressure.[9,13]

Any loss of protective airway reflexes (e.g., during induction of general anesthesia) is therefore associated with considerable risk of pulmonary aspiration of stomach contents. Measures such as preoperative antacid administration and rapid sequence induction with cricoid pressure are routinely used to prevent pulmonary aspiration. General anesthesia should be the last resort in a parturient beyond the middle of the second trimester and should never be conducted without an endotracheal tube securing the airway.

On the other hand, the risk of aspiration under regional anesthesia is negligible, with the mother being wide awake with intact upper airway reflexes; therefore this technique is preferred whenever possible.[14]

EFFECTS OF REGIONAL ANESTHESIA ON CARDIAC FUNCTION

A review on anesthetic management of the pregnant cardiac patient is incomplete without a brief discussion on the hemodynamic effects of regional anesthesia. In general, the effects of epidural and spinal anesthesia on cardiac function depend on the *extent* of sympathetic blockage.[15] The higher the level of block, the greater the effects. As noted earlier, satisfactory labor analgesia is achieved with epidural anesthesia extending to the tenth thoracic dermatome (T10), which is considered to be a "low" block. The hemodynamic perturbations resulting from such a low level are minimal and therefore acceptable in most pregnant cardiac patients.

For cesarean delivery, higher dermatome levels are needed. Therefore, local anesthetics of higher strength in larger volumes are administered to extend anesthesia all the way up to the sixth to the fourth thoracic dermatomal levels (T6–T4). Often, the sympathetic block extends several segments higher than the sensory and motor levels. Therefore, at T4 levels, most of the cardiac sympathetics may be blocked (T1–T4), causing profound hemodynamic changes. Despite such extensive sympathectomy induced by the local anesthetics, the hemodynamic changes are slower and occur in a more controlled fashion. Most pregnant women with cardiac diseases, including those with right-to-left shunts, readily tolerate a carefully administered epidural anesthesia for labor, vaginal delivery, and cesarean section.

In addition to the level of block, the speed of onset of the block determines the degree of hemodynamic changes.[16,17] For example, subarachnoid block causes the mean arterial pressure to fall precipitously as a result of the rapid onset of sympathetic blockade. Therefore, despite the simplicity and ease of the technique (compared to epidural), spinal anesthesia is not the appropriate anesthetic in most pregnant women with cardiac diseases. The following section briefly discusses the effects of regional anesthesia on cardiac function.

Cardiac Functions Affected by Regional Anesthesia

Preload   Various studies have shown that regional anesthesia decreases the preload as a result of the accompanying dilatation of venous capacitance vessels and sequestration of blood in the large peripheral vessels, with decreased venous return and cardiac output.[18–20] Often the hypotension due to regional block can be minimized by adequate hydration and strict avoidance of aortocaval compression. Needless to say, in the pregnant cardiac patient, any hydration that precedes regional blocks should be done judiciously, with the aid of invasive monitoring.

Afterload   Even with extensive sympathetic blockade, afterload decreases to a lesser degree than preload because the arteriolar tone is affected to a lesser extent than the tone of venous capacitance vessels.[21]

Heart Rate   Heart rate may decrease with high levels of regional anesthesia, partially because blockade of cardiac sympathetics has occurred. Recent studies have shown that in pregnant women, heart rate variability is significantly reduced compared to nonpregnant controls.[22–24] Power spectral analysis of heart rate variability of term parturients receiving regional anesthesia for cesarean section have shown that the total variability as well as high (mediated by parasympathetics) and low (mediated by both parasympathetic and sympathetic systems) spectral components of heart rate variability are further reduced from baseline. The significance of such findings in pregnant cardiac patients is yet to be defined.

Contractility   The effects of regional anesthesia on myocardial contractility are not studied in detail. A report published in 1993 showed that contractility may be adversely affected by regional anesthesia.[25]

REGIONAL ANESTHESIA AND AORTOCAVAL COMPRESSION

When a pregnant woman assumes the supine position, the inferior vena cava is almost completely occluded and the aorta is partially occluded, as shown by angiographic studies.[26,27] This effect is evident from the first trimester. Venous return occurs presumably by collateral blood flow through vertebral and azygous veins. However, studies have shown that the right atrial pressure falls significantly in the supine position, indicating a decrease in venous return.

Aortocaval compression has been shown in semirecumbent as well as standing positions.[28,29] Almost 10% of all pregnant women are unable to assume supine position because of symptoms of "supine hypotension" such as dizziness and lightheadedness. Such symptoms are due to sudden decrease in venous return and rapid fall in blood pressures. The syndrome is immediately recognized and therefore termed as "revealed caval compression." In the majority of pregnant women, however, despite the compression of the great vessels, the blood pressures are well maintained owing to compensatory vasoconstriction and increased heart rate. Such "concealed aortocaval compression" is seldom identified with routine monitoring.

The sympathetic blockade resulting from regional anesthesia interferes with the mother's ability to compensate, thereby causing severe hypotension. This underscores the importance of strict avoidance of supine position during labor and delivery. Also important are slow induction of the block, proper hydration before the institution of the block, careful monitoring, and appropriate use of vasopressors.

ANALGESIA AND ANESTHESIA IN OBSTETRICS

Systemic Medication

The use of systemic analgesics and inhalation agents modulates pain perception and simultaneously enhances systems that inhibit nociception.[30–32] Such methods of pain relief may be necessary in certain specific cardiac conditions in which regional anesthesia is neither feasible nor advisable.

The major drugs available for the relief of anxiety and pain during labor and delivery are sedatives, tranquilizers, opioids, and the dissociative agent ketamine. Sedatives and tranquilizers, which are useful in allaying anxiety and apprehension at the start of labor, may also potentiate the analgesic effect of opioids and reduce nausea and vomiting. Maternal respiratory depression, altered maternal hemodynamics, changes in fetal heart rate, and neonatal depression are the major risks associated with the use of systemic medication.[2,33,34] Pharmacologic effects on the maternal cardiovascular and respiratory systems as well as on the uterus and neonate are summarized in Table 24.1.

Inhalation Analgesia for Labor Pain

In a significant number of parturients, inhalation analgesia provides satisfactory and safe pain relief during labor and delivery. Inhaled agents are actually general anesthetics that are used in subanesthetic concentrations, continuously or intermittently during uterine contractions.[35–37] During contractions, the patient is taught to use specially built cylinders and breathing apparatus to self-administer a mixture of either nitrous oxide, trichloroethylene, methoxyflurane, enflurane, or isoflurane in oxygen. Theoretically, because volatile anesthetics are eliminated rapidly through the lungs, inhalation analgesia offers some advantage for the newborn compared to systemic administration of opioids.[2,33] However, the ease with which the mother can lose her protective airway reflexes has been alluded to and therefore, such techniques of analgesia should be used with caution and only at institutions where skillful nursing care is available.

General Anesthesia The use of general anesthesia for routine vaginal or forceps delivery is not recommended. General anesthesia is chosen for cesarean section when indicated, as in parturients with certain cardiac lesions. Highlights from recommended protocols for general anesthesia in *healthy* pregnant women include administration of nonparticulate antacid 1 hour prior to induction, left uterine displacement, preoxygenation followed by rapid sequence induction with cricoid pressure and tracheal intubation.[14] Rapid induction of general anesthesia as described above is seldom appropriate in the majority of critically ill cardiac patients because of severe hemodynamic perturbations such as tachycardia, hypertension, or hypotension that often accompany such induction techniques. A slow, controlled induction of anesthesia using large doses of narcotics along with the use of inotropes and vasodilators to "fine-tune" the hemodynamics using invasive monitoring is regarded as an acceptable alternative for these patients.[15] In this regard, the induction of general anesthesia for a severely ill pregnant cardiac patient scheduled for cesarean delivery is quite similar to that used in procedures such as cardiac surgery. Choice of a high dose narcotic anesthetic technique calls for thorough evaluation of the benefits versus the risks in each individual case. The advantages of such a technique are the remarkable cardiovascular stability and the smooth intraoperative course. The drawbacks are the loss of protective upper airway reflexes and the risk of pulmonary aspiration during the slow induction. Premedication with antacids and histamine receptor blockers may partially alleviate the problem. Another concern is neonatal depression due to large doses of narcotics administered to the mother. The need for postpartum mechanical ventilation of both the mother and the neonate should be anticipated.

Characteristics of drugs for analgesia and general anesthesia are summarized in Table 24.1. In addition to dose-related myocardial depression, potent inhaled agents may cause increased postpartum uterine bleeding by interfering with uterine contraction. Therefore, only low concentrations should be used.

TABLE 24.1   Pharmacologic Effects of Drugs Used for Analgesia and Anesthesia in Obstetrics

Drugs	Dose and Duration	Effects on Cardiovascular System	Effects on Uterine Contraction	Effects on Neonate	Comments
Benzodiazepines					
Diazepam	2.5–5 mg 1–2 h 10 mg 3–4 h	↓ BP	No effect	Hypothermia, hypotonia, respiratory depression (minimal)	Rarely used for labor anxiolysis Primarily for eclamptic seizures.
Midazolam	1–5 mg	↓ BP	No effect	Same as diazepam	Rarely used for labor. Used during cesarean section for amnesia and anxiolysis.
Opioids					
Butorphanol	1–2 mg IV/IM		No effect		Opiate agonist/antagonist with sedative qualities.
Fentanyl	0.3–0.5 µg/kg IV 1–1.5 µg/kg IM 1 µg/kg epidurally < 50 µg intrathecal	↓ HR	No effect	Respiratory depression	Rapidly crosses placenta. May be used via PCA. Excellent analgesia administered spinally with minimal sympathetic block.
Meperidine	0.3 mg/kg IV 0.5 mg/kg IM	Postural, hypotension, tachycardia	No effect	Respiratory, depression	Normeperidine is active metabolite with depressant effects on fetus. Most likely 1–4 h after administration.
Morphine	2–5 mg IV, 10 mg IM 3–4 mg epidural 0.25–0.5 mg intrathecal	Postural hypotension bradycardia	No effect	Marked respiratory depression	Less frequent use than meperidine; significant respiratory depression. Prolonged analgesia administered spinally.
Nalbuphine	10–20 mg	No effect	No effect	Minimal	Opiate agonist/antagonist with similar respiratory depression to morphine. Ceiling effect on maternal sedation.
Pentazocine	20–40 mg IV or IM	↑ HR		Respiratory depression	Opiate agonist/antagonist with significant CNS side effects.
Sufentanil	5–10 µg IV 10–25 µg epidural 5–10 µg intrathecal	No effect	No effect		
Induction Agents					
Barbiturates Thiopental Methohexital	4 mg/kg	Myocardial depression, vasodilation	No effect	Respiratory and CNS depression	Proven safety in healthy parturients. Use caution in cardiac patients; decrease dose if hypotension is deleterious.
Etomidate	0.2–0.4 mg/kg IV	Stable hemodynamics	No effect	Neonatal cortisol and possible mild hypoglycemia	Excellent CV stability, particularly when used with fentanyl 5 µg/kg for induction.
Ketamine	0.5–1.5 mg/kg IV for induction 0.2–0.3 mg/kg IV for analgesia	Sympathomimetic effect: ↑ HR ↑ BP ↑ SVR ↑ CO	Stimulation of uterine contraction at higher doses	No significant depression	Dissociative anesthesia, useful as adjunct to regional anesthesia. Appropriate for asthmatics due to bronchodilation.

(continued)

TABLE 24.1 (*Continued*)

Drugs	Dose and Duration	Effects on			Comments
		Cardiovascular System	Uterine Contraction	Neonate	
Propofol	2–2.5 mg/kg	Hypotension	No effect	Depressed neonate; lower Apgar and neurobehavioral scores	Infrequently used in pregnant cardiac patients.
Inhalation Agents					
Enflurane	0.5–1%	↓ CO ↓ BP ↓ SVR	Uterine relaxation		Used to provide uterine relaxation for retained placenta, uterine inversion.
Halothane	0.3–0.8%	↓ CO ↓ BP ↓ SVR	Uterine relaxation		Used to provide uterine relaxation for retained placenta, uterine inversion.
Isoflurane	0.5–0.75%	↓ CO ↓ BP ↓ SVR	Uterine relaxation		Used to provide uterine relaxation for retained placenta, uterine inversion.
N_2O	30–50%	↑ SVR ↑ HR	None	Respiratory depression if delivery time is prolonged	Commonly used adjunct to inhalation agents during general anesthesia. Increases pulmonary artery pressure.
Neuromuscular Blocking Agents					
Atracurium	0.2–0.5 mg/kg	↓ BP ↑ HR	No effect	No effect	Rapid elimination regardless of organ function.
Curare	0.2–0.5 mg/kg	↓ BP	No effect	No effect	Histamine release, hypotension, possible asthma.
Pancuronium	0.08–0.1 mg/kg	↑ BP ↑ HR	No effect	No effect	Long duration, tachycardia.
Succinylocholine	1–1.5 mg/kg	Bradyarrhythmia	No effect	No effect	Most common paralyzing agent for cesarean section. Prolonged effects with magnesium infusions.
Vecuronium	0.08–0.1 mg/kg	Stable hemodynamics	No effect	No effect	Drug of choice for cardiac patients.
Inotropic Agents					
Amrinone	Institute therapy with 750 μg/kg over 2–3 min, then 5–10 μg/kg/min	Loading dose may ↓ BP	May cause uterine relaxation	Not evaluated	
Dobutamine	1–100 μg/kg/min	↑ MAP	Direct effect UBF	No evaluated	Indirectly may ↑ UBF by stabilizing maternal hemodynamics.
Dopamine	1–10 μg/kg/min	↑ MAP			Increases uterine vascular resistance and may impair blood flow, indirectly my ↑ UBF by stabilizing maternal hemodynamics.
Epinephrine	0.5 mg bolus, 2–10 μg/kg/min	↑ MAP		Not evaluated	
Milrinone	Institute therapy with 50 μg/kg bolus over 10 min, then 0.375–0.75 μg/kg/min	↑ MAP	↑ UBF up to 20%	Not evaluated	

TABLE 24.1   (*Continued*)

Drugs	Dose and Duration	Effects on Cardiovascular System	Effects on Uterine Contraction	Neonate	Comments
Vasodilators					
Hydralazine	5–10 mg IV	↓ MAP	↑ UBF	Ample experience with few fetal side effects	Potent uterine relaxant.
Nitroglycerine	0.4–0.8 mg SL 0.5–40 μg/min IV	↓ MAP	↑ UBF		
Nitroprusside	0.5–3 μg/kg/min	↓ MAP	↑ UBF	Felal cyanide toxicity	Concern of cyanide toxicity in mother and fetus. Tachyphylaxis may occur. Do not increase dose above 3 μg/kg/min.
Vasoconstrictors					
Ephedrine	5–15 mg bolus	↑ HR ↑ BP	↑ UBF	No effect	Vasopressor of choice if tachycardia is not contraindicated. Loses effect with repeated doses.
Metaraminol	0.1–2 mg/min	↓ HR ↑ BP	↓ UBF	No effect	
Norepinephrine	0.05–0.15 μg/kg/min			No effect	Use when other methods to sustain BP have failed or when tachycardia is undesirable.
Phenylephrine	50–100 μg bolus 0.1–0.5 μg/kg/min infusion	↓ HR ↑ BP	↓ UBF	No effect	Same as norepinephrine.
Calcium Channel Blockers					
Nifedipine	10 mg SL 10–20 mg PO		↓ Uterine tone		No evidence of fetal side effects.
Verapamil	5–10 mg IV				No evidence of fetal side effects.
Antiarrhythmics					
Amiodarone	200–500 mg qd		No significant effect		All drugs cross the placenta, no significant fetal side effects.
Bretylium	5–10 mg/kg over 20 min, then 1–2 mg/min				
Lidocaine	1 mg/kg bolus; repeat as necessary 0.5 mg/kg; infuse 1–3 mg/min				
Phenytoin	100 mg over 5 min until arrhythmia is controlled; maximum of 1 g				Monitor blood levels.
Procainamide	100 mg every 5 min until arrhythmia is controlled, then 1–4 mg/min				Monitor blood levels.
Quinidine	200–400 mg PO				Monitor blood levels.

Abbreviations and symbols: BP, blood pressure; CNS, central nervous system; CV, cardiovascular; HR, heart rate; IV, intravenous; MAP, mean arterial pressure; PO, oral; qd, every day; PCA, patient controlled analgesia; SL, sublingual; SVR, systemic vascular resistance; UBF, uterine blood flow; ↑, increased; ↓ decreased.

Major Regional Blocks: Spinal, Epidural, and Caudal Analgesia and Anesthesia

The advantages of major regional blocks in obstetrics are as follows.

- Effective, unsurpassed pain relief during labor and delivery is assured, along with adequate anesthesia for obstetric interventions including abdominal delivery.
- Plasma concentrations of all stress-related hormones such as catecholamines, cortisol and β-endorphins decrease significantly in women receiving epidural anesthesia for labor and cesarean delivery.[38,39]
- When the mean arterial pressure is maintained, uteroplacental blood flow increases significantly from baseline measurements.[40]
- Maternal oxygen consumption decreases significantly.[41]
- The mother is able to participate in the birth of her child.
- Depression of the newborn is minimal to nonexistent.
- Pulmonary aspiration of stomach contents, being the major cause of maternal morbidity and mortality associated with general anesthesia, is practically eliminated under regional block.

The major contraindications to regional blocks are current anticoagulant therapy and blood dyscrasias, active neurological disease, local infection at the site of injection, severe hypovolemia, and patient's refusal or lack of cooperation.[42,43]

Intraspinal and Epidural Opioids

Another more recent and novel approach for providing pain relief for the pregnant cardiac patient is the direct application of low doses of opioids in the subarachnoid space or epidurally.[44] Compared with local anesthetics, spinally administered narcotics act on the opioid receptors located on the dorsal horn of the spinal cord in a selective manner to provide excellent labor analgesia. Moreover, the proprioceptive functions and, most importantly, the sympathetic functions, are spared. Therefore, the decrease in systemic vascular resistance, which is unavoidable with blocks induced by local anesthetics, is minimal or nonexistent with intraspinal narcotics.[45–49] Therein lies the safety of such a technique, which may be used in almost all cardiac patients regardless of the anatomic and functional classifications. Currently, the widely accepted technique is the epidural injection of opioids in combination with dilute solutions of local anesthetics to enhance the analgesic effect of the latter and to provide the same degree of pain relief while minimizing the degree of sympathetic blockade.[50] Severe, delayed respiratory depression is a major concern about the widespread use of spinal opioids. Respiratory depression has been reported with all

the spinally administered opioids, but morphine is associated with the highest risk.[51,52] Combined series of 25,000 patients receiving epidural morphine suggest that delayed respiratory depression is experienced by less than 1% of recipients, comparable to that of oral or parenteral morphine.[51,52]

More recently, the combined spinal–epidural technique (CSE) has become quite popular and is ideal for the parturient with cardiac disease.[53] In this technique, after the epidural needle has been correctly positioned in the epidural space, a long, thin spinal needle is introduced into the subarachnoid space through the epidural needle. When free flow of cerebrospinal fluid has been observed, a small dose of opioid is injected directly into the subarachnoid space and the spinal needle is withdrawn. An epidural catheter is then threaded into the epidural space in the usual manner and taped in place. Often the small dose of subarachnoid opioid will provide adequate analgesia for most of first stage and can be augmented with pudendal block for vaginal delivery. The epidural catheter can be used for injecting local anesthetic–opioid combinations epidurally if the duration of first stage outlasts the analgesia provided by intrathecal dose of narcotic.

MONITORING: GENERAL GUIDELINES

Pregnant women with cardiac disease require close cardiac monitoring during labor, delivery, and the immediate postpartum period. There is general agreement among anesthesiologists that all laboring patients with cardiac diseases, regardless of the New York Heart Association (NYHA) classification, should be monitored by means of standard monitors such as continuous electrocardiographic (EKG), automatic blood pressure cuffs, and pulse oximetry. Standard lead II is best for arrhythmia detection, while lead V5 (or modified CS5) is optimal for detection of myocardial ischemia.

At the University of Tennessee, all patients but those with very mild symptoms receive an indwelling arterial catheter. This is an invasive procedure with minimal risks that allows continuous monitoring of systolic and diastolic blood pressure as well as mean arterial pressure (important in patients with atrial fibrillation). In addition, frequent sampling of arterial blood gases is possible for early detection of hypoxemia, hypercarbia, and acidosis, all potent stimuli to pulmonary vasoconstriction.

Monitoring of pulmonary artery and central venous pressures may be warranted in the symptomatic patients with moderate and severe valvular, or myocardial disease (i.e., Mitral valve disease, aortic valve disease, coarctation of the aorta, hemodynamically important intracardiac shunts, pulmonary hypertension, cardiomyopathies, and ischemic heart disease). Use of the pulmonary artery catheter in patients with the Eisenmenger syndrome however is not recommended due to increased risk of complications (Chapter 4).

As mentioned earlier, noninvasive pulse oximetry may be a particularly valuable tool in parturients with intracardiac right-to-left shunts.

ANALGESIA AND ANESTHESIA FOR PARTURIENTS WITH VALVULAR HEART DISEASE

Mitral Stenosis

Fewer than 2% of pregnancies are complicated by cardiac disease, with the vast majority being of rheumatic origin (75%) and the remainder congenital.[54,55] Of those with rheumatic heart disease as the origin, approximately 90% have as their principal lesion mitral valve stenosis,[56–58] the most common valvular defect associated with maternal death in pregnancy.[59] Labor, delivery, and the early puerperium constitute the periods of maximal risk for the parturient.[60]

Goals of Anesthetic Management In planning the anesthetic approach, the following considerations should be taken into account:

1. Heart rate is of primary importance, since tachycardia (fear, pain, pushing) leads to decreases in diastolic filling time, left ventricular preload, and cardiac output.[55,61–64] In cases of severe stenosis, bradycardia also may be associated with lowering of cardiac output, unless there is a corresponding increase in preload. Therefore the optimal heart rate is 70–90 beats per minute.[65]

2. Factors that increase pulmonary vascular resistance (hypoxemia, hypercarbia, acidosis, hyperinflation of the lungs) should be avoided. Additionally, use of prostaglandin $F_{2\alpha}$ administered for uterine atony or bleeding should be avoided because it may cause increases in pulmonary vascular resistance.[66]

3. Hypotension caused by hypovolemia (bleeding) or reduced sympathetic tone (regional or general anesthesia) results in tachycardia, which is poorly tolerated.

4. Increased blood volume (uterine contractions, Trendelenburg position, aggressive hydration for regional anesthesia) may precipitate pulmonary edema.[54,63,67]

5. Sinus rhythm is essential to maintenance of cardiac output. If a patient develops atrial fibrillation, flutter, or any supraventricular tachydysrhythmia, the arrhythmia must be corrected immediately by cardioversion[68,69] or appropriate pharmacologic intervention, such as adenosine, β-adrenergic blockers or calcium channel blockers.[65,70,71]

Analgesia for Labor and Vaginal Delivery The use of epidural analgesia is recommended by most authors.[5,72–74]

By preventing the pain of contractions and the urge to bear down, it is possible to maintain cardiovascular stability throughout labor and delivery. Instrumental delivery, which is often advocated, can be painlessly performed.[75] Oxygen should be administered to all parturients with cardiac disease. Using invasive monitoring, Clark et al[5] studied the intrapartum hemodynamics in eight patients with severe mitral stenosis. Initiation of epidural analgesia in three of the parturients did not result in any significant hemodynamic changes. Furthermore, the authors commented that epidural analgesia minimized intrapartum fluctuations in cardiac output. Maintaining the increased venous capacitance by continuance of epidural analgesia into the postpartum period may help to avoid the danger of pulmonary edema related to autotransfusion from the contracting uterus. In a case report of a parturient with significant mitral stenosis, Hemmings et al[76] showed that epidural anesthesia for labor and vaginal delivery was associated with significant hemodynamic improvement. Hypotension, the primary complication associated with epidural analgesia, should be avoided by left uterine displacement and careful infusion of crystalloid. If blood pressure does not recover rapidly, metaraminol or phenylephrine, and not ephedrine, should be used.

Niv et al studied the analgesic effects of an epidural block using the combination of 0.25% bupivacaine with a low dose of morphine (2–3 mg) in 30 women in active labor.[34,50] The addition of morphine augmented the analgesic properties of low concentration bupivacaine with minimal influence on sympathetic tone. Subsequently, epidural analgesia and hemodynamic stability were achieved by an even lower concentration of bupivacaine: 0.2% combined again with 2–3 mg morphine in four parturients with mitral stenosis.[77] The addition of epidural opioids to allow lowering of the concentrations of local anesthetic solutions may merit further investigation in cardiac patients.

A second technique that may be used for labor is the combined spinal–epidural technique. Placing a small dose of opioid, such as fentanyl, sufentanil, or morphine, in the subarachnoid space and subsequently placing an epidural catheter, may serve to reduce the total dose and concentration of local anesthetic. Stage one of labor may require no further analgesics, or an infusion of dilute local anesthetic (0.06–0.125% bupivacaine) with or without opioid (2 μg/mL fentanyl) may be started. This technique offers the benefits of likelihood of hypotension from peripheral vasodilation and the presence of the epidural catheter for stages two and three of labor, where perineal anesthesia is necessary.

In seven of the eight patients with NYHA functional class III or IV disease monitored by Clark et al,[5] the behavior of the central venous pressure differed significantly from that of the pulmonary capillary wedge pressure. Therefore, pulmonary artery catheters are indicated in patients with moderate and severe mitral stenosis and should be inserted early. We have used continuous mixed venous saturation pulmonary artery catheters to monitor these patients, and the additional information proved to be helpful in determining the adequacy of cardiac output during labor and cesarean section.

To provide satisfactory analgesia for the second stage of labor without extending the epidural block and risking increased sympathetic blockade, additional bilateral pudendal blocks have been advocated.[78–80]

Anesthesia for Cesarean Section Although both regional and general anesthesia have been used successfully for cesarean section in parturients with mitral stenosis, many authors advocate continuous segmental epidural anesthesia as the technique of choice.[73,74,81–83]

An epidural catheter already in situ for analgesia during labor enables smooth and controllable transition to epidural anesthesia.[84] Since reduction in systemic vascular resistance is poorly tolerated and prophylactic fluid infusion may be hazardous, slow titration of the level of epidural block with incremental doses of local anesthetics is advisable. Local anesthetics should not contain epinephrine because the degree of vasodilation induced is more profound with this agent, as well as the likelihood of tachycardia. The level of sensory blockade should not exceed T5, since interruption of cardiac accelerator nerves at T1–T4 may result in bradycardia.[20,85] Ziskind et al[86] administered epidural anesthesia to seven patients with severe mitral stenosis and used varying angles of Trendelenburg position to control the pulmonary capillary wedge pressure (PCWP). These investigators were able to maintain a PCWP at 25 mmHg and maximize cardiac index.

Treatment of hypotension due to decreased preload during the administration of regional anesthetic techniques should be treated with α-adrenergic agonists such as phenylephrine or metaraminol. The potential for developing supine hypotensive syndrome should be kept in mind, and left uterine displacement be applied. Small doses of these agents act primarily on the venous vasculature and will increase preload. Tachycardia due to hypovolemia from regional anesthesia should be treated similarly.

Although epidural anesthesia is preferred to spinal anesthesia,[87] one case report[88] described the successful use of spinal anesthesia in a parturient with severe mitral stenosis and pulmonary edema when an emergency cesarean section was required.

In parturients with mitral stenosis, the disadvantages of general anesthesia for cesarean section may outweigh the advantages. Rapidity of administration, lower incidence of hypotension, and beneficial effects of intermittent positive pressure breathing on oxygenation and interstitial pulmonary edema are the major advantages of general anesthesia.[81,83] On the other hand, tracheal manipulation and mechanical ventilation may be associated with hypertension, tachycardia, arrhythmias, and pulmonary hypertension.[79,89,90] Addi-

tional disadvantages are myocardial depression from anesthetic agents[91,92] and neonatal depression induced by placental transfer of anesthetic drugs.[93] If general anesthesia is chosen, drugs that do not cause tachycardia are suggested (Table 24.1). In patients with very severe mitral stenosis, the high dose fentanyl technique, as used in cardiac anesthesia, may offer optimal cardiovascular stability, but its use commits the mother and neonate to prolonged postoperative ventilation.[94]

A second option is alfentanil, a very short-acting opioid that has been used for cesarean section in a parturient with severe mitral stenosis and pulmonary hypertension.[95] Because of the short duration of action, the mother was extubated at the end of the procedure, but the neonate required a brief period of intubation. Doses of 10 μg/kg will not adversely affect the fetus, but greater than 35 μg/kg will induce neonatal depression.[96] Excellent hemodynamic control can be maintained with this drug. β-Adrenergic blockade may also be necessary to prevent tachycardia in response to intubation. Anesthetic agents and neuromuscular blockers should be chosen for their lack of positive chronotropic or sympathomimetic effect.

Following delivery, attention must be paid to maintenance of stable hemodynamics and to the possibility of cardiac decompensation. Aggressive analgesic regimens should be instituted to avoid tachycardia, hyper- or hypotension, and pulmonary hypertension. Epidural administration of opioids should be continued and, in the more fragile patient, even the use of local anesthetic blockade.

Mitral Insufficiency

The second most common valvular malformation encountered in pregnancy is mitral regurgitation (MR).[55,63] This lesion seems to be better tolerated than mitral stenosis.[97,98] Hemodynamically, mitral insufficiency is characterized by a reduced forward stroke volume because a part of the total left ventricular stroke volume regurgitates through the incompetent mitral valve into the left atrium. It is thus a left ventricular volume overloaded state. The degree of regurgitation is determined by the size of the mitral orifice, duration of systole, and pressure gradient from the left ventricle to atrium.[65] Mitral regurgitation may be acute or chronic, and different pathophysiologies are possible. We will concentrate on chronic MR.

Pregnancy and Mitral Insufficiency Mitral regurgitation is generally well tolerated during pregnancy. The decrease in systemic vascular resistance associated with pregnancy may allow the patient to tolerate the increased blood volume. Because of the increased coagulability of pregnancy, the risk of systemic embolization is increased.[74] Szekely and Snaith reported an incidence of pulmonary edema in 5.5%, atrial tachycardia in 4%, and pulmonary embolism in 2.8%.[55] If the patient has a history of systemic or pulmonary embolization, anticoagulation should be continued throughout pregnancy. Also, all antiarrhythmic medications should be continued.

Goals of Anesthetic Management   The anesthetic technique for parturients with mitral regurgitation should be one that:

avoids or prevents increases in systemic vascular resistance (pain, anxiety, light anesthesia)

avoids myocardial depressant drugs

maintains sinus rhythm

avoids hypoxemia, hypercarbia, and acidosis, which may increase pulmonary vascular resistance

Most regional anesthetic techniques fulfill these goals.

Analgesia for Labor and Vaginal Delivery   There is no doubt that in mitral insufficiency, epidural analgesia is to be highly recommended.[73,80,99] In addition to providing analgesia, it results in a decrease in peripheral vascular resistance, thus reducing after load and improving cardiac output. The decrease in systemic vascular resistance is partially mediated by a decrease in maternal pain and therefore serum catecholamine levels, and partially by sympathetic blockade and direct reduction of the vascular tone. This sequence of events was documented by Lynch and Rizor[100] using invasive monitoring in a parturient with mitral insufficiency. Epidural blockade resulted in decreased systemic vascular resistance and pulmonary capillary wedge pressure as well as increased cardiac output. Epidural anesthesia may also result in dramatic declines in preload, necessitating fluid administration. Left uterine displacement must be assiduously maintained. If blood pressure should decline, ephedrine is the pressor of choice owing to its chronotropic and inotropic effects. Use of epidural opioids in combination with local anesthetics may decrease the potential for sudden changes in systemic vascular resistance while providing excellent analgesia.

Anesthesia for Cesarean Section   As for vaginal delivery, epidural anesthesia is the method of choice for cesarean section in parturients with mitral regurgitation.[73,74,80,99] Oxygen supplementation by mask, left uterine tilt, judicious fluid administration, and appropriate level of epidural blockade provide optimal conditions for a safe outcome.

Our anesthetic approach consists of injecting repeated low doses of 0.5% bupivacaine through the epidural catheter, to gradually extend and finally limit the block to T5 dermatome. With the block reaching T2 dermatome, all the cardiac accelerator nerves are blocked, resulting in bradycardia.[85,87] Cunningham et al[101] reported a fall in systolic blood pressure and cardiac index in a parturient with mitral insufficiency who developed bradycardia following an epidural blockade

reaching T2. If treatment becomes necessary, ephedrine is again the vasopressor of choice. If bradycardia is present without significant hypotension, atropine (0.5 mg) will suffice.

An additional problem associated with epidural anesthesia is the concomitant increase in venous capacitance. This increase requires cautious fluid administration to maintain adequate left ventricular volume. However, pulmonary edema may develop during the third stage of labor as the contracting uterus expels blood into the circulation simultaneously with the return of sympathetic tone, due to the fading epidural block.[54,63,102] We favor the approach of other authors[101,103,104] who advocate preload reduction with diuretics coupled with afterload reduction by continuing the epidural blockade.

If general anesthesia is chosen, a rise in peripheral vascular resistance may be expected, and measures such as deepening the anesthesia before intubation and the use of vasodilators (nitroglycerine or nitroprusside) should be considered. Provided there is good ventricular function, any of the commonly used induction agents are appropriate. In patients with good left ventricular function, potent inhalational agents may be carefully added to nitrous oxide and oxygen. In extremely sick patients, high dose fentanyl or alfentanil anesthesia should be considered.[94,95] Care should be taken to avoid those factors, including hypothermia, that increase the pulmonary artery pressure. Postoperative shivering will increase oxygen utilization, systemic vascular resistance, and pulmonary vascular resistance.[105] As with mitral stenosis, atrial fibrillation should be treated with direct cardioversion, β-adrenergic blockade or calcium channel blockers.

Mitral Valve Prolapse

Interaction with Pregnancy   Mitral valve prolapse (MVP) occurs in 3–5% of healthy individuals and is twice as frequent in females as in males.[106,107] Disease characteristics include elongated chordae tendineae and redundant mitral valve leaflets. Prolapse of the valve may or may not result in regurgitant flow, depending on the inotropic and volume state of the patient. Factors that increase the likelihood of regurgitation include hypovolemia, venodilation, increased airway pressure, and an increased inotropic state. Conversely, hypervolemia and bradycardia may decrease the severity of regurgitation or prolapse. Some patients may develop chest pain, palpitations, and anxiety. Arrhythmias are not uncommon, and paroxysmal supraventricular tachycardia is the most common.[108]

The majority of patients with MVP tolerate pregnancy well (Chapter 14) and, if there is no change in the murmur, may be treated in a routine but watchful manner. Patients with an increase of symptoms, murmur, or regurgitant volume should be treated more aggressively, in a manner similar to parturients with mitral insufficiency.

Goals of Anesthetic Management   The goals of anesthetic management include

avoidance of significant decreases in preload

avoidance of significant increases in afterload

continuation of beta blockers and antiarrhythmic medications

minimization of catecholamine response and bearing down with contractions

Analgesia for Labor and Vaginal Delivery   Lumbar epidural anesthesia is recommended by most authors.[73,74,80,109] When this mode of anesthesia is properly applied, the pain of contractions and the accompanying increase in circulating catecholamines can be blunted. The result is a decrease in the severity of increased peripheral resistance with pain, and obstruction to forward blood flow is lessened. The dermatomal level should maintained only high enough to provide analgesia, while not decreasing venous return. Opioids in low dose combined with low concentrations of local anesthetic will give excellent analgesia with minimal hemodynamic side effects. As labor progresses to the second stage and increased analgesia is required, the local anesthetic should be administered slowly to avoid sudden decreases in preload. Left uterine displacement should be maintained throughout. Additional intravenous fluids may need to be administered to maintain cardiac output. Should there be a sudden decline in preload, phenylephrine or methoxamine is the vasopressor of choice owing to the lack of chronotropic effect. Epinephrine should be avoided in the test dose and the air test dose performed to verify extravascular placement of the epidural catheter.

Anesthesia for Cesarean Section   Lumbar epidural (LEA) or spinal anesthesia would seem to be contraindicated for cesarean section, but LEA, properly administered is well tolerated.[109] Slow incremental dosing of local anesthetic without epinephrine to a T6 dermatomal level will allow surgery to proceed. Avoiding exteriorization of the uterus following delivery will allow a lower than normal level of anesthesia.[109] Trendelenburg position and uterine displacement will promote venous return.

Agents that have sympathomimetic effects (ketamine, pancuronium) should be avoided for general anesthesia. Induction using sodium thiopental, or a combination of ketamine (0.5 mg/kg) and thiopental (2 mg/kg), will provide stable hemodynamics.[110] If there is myocardial dysfunction, etomidate (0.2–0.4 mg/kg) can be safely used in the parturient with minimal risk to the neonate.[111–113] In patients with normal myocardial function, volatile anesthetic agents may be used. Nitrous oxide/oxygen/relaxant techniques may promote tachycardia and peripheral vasoconstriction, which should be avoided.

Aortic Stenosis

Interaction with Pregnancy   The incidence of aortic stenosis in parturients with valvular lesions ranges from 0.5 to 3%.[57,62,114] Maternal and fetal risks during pregnancy correlate with the severity of the stenosis.[102,115] Hemodynamically, the reduced area of the aortic orifice is associated with an increase in left ventricular end diastolic pressure and a fixed stroke volume. If signs or symptoms of left ventricular failure develop during pregnancy, invasive monitors such as pulmonary and redial arterial catheters are indicated during labor and delivery.

Goals of Anesthetic Management   The anesthetic technique that is chosen should

maintain adequate preload

avoid a significant decrease in afterload

avoid myocardial depression

maintain a heart rate of 70–90 bests per minute and sinus rhythm

Analgesia for Labor and Vaginal Delivery   The hemodynamic consequences of the pain and stress of labor are relatively well tolerated by parturients with aortic stenosis. Systemic medication or inhalation analgesia may therefore provide adequate conditions for the first stage of labor. Bilateral pudendal blocks may then be used for the second stage.

Regional anesthesia may be used, provided caution is exercised, because decreases in systemic vascular resistance are poorly tolerated.[116–118] Since stroke volume is usually fixed, the heart responds to afterload reduction mainly by an increase in rate.[119,120] If epidural analgesia is chosen, repeated small doses of local anesthetic must be carefully titrated to the desired level. Avoidance of epinephrine in both the test dose and use of subsequent volumes of local anesthetic is advisable. Alternatively, adding opioids to the local anesthetic allows a reduction in the concentration of the latter,[50] thus decreasing the degree of sympathetic blockade. Intrathecal injection of morphine may be another approach to pain relief with hemodynamic stability.[48,49,121] Epidural opioids alone will not provide adequate analgesia for the second stage of labor, and pudendal nerve block will allow for instrumental delivery.

Anesthesia for Cesarean Section   General anesthesia, induced with thiopental or ketamine/thiopental, followed by nitrous oxide/oxygen and muscle relaxants, remains the preferred technique for parturients with aortic stenosis. Etomidate may also be used. Marked depression of myocardial contractility or vascular tone by large doses of thiopental or inhalation agents should be avoided. Therefore, adequate depth of anesthesia may be achieved by the addition of intravenous opioids following umbilical cord clamping. Redfern et al[122] used etomidate and alfentanil to induce anesthesia with excellent hemodynamic stability. The neonate, however, required intubation and ventilatory support and naloxone. Hypotension should be treated promptly with α-adrenergic agonist (phenylephrine). If tachycardia develops, small incremental doses of propranolol or edrophonium should be used.[99,123]

Aortic Insufficiency

Interaction with Pregnancy   Over 90% of the parturients with aortic insufficiency are asymptomatic during pregnancy.[55,56,61,124] The patient who develops symptoms has failed to cope with the increased cardiac workload. Hemodynamically, blood regurgitates through the inefficient aortic orifice, overloads, and distends the left ventricle, which consequently hypertrophies. With mounting left heart failure, forward stroke volume decreases and diastolic volume expands.[125,126] There is an incidence of 3–9% of pregnant patients progressing to this level of valvular dysfunction during pregnancy.[55,127,128] The incidence of acute aortic insufficiency in pregnancy may rise as illicit intravenous drug use and subsequent bacterial endocarditis continue to be found in the childbearing population.

Goals of Anesthetic Management   The anesthetic technique administered should aim to:

    reduce systemic vascular resistance

    avoid myocardial depression

    maintain adequate preload

    maintain sinus rhythm and avoid bradycardia (heart rate goal 75–85 beats/min)

Analgesia for Labor and Vaginal Delivery   The same indications as described for mitral insufficiency are relevant for aortic insufficiency. Epidural analgesia with its peripheral vasodilating effect is indicated to reduce afterload, thus improving left ventricular performance in this pathology. Alderson[129] reported a case in which a fatality occurred following epidural placement with rapid administration of 26 mL of 0.5% bupivacaine in a parturient with aortic insufficiency. The patient became hypotensive and could not be resuscitated. This case highlights the need for prudent administration of local anesthetics and attentive monitoring of the volume status.

Anesthesia for Cesarean Section   As with mitral insufficiency, the anesthetic method of choice is epidural block, and a similar management plan should be employed. If general anesthesia is chosen, the same precautions should be taken. In case of severe left ventricular failure, afterload reduction with nitroprusside, combined, if necessary, with dobutamine

for inotropic support of the left ventricle, improves cardiac function.[98] Etomidate in combination with fentanyl (5–10 μg/kg) will provide stable hemodynamics during and after intubation.[130] Nitroprusside should be used only if its benefits are considered to outweigh any potential complications. Fetal toxicity may arise from extensive placental transfer of both nitroprusside and cyanide and because of the reduced ability of a neonate to metabolize cyanide.[131] Naulty et al[131] showed that low doses of nitroprusside were safe and did not harm the fetus or induce acidosis.

CONGENITAL HEART DISEASE

Coarctation of the Aorta

As a result of early detection and repair, fewer parturients are presenting to the delivery room with surgically uncorrected coarctation of the aorta. The primary hemodynamic problems are obstruction to blood flow, resulting in hypertension, and increased cardiac workload, causing concentric ventricular hypertrophy. Inadequacy of collateral circulation may result in decreased uterine and placental blood flow, endangering the fetus.

Pregnancy and Coarctation of Aorta   Pregnancy-related hemodynamic changes are poorly tolerated.[73] The decrease in systemic vascular resistance and increases in blood volume as well as cardiac output can place severe demands on these patients with fixed cardiac output. Left ventricular failure, aortic dissection, and rupture are potential risks.

Goals of Anesthetic Management   Because a fixed stroke volume is imposed by the coarctation, the ability to compensate for hypotension is compromised. Hypotension may be caused by a fall in systemic vascular resistance, aortocaval compression, or severe blood loss during delivery. Maintaining normal peripheral vascular resistance and adequate venous return and avoiding bradycardia are important.

Anesthetic management is similar to that recommended for parturients with valvular aortic stenosis. Epidural analgesia has been recommended and used without detriment to the mother or fetus.[57,73,132] Mangano,[73] on the other hand, recommended the use of systemic medication, inhalation analgesia, or pudendal block for labor and delivery, and light general anesthesia for cesarean section. Rosenthal et al[133] reported successful management of cesarean section under spinal anesthesia. This, however, is a poor choice for pregnant patients with cardiac diseases, because the associated hemodynamic changes are precipitous in nature.

Marfan's Syndrome

The Marfan syndrome is a hereditary autosomal disorder of connective tissue with cardiac, pulmonary, musculoskeletal, and ocular involvement. Mitral valve prolapse and dilatation of the ascending aorta are common features.[134] The life-threatening complications of this condition include formation of a saccular aneurysm of the ascending aorta with aortic incompetence and aortic dissection.

Pregnancy and Marfan's Syndrome The risk of aortic dissection increases with pregnancy. The cardiovascular changes of pregnancy such as expanded blood volume and increased cardiac output can cause significant stress on the aortic wall. In addition, the structural integrity of the dilated aortic wall is further compromised by hormonal changes of pregnancy. The increased pulsatile shear stress on the weakened aortic wall can thus lead to aortic dissection or rupture.[135]

Goals of Anesthetic Management

- Minimize the factors that increases myocardial contractility.
- Control blood pressure aggressively during anesthesia.

Monitoring

- Use a radial arterial line for accurate monitoring and control of blood pressures.
- Use a central venous line and two large-bore intravenous access lines for monitoring, as well as for rapid infusion of blood and fluids in case of aortic dissection or rupture.
- Use routine monitoring such as continuous EKG and pulse oximetry.

Anesthesia for Labor and Vaginal Delivery The presence of kyphoscoliosis may pose difficulties with the placement of epidural catheters. Nevertheless, for labor pain relief, epidural anesthesia is highly recommended.[136,137] After adequate hydration, continuous lumbar epidural anesthesia with 0.125% bupivacaine and fentanyl or sufentanil may be used. For treatment of hypotension, phenylephrine rather than ephedrine is preferred, since ephedrine increases myocardial contractility and heart rate. If the patient's medications include β-adrenergic blockers, this should be continued through the peripartum period. Additional intravenous doses of β-adrenergic blockers may be needed to prevent tachycardia and hypertension during labor. Labetalol, with its α/β-adrenergic blocking effects, is ideally suited for this purpose.

Anesthesia for Cesarean Delivery For nonemergency cesarean section, epidural anesthesia may be administered. For emergencies the only option is general anesthesia. Recently, Pinosky et al[137] described the anesthetic management of a patient with Marfan's syndrome at 35 weeks of gestation who had acute dissection of ascending aorta. These authors chose thiopental for induction of anesthesia for its transient myocardial depressant action, a highly desirable effect in such patients. Furthermore, to prevent the hypertensive and tachycardic responses to laryngoscopy and tracheal intubation, the patient was pretreated with intravenous labetalol and lidocaine. Labetalol can be safely used to attenuate the sympathetic response to tracheal intubation.[138]

Eisenmenger's Syndrome

A comprehensive review by Gleicher et al[139] showed that pregnancy and delivery in women with Eisenmenger's syndrome are associated with high mortality rates.

The syndrome is characterized by pulmonary hypertension with right-to-left or bidirectional blood shunting at the aortopulmonary, ventricular, or atrial level. The chronic right-sided volume overload results in right ventricular hypertrophy with increased and relatively fixed pulmonary vascular resistance. The shunt may be bidirectional; however, any acute changes in the pulmonary or systemic vascular resistance may change the direction and the degree of shunt. Polycythemia and cyanosis are the other common findings.

Pregnancy and Eisenmenger's Syndrome The cardiovascular changes of pregnancy are poorly tolerated. While the increase in cardiac output causes right-sided volume overload, the low systemic vascular resistance tends to exacerbate the right-to-left shunt. In addition, the hypercoagulable state of pregnancy increases the risk of thromboembolic events. The physiologic anemia of pregnancy may be beneficial in terms of alleviating the ill effects of polycythemia such as increased blood viscosity and decreased uterine blood flow. While pregnancy-related hemodynamic changes occur gradually, those related to labor, delivery, and postpartum are acute and more severe. It is no surprise that sudden deterioration and maternal death occur more often during such stressful periods.

Goals of Anesthetic Management

- Avoid or minimize any sudden fall in systemic vascular resistance or rise in pulmonary vascular resistance, which will exacerbate the right to left shunt.[140]
- Avoid or minimize any rise in systemic vascular resistance, which may result in left-to-right shunt with increased pulmonary blood flow and a further rise in pulmonary artery pressure.
- Avoid or plan to compensate for agents that induce tachycardia, which are not well tolerated.
- Avoid or minimize the factors that increase the pulmonary vascular resistance under anesthesia, which include hypoxia, hypercarbia, acidosis, and hyperinflation

of lungs during positive pressure ventilation. In the parturients, emotional stress associated with labor can cause an additional rise in pulmonary artery pressures.

Monitoring

1. *Pulse Oximetry*   Administration of supplemental oxygen is beneficial as increased inspired oxygen concentration (FIO_2) results in an increase in both maternal and fetal oxygen saturation. In addition, oxygen decreases pulmonary vascular resistance in some patients with cyanotic congenital heart diseases.[141,142] Pollack et al[143] described the intrapartum use of upper and lower extremity pulse oximetry in a patient with Eisenmenger's syndrome with patent ductus arteriosus. By simultaneous measurements of the differences in oxygen saturation in the right hand and the left foot, these authors were able to measure the changes in the shunt fractions in response to various anesthetic and obstetric interventions.[143]

2. *Arterial Lines*   Arterial lines are often necessary for accurate measurement of blood pressure and blood gas sampling.

3. *Central Venous Pressure (CVP) and Pulmonary Artery Pressure (PAP)*   There is consensus among anesthesiologists that monitoring the right-sided pressure is essential for early detection of right heart failure (or any change from baseline measurement), and therefore insertion of a CVP line is justified despite the considerable risks.

The use of PA catheter monitoring is controversial. Gleicher et al[139] considered such monitoring to be essential in all laboring women with Eisenmenger's syndrome. Others argued against its use in such patients, citing the increased risks of complications (Chapter 4).[74,143]

The following factors should be kept in mind.

- The correct positioning of the PA catheter within the pulmonary artery may be difficult without radiographic control.
- Wedging may be difficult if not impossible; the risk of pulmonary artery perforation is ever-present.
- Thermodilution cardiac output measurements and calculations of systemic vascular resistance are not valid in the presence of large, variable intracardiac shunts.
- Pulmonary artery pressures are often elevated and fixed, and therefore the information derived is of limited use.
- Other complications such as air embolism, pneumothorax, and arrhythmia, may be fatal to these women.

We believe the decision to monitor PA pressures should be made in consultation with the cardiologist and the obstetri-

cian and should be based on the patient's clinical presentation.

Analgesia for Labor and Vaginal Delivery   Several authors have successfully used epidural or intrathecal narcotics and local anesthetics for labor pain relief and cesarean delivery.[143–145] When there is adequate pain relief for labor, the excessive increases in oxygen consumption, cardiac output, and heart rate during contractions are effectively blunted. This combination of effects is highly beneficial for both the mother and her fetus. Epidural block was considered to be contraindicated in patients with right-to-left shunts for fear of decreasing the systemic vascular resistance, thereby worsening the shunt. However, by using invasive monitoring, Midwall et al[146] showed that neither pulmonary hemodynamics nor shunt flow was adversely affected by gradual epidural blockade. Pollack et al[143] reported the use of intrathecal morphine (1.5 mg) for labor analgesia in a parturient with Eisenmenger's syndrome. A pudendal block and small supplemental doses of intravenous fentanyl were used for providing analgesia for a forceps delivery in this patient. More recently, Smedstad et al[147] described the anesthetic management of a series of eight parturients with pulmonary hypertension. Five of these patients had Eisenmenger's syndrome, and all five received epidural anesthesia for vaginal delivery. The excellent outcome in this series can be attributed to the multidisciplinary approach from approximately week 25 of pregnancy, including appropriate planning, monitoring, meticulous anesthetic technique, and careful obstetric management.

We recommend the use of a combined spinal–epidural technique to provide labor analgesia as described earlier in this chapter. The use of such a technique offers excellent labor pain relief with minimal hemodynamic perturbations.

Anesthesia for Cesarean Section

EPIDURAL ANESTHESIA   Spinnato et al[144] reported the first successful management of an elective cesarean section under epidural block using 3% 2-chloroprocaine in 2 mL increments. Uneventful cesarean section under epidural anesthesia was later reported by Rosenberg et al[148] using 0.5% bupivacaine.

Briefly, our guidelines for epidural anesthesia are as follows.

1. Check coagulation status (maternal anticoagulation therapy is common in such patients).
2. Initiate appropriate invasive monitoring preferably under sedation. Hydrate cautiously.
3. Administer oxygen continuously by face mask.
4. Induce block slowly, segment by segment.
5. Avoid the use of air for loss-of-resistance technique.

6. Avoid the use of air or epinephrine for "test doses."
7. Maintain preload; avoid aortocaval compression; continue intravenous crystalloid. Use small doses of phenylephrine to prevent decreases in mean arterial pressures. Replace blood loss as needed.

GENERAL ANESTHESIA In the presence of a large right-to-left shunt, intravenous induction agents act unusually quickly, while the onset of action of inhalation agents is slowed.[149,150] Ogura et al[94] reported good hemodynamic stability with the use of ketamine (0.5 mg/kg) and high dose fentanyl (50 μg/kg). However, mechanical ventilation was required for both the mother and the newborn. Furuya et al,[151] on the other hand, reported using barbiturate induction followed by small doses of diazepam and fentanyl, also requiring mechanical ventilation of the newborn.

A high dose, narcotic-based induction of general anesthesia allows a controlled induction with the least hemodynamic perturbations. Needless to say, preoperative administration of oral antacids and H2-receptor antagonists, and application of cricoid pressure, are necessary to minimize the risk of pulmonary aspiration. Mechanical ventilation of the mother as well as the neonate may be necessary after delivery. Despite these problems, we believe that such a technique is safer than routine induction with intravenous and inhalation agents, which cause myocardial depression.

Primary Pulmonary Hypertension

In an extensive review of the literature, Elkayam and Gleicher[152] found a 40% overall mortality in patients with primary pulmonary hypertension during pregnancy and the early postpartum period. They suggested that this high rate of loss was due to the increased circulatory burden of parturition (Chapter 15).

Primary Pulmonary Hypertension and Pregnancy
Right ventricular hypertrophy, which develops as a response to pulmonary hypertension, may progress during late pregnancy to right ventricular failure with a decreased and relatively fixed cardiac output, elevated central venous pressure with passive liver congestion, and peripheral edema. The development of cyanosis, chest pain, and dyspnea has been found to lead to a grave prognosis.[153]

Anesthetic management of women with primary pulmonary hypertension can be a challenge for even the most experienced obstetric anesthesiologist.[73,154–156] Potential risks of epidural anesthesia include refractory hypotension associated with decreases in systemic vascular resistance. The major risks associated with general anesthesia are further rise in pulmonary artery pressure with rapid sequence induction, laryngoscopy and tracheal intubation, and the myocardial depressant effects of intravenous and inhalation agents. Intramyometrial prostaglandins should not be ad-

ministered if hemorrhage is encountered during either vaginal or cesarean delivery. Drugs of this class, particularly prostaglandin $F_{2\alpha}$, may cause pulmonary hypertension, bronchospasm, or systemic hypotension.[157,158] Thus, other means of hemostasis should be employed.

Goals of Anesthetic Management

- Avoid further increases in pulmonary artery pressure and pulmonary vascular resistance by avoiding stress, hypercapnia, hypoxemia, acidosis, hyperinflation of lungs, and vasoconstrictors.
- Maintain preload with early correction of fluid and blood loss, and avoid supine hypotension.
- Minimize changes in systemic vascular resistance with slow induction of epidural block.
- Avoid negative inotropes, to prevent acute refractory right-sided failure.
- Attend to monitoring considerations, which are similar to those discussed in connection with Eisenmenger's syndrome.

Analgesia during Labor and Delivery Mangano[73] recommended the use of systemic opioids, inhalation analgesia, intrathecal opioids, and paracervical or pudendal blocks. Conversely, published reports indicated the successful use of segmental epidural anesthesia with 2-chloroprocaine and 0.5% bupivacaine supplemented with pudendal block for delivery.[159] Abboud et al[160] reported good pain relief and hemodynamic stability with intrathecal injection of 1 mg of morphine.

Anesthesia for Cesarean Section Standard textbooks recommend general anesthesia for cesarean section with either a high dose opioid technique or inhalation agents such as halothane.[73,99] Right heart failure, the most dreaded complication, may respond to dobutamine combined with nitroprusside, titrated under hemodynamic monitoring to the desired end point. On the other hand, in 1991 Breen and Janzen[154] described the successful use of epidural anesthesia for cesarean delivery. These authors monitored a patient with an indwelling radial arterial line and a pulmonary artery catheter. For epidural anesthesia, 2% lidocaine mixed with fentanyl was injected in 3 mL increments. Adequate block was established gradually, over 30–40 minutes (instead of the usual 15 min in healthy women), which probably explains why minimal hemodynamic changes were observed. Both systemic and pulmonary pressures remained unchanged.

Tetralogy of Fallot

Tetralogy of Fallot is the most common cyanotic congenital heart defect encountered in pregnancy. This lesion is characterized by right ventricular outlet obstruction resulting in right ventricular hypertrophy, ventricular septal defect, and an overriding aorta. The degree of right-to-left shunting is determined by the relatively fixed right ventricular pressure, the degree of obstruction to pulmonary flow, and the variable systemic blood pressure.

Tetralogy of Fallot and Pregnancy   Most pregnant women with this lesion have undergone surgical treatment in childhood to close the septal defect and widen the pulmonary outflow tract.[74] In a number of women, pregnancy-related changes such as increased blood volume and cardiac output, and decreased systemic vascular resistance, can unmask residual symptoms of corrected tetralogy. Echocardiography is recommended in all pregnant patients with corrected tetralogy of Fallot.

Goals of Anesthetic Management   An increase in pulmonary vascular resistance or a decrease in systemic vascular resistance will exacerbate right-to-left shunt and therefore should be avoided. Triggering factors include airway obstruction, acidosis, high ventilating airway pressure and hypovolemia.

Analgesia for Labor and Vaginal Delivery   Ostheimer and Alper[83] reported 12 successful vaginal deliveries under three types of anesthesia: general in one, spinal in two, and epidural in nine parturients with corrected or uncorrected tetralogy of Fallot. All mothers and babies did well. Krivosic-Horber et al[161] reviewed the anesthetic course of labor and delivery in a group of 14 parturients with a congenital heart disease. Two of the women had tetralogy of Fallot. The authors suggested a vaginal delivery, preceded by continuous epidural block using a low concentration of bupivacaine as the method of choice for labor. Ferguson et al,[99] on the other hand, recommended the use of inhalation analgesia, systemic medication, and paracervical or pudendal block.

Major regional blocks should be used with extreme caution, since significant decreases in systemic vascular resistance may result. A segmental epidural block for the first stage of labor associated with a pudendal or caudal block for the second stage might result in greater hemodynamic stability. Alternatively, the addition of opioids to local anesthetics injected epidurally may allow a decrease in the concentration of the latter, thus reducing their hemodynamic effects.

Anesthesia for Cesarean Section   Before the administration of anesthesia, along with the anesthetic considerations cited above, one should estimate the degree of infundibular obstruction to right ventricular outflow. Light (O_2/N_2O plus relaxants) and deep (potent inhaled agents) general anesthesia is suggested for mild and severe obstruction, respectively.[73,99] Increases in cardiac rate and contractility can be successfully treated with propranolol.

Single Ventricle with Transposition of the Great Arteries

Single ventricle accounts for 0.5–3.0% of patients with congenital heart disease. There is only one common mixing chamber that, through a common or two separate atrioventricular (AV) valves, receives both pulmonary and systemic blood. Initially, when no obstruction to pulmonary flow exists, patients have clinical features of large left-to-right shunt with little or no cyanosis. When pulmonary vascular obstruction develops, right-to-left shunting with cyanosis appears. Pregnancy is then associated with increased morbidity and mortality, especially if arterial desaturation and polycythemia are present.[78]

Goals of Anesthetic Management   The principles of management are similar to those laid out for other cyanotic congenital cardiac lesions discussed earlier. The main objective is to maintain a favorable balance between systemic and pulmonary vascular pressures and resistance. As described earlier, a sudden and severe decrease in systemic vascular resistance or an increase in pulmonary vascular resistance will result in an increase in right-to-left shunting.

Monitoring   It is essential to provide intraarterial and central venous pressure monitoring. Pulse oximetry enables one to monitor the changes in the oxygen saturation with various anesthetic and obstetric interventions.

Analgesia for Labor and Vaginal Delivery   The subarachnoid injection of 1 mg of morphine for analgesia during labor and pudendal block for vaginal delivery in parturients with a single ventricle has been described.[78,162] Excellent analgesia without any hemodynamic changes was observed. Recently, Fong and others[163] reported the use of epidural analgesia for labor using 0.25% bupivacaine. The sensory block was maintained at T10 level, using continuous infusion of 0.125% bupivacaine. The epidural block was later extended to T4 dermatomal level for emergency cesarean delivery.

Anesthesia for Cesarean Section   Leibbrandt et al[164] reported two successful deliveries by cesarean section in a patient with a single ventricle and transposition of the great arteries managed with epidural anesthesia. With appropriate invasive monitoring and a slow induction, epidural anesthesia is a safe alternative to general anesthesia for cesarean deliveries.

On the other hand, traditional teaching recommends general anesthesia for cesarean section in patients with complex cyanotic heart diseases as described in two earlier reports.[165,166] More recently, Zavisca et al[167] described the use of general anesthesia for cesarean section in a patient with single ventricle and pulmonary atresia. Large doses of fentanyl and midazolam were administered for sedation before the insertion of invasive monitoring lines, and intravenous etomidate was used for induction of general anesthesia.

We consider that the basic principles of management of general anesthesia in such cases include avoidance of myocardial depressants and tachycardia, assurance of adequate oxygenation and venous return, prevention of aortocaval compression, and maintenance of a favorable balance of pulmonary and systemic vascular resistance.

Since the severity of the lesion and the adequacy of cardiac compensation vary from one parturient to another, the merits of general versus regional anesthesia must be decided for each patient.

HYPERTROPHIC CARDIOMYOPATHY

Hypertrophic cardiomyopathy (HC) is characterized by various degrees of left ventricular hypertrophy, either asymmetric or global.[73] Obstruction to left ventricular out flow may be present. The presence and degree of obstruction are affected by changing hemodynamic conditions as well as by medical manipulations. The degree of obstruction worsens with events that increase myocardial contractility (pain, light general anesthesia), cause tachycardia, decrease venous return, or induce peripheral vasodilatation (major regional blocks).

Pregnancy and Hypertrophic Cardiomyopathy

The hypervolemia of pregnancy increases the left ventricular chamber size, thereby decreasing the left ventricular outflow obstruction. On the other hand, the decrease in systemic vascular resistance, and the increase in other variables such as heart rate, myocardial contractility, and metabolic demands of pregnancy, worsen the obstruction. Thus, while some women with hypertrophic cardiomyopathy tolerate pregnancy-related cardiovascular changes well, others may have exacerbation of all their symptoms.

Goals of Anesthetic Management

Anesthetic management should be aimed at maintaining normo- to slight hypervolemia, continuing beta blockers during labor, and favoring anesthetic drugs that depress myocardial contractility.

Anesthesia for Labor Pain Relief Recommendations for pain relief during labor and delivery include systemic medication, inhalation analgesia, or paracervical and pudendal blocks.[73] Epidural anesthesia is safe when administered judiciously with careful maintenance of intravascular volume and avoidance of aortocaval compression. Use of dilute solutions of local anesthetics with narcotics is recommended,

along with slow induction of block, to avoid major hemodynamic perturbations. Epinephrine should not be used in local anesthetics. For treatment of hypotension, a pure α-adrenergic agonist such as phenylephrine is preferred. Ephedrine should be avoided because of its positive chronotropic qualities. β-Adrenergic blockers should be continued during labor and delivery. Additional doses of β-adrenergic blockers may be needed to slow the heart rate during labor and delivery.

Spinal anesthesia is perhaps the least desirable of all anesthetics in patients with hypertrophic cardiomyopathy. Kitamura and Fujimori[168] described the hemodynamic events during two different anesthetic techniques in a patient with HC undergoing dilatation and curettage (D & C). The first D & C was performed under a saddle block with marked hemodynamic instability despite the use of beta blockers. The second D & C, 8 months later, was performed under heavy premedication, thiopental induction, and followed by halothane with N_2O/O_2 by mask. Under these conditions, the patient remained hemodynamically stable. Loubser et al[169] also described the adverse effects of spinal anesthesia in a patient with HC.

Anesthesia for Cesarean Section For cesarean delivery, either epidural or general anesthesia may be used. Tessler et al[170] described the anesthetic management of two patients with hypertrophic cardiomyopathy; one patient received general anesthesia for cesarean section and the other received epidural anesthesia for labor and delivery. The PA pressures were not monitored. Despite what was considered to be an appropriate anesthetic management, both patients developed pulmonary edema. These authors correctly concluded that regardless of the anesthetic choice, monitoring of left ventricular filling pressure is essential for accurate fluid management in the peripartum period.

The successful management of general anesthesia for cesarean sections in parturients has been described in detail in various case reports.[171,172]

CORONARY ARTERY DISEASE

Coronary artery disease (CAD) occurs in about one in 10,000 parturients.[173] The present trend toward childbearing later in life, along with such other factors as increased tobacco and cocaine abuse among young women, may increase the frequency with which CAD is seen in the delivery room. Nevertheless the condition is still rare, and fewer than a hundred cases were reviewed in the literature in the last decade.

Pregnancy and CAD

Pregnancies undoubtedly increase the maternal morbidity and mortality in women with CAD. The precarious balance between myocardial oxygen supply and demand may be further worsened by the pregnancy-related hemodynamic changes, which include large increases in cardiac output, blood volume, and oxygen consumption. During labor and delivery, the additional increases in these parameters are coupled with fear, anxiety, and pain. The conditions are thus ripe for the onset of myocardial ischemia, infarction, and failure.

Goals of Anesthetic Management

Adequate labor analgesia is essential to prevent the adverse hemodynamic consequences of labor pains. Tachycardia and severe lowering in diastolic blood pressure results in reduced coronary perfusion and should be avoided.

Monitoring

At the University of Tennessee, all parturients with a history of myocardial infarction (MI) during the present pregnancy and those in congestive heart failure are admitted to the obstetric intensive care unit and monitored with radial and pulmonary arterial catheters. Others with a history of MI in the past are monitored closely, and decisions regarding ICU admission and invasive monitoring are based on the clinical course during peripartum period. All cardiac medications such as nitrates are continued throughout the peripartum period.

Analgesia for Labor and Vaginal Delivery   Since the pain, fear, and anxiety associated with labor can precipitate angina and worsen the situation, early administration of epidural anesthesia with liberal use of epidural narcotics is recommended. Besides providing pain relief, the increase in endogenous catecholamine secretion is blunted. In addition, epidural anesthesia primarily affects the preload, though afterload also decreases somewhat. The extent of decreases in the preload and afterload should be tightly controlled, to prevent interference with diastolic filling and coronary perfusion pressures. The monitoring of left ventricular filling pressures is vital for appropriate fluid management.

Several case reports describe the safety and benefits of epidural anesthesia in parturients with CAD.[174–177] One report described the successful administration of epidural anesthesia for labor and delivery in a patient who had sustained a myocardial infarction and cardiac arrest from which she was resuscitated only 48 hours earlier.[175] Unlike patients with other forms of cardiac disease, parturients with CAD may benefit from intense sensory block (extending to higher than T10 levels) that ensure an almost painless labor and provide adequate anesthesia for forceps delivery. Therefore, some authors recommend the use of higher concentrations of local anesthetics, such as 2% lidocaine with fentanyl in larger volumes.[176,177] With preexisting higher levels of intense sensory and motor blocks, further extension to T4 levels for an emergency cesarean section can be accomplished quickly, thus avoiding the need for a general anesthetic. As always,

the patient should be allowed to labor in the left lateral position, and oxygen should be administered through a face mask. For treatment of hypotension, small intravenous dose of phenylephrine is preferred.[176,177]

Anesthesia for Cesarean Section   Regional or general anesthesia may be used with invasive monitoring. Electrocardiographic lead V_5 or any other that is likely to demonstrate ischemic changes based on coronary anatomy and/or history should be monitored. Strict avoidance of increases in variables such as afterload and heart rate is essential, as is prevention of decreases in diastolic arterial pressure. For induction of general anesthesia, the use of high doses of fentanyl followed by an intermediate-acting muscle relaxant to facilitate intubation is recommended. Ventilation with air/oxygen mixture and nitroglycerin infusion during surgery ensures hemodynamic stability. Postoperatively, patients should be monitored in the ICU for a minimum of 24–48 hours. It must be remembered that intravenous nitroglycerin will promote uterine relaxation, particularly in the presence of volatile anesthetic agents and may potentially increase blood loss. Vigorous uterine massage and oxytocic agents may be required.

PERIPARTUM CARDIOMYOPATHY

Peripartum cardiomyopathy is a rare condition in which left ventricular failure occurs in the last month of pregnancy or the first 5 months postpartum. Other criteria for the diagnosis of peripartum cardiomyopathy include absence of prior history of heart disease and no obvious etiology.

Pregnancy and Peripartum Cardiomyopathy

There is controversy as to whether the condition is solely related to pregnancy or pregnancy simply exacerbates a preexisting cardiac disorder.[73] The normal cardiovascular changes of pregnancy increase the stress on the diseased, enlarged heart, causing progressive left ventricular failure. With the onset of labor, the cardiac status can deteriorate, causing florid pulmonary edema.

Goals of Anesthetic Management

The use of all myocardial depressants should be avoided. Measures of medical management such as administration of digoxin, use of diuretics, and afterload reduction should be continued. The hemodynamic status, with the aid of invasive monitoring, should be optimized before any major anesthetic interventions are attempted. Radial and pulmonary arterial pressure monitoring should be considered in all patients with persistent cardiomegaly following peripartum cardiomyopathy during a prior pregnancy. In addition, such monitoring is indicated in all patients presenting with left heart failure and pulmonary edema. Sudden increases in the afterload and heart rate are poorly tolerated and therefore should be avoided.

Anesthesia for Labor and Delivery Epidural anesthesia is recommended for labor analgesia.[178,179] The preload and afterload reductions are highly beneficial. Women who have peripartum cardiomyopathy usually also have high left ventricular filling pressures and reduced left ventricular stroke work index. Epidural anesthesia decreases afterload with minimal changes in myocardial contractility. A slow induction of epidural anesthesia with careful titration of fluid administration, based on left-sided filling pressures, is the technique of choice in such patients.

Anesthesia for Cesarean Delivery Most anesthesiologists favor the use of regional anesthesia to avoid the detrimental hemodynamic changes associated with the induction of general anesthesia, such as sudden increases in heart rate and afterload and the fetal depressant effects of narcotics. In patients requiring an emergency cesarean delivery for either maternal or fetal indications, general anesthesia is unavoidable because slow induction of epidural block is not feasible. For general anesthesia, a high dose narcotic induction technique is preferred. Afterload reduction with a nitroglycerin or nitroprusside infusion with dobutamine, depending on systolic blood pressure, is essential.

ANESTHESIA FOR CARDIAC SURGERY IN PREGNANCY

Cardiac disease during pregnancy is usually managed medically. Heart surgery is indicated only when the cardiac condition worsens under optimal medical treatment or complications supervene that can only be corrected surgically. Therefore, a parturient scheduled for cardiac surgery is frequently in an unstable hemodynamic condition, requiring meticulous anesthetic technique. Prior to anesthesia and surgery, every effort should be made to improve and stabilize the patient's condition. The anesthetic approach is dictated by the underlying cardiac pathology, except for the additional requirements of a rapid induction technique during the second and third trimesters. Left uterine displacement throughout the surgery and convalescence is essential, and there must be continuous intra- and postoperative monitoring of fetal heart rate and uterine activity.

Outcome studies in women undergoing cardiac surgery with cardiopulmonary bypass suggest no increase in maternal mortality over nonpregnant individuals, but the accompanying fetal mortality remains substantial.[180–183] Maternal mortality is quoted to be less than 2%, while fetal wastage is approximately 17%.[180–183] The reason for fetal demise remains speculative, but possible causes include the emergency nature of the surgery, precarious maternal status, poor placental perfusion during and after cardiopulmonary bypass, and actual destruction of the placental structure by microemboli, leukocytes, and complement activation.[183]

Monitoring

Monitoring the pregnant patient for cardiac surgery should include all the following: electrocardiogram, invasive arterial blood pressure, end-tidal carbon dioxide, pulse oximetry, core temperature, and continuous monitoring of fetal heart rate and uterine activity. Use of central venous pressure or pulmonary artery catheter is based on the severity and nature of the disease. Additionally, although not reported elsewhere, femoral arterial blood pressure may prove helpful in determining adequacy of uterine blood pressure in the event of fetal bradycardia.

Timing of surgery places the needs of the mother and fetus somewhat at odds. Ideally, surgery should be undertaken while the mother is in the optimal physical condition, before the major physiologic and hemodynamic changes of pregnancy occur: that is, during the first trimester. Conversely, the fetus should be at the point of significant extrauterine viability. Early surgery may put the fetus at risk during the phase of organogenesis, while later surgery stresses the maternal system. The consensus opinion is that surgery may be performed at any time to save the life of the mother, but preferably during the late second trimester when organogenesis is complete and the risk of premature labor is not as high.[180,182,184]

Anesthetic Management

The majority of the published literature does not address specific anesthetic induction or maintenance technique. The few articles that do are case reports, and no systematic study of the techniques is reported.[183,185–188] El Maraghy et al[189] detail the only technique applied on a large scale basis, in 42 pregnant patients of NYHA functional class IV, undergoing closed mitral valvulotomy. Premedication consisting of morphine (0.1 mg/kg) and scopolamine (0.4 mg) and preoxygenation were followed by thiopental induction (4 mg/kg), endotracheal intubation facilitated by succinylcholine, maintenance with O_2/N_2O (1:1), and muscle relaxation with pancuronium. At the end of surgery, neuromuscular block was reversed with atropine and neostigmine. Strickland et al[183] report techniques including isoflurane and fentanyl in combination, ketamine and fentanyl in combination, meperidine and nitrous oxide, and halothane and meperidine alone. Others report the use of sufentanil and vecuronium,[188] thiopental and succinylcholine,[185] and halothane in nitrous oxide.[186] Provided the hemodynamic, chronotropic, and inotropic goals are attained by appropriate drug dosing, there is little evidence that any one technique is superior to another. It must be remembered that after the first trimester, the airway is at risk of passive regurgitation, and aspiration, and cricoid pressure must be maintained until the airway is secure regardless of the anesthetic.

In a parturient at term, a combined operation (i.e., cesarean section/heart surgery) may be elected. Depending on the severity of the underlying cardiac condition, cesarean section either precedes or is performed while the patient is on cardiopulmonary bypass.[190] Provision for immediate intubation and mechanical ventilation of the neonate is essential. A second option for valvular disease is urgent balloon valvulopasty to temporize until the fetus has been delivered and the mother is stable.

The actual cardiopulmonary bypass technique is a matter of little controlled scientific study, and therefore decisions are based on case reports and combined series. Because of the increased cardiac output demands of pregnancy, the use of high flow, high pressure bypass is recommended. Flow rates of at least 2.5 L/min/m^2 are recommended as a start, with increases to 80 mL/kg/min as necessary to maintain normal fetal heart rate.[181,183,191] Mean arterial pressure should also be maintained at high levels, since the blood flow to the uteroplacental unit is dependent on perfusion pressure. Mean pressures of 70 mmHg or greater may be necessary, as determined by the fetal heart rate and variability.[181,191,192] If fetal bradycardia should develop, first-line therapy consists of increasing pump flow rate, which usually increases perfusion pressure.[191-193] Placental blood flow may also be decreased by uterine contractile activity. This change in hemodynamic status, with the already decreased placental perfusion, may result in fetal hypoxemia. Such contractions are frequently noted at two intraoperative events, during hypothermia and while rewarming.[180] Therefore, if fetal bradycardia or decelerations are noted, uterine contractions must be ruled out as a cause and terminated if present.[194] Therapy may include intravenous β$_2$-adrenergic agonists such as terbutaline or ritodrine, magnesium sulfate, or nifedipine.[195,196] The benefits of nifedipine are its rapid onset when administered sublingually (3–5 min), potent uterine relaxation, and lack of chronotropic or negative inotropic effects.[195] Further therapy of fetal bradycardia should include increasing the maternal hematocrit to 20–25%, assuring adequate left uterine displacement, and correction of alkalosis.

Hypothermia is commonly used during cardiopulmonary bypass for organ protection and to decrease corporal oxygen demands. In the pregnant patient this standard technique may introduce confounding variables if fetal bradycardia is manifested, and it may not be necessary for fetal or maternal protection. Studies in pregnant dogs cooled to 28°C revealed an increase in uterine tone and vascular resistance, and a decrease in uterine blood flow, but no change in fetal survival.[197] There are many reports of pregnant patients undergoing hypothermia, even deep hypothermia with circulatory

arrest, with no apparent fetal harm, and others cases in which the result was fetal demise.[183,198,199] Hypothermia may confer some protection on the fetus, but since uterine contractions and fetal bradycardia may be induced, hypothermia should be minimized or avoided unless it is necessary for long aortic cross-clamping.[180,181] Fetal tachycardia, often noted subsequent to weaning from bypass, has been reported to resolve over the succeeding several hours and is felt to be compensatory to mild fetal hypoxemia.[186,191] In summary, mild hypothermia, to no less than 32°C, appears to be well tolerated with minimal fetal side effects. Lower temperatures should be used only for specific indications, such as prolonged aortic cross-clamping.

Additional recommendations for cardiopulmonary bypass include the use of arterial filters on the inflow line of the circuit. This measure is particularly important if normothermic bypass will be used. The inferior vena cava cannula must be carefully placed. If venous drainage from the lower extremities is impeded, decreased placental perfusion may result.[200]

Vasoactive, inotropic, and antiarrhythmic drugs are often required during cardiac surgery. Their effects on uterine blood flow should be taken into account when choosing the appropriate one. The effects of these drugs are summarized in Table 24.1.

The literature is now replete with case reports and series of parturients with severe cardiac valvular disease having undergone balloon valvuloplasty.[201-205] These techniques are uniformly successful in decreasing the acuity of the cardiac disease and allowing the pregnancy to proceed to a natural conclusion. The pathophysiology of valvular disease in the young is congenital or rheumatic in nature and not of longstanding. Young females, therefore, are the ideal candidates for balloon procedures because their valves are not heavily calcified or thickened, there is minimal subvalvular involvement, and the leaflets are mobile.[206,207] Balloon plasty of each of the valves separately and in combination has been reported.[202,203,205] Risks to the mother include arterial, venous, or atrial perforation, cardiac tamponade, hemorrhage, arrhythmias, emboli, valvular regurgitation, hypotension, seizures, stroke, and death.[202,204] The fetus may exhibit heart rate decelerations due to transient hypoxemia during hemodynamic instability in the mother. An additional benefit of valvuloplasty is elimination of the potential need for maternal anticoagulation. In the future, the need for cardiopulmonary bypass for decompensated valvular disease in pregnancy may become even more uncommon.

REGIONAL ANESTHESIA IN PARTURIENTS RECEIVING ANTICOAGULANTS

Antithrombotic agents are administered during pregnancy in three clinical settings: for prevention or treatment of venous thrombosis, for the prevention of systemic embolization associated with the presence of mechanical heart valves or valvular heart disease, and for the prevention of fetal loss and growth retardation associated with antiphospholipid antibodies.[208] Anticoagulants that may be used include heparin, coumarin, and acetylsalicylic acid. These drugs may be administered singly or in combination throughout pregnancy up to and including the time of delivery.

The use of regional anesthesia in obstetric patients requiring anticoagulant therapy is controversial. Opinions vary from absolute condemnation of all regional anesthetic techniques if any anticoagulant is administered to very permissive recommendations.[73,209] To make a fully informed decision, the risks and benefits of the procedure must be weighed for each individual patient in light of the cardiac and systemic pathology. Damage to an epidural vein occurs in approximately 3–12% of cases,[210] with frequent formation of asymptomatic epidural hematoma[211] but rare neurologic injury.[212] In the majority of case reports of neurologic injury, patients were receiving anticoagulants or had coagulation disorders.[213–215] Despite these case reports, prospective trials and large retrospective studies of patients receiving antiplatelet therapy,[216,217] warfarin,[209] and a range of heparin doses[218–220] have proven that epidural analgesia and anesthesia may be safely administered.

Several authors have advised against regional blocks even if heparin is stopped when labor starts and protamine is given if required. The need for early resumption of heparin therapy soon after removal of the epidural catheter constitutes another possible reason for objection, since formation of an epidural hematoma may result, with possible neurological sequelae. Saka and Marx[221] described such a complication and recommended delaying reheparinization until 24 hours after removal of the catheter. Another more recent report described resumption of subcutaneous heparin therapy as early as 3 hours following removal of the epidural catheter.[222] Abouleish[223] concluded that when heparin has been discontinued for 6 hours and the coagulation tests are found to be normal, insertion of an epidural catheter can be considered to be safe. Heparin therapy may be restarted 6 hours after removal of the epidural catheter.[223]

Two frequently used anticoagulation protocols may be encountered in parturients. Heparin administered subcutaneously or intravenously to attain an activated partial thromboplastin time (APTT) of 1.5–2.5 times control or coumarin daily dosing to maintain a prothrombin time (PT) international normalized ratio (INR) of 2.0–2.5.[208,224] A third combination used for patients with antiphospholipid antibodies may include aspirin with prednisone, low dose aspirin, or heparin for full anticoagulation.[208] Regardless of regimen, the parturient who remains anticoagulated at the time of delivery is at risk of bleeding complications because heparin has prolonged anticoagulant effects in the parturient.[225] Elevated APTT was noted to persist for up to 28 hours after the last adjusted dose subcutaneous heparin injection.[225] Thus,

all patients receiving anticoagulation should have the drugs stopped at least 24 hours prior to labor induction and the APTT or PT verified at a normal level. Chronic heparin administration will result in 5–10% of individuals developing thrombocytopenia ($< 150,000$ platelets/mL blood).[226] Therefore, an adequate platelet count must also be assured.

The use of continuous epidural analgesia in a parturient with a triple-heart-valve prosthesis was reported by Duffy.[227] Sixteen hours following the last subcutaneous heparin dose, an epidural catheter was inserted and the patient had an uneventful labor. Instrumental delivery was performed under stable hemodynamic conditions. The first dose of heparin was erroneously administered 1 hour following removal of the epidural catheter, but there were no untoward effects. The authors suggested that anticoagulation therapy can be resumed in less than 24 hours.

Rao and El-Etr[219] followed up 4011 heparinized patients undergoing vascular surgery under continuous epidural or spinal anesthesia. Although all catheters were removed 1 hour before the next scheduled dose of heparin, no peridural hematomas leading to spinal cord compression were observed. To the best of our knowledge, no similar study in obstetrics has been reported. Odoom and Sih[209] prospectively studied 950 patients undergoing vascular surgery who had epidural catheters placed after having received oral anticoagulants with both the thrombotest and the partial thromboplastin time prolonged. No patient developed neurologic sequelae despite the coagulation status. Horlocker et al[216] have shown that it is feasible to place an epidural catheter in patients receiving antiplatelet drugs with no neurologic complications.

If an epidural or spinal is indicated while the patient is anticoagulated, reversal of the anticoagulating agent may be performed cautiously. Heparin reversal may be accomplished with small doses of protamine administered slowly, recalling the potential for a systemic reaction (e.g., peripheral vasodilation, pulmonary hypertension).[228] Coumarin effect will spontaneously diminish 24–48 hours following the last dose. Should more rapid reversal be required, vitamin K may be administered intravenously or subcutaneously with rapid effect. Doses of 0.5–1 mg will lower the INR within 8 hours,[229] while larger doses will decrease this time to 6 hours.[230] Larger doses will induce coumarin resistance for up to 7 days after reversal.[231] Fresh frozen plasma will also reverse coumarin effects immediately, but with the risk of blood-borne pathogen transmission and the need for redosing every 6 hours.[232]

The merits of regional anesthesia for parturients requiring anticoagulation must be carefully weighed against the possible risk of neurological sequelae. A thorough evaluation of ventricular function, the presence of pulmonary hypertension, and signs of cardiac decompensation should be considered when alternate analgesic and anesthetic techniques are weighed. The following recommendations pertain when a regional anesthetic technique is appropriate.

1. Regional anesthesia should be avoided in patients who are fully anticoagulated at the anticipated time of needle placement. Heparin should preferably be stopped 24 hours prior and coumarin stopped 48 hours prior to planned labor induction. Verification of anticoagulant reversal should be performed (APTT or PT), as well as platelet count.

2. Anticoagulation may be resumed 1 hour after needle placement if it is necessary to maintain a fully anticoagulated state.

3. Removal of an epidural catheter should occur following reversal of anticoagulation and at least 1 hour before redosing.

4. Antiplatelet drugs are not a contraindication to epidural or spinal needle placement.

REFERENCES

1. Lunn JN, Mushin WW. *Mortality Associated with Anesthesia.* Oxford: Nuffield Provincial Hospitals Trust; 1982.

2. Bonica JJ. Labor pain: mechanisms and pathways. In: Marx GF, Bassel GM, eds. *Obstetric Analgesia and Anesthesia.* Amsterdam: Elsevier/North-Holland; 1980;173–196.

3. Hunter S, Robson SC. Adaptation of the maternal heart in pregnancy. *Br Heart J* 1992;68:540–543.

4. Robson SC, Hunter S, Boys RJ. Serial study of factors influencing changes in cardiac output during human pregnancy. *Am J Physiol* 1989;256:1060–1065.

5. Clark SL, Cotton DB, Lee W, Bishop C, Hill T, Southwick J, Pivarnik J, Spillman T, De Vore GR, Phelan J, Hankins GDV, Benedetti TJ, Tolley D. Central hemodynamic assessment of normal term pregnancy. *Am J Obstet Gynecol* 1989;161:1439–1442.

6. Proctor AJM, White JB. Laryngeal edema in pregnancy. *Anaesthesia* 1983;38:167.

7. Archer GW, Marx GF. Arterial oxygen tension during apnoea in parturient women. *Br J Anaesth* 1974;46:358–360.

8. Cohen AM, Mulvein J. Obstetric anaesthetic management in a patient with the Fontan circulation. 1994;*Br J Anaesth* 73:252–255.

9. Marx GF, Bassell GM. Physiologic considerations of the mother. In: Marx GF, Bassel GM, eds. *Obstetric Analgesia and Anesthesia.* Amsterdam: Elsevier/North-Holland, 1980; 21–54.

10. Cheek TS, Gutsche BB. Maternal physiologic alterations during pregnancy. In: Shnider SM, Levinson G, eds. *Anesthesia for Obstetrics.* (2nd ed.) Baltimore: Williams & Wilkins; 1974;3–13.

11. Macfie AG, Magibes AD, Richmond MN, Reilly CS. Gastric emptying time during pregnancy. *Br J Anaesth* 1991;67:54–57.

12. O'Sullivan GM, Sutton AJ, Thompson SA, Carrie LE, Bullingham RE. Noninvasive measurement of gastric emptying in obstetric patients. *Anesth Analg* 1987;66:505–511.

13. Cohen SE. Why is the pregnant patient different? *Semin Anesth* 1982;2:73–82.

14. Joyce TH. Regional versus general anesthesia: any advantage? *Semin Anesth* 1982;2:125–132.

15. Hartigan PM. Cardiac problems. In: Datta S, ed. *Common Problems in Obstetric Anesthesia.* 2nd ed. St Louis: CV Mosby; 1994;321–346.

16. Caritis SN, Aboulish E, Edelstone DI. Fetal acid–base state following spinal and epidural anesthesia for cesarean section. *Obstet Gynecol* 1980;56:610–615.

17. Robson SC, Boys RJ, Rodeck C, Morgan B. Maternal and fetal haemodynamic effects of spinal and extradural anesthesia for elective caesarean section. *Br J Anaesth* 1992;68:54–59.

18. Chestnut DH, Laszewski LJ, Pollack KL, Bates JN, Manago NK, Choi WW. Continuous epidural infusion of 0.0625% bupivacaine–0.0002% fentanyl during the second stage of labor. *Anesthesiology* 1990;72:613–618.

19. Naulty JS. Epidural analgesia for labor. In: Norris MC, ed. *Obstetric Anaesthesia.* Philadelphia: JB Lippincott; 1993;319–340.

20. Green NM, Brull SJ. *Physiology of Spinal Anaesthesia.* 4th ed. Baltimore: Williams & Wilkins; 1993.

21. Mark JB, Steale SM. Cardiovascular effects of spinal anesthesia. *Int Anesthesiol Clin* 1989;27:31–39.

22. Eneroth-Grimfors E, Westgren M, Erikson M, Ihrman-Fandahl C, Lindblad LE. Autonomic cardiovascular control in normal and preeclamptic pregnancy. *Acta Obstet Gynecol Scand* 1994;73:680–684.

23. Landry DP, Bennett FM, Oriol NE. Analysis of heart rate dynamics as a measure of autonomic tone in obstetrical patients undergoing epidural or spinal anesthesia. *Reg Anesth* 1994;19:189–195.

24. Eisenach JC, Tuttle R, Stein A. Is ST segment depression of electrocardiogram during cesarean section merely due to cardiac sympathetic block? *Anesth Analg* 1994;78:287–292.

25. Goertz AN, Seeling W, Heilrich H, Lindner KH, Schirmer U. Influence of high thoracic epidural anesthesia on left ventricular contractility assessment using the end-systolic pressure length relationship. *Acta Anaesthesiol Scand* 1993;37:38–44.

26. Kerr MG, Scott DB, Samule E. Studies of the inferior vena cava in late pregnancy. *Br Med J* 1964;1:532–533.

27. Bieniarz I, Crottogini JJ, Curachet E. Aortocaval compression by the uterus in late human pregnancy. *Am J Obstet Gynecol* 1968;100:203–217.

28. Kinsella SM, Whitwam JG, Spencer JA. Reducing aortocaval compression: how much tilt is enough? *Br Med J* 1992;305:539–540.

29. Kinsella SM, Lohmann G. Supine hypotensive syndrome. *Obstet Gynecol* 1994;83:774–788.

30. Yaksh TI, Rudy TA. Narcotic analgesics: CNS sites and mechanisms of action as revealed by intracerebral injection techniques. *Pain* 1978;4:299–359.

31. Jones PI, Rosen M, Mushin WW, Jones EV. Methoxyflurane and nitrous oxide as obstetric analgesics. I. A comparison by continuous administration. *Br Med J* 1969;3:255–259.

32. Fields HL, Basbaum AI. Endogenous pain control mechanism. In: Wall RD, Melzack R, eds. *Textbook of Pain*. London: Churchill Livingstone; 1984;142–252.

33. Doughty A. The physiology of childbirth. In: Churchill-Davidson HC, ed. *A Practice of Anaesthesia*. 4th ed. London: Lloyd-Luke Medical Books, 1979;2:1287–1301.

34. Niv D, Rudick, V, Freedman M, Leykin Y, Geller E. Epidural 0.35% bupivacaine versus intravenous meperidine–promethazine for pain relief in labor. *Schmerz Pain Douleur* 1985;3:125–127.

35. Carstoniu J, Levytam S, Normal P. Nitrous oxide in labor: safety and efficacy assessed by double-blind placebo controlled study. *Anesthesiology* 1994;80:30–35.

36. Abboud T, Shnider S, Wright R. Enflurane analgesia in obstetrics. *Anesth Analg* 1981;60:133–137.

37. McLeod DD, Ramayya GP, Turnstall ME. Self-administered isoflurane in labour. *Anaesthesia* 1985;40:424–426.

38. Shnider SM, Abboud TK, Artal R, Henrikson EH, Stefani SJ, Levinson G. Maternal catecholamines decrease during labor after lumbar epidural analgesia. *Am J Obstet Gynecol* 1983;147:13–15.

39. Abboud TK, Sarkis F, Hung TT, Khoo SS, Varakian L, Henrik E, Noueihed R, Goebelsmann U. Effects of epidural anesthesia during labor on maternal plasma beta endorphin levels. *Anesthesiology* 1983;59:1–5.

40. Holleman A, Jouppila R, Jouppila P, Koivula A, Vierola H. Effect of extradural analgesia using bupivacaine and 2-chloroprocaine on intervillous blood flow during normal labour. *Br J Anaesth* 1982;54:837–842.

41. Hagedral M, Morgan CW, Sumner AE, Gutsche BB. Minute ventilation and oxygen consumption during labor with extradural analgesia. *Anesthesiology* 1983;59:425–427.

42. Cousins MJ, Bromage PR. Epidural neural blockade. In: Cousins MJ, Bridenbaugh PO, eds. *Neural Blockade*. Philadelphia: Lippincott; Neural Blockade 1988;253–360.

43. Bromage PR. *Epidural Analgesia*. Philadelphia: WB Saunders; 1978.

44. Forster R, Joyce TD. Spinal opioids and the treatment of the obstetric patient with cardiac disease. *Clin Perinatol* 1989;16:955–974.

45. Perriss BW. Epidural opiates in labour. *Lancet* 1979;2:422.

46. Booker PD, Wilkes RG, Bryson THL, Beddard J. Obstetric pain relief using epidural morphine. *Anaesthesia* 1980;35:377–379.

47. Niv D, Rudick V, Chayen MS, David MP. Variations in the effect of epidural morphine in gynecological and obstetric patients. *Acta Obstet Gynecol Scand* 1983;62:455–459.

48. Scott PV, Bowen FE, Cartwright P, Rao BCM, Deeley D, Wotherspoon HG, Sumrein IMA. Intrathecal morphine as a sole analgesic during labor. *Br Med J* 1980;281:351–353.

49. Baraka A, Noueihed R, Hajj S. Intrathecal injection of morphine for obstetric analgesia. *Anesthesiology* 1981;54:136–146.

50. Niv D, Rudick V, Golan A, Chayen MS. Augmentation of bupivacaine analgesia in labor by epidural morphine. *Obstet Gynecol* 1986;67:206–209.

51. Ready LB, Loper KA, Nessly M, Wild L. Postoperative epidural morphine is safe on surgical wards. *Anesthesiology* 1991;75:452–456.

52. Morgan M. The rational use of intrathecal and extradural opioids. *Br J Anaesth* 1989;63:165–188.

53. Carrie LES. Epidural versus combined spinal epidural block for cesarean section. *Acta Anaesthesiol Scand* 1988;32:595–596.

54. Szekely P, Turner R, Snaith L. Pregnancy and the changing pattern of rheumatic heart disease. *Br Heart J* 1973;35:1293–1303.

55. Szekely P, Snaith L. *Heart Disease and Pregnancy*. London: Churchill Livingstone; 1974.

56. Mendelson CL. *Cardiac Disease in Pregnancy*. Philadelphia: FA Davis; 1960.

57. Barnes CG. *Medical Disorders in Obstetric Practice*. 4th ed. Oxford: Blackwell Scientific; 1970.

58. Ueland K. Cardiac surgery and pregnancy. *Am J Obstet Gynecol* 1965;92:148–162.

59. Department of Health and Social Security. Report on confidential enquiries into maternal deaths in England and Wales, 1970–1972. London: Her Majesty's Stationery Office; 1975.

60. Ueland K. Intrapartum management of the cardiac patient. *Clin Perinatol* 1981;8:155–168.

61. Arani DT, Carleton RA. The deleterious role of tachycardia in mitral stenosis. *Circulation* 1967;36:511–516.

62. Hildner IJ. Myocardial dysfunction associated with valvular heart disease. *Am J Cardiol* 1972;30:319–326.

63. Metcalfe J. Rheumatic heart disease in pregnancy. *Clin Obstet Gynecol* 1968;11:1010–1025.

64. Selzer A, Cohen E. Natural history of mitral stenosis. A review. *Circulation* 1972;45:878–890.

65. DiNardo JA. Anesthesia for valve replacement in patients with acquired valvular heart disease. In: DiNardo JA, Schwartz MJ, eds. *Anesthesia for Cardiac Surgery*. Norwalk, CT: Appleton & Lange; 1990;85–115.

66. Secher NJ, Thayssen P, Arnsbro P, Olsen J. Effect of prostaglandin E_2 and F_2 on the systemic and pulmonary circulation in pregnant anesthetized women. *Acta Obstet Gynecol Scand* 1982;61:213–218.

67. Ueland K, Hansen JM. Maternal cardiovascular dynamics. III. Labor and delivery under local and caudal analgesia. *Am J Obstet Gynecol.* 1969;103:8–18.

68. Schroeder JS, Harrison DC. Repeated cardioversion during pregnancy: treatment of refractory paroxysmal atrial tachycardia during three successive pregnancies. *Am J Cardiol* 1971;27:445–446.

69. Vogel JHK, Pryor R, Blount SGJ. Direct-current defibrillation during pregnancy. *JAMA* 1965;193:970–971.

70. Elkayam U, Goodwin TM. Adenosine therapy for supraventricular tachycardia during pregnancy. *Am J Cardiol* 1995;75:521–523.

71. Hagley MT, Cole PL. Adenosine use in pregnant women with supraventricular tachycardia. *Ann Pharmacother* 1994;28:1241–1242.

72. McMurray TJ, Kenny NI. Extradural anesthesia in parturients with severe cardiovascular disease. Two case reports. *Anaesthesia* 1982;37:442–445.

73. Mangano DT. Anesthesia for the pregnant cardiac patient. In: Shnider SM, Levinson G, eds. *Anesthesia for Obstetrics.* Baltimore: Williams & Wilkins; 1993;485–524.

74. Thornhill ML, Camann WR. Cardiovascular disease. In: Chestnut DH, ed. *Obstetric Anesthesia: Principles and Practice.* St Louis: CV Mosby; 1994;746–779.

75. Adams JQ. Management of the pregnant cardiac patient. *Clin Obstet Gynecol* 1968;11:910–923.

76. Hemmings GT, Whalley DG, O'Connor PJ, Benjamin A, Dunn C. Invasive monitoring and anaesthetic management of a parturient with mitral stenosis. *Can J Anaesth* 1987;34:182–185.

77. Niv D, Wolman I, Rudick V, Geller E. Epidural analgesia in parturients with mitral stenosis: advantage of bupivacaine–morphine combination. *Schmerz Pain Douleur* 1987;3:130–131.

78. Shireen A, Hawes D, Dooley SH, Faure E, Brunner EA. Intrathecal morphine in a parturient with a single ventricle. *Anesthesiology* 1981;54:515–516.

79. Sorenson MB, Korshin JD, Fernandes A, Secher O. The use of epidural analgesia for delivery in a patient with pulmonary hypertension. *Acta Anesthesiol Scand* 1982;26:180–182.

80. McAnulty JH. Heart and other circulatory diseases. In: Bonica JJ, McDonald JS, eds. *Principles and Practice of Obstetric Analgesia and Anesthesia.* 2nd ed. Baltimore: Williams & Wilkins; 1995;1013–1039.

81. Marx GF, Hodgkinson R. Special considerations in complications of pregnancy. In: Marx GF, Bassell GM, eds. *Obstetric Analgesia and Anesthesia.* Amsterdam: Elsevier/North Holland; 1980;297–334.

82. Moir DD, Willocks J. Epidural analgesia in British obstetrics. *Br J Anaesth* 1968;40:129–138.

83. Ostheimer GU, Alper MH. Intrapartum anesthetic management of pregnant patient with heart disease. *Clin Obstet Gynecol* 1975;18:81–97.

84. Rudick V, Golan A, Niv D, Leykin Y, Baram A, Gelle E, Peyser MR. Anesthetic management of 646 consecutive cesarean section cases. *Isr J Med Sci* 1985;21:18–21.

85. Stanton-Hicks MDA. Cardiovascular effects of extradural anaesthesia. *Br J Anaesth* 1975;47:253–261.

86. Ziskind Z, Etchin A, Frenkel Y, Mashiach S, Lusky A, Goor DA, Smolinsky A. Epidural anesthesia with the Trendelenburg position for cesarean section with or without a cardiac surgical procedure in patients with severe mitral stenosis: a hemodynamic study. *J Cardiothorac Anesth* 1990;4:354–359.

87. Prince GD, Mostafa SM. Spinal anaesthesia and cardiac disease. *Br J Anaesth* 1986;58:683–684. Correspondence.

88. Mostafa SM. Spinal anesthesia for cesarean section. Management of a parturient with severe cardiovascular disease. *Br J Anaesth* 1984;56:1275–1277.

89. James FM, Crawford JS, Hopkinson R, Davies P, Nacem HA. A comparison of general anesthesia and lumbar epidural analgesia for elective cesarean section. *Anesth Analg* 1977;56:228–235.

90. Price HL, Cooperman LH, Warden JC, Morris JJ, Smith TC. Pulmonary hemodynamics during general anesthesia in man. *Anesthesiology* 1969;30:629–636.

91. Warren TM, Stoelting RK. Hemodynamic effects of general anesthetics. In: Altura BM, Halevy S, eds. *Cardiovascular Actions of Anesthetics Drugs Used in Anesthesia I: Basic Aspects.* Basel: S Karger 1986;3–50.

92. Fragen RJ. Cardiovascular effects of intravenous anesthetics. In: Altura BM, Halevy S, eds. *Cardiovascular Actions of Anaesthetics Drugs Used in Anesthesia I: Basic Aspects.* Basel: S. Karger; 1986;51–73.

93. Shnider SM, Levinson G, Cosmi EV. Obstetric anesthesia and uterine blood flow. In: Shnider SM, Levinson G, eds. *Anesthesia for Obstetrics.* 3rd ed. Baltimore: Williams & Wilkins; 1993;29–52.

94. Ogura M, Suzukawa M, Tasami M, Inada Y, Toyooka H, Ohgami Y, Kinoshita K, Mizuno M. High-dose fentanyl anesthesia in a pregnant patient with Eisenmenger's syndrome. *MASUI* 1985;34:241–246.

95. Batson MA, Longmire S, Csontos E. Alfentanil for urgent caesarean section in a patient with severe mitral stenosis and pulmonary hypertension. *Can J Anaesth* 1990;37:685–688.

96. Golub MS, Eisele JH, Donald JM. Obstetric analgesia and infant outcome in monkeys: neonatal measures after intrapartum exposure to meperidine or alfentanil. *Am J Obstet Gynecol* 1988;158:1219–1225.

97. McAnulty JH, Metcalfe J, Ueland K. General guidelines in the management of cardiac disease. *Clin Obstet Gynecol* 1981;24:773–778.

98. Sill JC, White RD. Valvular heart disease, cardiovascular performance, and anesthesia. In: Tarhan S, ed. *Cardiovascular Anesthesia and Postoperative Care.* Chicago: Year-Book Medical Publishing; 1983;204–209.

99. Ferguson JEI, Wyner J, Albright GA, Brodsky JB. Maternal health complications. In: Albright GA, Ferguson JE, Joyce TH, Stevenson DK, eds. *Anesthesia in Obstetrics Maternal Fetal Neonatal Aspects.* London: Butterworths; 1986;374–390.

100. Lynch C, Rizor RF. Anesthetic management and monitoring of a parturient with mitral and aortic valvular disease. *Anesth Analg* 1982;61:788–792.

101. Cunningham AJ, Crowley KJ, Tierney E. Elderly parturient with rheumatic heart disease presents for cesarean section: haemodynamic monitoring and anesthesia management. *Ir Med J* 1985;78:333–341.

102. Burwell CS, Metcalfe J. *Heart Disease and Pregnancy.* Boston: Little Brown; 1958.

103. Harshaw CW, Grossman W, Munro AB. Reduced systemic vascular resistance as therapy for severe mitral regurgitation of valvular origin. *Ann Intern Med* 1975;83:312–316.

104. Stone JG, Hoar PE, Calabro JR, De Petrillo MA, Bendixen HH. Afterload reduction and preload augmentatiion improve the anesthetic management of patients with cardiac failure and valvular regurgitation. *Anesth Analg* 1980;59:737–742.

105. Sessler DI, Rubinstein EH, Moayeri A. Physiological responses to mild perianesthetic hypothermia in humans. *Anesthesiology* 1991;75:594–610.

106. Levy D, Savage DD. Prevalence and clinical features of mitral valve prolapse. *Am Heart J* 1987;113;1281–1290.

107. Rayburn WF, Fontana ME. Mitral valve prolapse and pregnancy. *Am J Obstet Gynecol* 1981;141:9–11.

108. Fuenzalida CE. A selective advantage with mitral valve prolapse. *Ann Intern Med* 1983;98:670–671.

109. Alcantara LG, Marx GF. Cesarean section under epidural analgesia in a parturient with mitral valve prolapse. *Anesth Analg* 1987;66:902–903.

110. Krissel J, Dick WF, Leyser KH, Gervais H, Brockerhoff P, Schranz D. Thiopentone, thiopentone/ketamine, and ketamine for induction of anaesthesia in caesarean section. *Eur J Anaesthesiol* 1994;11:115–122.

111. Crozier TA, Flamm C, Speer CP, Rath W, Wuttke W, Kuhn W, Kettler D. Effects of etomidate on the adrenocortical and metabolic adaptation of the neonate. *Br J Anaesth* 1993;70:47–53.

112. Esener Z, Sarihasan B, Guven H, Ustun E. Thiopentone and etomidate concentrations in maternal and umbilical plasma, and in colostrum. *Br J Anaesth* 1992;69:586–588.

113. Gregory MA, DAvidson DG. Plasma etomidate levels in mother and fetus. *Anaesthesia* 1991;46:716–718.

114. Clark SL, Phelan JP, Greenspoon J, Aldahl D, Horenstein J. Labor and delivery in the presence of mitral stenosis: central hemodynamic observations. *Am J Obstet Gynecol* 1985;152:984–988.

115. Chayen MS, Rudick V, Borvine A. Pain control with epidural injection of morphine. *Anesthesiology* 1980;53:388–391.

116. Brian JE Jr., Seifen AB, Clark RB, Robertson DM, Quirk JG. Aortic stenosis, cesarean delivery, and epidural anesthesia. *J Clin Anesth* 1993;5:154–157.

117. Colclough GW, Ackerman WE, Walmsley PN, Hessel EA, Colclough G. Epidural anesthesia for cesarean delivery in a parturient with aortic stenosis. *Reg Anesth* 1990;15:273–274.

118. Easterling TR, Chadwick HS, Otto CM, Benedetti TJ. Aortic stenosis in pregnancy. *Obstet Gynecol* 1988;72:113–118.

119. Gorlin R, McMillan IKR, Medd WE, Matthews MB, Daley R. Dynamics of the circulation in aortic valvular disease. *Am J Med* 1955;18:855–870.

120. Trenouth RS, Phelps NC, Neill WA. Determinants of left ventricular hypertrophy and oxygen supply in chronic aortic valvular disease. *Circulation* 1976;53:644–650.

121. Abboud TK, Shnider SM, Dailey PA, Raya JA, Sarkis F, Grobler NM, Sadri S, Khoo SS, De Sousa B, Baysinger CL, Miller F. Intrathecal administration of hyperbaric morphine for the relief of pain in labor. *Br J Anaesth* 1984;56:1351–1360.

122. Redfern N, Bower S, Bullock RE, Hull CJ. Alfentanil for caesarean section complicated by severe aortic stenosis. A case report. *Br J Anaesth* 1987;59:1309–1312.

123. Jackson JM. Valvular heart disease. In: Thomas SJ, ed. *Manual of Cardiac Anesthesia*. 2nd ed. London: Churchill Livingstone; 1993;81–128.

124. James MF. Rapid sequence induction in pregnancy-associated hypertension—the role of magnesium. *Br J Anaesth* 1988;61:239–240. Letter.

125. Dodge HT, Kennedy JW, Peterson JL. Quantitative angio-cardiographic methods in the evaluation of valvular heart disease. *Prog Cardiovasc Dis* 1973;16:1–23.

126. Rackley CE, Hood WPJ. Aortic valve disease. In: Levine HJ, ed. *Clinical Cardiovascular Physiology*. New York: Grune & Stratton; 1976.

127. Baxley WA, Kennedy JW, Field B, Dodge HT. Hemodynamics in ruptured chordae tendineae and chronic rheumatic mitral regurgitation. *Circulation* 1973;48:1288–1294.

128. Mendelson MA, Chandler J. Postpartum cardiomyopathy associated with maternal cocaine abuse. *Am J Cardiol* 1992;70:1092–1094.

129. Alderson JD. Cardiovascular collapse following epidural anaesthesia for caesarean section in a patient with aortic incompetence. *Anaesthesia* 1987;42:643–645.

130. Weiss-Bloom LJ, Reich DL. Haemodynamic responses to tracheal intubation following etomidate and fentanyl for anaesthetic induction. *Can J Anaesth* 1992;39:780–785.

131. Naulty J, Cefalo RC, Lewis PE. Fetal toxicity of nitroprusside in the pregnant ewe. *Am J Obstet Gynecol* 1981;139:708–711.

132. Benny PS, Prasad J, MacVicar J. Pregnancy and coarctation of the aorta. Case report. *Br J Obstet Gynaecol* 1980;87:1159–1161.

133. Rosenthal L. Coarctation of the aorta and pregnancy: report of five cases. *Br Med J* 1955;1:16–17.

134. Elkayam U, Ostrzega E, Shotan A, Mehra A. Cardiovascular problems in the pregnant women with the Marfan syndrome. *Ann Intern Med* 1995;123:117–122.

135. Williams GM, Gott VL, Brawley KK. Aortic disease associated with pregnancy. *J Vasc Surg* 1988;8:470–475.

136. Gordon CF, Johnson MD. Anesthetic management of the pregnant patient with Marfan syndrome. *J Clin Anesth* 1993;5:248–251.

137. Pinosky ML, Hopkins RA, Pinckert TL, Suyderhood JP. Anesthesia for simultaneous cesarean section and acute aortic dissection repair in a patient with Marfan's syndrome. *J Cardiothorac Anesth* 1994;8:451–454.

138. Ramanathan J, Sibai BM, Mabie WC, Chauhan D, Ruiz AG. The use of labetalol for attenuation of the hypertensive response to endotracheal intubation in preeclampsia. *Am J Obstet Gynecol* 1988;159:650–654.

139. Gleicher N, Midwall J, Hochberger D, Jaffin H. Eisenmenger's syndrome in pregnancy. *Obstet Gynecol Survey* 1979;3:721–741.

140. Foster R, Jones RM. Spinal opioids and the treatment of the obstetric patient with cardiac disease. *Clin Perinatol* 1989;16:955–974.

141. Swan HJC, Burchell HB, Wood EH. Effect of oxygen on pulmonary vascular resistance in patients with pulmonary hypertension associated with atrial septal defect. *Circulation* 1959;20:66–73.

142. Marshall HW, Swan HJC, Burchell HB. Effect of breathing oxygen on pulmonary arterial pressure and pulmonary vascu-

lar resistance in patients with ventricular septal deect. *Circulation* 1961;23:241–252.

143. Pollack KL, Chestnut DH, Wenstrom KD. Anesthetic management of a parturient with Eisenmenger's syndrome. *Anesth Analg* 1990;70:212–215.

144. Spinnato JA, Kraynack BJ, Cooper MW. Eisenmenger's syndrome in pregnancy: epidural anesthesia for elective cesarean section. *N Engl J Med* 1981;20:1215–1217.

145. Crawford JS, Mills WG, Pentecost BL. A pregnant patient with Eisenmenger's syndrome. Case report. *Br J Anaesth* 1971;43:1091–1094.

146. Midwall J, Jaffin H, Herman MV, Kupersmith J. Shunt flow and pulmonary hemodynamics during labor and delivery in the Eisenmenger syndrome. *Am J Cardiol* 1978;42:299–303.

147. Smedstad KG, Cramb R, Morison DH. Pulmonary hypertension and pregnancy: a series of eight cases. *Can J Anaesth* 1994;41:502–512.

148. Rosenberg B, Simon K, Peretz BA, Rougin N, Birkhan HJ. Eisenmenger's syndrome in pregnancy. Controlled segmental epidural block for cesarean section. *Reg Anaesth* 1984;7:131–133.

149. Stoelting B, Longnecker D. Effect of right to left shunt on rate of increase of arterial anesthetic concentration. *Anesthesiology* 1972;36:352–354.

150. Bland JW, Williams WH. Anesthesia for treatment of congenital heart defects. In: Kaplan JA, ed. *Cardiac Anesthesia.* 2nd ed., New York: Grune & Stratton; 1979;281–346.

151. Furuya H, Okumura F, Ishida T, Chiba Y. General anesthesia for cesarean section on the patient with Eisenmenger's syndrome. *MASUI* 1983;32:1269–1273.

152. Elkayam U, Gleicher N. Primary pulmonary hypertension and pregnancy. In: Elkayam U, Gleicher N, eds. *Cardiac Problems in Pregnancy.* 2nd ed. New York: Alan R. Liss; 1990;189–197.

153. McCaffrey RM, Dunn LJ. Primary pulmonary hypertension in pregnancy. *Obstet Gynecol Survey* 1964;19:567–591.

154. Breen TW, Janzen JA. Pulmonary hypertension and cardiomyopathy: anaesthetic management for caesarean section. *Can J Anaesth* 1991;38:895–899.

155. Slomka F, Salmeron S, Zetlaoui P, Cohen H, Simonneau G, Samii K. Primary pulmonary hypertension and pregnancy: anesthetic management for delivery. *Anesthesiology* 1988;69:959–961.

156. Myles PS. Anaesthetic management for laparoscopic sterilisation and termination of pregnancy in a patient with severe primary pulmonary hypertension. *Anaesth Intensive Care* 1994;22:465–469.

157. Eklund B, Carlson LA. Central and peripheral circulatory effects and metabolic effects of different prostaglandins given IV to man. *Prostaglandins* 1980;20:333–338.

158. Buttino L, Garite TJ. The use of 15-methyl $F_{2\alpha}$-prostaglandin (Prostin 15 M) for the control of postpartum hemorrhage. *Am J Perinatol* 1986;3:241–243.

159. Nelson DM, Main E, Crafford W, Ahumada GG. Peripartum heart failure due to primary pulmonary hypertension. *Obstet Gynecol* 1983;3:58S–63S.

160. Abboud TK, Raya J, Noueihed R, Daniel J. Intrathecal morphine for relief of labor pain in a parturient with severe pulmonary hypertension. *Anesthesiology* 1983;5:477–479.

161. Krivosic-Horber R, Ducroux G, Beague D. L'anesthésie chez la parturiente cardiaque. Trente-huit cas. *Anesth Anal Reanim* 1980;37:681–684.

162. Copel JA, Harrison D, Whittemore R, Hobbins JC. Intrathecal morphine analgesia for vaginal delivery in a woman with a single ventricle. A case report. *J Reprod Med* 1986;31:274–276.

163. Fong J, Druzin M, Gimbel AA, Fisher J. Epidural anaesthesia for labour and caesarean section in a parturient with a single ventricle and transposition of the great arteries. *Can J Anaesth* 1990;37:680–684.

164. Leibbrandt G, Munch V, Gander M. Two successful pregnancies in a parturient with single ventricle and transposition of the great arteries. *Int J Cardiol* 1982;1:257–262.

165. Yuzpe AA, Sanghvi VR, Johnson FL. Successful pregnancy in a patient with a single ventricle and other congenital cardiac anomalies. *Can Med Assoc J* 1970;104:1076.

166. Stiller RJ, Vintzileos AM, Nochimson DJ, Clement D, Campbell WA, Leach C Jr. Single ventricle in pregnancy: case report and review of the literature. *Obstet Gynecol* 1984;64:18S–20S.

167. Zavisca FG, Johnson MD, Holubec JT, Kao YJ, Racz GB. General anesthesia for cesarean section in a parturient with a single ventricle and pulmonary atresia. *J Clin Anesth* 1993;5:315–320.

168. Kitamura E, Fujimori M. IHSS and anesthesia. *MASUI* 1977;26:1632–1639.

169. Loubser P, Suh K, Cohen SH. Adverse effects of spinal anesthesia in a patient with idiopathic hypertrophic subaortic stenosis. *Anesthesiology* 1984;60:228–230.

170. Tessler MJ, Hudson R, Naugler-Colville M, Biehl DR. Pulmonary oedema in two parturients with hypertrophic obstructive cardiomyopathy (HOCM). *Can J Anaesth* 1990;37:469–473.

171. Boccio RV, Chung JH, Harrison DM. Anesthetic management of cesarean section in a patient with idiopathic hypertrophic subaortic stenosis. *Anesthesiology* 1986;65:663–665.

172. Kobori M, Suzuki T, Masuda Y, Namiki M, Hatanaka S, Ban M, Hosoyamada A. Anesthesia for a cesarean section on a patient with hypertrophic obstructive cardiomyopathy (HOCM). *MASUI* 1985;39:1530–1534.

173. Speroff L. Toxemia of pregnancy: mechanism and therapeutic management. *Am J Cardiol* 1973;32:582–591.

174. Soderlin MK, Purhonen S, Haring P, Hietakorpi S, Koski E, Nuutinen LS. Myocardial infarction in a parturient. A case report with emphasis on medication and management. 1994;49:870–872.

175. Bembridge M, Lyons G. Myocardial infarction in the third trimester of pregnancy. *Anaesthesia* 1988;43:202–204.

176. Hands ME, Johnson MD, Saltzman DH, Rutherford JD. The cardiac, obstetric, and anesthetic management of pregnancy complicated by acute myocardial infarction. *J Clin Anesth* 1990;2:258–268.

177. Aglio LS, Johnson MD. Anaesthetic management of myocardial infarction in a parturient. *Br J Anaesth* 1990;65:258–261.

178. Johnson M, Saltzman D. Peripartum cardiomyopathy. In: Datta S, ed. *Anesthetic and Obstetric Management of High-Risk Pregnancy.* St Louis: CV Mosby; 1991;229–231.

179. Hutchinson RC, Ross AW. Severe peripartum cardiomyopathy. *Anaesth Intensive Care* 1992;20:398.

180. Becker RM. Intracardiac surgery in pregnant women. *Ann Thorac Surg* 1983;36:453–458.

181. Rossouw GJ, Knott-Craig CJ, Barnard PM, Macgregor LA, Van Zyl WP. Intracardiac operations in seven pregnant women. *Ann Thorac Surg* 1993;55:1172–1174.

182. Bernal JM, Miralles PJ. Cardiac surgery with cardiopulmonary bypass during pregnancy. *Obstet Gynecol Survey* 1986;41:1–6.

183. Strickland RA, Oliver WC Jr., Chantigian RC, Ney JA, Danielson GK. Anesthesia, cardiopulmonary bypass, and the pregnant patient. *Mayo Clin Proc* 1991;66:411–429.

184. Zitnik RS, Brandenburg RO, Sheldon R, Wallace RB. Pregnancy and open heart surgery. *Circulation* 1969;39:1257–1262.

185. Whitburn RH, Laishley RS, Jewkes DA. Anaesthesia for simultaneous caesarean section and clipping of intracerebral aneurysm. *Br J Anaesth* 1990;64:642–645.

186. Trimakas AP, Maxwell KD, Berkay S, Gardner TJ, Achuff SC. Fetal monitoring during cardiopulmonary bypass for removal of a left atrial myxoma during pregnancy. *Johns Hopkins Med* 1979;144:156–160.

187. Estafanous FG, Buckley S. Management of anesthesia for open heart surgery during pregnancy. *Cleveland Clin Q* 1976; 3:121–124.

188. Conroy JM, Bailey MK, Hollon MF, Cooke JE, Baker JD. Anesthesia for open heart surgery in the pregnant patient. *South Med J* 1989;82:492–495.

189. El-Maraghy M, Abou Senna I, El-Tehewy F, Bassiouni M, Ayoub A, El-Sayed H. Mitral valvotomy in pregnancy. *Am J Obstet Gynecol* 1983;145:708–710.

190. Martin MC, Pernoll ML, Boruszak AN, Jones JW, Locicero JI. Cesarean section while on cardiac bypass. Report of a case. *Obstet Gynecol* 1981;6:41S–45S.

191. Koh KS, Friesen RM, Livingstone RA. Fetal monitoring during maternal cardiac surgery with cardiopulmonary bypass. *Can Med Assoc J* 1975;112:1102–1104.

192. Lamb MP, Ross SK, Johnstone AM, Manners JM. Fetal heart rate monitoring during open heart surgery. *Br J Obstet Gynaecol* 1981;88:669–674.

193. Werch A, Lambert HM. Fetal monitoring and maternal open heart surgery. *South Med J* 1977;70:1024–1029.

194. Pederson H, Finster M. Anesthetic risk in the pregnant surgical patient. *Anesthesiology* 1979;51:439–451.

195. Childress CH, Katz VL. Nifedipine and its indications in obstetrics and gynecology. *Obstet Gynecol* 1994;83:616–624.

196. Glock JL, Morales WJ. Efficacy and safety of nifedipine versus magnesium sulfate in the management of preterm labor: a randomized study. *Am J Obstet Gynecol* 1993;169:960–964.

197. Assali NS, Westin B. Effects of hypothermia on uterine circulation and on the fetus. *Proc Soc Exp Biol Med* 1962;109:485–488.

198. Boatman KK, Bradford VA. Excision of an internal carotid aneurysm during pregnancy employing hypothermia and a vascular shunt. *Ann Surg* 1958;148:271–275.

199. Matsuki A, Oyama T. Operation under hypothermia in a pregnant woman with an intracranial arteriovenous malformation. *Can Anaesth Soc J* 1972;19:184–191.

200. Harrison EC,. Roschke EJ. Pregnancy in patients with cardiac valve prostheses. *Clin Obstet Gynecol* 1975;18:107–123.

201. Banning AP, Pearson JF, Hall RJ. Role of balloon dilatation of the aortic valve in pregnant patients with severe aortic stenosis. *Br Heart J* 1993;70:544–545.

202. Lao TT, Adelman AG, Sermer M, Colman JM. Balloon valvuloplasty for congenital aortic stenosis in pregnancy. *Br J Obstet Gynaecol* 1993;100:1141–1142.

203. Ben Farhat M, Maatouk F, Betbout F, Ayari M, Brahim H, Souissi M, Sghairi K, Gamra H. Percutaneous balloon mitral valvuloplasty in eight pregnant women with severe mitral stenosis. *Eur Heart J* 1992;13:1658–1664.

204. Glantz JC, Pomerantz RM, Cunningham MJ, Woods JR Jr. Percutaneous balloon valvuloplasty for severe mitral stenosis during pregnancy: a review of therapeutic options. *Obstet Gynecol Survey* 1993;48:503–508.

205. Savas V, Grines CL, O'Neill WW. Percutaneous triple-valve balloon valvuloplasty in a pregnant woman. *Cathet Cardiovasc Diagn* 1991;24:288–294.

206. Reyes VP, Raju BS, Wynne J, Stephenson LW, Raju R, Fromm BS, Rajagopal P, Mehta P, Singh S, Rao DP, et al. Percutaneous balloon valvuloplasty compared with open surgical commissurotomy for mitral stenosis. *N Engl J Med* 1994;331:961–967.

207. Gangbar EW, Watson KR, Howard RJ, Chisholm RJ. Mitral balloon valvuloplasty in pregnancy: advantages of a unique balloon. *Cathet Cardiovasc Diagnosis* 1992;25:313–316.

208. Ginsberg JS, Hirsh J. Use of antithrombotic agents during pregnancy. *Chest* 1992;102:385S–390S.

209. Odoom JA, Sih IL. Epidural analgesia and anticoagulant therapy. *Anaesthesia* 1983;38:254–259.

210. Schwander D, Bachmann F. Heparin and spinal or epidural anesthesia: decision analysis. *Ann Fr Anesth Reanim* 1991;10: 284–296.

211. Wulf H, Streipling E. Postmortem findings after epidural anaesthesia. *Anaesthesia* 1990;45:357–361.

212. Sage DJ. Epidurals, spinals and bleeding disorders in pregnancy: a review. *Anaesth Intensive Care* 1990;18:319–326.

213. Kane RF. Neurodeficits following epidural or spinal anesthesia. *Anesth Analg* 1981;60:150–161.

214. Schmidt A, Nolte H. Subdural and epidural hematomas following epidural anesthesia: a literature review. *Anaesthetist* 1992;41:276–284.

215. Dickman CA, Shedd SA, Spetzler RF, Shetter AG, Sonntag VK. Spinal epidural hematoma associated with epidural anesthesia: complications of systemic heparinization in patients receiving peripheral vascular thrombolytic therapy. *Anesthesiology* 1990;72:947–950.

216. Horlocker TT, Wedel DJ, Offord KP. Does preoperative antiplatelet therapy increase risk of hemorrhagic complications associated with regional anesthesia? *Anesth Analg* 1990;70:631–634.

217. Horlocker TT, Wedel DJ. Anticoagulation, antiplatelet therapy, and neuraxis blockade. Epidural and spinal analgesia and anesthesia: contemporary issues. In: Batra MS, Benumof J, eds. *Anesthesiology Clinics of North America.* Philadelphia: WB Saunders; 1992;1–11.

218. Wille JP, Jorgensen LN, Rasmussen LS. Lumbar regional anaesthesia and prophylactic anticoagulant therapy: is the combination safe? *Anaesthesia* 1991;46:623–627.

219. Rao TK, El-Etr AA. Anticoagulation following placement of epidural and subarachnoid catheters. *Anesthesiology* 1981;55:618–620.

220. Bergqvist D, Linblad B, Matzsch T. Low molecular weight heparin for thromboprophylaxis and epidural/spinal anesthesia: is there a risk? *Acta Anaesthesiol Scand* 1992;36:605–609.

221. Saka DM, Marx GF. Management of the parturient with cardiac valve prosthesis. *Anesth Analg* 1976;55:214–216.

222. Gothard JWW. Heart disease in pregnancy. *Anaesthesia* 1978;33:523–526.

223. Abouleish A. Anesthesia for the high-risk parturient. *Semin Anesth* 1982;2:154.

224. Saour JN, Sieck JO, Mamo LAR, Gallus AS. Trial of different intensities of anticoagulation in patients with prosthetic heart valves. *N Engl J Med* 1990;322:428–432.

225. Anderson DR, Ginsberg JS, Burrows R. Subcutaneous heparin therapy during pregnancy: a need for concern at the time of delivery. *Thomb Haemostasis* 1991;65:248–250.

226. Warkentin TE, Kelton JG. Heparin-induced thrombocytopenia. *Prog Hemostasis Thromb* 1991;10:1–34.

227. Duffy BL. Pregnancy and triple heart valve prosthesis. *Anaesth Intensive Care* 1982;1:59–61.

228. Levy JH. *Anaphylactic Reactions in Anesthesia and Intensive Care.* 2nd ed. Boston: Butterworth-Heinemann; 1992.

229. Shetty HG, Backhouse G, Bently DP, Routledge PA. Effective reversal of warfarin-induced excessive anticoagulation with low dose vitamin K_1. *Thromb Haemostasis* 1992;67:13–15.

230. Hirsh J, Fuster V. Guide to anticoagulant therapy. 2: oral anticoagulants. American Heart Association. *Circulation* 1994;89:1469–1480.

231. Hirsh J, Dalen JE, Deykin D, Poller L. Oral anticoagulants. Mechanism of action, clinical effectiveness, and optimal therapeutic range. *Chest* 1992;102:312S–326S.

232. Litin SC, Gastineau DA. Current concepts in anticoagulant therapy. *Mayo Clin Proc* 1995;70:266–272.

25

CARDIOPULMONARY RESUSCITATION OF PREGNANT WOMEN

RICHARD V. LEE, MD, FACP

INTRODUCTION

Cardiac and respiratory arrest are unusual events during pregnancy. Cardiopulmonary resuscitation (CPR) of the pregnant woman is unlike the more usual medical and surgical situations in which management focuses on a single patient. The need for CPR in pregnant women is rare but, when required, is attended by unique ethical and emotional concerns and must be applied with special intensity and caution.[1–5]

CPR during pregnancy attempts to restore the stricken mother and to salvage the pregnancy or to salvage the child. In growing numbers of cases of maternal brain death or vegetative coma, the mother survives long enough to allow salvage and survival of the fetus.[6,7] Gestational anatomy and physiology alter the effectiveness and practicality of standard CPR methods and require modifications in technique and urgency in decision making. Converting the mother from the pregnant to the nonpregnant state by emergent operative delivery may be life-saving for her, her infant, or both, and should be considered a part of maternal CPR.[8] The literature on maternal resuscitation is replete with case reports or series discussing perimortem or postmortem cesarean section.[5,9–13] It may be more appropriate when caring for the individual patient to talk about resuscitation, stabilization, and life support rather than perimortem or postmortem cesarean section, which are usually "after the fact" designations.

Social trends and medical progress have expanded the numbers of pregnant women with medical illness, the variety of medical illnesses among pregnant women, and the sophistication of reproductive, obstetric, surgical, and anesthetic techniques used in their care. Before World War II,

three-fourths of maternal deaths were caused by infection and hypertensive disease.[5] Following World War II, hypertensive and infectious diseases declined as causes of maternal mortality, to be replaced by anesthetic events, embolism, diabetes, cerebrovascular accidents, asthma, cardiac disease, trauma, and neoplastic disease.[5] In my practice over the past 20 years, a growing number of women with serious medical disease, such as type I diabetes, cystic fibrosis, hemoglobinopaties, steroid-dependent asthma, congenital and acquired heart disease, cancer, and transplanted organs, live well enough to conceive and to survive pregnancy, labor, and delivery. Many more than once. The past 20 years have seen an expansion of reproductive age as more women postpone pregnancy to their thirties and forties. Contemporary reproductive technology has made it possible for older, postmenopausal women to become pregnant: these women in the declining period of reproductive activity have a variety of acquired medical and surgical conditions, including wear and weathering. The need for nursing, medical, and obstetric clinicians familiar with the special anatomic and physiologic changes of pregnancy that affect the performance of CPR is growing commensurately with the number of pregnant women with conditions that place them at risk.

HISTORICAL BACKGROUND

Resuscitation has been practiced for time out of mind. The Old Testament has references to mouth-to-mouth ventilation. In the eighteenth century, William Hunter spoke of mouth-to-mouth respiration as a method used by the vulgar to re-

Cardiac Problems in Pregnancy, Third Edition
Edited by Uri Elkayam, MD, and Norbert Gleicher, MD
Copyright © 1998 by Wiley-Liss, Inc. ISBN 0-471-16358-9

store stillborn children. Electric shocks and a vast array of medicines delivered intravenously or rectally were widely used in the seventeenth, eighteenth, and nineteenth centuries.[4] Assisted respiration by mouth-to-mouth ventilation, tracheal intubation, or external thoracic compression were the mainstays of resuscitation until the close of nineteenth century when open-chest CPR became technically possible.

Cesarean section to extract the baby from a dead mother has a history as old as resuscitation.[5,11–14] For centuries, operative delivery of a dead mother was performed as much for religious as for medical reasons. During the nineteenth century, as surgical daring increased and techniques improved, postmortem cesarean section became more common. Despite surgical advances, however, the survival of infants so delivered remained less than 5%.

Over the past century the epidemiology of maternal death has changed, and advances in life support techniques have altered the meaning of "postmortem" cesarean section. Between 1879 and 1986, 269 postmortem cesarean sections with survival of 188 infants (70%) had been reported.[5] Survival of the infant was directly proportional to the interval between the death of the mother and the delivery. Delivery more than 15 minutes after maternal death rarely produced a viable infant; of the infants surviving, virtually all had some neurologic sequelae. All surviving infants delivered within 5 minutes after maternal death were healthy. If the interval was between 6 and 15 minutes, fewer infants were live-born, and 15% of the survivors suffered neurologic sequelae. Successful rescue and long-term maintenance of "brain dead" and comatose mothers allows for delivery at times more beneficial for the fetus. But such successes add new dimensions to contemporary ethical and obstetrical debates and to the information and skills required of the clinician.

Open-chest heart massage and direct electrical defibrillation were used as desperate measures until the 1950s. During studies on external defibrillation, Kouwenhoven et al[15] noted an increase in intraarterial pressure following firm application of defibrillator electrodes to the chest wall of an experimental animal. Their experimental and clinical studies on closed-chest CPR were publicized and adopted as the standard CPR techniques between 1958 and 1960. Sternal compression was thought to produce forward flow of blood and emptying of the ventricles by compressing the heart contained in the inelastic pericardium between the sternum and the vertebral column. It is clear now that this simple explanation is inadequate. Rhythmic increases in intrathoracic pressure, as well as cardiac compression, are essential for maintaining forward flow and circulation of the blood.[16–19]

PHYSIOLOGIC CHANGES OF PREGNANCY IMPORTANT FOR CPR

Pregnancy produces dramatic changes in cardiovascular and pulmonary physiology (Table 25.1). This chapter briefly re-

TABLE 25.1   Anatomic and Physiologic Effects of Pregnancy Affecting Cardiopulmonary Resuscitation

Increased blood volume
Increased cardiac output
Decreased peripheral vascular resistance, except in toxemic
   syndromes
Increased oxygen consumption
Increased rate of acid metabolite production
Decreased arterial P_{CO_2}
Increased clotting factors
Decreased colloid osmotic pressure
Mechanical effects of enlarging uterus, especially in supine
      position
   Decreased compliance for artificial ventilation
   Decreased compliance for thoracic compression
   Compression of aorta and inferior vena cava, causing decreased
      venous return
   Aortoiliac arterial compression, causing decreased venal and
      uterine arterial flow

views only the changes having prominent effects on the emergent care of a pregnant woman suffering cardiopulmonary collapse. Most studies of the physiology of CPR have been carried out using nonpregnant quadrupeds or nonpregnant, nonhuman primates. Human pregnancy produces anatomic and physiologic effects not found in quadrupeds. The applicability to pregnant women of contemporary recommendations for CPR is, therefore, not clearly defined.

Hemodynamics

Maternal blood volume and cardiac output increase to about 130–150% of nonpregnant values. The increase in plasma is greater than the increase in red blood cells; there is a decrease in the hematocrit and in the concentration of albumin. Decreased colloid osmotic pressure makes the pregnant patient susceptible to extravasation of plasma into extravascular compartments: peripheral and pulmonary edema.

Redistribution of the expanded blood volume follows changes in peripheral vascular resistance and the enlargement of the uterus and its contents. In the nonpregnant state, the uterus receives less than 2% of the cardiac output. During pregnancy, the proportion of cardiac output flowing to the uterus is 20–30%. Peripheral vascular resistance and maternal blood pressure decline during the second trimester, a time when the uteroplacental mass is growing most rapidly. Vasodilatory prostaglandins, progesterone, atrial natriuretic factors, and endothelial cell production of nitric oxide increase during pregnancy and foster relaxation of tubular structures and a reduction in peripheral vascular resistance. Pregnancy is a high flow, low resistance state of cardiovascular homeostasis. Obstructions to flow, such as valvular stenosis or hypertension, and reductions in flow, such as blood loss, venous sequestration, or ventricular failure, are poorly tolerated by both mother and fetus.[20,21]

Decades ago, α- and β-adrenergic receptors were demonstrated in the uterine vasculature.[21–23] In pregnant sheep, adrenergic stimulation at different perfusion pressures revealed no autoregulation of blood flow. The uteroplacental vascular bed functions as a maximally dilated, passive, low resistance system so that uterine flow is determined by perfusion pressure. In normal pregnancy, β-adrenergic agonists and combined α- and β-adrenergic agonists do not cause uteroplacental vasoconstriction and do not impair uteroplacental blood flow. Under abnormal conditions—hypoxia, hypotension, and toxemia—the maternal cardiovascular system, including the uteroplacental vasculature, has enhanced sensitivity to the vasoconstrictive action of epinephrine and norepinephrine (Table 25.2).[22-24]

During the second half of pregnancy, the uterus fills and expands out of the pelvis (Fig. 25.1). The supine posture allows the gravid uterus to exert pressure on the iliac veins and arteries, the inferior vena cava, and the abdominal aorta. Hypotension may develop in the supine position because compression of the inferior vena cava and major pelvic veins by the uterus can sequester as much as 30% of the circulating blood volume.[20,25,26] A 25% increase in cardiac output occurred when term patients were changed from the supine to the lateral recumbent position.[25] If intraarterial pressures are diminished when a pregnant woman is flat on her back, compression of the abdominal aorta causing reduced uteroplacental blood flow is likely to occur.[26] Hypotensive pregnant patients should not be kept supine. The decubitus posture minimizes the hemodynamic effects of the uterus.

Reduction in uteroplacental blood flow because of hypovolemia from any cause is managed by restoring and maintaining circulating blood volume; the administration of vasopressors will not help and may make things worse. In the hypoxic, hypotensive gravida, vasopressors may further impair uteroplacental blood flow. The preservation of circulating blood volume and high flow is important during hypotension associated with sepsis and cardiopulmonary failure because of pregnancy-enhanced clotting factors and the risk of intravascular coagulopathy. The management of critically ill pregnant patients must balance the necessity to provide sufficient volume to preserve uteroplacental blood flow with the propensity for the capillaries to leak because of re-

TABLE 25.2   Maternal Conditions Adversely Affecting Uteroplacental Blood Flow

Toxemia of pregnancy (preeclampsia)	
Hypovolemia	
Hypoxia:	Enhances sensitivity of uteroplacental vasculature to vasoconstriction by α-adrenergic agonists
Acidosis	
Alkalosis:	Induces uteroplacental vasoconstriction

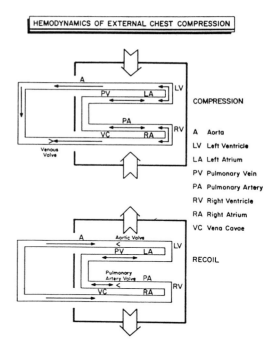

Figure 25.1   Effects of the gravid uterus on the pathophysiology of cardiopulmonary arrest and resuscitation.

duced colloid oncotic pressure. Using large volumes of fluid to maintain adequate blood pressure may precipitate acute pulmonary edema. Peripheral and pulmonary edema not uncommonly follow spinal conduction anesthesia because of the additional fluid volume needed to replace the blood volume sequestered in dilated vascular beds and to stabilize maternal blood pressure.[27]

Ventilation and Acid–Base Balance

Increased ventilation, due to central stimulation by progesterone, begins in the first trimester and by late pregnancy is about 50% greater than in the nonpregnant state.[28] The arterial PCO_2 declines to about 30–35 torr, but renal compensation for the respiratory alkalosis maintains a normal maternal arterial blood pH.[29] Maternal hypocapnea and respiratory alkalosis enhance the removal of carbon dioxide and buffer hydrogen ion and acidic metabolites produced by the fetus and placenta; they constitute an essential component of fetoplacental acid–base balance. The arterial PO_2 of healthy pregnant women in upright posture is in the range of 100 torr, not very different from nonpregnant patients. However, the arterial PO_2 may decline when the patient is supine.[29]

By the end of the first trimester, maternal basal metabolic rate and oxygen consumption begin to rise progressively until close to term. Oxygen consumption increases to meet the metabolic demands of breast, uterine, placental, and fetal growth, and the increased work of moving and breathing attendant to changing shape and size. The gravid uterus and hypertrophied breasts appear to increase the work of ventilation, especially when the patient is supine. A progressive increase in the oxygen cost of breathing during the last 4 months of pregnancy has been attributed to an increase in diaphragmatic work.[30] The thorax is less compressible by external pressure because of the cephalad displacement of abdominal contents and the presence of the gravid uterus. It is more difficult to ventilate a flaccid pregnant patient by mouth-to-mouth respiration or via an endotracheal tube than to perform the same procedure on a nonpregnant patient.

Respiratory volumes and mechanics are altered by displacement of the diaphragm by the enlarging uterus. Total lung capacity is reduced 4–6%, and function residual capacity is reduced by as much as 25%.[31] Studies conducted 50 years ago using chest X-rays reported that pregnancy produced a 4 cm elevation of the diaphragm and a 2 cm increase in the transverse diameter of the thorax.[32] The diminution in residual volumes is more dramatic in the supine than in the sitting and upright postures.

The combination of diminished residual capacity and increased oxygen consumption predisposes the pregnant patient to steep drops in arterial PO_2 with reduced ventilation.[33,34] Supine posture and reduced cardiac output magnify the rate and severity of the decline in oxygenation. The pregnant patient and her fetus are exquisitely sensitive to acute hypoxia (Table 25.2). Acute maternal hypoxia produces a substantial reduction in uteroplacental perfusion. Pregnant ewes had a 17% decrease in uteroplacental blood flow at an arterial oxygen tension of 55 torr and a 22% decrease at an arterial oxygen tension of 30 torr.[21] The decrease in uteroplacental blood flow induced by hypoxia can be minimized by α-adrenergic blockage, indicating that α-adrenergic stimulation under hypoxic conditions may exaggerate vasoconstriction and exacerbate reduction of the uteroplacental blood supply. Maternal alkalosis, associated with hyperventilation in excess of the physiologic hypocapnea of pregnancy or with metabolic alkalosis, correlates with decreases in fetal oxygen tension, possibly because hypocarbia induces vasoconstriction of the uterine arteries and/or because of alkalosis-induced shifts in the oxyhemoglobin dissociation curve.

Data from sheep and human studies demonstrate that at all levels of maternal oxygenation the oxygen tension in the umbilical vein is always less than the oxygenation in the uterine vein.[35] The fetus is, in other words, always hungry for oxygen. There is at best a 2-minute reserve of oxygen in the fetoplacental unit. The incidence of teratogenesis can be increased in the children of mothers undergoing cardiac surgery requiring cardiopulmonary bypass during the first trimester if standard cardiopulmonary bypass techniques are used. Maintenance of supernormal maternal oxygenation and high flow rates with cardiopulmonary bypass is the most effective way to minimize fetal risk during open-heart surgery on pregnant patients.[36] These clinical experiences emphasize the importance of maintaining adequate uteroplacental blood flow and normal-for-pregnancy arterial pH, PO_2 and PCO_2.

The time limit for successful resuscitation of nonpregnant adults is 5–6 minutes of apnea and asystole. During pregnancy, maternal apnea is followed by precipitous declines in arterial pH and PO_2 and an abrupt rise in PCO_2. The fetus of an apneic and asystolic mother has 2 minutes or less of oxygen reserve. The tolerable duration of apnea and/or asystole for a pregnant woman is only 2–4 minutes; beyond this time the chances of successful resuscitation of the mother and/or fetus diminish. In essence, the clinician has 4 minutes to restore vital activity in the mother and to decide what to do if resuscitation fails—the so-called four-minute rule.[5]

PHYSIOLOGY OF CPR

The procedure of closed-chest CPR has changed little in the 35 years the technique has been used. Many studies have documented that although contemporary closed-chest CPR is reasonably successful for rescuing patients from responsive arrhythmias, it is less effective for resuscitation from refractory dysrhythmias, asystole, and electromechanical dissociation.[15–19]

Observations in animals and humans indicate that blood flow and systemic perfusion during closed-chest CPR are produced by phasic fluctuations in intrathoracic pressure, not simply by compression of the heart between the sternum and the spine.[16–19] To produce forward flow of blood, a pressure gradient from the arterial to the venous circulation must be generated (Fig. 25.2). Changes in intrathoracic pressure generated by external compression are transmitted equally to the intrathoracic great vessels and cardiac chambers. The peripheral arterial-to-venous pressure gradients needed for systemic perfusion are found only in vasculature supplied with competent venous valves, which inhibit retrograde flow from the intrathoracic veins and permit forward flow into the arteries.

Increasing intrathoric pressures augment the arterial pressure and flow produced by closed-chest massage.[18] In experimental animals, simultaneous chest compression and ventilation generate higher arterial pressures than alternating compression and ventilation.[37] In human subjects, simultaneous ventilation and chest compression have produced greater carotid artery blood flow and higher radial artery systolic pressure than conventional chest compression and ventilation.[38] Effective systemic perfusion produced by pulses of increased intrathoracic pressure explains the observation of Niemann et al[39] that patients who coughed during ventricular filbrillation were able to maintain consciousness until definitive management could be initiated.

Attempts to improve closed-chest CPR by increasing intrathoracic pressure by abdominal binding have proved less successful.[38] Sanders et al[18] failed to resuscitate dogs using

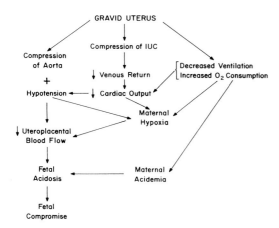

GRAVID UTERUS

Figure 25.2   For closed-chest massage to work, there must be unimpeded flow of blood through the intrathoracic vasculature. The heart as the limiting lumen or vessel through which the blood must flow must be compliant. Closed-chest cardiopulmonary resuscitation, for example, is ineffective with pericardial tamponade or constrictive pericarditis. With compression of the thorax, pressure increases in all intrathoracic vessels with extrusion of blood anterograde in the aorta and retrograde in the vena cavae. Competent venous valves restrict the retrograde venous flow so that forward arterial flow results. When the chest recoils and expands, blood flows into the thorax anterograde from the vena cavae and retrograde from the aorta, subclavian, and carotid arteries. Retrograde arterial flow is arrested by the aortic and pulmonary valves. Obstruction to arterial outflow such as aortic stenosis and reductions in venous inflow limit the effectiveness of closed-chest massage.

simultaneous chest compression/ventilation and abdominal binding, in contrast to successful resuscitation of dogs using standard closed-chest CPR. Increasing intrathoracic pressure by manipulation of extrathoracic structures interferes with the free flow of blood into and out of the thorax, thus destroying the utility of chest compression.

Although no systematic studies on open- or closed-chest CPR have been performed in pregnant animals or humans, it is obvious that the physiology of human pregnancy is likely to impede the success of standard closed-chest CPR.[1,3–5] The mechanical effects of the gravid uterus in a supine woman suffering cardiac or ventilatory arrest act like abdominal binding, producing increased intrathoracic pressure, diminished venuous return, and obstructed forward flow of blood in the abdominal aorta. The effect of the pregnant uterus on closed-chest CPR was dramatized by the report by DePace et al[40] of a young woman who suffered a respiratory arrest during massive hemoptysis in her 36th week of gestation. Although the patient never had cardiac standstill or ventricular fibrillation, her physicians were unable to generate blood pressure despite endotracheal intubation, closed-chest cardiac message, and vigorous fluid and electrolyte therapy. The patient's blood pressure rose from 0 to 80 torr immediately upon evacuation of the uterus by bedside cesarean section.

The pressure gradients generated by standard closed-chest CPR may be adequate to sustain fetal life; the survival of infants delivered from patients such as the one described by DePace et al[40] suggest that even compromised closed-chest CPR is of value. Fortunately, the uteroplacental circulation offers minimal vascular resistance as long as adequate oxygenation and acceptable acid–base balance are maintained. However, hypoxia and acidosis produce vasoconstriction and increased resistance in the uteroplacental vasculature. Despite seemingly adequate maternal responses to closed-chest CPR, reduced uteroplacental circulation due to the increased oxygen consumption and increased carbon dioxide and hydrogen ion production accompanying fetoplacental metabolism may result in regional hypoxia and acidosis, with disastrous effects on the fetus. Delays in establishing effective ventilation or problems in maintaining normal pH magnify the circulatory comprise of the uteroplacental unit and accelerate the rate at which the mother and fetus become unresuscitatable despite adequate chest compression.

Open-Chest Cardiac Massage (Table 25.3)

The anatomic and physiologic changes of pregnancy and their adverse effect on standard resuscitation procedures encourage reconsideration of open-chest cardiac massage in the resuscitation of pregnant women. Thoracotomy and open-chest heart massage are often the only effective measures in patients with chest trauma, tension pneumothorax, massive pulmonary embolism, pericardial tamponade, chest or spine deformities, and profound hypovolemia.[41–45] Human and

TABLE 25.3   Technique of Open-Chest Cardiac Massage

1.   Open the chest and pericardium with an incision through the left fifth intercostal space.
2.   One hand: the ventricles are cupped by the fingers and palm of the right hand and the heart is compressed against the sternum and squeezed by the fingers.
3.   Two hands: if there is sufficient exposure, the heart is enclosed, one hand below, the other hand above the heart; compression is produced by squeezing the hands together and squeezing the fingers.
4.   One-handed massage without a firm opposing force (either the sternum or the other hand) is less effective.
5.   Sixty compressions per minute is adequate if good filling and emptying of the ventricles are achieved.
6.   Cross-clamping the aorta is contraindicated unless or until the fetus is nonviable or delivered.
7.   Endotracheal intubation is essential to maintain adequate ventilation.
8.   Broad spectrum antibiotic coverage should be initiated immediately.
9.   Open-chest massage can be a bloody business: today, precautions for hepatitis B virus and human immunodeficiency virus must be observed.

animal studies have demonstrated superior hemodynamic effects using open-chest cardiac massage compared with closed-chest techniques. DelGuercio et al[41] reported that internal cardiac massage doubled the cardiac index and shortened the circulation time in 11 patients. Animal studies indicate that open-chest massage improves cardiac output, arterial pressures, and cartoid, coronary, and aortic blood flow. The benefits of open-chest cardiac massage decline the longer unsuccessful closed-chest CPR is utilized: after 25 minutes of closed-chest massage in experimental animals, there was no survival advantage in performing thoracotomy and internal massage. Cross-clamping the descending aorta has been advocated as a way to improve blood flow to the heart, lungs, and brain during open-chest cardiac massage. Obviously this procedure is contraindicated because it would stop the uteroplacental blood flow. Cross-clamping the aorta could be employed after the fetus has been delivered, or if the fetus is nonviable.

No studies comparing closed- and open-chest cardiac massage on the hemodynamics of the human uterus and placenta have been performed. Open-chest resuscitation is a formidable procedure probably best reserved for specific indications and as a last resort. Operative delivery to rapidly return the mother to nonpregnant hemodynamics and status remains the first surgical priority.

CARDIOPULMONARY CRISIS IN PREGNANT PATIENTS

The causes of maternal cardiopulmonary arrest are legion (Table 25.4).[46–52] Because the pregnant patient is not a likely candidate for successful closed-chest CPR,[53,54] clinicians will be forced to make decisions to perform emergency procedures with discomfiting celerity. Unless the stricken mother shows a favorable response to resuscitative efforts within 4 minutes, an operation—bedside cesarean section and/or open-chest cardiac massage—is mandatory. The duration of gestation, predisposing acute or chronic maternal conditions, and logistical factors influence the specifics of emergent management but do not alter the need for difficult decisions in the first 4 or 5 minutes after maternal cardiopulmonary arrest.

Management of maternal cardiopulmonary arrest will be directed by many factors (Table 25.5, Figure 25.3). The most important are the medical and gestational status of the mother, the cause of the cardiorespiratory failure, and the location of the patient at the time of the arrest. A patient brought to emergency facilities after an unwitnessed cardiorespiratory arrest at a distant site and a patient arresting in the operating room present very different problems. Cardiopulmonary arrest in a patient with rheumatic mitral stenosis has different implications from cardiopulmonary arrest in a woman with a normal heart.

TABLE 25.4   Some Causes of Cardiopulmonary Collapse During Pregnancy

Preexisting heart disease
   Congenital heart disease
   Acquired valvular disease
   Coronary artery disease, myocardial infarction
   Arrhythmia
Acute heart disease
   Drug-induced arrhythmia—iatrogenic (tocolysis)
   Drug-induced arrhythmia—illicit drugs, especially cocaine
   Pericardial tamponade—iatrogenic (following perforation of the heart by central catheters or trauma)
Pregnancy-associated cardiomyopathy
Pregnancy-induced hypertension/toxemia
Anaphylaxis/angioedema of larynx
Envenomation
Lightning
Asthma
Aspiration pneumonia
Pulmonary embolus/amniotic fluid embolism
Cerebral vascular accident
Overwhelming infection/septicemia
Iatrogenic (e.g., hypermagnesemia, anesthesia)
Trauma
Poisoning and drug overdose

Special emphasis should be given to the gestational age of the fetus (Figure 25.4). Before the onset of fetal viability, about the 24th gestational week, the objectives of CPR can be directed almost exclusively to maternal considerations. Although emergency cesarean section is not indicated to rescue the fetus, on some occasions emptying the uterus is essential to preserve the mother. After the 24th week of gestation, management must include delivering the child at the most propitious time for both mother and infant. Immediate resuscitation of the mother without emergent delivery of a premature or asphyxiated infant is the ideal goal for any pregnant woman remote from term, but clinical reality is often cruel.

The more remote the patient is from term, the more cautious the clinician should be about emergent delivery. Restoration of maternal function sufficient to maintain the pregnancy, even if recovery is incomplete in terms of independence and/or consciousness, may be of value for the fetus and the family.

TABLE 25.5   Factors Influencing Management of CPR and Timing of Cesarean Section in Pregnant Women

Maternal health: preexisting and pregnancy-related conditions
Gestational age
Duration of cardiopulmonary arrest
Duration of effective CPR/life support
Fetal status
Location of the patient (in hospital, out of hospital)

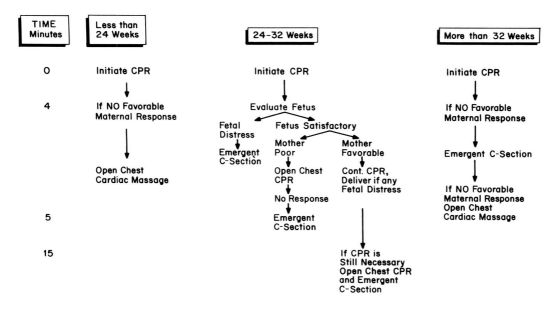

Figure 25.3   Resuscitation strategy for pregnant patients.

The closer the patient is to term, the more aggressive the clinician should be about delivering the infant. After 32–34 weeks gestation, the chances of successful resuscitation of both the mother and fetus are enhanced by prompt emergency delivery.

Management of the fetus independent of the mother is more likely to produce successful resuscitation for both. The availability of surfactant insufflation has reduced some of the morbidity from hyaline membrane disease in premature infants. When emergency delivery of a fetus in the 24th or later gestational week is unavoidable, the use of surfactant offers an important advantage in enhancing the child's survival.

Restoration of maternal vital signs—cardiac rhythm, blood pressure, respiratory effort—even when vigorous support is required, reduces the urgency for delivery and allows for appropriate positional, medicinal, and ventilatory management. Except for the term patient arresting on the operating room table, immediate cesarean section is not desirable without careful assessment of maternal and fetus status and evidence of fetal compromise. Even mothers sustaining irreparable trauma and those suffering unwitnessed cardiopulmonary collapse deserve attentive assessment and institution of life support.

I believe it is important to establish uniform definitions for operative delivery during maternal cardiorespiratory crisis. For the purposes of this chapter, "postmortem" refers to events after maternal cardiorespiratory function has ceased and artificial life support is ineffective or has ceased. "Perimortem" refers to events occurring after maternal cardiorespiratory function has failed, while artificial life support sustains ventilation and circulation. Recommendations about the timing of cesarean section have been based on the premise that cardiopulmonary arrest means sure death, that CPR during pregnancy, especially close to term, is ineffective, and that delivery is essential to maternal and fetal resuscitation and survival. Reviews of outcome following maternal cardiopulmonary arrest have not stratified the clinical material according to the effect of CPR and life support. Cesarean section performed 10 minutes after cessation of cardiorespiratory function would be expected to have a different outcome for mother and child from cesarean section after 10 minutes of effective CPR and maternal life support. There are sufficient numbers of reports describing the rescue of the mother[55] and/or survival of the infant[8–10] after prolonged episodes of presumed inadequate maternal cardiorespiratory function or prolonged maternal CPR to indicate the need to establish definitions and guidelines for prospective studies.

Although no legal action has been brought for true postmortem cesarean section by conscientious practitioners, overzealous bedside cesarean section on a viable mother remote from term would be suspect in the contemporary medicolegal climate. On the other hand, a mother still requiring open- or closed-chest cardiac massage after 5 minutes of resuscitative effort should be delivered regardless of how viable the fetus may seem.

CPR FOR PREGNANT WOMEN

Cardiopulmonary arrest in a pregnant woman should set in motion standard resuscitative measures and procedures.[56]

TIME
(minutes)

```
0        Witnessed arrest                        Unwitnessed arrest
              |                                         |
         Check pulse/respiration                  Check pulse
              |                                         |
         If no pulse/respiration              If no pulse/respiration
              |                                         |
         Precordial thump/intubate            Intubate
              |
         Check pulse - if no pulse
                                    ↓ ←
              Initiate CPR
                   |
1        Obtain ABG/evaluate fetus[a]
                   |
         Check monitor for rhythm (if VT or VF)
                   |
         Defibrillate, 200 Joules[b]
                   |
         Defibrillate, 200-300 Joules
                   |
         Defibrillate with up to 360 Joules
                   |
         Epinephrine 1:10,000, 0.5-1 mg IV push[c]
                   |
         Defibrillate with up to 360 Joules[b]
                   |
         Lidocaine, 1 mg/kg IV push
                   |
4        Uterine evacuation[d]
                   |
         Defibrillate with up to 360 Joules
                   |
         Bretylium 5 mg/kg IV push
                   |
         Defibrillate with up to 360 Joules
                   |
         Bretylium 10 mg/kg IV push
                   |
         Defibrillate with up to 360 Joules
                   |
         Repeat Lidocaine or Bretylium
                   ↓
         Defibrillate with up to 360 Joules
```

a Maintain pH approximately 7.4 - see text for fetal evaluation.
b Check pulse and rhythm after each shock.
c Epinephrine should be given every 5 minutes if pH is maintained.
d See text regarding open cardiac massage. Fetal evaluation is
   at or before 4 minutes is required to ensure fetal and
   maternal outcome.

```
Intubate - continue CPR
        |
ABG, Establish IV access[a]
        |
Epinephrine 1:10000, 0.5-1 mg IV push
        |
Atropine 1 mg and repeat in 5 minutes
        |
Evacuate uterus[b,c]
        |
Continue maternal CPR
```

a Goal to maintain pH at 7.4.

b Regardless of viability and gestational
   age. Hopefully with maintenance of
   normal pH and within 4 minutes.

A c See text regarding open cardiac massage.

```
Establish IV, intubate, initiate CPR
        |
Epinephrine 1:10000, 0.5-1 mg IV push
        |
Consider:  hypovolemic cardiac tamponade,
           tension pneumothorax, hypoxemic
           acidosis, pulmonary embolus
        |
Evacuate uterus
        |
```
B Continue maternal CPR

The algorithms developed by the American Heart Association in its Guidelines for Cardiopulmonary Resuscitation and Emergency Cardiac Care[57] should be followed with only minor modification. The flowsheet diagrams provided in this publication are widely available and should be the standard procedure in every obstetric care facility. The greatest risk lies in hesitating to institute for a pregnant patient the established guidelines for nonpregnant patients.

Monitoring Fetal Status

Management of cardiopulmonary arrest in pregnant women requires monitoring of both the mother and fetus. Because the cervix is usually closed and the fetal membranes are intact in women not in active labor, external fetal monitoring, real-time ultrasound, and careful auscultation of the fetal heart provide the only reasonable indication of fetus status. Parturient patients in labor with dilated cervix afford the option of internal fetal monitoring. Considerable noise and motion interference are invariably a part of resuscitation efforts. The physicians directing the resuscitation must ensure that there are pauses to ascertain the presence and status of the fetal heartbeat. When available, real-time ultrasound to examine the fetal heart, fetal motion, tone, and breathing movements is the most useful technique. In the absence of such sophisticated equipment, auscultation retains its time-honored utility.

Ventilation and Acid–Base Balance

Prompt endotracheal intubation of the mother and frequent monitoring of arterial blood gases and pH are essential. The mechanics of ventilation as pregnancy progresses to term require increasing effort. Endotracheal intubation and aggressive management of the airway are perhaps the most important parts of successful resuscitation for the mother and rescue of the infant. Mouth-to-mouth or face mask Ambu bag ventilation are less effective. A common theme in cases of successful fetal rescue despite maternal catastrophe is the maintenance of maternal ventilation. The goal of ventilation is to maintain a minimal arterial PO_2 of 80–90 torr and of arterial PCO_2 of 30–35 torr. The pH should be kept as close to 7.4 as possible. Both acidosis and alkalosis are injurious to uteroplacental perfusion. Judicious use of bicarbonate and careful ventilation are essential; this is not the place to manage metabolic acidosis by respiratory alkalosis induced by overvigorous ventilation or metabolic alkalosis caused by overvigorous administration of bicarbonate.

Hemodynamics

The resuscitators are supposed to deliver 60 lb of force and to depress the sternum 1.5–2 inches.[56,57] If adequate chest compression is not generating palpable arterial pulses, simultaneous ventilation and compression may be tried. The uterus must be displaced from resting on the abdominal and pelvic great vessels. The use of a wedge, inflatable or solid, under the right flank and hip may help, as can simply pushing and holding the uterus to the left side.[53,54] Placing the patient on an operating room table to produce favorable positioning and a strong surface for closed-chest massage may facilitate management. The left lateral decubitus position makes resuscitative efforts clumsy and ineffective, and closed-chest massage impossible.

There is no contraindication to external defibrillation during pregnancy.[48] If the patient has experienced cardiac arrest from ventricular fibrillation, prompt electrical countershock, at maximum recommended levels, should be used.

Lidocaine crosses the placenta but has been used safely in many pregnancies.[58,59] At therapeutic maternal blood levels, there is no evidence of adverse effects on the fetal heart rate or the uteroplacental unit. Toxic maternal blood levels have been associated with cardiac and central nervous system depression in the neonate. Intravenous β-adrenergic blocking agents and quinidine may precipitate uterine contractions. Rapid intravenous administration of calcium channel blocking agents such as verapamil may exacerbate maternal hypotension and may cause uterine atony.[59] Bretylium has been rarely used in pregnant patients, and there are no data about its efficacy and safety in this setting.[59] This agent should not be used except as a last resort when lidocaine, procainamide, and electrical pacing have failed. The use of epinephrine intravenously via a central catheter or an intracardiac injection is common when cardiac standstill or electromechanical dissociation occurs. Because α-adrenergic drugs cause uteroplacental vasoconstriction in hypoxic, acidemic women, we do not encourage their use except with extreme caution or unless delivery of the fetus is imminent. The use of adrenergic drugs and glucose-containing solutions during CPR stimulates fetal insulin secretion and may set the stage for profound neonatal hypoglycemia. Antiarrhythmic agents may produce therapeutic and toxic effects in neonates.

After 4 minutes, or at any time if resuscitative efforts are without obvious benefit and the fetal status deteriorates, the clinician must act. If gestation is past 32 weeks, emergency cesarean section is the first priority. Delivery of an asphyxiated, premature fetus after unsuccessful maternal CPR poses special risks and problems. A neonatologist is an essential member of the CPR team for pregnant patients.

Immediate Cesarean Section (Table 25.6)

After 24 weeks of gestation, injury or disease of the mother's heart and lungs that will hinder resuscitation and life support are indications for immediate cesarean section in women sustaining cardiopulmonary arrest after the fetus has attained extrauterine viability. Cardiac compliance is essential for successful closed-chest massage. The ventricle must be supple enough to fill adequately during the relaxation phase and to impose minimal obstruction to outflow during the compression phase. Mitral and aortic valve stenosis and decreased compliance caused by cardiomyopathy or pericardial disease interfere with closed-chest cardiac massage. Maintenance of the fetoplacental unit would be unlikely even with successful restoration of maternal heart action. Cardiopulmonary arrest in such patients should prompt immediate, simultaneous institution of CPR and cesarean section. In unwitnessed cardiopulmonary arrest, if there is no maternal or fetal response

TABLE 25.6 Maternal Health Conditions Indicating Rapid Delivery in Women Suffering Cardiopulmonary Arrest Past 24 Weeks of Gestation

Carbon monoxide poisoning
Hypothermia (< 34°C)
Pulmonary injury or disease
    Lung parenchymal injury secondary to trauma
    Multilobe pneumonia
    Massive pulmonary embolism
    Inhalation of corrosive gases
    Aspiration of solvents or corrosives
    Drowning
Cardiac injury or disease
    Dilated cardiomyopathy
    Massive myocardial infarction
    Severe aortic and/or mitral valve stenosis
    Pericardial tamponade secondary to trauma
Unwitnessed cardiopulmonary arrest
Failed resuscitation
Prolonged resuscitation

to CPR within one minute, the infant should be immediately delivered.

Severe hypothermia,[57] core temperature less than 34°, and carbon monoxide poisoning[60] are indications for prompt delivery, because the fetoplacental unit can interfere with maternal management and because the infant may be more effectively managed when separated from the mother. Pulmonary injury interfering with ventilation, with resulting impairment of efforts to achieve and maintain arterial blood gases appropriate for pregnancy, requires prompt cesarean section. Indeed, declining maternal ventilatory function in this setting may dictate cesarean section before cardiopulmonary arrest occurs. Liquid ventilation has been used successfully in children and adults, but not during pregnancy.

Complications of Closed-Chest CPR

Vigorous thoracic compressions can produce a variety of maternal injuries including fractures (especially of the ribs but also of the sternum); separation of the costal cartilages from the sternum; laceration or rupture of the liver, spleen, uterus, and pericardium; and hemothorax, hemopericardium, and hemoperitoneum.[61,62] Toxemia of pregnancy predisposes to bleeding because of thrombocytopenia and because of specific organ injury, such as spontaneous hematomas of the liver.[63] Pneumothorax and pneumomediastinum can be associated with endotracheal intubation, subclavian catheterization, and intracardiac injections.

For the fetus, the risk of injury or toxicity increases the longer maternal closed-chest CPR and emergent use of drugs continue.

Maternal complications of CPR jeopardize the fetus as well as the mother and must influence the decision to deliver. As resuscitative efforts extend, there is an increase in the number of maternal complications and uses of medication, and the chances of survival of the mother, without major life support, decline. Common complications of standard CPR become an important factor in the decision to perform emergency cesarean section. It would be prudent, for example, to proceed with delivery in a patient sustaining rib fractures and a penumothorax during CPR at 32 weeks of gestation, even though the fetus had no evidence of distress.

Post delivery Care of the Mother Suffering Cardiopulmonary Arrest

Once an infant has been delivered, attention focuses on the newborn, and there is a risk that successful emergency cesarean section can become a death sentence for the mother. Cardiopulmonary crisis during pregnancy requires a multidisciplinary team at the onset of the crisis. The internist or cardiologist or intensivist must be involved at the beginning of the resuscitation effort, not at the end.

A mother emergently delivered of a viable fetus 5–6 minutes after collapsing is still resuscitatable; indeed success may be enhanced by the delivery. The empty uterus allows free use of many drugs and procedures prescribed or used only sparingly during pregnancy. Thoracotomy and open-chest massage have a place in this setting if the mother is still not responding after 15 minutes of resuscitation.

Open-Chest Cardiac Massage

I believe that thoracotomy and open-chest cardiac massage should be considered between the 24th and 32nd weeks of gestation. If open-chest massage is without effect in 60–90 seconds, emergency cesarean section is mandatory. If open-chest massage is successful, the mother may be supported, despite severe residua, until delivery of the fetus is necessary or desirable. Antibiotic therapy and wound management directed at minimizing the potential infectious, hemostatic, and mechanical effects of emergency bedside surgery will be necessary if the mother survives regardless of whether the chest and/or abdomen are opened.

In severe preeclampsia, cardiopulmonary arrest may be precipitated by arrhythmia, congestive heart failure, myocardial infarct, intracranial bleeding, or iatrogenic events such as hypermagnesemia. The vascular changes of toxemia can produce substantial interference with uteroplacental blood flow even with otherwise normal cardiac function. The use of vasoconstricting vasopressor agents may exacerbate the vasospasm that characterizes preeclampsia. Open-chest cardiac massage by preserving uteroplacental blood flow while simultaneously increasing cardiac output would seem to offer a rational alternative to desperate polypharmacy. Internal cardiac massage can be combined with vasodilators to maintain or improve uteroplacental and visceral perfusion that may not be possible with closed-chest cardiac massage.

SUMMARY

Pregnancy alters the approach to cardiopulmonary resuscitation, not only because of the need to accommodate the presence of the fetus but because of the anatomy and physiology of gestation. Differences in knowledge and attitudes of the resuscitators about pregnancy are also a factor. Managing cardiopulmonary crisis in a pregnant woman must avoid inertia: (1) the inertia of fear that proven procedures and medications in nonpregnant patients will adversely affect the fetus, (2) the inertia of indecision about emergent surgical delivery, (3) the inertia of hopelessness for the desperately ill mother, delivered or undelivered, and (4) the peculiarly American condition of medicolegal dystocia.

REFERENCES

1. Lee RV, Rodgers BD, White LM, Harvey RC. Cardiopulmonary resuscitation of pregnant women. *Am J Med* 1986;81:311–318.

2. Songster GS, Clark SL. Cardiac arrest in pregnancy. What to do? *Contemp Obstet Gynecol* 1985;27:141–155.

3. Strong TH, Lowe RA. Postmortem cesarean section. *Am J Emergency Med* 1989;7:489–494.

4. Satin AJ, Hankins GDV. Cardiopulmonary resuscitation in pregnancy. In: Clark SL, Cotton DB, Hankins GDV, Phelan JP, eds *Critical Care Obstetrics.* 2nd ed. Boston: Blackwell Scientific Publications; 1991;579–598.

5. Katz VL, Dotters DJ, Droegemueller W. Perimortem cesarean delivery. *Obstet Gynecol* 1986;68:571–576.

6. Dillon WP, Lee RV, Tronolone MJ, Buckwald S, Foote RJ. Life support and maternal brain death during pregnancy. *JAMA* 1982;248:1089–1091.

7. Hill LM, Parker D, O'Neill BP. Management of maternal vegetative state during pregnancy. *Mayo Clin Proc* 1985;60:469–472.

8. O'Connor RL, Savarino FB. Cardiopulmonary arrest in the pregnant patient: a report of successful resuscitation. *J Clin Anesth* 1994;6:66–68.

9. Lopez-Zeno JA, Carlo WA, O'Grady JP, Fanaroff AA. Infant survival following delayed postmortem cesarean delivery. *Obstet Gynecol* 1990;76:991–992.

10. Awwad JT, Azar GB, Aouad AT, Raad J, Karam KS. Postmortem cesarean section following maternal blast injury. *J Trauma* 1994;36:260–261.

11. Weber CE. Postmortem cesarean section: review of the literature and case reports. *Am J Obstet Gynecol* 1971;110:158–165.

12. Arthur RK. Postmortem cesarean section. *Am J Obstet Gynecol* 1978;132:175–179.

13. Buchsbaum HJ, Cruikshank DP. Postmortem cesarean section. In: Buchsbaum HJ, ed *Trauma in Pregnancy.* Philadelphia : WB Saunders, 1979;236–249.

14. Lee RV. Cardiopulmonary resuscitation in the 18th century. *J Hist Med Allied Sci* 1972;27:418–433.

15. Kouwenhoven WB, Jude JR, Knickerbocker GG. Closed chest cardiac massage. *JAMA* 1960;173:1064–1067.

16. Sladen A, Kouwenhoven WB, Jude JR, Knickerbocker GG. Closed chest massage. *JAMA* 1984;251:3137–3140.

17. Weisfeldt ML, Chandra N. Physiology of cardiopulmonary resuscitation. *Annu Rev Med* 1981;32:435–442.

18. Sanders AB, Meislin HW, Ewy GA. The physiology of cardiopulmonary resuscitation. *JAMA* 1984;252:3283–3286.

19. Niemann JT. Artificial perfusion techniques during cardiac arrest: questions of experimental focus versus clinical need. *Ann Emergency Med* 1985;14:761–768.

20. Ueland K, Novy MJ, Peterson EN, Metcalfe J. Maternal cardiovascular dynamics. *Am J Obstet Gynecol* 1969;104:856–864.

21. Sullivan JM, Ramanathan KB. Management of medical problems in pregnancy: severe cardiac disease. *N Engl J Med* 1985;313:304–309.

22. Dilts PV, Brinkman CR, Kirschbaum TH, Assali NS. Uterine and systemic hemodynamic interrelationships and their response to hypoxia. *Am J Obstet Gynecol* 1969;103:138–157.

23. Brinkman CR III, Woods JR. Effects of hypovolemia and hypoxia upon the conceptus. In: Buchsbaum HJ, ed. *Trauma in Pregnancy.* Philadelphia: WB Saunders, 1979;52–81.

24. Karlsson K. The influence of hypoxia on uterine and maternal placental blood flow, and the effect of alpha-adrenergic blockade. *J Perinat Med* 1974;2:176–184.

25. Kerr MG. The mechanical effects of the gravid uterus in late pregnancy. *J Obstet Gynaecol Br Commonw* 1965;72:513–529.

26. Bieniarz J, Crottogini JJ, Curuchet E, Romero Salimas G, Yashida T, Poseiro JJ, Caldeyro Barcia R. Aortocaval compression by the uterus in late human pregnancy. *Am J Obstet Gynecol* 1968;100:203–217.

27. Hawkins JL. What's new in obstetric anesthesia? *Curr Obstet Med* 1991;1:275–299.

28. Weinberger SE, Weiss ST, Cohen WR, Weiss JW, Johnson TS. Pregnancy and the lung. *Am Rev Respir Dis* 1980;121:559–581.

29. Andersen GJ, James GB, Mathers NM, Smith EL, Walker J. The maternal oxygen tension and acid base status during pregnancy. *J Obstet Gynaecol Br Commonw* 1969;76:16–19.

30. Gee JBL, Packer BS, Millen JE, Robin ED. Pulmonary mechanics during pregnancy. *J Clin Invest* 1967;46:945–952.

31. Baldwin GR, Moorthi DS, Whelton JA, MacDonnell KF. New lung functions and pregnancy. *Am J Obstet Gynecol* 1977;127:235–239.

32. Rubin A, Russo N, Goucher D. The effect of pregnancy upon pulmonary function in normal women. *Am J Obstet Gynecol* 1956;72:963–969.

33. Archer GW, Marx GF. Arterial oxygen tension during apnoea in parturient women. *Br J Anaesth* 1974;46:358–360.

34. Awe RJ, Nicotta MB, Newsom TD, Viles R. Arterial oxygenation and alveolar-arterial gradients in term pregnancy. *Obstet Gynecol* 1979;53:182–186.

35. Greenburger PA, Patterson R. Management of asthma during pregnancy. *N Engl J Med* 1985;312:897–902.

36. Bernal JM, Miralles PJ. Cardiac surgery with cardiopulmonary bypass during pregnancy. *Obstet Gynecol Survey* 1986;41:1–6.

37. Wilder RJ, Weir D, Rush BF, Ravitch MM. Methods of coordinating ventilation and closed chest cardiac massage in the dog. *Surgery* 1963;53:186–194.

38. Chandra N, Snyder LD, Weisfeldt ML. Abdominal binding during cardiopulmonary resuscitation in man. *JAMA* 1981; 246:351–353.

39. Niemann JR, Rosenborough JR, Hausknecht M. Cough-CPR. *Crit Care Med* 1980;8:141–146.

40. DePace NL, Betesh JS, Kotler MN. Postmortem cesarean section with recovery of both mother and offspring. *JAMA* 1982;248:971–973.

41. DelGuercio LRM, Feins NR, Cohn JD, Coomazaswamy RP, Wollman SB, Stake D. Comparison of blood flow during external and internal cardiac massage in man. *Circulation* 1965;31 (suppl):171–180.

42. Stephenson HE Jr. Pathophysiological considerations that warrant open-chest cardiac resuscitation. *Crit Care Med* 1980;8:185–187.

43. Sanders AB, Kern KB, Ewy GA. Improved survival from cardiac arrest with open chest massage. *Ann Emergency Med* 1983;12:138, Abstract.

44. Barnett WM, Alifimoff JK, Paris PM, Stewart RD, Safar P. Comparison of open-chest cardiac massage techniques in dogs. *Ann Emergency Med* 1986;15:408–411.

45. Jacobson S. Current status of open chest procedures. *Clin Emergency Med* 1983;2:121–128.

46. Curry JJ, Quintana FJ. Myocardial infarction with ventricular fibrillation during pregnancy treated by direct current debrillation with fetal survival. *Chest* 1970;58:82–84.

47. Clark SL. Structural cardiac disease in pregnancy. *Curr Obstet Med* 1991;1:179–196.

48. Lee W, Cotton DB. Peripartum cardiomyopathy. *Curr Obstet Med* 1991;1:329–348.

49. Hankins DVM. Complications of tocolytic therapy. *Curr Obstet Med* 1991;1:301–328.

50. Swartjes JM, Schutte MF, Bleker OP. Management of eclampsia: cardiopulmonary arrest resulting from magnesium sulfate overdose. *Eur J Obstet Gynecol Reprod Biol* 1992;47:73–75.

51. Myint Y, Bailey PW, Milne BR. Cardiorespiratory arrest following combined spinal epidural anaesthesia for cesarean section. *Anaesthesia* 1993;48:684–686.

52. Ravindran J. Sudden maternal deaths probably due to obstetrical pulmonary embolism in Malaysia for 1991. *Med J Malaysia* 1994;49:53–61.

53. Marx GF. Cardiopulmonary resuscitation of late-pregnant women. *Anesthesiology* 1982;56:156.

54. Rees GAD, Willis BA. Resuscitation in late pregnancy. *Anaesthesia* 1988;43:347–349.

55. Selden BS, Burke TJ. Complete maternal and fetal recovery after prolonged cardiac arrest. *Ann Emergency Med* 1988;17:346–349.

56. Baird SM, McCoy G. Cardiopulmonary resuscitation during pregnancy. *Clin Issues Perinat Women's Health Nurs (NAACOGS)* 1992;3:538–548.

57. Guidelines for Cardiopulmonary Resuscitation and Emergency Cardiac Care. *JAMA* 1992;268:2171–2295.

58. Rotmensch HH, Elkayam U, Frishman W. Antiarrhythmic drug therapy during pregnancy. *Ann Intern Med* 1983;98: 487–497.

59. Widerhorn J, Shotan A, Widerhorn ALM, Elkayam U. Antiarrhythmics. *Curr Obstet Med* 1995;3:95–116.

60. Longo LD. The biological effects of carbon monoxide on the pregnant woman, fetus, and newborn infant. *Am J Obstet Gynecol* 1977;129:69–103.

61. Adler SN, Klein RA, Pellecchia C, Lyon DT. Massive hepatic hemorrhage associated with cardiopulmonary resuscitation. *Arch Intern Med* 1983;143:813–814.

62. Lau G. A case of sudden maternal death associated with resuscitative liver injury. *Forensic Sci Int* 1994;67:127–132.

63. Manas KJ, Welsh JD, Rankin RA, Miller DD. Hepatic hemorrhage without rupture in preeclampsia. *N Engl J Med* 1985; 312:424–426.

26

PREGNANCY AFTER CARDIAC TRANSPLANTATION

Walid S. Alami, md, and James B. Young, md

INTRODUCTION

Cardiac transplantation has become a widely accepted, feasible, and successful treatment modality for selected patients with end stage heart disease. As the number and survival time of heart transplant recipients continues to increase, quality of life, including sexuality and childbearing, have become important issues for these individuals. Many patients with end organ damage to the heart, lung, kidney, liver, bone marrow, or pancreas suffer from infertility. The restoration of normal function to any of those systems via transplantation has led, in many cases, to states conducive to conception and pregnancy. From data available since the first pregnancy of a renal transplant recipient in 1958,[1] it is evident that reproduction after organ transplantation is possible for both females and males. The desire to procreate is normal in women of childbearing age, including those who are heart transplant recipients. The transplant recipient attempting successful conception, pregnancy, and delivery presents a rare challenge to those participating in her care. Furthermore, the issues relevant to males wishing to procreate after transplantation are entirely different.

In the United States, more than 2500 heart transplants are performed per year, with an expected one-year survival rate of around 80% and a 5-year survival rate of about 65%.[2,3] The female recipient heart transplant population represents about 21%[4] to 38%[5] of heart transplants, of which a considerable percent are of childbearing age. From the renal transplant population, it was estimated that at least 1 in 50 women of childbearing age will become pregnant after transplantation.[6] From 1958 to date, more than 2400 pregnancies have occurred in organ transplant recipients. As would be anticipated, the largest number reported is in the renal transplant population, with about 2300 pregnancies reported worldwide

by 1991.[7] Successful pregnancies have also occurred in liver[8–10] and bone marrow[12] transplant recipients. The largest series of pregnancies in the heart transplant recipient population was reported by Wagoner et al.[13]: 35 pregnancies in 29 transplant recipients.

Pregnancy after heart transplant involves delicate circumstances not encountered in pregnancies with other organ allograft recipients. The denervated cardiac allograft must respond to hemodynamic alterations associated with pregnancy, and surveillance for allograft rejection requires serial endomyocardial biopsies and invasive procedures for hemodynamic monitoring.

This chapter presents an overview of the successful pregnancies in the renal and liver transplant populations. Data from the available pregnancies in heart transplant patients, along with maternal and fetal outcomes, will then be analyzed and compared to this experience. Immunosuppressive therapy, its effects on fertility, the recipient, and the fetus will also be discussed. Counseling guidelines regarding pre-, peri-, and postpartal care will be outlined. Anecdotally, it appears that in the United States today, many transplant centers discourage pregnancy after heart transplantation, and strict contraception is often preached to the heart recipient, whether male or female. We will try to draw conclusions about the advisability of avoiding pregnancy postheart transplant.

PREGNANCY AFTER SOLID ORGAN TRANSPLANTATION

Kidney

As mentioned earlier, the largest number of pregnancies after solid organ transplantation is in the renal recipient popu-

Cardiac Problems in Pregnancy, Third Edition
Edited by Uri Elkayam, MD, and Norbert Gleicher, MD

lation: more than 2300 pregnancies reported worldwide. Most of the data on use of immunosuppression, and maternal and fetal outcome, were extrapolated from this population. The largest series reported is by Davison[14]: 2309 pregnancies in 1594 recipients. Table 26.1[8,9,14–27] outlines the outcomes in that series, in addition to others. Of the estimated 1 in 50 women of childbearing age in the renal transplant population becoming pregnant, 40% do not go beyond the first trimester secondary to spontaneous and therapeutic abortion. Of the pregnancies that continue, 90% have successful outcomes.[28]

Liver

There were 48 pregnancies in 34 female liver recipients reported at the 1994 meeting of the American Association for the Study of Liver Diseases.[27] The first successful pregnancy was noted in 1976.[29] The outcomes in those patients have been encouraging. Table 26.1 lists four series reported in the literature with outcomes detailed after liver transplant.[8,9,26,27]

Heart

The first pregnancy in a heart transplant recipient was reported in 1988.[30] Since then, more than 35 pregnancies have been reported. In the largest series, which comes from the University of Utah,[13] data accumulated from 194 heart transplant centers reported 32 pregnancies in heart recipients and 3 in heart/lung recipients that resulted in 29 children, including two sets of twins. This series detailed methods of delivery, maternal complications, number of rejection episodes, infant outcomes, and immunosuppressive regimes and alterations to them during pregnancy. Finally, the study cohort was compared to another high risk obstetrical group—diabetic mothers.

The cesarean section rate was 33% (it is 23% in the general population) versus 67% vaginal deliveries. Premature delivery occurred in 11 patients (41%). The range of time of conception posttransplant was 6 weeks to 6.5 years (average 2.6 years). Age at conception was between 19 and 35 years. Hypertension occurred in 44% (7% reported in the nontransplant population), premature labor was seen in 30% (5%–10% in the nontransplant population), and preeclampsia developed in 22% (5% reported in the nontransplant population). These were the most frequent maternal complications reported. Other infrequent complications are reported in Table 26.2. Six patients (22%) experienced allograft rejection during pregnancy, ranging from mild focal to diffuse moderate cell-mediated rejection, all cases of which were successfully treated by increasing the doses of conventional regimens without using antilymphocyte preparations. One patient died 2 years postdelivery of cryptococcal meningitis. Two patients died, one at 5 months and one at 2.5 years postpartum, possibly secondary to medicine noncompliance. In

terms of infant outcome (Table 26.3), no fetal anomalies or deaths were reported. However, prematurity was noted in 41% and low birth weight in 17%. No adrenal insufficiency, neonatal infections, or presumed teratogenicities occurred. By the time this series was submitted for publication, the average age of the 29 healthy children was 3.4 ± 0.4 years (0.4–6.5 years). Most of the mothers were on triple-drug immunosuppressive regimens before, during, and after pregnancy (59% on cyclosporine, azathioprine, and prednisone). One patient was on cyclosporine alone, and those remaining were on combinations of two drugs. Some medication adjustments had to be made during the course of pregnancy. In 11 patients (41%) cyclosporine dose was increased by 13–227% to maintain adequate levels. Six patients underwent dose-lowering to decrease the risks of nephrotoxicity and teratogenicity. Among those patients, 2 experienced rejection episodes. Corticosteroids were increased in 4 patients because of rejection. Three patients were taken off azathioprine for medical reasons: 1 for severe anemia and the other 2 for cholestatic jaundice. The mean doses were as follows: cyclosporine, 392 mg/day (200–650 mg/d); prednisone, 12 mg/day (5–30 mg/d); and azathioprine, 105 mg/day (25–250 mg/d). The complication rate in the heart transplant recipient population was compared to a diabetic population (Table 26.4).[32]

Maternal and fetal outcomes after solid organ transplantation in general are compared to that of the population at large in Table 26.5. Results of the liver and heart series should be interpreted with caution in view of the small number of patients. The outcomes, however, appear to be favorable. The rates of spontaneous abortion and congenital anomalies are similar. The rate of preeclampsia is higher, and that result may be explained by increased incidence of hypertension in the face of possible azotemia, as well as cyclosporine and steroid use. The incidence of premature deliveries is higher, too, most likely secondary to increased rate of premature rupture of membranes noted more frequently with steroid use. The indications for cesarean section were mainly obstetrical and were higher in the transplant population. Armenti,[33] who reported the outcomes of 500 pregnancies in female transplant recipients (kidney, liver, and heart), noted allograft loss within 2 years of delivery as 4.5, 8.9, 6.9, and 0.0 in the kidney (non cyclosporine), kidney (cyclosporine), liver, and heart groups, respectively.

PATERNITY BY HEART TRANSPLANT RECIPIENTS

Wagoner[32] reported 42 paternities after heart transplantation. Term delivery occurred in 93%, and 7% of the infants were pre term. One newborn had a cleft palate; another died from umbilical cord circulation interruption at 24 weeks of gestation. Father's age at conception was less than 45 years in 95%

TABLE 26.1   Maternal and Fetal Outcome After Solid Organ Transplantation

Ref: First Author (year)	Organ TP	Number of Patients/ Number of Pregnancies	TA	SA	PreE	Still	Csect	Live Birth	Premature	LBW	Cong Anom	Neo Death
Rifle[15] (1975)	Kidney	103/120	18	7		0	57	72			0	
Rudolph[16] (1979)	Kidney	406/440	24	5		1	63	63	19		3	2
Penn[17] (1980)	Kidney	37/56	12	2		2	20	78	50	13	9	
O'Donell[18] (1985)	Kidney	21/38	15	23		2	75		59	32	4	
Marushak[19] (1986)	Kidney	20/24	0	0				100	33	16	0	
Davison[20] (1987)	Kidney	1004/1569	22	16	30				50	20		
Muirhead[21] (1991)	Kidney	22/22				4	59	85	59	45	0	
Cararach[22] (1993)	Kidney	/133	16	10					46	25	4	0.01
Cararach[22] (1993)	Kidney	/66	0	12					48	29	0	0.06
Pahl[23] (1993)	Kidney	21/32			32		79	100	34		4	
Davison[14] (1994)	Kidney	1594/2309	27	14	30				45–60	20		
Armenti[24] (1994)	Kidney	264/394			24				53	43		2
Jimenez[25] (1995)							Triplets, all alive and well					
Laifer[26] (1990)	Liver	7/7	14		37		62	85				14
Scatleber[8] (1992)	Liver	17/17					76	100	55	1	0	
Ville[9] (1994)	Liver	19/19	15	21			40	65	0	8	0	0
Radomski[27] (1994)	Liver	34/48	8	18	21	0	47	74	39	31	0	0
Wagoner[13] (1993)	Heart	32/32	11	7	22	0	33	90	41	17	0	0

Abbreviations: TA, therapeutic abortions; SA, spontaneous abortions; PreE, preeclampsia; Still, still births; Csect, casearan section; LBW, low birth weight; Cong Anom, congenital anomalies; Neo Death, neonatal death.

329

TABLE 26.2 Maternal Characteristics and Complications (*n* = 27) in a Heart Transplant Population

Characteristic/Complication	Number of Occurrences
Onset of pregnancy from transplantation (years)[a]	2.6 ± 0.3
History of peripartem cardiomyopathy	3
Hypertension	12
Premature labor	8
Preeclampsia	6
Premature rupture of membranes	3
Cholestatic jaundice	4
Postpartum hemorrhage	2
Postpartum depression	1
Diabetes	1
Worsening chronic kidney failure	4
Rejection during pregnancy	6
Infections during pregnancy	4
Maternal deaths	
Early	0
Late	3
Information unavailable	2

[a]Reported as mean ± SEM.

Source: Wagoner et al,[13] used with permission.

of the cases. Immunosuppression regimens were reported for 37 paternities, with 60% on cyclosporine/azathioprine/prednisone combination, 14% on cyclosporine and prednisone, 10% on cyclosporine and azathioprine, and 5% on azathioprine and prednisone. In this small cohort, no serious fetal anomalies have been reported. Although long-term follow-up of children may be lacking, it can be assumed that paternity by cardiac transplant recipients carries only slightly higher risk.

TABLE 26.3 Characteristics and Complications (*n* = 29)* in Infants Born to Female Heart Transplant Recipients

Characteristic/Complication	Number of Occurrences
Age (years)[a]	3.4 ± 0.4
Number of sets of twins	2
Premature	12
Low birth weight	5
Respiratory distress	4
Patent ductus arteriosus	2
Anemia	1
Polycythemia	1
Jaundice	1
Hypoglycemia	1
Anomalies	0
Intrauterine deaths	0
Neonatal deaths	0

[a]Reported as mean ± SEM.

Source: Wagoner et al,[13] used with permission.

TABLE 26.4 Statistical Comparison to Another High Risk Group

Charicteristic/Complication	High Risk Groups (%)	
	Heart Transplant	Diabetic
Hypertension	44	15–30
Premature delivery	41	19–50
Preeclampsia	22	16
Low birth weight	17	50
Fetal anomalies	0	9–15
Fetal respiratory distress	14	3
Cesarean delivery	33	50–81

Source: Wagoner,[31] used with permission.

THE DENERVATED HEART: PHYSIOLOGY, FUNCTION, AND ADAPTIVE MECHANISMS TO THE STATE OF PREGNANCY

Pregnancy is associated with substantial physiologic changes that require adaptation of the cardiovascular system. Those hemodynamic changes are discussed in detail in Chapter 1 and 2. In this section we give an overview of physiology and function of the denervated heart and discuss the changes to which the implanted heart must adapt in its new milieu. The function of the orthotopically transplanted heart is a complicated interplay of ventricular loading conditions, intrinsic myocardial contractile capability, circulatory catecholamine levels, denervation, donor/recipient size relation, pulmonary performance, and atrial function. Table 26.6 summarizes many issues relevant to function of the transplanted heart. Early reports[33] suggested that cardiac output (CO) was usually depressed soon after transplant and that maintenance of high central venous pressure (CVP) was essential to maintain CO. Atrial dynamics have been noted to be abnormal.[34] Because of midatrial anastomoses between donor and recipient hearts, varying portions of the donor and recipient atria are present, and the native atria do not contract synchronously with the allograft atria because native sinus node electrical activity is not transmitted across the atrial suture lines. Consequently, less than the expected 15–20% normal contribution to net stroke volume is often noted. It is also reported[35,36] that intracardiac pressures were normal at rest, but ventricular diastolic pressures increased dramatically with exertion. Additionally, a restrictive hemodynamic pattern that resolves within days to weeks was documented early after transplant.[37] Donor/recipient size mismatch may also account for the restrictive pattern. In the absence of rejection, the ejection fraction remains within normal limits for at least a 4-year follow-up period, and substantial increase in cardiac volume and end diastolic wall stress are noted. An appropriate increase in CO during low intensity exercise, resulting from increase in end diastolic volume and stroke volume, has

TABLE 26.5   Maternal and Fetal Outcomes After Solid Organ Transplant Compared to That of the Population at Large

Outcome	Transplant Population			Nontransplant Population
	Kidney	Liver	Heart	
Spontaneous abortions (%)	2–23	18–21	7	15
Preeclampsia (%)	24–32	21–37	22	7
Still births (%)	0–4	0	0	
Premature (%)	19–60	39–55	41	7–10
Low birth weight (%)	13–45	1–31	17	4–8
Congenital anomalies (%)	0–9	0	0	2

Source: Creasy and Resnik.[28]

been observed. At more intense exercise levels, heart rate and contractility are increased as well, probably because of an increase in circulating catecholamines.[38] One characteristic of the denervated transplanted heart without tonic vagal input is a high resting heart rate (95–115 beats/min) versus that in the innervated heart (60–100 beats/min). The rate accelerates more slowly than normal during exercise and tends to be lower at the same level of exercise, compared to the normal pop-

TABLE 26.6   Factors Affecting Function of the Transplanted Heart

HEMODYNAMIC

Donor/recipient body size relation
Donor/recipient atrial asynchrony
Early postoperative restrictive physiology
Late postoperative restrictive physiology

DENERVATION

Afferent denervation
  Altered reflex control of peripheral vasoconstriction/
    vasodilation
  Altered Na^+/H_2O regulation via central nervous system–
    dependent vasopressin, renin, angiotensin, aldosterone
    secretion
  Absence of anginal syndrome during ischemia
Efferent denervation
  Absent vagal nerve control
  Rapid heart rate at rest
  Attenuated heart rate response to exercise
  Hypersensitivity to circulating catecholamines

ALTERED HORMONAL MILIEU

Atrial natriuretic peptide secretion changed
Elevated exercise circulating catecholamines

MYOCARDIAL INJURY/MALADAPTATION

Organ preservation/recovery injury
Intraoperative complications
Rejection
Ventricular hypertrophy
Hypertension (increased ventricular wall stress)
Allograft arteriopathy (ischemia)

ulation. The rate does not respond to physiologic stimuli such as carotid sinus massage or innervation-dependent pharmacological stimuli. As suggested, heart transplant recipients have decreased maximal exercise tolerance compared to normal subjects. This abnormality results from submaximal increase in ejection fraction and cardiac output augmentation in response to exercise, as well as an exaggerated increase in intracardiac filling pressure.[39–41] Thus, the transplant ventricles are less compliant than normal ventricles. A denervated heart is well understood once we keep in mind that both afferent and efferent nerves are interrupted. Afferent nerve interruption alters cardiobaroreceptor homeostatis by impairing renin–angiotensin–aldosterone regulation and impeding normal vasomotor response to changing cardiac filling pressures. The absence of afferent signaling eliminates the subjective experience of angina pectoris during periods of ischemia. Cardiac efferent innervation mediates the sympathetic and parasympathetic nervous systems of the heart. The absence of afferent-mediated parasympathetic influences causes a higher heart rate at rest, as mentioned earlier, and eliminates the influence on the heart of vagal nerve stimulation from the central nervous system.[42] Loss of autonomic innervation blunts the usual rapid changes in the heart rate and contractility seen during exercise, volume depletion, or vasodilation. In summary, the denervated heart performs similarly but not identically to that of a normal heart at rest. Diastolic dysfunction is common early after transplant and may recur at a later stage in some patients. Cardiac reserve during stress or exercise is adequate but less than normal. Increase of cardiac performance does occur and seems to result from endogenous increase in catecholamines and changes in diastolic loading conditions. In the normal pregnant patient, blood volume increases by about 40%, thus increasing preload, with a resulting increase in stroke volume. Heart rate increases secondary to increased catecholamines, resulting in further increase in cardiac output. Systemic vascular resistance decreases, also contributing to augmented cardiac output.

It would be anticipated that the denervated heart during pregnancy would display increase in stroke volume in response to increased central venous pressure through Frank/Starling mechanisms, similar to what is seen in normals. Increased contractility may also be noted secondary to increased catecholamines. Thus, because of these adaptive mechanisms, there may be nothing preventing a normally functioning cardiac allograft from withstanding the hemodynamic demands of pregnancy. In the presence of rejection, even more compromised systolic and/or diastolic dysfunction can occur, and a restrictive physiology may become overt instead of covert, all of which interferes with the ability to increase stroke volume in response to increased preload. This compromise in cardiac function might predispose a patient to difficulties in meeting the hemodynamic demands of pregnancy. Finally, allograft arteriopathy is a frustrating problem after heart transplant. There is an incidence of 30–50% at 5 years, and some patients can have significant diastolic and systolic ventricular dysfunction because of it. If pregnancy occurs at a time when this problem exists, often in occult fashion, theoretically, even more difficulties could occur.[38]

IMMUNOSUPPRESSIVE THERAPY: EFFECTS ON FERTILITY, THE PREGNANT FEMALE, AND THE FETUS

Stable heart transplant recipients 1–2 years after transplantation are maintained on different combinations of immunosuppressive medications. Those medications most often include cyclosporine, azathioprine, prednisone, and tacrolimus. Most pregnancies reported in different recipients have occurred as early as 1.5–2 years posttransplant. One author, however,[43] reported a successful term pregnancy by a 23-year-old heart recipient who conceived 4 months after her transplant. Data available to date, primarily from the renal transplant population, have again provided most of the information regarding the use of immunosuppressive therapy and its effect on fertility, the mother, and the fetus. These data are little different from the observations reported earlier regarding pregnancy in this group, in general.

Cyclosporine

Cyclosporine, a fungal metabolite, is a cyclic endecapeptide with several N-methylated amino acids and a characteristic unsaturated C-9 amino acid that is unique to this substance. A property that distinguishes cyclosporine from other immunosuppressants is the ability to decrease the immune response without significant myelotoxicity. This agent acts on T lymphocytes rather than by a cytotoxic mechanism. It does cross the placenta readily and is found in concentrations in the fetal circulation similar to those measured in the mother.[44] In many of the reported series, no adverse effects on fetal outcome was observed. Cyclosporine has been noted to be teratogenic in animals only when given in very high doses.[45] In a study conducted by Sandoz Pharmaceuticals, no chromosomal abnormalities were produced in research animals given cyclosporine.[5] Sandoz also collected data on 51 pregnancies in 48 women treated with cyclosporine. The 51 pregnancies resulted in 43 live births, 1 spontaneous abortion, 1 missed abortion, and 6 induced abortions. Two live-born infants and one aborted fetus had anomalies. Forty-five percent of infants were born between 28 and 35 weeks of gestation. Thus, prematurity and birth defects were not more common than in published reports of women treated with prednisone and azathioprine in the renal transplant population.

The National Transplant Pregnancy Registry reported 394[46] pregnancies in 264 female recipients.[46] All were immunosuppressed before, during, and after pregnancy; 43.5% were on cyclosporine regimens. There were fewer reported newborn complications (21.7%) in offspring of cyclosporine recipients than in the noncyclosporine group (29.6%). One of 6 neonatal deaths occurred in the cyclosporine group.

Maternal factors associated with lower birth weight in infants included the presence of drug-treated hypertension and serum creatinine of 1.5 mg/Dl or higher. More cases of hypertension, preeclampsia, and premature births were seen with cyclosporine, more likely secondary to preexisting hypertension and nephrotoxicity with chronic cyclosporine use. In a study by Pahl, et al,[23] preeclampsia was seen in as many as 30% of the women.

The 1995 *Physician Desk Reference* (PDR)[47] states the following about cyclosporine. On carcinogenesis, mutagenesis, and impairment of fertility:

> Cyclosporine gave no evidence of mutagenic or teratogenic effects in appropriate test systems. Only at dose levels toxic to man were adverse effects seen in reproduction in rats. . . . No impairment in fertility was demonstrated in studies in male or female rats. . . . [On pregnancy:] There are no adequate and well controlled studies in pregnant women. Cyclosporine should be used during pregnancy only if the potential benefit justifies the potential risk to the fetus.

Azathioprine

Azathioprine is an imidazole derivative of 6-mercaptopurine. Its active metabolites cross the placenta, and the fetus lacks the enzyme inosinate pyrophosphorylase that converts azathioprine to its active metabolites.[45] Theoretically, the fetus is, therefore, protected from potential teratogenic effects, and, actually, none have been reported. Teratogenicity in animals has been noted at doses greater than 6 mg/kg. Azathioprine has no apparent effects on fertility. Its main side effects are bone marrow suppression and hepatotoxicity. No difference in gestational birth was noted between infants exposed to cyclosporine and those exposed to azathioprine.[23] Congenital anomalies were reported in 7 of 103 children in one series.[23] The authors noted that mothers of children with anomalies had received higher doses of azathioprine than those who had normal infants. A retrospective analysis of many reported pregnancies posttransplant revealed a congenital malformation rate of less than 3% in the face of azathioprine therapy. Lymphocyte chromosomal abnormalities have been reported in infants of transplant patients. Although the effects were reportedly transient, information on the chromosomal effects on other tissues is lacking. These changes can potentially lead to neoplasms, infertility, or congenital malformation in subsequent generations. The series by Pahl, et al.[23] cited earlier includes offspring up to 18 years of age and, by the time the study was submitted for publication, no azathioprine-related difficulties seemed to have appeared. However, one hepatoblastoma, a type of tumor that is not thought to be associated with azathioprine or cyclosporine, was noted. The safety of azathioprine in pregnancy has also been reviewed in patients treated for inflammatory bowel disease. Alstead, et al[48] conducted a retrospective analysis of the outcome of 16 pregnancies in 14 women receiving azathioprine for this difficulty. There was one infectious complication with hepatitis B virus, but there were no congenital anomalies or subsequent health problems in those children, whose ages ranged from 6 months to 16 years when the study was reported. Although lymphopenia, hypogammaglobulinimia, thrombocytopenia, and thymic hypoplasia have been reported in children of mothers who took azathioprine in addition to prednisone during pregnancy, those changes were transient and reversible.

The PDR of 1995 states the following on the Imuran brand of azathioprine[47]:

> Imuran has been reported to cause temporary depression in spermatogenesis and reduction in sperm viability and sperm count in mice at doses 10 times the human therapeutic dose. . . . Imuran can cause fetal harm when administered to a pregnant woman. Imuran should not be given during pregnancy without carefully weighing the risks versus benefits.

Prednisone

Prednisone impairs cell-mediated immune activity by decreasing the number of circulating monocytes and lymphocytes. It also blocks antigenic sensitization and inhibits responsiveness of monocytes to chemotactic factors. There has been vast experience with the use of steroids during pregnancy. It is desirable that prednisone be used at the lowest possible doses during pregnancy, and this is the case in most instances 1–2 years posttransplant, when the dose can be as low as 2.5 mg/day. The ratio of fetal-to-maternal blood levels is 1:10. It is expected that at times doses may be as high as 35 mg/day if the recipient is being treated for allograft rejection. Animal studies have suggested an increased incidence in cleft lip, cleft palate, and intrauterine growth retardation; however, the experience in humans has been reassuring.[1] Adrenal insufficiency has been reported in two infants born to mothers taking 10–20 mg/day of prednisone.[17] An increased frequency of premature rupture of membranes also has been observed. Other side effects include aggravation of hypertension in the pregnant females, gestational diabetes, and increased risk of maternal infections. No teratogenic effects have been reported.

The PDR of 1995[49] states:

> Use of these drugs [prednisone] in pregnancy and nursing mothers . . . requires that the possible benefits of the drug be weighed against the potential hazards to the mother or fetus. Infants born of mothers who have received substantial doses of corticosteroids during pregnancy should be carefully observed for signs of hypoadrenalism.

Tacrolimus

Tacrolimus is a macrolide antibiotic that has similar, but more potent, immunosuppressive effects than cyclosporine with, possibly, fewer side effects. Information from the University of Pittsburgh indicates that tacrolimus crosses the placenta and is found in fetal blood and breast milk at concentrations similar to that of the mother. Little experience is available with the use of tacrolimus during pregnancy, especially in the heart transplant population. Laifer[49] reported on a 39-year-old female heart transplant recipient who conceived 2 years postoperatively while on tacrolimus and gave birth to a healthy, 2093 g female. The pregnancy was terminated at 33 weeks of gestation secondary to preeclampsia.

More data are available from the liver transplant population. There have been 9 pregnancies reported in 9 patients on tacrolimus.[50] Four patients were initially on this drug and the other 5 were switched to tacrolimus after chronic rejection while on cyclosporine. Eight infants born were normal for gestational age. One infant was born at 22 weeks and died 2 hours later; his mother had conceived one month posttransplant and was found to have cytomegalovirus in her gastrointestinal tract and blood. The other 8 infants continued to do well. The PDR of 1995[47] states:

> In reproduction studies in rats and rabbits, adverse effects on the fetus were observed mainly at dose levels that were toxic to man. . . . No reduction in male or female fertility was evident. . . . There are no adequate and well controlled studies in pregnant women. . . . The use of Tacrolimus during pregnancy has been associated with neonatal hyperkalemia and renal dysfunction. Tacrolimus should be used during pregnancy only if the potential benefit to the mother justifies potential risk to the fetus.

In summary, the current immunosuppression regimens used during pregnancy may be relatively safe as long as levels and potential adverse effects are carefully screened for and dosage adjustments made accordingly. The higher incidence of preeclampsia and hypertension in the cyclosporine population is not surprising in view of underlying renal effects of this drug and hypertension, which may contribute to premature birth. Although "safe" drug administration levels are not strictly known, it is recommended that the dose of prednisone be less than 10 mg/day, azathioprine less than 2 mg/kg/day, and cyclosporine 2–4 mg/kg/day.

COUNSELING GUIDELINES

Pregnancy after heart transplant heightens psychological stress because one is simultaneously a transplant recipient and an expectant mother or father. Pregnancy in this situation should be undertaken with utmost caution. Risks to the mother and fetus are clearly higher than pregnancy in nontransplant populations. However, these risks possibly are not high enough to completely rule out conception. Prospective parents need to work in concert with a team consisting of a high risk obstetrician, a transplant cardiologist, a psychiatrist, and a neonatalogist. The course of contraception, pregnancy, delivery, and postpartum care should be closely monitored, and access to a high risk obstetrical facility should be available. Importantly, heart transplant recipients who wish to become parents need to keep in mind that they may not live long enough to raise their children; the proportion of those who do not survive past 5 years posttransplant may be as high as 25%. The fear of possible side effects of immunosuppressive drugs, potential teratogenicity, risks of rejection, increased infection, gestational diabetes, and other outcomes have led to some planned abortions. Certain guidelines should be followed by the allograft recipient and caregivers.

Contraception

Most transplant centers initially recommended strict contraception to female heart recipients of childbearing age, to avoid any additional risk to the transplant in the early postoperative months. As more successful pregnancies and outcomes are being reported, liberalization of that view may be developing. Menstrual cycles can recur as early as 2 months posttransplant. The majority of patients return to regular cycles within a year. Until the woman is ready to become pregnant, she must choose a form of birth control. Intrauterine devices are not an option secondary to the increased risk of infection in the innumocompromised host. Use of oral contraceptives are not desirable owing to increased risk of hypertension via action on the renin–angiotensin system, especially with concommitant use of cyclosporine. Risks of depression, thromboembolism, edema, and gastrointerstinal disturbances may also be increased by simultaneous use of corticosteroids. Barrier methods, such as condoms, diaphragms, sponges, and foams, are the safest forms of birth control in the transplant patient, yet not the most effective.

Tubal ligation or vasectomy may be the best options, but reversibility can be difficult.

Fertility

Reports have concluded that the currently used immunosuppressive regimens in allograft recipients do not decrease fertility.[51] Good gynecological care should be ensured with biannual screening. Increased risk of genital tract cancer has been associated with immunosuppressive treatment. In the renal transplant population, Creasy and Resnik[28] reported that the rate of female genital tract malignancy is estimated to be 100 times greater than normal. Plasma calcium should be routinely monitored because hypercalciuria is induced by prednisone.[5] Prior to considering pregnancy after heart transplant, the female recipient should ideally be at least one year postsurgery, a time frame that allows recovery from the primary and secondary disease processes as well as graft stabilization. By 1–2 years posttransplant, recipients generally have achieved optimal immunosuppression at lowest dose possible.[5] Cardiac catheterization should reveal normal coronary anatomy, normal wall motion and ejection fraction, and acceptable intracardiac pressures and cardiac output. A right ventricular endomyocardial biopsy should reveal absence of rejection. Renal function should be as close to normal as possible, keeping in mind that those parameters may be hard to control secondary to progressive nephrotoxicity caused by cyclosporine. Creatinine clearance should be above 70 mL/h. Blood pressure should be well controlled prior to conception in view of increased risk from preeclampsia in that population. The use of low dose aspirin has been proposed to decrease the incidence of this problem[52] (see Chapter 22). Table 26.7 summarizes recommendations for preconception condition in the prudent heart transplant patient.

Antepartal Care

If pregnancy is achieved, close follow-up is important. Current literature, mostly from renal transplant data, supports the contention that pregnancy does not increase the chance of acute rejection. Indeed, pregnancy is considered to be an im-

---

TABLE 26.7 Recommended Criteria for Optimal Preconception Condition in Heart Transplant Recipients

General good health
Conception at least one year posttransplant
Normal blood pressure or easily controlled hypertension
Reasonably normal renal function
Lowest dose of immunosuppression medicines possible
Absence of allograft rejection
Acceptable cardiac pressures and flows
Psychological stability

mune privileged state, in some senses. That does not mean that rejection does not occur, however. The fetus is an allograft, of sorts, with paternal human leukocyte antigens that can stimulate an immunologic rejection against the transplanted organ; yet the incidence of serious rejection episodes described by Gaudier et al.[53] was only 9% in the renal transplant population, which is similar to that of a nonpregnant state. After heart transplant, right ventricular endomyocardial biopsies and right heart catheterizations should continue as planned or if rejection is suspected. The use of fluoroscopy for guidance may have deleterious effects on the fetus, especially during the first two trimesters (see Chapter 3). One group reported the occurrence of supine hypotension in a patient undergoing fluorocopically guided biopsy at 7 months of gestation, which was believed to be aggravated by the weight of the lead apron placed over the patient's abdomen.[56] The use of echocardiography is thus recommended for endomyocardial biopsy guidance and estimation of hemodynamic parameters.

Antepartal risks to the fetus are increased and include prematurity, possible anomalies, infection, carcinogenicity, bone marrow suppression, and adrenal insufficiency. Prematurity is frequent because of premature rupture of membranes thought to be aggravated by the use of steroids; in addition, premature labor may occur, or intervention may be necessary for obstetrical reasons. To date, there has been no increase in the incidence of stillbirth in the heart transplant population. Spontaneous abortion may occur more frequently because of increased risk of infection (e.g., *Listeria,* cytomegalovirus, herpes, and rubella).[54] It is important that women who desire to become pregnant receive immunization prior to transplantation. The risk of infection may decrease with use of noninvasive monitoring techniques. Biweekly obstetric examination under sterile conditions is recommended until the 32nd week; thereafter, such assessments should be performed weekly. Screening for gestational diabetes is important, especially with the use of corticosteroids. Surveillance for cytomegalovirus and herpesvirus infections should be performed routinely every 3 months. Cytomegalovirus infections are reported in up to 2.2% of newborns.[55] Only 10% of affected infants are symptomatic, and 90% of these either die or have long-term sequelae.[1] Pregnancy termination is generally not recommended when primary cytomegalovirus infection is documented in a pregnant woman because only a small number of infants are seriously affected. Cyclosporine levels, leukocyte and platelet counts, and electrolyte levels should be closely monitored. Urinary estriol tests are not valid because of steroid therapy. Oxytocin challenge tests are not used because of the increased risk of premature labor.[1] An initial and ongoing evaluation of Rhesus titers is needed in this population to determine compatibility because of donor/recipient mismatch.[45] Transplants may be done from Rh+ donor to an Rh− recipient as Rh antibodies do not generally precipitate rejection.[1] Such a recipient should be

TABLE 26.8   Antepartal Considerations in Pregnant Heart Transplant Recipients

MATERNAL
Gestational diabetes
Hypertension
Preeclampsia
Infection
Allograft rejection
Increased risk of genital tract malignancy
Death

FETAL
Teratogenicity from immunosuppressive drugs
Spontaneous abortion
Prematurity
Low birth weight
Infection
Radiation exposure during endomyocardial biopsy surveillance
Adrenal insufficiency
Bone marrow suppression

monitored for rising titers of Rh antibodies when there is a possibility that she is carry an Rh− fetus. Table 26.8 summarizes anterpartal considerations in pregnant heart transplant recipients.

Peripartal Care

The goal of most women during labor is to undergo vaginal delivery.[56] However, the need for cesarean section is increasing in transplant recipients, and those patients should not undergo a torturous labor. The incidence of rejection has been reported higher in females who undergo stressful labor.[53] Wagoner et al[13] reported the rate of cesarean section to be 33% (vs. 23% in the nontransplant population). Use of broad spectrum antibiotics is recommended after membrane rupture. A pulmonary artery catheter may also be helpful in monitoring volume status during the labor period. An anesthesiologist who has experience with the function of the denervated heart should be on hand to administer the anesthetics.

Postpartal Care

Care should continue as usual, since the transplant recipient is also at risk of infection and rejection postpartum. In terms of infant outcomes, data from the renal transplant population show that the incidence of congenital anomalies is no different from that in the nontransplant population. There is an increased incidence of growth retardation, mainly because of babies small for gestational age. Fetal adrenocortical insufficiency has been reported in rare instances as a result of chronic use of steroids by the mother, and perhaps in these cases the infant may be at increased risk for infection and hypotension after delivery.[1]

Many studies have looked at the issue of breast feeding. Human milk offers an infant protection against infections, particularly those of respiratory and gastrointestinal tract. So can the breast milk of an immunocompromised mother be protective? Levels of immunoglobulin A have been found to be the same in immunosuppressed transplant recipients and in nonimmunosuppressed subjects. Breast-fed infants were found to have normal cell counts and no increased incidence of infections. Cyclosporine has been found in fetal circulation at birth in concentrations similar to maternal concentrations and was undetectable by 1 week postdelivery. In a study by Flechner et al,[57] cyclosporine was noted to be present in lower concentrations in breast milk than in serum. Measurements of breast milk levels in cases reported by Sandoz Pharmaceuticals were 214–263 ng/mL at their highest. Assuming breast milk intake of about 225 mg/kg/day, a breast-fed infant will receive 0.06 mg/kg/day of cyclosporine. Azathioprine and its metabolites have, likewise, been found in mother's milk in very low concentrations. In a woman taking 25 mg/day of azathioprine, the highest level in breast milk detected was 18 ng/Ml.[58] Although gestational exposure to immunosuppressants cannot be avoided, unnecessary postpartum exposure by the infant should be avoided. Therefore, breast feeding of infants by mothers receiving cyclosporine and/or azathioprine is not recommended. Finally, psychological support for mothers is important, since postpartum depression may be exaggerated by steroid use.

CONCLUSION

The risk of pregnancy after heart transplantation may have been overstated in the past. The transplanted heart, in the absence of dysfunction secondary to arterioptathy or rejection, can withstand the physiological demands imposed by the state of pregnancy. Premature labor, low birth weight, preeclampsia, hypertension, and premature rupture of membranes are encountered more frequently in heart transplant recipients than in the low risk obstetrical nontransplant population. Allograft rejection, infection, and congenital malformations, however, are not. With modern advances, the rate of survival after heart transplantation has improved dramatically. The recipient expects to conduct a relatively normal life after transplant, and the notion of conception and bearing children appears to be an attractive situation for many women posttransplant.

We believe the female heart transplant recipient should not be discouraged from procreating; however, the moderate increase in risk to the mother and the infant needs to be carefully outlined, and a high risk obstetrical facility should be accessible. Consideration must be given to the responsibility of parenting, in the event of premature death of the post transplant parent.

REFERENCES

1. Hou S. Pregnancy in organ transplant recipients. *Med Clin North Am* 1989;73:667–683.

2. Bourge RC, Naftel DC, Costanzo-Nordin M, Kirklin JK, Young JB, Kubo SH, Olivari MT, Kasper EK, and the Transplant Cardiologists Research Database Group. Pre-transplant risk factors for death after cardiac transplantation: a multi-institutional study. *J Heart Lung Transplant* 1993;12:549–562.

3. Young JB, Naftel DC, Bourge RC, Kirklin JK, Clemson BS, Porter CB, Rodeheffer RJ, Kenzora JL, and the Cardiac Transplant Research Database Group. Matching the heart donor and heart transplant recipient. Clues for successful expansion of the donor pool: a multivariable, multinstitutional report. *J Heart Lung Transplant* 1994;13:353–365.

4. UNOS. Report of Center-Specific Graft and Patient Survival Rate. Heart Volume. US Department of Health and Human Services Administration, Bureau of Health Resources Development, Division of Organ Transportation, Rockville, MD, 1994.

5. Akin S. Pregnancy after heart transplantation. *Prog Cardiovasc Nurs* 1992;7:2–5.

6. Kirk EP. Organ transplantation and pregnancy. *Am J Obstet Gynecol* 1991;164:1629–1634.

7. Davison JM. Dialysis, transplantation and pregnancy. *Am J Kidney Dis* 1991;17:127–132.

8. Scantelbury V, Gordon R, Tzakis A, Korem B, Bowman J, Mazzatero V, Stevenson WC, Todo S, Iwatsuki S, Starzl TE. Childbearing after liver transplantation. *Transplantation* 1990;49:317–21.

9. Ville Y, Fernandez H, Samuel D, Bismuth H, Frydman R. Pregnancy in liver transplant recipients. *Am J Obstet Gynecol* 1993;168:896–902.

10. Grow D, Simson N, Liss J, Delp W. Twin pregnancy in liver transplantation. *Am J Perinatol* 1991;8:135–138.

11. Calve RY, Brons IGM, Williams PF, Evans DB, Robinson RE, Dossa M. Successful pregnancy after paratopic segmental pancreas and kidney transplantation. *Br Med J* 1988;296:1709.

12. Schmidt H, Ehninger G, Popfer R, Walker HD. Pregnancy after bone marrow transplantation for severe aplastic anemia. *Bone Marrow Transplant* 1987;2:329–323.

13. Wagoner L, Taylor D, Olson S, Price G, Rasmussen L, Larsen C, Scott J, Renlund D. Immunosuppressive therapy, management and outcomes of heart transplant recipients during pregnancy. *J Heart Lung Transplant* 1993;12:993–1000.

14. Davison JM. Pregnancy in renal allograft recipients: problems, prognosis and practicalities. *Baillieres Clin Obstet Gynaecol* 1994;8:501–525.

15. Rifle G, Traeger J. Pregnancy after renal transplantation. An international survey. *Transplant Proc* 1975;7:723.

16. Rudolph JE, Schweizer RT, Bar SA. Pregnancy in renal transplant recipient. *Transplantation* 1979;27:26.

17. Penn I, Makowski EL, Harris P. Parenthood following renal transplantation. *Kidney Int* 1980;18:221.

18. ODonnell D, Sevitz H, Seggie JL. Pregnancy after renal transplantation. *Aust N Z J Med* 1985;15:320.

19. Marushak A, Weber T, Bock J. Pregnancy following kidney transplantation. *Acta Obstet Gynecol Scand* 1986;65:557.

20. Davison JM. Renal transplantation in pregnancy. *Am J Kidney Dis* 1987;9:374.

21. Muirhead N, Sabharwal AR, Reider MJ, Lazarovits A, Hollomby D. The outcome of pregnancy following renal transplanation. The experience of a single center. *Transplantation* 1991;54:429–432.

22. Cararach V, Carmona F, Monlean F, Andrew J. Pregnancy after renal transplantation. *Br J Obstet Bynaecol* 1993;100:122–125.

23. Pahl MV, Vaziri ND, Kaufman DJ, Martin DC. Childbirth after renal transplantation. *Transplant Proc* 1993;25:2727–2731.

24. Armenti VT. Pregnancy in transplant recipients. *Transplant Immunol Let* 1995;11:4–14.

25. Jimenez E, Gonzalez-Ceraballo Z, Morales-Otero L, Santiago-Delpin E. Triplets born to a kidney transplant recipient. *Transplantation* 1995;54:435–436.

26. Laifer S, Marilyn D, Scantlebury V, Harger A, Caritis S. Pregnancy and liver transplantation. *Obstet Gynecol* 1990;76:1083–1088.

27. Radomsri JS, Moritz MJ, Munoz SJ, Ahlswede BA, Cater JR, Jarrell BE. National Transplantation Pregnancy Registry. Analysis of pregnancy outcomes in female liver transplant recipients. *Hepatology* 1994;20:142A.

28. Creasy R, Resnik R. *Maternal–Fetal Medicine. Principles and Practices.* 3rd ed. Philadelphia: WB Saunders; 1994.

29. Walcott WO, Derick DE, Jolly JJ, Snyder OL. Successful pregnancy in a liver transplant patient. *Am J Obstet Gynecol* 1978;132:340–341.

30. Lowenstein BR, Vain NW, Perron SV. Successful pregnancy and vaginal delivery after heart transplantation. *Am J Obstet Gynecol* 1988;158:589–590.

31. Wagoner L. Erratum. *J Heart Lung Transplant* 1994;13:342.

32. Wagoner L, Taylor D, Price G, Hagun M. Holland C, Olsen S, Renlund D. Paternity by cardiac transplant recipients. *Transplantation* 1994;57:1337–1340.

33. Stinson EB, Dong E, Schroeder J, Harrison DC, Shumway NE. Initial clinical experience with heart transplantation. *Am J Cardiol* 1968;22:791–803.

34. Valantine HA, Appleton CP, Hatle LV, Hunt SA, Stinson EB, Popp RL. Influence of recipient atrial contraction on left ventricular filling dynamics of the transplanted heart assessed by echocardiography. *Am J Cardiol* 1987;59:1159–1163.

35. Shaver JA, Leon EF, Gray S, Leonard JJ, Bahnson HT. Hemodynamic observations after cardiac transplantation. *N Engl J Med* 1969;281:822–824.

36. Stinson EB, Griepp RB, Schroeder J, Dong E, Shumway NE. Hemodynamic observations one and two years after cardiac transplantation in man. *Circulation* 1972;65:1183–1193.

37. Tischler MD, Lee RT, Plappert T, Mudge GH, St John-Sutton M, Parker JD. Serial assessment of left ventricular function and mass after orthotopic heart transplantation; a four year longitudinal study. *J Am College Cardiol* 1992;19:60–66.

38. Young JB, Winters W, Bourge R, Uretsky B. Task Force 4: Function of the heart transplant recipient. In: Hunt SA, ed. American College of Cardiology 24th Bethesda Conference: Cardiac Transplantation. *J Am College Cardiol* 1993;22: 31–41.

39. Verani MS, George SE, Leon CA. Systolic and diastolic performance at rest and during exercise in heart transplant recipients. *J Heart Lung Transplant* 1988;7:145–151.

40. Plugfelder PW, Purves PD, McKenzie FN, Costuk WJ. Cardiac dynamics during supine exercise in cyclosporine treated orthotopic heart transplant recipients. Assessment by radionuclide angiography. *J Am College Cardiol* 1987;10:336–341.

41. Rudas L, Plugfelder PW, Costuk JW. Comparison of hemodynamic responses during dynamic exercise in the upright and supine postures after orthotopic cardiac transplantation. *J Am College Cardiol* 1990;16:1367–1373.

42. Uretsky BF. Physiology of the transplanted heart. *Cardiovasc Clin* 1990;20:23–56.

43. Ahner R. Pregnancy and delivery after heart transplantation. *Am J Obstet Gynecol* 1994;170:1476–1477.

44. Venkataramanan R, Koneru B, Wang CCP, Burckart GJ, Caritis SN, Starzl TE. Cyclosporine and its metabolites in mother and baby. *Transplantation* 1988;46:468–469.

45. Hunt S. Pregnancy in heart transplant recipients. A good idea? *J Heart Lung Transplant* 1991;10:499–503.

46. Armenti VT, Ahlswede KM, Ahlswede BA, Cater JR, Moritz MJ, Burke JF. National Transplantation Pregnancy Registry: analysis of outcome/risks of 394 pregnancies in kidney transplant recipients. *Transplant Proc* 1994;26:2535.

47. *Physicians' Desk Reference.* 49th ed. Oradell, NJ: Medical Economic Data; 1995.

48. Alstead EM, Ritchie JK, Lennard-Jones JG, Farthing MJG, Clark MK. Safety of azathioprine in pregnancy in inflammatory bowel disease. *Gastroenterology* 1990;99:443–446.

49. Laifer S, Yeagley C, Armitage J. Pregnancy after cardiac transplantation. *Am J Perinatol* 1994;11:217–219.

50. Starzl TE, Satoru T, Fung J, Warty V. FK-506 and pregnancy in liver transplant recipients. *Transplantation* 1993;56:1588–1589.

51. Kossoy L, Herbert C, Wentz A. Management of heart transplant recipients. *Am J Obstet Gynceol* 1988;159:490–497.

52. Cunningham FG, Grant NF. Prevention of preeclampsia, a reality? *N Engl J Med* 1989;321:606–607.

53. Gaudier F, Santiago-Delpin E, Rivera J, Gonzales Z. Pregnancy after renal transplantation. *Surg Gynecol Obstet* 1988; 6:533–542.

54. Dick J, Paltramann A, Hamilton D. Listenosis and recurrent abortion in a renal transplant recipient. *J Infect* 1988;16: 274–276.

55. Stagno S, Whitley RJ. Herpes virus infection in pregnancy. *N Engl J Med* 1985;313:1270–1274.

56. Camman WR, Janachs JS, Mintz KJ, Greene MF. Uncomplicated vaginal delivery 14 months after cardiac transplantation. *Am Heart J* 1991;121:939–941.

57. Flechner SM, Katz AR, Rogers AJ. The presence of cyclosporine in body tissues and fluids during pregnancy. *Am J Kidney Dis* 1985;5:60–63.

58. Coulman CB, Moyer TP, Kain NS. Breast feeding after renal transplantation. *Transplant Proc* 1982;14:605.

PART VI

CARDIOVASCULAR DRUGS IN PREGNANCY

27

PHARMACOKINETICS OF DRUGS IN PREGNANCY AND LACTATION

IRVING STEINBERG, PHARM D, GLADYS MORIGUCHI MITANI, PHARM D,
EARL C. HARRISON, MD, AND URI ELKAYAM, MD

INTRODUCTION

The pharmacokinetic behavior of drugs in pregnancy and lactation is a major concern to the clinician, not only because of the potentially unintended exposure of the fetus to the pharmacologic agent, but because of the uncertainty of drug response and toxicity during the course of pregnancy. The physiologic changes that develop during the different stages of pregnancy, labor, and the postpartum period, as well as the complex nature of the maternal/placental/fetal compartments, significantly alter the absorption, distribution, and elimination of various drugs. Close monitoring of the pharmacokinetics and pharmacodynamics of drugs throughout pregnancy is required to properly adjust dosage, to provide safe and effective therapy to the mother while limiting risk to the fetus.[1] These considerations are extended to the postpartum period when return to baseline pharmacokinetic disposition may occur slowly or rapidly, and when exposure of the neonate and infant to drugs via the breast milk creates potential risk. New opportunities for improved maternal and fetal therapy have developed over the last decade,[2] demanding an understanding of the factors that allow transplacental passage of drugs. A working knowledge of pharmacokinetic concepts applicable to the pregnant patient with cardiac disease, and the fetus/newborn, should assist the clinician in the critical choices and monitoring of pharmacotherapy.

PHYSIOLOGIC CHANGES AND DRUG DISPOSITION IN PREGNANCY

Absorption

Changes in extent and rate of absorption due to pregnancy require consideration. The absorption of orally administered drugs undergoes relatively small changes during pregnancy. With the increase in emesis seen in early pregnancy, the bioavailability and compliance with medication may be reduced. Prolonged gastric emptying time may delay the expected onset of effect of some drugs, since the time to peak concentration will be delayed. This may also reduce the peak concentration, particularly for rapidly cleared drugs and for those undergoing inactivation in the stomach. Further delay may occur if patients consume meals with a higher fat content. However, the delayed gastrointestinal transit time, with resultant prolonged drug retention, may enhance the bioavailability of some incompletely absorbed sustained-release medications. During labor, oral absorption is further compromised. The bioavailability of drugs with high first-pass metabolism (e.g., nifedipine, propranolol) is subject to large variations during pregnancy.[3,4] The intestinal wall may metabolize some drugs, limiting the bioavailability of some and enhancing the enterohepatic circulation of others. Additionally, drug interactions that may reduce drug absorption must be considered. The administration of iron supplements in pregnancy, with consequent reduction of methyldopa ab-

Cardiac Problems in Pregnancy, Third Edition
Edited by Uri Elkayam, MD, and Norbert Gleicher, MD
Copyright © 1998 by Wiley-Liss, Inc. ISBN 0-471-16358-9

sorption and blood pressure response, is one example.[5] Other routes of administration generally retain their rates of absorption as for nonpregnant patients, although some changes may be seen with augmented regional blood flow.

Volume of Distribution

The volume of distribution of drugs is usually referred in its pharmacokinetic sense as an "apparent" volume. Body composition plays a large role in the differences in volume of distribution among patients.[6] Although some drugs may conform to a volume that is consistent with an actual physiologic volume (e.g., warfarin and intravascular volume, aminoglycosides and extracellular volume, heparin and total body water), many drugs distribute to spaces much larger than any physiologic volume due to extensive tissue binding (e.g., digoxin, amiodarone). Blood and extracellular and total body water volumes increase greatly during pregnancy, enlarging the distribution volume of many drugs. The plasma volume increases 20% by midgestation and 50% at term. There is a 50–80% increase in extracellular and total body volume in concert with the development of the conceptus and the enlargement of the uterus and breasts. This will increase the volume of distribution of polar compounds such as penicillins, cephalosporins, and aminoglycoside antibiotics.[7] The blood volume increases to a lesser degree in pregnancy-induced hypertension and preeclampsia, and may provide values for volume of distribution and peak plasma concentrations of antihypertensive agents that are closer to nonpregnant patient values.[8] Distribution volumes greater than total body water indicate drug binding to lean or adipose tissue (pharmacologic receptor and nonreceptor binding). The relatively greater added contribution of body water compared to tissue to the overall gain in body weight explains why an extensively tissue-bound drug such as digoxin has a reduced relative volume of distribution in pregnancy (5.7 L/kg compared to 7 L/kg in controls).[9] The body fat increases in pregnancy may expand the volume of distribution of highly lipid-soluble drugs (e.g., diazepam), creating a potential repository of drug for prolonged activity. However, the volume normalized to weight for more rapidly cleared lipophilic agents (e.g., morphine)[10] may be comparatively reduced, since the contribution to the weight gain in pregnancy is larger for water and lean tissue than for fat mass.

The volume of distribution is also greatly influenced by the degree of plasma protein binding of the drug, since under conditions of normal vascular integrity, the unbound drug is the entity that can leave the intravascular space to interact with receptor and nonreceptor binding sites. Conceptually, the volume of distribution V_d has been described by Oie and Tozer[11] as follows:

$$V_d = V_P + V_T \times \frac{f_{up}}{f_{uT}}$$

where V_P is plasma volume, V_T is nonplasma water and tissue volume, and f_{up} and f_{uT} are the fraction unbound in the plasma and tissue, respectively. Drugs for which f_{up} greatly exceeds f_{uT} will not be restricted to the plasma space, and the volume of distribution may be equal to or greater than total body water (≥ 0.6 L/kg; e.g., phenytoin, tricyclic antidepressants, amiodarone). However, when the protein binding in the serum is higher than that in the tissue ($f_{up} \ll f_{uT}$), the volume of distribution will be restricted and will approach 0.1 L/kg, or the volume of distribution of albumin itself (e.g., furosemide, warfarin).[12] This equation is also useful in demonstrating the reduced volume of distribution of digoxin in renal failure, heart failure, and hypothyroidism, where the diminished tissue binding is suggested.[13] The V_T can be further resolved into other pharmacokinetic "spaces" via classical compartment modeling. Finally, it is important to standardize or normalize volume of distribution values to body weight or surface area, to compare patients of different disease states/conditions, body habitus, or ages.

Plasma Protein Binding

Alterations in drug disposition may result from changes in plasma protein binding during the course of pregnancy, labor, or delivery, and the puerperium. Protein binding alterations may occur secondary to changes in the concentration of specific proteins and the available number of binding sites that bind various drugs (binding capacity), as well as changes in the ability of these proteins to bind drugs (binding affinity).[12] Variation in the protein binding of drugs is significant for the impact that it makes on pharmacokinetics and pharmacodynamics (as the moiety that binds to receptors is the unbound drug). The major proteins involved in plasma binding of drugs are albumin and α_1-acid glycoprotein (AAG). Other proteins and blood components play a more minor role in drug binding during pregnancy, with cyclosporin and its binding to lipoproteins a notable exception.[14]

Progressive decreases in maternal serum albumin occur through each trimester of gestation, with levels falling to 3–3.5 g/dL, potentially lower in preeclampsia. Hypoalbuminemia will lower the plasma binding of mainly acidic drugs, with the most clinically important changes occurring for drugs that are typically highly ($\geq 90\%$) bound. For example, the unbound fraction of phenytoin increases by 40% from baseline to third trimester,[15] increasing the free fraction available for distribution, receptor interaction, and clearance from the body.[16] The unbound fraction negatively correlates with the albumin concentration. In general, the drug affinity of albumin binding sites is not changed due to pregnancy.[17] However, endogenous displacers such as free fatty acids (increased during gestation), bilirubin, and nitrogenous compounds in uremia,[18] as well as drugs with high competitive binding affinity (oral hypoglycemic agents, valproic acid), lead to disruption of binding affinity and increases in unbound fraction for a variety of displacement interactions. Such binding displacement during pregnancy may make more drug available not only for pharmacodynamic effect, but also for delivery to the fetal compartment. This modification in availability is magnified by the increased albumin concentration in the fetus with gestation (opposite to the maternal pattern),[18,19] thus allowing for greater binding in the fetal compartment and increasing the fetal/maternal concentration ratio of highly bound drugs with advancing gestation.[20]

The other major binding protein is α_1-acid glycoprotein. This heavy protein (MW 44,000) is synthesized by the liver; it is an acute phase reactant (rising with trauma, cancer, myocardial infarction, etc.), and it mostly binds basic drugs. Among those bound are lidocaine (and other "-caine" anesthetics), disopyramide, quinidine, propranolol, nadolol and other β-adrenergic blocking agents. At any given total drug concentration, the free level will negatively correlate with the concentrations of AAG. The protein binding of lidocaine and disopyramide exhibits concentration-dependence, with the free fraction ranging severalfold within the therapeutic range for each drug. As the concentration of this protein is more than one log-fold below that of albumin, the molar therapeutic concentration of these antiarrhythmics approaches/exceeds the molar concentration of AAG, yielding saturability. Therefore, the pharmacodynamics of these agents may be expected to vary beyond the observed variability of the dose/serum concentration relationship. During pregnancy, concentrations of AAG are slightly lower than average, and may fall during the first trimester and stabilize until delivery.[21,22] Since somewhat higher values are found in preeclampsia,[8] binding studies and the resultant pharmacodynamic variability must be specifically evaluated in these patients. With labor, birth trauma, or cesarian section, the concentration of AAG dramatically rises, and the free fraction of basic drugs will fall. This drop has been demonstrated in a well-designed study of maternal disopyramide binding in each trimester and postpartum.[22] Competitive binding interactions can occur between basic drugs for sites on this protein. Monitoring of free drug concentration may be needed if interpretation of total levels is made difficult by the complexity of these drug–protein binding relationships and changes.[1] As with albumin, the concentration of AAG increases in the fetus during gestation, and this increases the fetal-to maternal concentration ratio for propranolol into the third trimester.[20] However, basic drugs that are transmitted to the fetus will have a lower free fraction, and this may sustain pharmacodynamic effects in the newborn after delivery for drugs given during labor (e.g., meperidine and neonatal depression).[23]

Clearance Concepts

The clearance of a drug is defined as the volume of blood completely purged of drug per unit time. The total body clearance of a drug combines all the available routes of elimination (hepatic, renal, lung, skin, intestinal, etc.). The clearance can be measured directly (e.g., urine collection over time), calculated assuming a single- or multicompartment model, or evaluated using a noncompartmental analysis that assumes no a priori model constraint. The latter approach involves evaluation of the area under the curve (AUC) for serum concentration versus time, usually demanding intensive serum sampling. The clearance CL can then be calculated as follows:

$$CL = \frac{\text{dose} \times \text{bioavailability}}{\text{AUC}}$$

This can be converted to rates per unit time in minutes or hours or per day. Compartmental analysis allows fitting of the serum concentration–time data to a specified model, and clearance is derived. A simplified version of analysis is:

$$CL = kV_d$$

where k is elimination rate constant in reciprocal hours. Finally if a steady state (ss) blood concentration is available for a drug that does not show large perturbations in blood levels during a dosage interval, the clearance can be evaluated as follows:

$$CL = \frac{\text{dose} \times \text{bioavailability}}{C_{ss}}$$

As with volume of distribution, this value is standardized to body weight or surface area for appropriate pharmacokinetic comparisons. The elimination half-life is the time taken for the plasma or body fluid concentration to be halved, and is related to clearance and distribution volume:

$$t_{1/2} = \frac{0.693\ V_d}{CL}$$

Although most clinicians recognize the impact of reduced clearance on prolonging the half-life, it is often less appreciated that changes in half-life may be proportional to changes in volume of distribution, assuming linear kinetics. Therefore, when third-spacing of fluid or drug occurs and the volume of distribution expands, the elimination half-life will rise if clearance remains stable. This effect may require increasing the dose, but lengthening the dosage interval, if peak and trough levels are critical to control.

Renal Clearance

Cardiac output increases 40–50% by the middle of gestation, as mirrored by the increase in glomerular filtration rate (GFR), increasing the clearance and shortening the elimination half-life of polar drugs such as β-lactam antibiotics. The renal clearance can be correlated with the increase in inulin and creatinine clearance, as shown for the antibiotic ceftazidime.[24] Renal blood flow increases 25–50%, augmenting the filtration and tubular secretion of drugs. Delivery of drugs with local action in the kidney (e.g., antibiotics, loop diuretics) is enhanced. Peak renal clearances are observed at 26–28 weeks of gestation and may fall somewhat afterward, given the protuberance of the abdomen and the increased mechanical pressure of the conceptus on blood flow to the kidney.[25] However, renal clearance remains well above nonpregnant values. The more rapid clearance and the larger distribution volume of polar agents demand dosage regimen adjustments (shortening the dosage interval, increasing the dose, or both), to maintain adequate pharmacodynamic effect.[7] These physiologic changes augmenting renal clearance may be muted in pregnancy-induced hypertension and preeclampsia, since the renal blood flow and GFR will be negatively affected. With pregnancy-mediated decreases in plasma protein binding and higher free fraction, more unbound drug is available to be cleared by the kidney. An offset of effect, however, may be observed for furosemide in preeclampsia, when the drug may be more unbound in the hypoalbuminemic plasma and delivered more readily to the kidney, but have higher binding within the tubular filtrate, keeping it from the active site in the loop of Henle. A comprehensive physiologic approach to evaluating renal drug clearance suggests:

$$CL_{renal} = fu \times GFR\,(1 - f_{reabsorbed}) + CL_{tubular\ secretion}$$
$$(1 - f_{reabsorbed})$$

One can observe that the changing elements during pregnancy of decreased protein binding, and increased glomerular filtration and renal blood flow contribute to the increase in renal clearance.

Hepatic Clearance

Despite the large increase in cardiac output in the pregnant patient, liver blood flow is not increased.[8] The efficiency of metabolism mediated by hepatic enzymes varies by drug and pathway considered. Overall, hepatic clearance is dependent on liver blood flow (Q), plasma protein binding (as the fraction unbound, f_{up}), and the intrinsic microsomal enzymatic clearance (CL_{int}):

$$CL_{hepatic} = \frac{Q(f_{up} \times CL_{int})}{Q + (f_{up} \times CL_{int})}$$

The equation suggests that for drugs with a very high intrinsic clearance that exceeds liver blood flow—that is, having a high extraction ratio (e.g., propranolol, flecainide, nifedipine, lidocaine)—$CL_{hepatic} \approx Q$. Therefore, hepatic clearance is "blood-flow-limited," and changes in protein binding does not significantly change clearance, but adjusts the relationship between free and total drug concentration, as discussed earlier. The pharmacokinetics of propranolol and labetalol differ little in the pregnant and nonpregnant states.[4,26]

However, nifedipine may vasodilate the portal system and increase flow. It follows then that the pharmacodynamics of the dihydropyridine calcium channel blockers may affect their pharmacokinetics. Nifedipine has shown a greater clearance in pregnant patients than in nonpregnant volunteers.[3] The high intrinsic clearance of these drugs helps explain their extensive first-pass effect and reduced (relative to intravenous dose) oral bioavailability. These drugs are also subject to reduced clearance when heart failure is present. Variability in metabolism and pharmacodynamic response is also influenced by genetic polymorphism and ethnicity, and, potentially, by pregnancy itself.[27–29]

For drugs with a low extraction ratio, where liver blood flow is much greater than the intrinsic clearance, the $CL_{hepatic}$ roughly equals $f_{up} \times CL_{int}$. Theophylline and phenytoin are examples of drugs in which an increase in the fraction unbound will increase the clearance of the drug. Since the steady-state total drug concentration will decrease as a function of increased f_{up} and clearance, the free concentration at steady-state should remain approximately the same. It is important for the clinician to recognize this "shift" in the total concentration therapeutic range and not spontaneously change the dose based on a lowered drug level, if therapeutic efficacy is being maintained. However, peak-to-trough variability may increase. The CL_{int} during pregnancy may show varied patterns, not always demonstrating the expected increases in clearance.[30] Using antipyrine as a marker of P-450 enzyme metabolism, Loock et al.[31] demonstrated the impact of estradiol and progesterone on hepatic elimination in a matched-control study. The pregnant/nonpregnant antipyrine clearance ratio was negatively correlated with the estradiol-to-progesterone concentration ratio in pregnant versus nonpregnant subjects. Therefore, the balance between estrogen (inhibiting metabolism) and progesterone (stimulating metabolism) hormones that rise during early gestation may regulate the efficiency of hepatic clearance.

PHARMACOKINETICS OF THE FETOPLACENTAL UNIT

The placenta is a dynamic organ that controls environmental exposure. However, protection from drug exposure, intended[32] or unintended, is certainly not fail-safe. Although a full discussion of teratogenic effects of drugs is beyond the scope of this chapter, noteworthy fetopathy due to cardiovascular drugs such as angiotensin-converting enzyme inhibitors[33] and warfarin[34] contraindicates the use of these cardiovascular agents during pregnancy. Other agents may present a significant risk/benefit profile that must be weighted by the clinician in light of fetal risk versus maternal risk, and if possible, potential safer choices. Examples such as beta-blockers and intrauterine growth retardation[1,29,35] and amiodarone and neonatal hypothyroidism[36] present dilemmas for the clinician choosing agents for the management of cardiac and vascular disease. An understanding of the transplacental kinetics is important to supplement knowledge regarding appropriate drug selection for the pregnant patient with cardiovascular disease.

Trophoblast tissue appears at 1 week of gestation, and the formation of a villous circulation begins in the third week and progresses to form the eventual contact point for the maternal and fetal circulations, which are established by the fourth week. The main transfer mode for almost all drugs is passive diffusion.

$$\text{rate of diffusion} = \frac{kxA(C_m - C_f)}{l}$$

where k = diffusion constant denoting the physicochemical features of the drug
A = surface area of the placental membrane
C_m, C_t = maternal and fetal blood drug concentrations
l = thickness of the placental membrane

Progressive surface area increase and placental membrane thinning occur during gestation, causing the rate of transfer to be greatest toward term. However, in the face of fetal hydrops, with edema and thickening of the fetoplacental interface, a decreased fetal/maternal ratio is evidenced as observed for cefuroxime and digoxin.[9,37] The placental membrane behaves like other semipermeable lipid biologic membranes with respect to diffusional drug transfer. As expected, low molecular weight, lipid-soluble, and nonionized molecules will more easily pass to the fetus, and rapid equilibrium between maternal and fetal compartments occurs. The following conditions assist the transfer process of drugs across the placenta toward term[38]: increased uteroplacental blood flow, increased maternal unbound fraction (leading to more free drug available for passage), greater physical trauma/disruption of placental membranes, and fetal compartment acidic relative to the maternal blood pH (leading to "ion trapping" of basic drugs)—this is of particular relevance to antihypertensives and antiarrhythmics, most of which are basic. The concentration gradient will vary with gestation, since the free fraction in the maternal and fetal compartments changes with alteration in albumin and AAG concentrations.[19,23] Unlike the situation with breast milk transfer, it is suggested that the ionic state of the drug may be more important than the unbound fraction in the maternal plasma in determining the rate of placental transfer. This primacy of the ionic state is likely due to the initial binding to placental binding sites that then controls the rate of release of drugs to the fetal circulation. Much more relatively restricted penetration, therefore, is observed for cardiovascular agents comparing transplacental and breast milk passage. Low plasma protein-

bound agents that would typically have milk/plasma concentration ratios of 2–7 will be less than unity for fetal/maternal ratio (e.g., flecainide[39]) and sotalol[40]). The differences in pK_a and fetal/maternal pH are the main factors in the greater-than-unity fetal/maternal ratio of procainamide.[41] The pH difference may be accentuated at delivery with fetal distress and acidosis, leading to greater passage and retention of lidocaine[42,43] and meperidine.[44] Other mechanisms of placental transport include facilitated diffusion (carrier molecule but no energy expenditure) for glucose, active transport (carrier + energy) for methyldopa, and pinocytosis for IgG.

The fetal/maternal concentration ratio is the major expression of quantitative transfer of drugs. However, since these are usually single-point estimates with small numbers of subjects studied, gestational physiologic changes between and within women are not easily captured. This ambiguity in part contributes to the overlap across unity fetal/maternal concentration ratio seen with individual cardiovascular drugs (e.g., atenolol).[45] Drug that is swallowed by the fetus after excretion into the amniotic fluid may increase the concentration in the fetal circulation (if absorbed), and potentially prolong the pharmacodynamic effect. Fetal and placental tissue uptake may reduce the measured concentration ratio from cord sampling at term, when most evaluations occur. The placenta itself is capable of limited enzymatic drug metabolism and conjugation,[46] including cocaine[47] and norepinephrine,[48] which may be protective against catecholamine excess. Other factors that may affect the interpretation of the fetal/maternal concentration ratio include the timing of the cord sample relative to the time the last dose was administered to the mother, maternal pharmacokinetic variability, single-dose versus steady state determination, and umbilical venous versus arterial sampling (differences may indicate fetal/placental metabolism or binding).

Studies in premature births and repeated blood/amniotic fluid sampling during fetal therapy allow much important information to be gained over the broader range of gestational ages. Further advancing the study of placental transfer of drugs is the use of in vitro systems such as the isolated perfused cotyledon model.[49] Viable, intact cotyledons are harvested immediately after birth, then perfused through the maternal and fetal circulations at a defined pressure and flow rate. Drug transfer rates from maternal-to-fetal and fetal-to-maternal directions, and placental binding and metabolism, can be studied with appropriate sampling intensity. The "fetal/maternal" concentration ratio can be assessed, and the time to equilibrium determined; antipyrine is used as a freely diffusible, rapidly equilibrating marker. Studies applying this technique to more than 50 drugs and compounds have been published since 1972. Although this method confirms the human in vivo data for drugs like digoxin,[50] this is a metabolically static system that gives drug transfer information only in late gestation; since the viability of the cotyledon lasts but a few hours, the method may not reflect the maternal use of drugs throughout gestation. Despite the limitations of technique and extrapolation to in vivo data, this method should prove a useful adjunct in evaluating fetal risk for less studied older and newer drugs.

PHARMACOKINETICS OF DRUGS IN BREAST MILK

The emphasis on the benefits of breast feeding that increased the popularity of this practice during the 1970s and 1980s has plateaued in the 1990s, with about 50–60% of newborns being breast-fed. This route of drug exposures is unintended, but engenders potential harm to the infant depending on the drug's physicochemical and pharmacokinetic features and inherent toxicity.[51] The seminal work of Fleishaker and colleagues[52–55] and Atkinson and Begg[56–61] have extended the earlier work of Meskin and Lien[62] to better define the factors that influence the passage of drugs from maternal circulation to the breast milk and demonstrate the dynamic nature of drug transfer in milk. Further evaluations of risk include usual or unique drug effects in the exposed infant and the pharmacokinetic disposition of the acquired drug in the infant. Excretion of the drug into milk may require cessation of breast feeding for prolonged periods of time (e.g., in the case of gallium citrate), or be contraindicated altogether (e.g., methotrexate, phenindione, lithium). Attention to proper precautions against breast feeding when contraindicated provides an overall lower risk profile to infants.[63] Exposures of drugs deemed relatively compatible with breast feeding[64] can be reduced by timing the feeds at the expected trough of the maternal serum concentration (typically predose).

Breast milk is composed of 4–9% fat, promoting binding of the partitioned lipid-soluble drugs. Milk protein concentration decreases with time postpartum, with the highest content in the lower fat colostrum.[55] Additionally, the balance of lipid and proteins varies with time of day of breast feeding, maternal diet, and the duration of an individual feed (with the foremilk having more protein and the hindmilk more fat). The proteins in breast milk include albumin, lactoferrin, and α-lactalbumin, and a minor (clinically, but not pharmacokinetically, relevant) amount of immunoglobulins. However, no binding occurs to α-lactalbumin, despite its being the most abundant.[56] Overall, protein binding in breast milk is less than one-third that of plasma binding even for the most highly plasma-bound drugs. The protein binding in milk can be successfully predicted from the plasma protein binding by an equation relating the two components for acidic and basic drugs[57]:

$$f_{um} = \frac{f_{up}^{0.448}}{0.038 + f_{up}^{0.448}}$$

where f_{um} is fraction unbound in milk and f_{up} is fraction unbound in plasma. This would indicate that for any drug with plasma protein binding less than 90%, the unbound fraction in milk will be more than 90%. Several studies point to the protein binding in milk and plasma as the most important quantitative determinants of the milk-to-plasma concentration ratio (M/P).[59] As with partitioning of drugs out of the intravascular space, the higher the plasma protein binding, the more limited the drug delivery into breast milk. This has been demonstrated well for beta blockers.[65] Whereas the M/P for highly bound propranolol is 0.4 (despite high lipid solubility), the M/P for the low plasma protein bound atenolol and acebutolol is 4.5 to 7.1, respectively.[66,67] This linkage is confirmed by reports of infant toxicity after ingestion of breast milk following maternal consumption of these beta blockers.[67,68] The increase in maternal serum α_1-acid glycoprotein after delivery coupled with the decreased fat content in the early postpartum period predict lower milk/plasma concentration ratio for highly serum-bound propranolol.[52] However, this ratio will increase as the serum binding lessens and the percentage of milk fat increases later in the postpartum lactating period.[55]

The other factors affecting the quantitative excretion of drugs into breast milk include drug lipid solubility (as explained by the partition coefficient value or lipid phase/aqueous phase concentration ratio); ionization constant (pK_a) of the drug, pH difference between the maternal plasma and milk, molecular weight of the drug, blood flow to the breasts, and maternal drug clearance and half-life. In general, lipid-soluble drugs partition across biological membranes more readily than water-soluble drugs and will solubilize in the milk fat. However, the partition coefficient has been reported to have a negative correlation with the milk/plasma ratios.[62] This paradoxical observation is, in part, explained by the generally greater degree of plasma protein binding associated with drugs having a higher partition coefficient value (i.e., greater lipid solubility). Additionally, in breast milk, drugs may associate more closely with milk fat globules as a function of protein binding to the membrane surrounding glycoproteins and proteinaceous coat. Experiments altering the fat and protein content of milk demonstrate this more-than-additive, complex interaction.[69] The pH differential and the ionization constant for a drug (pK_a) suggest that weak bases will be more un-ionized in serum (and more available for passive diffusion) and will be "ion-trapped" in the more acidic breast milk. Therefore, based on the Henderson–Hasselbalch equation for ionic equilibrium, weak bases are predicted to have a milk/plasma ratio greater than one, while for acidic drugs the ratio would be below unity. The degree of ionization in breast milk compared with plasma $= 10^{(pH\ difference)}$.[70] Therefore, if pH of the milk is 7.1 and the blood pH is 7.4, the weak base will be twice as ionized in milk than in plasma. The pK_a and pH differential helps explain the high milk/plasma ratios of weak bases such as low serum bound beta blockers atenolol,[68] sotalol,[40] and acebutolol,[67] and for the class 1c antiarrhythmic agent flecainide.[40,71]

Meskin and Lien[62] analyzed milk/plasma ratios for human data and made quantitative correlations with the physicochemical drug parameters of molecular weight, partition coefficient values, and ionization. They observed that molecular weight did not significantly impact partitioning of basic drugs and that ionization did not affect acids. However, the two predictive equations developed explained only 65% of the variance in milk/plasma ratio. Utilizing only factors associated with passive membrane diffusion, without regard for the influence of breast milk and plasma constituents, limits the application of this modeling effort.[60] Fleishaker and colleagues[53] developed a model for milk/plasma concentration ratio that incorporates ionization, plasma and milk protein binding, milk fat fraction, and the drug partition coefficient. The latter two factors were merged to describe the ratio of skim to whole milk:

$$M/P = \frac{f_p \times f_{p,un}}{f_m \times f_{m,un} (S/M)}$$

where f_p and f_m are the unbound fractions in plasma and milk, $f_{p,un}$ and $f_{m,un}$ are the un-ionized fractions, and S/M is the ratio of skim to whole milk. This equation has been applied to several drugs of differing physicochemical properties with good predictive value in an animal model,[53,54] but poorer results using human data, particularly for basic cardiovascular agents. Better overall predictive performance is evidenced by the method of Atkinson and Begg.[59,61] This method incorporates features similar to those evaluated by Fleishaker and colleagues[53] but relies on prior assessment of the relationship of milk protein binding to plasma protein binding as illustrated above[57] and a derived relationship between the milk–lipid/ultrafiltrate and octanol/water partition coefficients.[58] Human data were used to build and refine the model,[59,61] and the authors were careful to accept only data derived from area-under-the-curve (AUC) evaluations of milk/plasma concentrations. This is most important, since evaluation of spot simultaneous samples of breast milk and serum levels only is often misleading. This is because the peak time and half-life may be different for breast milk and serum,[72] as is the case for captopril. These authors modified their phase model to allow for a stepwise multiple regression analysis to determine regression coefficients.[60,61]

acidic drugs: $\ln M/P = -0.41 + 9.36 \ln (M_u/P_u)$
$- 0.69 \ln f_{up} - 1.54 \ln K;$ $(R^2 = 0.93)$
basic drugs: $\ln M/P = -0.09 + 2.54 \ln (M_u/P_u) + 0.79$
$\ln f_{up} + 0.46 \ln K;$ $(R^2 = 0.87)$

where M_u/P_u = milk/plasma unbound concentration ratio
(from Henderson–Hasselbalch equation)
f_{up} = fraction unbound in plasma
$K = (0.955/f_{um}) + 0.045$ (milk/lipid partition coefficient)

These equations give superior predictions of the milk/plasma concentration ratio, particularly improving prediction over other published models for basic drugs,[60,61] including cardiovascular agents. This model should prove useful in assessing predicted breast milk levels and potential infant risk/safety profiles of breast feeding for newer and less-studied cardiovascular drugs, or those yet to be released.

Finally, the quantitative exposure risk to the infant is based on the amount of the drug ingested via the breast milk and the pharmacokinetics of the drug in the infant.[73] The dose can be calculated as follows:

dose/day = maternal steady state concentration × M/P ×
volume of milk ingested

The volume of milk ingested daily averages 150–200 mL/kg. The serum concentration obtained in the infant will depend on the oral bioavailability (F) and the infant's total body clearance (CL):

$$C_{ss} \text{ (mg/L)} = \frac{\text{dose (mg/day) } (F)}{CL \text{ (L/day)}}$$

Using flecainide as an example, if the maternal level is at the high end of the therapeutic concentration range (0.2–1 mg/L), and the M/P is 2.6,[71] then for a 4 kg infant ingesting 150 mL/kg/day, the daily dose is 1 mcg/ml × 2.6 × 600 ml = 1560 mcg or 1.56 mg. Using a neonatal clearance of 3 mL/min/kg, the steady state level in the neonate would be calculated as .09 mg/L, which is less than half the lower end of the therapeutic range. This, of course, does not assure a nontoxic exposure, but it can be seen to be relatively safe.[65] Again, the exposure can be further reduced if feeds are timed at predose. It can be demonstrated that the higher the infant drug clearance, particularly with maturation of clearance pathways, the lower the quantitative exposure relative to the infant of maternal therapeutic dose.[73] In contrast, the premature infant with extremely limited renal and hepatic clearance may be at theoretically greater risk, although some of this risk may be offset by the reduced volume of milk ingested.

Although refined pharmacokinetic models for distribution of drugs into breast milk are highly predictive of quantitative infant exposure, the individual pharmacodynamic response of the infant, particularly for drugs that not used therapeutically in the neonatal period, may be more difficult to predict. Therefore, excellent quantitative prediction cannot replace adequate clinical observation and follow-up of the infant exposed to drugs via this "route of administration."

REFERENCES

1. Knott C, Reynolds F. Therapeutic drug monitoring in pregnancy: rationale and current status. *Clin Pharmacokinet* 1990;19: 425–433.

2. Schneider H. Drug treatment in pregnancy. *Curr Opin Obstet Gynecol* 1994;6:50–57.

3. Prevost RR, Aki SA, Whybrew WD, Sibai BM. Oral nifedipine pharmacokinetics in pregnancy-induced hypertension. *Pharmacotherapy* 1992;12:174–177.

4. O'Hare MF, Kinney CD, Murnaghan GA, McDevitt DG. Pharmacokinetics of propranolol during pregnancy. *Eur J Clin Pharmacol* 1984;27:583–587.

5. Campbell N, Paddock V, Sundaram R. Alteration of methyldopa absorption, metabolism, and blood pressure control caused by ferrous sulfate and ferrous gluconate. *Clin Pharmacol Ther* 1988;43:381–386.

6. Steinberg I, Zaska DE. Body composition and pharmacokinetics. In: Roche AF, ed. *Body Composition Assessment in Youth and Adults.* Columbus, OH: Ross Laboratories; 1985;96–102.

7. Heikkila A, Erkkola R. Review of beta-lactam antibiotics in pregnancy: the need for adjustment of dosage schedules. *Clin Pharmacokinet* 1994;27:49–62.

8. Knott C. The treatment of hypertension in pregnancy: clinical pharmacokinetic considerations. *Clin Pharmacokinet* 1991;21: 233–241.

9. Azancot-Benisty A, Aigrain EJ, Guirgis NM, Decrepy A, Oury JF, Blot P. Clinical and pharmacologic study of fetal supraventricular tachyarrythmias. *J Pediatr* 1992;121:608–613.

10. Gerdin E, Salmonson T, Lindberg B, Rane A. Maternal kinetics of morphine during labor. *J Perinat Med* 1990;18:479–487.

11. Oie S, Tozer TN. Effect of altered plasma protein binding on apparent volume of distribution. *J Pharm Sci* 1979;68: 1203–1205.

12. Herve F, Urien S, Albengres E, Duche JC, Tillement JP. Drug binding in plasma: a summary of recent trends in the study of drug and hormone binding. *Clin Pharmacokinet,* 1994;26: 44–58.

13. Mutnick AH. Digoxin. In: Schumacher GE, ed. *Therapeutic Drug Monitoring.* Norwalk, CT: Appleton & Lange; 1995; 469–491.

14. Roberts M, Brown AStJ, James OFW, Davison JM. Interpretation of cyclosporin A levels in pregnancy following orthotopic liver transplantation. *Br J Obstet Gynaecol* 1995;102:570–572.

15. Tomson T, Lindbom U, Ekqvist B, Sundqvist A. Disposition of carbamazepine and phenytoin in pregnancy. *Epilepsia* 1994;35: 131–135.

16. Dickinson RG, Hooper WD, Wood B, Lander CM, Eadie MJ. The effect of pregnancy in humans on the pharmacokinetics of stable isotope labelled phenytoin. *Br J Clin Pharmacol* 1989;28:17–27.

17. Yoshikawa T, Sugiyama Y, Sawada Y, Iga T, Hanano M, Kawasaki S, Yanagida M. Effect of late pregnancy on salicylate, diazepam, warfarin, and propranolol binding: use of fluorescent probes. *Clin Pharmacol Ther* 1986;36:201–208.

18. Notarianni LJ. Plasma protein binding of drugs in pregnancy and in neonates. *Clin Pharmacokinet* 1990;18:20–36.

19. Fryer AA, Jones P, Strange R, Hume R, Bell JE. Plasma protein levels in normal human fetuses: 13 to 41 weeks gestation. *Br J Obstet Gynaecol* 1993;100:850–855.

20. Krauer B, Nau H, Dayer P, Bischof P, Anner R. Serum protein binding of diazepam and propranolol in the feto-maternal unit from early to late pregnancy. *Br J Obstet Gynaecol* 1986;93: 322–328.

21. Wood M, Wood AJJ. Changes in plasma drug binding and alpha-1-acid glycoprotein in mother and newborn infant. *Clin Pharmacol Ther* 1981;29:522–526.

22. Echizen H, Nakaura M, Saotome T, Minoura S, Ishizaki T. Plasma protein binding of disopyramide in pregnant and postpartum women, and in neonates and their mothers. *Br J. Clin Pharmacol* 1990;29:423–430.

23. Hill MD, Abramson FP. The significance of plasma protein binding on the fetal/maternal distribution of drugs at steady-state. *Clin Pharmacokinet* 1988;14:156–170.

24. Nathorst-Boos J, Philipson, A, Hedman A, Arvisson A. Renal elimination of ceftazidime during pregnancy. *Am J Obstet Gynecol* 1995;172:163–166.

25. Bourget P, Fernandez H, Delouis C, Taburet AM. Pharmacokinetics of tobramycin in pregnant women: safety and efficacy of a once-daily dose regimen. *J Clin Pharm Ther* 1991;16: 167–176.

26. Rogers RC, Sibai BM, Whybrew WD. Labetalol pharmacokinetics in pregnancy-induced hypertension. *Am J Obstet Gynecol* 1990;162:362–366.

27. Wood AJJ, Zhou HH. Ethnic differences in drug disposition and responsiveness. *Clin Pharmacokinet* 1991;20:350–373.

28. Rubin PC, Butters L, McCabe R, Kelman A. The influence of pregnancy on drug action: concentration-effect modelling with propranolol. *Clin Sci* 1987;73:47–52.

29. Saotome T, Minoura S, Terashi K, Sato T, Echizen H, Isizaki T. Labetalol in hypertension during the third-trimester of pregnancy: its hypertensive effect and pharmacokinetic–dynamic analysis. *J Clin Pharmacol* 1993;33:979–988.

30. Carter BL, Driscoll CE, Smith GD. Theophylline clearance during pregnancy. *Obstet Gynecol* 1986;68:555–559.

31. Loock W, Nau H, Schmidt-Gollwitzer M, Dvorchik BH. Pregnancy-specific changes of antipyrine pharmacokinetics correlate inversely with changes of estradiol/protesterone plasma concentration ratios. *J Clin Pharmacol* 1988;28:216–221.

32. Simpson LL, Marx GR, D'Alton. Management of supraventricular tachycardia in the fetus. *Curr Opin Obstet Gynecol* 1995;7:409–413.

33. Shotan A, Widenhorn J, Hurst A, Elkayam U. Risks of angiotensin-converting enzyme inhibition during pregnancy: experimental and clinical evidence, potential mechanisms, and recommendations for use. *Am J Med* 1994;96:451–456.

34. Wong, V, Cheng CH, Chan KC. Fetal and neonatal outcome of exposure to anticoagulants during pregnancy. *Am J Med Genet* 1993;45:17–21.

35. Page RL. Treatment of arrhythmias during pregnancy. *Am Heart J* 1995;130:871–876.

36. Widerhorn J, Bhandari AK, Bughi S, Rahimtoola SH, Elkayam U. Fetal and neonatal adverse effects profile of amiodarone treatment during pregnancy. *Am Heart J* 1991;122:1162–1166.

37. Holt DE, Fisk NM, Spencer JAD, de Louvois J, Hurley R, Harvey D. Transplacental transfer of cefuroxime in uncomplicated

pregnancies and those complicated by hydrops or changes in amniotic fluid volume. *Arch Dis Child* 1993;68:54–57.

38. Livezey GT, Rayburn WF. Principles of perinatal pharmacology. In: Rayburn WF, Zuspan FP, eds. *Drug Therapy in Obstetrics and Gynecology.* 3rd ed. St. Louis: Mosby-Year Book; 1992;3–12.

39. Bourget P, Pons JC, Delouis C, Fermont L, Frydman R. Flecainide distribution, transplacental passage, and accumulation in the amniotic fluid during the third trimester of pregnancy. *Ann Pharmacother* 1994;28:1031–1034.

40. Wagner X, Jouglard J, Moulin M, Miller AM, Petitjean J, Pisapia A. Coadministration of flecainide and sotolol during pregnancy: lack of teratogenic effects, passage across the placenta, and excretion in human milk. *Am Heart J* 1990;199:700–702.

41. Ward RM. Drug therapy of the fetus. *J Clin Pharmacol* 1993;33:780–789.

42. Biehl D, Shnider SM, Levinson G, Callender K. Placental transfer of lidocaine: effects of acidosis. *Anesthesiology* 1978; 48:409–412.

43. O'Brien WF, Cefalo RC, Grisson MP. The influence of asphyxia on fetal lidocaine toxicity. *Am J Obstet Gynecol* 1982;142:205–208.

44. Simone C, Derewlany LO, Koren G. Drug transfer across the placenta: considerations in treatment and research. *Clin Perinatol* 1994;21(3):463–481.

45. Pacifici GM, Nottoli R. Placental transfer of drugs administered to the mother. *Clin Pharmacokinet* 1995;28:235–269.

46. Krauer B, Dayer P. Fetal drug metabolism and its possible clinical implications. *Clin Pharmacokinet* 1991;21:70–80.

47. Roe DA, Little BB, Bawdon RE, Gilstrap LC. Metabolism of cocaine by human placentas: implications for fetal exposure. *Am J Obstet Gynecol* 1990;163:715–718.

48. Bzoskie L, Bount L, Kashiwai K, Tseng YT, Kay WW Jr, Padbury JF. Placental norepinephrine clearance: in vivo measurement and physiologic role. *Am J Physiol* 1995;269:E145–E149.

49. Bourget P, Roulet C, Fernandez H. Models for placental transfer studies of drugs. *Clin Pharmacokinet* 1995;28:161–180.

50. Derewlany LO, Leeder JS, Kumar R, Radde I, Knie B, Koren G. The transport of digoxin across the perfused human placental lobule. *J Pharmacol Exp Ther* 1991;256:1107–1111.

51. Kacew S. Adverse effects of drugs and chemicals in breast milk on the nursing infant. *J Clin Pharmacol* 1993;33:213–221.

52. Fleishaker JC, McNamara PG. Effect of altered protein binding on propranolol distribution into milk in the lactating rabbit. *J Pharmacol Exp Ther* 188;244:925–928.

53. Fleishaker JC, Desai N, McNamara PJ. Factors affecting the milk-to-plasma concentration ratio in lactating women: physical interactions with protein and fat. *J Pharm Sci* 1987;76: 189–193.

54. Fleishaker JC, McNamara PJ. In-vivo evaluation in the lactating rabbit of a model for xenobiotic distribution into breast milk. *J Pharmacol Exp Ther* 1988;244:919–924.

55. Fleishaker JC, Desai N, McNamara PJ. Possible effect of lactation period on the milk-to-plasma drug concentration ratio in lactating women: results of an in-vitro evaluation. *J Pharm Sci* 1989;78:137–141.

56. Atkinson HC, Begg EJ. The binding of drugs to major human milk whey proteins. *Br J Clin Pharmacol* 1988;26:107–109.

57. Atkinson HC, Begg EJ. Prediction of drug concentrations in human milk from human skim milk from plasma protein binding and acid–base characteristics. *Br J Clin Pharmacol* 1988;25: 495–503.

58. Atkinson HC, Begg EJ. Relationship between human milk:ultrafiltrate and octanol:water partition coefficients. *J Pharm Sci* 1988;77:796–798.

59. Atkinson HC, Begg EJ. Prediction of drug distribution into human milk from physicochemical characteristics. *Clin Pharmacokinet* 1990;18:151–167.

60. Begg EJ, Atkinson HC. Modelling of the passage of drugs into milk. *Pharmacol Ther* 1993;59:301–310.

61. Begg EJ, Atkinson HC, Duffull SB. Prospective evaluation of a model for the prediction of milk:plasma drug concentrations from physicochemical characteristics. *Br J Clin Pharmacol* 1992;33:501–505.

62. Meskin M, Lien EJ. QSAR analysis of drug excretion into human milk. *J Clin Hosp Pharm* 1985;10:269–278.

63. Ito S, Blajchman A, Stephenson M, Eliopoulos C, Koren G. Prospective follow-up of adverse reactions in breast-fed infants exposed to maternal medication. *Am J Obstet Gynecol* 1993; 168:1393–1399.

64. Committee on Drugs, American Academy of Pediatrics. The transfer of drugs and other chemicals in to human milk. *Pediatrics* 1994;93:137–150.

65. Riant P, Urien S, Albengres E, Duche JC, Tillement JP. High plasma protein binding as a parameter in the selection of beta blockers for lactating women. *Biochem Pharmacol* 1986; 35(24):4579–4581.

66. Liedholm H, Melander A, Bitzen PO, Helm G, Lonnerholm G, Mattiasson I, Nilsson B, Wahlin-Boll E. Accumulation of atenolol and metoprolol in human breast milk. *Eur J Clin Pharmacol* 1981;20:229–231.

67. Boutroy MJ, Bianchetti G, Dubruc C, Vert P, Morselli PL. To nurse when receiving acebutolol: is it dangerous for the neonate? *Eur J Clin Pharmacol* 1986;30:737–739.

68. Schimmel MS, Eidelman AJ, Wilshanski MA, Shaw D Jr, Ogilvie RJ, Koren G. Toxic effects of atenolol consumed during breast feeding. *J Pediatr* 1989;114:476–478.

69. Notarianni LJ, Belk D, Aird SA, Bennett PA. An in-vitro technique for the rapid determination of drug entry into breast milk. *Br J Clin Pharmacol* 1995;40:333–337.

70. Scialli AR. *A Clinical Guide to Reproductive and Developmental Toxicology.* Boca Raton, FL: CRC Press; 1994; 193–208.

71. Mcquinn RL, Pisani A, Wafa S, Chang SF, Miller AM, Frappell JM, Chamberlain GVP, Camm AJ. Flecainide excretion in human breast milk. *Clin Pharmacol Ther* 1990;48:262–267.

72. Wilson JT, Brown RD, Hinson JL, Dailey JW. Pharmacokinetic pitfalls in the estimation of the breast milk/plasma ratio for drugs. *Annu Rev Pharmacol Toxicol* 1985;25:667–689.

73. Ito S, Koren G. A novel index for expressing exposure of the infant to drugs in breast milk. *Br J Clin Pharmacol* 1994; 38:99–102.

28

DIURETICS IN PREGNANCY

EYTAN COHEN, MD, AND MOSHE GARTY, MD

INTRODUCTION

The use of diuretic treatment during pregnancy is controversial, especially because of insufficient data concerning the teratogenesis of these drugs in the first half of pregnancy, and also because our understanding of their effect on maternal and fetal hemodynamics is incomplete. Apart from their conventional use in hypertension and heart failure, until the 1970s, diuretics were also commonly prescribed for generalized edema and in the prevention of preeclampsia. Routine prophylactic use of diuretics was particularly stimulated by a report[1] indicating that the daily use of diuretics reduced the frequency of preeclampsia. In the two decades that followed, however, the role of diuretics in pregnancy was seriously challenged. It became apparent that dependent edema is a normal physiological accompaniment of pregnancy and does not require therapy.[2] Moreover, treatment of edema by diuretics in the last half of the third trimester has been associated with higher rates of induction of labor, uterine inertia, meconium staining, and perinatal mortality.[3] Preeclampsia was also found to be associated with a reduction of plasma volume,[4] and since diuretics lower plasma volume even further,[5] their use for this purpose was abandoned. Furthermore, a meta-analysis of nine randomized studies conducted in the 1960s and 1970s showed that treatment with diuretics did not prevent preeclampsia or reduce perinatal mortality.[6] Therefore, as early as 1973, a review concerning diuretics in pregnancy[7] stated that "the only patients in whom saliuretics should be prescribed are gravidas with heart disease."

The avoidance of diuretics during pregnancy is currently the common practice by most obstetricians.[8] However, both because of and despite the incompleteness of our knowledge concerning diuretic treatment in obstetric practice, we review the current indications and contraindications for the use of these drugs during pregnancy.

PHARMACOLOGY OF DIURETICS

Remarkable physiological changes in salt and water homeostasis occur during a normal pregnancy. Plasma volume begins to increase during the first trimester, is most marked during the second, and thereafter is sustained to term. On the other hand, the greatest gain in interstitial volume occurs in the third trimester. These changes in fluid volume during pregnancy are due to the complex renal handling of sodium influenced by hemodynamic, humoral and physical changes (Table 28.1). Their net effect is a cumulative retention of 500–900 mEq of sodium and an increase in total body water of 6–8 L till the end of the pregnancy.[7] Cardiac output begins to increase by the 10th week of pregnancy and plateaus, at 40% above baseline, by the 20th week. Increased stroke volume accounts for the initial rise in cardiac output, which is later maintained by an increase in heart rate. Arterial blood pressure normally falls in the first half of the pregnancy as a result of a reduction in peripheral resistance. Later, blood pressure rises and normally approaches nonpregnant values by term or may even transiently exceed them.[9]

In contrast to the normal pregnancy, preeclampsia is associated with vasospasm that is partly the result of an exaggerated vascular responsiveness to circulating angiotensin II and catecholamines[10] and possibly to an imbalance between thromboxane and prostacyclin production.[11] As a result, pregnancy-induced hypervolemia either never develops or is significantly reduced when preeclampsia ensues.

Diuretics have an acute and a chronic effect. Acutely they cause a 5–10% decrease in plasma volume during the initial

Cardiac Problems in Pregnancy, Third Edition
Edited by Uri Elkayam, MD, and Norbert Gleicher, MD
Copyright © 1998 by Wiley-Liss, Inc. ISBN 0-471-16358-9

TABLE 28.1   Factors Affecting Sodium Handling in Pregnancy

Increased Sodium Excretion	Decreased Sodium Excretion
HEMODYNAMIC FACTORS	
Increase in glomerular filtration rate	Increase in renal tubular sodium reabsorption
HORMONAL FACTORS	
Progesterone	Aldosterone
Antidiuretic hormone	Estrogen
Prostaglandins	Placental lactogen
Oxytocin	Prolactin
Melanocyte-stimulating hormone	Renin–angiotensin
	Suppresssion of atrial natriuretic factor
PHYSICAL FACTORS	
Decrease in plasma albumin	Increase in ureteral pressure
Decrease in renal vascular resistance	Uteroplacental shunt

days of therapy. This in turn lowers cardiac output and blood pressure. Over the ensuing 4–6 weeks, compensatory mechanisms return the plasma volume toward normal, and at the same time cardiac output returns to pretreatment levels. However, total peripheral resistance remains low because mobilization of excess sodium from the arteriolar wall leads to widening of the vascular lumen and possibly to a decrease in vascular responsiveness to endogenous catecholamines. Thus, the acute blood pressure lowering effect is due to volume contraction, while the sustained effect is due to a combination of volume contraction and a decrease in total peripheral resistance.[12]

Loop Diuretics

Loop diuretics are among the most potent diuretic agents known, capable of inducing a natriuresis of up to 20% of the filtered load of sodium and an increase in free water clearance. They produce their effect by inhibiting the Na/K/2Cl transport system at the thick ascending part of Henle's loop. Furosemide is the most commonly used agent in this class. Normal doses are between 20 and 120 mg/day, and duration of effect is between 4 and 6 hours. Ototoxicity and conditions of electrolyte imbalance such as hypo- and hypernatremia, hypokalemia, and hypomagnesemia are the most common side effects. Hypokalemia resistant to replacement therapy may be due to concomitant and unrecognized hypomagnesemia, which must be corrected before potassium levels can start to rise.

During pregnancy furosemide crosses the placenta.[13] Following oral doses of 25–40 mg, peak concentrations in cord serum of 330 ng/mL have been recorded 9 hours later. Maternal and cord levels were equal at 8 hours. Administration of furosemide during pregnancy did not significantly alter amniotic fluid volume,[14] but intervillous blood flow was sig-

nificantly reduced.[15] Administration of furosemide to the mother has been used to assess fetal kidney function by provoking urine production that can then be visualized by ultrasonic techniques.[16,17] Diuresis has been found more often in newborns exposed to furosemide shortly before birth than in controls.[18]

There is no evidence of a teratogenic effect of furosemide. However, a possible association between the use of this agent in pregnancy and the development of hypospadias in the fetus has been described.[19] According to the classification of teratogenesis established by the U.S. Food and Drug Administration (FDA), furosemide is in category C, so its use should be limited in the first trimester. Furosemide can be given in the second and third trimesters but close fetal monitoring is necessary during acute use of this drug, since a sudden decrease in blood pressure and placental perfusion pressure may cause fetal distress.

Thiazides

Thiazides can induce a natriuresis of up to 10% of the filtered load of sodium. They produce their effect by inhibiting sodium reabsorption in the early portion of the distal tubule. Increased delivery of sodium to the distal nephron enhances sodium/potassium ion exchange and kaliuresis results. Differences in relative potency and duration of action are related to differences in lipid solubility. Chlorothiazide and hydrochlorothiazide are most commonly used. Normal doses are 0.5–2 grams/day and 25-100 mg/day respectively.

Side effects in obstetric patients are similar to those in nonpregnant women. These include hypovolemia, hypokalemia, and metabolic alkalosis,[20] hyperuricemia,[21] and impaired carbohydrate tolerance.[22,23] Complications include fatal hemorrhagic pancreatitis[24] and death.[25] Effects on the fetus include possible hypoglycemia,[26] thrombocytopenia by transfer of platelet antibodies from the mother to the fetus,[27] hemolytic anemia,[28] hyponatremia,[29] and fetal bradycardia due to chlorothiazide-induced maternal hypokalemia.[30] Thiazides may also decrease the endocrine function of the placenta by impairing uterine blood flow and placental perfusion. This impairment has been shown by a decrease in placental clearance of estradiol[31] and dehydroisoandrosterone.[32]

The Collaborative Perinatal Project found an increased risk of neonatal malformation in women treated with chlorthalidone and other thiazides excluding chlorothiazide and hydrochlorothiazide.[33] According to the FDA classification, teratogenesis thiazides are rated class D, and their use should be avoided in the first trimester. Thiazides may be given in the last two trimesters. However, since their diuretic effect is mild and since their use is associated with more side effects than typically accompany furosemide, the latter drug is more commonly used.

Potassium-Sparing Diuretics

Potassium-sparing diuretics block the sodium/potassium and sodium/hydrogen pumps in the distal tubule and cortical collecting ducts. These agents produce sodium diuresis, but in contrast to the thiazide and loop diuretics, there is potassium retention. Spironolactone acts by competitive inhibition of aldosterone, while triamterene and amiloride have the same effect but are not dependent on aldosterone presence. Potassium-sparing diuretics are often used to counteract the potassium loss that attends the use of thiazides and loop diuretics. Normal dosages are between 50 and 400 mg/day.

No reports linking these drugs with congenital defects have been found. Some authors, however, have commented that spironolactone may be contraindicated during pregnancy based on known antiandrogenic effect in humans and the feminization observed in male rat fetuses.[34] According to the FDA classification of teratogenesis spironolactone is rated D, and its use should be avoided in the first trimester. In the last two trimesters these agents may be used when the risk/benefit ratio is low.

Carbonic Anhydrase Inhibitors

Acetazolamide is the prototype of the group of drugs that are potent inhibitors of carbonic anhydrase. Their action at the proximal tubule decreases the rate of carbonic acid formation, hence H^+ production. Renal tubular secretion of H^+ and reabsorption of HCO_3^- and Na^+ are thereby inhibited. Urinary excretion is increased because of large excretions of solutes. The main use of these drugs is in glaucoma; they are rarely administered as a diuretic. During pregnancy they have been used in the treatment of pseudotumor cerebri.[35] A possible association between acetazolamide administration during pregnancy and metabolic acidosis, hypocalcemia, and hypomagnesemia in the infant has been described.[36]

No reports linking the usage of acetazolamide with congenital defects have been located. A single case of a neonatal sacrococcygeal teratoma was described in 1978.[37] According to the FDA classification of teratogenesis, acetazolamide is in class D, and its use should be avoided in the first trimester. In the last two trimesters the drug may be used when necessary in treating glaucoma.

Osmotic Diuretics

Mannitol is the prototype of the osmotic diuretics, which are freely filterable at the glomerulus and undergo limited reabsorption by the renal tubules. Their presence in the proximal tubule and loop of Henle reduces the reabsorption of Na^+ and water. Their main use is for prophylaxis against acute renal failure in conditions of severe hemodynamic changes and for reduction of both pressure and volume in the cerebrospinal fluid. Mannitol, given by intraamniotic injection, has been used for induction of abortion.[38] Osmotic diuretics have been used in pregnancy in a patient with water intoxication following oxytocin perfusion.[39]

There are no reports of teratogenesis concerning the treatment with mannitol. Mannitol is in class D of the FDA classification of teratogenesis, and its use should be avoided in the first trimester.

INDICATIONS FOR USE OF DIURETICS IN PREGNANCY

Hypertension

High blood pressure complicates approximately 10% of all pregnancies and remains a major cause of both fetal and maternal morbidity and mortality.[40] The recent working group on high blood pressure in pregnancy[41] suggested abandoning the term "pregnancy-induced hypertension" (PIH), which fails to differentiate transient hypertension with a benign prognosis from the more ominous preeclampsia. These authors adopted the classification proposed in 1972 by the American College of Obstetricians and Gynecologists, which identifies four categories of hypertension associated with pregnancy:

1. Chronic hypertension, defined as a blood pressure equal to or greater than 140/90 mmHg that is present and observable before pregnancy or diagnosed before the 20th week of gestation. Hypertension diagnosed for the first time during pregnancy and persisting beyond the 42nd day postpartum is also classified as chronic hypertension.
2. Preeclampsia/eclampsia, defined as increments in blood pressure of 30 and 15 mmHg over previous systolic and diastolic levels, respectively, that usually oc-

cur after the 20th week of gestation. The hypertension can be accompanied by proteinuria of 0.3 gram or greater in a 24-hour specimen and by edema.

3. Preeclampsia superimposed on chronic hypertension.

4. Transient hypertension, defined as development of elevated blood pressure during pregnancy or in the first 24 hours postpartum without other signs of or preexisting hypertension. The blood pressure returns to normal within 10 days after delivery.

The differential diagnosis may be difficult because there are no reliable tests for distinguishing between the different categories of hypertension. The need to distinguish preeclampsia from other disorders is particularly important in women in midpregnancy (before gestational week 28), since elevated blood pressure due to essential hypertension may be managed conservatively, while in case of severe preeclampsia, conservative treatment may be disastrous.[42]

Sodium restriction or diuretic therapy has no role in the prevention or treatment of preeclampsia. It is known that preeclampsia is associated with reduction of plasma volume,[4] and any further reduction in plasma volume may be detrimental to the mother but even more to the fetus. For example, fetal outcome is worse in women with chronic hypertension who do not have expanded plasma volume.[43] This theoretical concern must be tempered by extensive experience in several well-controlled studies with the prophylactic use of diuretics in normotensive gravid women in whom no excess of perinatal death or morbidity was evident.[44] There is no conclusive answer to the question, "Does treatment of chronic hypertension prevent preeclampsia?" A meta-analysis of nine randomized trials with diuretics including more than 7000 subjects revealed a decrease in edema and hypertension but not prevention of preeclampsia or reduction of perinatal mortality.[6]

The hypertension of preeclampsia should be treated to try and avoid overt eclampsia and the dreaded HELLP (hemolysis, elevated liver enzymes, low platelet count) syndrome. However, aggressive antihypertensive therapy in preeclampsia is of questionable advisability because of the disagreement about the uteroplacental blood flow autoregulation. Even the aggressive therapist will select methyldopa, hydralazine, β-adrenergic blockers, and calcium blockers, but not diuretics. No evidence is provided for the advantage of aggressive antihypertensive therapy, although a small study claims a reduction of proteinuria by intensive anti-hypertensive treatment.[45] Invasive monitoring of central pressures in patients with severe preeclampsia may optimize treatment and clinical status before delivery.[46]

Although data concerning the use of diuretics in pregnant women with chronic hypertension is sparse, diuretics can be used safely if indicated but not as first-line antihypertensive agents. The beneficial effect of antihypertensive drugs in preexisting chronic hypertension was proved with methyldopa,

which is recommended as drug of choice,[47] hydralazine, β-adrenergic blockers,[48] and labetalol.[49] Because of teratogenesis in rats, calcium channel blockers are not recommended apart from preterm labor.[50] Angiotensin-converting enzyme inhibitors are contraindicated in pregnancy because of their possible adverse effect on fetal kidney. Their use has been associated with oligohydramnios and neonatal death from renal failure.[51] They may be used in pregnancy in hypertensive patients with scleroderma.[52]

Transient hypertension develops after midpregnancy, often near term or in puerperium. This condition is often predictive of the eventual development of essential hypertension. Intravenous hydralazine can be used to control severe postpartum hypertension, to be replaced later by standard oral antihypertensive agents.

In summary, diuretics do not prevent preeclampsia or perinatal death and are hazardous in preeclampsia. They may occasionally be useful in the treatment of chronic hypertension but not as first-line drugs, and only in combination with antiadrenergic agents and vasodilators, especially if refractoriness to the latter is due to excessive sodium retention.

Congestive Heart Failure

Furosemide and thiazides, with or without digoxin, remain the best treatments for congestive heart failure and pulmonary edema in pregnancy.[9] Angiotensin-converting enzyme inhibitors are contraindicated in pregnancy because of their possible adverse effect on fetal kidney: The use of these agents has been associated with oligohydramnios and neonatal death from renal failure.[51] Recently, three groups of pulmonary edema associated with pregnancy were identified by echocardiographic studies: patients with decreased systolic function, patients with normal systolic function but impaired diastolic function, and patients with normal hearts in whom pulmonary edema was due to tocolytic therapy and iatrogenic volume overload. Diuretics may be used in all three groups. In patients with diastolic dysfunction, however, diuresis must be closely monitored because excessive reduction in central blood volume may reduce preload below that necessary to fill the stiff ventricle adequately and thereby maintain forward cardiac output.[53]

Miscellaneous

Diuretics have been used in left heart failure due to amniotic fluid embolism,[54] in renal failure due to acute fatty liver of pregnancy,[55] and to reduce hypercalciuria in a pregnant woman with idiopathic hypoparathyroidism.[56]

CONTRAINDICATIONS

Diuretics are contraindicated in the setting in which uteroplacental perfusion is already reduced, that is, in patients with preeclampsia and in cases of intrauterine growth retardation.

According to the FDA classification of teratogenesis, furosemide is in group C, while thiazides, potassium-sparing agents, carbonic anhydrase inhibitors, and osmotic diuretics are classed as D. Detailed description on teratogenesis of each drug may be found in the FDA's listing in the section Pharmacology of Diuretics. In a surveillance study of Michigan Medicaid recipients involving 229,191 completed pregnancies conducted between 1985 and 1992, a number of newborns were exposed to diuretics: 635 to thiazides, 350 to furosemide, and 31 to spironolactone. No association was found between diuretics and congenital defects. There was only a suggestion of a connection between use of furosemide and hypospadias.[19]

LACTATION

Thiazides,[57] furosemide, and acetazolamide are excreted into breast milk. However, the risk of pharmacological effect on the nursing infant are remote. The administration of thiazides is not recommended in the first month of lactation because these agents may inhibit milk formation.[58] It is not known whether unmetabolized spirononlactone is excreted in breast milk. However, canrenone, the principal metabolite, has been found in breast milk.[59] The effect on the infant from this ingestion in unknown. There are no data concerning mannitol and lactation. The American Academy of Pediatrics considers the use of these drugs to be compatible with breast feeding.[60]

REFERENCES

1. Finnerty FA Jr, Bepko FJ Jr. Lowering the perinatal mortality and the prematurity rate: the value of prophylactic thiazides in juveniles. *JAMA* 1966;195:429–432.

2. Robertson EG. The natural history of oedema during pregnancy. *J Obstet Gynaecol Br Commonw* 1971;78:520–529.

3. Christianson R, Page EW. Diuretic drugs and pregnancy. *Obstet Gynecol* 1976;48:647–652.

4. Hays PM, Cruikshank DP, Dunn LJ. Plasma volume determination in normal and preeclamptic pregnancies. *Am J Obstet Gynecol* 1985;151:958–966.

5. Sibai BM, Grossman RA, Grossman HG. Effects of diuretics on plasma volume in pregnancies with long-term hypertension. *Am J Obstet Gynecol* 1984;150:831–835.

6. Collins R, Yusuf S, Peto R. Overview of randomized trials in pregnancy. *Br Med J* 1985;290:17–23.

7. Lindheimer MD, Katz AI. Sodium and diuretics in pregnancy. *N Engl J Med* 1973;288:891–894.

8. Wide-Swensson D, Montal S. Ingemarsson I. How do Swedish obstetricians manage hypertensive disorders in pregnancy? *Acta Obstet Gynecol Scand* 1994;73:619–624.

9. Raymond R, Underwood DA, Moodie DS. Cardiovascular problems in pregnancy. *Cleveland Clin J Med* 1987;54:95–104.

10. Gant NF, Daley GL, Chand S, Whalley PJ, MacDonald PC. A study of angiotensin II pressor response throughout primigravid pregnancy. *J Clin Invest* 1973;52:2682–2689.

11. Walsh SW. Preeclampsia: an imbalance in placental prostacyclin and thromboxane production. *Am J Obstet Gynecol* 1985;152:335–340.

12. Mabie WC, Pernoll ML, Biswas MK. Chronic hypertension in pregnancy. *Obstet Gynecol* 1986;67:197–205.

13. Beermann B, Groschinsky-Grind M, Fahraeus L, Lindstrom B. Placental transfer of furosemide. *Clin Pharmacol Ther* 1978;24:560–562.

14. Votta RA, Parada OH, Winogard RH, Alvarez OH, Tomassinni TL, Pastori AA. Furosemide action on the creatinine concentration of amniotic fluid. *Am J Obstet Gynecol* 1975;123:621–624.

15. Suonio S, Saarikoski S, Tahvanainen K, Paakkonen A, Olkkonen H. Acute effects of dihydralazine mesylate, furosemide, and metoprolol on maternal hemodynamics in pregnancy-induced hypertension. *Am J Obstet Gynecol* 1985;155:122–125.

16. Barrett RJ, Rayburn WF, Barr M Jr. Furosemide (Lasix) challenge test in assessing bilateral fetal hydronephrosis. *Am J Obstet Gynecol* 1983;147:846–847.

17. Harman CR. Maternal furosemide may not provoke urine production in the compromised fetus. *Am J Obstet Gynecol* 1984;150:322–323.

18. Pecorari D, Rangi N, Autera C. Administration of furosemide to women during confinement, and its action on the newborn infants. *Acta Biomed (Italy)* 1969;40:2–11.

19. Briggs GG, Freeman RK, Yaffe SJ. *Drugs in Pregnancy and Lactation.* 4th ed. Baltimore: Williams & Williams; 1994.

20. Prichard JA, Walley PJ. Severe hypokalemia due to prolonged administration of chlorothiazide during pregnancy. *Am J Obstet Gynecol* 1961;81:1241–1244.

21. McAllister CJ, Stull CG, Courey NG. Amniotic fluid levels of uric acid and creatinine in toxemic patients. Possible relation to diuretic use. *Am J Obstet Gynecol* 1973;115:560–563.

22. Goldman JA, Neri A, Ovadia J. Eckerling B, DeVries A. Effect of chlorothiazide on intravenous glucose tolerance in pregnancy. *Am J Obstet Gynecol* 1969;105:556–560.

23. Lander CN, Pearson JW, Herrick CN, Harrison HE. The effect of chlorothiazide on blood glucose in the third trimester of pregnancy. *Obstet Gynecol* 1964;23:555–560.

24. Minkowitz S, Soloway HB, Hall JE, Yermakov V. Fatal hemorrhagic pancreatitis following chlorothiazide administration in pregnancy. *Obstet Gynecol* 1964;24:337–342.

25. Schifrin BS, Spellacy WN, Little WA. Maternal death associated with excessive ingestion of a chlorothiazide diuretic. *Obstet Gynecol* 1969;34:215–220.

26. Senior B, Slone D, Shapiro S, Mitchell AA, Heinonen OP. Benzothiazides and neonatal hypoglycaemia. *Lancet* 1976;2:377.

27. Rodrigues SU, Leikin SL, Hiller MC. Neonatal thrombocytopenia associated with ante-partum administration of thiazide drugs. *N Engl J Med* 1964;270:881–884.

28. Harley JD, Robin H, Robertson SEJ. Thiazide-induced neonatal haemolysis? *Br Med J* 1964;1:696–697.

29. Alstatt LB. Transplacental hyponatremia in the newborn infant. *J Pediatr* 1965;66:985–988.

30. Anderson GG, Hanson TM. Chronic fetal bradycardia: possible association with hypokalemia. *Obstet Gynecol* 1974;44: 896–898.

31. Shoemaker ES, Gant NF, Madden JD, MacDonald PC. The effect of thiazide diuretics on placental function. *Texas Med* 1973;69:109–115.

32. Gant NF, Madden JD, Siteri PK, MacDonald PC. The metabolic clearance rate of dehydroisoandrosterone sulfate. The effect of thiazide diuretics in normal and future preeclamptic pregnancies. *Am J Obstet Gynecol* 1975;123:159–163.

33. Heinonen OP, Slone D, Shapiro S. *Birth Defects and Drugs in Pregnancy.* Littleton, MA: Publishing Sciences Group, 1977;371–373.

34. Messina M, Biffignandi P, Ghigo E, Jeantet MG, Molinatti GM. Possible contraindication or spironolactone during pregnancy. *J Endocrinol Invest* 1990;2:222. Letter.

35. Meeker DP, Barnett GH. Right pleural effusion due to a migrating ventriculoperitoneal shunt. *Cleveland Clin J Med* 1994;61:144–146.

36. Merlob P, Litwin A, Mor N. Possible association between acetazolamide administration during pregnancy and metabolic disorders in the newborn. *Eur J Obstet Gynecol Reprod Biol* 1990;35:85–88.

37. Worsham F Jr, Beckman EN, Mitchell EH. Sacrococcygeal teratoma in a neonate. Association with maternal use of acetazolamide. *JAMA* 1978;240:251–252.

38. Craft IL, Musa BD. Hypertonic solutions to induce abortion. *Br Med J* 1971;2:49.

39. Borg G, Seligmann G, Sournies G, Thoulon JM. Water intoxication following oxytocin perfusion. *J Gynecol Obstet Biol Reprod Paris* 1983;12:51–53.

40. Lindheimer MD. Hypertension in pregnancy. *Hypertension* 1993;22:127–137.

41. National High Blood Pressure Education Program Working Group Report on High Blood Pressure in Pregnancy. *Am J Obstet Gynecol* 1990;163:1689–1712.

42. Sibai BM, Taslimi M, Abdella TN, Brooks TF, Spinnato JA, Anderson GD. Maternal and perinatal outcome of conservative management of severe pre-eclampsia in midtrimester. *Am J Obstet Gynecol* 1985;152:32–37.

43. Arias F, Zamora J. Antihypertensive treatment and pregnancy outcome in patients with mild chronic hypertension. *Obstet Gynecol* 1979;53:489–494.

44. Kraus GW, Marchese JR, Yen SSC. Prophylactic use of hydrochlorothiazide in pregnancy. *JAMA* 1966;198:1150–1154.

45. Blake S, MacDonald D. The prevention of the maternal manifestations of preeclampsia by intensive antihypertensive treatment. *Br J Obstet Gynaecol* 1991;98:244–248.

46. Hjertberg R, Belfrage P, Hagnevik K. Hemodynamic measurements with Swan–Ganz catheter in women with severe proteinuric gestational hypertension (pre-eclampsia). *Acta Obstet Gynecol Scand* 1991;70:193–198.

47. Redman CW. Fetal outcome in trial of antihypertensive treatment in pregnancy. *Lancet* 1976;2:753–756.

48. Fletcher AE, Bulpitt CJ. A review of clinical trials in pregnancy. In: Rubin PC, ed. *Hypertension in Pregnancy.* New York: Elsevier, 1988;186–201.

49. Sibai BM, Mabie WC, Villar M, Shamsa F, Anderson GD. A comparison of no medication versus methyldopa or labetalol in chronic hypertension during pregnancy. *Am J Obstet Gynecol* 1990;162:960–966.

50. Constantine G, Beevers DG, Reynolds AL, Luesley DM. Nifedipine as a second line antihypertensive drug in pregnancy. *Br J Obstet Gynaecol* 1987;94:1136–1142.

51. Hanssens M, Keirse MJ, Vankelecom F, Van-Assche FA. Fetal and neonatal effects of treatment with angiotensin-converting enzyme inhibitors in pregnancy. *Obstet Gynecol* 1991;78: 128–135.

52. Baethge BA, Wolf RE. Successful pregnancy with scleroderma renal disease and pulmonary hypertension in a patient using angiotensin converting enzyme inhibitors. *Ann Rheum Dis* 1989;48:776–778.

53. Mabie WC, Hackman BB, Sibai BM. Pulmonary edema associated with pregnancy. Echocardiographic insights and implications for treatment. *Obstet Gynecol* 1993;81:227–234.

54. Vanmaele L, Noppen M, Vincken W, De-Catte L, Huyghens L. Transient left heart failure in amniotic fluid embolism. *Intensive Care Med* 1990;16:269–271.

55. Mabie WC. Acute fatty liver of pregnancy. *Gastroenterol Clin North Am* 1992;21:951–960.

56. Kurzel PB, Hagen GA. Use of thiazide diuretics to reduce the hypercalciuria of hypoparathyroidism during pregnancy. *Am J Perinatol* 1990;7:333–336.

57. Werthmann MW, Krees SV. Excretion of chlorothiazide in human breast milk. *J Pediatr* 1972;81:781–783.

58. Healy M. Suppressing lactation with oral diuretics. *Lancet* 1961;1:1353–1354.

59. Phelps DL, Karim Z. Spironolactone: relationship between concentrations of dethioacetylated metabolite in human serum and milk. *J Pharm Sci* 1977;66:1203.

60. American Academy of Pediatrics Committee on Drugs. The transfer of drugs and other chemicals into breast milk. *Pediatrics* 1994;93:137–150.

29

THE USE OF β-ADRENERGIC BLOCKING AGENTS IN PREGNANCY AND LACTATION

AGNETA K. HURST, PHARMD, KRISTINA HOFFMAN, PHARMD, WILLIAM H. FRISHMAN, MD, AND URI ELKAYAM, MD

INTRODUCTION

The therapeutic indications for β-adrenergic blocking drugs are varied. These drugs have proven their efficacy in the treatment of hypertension, arrhythmias, hyperthyroidism, atherosclerotic heart disease, essential tremor, migraine headache, and glaucoma.[1] Many of these conditions will manifest themselves during the reproductive years of the female patient.

This chapter first describes the unique pharmacologic properties of different beta blockers and their pharmacokinetic behavior during pregnancy. The world experience with beta-blocker treatment during pregnancy and lactation is then assessed. Finally, recommendations concerning administration of these agents during pregnancy are proposed in light of this world experience.

ADRENERGIC INFLUENCES ON MATERNAL–FETAL PHYSIOLOGY

α-Adrenergic agonists influence umbilical blood flow indirectly, through their action on uterine blood vessels. When a low dose of norepinephrine was infused directly into the uterine artery, a profound reduction in uteroplacental blood flow developed.[2] A direct action of norepinephrine on the umbilical circulation has not been demonstrated.[3,4]

In the myometrium, there are adrenergic receptors of the α and β types (Table 29.1). Stimulation of the β-adrenergic receptors results in myometrial relaxation, whereas increased

α-adrenergic stimulation potentiates contractility.[5] In animal studies, propranolol has been shown to reverse the myometrial depressant action of β-adrenergic stimulation.[6] Barden and Stander[7] also demonstrated this effect of propranolol in pregnant humans. In their study, pregnant women at term were selected for elective induction of labor. Maternal and fetal heart rates, maternal blood pressure, and intrauterine pressure were measured in all patients. After an infusion of oxytocin to eight patients, epinephrine was administered; the result was a consistent inhibition of uterine activity accompanied by an accelerating maternal heart rate. These effects were completely reversed if the epinephrine was preceded by treatment with propranolol. Norepinephrine infusion potentiated uterine activity while decreasing maternal heart rate and increasing blood pressure. Prior propranolol treatment had no effect, whereas the α-adrenergic blocker phentolamine significantly attenuated the actions of norepinephrine. After these studies, all the subjects had normal term vaginal deliveries.

The influence of the sympathetic nervous system on normal fetal circulation has also been studied in the fetal lamb preparation. In a report by Joelson and Barton,[8] isoproterenol administered to the fetus caused an increase in heart rate and a decrease in blood pressure, whereas propranolol caused only a slight drop in heart rate. It was apparent that the effects of β-adrenergic blockade in the unstressed and undisturbed fetus were minimal. However when the fetus is stressed, stimulation of the β-adrenergic receptor may provide an important reserve for neonatal adaptation. Thus, maternal treatment with beta blockers may impair the response to fetal distress.

Cardiac Problems in Pregnancy, Third Edition
Edited by Uri Elkayam, MD, and Norbert Gleicher, MD
Copyright © 1998 by Wiley-Liss, Inc. ISBN 0-471-16358-9

TABLE 29.1 Effects of α- and β-Adrenergic Receptor Stimulation and Blockade on Maternal–Fetal Physiology

Physiologic Characteristic	Stimulation		Blockade	
	α-Receptor	β-Receptor	α-Receptor	β-Receptor
Fetal heart rate	↔	↑	↔	↔ ↓
Maternal heart rate	↔	↑	↔	↓
Umbilical blood flow	↔	↑	↔	↓
Myometrial activity	↑	↓	↓	↑

Symbols: ↔, no effect; ↑, increase; ↓, decrease.

GENERAL CONSIDERATIONS WHEN β-ADRENERGIC BLOCKERS ARE USED DURING PREGNANCY AND LACTATION

Beta blockers can be divided into several categories based on beta-receptor specificity, intrinsic sympathomimetic activity (ISA), and the presence or absence of alpha receptor effects (Table 29.2).

In general, selectivity for β_1-adrenergic receptors is a desirable feature in cardiac patients, since effects on respiratory and uterine systems are to be avoided. Drugs with ISA may also have an advantage in pregnant patients treated for hypertension (but not for rhythm disturbances), since there may be fewer changes in the uteroplacental circulation, in uterine activity, and in the fetal heart rate.

All beta blockers cross the placenta and have been found in the fetal circulation (Table 29.3). At birth, neonatal plasma concentration is very similar to that in the maternal circulation but may transiently rise after delivery.[9–12] Although the exact cause of this finding is not known, redistribution of the drug secondary to the changing hemodynamic status of the neonate may be responsible.

The American Academy of Pediatrics considers maternal beta-blocker administration to be compatible with breast feeding.[13] All beta blockers are secreted into breast milk in lactating women (Table 29.3). Milk is slightly acidic, and basic compounds such as the beta-blocking drugs will become ionized and trapped. As a result, milk concentrations may be much higher than plasma concentrations. Since the amount of drug secreted into milk depends on maternal plasma concentrations, which are constantly fluctuating, the amount of drug ingested by the nursing infant is difficult to assess. Nursing at times of the minimum concentrations should, therefore, be encouraged (or conversely, the time of maxi-

TABLE 29.2 β-Adrenergic Blockers Used in Pregnancy and Lactation

Generic Name	Trade Name	FDA Risk Category	Experience in Pregnancy	Predominant Receptor Blocked	ISA
Acebutolol	Sectral	B	Hypertension	β_1	Yes
Atenolol	Tenormin	C	Hypertension[a] Arrhythmias[a]	β_1	No
Betaxolol	Kerlone		Hypertension	β_1	No
Celiprolol	Selecor	B	Hypertension[a]	β_1	Yes[b]
Esmolol	Brevibloc	C	Hypertension[c] Arrhythmias[c]	β_1	No
Labetalol	Normodyne Trandate	C	Hypertension[a]	$\beta_1, \beta_2, \alpha_1$	No
Metoprolol	Lopressor	B	Hypertension[a]	β_1	No
Nadolol	Corgard	C	Hypertension[c]	β_1, β_2	No
Oxprenolol		C	Hypertension[a]	β_1, β_2	Yes
Pindolol	Visken	B	Hypertension[a]	β_1, β_2	Yes
Propranolol	Inderal Ipran	C	Hypertension[a] Arrhythmias	β_1, β_2	No
Sotalol	Betapace	B	Hypertension[a] Arrhythmias[c]	β_1, β_2	No

[a]Clinical trial.
[b]β_2-specific.
[c]Case report.

TABLE 29.3   Concentration Ratios of β-Adrenergic Blocking Drugs During Pregnancy and Lactation

Drug	Ratios	
	Cord Blood/Maternal Blood	Breast Milk/Maternal Blood
Acebutolol	0.8	2.3–9.2
(diacetalol)[a]	(0.6)	(1.5–13.5)
Atenolol	≈1	1.5–6.8
Betaxolol	0.6–1.2	>2
Celiprolol	0.2–0.5	
Esmolol		
Labetalol	0.3–0.5	0.8–2.6
Metoprolol	≈1	2–4
Nadolol		4.6
Oxprenolol	0.2–0.4	0.2–0.4
Pindolol	0.4–0.7	
Propranolol	0.2–1.3	0.3–1.7
Sotalol	0.5–1.4	2.4–5.6

[a]Active metabolite of acebutolol.

mum concentrations, which usually occurs within 3 hours of the dose, should be avoided) to minimize drug ingestion by the child.

CLINICAL EXPERIENCE

Propranolol

Propranolol was the first beta blocker to be used in pregnant patients and is classified in the pregnancy risk category C of the U.S. Food and Drug Administration (FDA). The drug has been employed successfully in the treatment of gestational hypertension,[14] thyrotoxicosis,[15] obstructive cardiomyopathy,[16] paroxysmal atrial tachycardia,[17,18] dysfunctional uterine activity,[19] and fetal tachycardia.[20]

Propranolol is a lipophilic compound, well absorbed from the gastrointestinal tract, but with a low absolute bioavailability due to extensive first-pass metabolism in the liver. The absolute bioavailability has been measured in pregnant patients at 32 and 36 weeks of gestation and postpartum. Although bioavailability of the drug was not significantly different during pregnancy and in the postpartum period, there were large interindividual differences, and the bioavailability ranged between 7 and 77%.[21] Propranolol is extensively protein bound (about 90%); its binding, however, may be slightly reduced during pregnancy, resulting in higher concentrations of free drug.[22,23] In the neonate, protein binding may be much lower (43%), possibly due to altered α_1-acid glycoprotein concentrations.[22,24] Rubin[25] and O'Hare[21] evaluated the disposition of propranolol during pregnancy and concluded that pregnancy has no effect on the maternal clearance, volume of distribution, area under the concentra-

tion–time curve, and the elimination half-life of the drug. At birth, cord serum propranolol concentrations have been reported to vary from 19% to 127% of maternal concentrations.[26] Comparisons of cord and maternal plasma concentrations and protein binding of propranolol and a major metabolite, naphthoxylactic acid, suggest that metabolism of propranolol occurs in the placenta and fetus.[27] There appear to be significant changes in the drug disposition in the newborn shortly after birth. It has been observed that 4 hours after delivery, the serum concentration in the newborn significantly increases, with the levels approximately doubling, possibly secondary to redistribution.[11] In addition, the half-life of propranolol is increased, probably because of the neonate's immature hepatic function.[24]

Despite the predominantly encouraging experience with propranolol therapy, many severe adverse reactions have also been reported (Table 29.4). The most consistent observation has been intrauterine fetal growth retardation. In a long-term study of 12 pregnant women receiving chronic propranolol, Pruyn et al.[28] demonstrated poor intrauterine growth in half their cases. Decreased umbilical blood flow reported in the ewe after chronic propranolol administration may explain these findings.

In contrast to the findings of Pruyn et al, the incidence of fetal growth retardation in five prospective studies with propranolol and oxprenolol in 94 pregnancies was only 4%.[14,29–32] In addition, two of the mothers whose babies were small for gestational age had normal-sized babies in subsequent pregnancies despite continued propranolol therapy.[32] Furthermore, Livingstone et al,[33] who compared methyldopa to propranolol in a 3-year randomized prospective study in 28 women with pregnancy-associated hypertension, found the two drugs to be equally effective and in the

TABLE 29.4 Reported Adverse Effects of β-Adrenergic Blocking Drugs During Pregnancy and in the Neonate

Adverse Effects	Drugs										
	Acebutolol	Atenolol	Betaxolol	Esmolol	Labetalol	Metoprolol	Nadolol	Oxprenolol	Pindolol	Propranolol	Sotalol
IN UTERO											
Fetal bradycardia		X	X	X	X		X			X	X
Low placental weight		X									
Premature labor											X
Prolonged labor										X	
Fetal distress leading to cesarean section				X		X					
Decreased response to sound stimulus										X	
NEONATAL											
Low birth weight	X	X					X			X	X
Hypoglycemia	X	X					X			X	
Respiratory dysfunction				X	X		X			X	X
Hyperbilirubinemia					X					X	
Circulatory collapse					X						
Hypothermia							X				
Poor muscle tone				X							

treatment of maternal hypertension and no significant difference in the birth weights of the babies in the two groups.

Fetal side effects associated with propranolol during pregnancy include hypoglycemia in the newborn,[33] decreased fetal heart rate response to sound stimulus,[34] birth apnea,[35] bradycardia,[36] polycythemia,[37] hyperbilirubinemia,[28] and prolonged labor,[36] as well as a case report of fetal death associated with propranolol administration.[38] None of the foregoing reactions were reported consistently in chronic therapy studies. Many of these reactions may represent consequences of fetal distress occurring in high risk obstetrical patients. However, these isolated case reports deserve close attention and consideration.

Propranolol is excreted into breast milk.[27,39,40] A milk/maternal plasma concentration ratio of approximately 1 was observed 3 hours after single oral doses of 20–160 mg given several days apart in two nursing mothers.[40] The drug appears to be secreted into breast milk in a dose-dependent manner, and the milk-to-plasma ratio varies with the fluctuations of the plasma concentrations.[40] In three lactating women receiving chronic propranolol therapy, breast milk/whole plasma ratios of propranolol ranged from 0.33 to 1.65.[40a] The increase in ratio appeared to correlate with a longer time interval since the last dose. The half-life of propranolol in breast milk was 6.5 ± 3.4 hours in breast milk and 2.6 ± 1.2 hours in maternal plasma.[40a] Two of propranolol's major metabolites, propranolol glucuronide and naphthoxylactic acid, were excreted into the breast milk but to a lesser extent than propranolol.[27] In another case, breast milk concentrations were less than 40% of the peak maternal plasma concentrations after a single propranolol dose of 40 mg and less than 64% after chronic dosing (60 mg, four times daily). Breast milk and plasma concentrations were maximal 3 hours after a dose. While plasma concentrations were higher than breast milk concentrations at 3 hours during chronic dosing, these concentrations were equal 8 hours after the last dose. After 30 days of chronic dosing, breast milk concentrations were 64 mg/L 3 hours after the dose and 26 mg/L predose. It was estimated that a nursing infant would ingest 32 µg in a 24-hour period (assuming a total milk ingestion not exceeding 500 mL/day and maternal propranolol doses of 240 mg/day). This dose would be only 1% of the pediatric dose used for treatment. Because neonates have immature hepatic metabolism, however, close observation of nursing infants is recommended.[39]

Nadolol

Nadolol is a nonselective β-adrenergic blocking drug with no intrinsic sympathomimetic activity; it is low in lipid solubility and in protein binding.[41] The drug is indicated for the treatment of hypertension and angina. The serum half-life is long (20–24 hours), and the drug is excreted unchanged by the kidneys.[41]

Experience with nadolol in pregnancy is limited to one report of an infant whose mother was treated throughout the pregnancy with 20 mg of nadolol a day; at delivery, the cord nadolol concentration was 43 ng/mL.[12] In addition to nadolol, the mother was receiving triamterene and hydrochlorothiazide for IgA nephropathy and hypertension. Delivery was by emergency cesarean section at 35 weeks of gestation. The infant was small for gestational age and experienced respiratory dysfunction (initially tachypnea and then depressed respiration), bradycardia, hypoglycemia, and hypothermia. The infant's serum concentration increased 12 hours after delivery from 43 ng/mL to 145 ng/mL and at 38 hours was 80 ng/mL. Respiratory and cardiac effects in the neonate persisted for 72 hours. Although the maternal disease could account for fetal growth retardation and, along with the diuretic therapy, could also cause hypoglycemia, nadolol's long serum half-life, renal elimination, and low protein binding may predispose the fetus and the newborn to toxic side effects.[12,26]

Nadolol is excreted into breast milk.[42] In 12 lactating normotensive women receiving 80 mg of nadolol daily, the mean steady state breast milk concentration was 4.6 times the mean serum concentration. It was estimated that 2–7% of the therapeutic pediatric dose of drug would be ingested daily by the infant.

Sotalol

Sotalol is a noncardioselective beta-blocking drug without ISA. Independent of the effects on the beta-receptors, sotalol prolongs the action potential duration in the atria, the ventricle, and the His–Purkinje fibers and has class III antiarrhythmic effects.[43] It does not have the myocardial depressant effect seen with most other beta-blocking drugs.[43,44] The drug is a hydrophilic compound, with low plasma protein binding.[45] It is 100% bioavailable, with peak plasma concentrations occurring 2–4 hours after a dose.[44] It is primarily excreted unchanged in the urine, and clearance is linearly correlated with creatinine clearance. Dosage adjustment is necessary for patients with impaired renal function.[44,46]

In pregnancy, sotalol has been used to manage patients with chronic hypertension and maternal and fetal arrhythmias. This drug is classified in FDA pregnancy risk category B and is FDA-approved for use in the treatment of ventricular arrhythmias.

A study of the pharmacokinetics of sotalol in the third trimester of pregnant healthy patients[46] demonstrated a plasma half-life of about 11 hours after a single oral dose and about 7 hours after a single intravenous dose. Similar results were obtained in the same women 6 weeks postpartum. The drug clearance was significantly greater in the third trimester: 2.4 mL/min/kg, compared to 1.5 mL/min/kg in the postpartum. The volume of distribution did not change significantly. Sotalol rapidly crosses the placenta, with the maternal-to-cord ratio at birth between 0.7 and 2.1.[11,47,48] Amniotic fluid concentration is higher than the plasma concentration.[47]

There are several case reports of the successful use of sotalol during pregnancy in patients with arrhythmias. Wagner et al[48] described a patient with ventricular tachycardia associated with a left ventricular aneurysm who became pregnant while receiving flecainide (100 mg twice a day) and sotalol (80 mg twice a day). The drugs were continued throughout the pregnancy. A cesarean section was performed at 37 weeks and a normal baby delivered. The fetal heart rate during delivery remained between 130 and 140 beats per minute. One year later the baby was well and normal. In another report, 80 mg sotalol three times daily was used chronically to maintain normal sinus rhythm in a patient with symptomatic supraventricular tachycardia who was first cardioverted with adenosine and atenolol.[49] In another case, a woman with palpitations due to cardiomyopathy received sotalol (80 mg, three times daily) during her pregnancy. She successfully delivered a healthy 3.33 kg infant at 42 weeks of gestation.[50]

Sotalol has also been used for treatment of hypertension during pregnancy. O'Hare et al[47] reported using sotalol in 12 patients from 10 weeks of gestation up to 32 weeks. Therapy with 200–800 mg of the drug daily resulted in control of blood pressure. There were 2 spontaneous preterm deliveries. In both cases, however, there were other predisposing factors, including cervical incompetence in one patient and polyhydramnios in the second. Six of the newborns were bradycardic, with heart rates between 60 an 120 beats per minute at birth and persisting for up to 24 hours postpartum. One of the infants suffered severe distress during labor, resulting in an emergency cesarean section, and was asphyxiated at birth but recovered following resuscitation. Four babies were small for gestational age and two had congenital malformations: a large diaphragmatic hernia and the Down syndrome with duodenal atresia. In the latter cases, sotalol was instituted in the 21st and 28th week of gestation, respectively, and was therefore not a likely etiology of these malformations.

Since sotalol fetal blood levels were found to be comparable to the maternal levels, maternal administration of the drug has been used to treat fetal tachyarrhythmias. In six different cases,[51–54] transplacental therapy with sotalol was used to treat supraventricular tachycardia. Concurrent therapy with digoxin, verapamil, and amiodarone was also given. In these cases, at least two patients responded with cardioversion and two had partial responses to therapy.

Sotalol, which has low plasma binding, has been found in significant quantities in breast milk, usually in higher concentrations than in the blood.[47,48,50] In one patient receiving 240 mg daily, the milk-to-serum ratio ranged from 2.43 to 5.64.[50] It was estimated that the infant would have received 20–23% of the maternal dose, or approximately 0.41–0.58 mg/kg. In spite of this significant exposure, no side effects were evident in the infant. However, it is probably wise to carefully monitor babies who are breast-fed by mothers treated with sotalol.

In conclusion, sotalol has been used in a small number of pregnant women to control maternal blood pressure and maternal and fetal arrhythmias. In view of its potential maternal proarrhythmic side effects, and the perinatal complications experienced in patients with chronic hypertension, sotalol is best reserved for the treatment of serious maternal or fetal arrhythmias not responding to drugs with more established safety profiles.

Labetalol

Labetalol is a unique antihypertensive drug with β_1-, β_2-, and postsynaptic α_1-adrenoreceptor-blocking activity. In general, the β-adrenergic receptor effects predominate and the relative potencies of α- to β-receptor effects vary depending on the route of administration.[41] When labetalol is given orally, the α:β effects ratio is about 1:3; when given intravenously it is about 1:7.

Labetalol has been used in pregnancy to control blood pressure in essential hypertension, pregnancy-induced hypertension, preeclampsia, and eclampsia. It is classified in FDA pregnancy risk category C. Labetalol is rapidly absorbed when taken orally, with peak blood concentrations occurring in one hour in pregnant patients.[55] It is metabolized in the liver and has an extensive first-pass effect. Bioavailability ranges from 11 to 68%. The plasma half-life in the third trimester ranges from 1.7 to 5.8 hours.[55,56] During the third trimester, clearance after oral dosing is between 20–39 mL/min/kg.[57] Labetalol crosses the placenta, and fetal cord/maternal concentrations ratio at birth have been reported to be in the range of 0.3–0.5.[55,56,58] Amniotic fluid and the maternal blood contain approximately equivalent labetalol concentrations.[56,59]

The blood pressure response to labetalol in pregnant patients is similar to that in nonpregnant patients. The maximum effect on the systolic and diastolic blood pressure after an oral dose occurs at 4 and 2 hours respectively, and in 30 minutes after an intravenous dose.[55,60] The changes in blood pressure and the plasma concentration have been evaluated, and there appears to be a five- to six-fold interpatient variability in the sensitivity to the drug.[55] The effect on the maternal heart rate is modest, with a change from baseline of approximately 10 beats per minute.[55] Beneficial effects have been observed in patients with pregnancy-induced hypertension treated with labetalol. In a randomized, placebo-controlled evaluation of 144 patients with mild to moderate hypertension, 70 patients received 300–600 mg of labetalol. A decrease in proteinuria was observed when the labetalol therapy was initiated before 32 weeks of gestation.[61] These findings may suggest that labetalol induces a decrease in progression to preeclampsia and eclampsia in patients with pregnancy-induced hypertension. There was no evidence of benefit in this respect when the drug was initiated later than 32 weeks.

In an additional study, labetalol was effective in managing pregnant patients with essential hypertension. The effect of labetalol was compared to methyldopa and placebo in 300 patients with mild chronic hypertension.[62] Labetalol was given in doses between 300 and 2400 mg a day, starting in the first trimester. The blood pressure was effectively controlled with either drug compared to placebo. There were no congenital abnormalities nor intrauterine growth retardation, and neonatal glucose concentrations were normal. No difference was found in the perinatal outcome between drug therapy and placebo when Apgar scores, birth weight, and premature deliveries were evaluated. The authors concluded that treatment of mild essential hypertension provides no benefit during pregnancy and drug therapy should be reserved for severe hypertension.

Another study,[63] evaluated the effect of labetalol on eclampsia-related ventricular arrhythmias. When compared to dihydralazine, a continuous infusion of labetalol (20–160 mg/h) for 24 hours after delivery decreased the incidence of ventricular arrhythmias and effectively controlled the blood pressure in 18 women. Neonatal outcome, however, was poor with both therapies: 4 stillbirths in the labetalol group and 5 in the dihydralazine group. Three infants in the labetalol group had transient bradycardia at birth.

Pirhonen et al[60] found the effect of labetalol (0.8 mg/kg) on the uterine artery to be related to its effect on mean arterial pressure and was unchanged in 8 out of 10 patients studied in whom arterial pressure decreased by no more than 18%. In the remaining 2 patients who had a 31 and 34% decrease of the mean arterial pressure, there was, however, a decrease in the uterine blood flow. Fetal blood flow, which was measured in the umbilical and middle cerebral arteries, remained unchanged even when the maternal blood flow decreased. Neither the maternal nor the fetal heart rates were affected.[60] In another study 100 mg of labetalol was given intravenously to each of 15 patients. The umbilical artery blood flow and the fetal heart rate were noted to decrease, even though the fetal heart rate remained in the normal range. It was suggested that in fetuses with increased placental vascular resistance (i.e., stressed infants), labetalol's effects are pronounced and may result in decreased blood flow.

In another study, labetalol was compared to hydralazine in 22 very low birth weight babies, of 27–30 weeks gestation, born to preeclamptic mothers. The drug therapy ranged from 1 to 91 days, and no difference was observed in neonatal adaptation to stress between the two different treatments.[65,65a]

Complications with the use of labetalol immediately before cesarean section in preeclamptic patients have been reported. Hemodynamic collapse was observed in one premature (26–27 weeks of gestation) infant whose mother was treated for preeclampsia and given 50 mg of labetalol intravenously prior to cesarean section.[66,66a] Bradycardia, with inadequate breathing and hypotonia immediately after delivery, was reported in another infant; in this case, premature delivery at 33 weeks of gestation had been necessitated by preeclampsia.[9] Intravenous labetalol (50 mg) was given to the mother some hours prior to the cesarean section. The infant had persistent ductus arteriosus and experienced circulatory collapse but recovered. Labetalol blood levels in the neonate were higher on days 3 and 4 compared to day 2, indicating attenuated drug clearance.

Labetalol is excreted into breast milk. The ratio of drug concentration–time curve in milk compared to plasma ranged from 0.8 to 2.6 in three lactating patients.[59] Peak milk concentrations occurred within 3 hours after a dose. Measurable labetalol concentrations were found in one out of three nursing infants, and in that baby the plasma concentration was similar to that of the mother.

In summary, labetalol is effective in controlling maternal blood pressure, and its effects on both maternal and fetal heart rate are very modest. When given in the early stages of pregnancy-induced hypertension, labetalol may slow progression to preeclampsia. The intravenous use of labetalol for the treatment of preeclampsia shortly prior to delivery has been associated in a few cases with bradycardia, inadequate breathing, and circulating collapse in the newborn.

Pindolol

Pindolol has been used to treat pregnancy-induced hypertension and preeclampsia. The FDA has labeled pindolol as a pregnancy risk category B drug.

Pindolol is a nonselective beta-receptor blocking agent with pronounced intrinsic sympathomimetic activity. The pharmacokinetics of pindolol has not been evaluated in pregnant patients. In nonpregnant adults, however, pindolol possesses moderate lipid solubility, is well absorbed, and has an oral bioavailability of almost 100%. The half-life is 3–4 hours with 40% protein binding. About two-thirds of the dose is metabolized in the liver, with urinary excretion of the metabolites and unchanged drug. Poor hepatic function may substantially increase pindolol blood concentrations.[41]

The efficacy of pindolol in pregnancy-induced hypertension was evaluated in a comparative study with methyldopa in the treatment of 32 women.[67] The blood pressure decreased significantly more in the pindolol group, and less adjunct therapy was required. Furthermore, serum creatinine decreased in the pindolol-treated group. There was no difference in the two groups with regard to fetal intrauterine growth, Apgar scores at 1 and 5 minutes, and fetal morbidity. In another trial pindolol was compared with propranolol in the treatment of mild preeclampsia. In this randomized, double-blind study, 20 pregnant patients received either 40 mg of propranolol or 5 mg of pindolol orally, three times a day for 7 days.[68] Both beta-blockers reduced blood pressure significantly. The uteroplacental circulation and umbilical blood flow were evaluated by means of Doppler ultrasound. The lower resistance to flow measured in patients treated with pindolol than in those treated with propranolol is tentatively attributed to the intrinsic sympathomimetic activity of pindolol.

Oxprenolol

Oxprenolol, a nonselective β-adrenergic blocking drug with ISA, is classified by the FDA as a pregnancy risk class C drug. It is moderately lipid soluble and is highly protein bound (80%).[24,26] There is a significant first-pass effect, and the plasma half-life is approximately 2 hours. Oxprenolol crosses the placenta, and the fetal serum concentration at delivery is between 25 and 37% of the maternal serum concentration.[26]

The benefit of oxprenolol when used to manage pregnancy-induced hypertension occurring after 20 weeks of gestation was evaluated in a study by Plouin et al.[69] One hundred fifty-six patients with pregnancy-induced hypertension after the 20th gestational week were randomized to receive either placebo or oxprenolol (160–320 mg, twice daily). All patients had diastolic blood pressures exceeding 85 mmHg and received additional antihypertensive drugs if the diastolic blood pressure went above 105 mmHg. There was a decrease in the number of patients progressing to a diastolic blood pressure exceeding 105 mmHg in the oxprenolol group compared to placebo. In addition, oxprenolol reduced the incidence of cesarean sections and induction of labor due to fetal or maternal distress. Infant birth weights were the same, and incidence of Apgar scores less than 7 at one minute and neonatal respiratory distress were significantly reduced in the oxprenolol group.

Oxprenolol was compared to methyldopa in two different trials.[31,70] In the first trial, birth weight of babies exposed to oxprenolol was significantly higher than that for those exposed to methyldopa. However, the difference resolved by the 10th week postpartum.[31,71] The second study failed to show any differences in birth weight, placental weight, head size, and Apgar scores that were attributable to the two drugs.[70] Oxprenolol was used in combination with prazosin to control blood pressure in 25 patients with severe essential hypertension and in 19 with pregnancy-induced hypertension.[72] Blood pressure was successfully controlled in the first but not in the latter group.

As with other beta blockers, oxprenolol is excreted into breast milk. In a study of 25 lactating hypertensive women receiving oxprenolol, the milk-to-plasma ratio was 0.29 ±0.14.[70] It was estimated that a nursing infant would ingest only between 0.019 and 0.071 mg twice daily, which is less than one-tenth of the recommended pediatric dose.

In conclusion, the majority of available data demonstrate efficacy of oxprenolol in blood pressure control during pregnancy. There is some evidence that its use in pregnancy-induced hypertension is associated with a decreased rate of complicated deliveries and perinatal morbidity.

Metoprolol

Metoprolol is a β$_1$-selective adrenoreceptor blocking drug, and the FDA has placed it in pregnancy risk category C. Metoprolol is approved for the treatment of hypertension, angina, and myocardial infarction.[41] It has been used to treat pregnant patients with gestational hypertension.

The pharmacokinetics of metoprolol has been studied in pregnant patients.[10,73,74,74a] Metoprolol is moderately lipid soluble, has low protein binding, and readily enters the central nervous system. The drug is well absorbed, but oral bioavailability is low because of a first-pass effect that may vary between 40 and 77%, depending on the dosage form. Bioavailability increases when the drug is given with food. Serum concentration and systemic bioavailability of oral metoprolol have been found to be significantly lower in pregnancy than in nonpregnant patients.[74] Metoprolol is oxidatively metabolized in the liver, with less than 5% of the dose excreted unchanged in the urine. During pregnancy an increase in the concentration of metabolites is found in the urine, suggesting an enhanced absorption and an increase in the hepatic clearance.[10,73,74] In nonpregnant subjects, metoprolol's half-life ranges between 3 and 7 hours.

In patients with gestational hypertension, hydralazine and metoprolol may be used in combination. Hydralazine increases the peak plasma concentration, and the area under the concentration–time curve of metoprolol by 88 and 38%, respectively, and decreases the time to maximum concentration of metoprolol from 1.5 hours to 1.0 hour. This effect is most likely due to a reduction in metoprolol's first-pass metabolism by hydralazine.[73] Metoprolol crosses the placenta with drug concentrations in the umbilical cord approximately the same as the maternal plasma concentrations.[24] Amniotic concentrations of both metoprolol and its major metabolite, α-OH-metoprolol, exceed those in maternal plasma. After birth, neonatal blood levels of metoprolol and its metabolite may be higher than cord levels, suggesting a redistribution at birth. In addition, the ratio of metabolite to parent drug concentration is increased in the neonate[10] possibly because renal elimination is slower in the neonate.

There have been several clinical trials demonstrating metoprolol's efficacy in pregnant hypertensive patients. In one large-scale clinical study,[75,76] 101 pregnant patients with systemic hypertension were treated with one of two regimens: metoprolol alone or metoprolol in combination with hydralazine and a diuretic, for a mean period of 4 weeks. These groups were compared with 97 hypertensive gravidae treated with hydralazine alone. Perinatal mortality was lower in the metoprolol groups, as was the rate of fetal growth retardation. No significant adverse effects were reported in

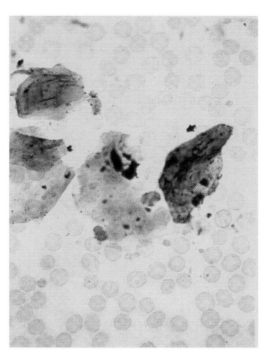

Figure 21.3 Squamous cells recovered from the pulmonary arterial circulation of a pregnant woman with New York Heart Association functional class IV rheumatic mitral stenosis. (Reproduced from SL Clark, Amniotic fluid embolism in critical care obstetrics, SL Clark, JP Phelan, DB Cotton, eds., *Critical Care Obstetrics*. Oradell, NJ: Medical Economics Books; 1987; pp. 393–411, with permission of the publisher.)

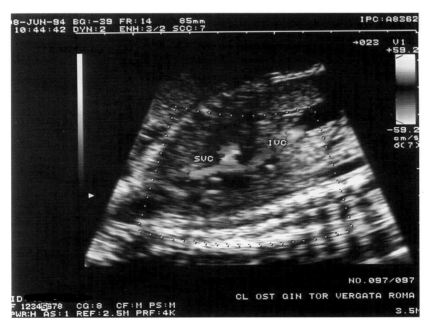

Figure 41.2 Parasigittal view of the fetal trunk showing the inferior vena cava (IVC) and superior vena cava (SVC) entering in the right atrium.

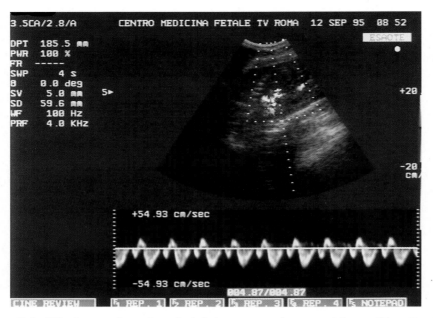

Figure 41.3 Velocity waveforms from the inferior vena cava in a normal fetus at 34 weeks of gestation. Note the small amount of reverse flow during atrial contraction (upper panel).

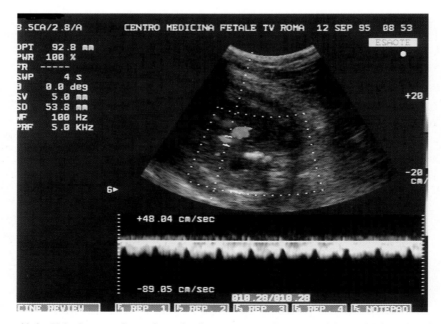

Figure 41.4 Velocity waveforms from the ductus venosus in a normal fetus at 36 weeks of gestation. Note the presence of forward flow during atrial contraction.

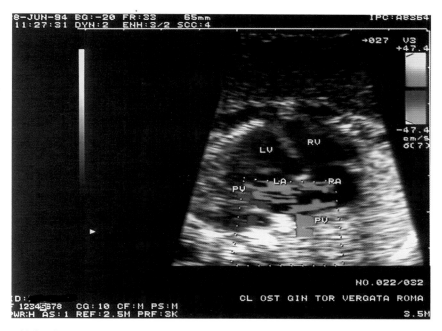

Figure 41.5 Cross-sectional section of the fetal chest showing the pulmonary veins (PV) entering in the left atrium (LA): RA, right atrium; LV, left ventricle, RV, right ventricle.

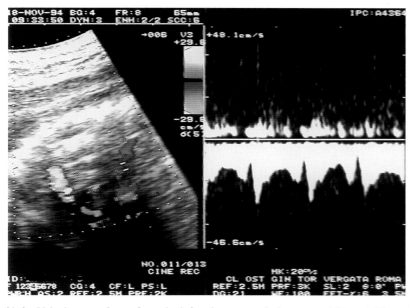

Figure 41.6 Velocity waveforms from the left pulmonary vein in a normal fetus at 36 weeks of gestation. Note the presence of forward flow during atrial contraction.

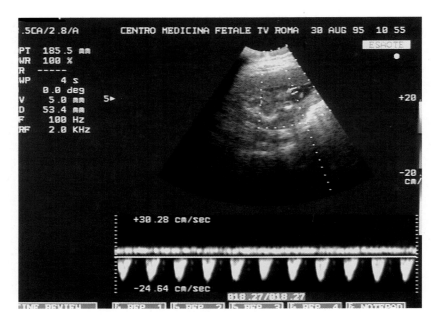

Figure 41.7 Velocity waveforms from the umbilical artery and vein in a normal fetus at 14 weeks of gestation. Note the presence of continuous flow in the umbilical vein.

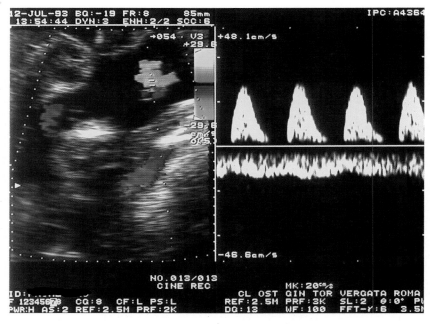

Figure 41.8 Velocity waveforms from the umbilical artery and vein in a severely growth-retarded fetus at 28 weeks of gestation. Note the absence of end-diastolic velocity in umbilical artery and presence of end-diastolic pulsations in the umbilical vein.

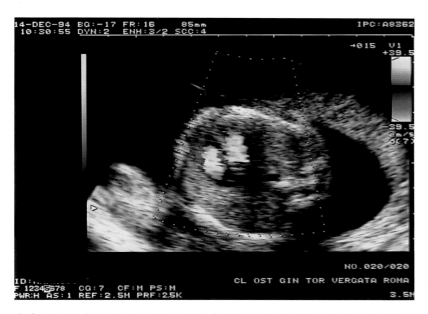

Figure 41.9 Apical four-chamber view of the fetal heart during diastole, showing the ventricular filling.

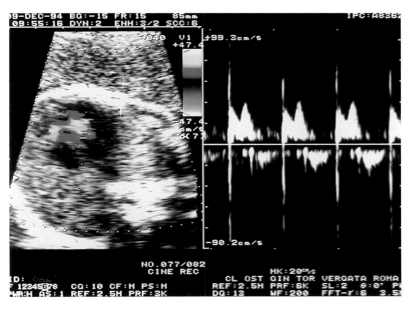

Figure 41.10 Velocity waveforms from the mitral valve in a normal fetus at 38 weeks of gestation. The E/A ratio is 0.81.

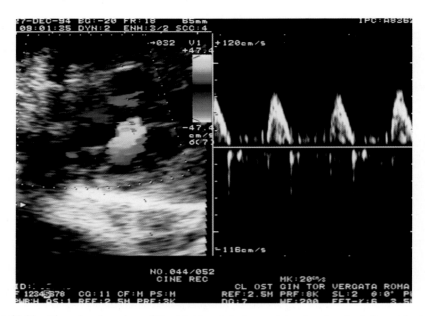

Figure 41.11 Five-chamber view of the fetal heart during systole, showing the left ventricular ejection into aorta and the corresponding velocity waveforms.

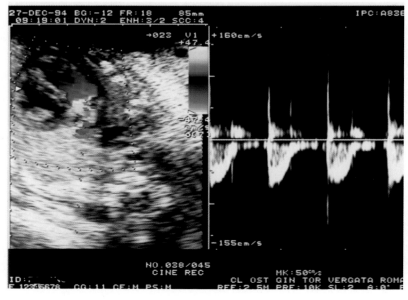

Figure 41.12 Short-axis view of the fetal heart during systole, showing the right ventricular ejection into the pulmonary artery and the corresponding velocity waveforms.

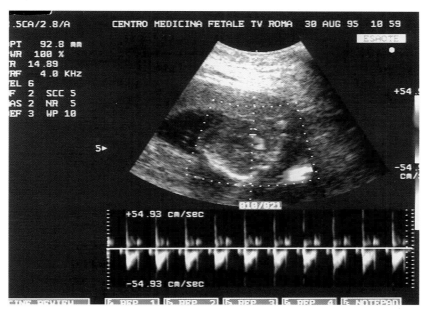

Figure 41.13 Velocity waveforms in a severely growth-retarded fetus at 28 weeks of gestation from pulmonary artery velocity waveforms. The PV is 34 cm/s (normal mean for gestation, 62 cm/s) and the TPV is 14 ms (normal mean for gestation 34.7 ms).

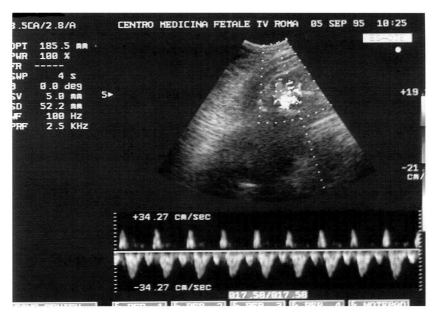

Figure 41.14 Velocity waveforms in a severely growth-retarded fetus at 30 weeks of gestation from inferior vena cava. The percentage reverse flow during atrial contraction is 29% (normal mean for gestation, 12%).

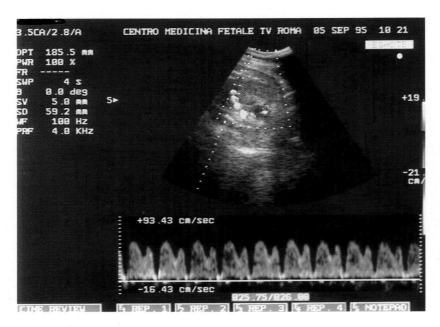

Figure 41.15 Velocity waveforms in a severely growth-retarded fetus at 32 weeks of gestation from the ductus venosus. The S/A is 9 (normal mena for gestation, 1.8).

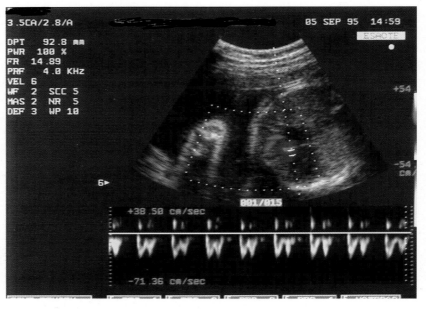

Figure 41.18 Velocity waveforms from the tricuspid valve at 30 weeks of gestation in a pregnancy complicated by rhesus isoimmunization 30 minutes after intravascular transfusion. The E/A is 1.4 (normal mean for gestation, 0.74).

the fetus. More recently, efficacy and safety of metoprolol were evaluated in a randomized study in which metoprolol (200 mg, slow-release daily) was compared with nicardipine (20 mg, three times daily) in the treatment of 100 pregnant women with mild to moderate gestational or chronic hypertension (systolic blood pressure ≥ 140 mmHg and/or diastolic blood pressure ≥ 90 mmHg).[77] Both groups had significant reductions in blood pressure and heart rates; however, blood pressure reduction was superior with nicardipine, while metoprolol resulted in a larger effect on heart rate. Seven nicardipine-treated patients and 15 metoprolol-treated patients needed additional drug therapy to control blood pressure. There were no significant differences in incidence of premature labor, mean gestational age at delivery, and reported side effects. Plasma creatinine increased significantly during metoprolol therapy, but did not change significantly during nicardipine therapy. Metoprolol patients had higher umbilical artery vascular resistance as evaluated by Doppler velocimetry. There were more cesarean sections for fetal distress in the metoprolol group, (14 vs. 3). No difference was found between the two groups in birth weights and placental weights.

Kaaja et al[78] evaluated the effect of metoprolol and atenolol on outcome of very low birth weight infants. A retrospective study of 36 infants, weighing 1500 g or less and born to mothers with pregnancy-induced hypertension or preeclampsia on combination therapy with clonidine, methyldopa, or diuretics, revealed 7 deaths and 19 instances of pulmonary or cerebrovascular complications within 7–218 days in patients receiving beta-blockers, and no deaths in 16 patients not receiving beta-blockers. Based on these data, the authors suggested use of antihypertensives other than beta-blockers or very low dosages of beta-blockers in hypertensive mothers who are likely to give birth to very low birth weight infants.

There are reports of metoprolol overdoses, including a case report of a massive overdose of metoprolol (15.2 g) in a 23-year-old woman of 20 weeks gestation.[79] Although the mother survived with resuscitation and treatment, intrauterine fetal death resulted.

Metoprolol is secreted into breast milk, and milk/plasma concentration ratios have been reported to be 2–4.[24] In spite of this, the amount of drug estimated to be ingested by the infant is considerably lower than the usual mg/kg dose in pediatric patients. Measured infant drug concentrations were either negligible or undetectable, and no clinical effects have been reported in nursing infants.

In conclusion, early studies confirmed the efficacy of metoprolol in controlling blood pressure during pregnancy and showed improvement of fetal outcome on metoprolol compared to hydralazine or diuretic therapy. More recently, however, the safety of metoprolol has come under question in very low birth weight infants, whose outcome may be affected unfavorably by this drug.

Atenolol

Atenolol is efficacious in the treatment of pregnant patients with essential hypertension when treatment is started in the first or second trimester[80–82] in pregnancy-induced hypertension[83,84] with therapy initiated in the third trimester, and in preeclampsia.[85,86] Atenolol is classified in FDA pregnancy risk category C.

Atenolol is β_1-adrenergic selective agent without ISA. Bioavailability of atenolol is unaltered during pregnancy and is 50%.[87] The maximum plasma concentrations are 2–4 hours after an oral dose in pregnant patients.[85,87] Atenolol crosses the placenta, and the maternal/cord blood ratio at delivery is approximately 1.[85] The drug is relatively polar and is excreted unchanged in the urine, with an elimination half-life of 4–8 hours.[85,87] Therefore, patients with renal impairment will accumulate atenolol. The effects on the blood pressure and heart rate are dose-related[87] and last for at least 24 hours when the drug is given as a single daily oral dose.[87]

Several controlled studies have demonstrated that the birth weights of newborns of mothers taking atenolol are reduced compared to those of patients given placebo, or other beta-blocking drugs such as pindolol, acebutolol, or labetalol.[80–83] The mechanism for this reduction is yet to be determined, but hemodynamic effects have been implicated. Doppler studies of fetal and maternal vascular systems have suggested that atenolol decreases the peripheral vascular resistance of both sides of the uteroplacental circulation,[88,89] possibly resulting in decreased placental perfusion, which thus may lead to growth retardation. In addition, placental weight[89] and placental lactogen concentration, a marker for placental well-being, have been shown to be decreased with atenolol therapy.[84] These observations have led to suggestions that atenolol be avoided, especially early in pregnancy and in situations when the fetal circulation may be compromised.

There is a substantial experience with the use of atenolol in pregnancy-induced hypertension. In one study,[57,85] 120 patients with pregnancy-induced hypertension were enrolled in the third trimester and received placebo or 100–200 mg of oral atenolol daily. Atenolol was found to effectively reduce diastolic blood pressure compared to placebo and was associated with a significantly lower incidence of developing proteinuria. In addition, use of atenolol enabled outpatient treatment in 65% of the patients compared to only 15% of patients in the placebo group. Premature labor with delivery did not occur in the atenolol group but occurred in 5 patients in the placebo group. Hypoglycemia occurred in 1 atenolol-treated baby and in 4 babies who received placebo. Transient bradycardia was observed in 18 out of 46 babies at delivery in the atenolol group and in 4 out of 39 in the placebo group. No significant difference was found in birth weight, placental weight, Apgar score, or respiratory function. At one-year follow-up, all babies were found to be normal. In another study, atenolol (100 mg daily for at least 3 days) was used in conjunction with methyldopa or hydralazine to control blood pressure in severely preeclamptic patients. Therapy resulted in modest reductions in maternal blood pressure (6%) and fetal heart rate (5%).[85] Frequent cardiotocographic evaluations were performed, and no adverse effects on the fetal response to stress were observed. At birth, all babies, except for one who was 7 weeks premature and had 5-minute Apgar scores of 8 or more. Birth weights were low, which was consistent with severe preeclampsia.

Rubin et al[82] reported on 10 patients with essential hypertension managed with chronic atenolol therapy during pregnancy. Two patients received the drug in the first, seven in the second, and one in the third trimester. Blood pressure was maintained at 140/90 mmHg or less with atenolol (100–200 mg/day). Two patients required additional therapy with methyldopa and prazosin. Nine babies were successfully delivered, but there was one intrauterine death at 41 weeks of gestation. Two neonates were hypoglycemic, and the mean birth weight was 82% of the gestational mean. Another report compared atenolol, pindolol, and acebutolol in 121 patients.[81] Fifty-six percent of the patients were hypertensive prior to pregnancy and had histories of complicated pregnancies with a 36% intrauterine death rate. Eleven patients received therapy starting in the first two trimesters. Blood pressure was satisfactorily controlled in 95% of the patients in all three treatment groups. There were no fetal deaths. One neonate of 35 weeks' gestation was hypotrophic. Four of 125 children had malformations. In 3 of these cases, atenolol had been started after the 24th week of pregnancy and thus not a likely cause. In the fourth case, the mother had received pindolol and the malformation was a vesicoureteral reflux. The mother of this infant had asymmetrical segmented renal hypoplasia. It was, therefore, concluded that none of the malformations were related to the use of beta blockers. Apgar scores were similar in all three groups. Birth weights of the atenolol group, however, were significantly reduced compared to the recipients of pindolol or acebutolol. In conclusion, this study demonstrated a good blood pressure control and good tolerance of beta-blockade both in the mothers and fetuses. Fetal outcome seemed to improve with therapy. However, the authors suggested that chronic therapy with atenolol should be avoided because it results in low birth weight.

Butters et al[80] reported a significant atenolol-mediated effect on diastolic blood pressure in a placebo-controlled trial of 33 pregnant women with mild essential hypertension who were started on atenolol in the first trimester.[81] There was one stillborn in the atenolol group. However that mother had a prior stillbirth without any drug therapy. Mean birth weight of babies in the atenolol group was 2620 g (vs. 3530 g for the placebo group); placental weight was also reduced in the atenolol group. The difference in weight of the babies had resolved after 1 year of age. The study concluded that atenolol was associated with intrauterine growth retardation when initiated in the first trimester in patients with essential hypertension. Kasab et al[90] used atenolol (100–200 mg/day) and propranolol (30–240 mg/day) to manage 25 pregnant patients with mitral stenosis who were in sinus rhythm and had symptoms of shortness of breath and palpitations. In 9 patients who received either drug prior to pregnancy, the dose was increased to maintain a ventricular rate below 90 beats per minute. Two-thirds of the patients also received digoxin and diuretics. Twenty-three of the patients demonstrated significant improvement of their functional capacity, while two patients required closed mitral valve valvotomy. Fetal heart rate during therapy remained between 130 and 154 beats per minute. Length of gestation was between 37 and 39 weeks, mean birth weight was 2.8 ±0.4 kg, mean Apgar score was 9, and the mean neonatal heart rate was 120–140 beats per minute. The authors attributed the tendency for low birth weight to a decreased cardiac output due to mitral stenosis.

Atenolol is secreted into breast milk at a concentration of 1.5–6.8 times greater than in the maternal plasma.[24] The drug first appears in milk after 4 hours, and peak concentrations occur about 8 hours after the oral dose.[24] Several reports indicate that most breast-fed infants have no adverse effects, negligible plasma levels, and no signs of beta-blockade.[24] In contrast, a significant concentration, leading to bradycardia and cyanosis, was reported in one nursing neonate.[91] The atenolol concentration in this milk was 469 ng/mL when measured 1.5 hours after a 50 mg oral dose. The infant's blood concentration 48 and 72 hours after discontinuing breast feeding was 2010 and 140 ng/mL, respectively, and the estimated atenolol ingested by the baby was at least 9 mg/day of the maternal daily dose of 100 mg.

In summary, clinical experience with atenolol indicates that this agent is efficacious in managing pregnant patients with hypertension, mitral stenosis, and palpitations. However, recent studies strongly suggest that atenolol is associated with fetal growth retardation, resulting in decreased birth weight.

Esmolol

Esmolol is a short-acting β_1-adrenergic receptor antagonist indicated for short-term use in treating supraventricular tachycardia. The drug is of interest in pregnancy mainly because of its rapid onset of action and maximum effect, which occurs in 5–10 minutes, a short plasma half-life of 9 minutes, and duration of action of ~20 minutes.[24,92] Because it is rapidly hydrolyzed to an inactive metabolite by esterases found in red blood cells, clearance is independent of hepatic or renal function.[92]

The clinical effects of esmolol on the fetus have been studied in the pregnant sheep model. Such studies indicate that there is rapid transplacental passage of esmolol and that maternal administration may decrease the fetal heart rate and mean arterial pressure.[93,94] In the sheep model, the fetal blood concentrations were approximately 13% of the maternal blood concentrations.[93,94] In the study by Eisenach, esmolol resulted in fetal hypoxemia and acidemia, which resolved 30 minutes after the drug was discontinued, lending support to the concern that beta-blockade may impair the fetal response to hypoxia.

The experience with esmolol during human pregnancy is limited to case reports. Esmolol has been used to control heart rate in a thyrotoxic patient,[95] to control blood pressure perioperatively in the second trimester,[96,97] and to manage supraventricular arrhythmias.[98,99] Isley et al[95] reported using esmolol at doses ranging from 250 to 500 μg/kg/min in a patient with hyperthyroidism who was undergoing laparotomy for appendicitis at 14 weeks of gestation. No information regarding fetal consequences was reported; but the patient's postoperative recovery was unremarkable. There are two reports of esmolol used to control blood pressure during surgery. In the first case,[96] esmolol and nitroprusside, used in the second gestational trimester to control blood pressure during surgery on a cerebral aneurysm, were associated with mild decreases in both the maternal and fetal heart rates. In the second case,[97] surgical repair was done in the 22nd week of gestation. Four boluses of esmolol (500 μg/kg), followed by a continuous infusion of 200 μg/kg/min, were given during the induction of anesthesia. In addition, 2 mg/kg boluses of esmolol were given during the intubation. When the patient emerged from anesthesia, sodium nitroprusside was given along with esmolol. The fetal heart rate remained between 112 and 120 beats per minute throughout the surgery and returned to a baseline value of 132–137 beats per minute after discontinuation of esmolol. At 37 weeks of gestation, the patient had an emergency cesarean section, prompted by uterine rupture and fetal distress. A 2880 g boy was delivered with Apgar score of 2 and 7 at 1 and 5 minutes. Follow-up at 9 months showed that mother and child were well.

There are two case reports of the use of esmolol at term for maternal supraventricular arrhythmias. The first case presented with mild preeclampsia and symptomatic paroxysmal supraventricular tachycardia during labor in the 39th week of pregnancy.[98] During labor, the maternal heart rate increased to 235 beats per minute and was associated with a marked fetal heart rate and pH decrease. The use of two boluses of esmolol (500 μg/kg/min) converted the rhythm to normal sinus rhythm. A continuous intravenous infusion was then given for 6.5 hours until the patient delivered. At the time of delivery, a total of 1060 mg esmolol had been given. The newborn was noted to have an Apgar score of 7 and 9 at 1 and 5 minutes, a weak cry, poor muscle tone, a heart rate of 120 beats per minute, and a respiration rate of 40 per minute. Forty-eight hours postpartum the infant was mildly jaundiced; but at 60 hours the muscle tone, cry, and respiration rate were normal. Follow up at 6 weeks and 6 months showed that the baby was healthy. A second case was reported by Ducey et

al,[99] who described a patient presenting with sudden onset of supraventricular tachycardia in the 38th week of gestation. A 500 μg/kg loading dose and then 50 μg/kg/min continuous intravenous infusion were given without conversion to normal sinus rhythm. Twenty minutes later, fetal heart rate increased to 175 beats per minute and 4 minutes later decreased to 60 beats per minute. Esmolol was discontinued, but fetal heart rate remained at 60 beats per minute and the pH was 7.09. An emergency cesarean section was performed. On administration of oxygen at delivery, the fetal heart rate increased to 140 beats per minute.

Although a compromised perfusion in both cases could have been secondary to maternal arrhythmia, esmolol-mediated aggravation of fetal hypoperfusion and distress cannot be ruled out. Caution and fetal monitoring should be used when esmolol is given to pregnant patients at term.

Betaxolol

Betaxolol has been used to treat pregnant patients with preexisting hypertension and pregnancy-induced hypertension.

Betaxolol is a β_1-adrenoreceptor blocking agent that is rapidly absorbed with almost 100% bioavailability in nonpregnant as well as pregnant patients.[100,101] The drug is 50% protein bound and has low liposolubility. Betaxolol is more than 80% metabolized in the liver to inactive metabolites, which are excreted in the urine. The half-life in both pregnant and nonpregnant women is 16–22 hours.[41,100–104]

Betaxolol crosses the placenta rapidly, and at delivery, Morselli et al[100] found the ratio of umbilical cord venous blood to maternal venous blood to be 0.56–1.20, with a mean of 0.93 ±0.04. Concentrations of betaxolol in the amniotic fluid were close to the maternal and umbilical venous concentrations at delivery. Morselli et al also reported an increase in blood concentrations during the first 12 hours following delivery in two-thirds of the infants. Neonatal half-life ranged from 14.8 to 38.5 hours and was negatively correlated with gestational age. Careful monitoring of the neonates' blood concentration may be warranted for 72–97 hours after delivery.

The efficacy of betaxolol in the treatment of pregnant women with hypertension and nonpregnant patients with essential hypertension is comparable.[105] Boutroy et al reported good tolerance of betaxolol in 22 pregnant women, and proteinuria was noted to decrease in 3 of 5 patients.[105]

No adverse fetal effects due to betaxolol have been described.[105] In the study cited, betaxolol resulted in a significant decrease of fetal heart rate; spontaneous changes in heart rate (acceleration/deceleration) were not prevented, however. No differences in the incidence of prematurity, cesarean section, or low birth weight were observed when betaxolol-treated patients were compared with hypertensive mothers from the same region at the same gestational age. Mean Apgar score of 23 newborns to mothers treated with betaxolol during gestation and delivery was 8 and 9 at 1 and 5 minutes. All 23 babies were in good health at a 9-month follow-up.[105]

Betaxolol accumulates in breast milk. The milk-to-blood concentration is above 2 at 24–72 hours after delivery. In spite of this, the amount of betaxolol that may be ingested by breast-fed newborns is low.

Celiprolol

Celiprolol is a β_1-adrenergic blocking agent[41] that has been effective in the treatment of angina and hypertension, including pregnancy-induced hypertension.[106]

As a result of partial, selective β_2-adrenergic agonist activity, and possibly direct papaverine-like smooth muscle relaxation, celiprolol has weak vasodilating and bronchodilating effects. In nonpregnant adult patients, celiprolol has a nonlinear, dose-dependent absorption, and a variable bioavailability ranging from 30 to 74%. The drug is hydrophilic, 25% bound to plasma proteins, and excreted unchanged in urine and feces. Serum half-life is relatively short (4–5 h), but the pharmacological effects last 24 hours. At steady state, the placental transfer averages 3% for celiprolol, compared to 18% for propranolol and 6% for atenolol.

There is one report of celiprolol used in pregnant women.[107] In this evaluation, four hypertensive pregnant patients received a single daily oral dose of celiprolol (200 mg). At delivery, the fetal plasma concentrations were 25–50% of the maternal concentrations.

Acebutolol

Acebutolol has been used to treat hypertension during pregnancy.[81,108–110] The FDA has classified acebutolol in pregnancy risk category B.

Acebutolol is a β_1-adrenergic selective adrenoreceptor antagonist with some intrinsic sympathomimetic activity. The drug is well absorbed and exhibits low lipid solubility and plasma protein binding. Bioavailability in nonpregnant adults is low, at 35–45%,[41,111] owing to a first-pass effect. However, the majority of the drug metabolism results in an equipotent β_1-adrenergic selective active metabolite, diacetolol.[41,111] Thus the pharmacologic effect of acebutolol is a composite of those of the parent drug and the metabolite. Acebutolol and diacetolol are excreted in both the urine and feces.[41,109] About 30–40% of an oral dose is found unchanged in the urine, and the plasma half-life of acebutolol and diacetolol in nonpregnant adults is 3–7 and 7–12 hours, respectively.[41,111] Plasma half-life is longer in neonates, however: 10–12 and 20 ±2 hours, respectively.[109] There is evidence that the fetus metabolizes acebutolol to diacetolol in utero.[113] Acebutolol crosses the placenta, and in a study of 20 hypertensive patients, concentration ratios of maternal plasma to umbilical plasma at delivery were 0.8 ±0.07 for acebutolol and 0.6 ±0.09 for diacetolol.[113]

The use of acebutolol in the treatment of pregnant hypertensive patients has been evaluated in several uncontrolled trials.[81,108,110] In one study the drug regimens were adjusted to achieve diastolic blood pressures less than 80 mmHg, and 9 patients received acebutolol (300–600mg/day) and 11 patients received methyldopa (500–1500 mg/day).[108] No difference was found between the two drug regimens with respect to premature labor, live births, birth weight, placental weight, or fetal distress. There was no incidence of bradycardia or hypoglycemia. In an earlier trial of 20 patients, acebutolol was compared to methyldopa.[110] In this trial, acebutolol was associated with lower birth weight, systolic blood pressure, heart rate, and mean blood glucose. Six out of 10 acebutolol neonates were noted to have hypoglycemia. The value of these findings is limited, however, by the open design of the study and because mean duration of acebutolol treatment was twice as long as the methyldopa treatment. In a study mentioned earlier, Dubois et al[81] compared 56 high risk hypertensive patients who received acebutolol to 38 patients receiving pindolol and 31 receiving atenolol. Acebutolol was given throughout pregnancy in 3 patients, at the 24th week of gestation in 14 patients, between the 24th and 32nd weeks in 15 patients, and after the 32nd week in 24 patients. Maternal blood pressure was well controlled. Acebutolol did not differ significantly from the other two beta blockers with respect to Apgar score or neonatal complications. The mean birth weight of babies exposed to acebutolol was not significantly different from that in the pindolol group and was somewhat higher than that for the atenolol group.

Acebutolol is secreted into breast milk and the measured concentration ratios of milk to maternal plasma of acebutolol and diacetolol are 2.3–9.2 and 1.5–13.5, respectively.[112] Seven lactating women receiving acebutolol were evaluated by Boutroy et al. One infant, whose mother had high breast milk concentrations, experienced decreased blood pressure and heart rate with transient tachypnea. It was estimated that if the milk contained at least 4 μg/mL of acebutolol, and 750 mL was ingested, an average neonate would receive doses between 0.5 and 1 mg/kg, which would result in pharmacologic effects. In this evaluation 2 out of the 7 women had such concentrations.

In conclusion acebutolol has been successfully used to control maternal blood pressure during pregnancy without teratogenic effects, and with little to no reduction in the birth weight. The pharmacologic effects are long-lasting due to the prolonged plasma half-life of the metabolite. This is especially the case in the newborn infant, and careful monitoring of the neonate is necessary. The effects on blood pressure and respiration may last for up to 3 days after delivery,[109] and this may be particularly significant in a "stressed" infant. Because acebutolol is concentrated in breast milk, and significant amounts may be ingested by the nursing infant, it is best to avoid breast feeding the neonate.

CONCLUSION

Clinical research using drug therapy during pregnancy is limited by ethical and practical considerations. However, the amount of available information regarding β-adrenergic blocking agents in pregnancy is equivalent to what is available for many antihypertensive drugs that are commonly used during gestation. The current evidence would suggest that beta- blockers are relatively safe when used during pregnancy, posing little risk to the fetus and possibly benefiting the mother. However, until data from definitive studies are available, it would be advisable to adhere to the following guidelines:

1. Avoid, whenever possible, initiating long-term beta-blocker therapy during the first trimester of pregnancy.

2. Use the lowest possible beta-blocker dose. Combination of low doses of beta-blockers and low doses of other agents might provide optimal drug therapy.

3. If possible, discontinue beta-blocker therapy at least 2–3 days prior to delivery, both as a way of limiting the effects of these drugs on uterine contractility and to prevent possible neonatal complications secondary to beta-blockade.

4. Closely observe neonates born to mothers treated with beta-blockers for 72–96 hours after parturition unless the drug was stopped well before delivery.

5. Use of beta-blockers with β_1-adrenergic selectivity, intrinsic sympathetic activity, or α-adrenergic blocking activity may be preferable in that these agents would be less likely to interfere with β_2-mediated uterine relaxation and peripheral vasodilation.

6. Lactating mothers should avoid nursing their infants at the time of the expected highest plasma concentration, which usually occurs within 3–4 hours after a dose.

REFERENCES

1. Frishman WH. Sonnenblick EH: β-adrenergic blocking drugs. In The Heart, edn 8. Schlant RC, Alexander RW (editors). New York: McGraw Hill, 1994;1271–1280.

2. Ladner E, Brinkman CR, Weston P, Assali NS. Dynamics of uterine circulation in pregnant and non-pregnant sheep. *Am J Physiol* 1970;218:257–263.

3. Adams FH, Assali NS, Cushman M, Westerstern A. Interrelationships of maternal and fetal circulations. I. Flow pressure response to vasocative drugs in sheep. *Pediatrics* 1961;27:627–635.

4. Chez RA, Ehrenkranz RA, Oaks GH, Walke AM, Hamilton LA, Vrennan SC, McLaughlin MK. Effects of adrenergic agents on bovine umbilical and uterine blood flows. In: Longo L, Reneau DD eds. *Fetal and Newborn Cardiovascular Physiology*. New York: Garland; 1978;2:1–16.

5. Maughan GB, Shabanah EH, Toth A. Experiments with pharmacologic sympatholysis in the gravid. *Am J Obstet Gynecol* 1967;97:764–776.

6. Wansbrough H, Nakanishi H, Wood C. Effect of epinephrine on human uterine activity in vitro and in vivo. *Obstet Gynecol* 1967;30:779–789.

7. Barden TP, Stander RW. Effects of adrenergic blocking agents and catecholamines in human pregnancy. *Am J Obstet Gynecol* 1968;102:226–235.

8. Joelson I, Barton MD. The effect of blockade of the beta-receptors of the sympathetic nervous system of the fetus. *Acta Obstet Gynecol Scand* 1969;48(suppl 3):75–79.

9. Haraldsson A, Geven W. Severe adverse effects of maternal labetalol in a premature infant. *Acta Paediatr Scand* 1989;78:956–958.

10. Lindeberg S, Lundborg P, Regardh C, Sandstrom B. Disposition of the adrenergic blocker metoprolol and its metabolite OH-metoprolol in maternal plasma, amniotic fluid and capillary blood of the neonate. *Eur J Clin Pharmacol* 1987;33:363–368.

11. Erkkola R, Lammintausta R, Liukko P, Anttila M. Transfer of propranolol and sotalol across the human placenta. *Acta Obstet Gynecol Scand* 1982;61:31–34.

12. Fox RE, Marx C, Stark AR. Neonatal effects of maternal nadolol therapy. *Am J Obstet Gynecol* 1985;152:1045–1046.

13. Roberts JR, Blumer JL, Gorman RL, Lambert GH, Rumack BH, Snodgrass W. American Academy of Pediatrics; Committee on Drugs; Transfer of drugs and other chemicals into human milk. *Pediatrics* 1989;84:924–936.

14. Eliahou HE, Silverber DS, Reisen E, Romem I, Mashiach S, Serr DM. Propranolol for the treatment of hypertension in pregnancy. *Br J Obstet Gynaecol* 1978;85:431–436.

15. Bullock JL, Harris RE, Young R. Treatment of thyrotoxicosis during pregnancy with propranolol. *Am J Obstet Gynecol* 1975;121:242–245.

16. Turner GM, Oakley CM, Dixon HG. Management of pregnancy complicated by hypertrophic obstructive cardiomyopathy. *Br Med J* 1968;4:281–284.

17. Schroeder JS, Harrison DC. Repeated cardioversion during pregnancy: treatment of refractory paroxysmal atrial tachycardia during three successive pregnancies. *Am J Cardiol* 1971;27:445–446.

18. Treakle K, Kostice B, Hulkower S. Supraventricular tachycardia resistant to treatment in a pregnant woman. *J Fam Pract* 1992;35:581–584.

19. Mitrani A, Oettinger M, Abinader EG. Use of propranolol in dysfunctional labor. *J Obstet Gynaecol* 1975;82:651–655.

20. Teuscher A, Bossi E, Imhof P, Erb E, Stocker F, Weber J. Effect of propranolol on fetal tachycardia in diabetic pregnancy. *Am J Cardiol* 1978;42:304–307.

21. O'Hare MF, Kinney CD, Murnaghan GA, McDevitt DG. Pharmacokinetics of propranolol during pregnancy. *Eur J Clin Pharmacol* 1984;27:583–587.

22. Mitani GHM, Steinberg I, Lien EJ, Harrison EC, Elkayam U. The pharmacokinetics of antiarrhythmic agents in pregnancy and lactation. *Clin Pharmacokinet* 1987;12:253–291.

23. Yoshikawa T, Sugiyama Y, Sawada Y, Iga T, Hanano M, Kawasaki S, Yanagida M. Effect of late pregnancy on salicylates, diazepam, warfarin, and propranolol binding: Use of fluorescent probes. *Clin Pharmacol Ther* 1984;36:201–208.

24. Cox JL, Gardner MJ. Treatment of cardiac arrhythmias during pregnancy. *Prog Cardiovasc Dis* 1993;36:137–178.

25. Rubin PC, Butters L, McCabe R, Kelman A. The influence of pregnancy on drug action: concentration–effect modelling with propranolol. *Clin Sci* 1987;73:47–52.

26. Briggs GG, Freeman RK, Yaffee SJ. *Drugs in Pregnancy and Lactation: A Reference Guide to Fetal and Neonatal Risk.* 4th ed. Baltimore: Williams & Wilkins; 1994.

27. Smith MT, Livingstone I, Hooper WD, Eadie MJ, Triggs EJ. Propranolol glucuronide, and naphthoxylactic acid in breast milk and plasma. *Ther Drug Monit* 1983;5:87–93.

28. Pruyn SC, Phelan JP, Buchanan GC. Long-term propranolol therapy in pregnancy: maternal and fetal outcome. *Am J Obstet Gynecol* 1979;135:485–489.

29. Bott-Kanner G, Schweitzer A, Reisner SH. Propranolol and hydralazine in the management of essential hypertension in pregnancy. *Br J Obstet Gynaecol* 1980;87:110–114.

30. Tcherdakoff PH, Colliard M, Berrard E. Propranolol in hypertension during pregnancy. *Br Med J* 1978;2:670.

31. Gallery EDM, Saunders DM, Hunyor SN, Gyory AZ. Randomized comparison of methyldopa and oxprenolol for treatment of hypertension in pregnancy. *Br Med J* 1979;1:1591–1594.

32. Oakley CDG, McGary K, Limb DG, Oakley CM. Management of pregnancy in patients with hypertrophic cardiomyopathy. *Br Med J* 1979;1:1749–1750.

33. Livingstone I, Craswell PW, Bevan EB, Smith MT, Eadie MJ. Propranolol in pregnancy: three-year prospective study. *Clin Exp Hypertension* 1983;2:341–350.

34. Jensen OH. Fetal heart rate response to a controlled sound stimulus after propranolol administration to the mother. *Acta Obstet Gynecol Scand* 1984;63:199–202.

35. Tunstall ME. The effect of propranolol on the onset of breathing at birth. *Br J Anesth* 1969;41:792.

36. Habib A, McCarthy JS. Effects on the neonate of propranolol administered during pregnancy. *J Pediatr* 1977;91:808.

37. Gladstone GR, Hordof A, Gersong WM. Propranolol administration during pregnancy: effects on the fetus. *J Pediatr* 1975;86:962–964.

38. Buechier AA, Palmer SK. Intrapartum fetal death associated with propranolol: case report and review of physiology. *Wisconsin Med J* 1982;81:23–25.

39. Bauer JH, Pape B, Zajicek J, Groshong T. Propranolol in human plasma and breast milk. *Am J Cardiol* 1979;43:860–862.

40. Karlberg B, Lundberg D, Aberg H. Excretion of propranolol in human breast milk. *Acta Pharmacol Toxicol* 1974;34:222–223.

41. *Drug Facts and Comparisons.* St. Louis: Facts and Comparisons, 1995.

42. Delvin RG, Duchin KL, Fleiss PM. Nadolol in human serum and breast milk. *Br J Clin Pharmacol* 1981;12:393–396.

43. Singh BN, Deedwania P, Nademanee K, Ward A, Sorkin EM. Sotalol. A review of its pharmacodynamic and pharmacokinetic properties, and therapeutic use. *Drugs* 1987;34: 311–349.

44. Antonaccio MJ, Gomoll A. Pharmacology, pharmacodynamics and pharmacokinetics of sotalol. *Am J Cardiol* 1990;65:12A–21A.

45. Riant P, Urien S, Albengres E, Duche JC, Tillement JP. High plasma protein binding as a parameter in the selection of beta blockers for lactating women. *Biochem Pharmacol* 1986;35: 4579–4581.

46. O'Hare ML, Leahey W, Murnaghan GA, McDevitt DG. Pharmacokinetics of sotalol during pregnancy. *Eur J Clin Pharmacol* 1983;24:521–524.

47. O'Hare MF, Murnaghan GA, Russell CJ, Leahey WJ, Varma MPS, McDevitt DG. Sotalol as a hypotensive agent in pregnancy. *Br J Obstet Gynaecol* 1980;87:814–820.

48. Wagner X, Jouglard J, Moulin M, Miller AM, Petitjean J, Pisapia A. Co-administration of flecainide acetate and sotalol during pregnancy: lack of teratogenic effects, passage across the placenta, and excretion in human breast milk. *Am Heart J* 1990;119:700–702.

49. Pearce SHS, Rees CJ, Smith RH. Fetal monitoring during maternal antiarrhythmic therapy. *Eur Heart J* 1993;14:1438.

50. Hackett LP, Wojnar-Horton RE, Dusci LJ, Ilett KF, Roberts MJ. Excretion of sotalol in breast milk. *Br J Clin Pharmacol* 1990;29:277–278.

51. Amiel C, Chau C, Millet V, Agher JP, Gamerre M. [Fetal supraventricular tachycardia. Management.] *J Gynecol Obstet Biol Reprod Paris* 1993;22:2284–2288.

52. Darwiche A, Vanlieferinghen P, Lemery D, Paire M, Lusson JR. [Amiodarone and fetal supraventricular tachycardia. àpropos of a case with neonatal hypothyroidism.] *Arch Fr Pediatr* 1992;49:729–731.

53. Meden H, Neeb U. [Transplacental cardioversion of fetal supraventricular tachycardia using sotalol.] *Z Geburtshilfe Perinatol* 1990;194:182–184.

54. Auzelle MP, Mensire A, Lachassine E, Caldera R, Boccara JF, Chavinie J, Badoual J. [In utero treatment of fetal tachycardias with a digitalis–beta blocker combination. àpropos of 2 cases.] *J Gynecol Obstet Biol Reprod Paris* 1987;16:383–391.

55. Saotome T, Minoura S, Terashi K, Sato T, Echizen H, Ishizaki T. Labetalol in hypertension during the third trimester of pregnancy: its antihypertensive effect and pharmacokinetic–dynamic analysis. *J Clin Pharmacol* 1993;33:979–988.

56. Rogers RC, Sibai BM, Whybrew WD. Labetalol pharmacokinetics in pregnancy-induced hypertension. *Am J Obstet Gynecol* 1990;162:362–366.

57. Rubin PC, Butters L, Kelman AW, Fitzsimons C, Reid JL. Labetalol disposition and concentration–effect relationships during pregnancy. *Br J Clin Pharmacol* 1983;15:465–470.

58. Michael CA. Use of labetalol in the treatment of severe hypertension during pregnancy. *Br J Clin Pharmacol* 1979;8 (suppl 2):211S–215S.

59. Lunell N, Kulas J, Rane A. Transfer of labetalol into amniotic fluid and breast milk of lactating women, *Eur J Clin Pharmacol* 28:597–599.

60. Pirhonen JP, Erkkola RU, Makinen JI, Ekblad U. Single dose of labetalol in hypertensive pregnancy: effects of maternal hemodynamics and uterine and fetal flow velocity waveforms. *J Perinat Med* 1991;19:167–171.

61. Pickles CJ, Pipkin FB, Symons EM. A randomised placebo controlled trial of labetalol in the treatment of mild to moderate pregnancy induced hypertension. *Br J Obstet Gynaecol* 1992;99:964–968.

62. Sibai BM, Mabie WC, Shamsa F, Villar MA, Anderson GD. A comparison of no medication versus methyldopa or labetalol in chronic hypertension during pregnancy. *Am J Obstet Gynecol* 1990;162:960–967.

63. Bhorat IE, Naidoo DP, Rout CC, Moodley J. Malignant ventricular arrhythmias in eclampsia: a comparison of labetalol with dihydralazine. *Am J Obstet Gynecol* 1993;168: 1292–1296.

64. Harper A, Murnaghan GA. Maternal and fetal haemodynamics in hypertensive pregnancies during maternal treatment with intravenous hydralazine or labetalol. *Br J Obstet Gynaecol* 1991;98:453–459.

65. Hjertberg R, Faxelius G, Belfrage P. Comparison of outcome of labetalol or hydralazine therapy during hypertension in pregnancy in very low birth weight infants. *Acta Obstet Gynecol Scand* 1993;72:611–615.

65a. Hjertberg R, Faxelius G, Lagercrantz H. Neonatal adaptation in hypertensive pregnancy—a study of labetalol vs hydralazine treatment. *J Perinat Med* 1993;21:69–75.

66. Olsen KS, Beier-Holgersen R. Fetal death following labetalol administration in preeclampsia. *Acta Obstet Gynecol Scand* 1992;71:145–147, 151–152.

67. Ellenbogen A, Jaschevatzky O, Davidson S, Anderman S, Grunstein S. Management of pregnancy-induced hypertension with pindolol—comparative study with methyldopa. *Int J Gynaecol Obstet* 1986;24:3–7.

68. Meizner I, Paran E, Katz M. Holcberg G, Insler V. Flow velocity analysis of umbilical and uterine artery flow in preeclampsia treated with propranolol or pindolol. *J Clin Ultrasound* 1992;20:115–119.

69. Plouin PF, Breart G, Llado J, Dalle M, Keller ME, Goiyon H, Berchel C. *Br J Obstet Gynaecol* 1990;97:134–141.

70. Fidler J, Smith V, Fayers P, deSwiet M. Randomized controlled comparative study of methyldopa and oxprenolol in treatment of hypertension in pregnancy. *Br Med J* 1983;286: 1927–1930.

71. Gallery EDM, Ross MR, Gyory AZ. Antihypertensive treatment in pregnancy: analysis of different responses to oxprenolol and methyldopa. *Br Med J* 1985;291:563–566.

72. Lubbe WF, Hodge JV. Combined α- and β-adrenoceptor antagonism with prazosin and oxprenolol in control of severe hypertension in pregnancy. *N Z Med J* 1981;94:169–172.

73. Lindeberg S, Holm B, Lundborg P, Regardh C, Sandstrom B. The effect of hydralazine on steady state plasma concentrations of metoprolol in pregnant hypertensive women. *Eur J Clin Pharmacol* 1988;35:131–135.

74. Hogstedt S, Lindberg B, Ren Peng D, Regardh C, Rane A. Pregnancy-induced increase in metoprolol metabolism. *Clin Pharmacol Ther* 1985;37:688–692.

74a. Hogstedt S, Rane A. Plasma concentrations—effect relationship of metoprolol during and after pregnancy. *Eur J Clin Pharmacol* 1993;44:243–246.

75. Sandstrom B. Antihypertensive treatment with the adrenergic beta-receptor blocker metoprolol during pregnancy. *Gynecol Obstet Invest* 1978;9:195–204.

76. Sandstrom B. Adrenergic β-receptor blockers in hypertension of pregnancy. *Clin Exp Hypertension* 1982;1:127–141.

77. Jannet D, Carbonne B, Sebban E, Milliez J. Nicardipine versus metoprol in the treatment of hypertension during pregnancy: a randomized comparative trial. *Obstet Gynecol* 1994;84:354–359.

78. Kaaja R, Hiilesmaa V, Holma K, Jarvenpaa A. Maternal antihypertensive therapy with beta-blockers associated with poor outcome in very low-birth weight infants. *Int J Gynecol Obstet* 1992;38:195–199.

79. Tai Y, Lo C, Chow W, Cheng C. Successful resuscitation and survival following massive overdose of metoprolol. *Br J Clin Pharmacol* 1990;44:746–747.

80. Butters L, Kennedy S, Rubin PC. Atenolol in essential hypertension during pregnancy. *Br Med J* 1990;301:587–589.

81. Dubois D, Petitcolas J, Temperville B, Klepper A, Catherine P. Treatment of hypertension in pregnancy with β-adrenoceptor antagonists. *Br J Clin Pharmacol* 1982;13:375S–378S.

82. Rubin PC, Butters L, Low R, Reid JL. Atenolol in the treatment of essential hypertension during pregnancy. *Br J Clin Pharmacol* 1982;14:279–281.

83. Lardoux H, Gerard J, Blazquez G, Flouvat B. Which beta-blocker in pregnancy-induced hypertension? *Lancet* 1983;i: 1194.

84. Rubin PC, Butters L, Clark D, Sumner D, Belfield A, Pledger D, Low RA, Reid JL. Obstetric aspects of the use in pregnancy-associated hypertension of the β-adrenoceptor antagonist atenolol. *Am J Obstet Gynecol* 1984;150:389–392.

85. Thorley KJ, McAinsh J, Cruickshank JM. Atenolol in the treatment of pregnancy-induced hypertension. *Br J Clin Pharmacol* 1981;12:725–730.

86. Fabregues G, Alvarez L, Varas Juri P, Drisaldi S, Cerrato C, Moschettoni C, Pituelo D, Baglivo HP, Esper RJ. Effectiveness of atenolol in the treatment of hypertension during pregnancy. *Hypertension* 1992;19:II129–II131.

87. Wadworth AN, Murdoch D, Brogden RN. Atenolol. A re-appraisal of its pharmacological properties and therapeutic use in cardiovascular disorders. *Drugs* 1991;42:468–510.

88. Montan S, Liedholm H, Lingman G, Marsal K, Sjoberg N, Solum T. Fetal and uteroplacental haemodynamics during short-term atenolol treatment of hypertension in pregnancy. *Br J Obstet Gynaecol* 1987;94:312–317.

89. Montan S, Ingemarsson I, Marsal K, Sjoeberg NO. Randomized controlled trial of atenolol and pindolol in human pregnancy: effects on fetal haemodynamics. *Br Med J* 1992;304: 946–949.

90. Kasab SM, Sabag T, Zaibag M, Awaad M, Bitar I, Halim M, Abdullah M, Shahed M, Rajendran V, Sawyer W. β-Adrenergic receptor blockade in the management of pregnant women with mitral stenosis. *Am J Obstet Gynecol* 1990;163:37–40.

91. Schmimmel MS, Eidelman AJ, Wilschanski MA, Shaw D, Ogilvie RJ, Loren G. Toxic effects of atenolol consumed during breast feeding. *J Pediatr* 1989;114:476–478.

92. Angaran DM, Schultz NJ, Tschida VH. Esmolol hydrochloride: an ultrashort-acting, β-adrenergic blocking agent. *Clin Pharm* 1986;5:288–303.

93. Ostman PL, Chestnut DH, Robillard JE, Weiner CP, Hdez MJ. Transplacental passage and hemodynamic effects of esmolol in the gravid ewe. *Anesthesiology* 1988;69:738–741.

94. Eisenach JC, Castro MI. Maternal administered esmolol produces fetal β-adrenergic blockade and hypoxemia in sheep. *Anesthesiology* 1989;71:718–722.

95. Isley WL, Dahl S, Gibbs H. Use of esmolol in managing a thyrotoxic patient needing emergency surgery. *Am J Med* 1990;89:122–123.

96. Larson CP Jr, Shuer LM, Cohen SE. Maternally administered esmolol decreases fetal as well as maternal heart rate. *J Clin Anesth* 1990;2:427–429.

97. Losasso TJ, Muzzi DA, Cucchiara RF. Response of fetal heart rate to maternal administration of esmolol. *Anesthesiology* 1991;74:782–784.

98. Gilson GJ, Knieriem KJ, Smith JF, Izquierdo L, Chatterjee MS, Curet LB. Short-acting beta-adrenergic blockade and the fetus. A case report. *J Reprod Med* 1992;37:277–279.

99. Ducey JP, Knape KG. Maternal esmolol administration resulting in fetal distress and cesarean section in a term pregnancy. *Anesthesiology* 1992;77:829–832.

100. Morselli PL, Boutroy MJ, Bianchetti G, Zipfel A, Boutroy JL, Vert P. Placental transfer and perinatal pharmacokinetics of betaxolol. *Eur J Clin Pharmacol* 1990;38:477–483.

101. Bianchetti G, Thiercelin JF, Thenot JP. Pharmacokinetics of betaxolol in middle aged patients. *Eur J. Clin Pharmacol* 1986;31:231–233.

102. Morselli PL, Kilborn JR, Cavero I, Harrison DC, Langer SZ. *Betaxolol and Other Beta-Adrenoceptor Antagonists.* L.E.R.S. monograph series. New York: Raven Press; 1983:1.

103. Beresford R, Heel RC. Betaxolol. *Drugs* 1986;31:6–28.

104. Cavero I, Lefevre-Borg F, Manoury P, Roach AG. In vitro and in vivo pharmacological evaluation of betaxolol, a new, potent, and selective beta-adrenoceptor antagonist. In: Morselli PL, Kilbourn JR, Cavro I, Harrison DC, Langer SZ, eds. *Betaxolol and Other Beta-Adrenoceptor Antagonists.* L.E.R.S. monograph series. New York: Raven Press; 1983;1:31–42.

105. Boutroy MJ, Morselli PL, Bianchetti G, Boutroy JL, Pepin L, Zipfel A. Betaxolol: a pilot study of its pharmacological and therapeutic properties in pregnancy. *Eur J Clin Pharmacol* 1990;38:535–539.

106. Briggs GG, Freeman RK, Yaffee SJ. Celiprolol, *Update: drugs in pregnancy and lactation.* 1991;7:17–18.

107. Kofahl B, Henke D, Hettenbach A, Mutschler E. Studies on placental transfer of celiprolol. *Eur J Clin Pharmacol* 1993;44:381–382.

108. Williams E, Morrissey J. A comparison of acebutolol with methyldopa in hypertensive pregnancy. *Pharmacotherapeutica* 1983;3:487–491.

109. Boutroy M. Fetal and neonatal effects of beta-adrenoreceptor blocking agents. *Dev Pharmacol Ther* 1987;10:224–231.

110. Dumez Y, Chobroutsky T, Hornych H, Amiel-Tison C. Neonatal effects of maternal administration of acebutolol. *Br Med J* 1981;283:1077–1079.

111. DeBono G, Kaye C, Roland E, Summers A. Acebutolol: ten years of experience. *Am Heart J* 1985;109:1221–1223.

112. Boutroy M, Bianchetti G, Dubrue C, Vert P, Morselli P. To nurse when receiving acebutolol: is it dangerous for the neonate? *Eur J Clin Pharmacol* 1986;30:737–739.

113. Bianchetti G, Dubroc C, Vert P, Boutroy M, Morselli P. Placental transfer and pharmacokinetics of acebutolol in newborn infants. *Clin Pharmacol Ther* 1981;29:233–234. Abstract.

30

ANTIARRHYTHMIC DRUGS DURING PREGNANCY AND LACTATION

AVRAHAM SHOTAN, MD, AGNETA HURST, PHARMD, JOSEF WIDERHORN, MD,
YAIR FRENKEL, MD, AND URI ELKAYAM, MD

CLASS IA ANTIARRHYTHMIC DRUGS

Quinidine

Quinidine, a class Ia antiarrhythmic medication, is a dextro-isomer of quinine. It is effective in suppressing both supraventricular and ventricular arrhythmias and has been used during pregnancy since 1930.[1] Because the drug is 60–80% bound to protein, hypoalbuminemia during pregnancy may result in a lower measured serum drug concentration, but the unbound and readily available fraction may increase. Transplacental passage of quinidine has been demonstrated in several reports with fetal–maternal serum concentration ratios ranging from 0.25 to 0.8.[2–4] Hill and Malkasian[3] reported a case of treatment with 2700 mg of quinidine daily throughout the pregnancy to prevent maternal ventricular tachycardia. Maternal quinidine levels were fairly constant during pregnancy, ranging between 5.1 and 7.8 μg/mL. At delivery, serum quinidine levels were 3.4 μg/mL in the mother, 2.8 μg/mL in the neonate, and 9.3 μg/mL in the amniotic fluid. Spinnato et al[2] described three cases of fetal supraventricular tachycardia successfully treated with digoxin and quinidine. In two of the fetuses, the drug combination also controlled tachycardia-induced ascites. Guntheroth et al[5] described a successful case of quinidine cardioversion of fetal supraventricular tachycardia resistant to digoxin and propranolol. On a dose of 1600 mg/day, the maternal quinidine level was 4.5 μg/mL and cord blood level was 0.8 μg/mL (fetomaternal ratio 0.18). However, the drug levels were not collected simultaneously, and the last maternal dose was given 18 hours prior to delivery. Johnson

et al[6] reported another successful case of cardioversion of fetal atrial flutter at 27 weeks of gestation with an oral maternal dose of quinidine of 3600 mg/day. The fetal arrhythmia cardioverted at a maternal quinidine serum concentration of 5.2 mg/L. Quinidine therapy was maintained until 36 weeks of pregnancy with no further recurrences of fetal tachycardia. Fetal heart enlargement and ascites recovered 2 weeks postcardioversion. At term, a 4500 g male infant with a congenital hip dislocation was delivered; a month later he was diagnosed as having a left lateral accessory pathway. Killeen and Bowers[7] reported a case of 3-hydroxyquinidine (a metabolite of quinidine with antiarrhythmic activity) toxicity in a pregnant patient in the 33rd week of gestation who was given very large doses of quinidine (≤4500 mg/day) to treat fetal supraventricular tachycardia. The quinidine blood level was within low to midtherapeutic level, but 3-hydroxyquinidine levels were substantially elevated. This patient demonstrated an unusually fast metabolism of quinidine to 3-hydroxy-quinidine with subsequent quinidine. Simultaneous blood and amniotic fluid sampling revealed similar quinidine concentrations at 2.6 and 2.2 μg/mL, respectively. At delivery (2 days after discontinuation of quinidine), the cord blood quinidine level was only 37% of the maternal level. The infant, who later was diagnosed as having an accessory atrioventricular bypass tract, tolerated the delivery well (Apgar score 8/9) and had no signs of quinidine toxicity. In another case quinidine was given parenterally to a 21-year-old pregnant woman for chloroquine-resistant malaria.[8] There was a premature labor at 31 weeks of gestation, with only transient neonatal respiratory difficulty.

Cardiac Problems in Pregnancy, Third Edition
Edited by Uri Elkayam, MD, and Norbert Gleicher, MD
Copyright © 1998 by Wiley-Liss, Inc. ISBN 0-471-16358-9

From the preceding reports, it appears that fetal quinidine blood levels are lower than maternal levels. However, the fetomaternal ratio is variable. The quinidine dosage for treatment of fetal tachyarrhythmias should be adjusted according to clinical response, and careful monitoring of quinidine and its metabolites serum levels as well as clinical response is recommended. Quinidine has been mostly effective when used for fetal supraventricular tachycardias. Sherer et al,[9] however, reported one unsuccessful attempt to use it for cardioversion of fetal ventricular tachycardia associated with nonimmunologic hydrops fetalis. Because of severe maternal preeclampsia, severe fetal condition, and breech presentation, cesarian section was performed at 30 weeks, 3 days after the treatment with 800 mg/day of quinidine was begun. Therapeutic maternal quinidine levels were not obtained. The hydropic infant, weighing only 1950 g, continued to have runs of ventricular tachycardia and died 5 hours later from cardiac and respiratory insufficiency. Braverman et al[10] added quinidine to metoprolol (100 mg/day) and successfully controlled sustained ventricular tachycardia in a 33-year-old woman in her 26th week of gestation. Therapeutic quinidine levels were achieved, and the combination therapy was maintained to term. A healthy but small for date (2240 g) infant was delivered.

Potential quinidine side effects during pregnancy include minimal oxytocic activity, an effect manifested mostly during development of spontaneous uterine contractions.[1,11] Toxic doses may cause premature labor[12] and abortion.[13] Also, transient neonatal thrombocytopenia[14] and damage to the eighth cranial nerve[15] have been reported. Quinidine in therapeutic concentrations depresses pseudocholinesterase activity by 60–70%.[11] This additional effect on the level of pseudocholinesterase activity, already low due to gestation, may affect the hydrolysis of esther-type anesthetics (procaine, tetracaine, chloroprocaine) and the duration of action of succinylcholine, with potential toxicity during epidural or general anesthesia.[16–18] Although these side effects are of concern, they have been rare during the large clinical experience with quinidine during gestation, supporting the drug's safety for the short-term treatment of both maternal and fetal arrhythmias. A surveillance study of Michigan Medicaid recipients involving 229,101 completed pregnancies conducted between 1985 and 1992 reports on 17 newborns exposed to quinidine during the first trimester. One major birth defect (5.9%) was observed. However no anomaly was observed in six categories specified (cardiovascular defect, oral clefts, spina bifida, polydactyly, limb reduction defect, and hypospadias).[19]

Recent data from two meta-analyses of studies performed in nonpregnant patients for atrial fibrillation as well as for ventricular arrhythmias revealed an increased risk of sudden death in patients treated with quinidine, probably due to QT interval prolongation and proarrhythmia.[20,21] Therefore, quinidine should be started in the hospital with cardiac monitoring and should be used for the shortest possible amount of time. Quinidine therapy should be carefully monitored (ECG, blood levels), and particular attention should be given to drug interactions, correction of electrolyte abnormalities, and rectification of any other condition that may potentially increase proarrhythmic events.

Quinidine is currently considered a risk category C by the U.S. Food and Drug Administration.[22] It is secreted in breast milk, with a milk/plasma ratio of 0.31–0.71.[3,7] The calculated total amount of quinidine likely to be ingested by the infant is far below the drug's recommended therapeutic daily pediatric dose. The Committee on Drugs of the American Academy of Pediatrics considers the use of quinidine compatible with breast feeding.[23]

Procainamide

Procainamide can be given both orally and parenterally and is effective in treating supraventricular as well as ventricular arrhythmias. Procainamide may be given orally and parenterally. Following oral administration, 75–95% of the dose is absorbed, and peak blood levels are reached in 45–75 minutes. The drug is 15–20% bound to plasma proteins, and its half-life is 2.5–5 hours. Approximately 40–70% of procainamide is eliminated unchanged by the kidneys, and 10–34% of the drug undergoes hepatic acetylation to N-acetylprocainamide (NAPA). This metabolite has also some antiarrhythmic activity. Congestive heart failure and renal impairment prolong both procainamide and NAPA half-lives.[24]

Chronic oral treatment may cause nausea, vomiting and diarrhea, mental depression, hallucination, psychosis, rash, fever, arthralgia, and agranulocytosis. Lupuslike syndrome may develop in as much as a third of patients treated longer than 6 months and is more common in slow acetylators. NAPA's proarrhythmic effects are associated with QT interval prolongation.

Onset of action following parenteral administration is almost immediate. Intravenous procainamide may cause hypotension and proarrhythmia.

Since it is a small molecule and a weak base, procainamide is expected to freely cross the placental barrier and be subject to ion trapping. Transplacental procainamide passage has been documented in several reports.[25–30] Dumesic et al[25] described a case of fetal supraventricular tachycardia resistant to digoxin alone and in combination with propranolol. The arrhythmia was successfully treated by adding procainamide to digoxin. At delivery, while digoxin levels were equal in maternal and fetal blood, procainamide levels were higher in maternal blood (15.6 vs. 4.3 μg/mL). In another report[26] fetal supraventricular tachycardia resistant to the combination therapy with digoxin and propranolol was cardioverted with digoxin and procainamide. However, in this report digoxin and procainamide levels found at delivery were discordant with those found by Dumesic et al.[25] Fetal levels of procainamide were 30% higher (8.3 vs. 6.3 μg/mL), while those of digoxin were 50% lower. Levels of NAPA in the maternal and fetal blood were 3.0 and 3.7 μg/mL, respectively. Lima et al[27] reported a case of maternal ventricular tachycardia treated at 40 weeks of gestation with procainamide (1.5 g/day) followed by 2.25 g of procainamide and 40 mg daily of propranolol. Also in this report, the fetal levels were higher than maternal levels.

Procainamide appears to be safe for use during pregnancy, and there have been no teratogenic effects reported to date.[28,29] However, because of the limited data available and the potential for unexpected side effects, especially the relatively high incidence of antinuclear antibodies and lupuslike syndrome associated with chronic therapy, caution is recommended. Currently the FDA pregnancy risk category of procainamide is C.[22] Both procainamide and NAPA are secreted and accumulated in breast milk[31]; the milk/plasma ratio has been found to be elevated (4.3 ± 2.4 for procainamide and 3.8 ± 1.8 for NAPA). The amount of procainamide ingested by the newborn is not expected to produce significant plasma levels.

The Committee on Drugs of the American Academy of Pediatrics considers the use of procainamide compatible with breast feeding.[23]

Disopyramide

Disopyramide is useful for suppressing premature ventricular beats and for the treatment and prevention of supraventricular and ventricular tachyarrhythmias. It has a marked negative inotropic effect that may cause cardiac decompensation, especially in patients with systolic ventricular dysfunction. In addition, disopyramide, like the other class Ia antiarrhythmic medications, may have proarrhythmic effects. Disopyramide has approximately 10% of the anticholinergic properties of atropine. Therefore it may cause dry mouth, constipation, or blurred vision; although rarely seen in this age group, urinary retention or closed-angle glaucoma may result, as well.

Following oral administration, 60–83% of the dose is absorbed with peak concentration within 3 hours. The half-life of disopyramide is 4–10 hours (average 6.5 h). About 40–60% of oral disopyramide is excreted unchanged in urine; an additional 15–25% undergoes liver metabolism to mono-*N*-desalkylated metabolite, which has mild antiarrhythmic properties.

Animal studies demonstrate passage of the drug across the placenta and its presence in breast milk. Decreased neonatal birth weight has been observed at very high doses, but without further teratogenic effects.[32,33]

Shaxted and Milton[34] administered disopyramide (600 mg/day) to a woman 26 weeks pregnant who had symptomatic ventricular tachycardia. The delivery was at term, and

there were no congenital abnormalities and no growth retardation. The fetal/maternal ratio of serum disopyramide concentrations 6 hours following the last maternal dose was 0.39. In a longitudinal study of disopyramide protein binding throughout the pregnancy, Echizen et al[35] showed that the protein binding of disopyramide is significantly decreased during the third trimester, with a consequent increase of its antiarrhythmic activity at the same therapeutic plasma concentration. The mean fetal/maternal plasma disopyramide concentration ratio at term was 0.78 at a therapeutic maternal plasma concentration of 2.0–5.0 μg/mL. Elsworth et al[36] treated a 27-year-old woman throughout her pregnancy because there had been prior exertional ventricular fibrillation. The course was uneventful, and at delivery fetal/maternal plasma concentration ratio was 0.26.

Leonard et al[37] reported that the use of disopyramide for refractory supraventricular tachycardia in a pregnant patient with mitral valve prolapse was associated with uterine contractions that abated on withdrawal of the drug. To further investigate this effect, Tadmor et al[38] performed a placebo-controlled, randomized, double-blind study in 20 pregnant women. Disopyramide (600 mg/day) was given for 48 hours to 10 women with indication for labor induction. The other 10 women received placebo. Regular uterine contraction occurred in all 10 women receiving the active drug, versus none in the control group. Eight women on the active drug delivered within 48 hours, versus none in the control group. At delivery, the fetomaternal concentration ratio was 0.36.

Currently the FDA pregnancy risk category of disopyramide is C.[22] From the data above, however, it appears that disopyramide may induce uterine contraction and delivery. Therefore, until sufficient information regarding its safety has accumulated as a result of further investigation, disopyramide should be avoided during pregnancy, especially at the third trimester.[38,39]

Disopyramide has been found in human breast milk in concentrations similar to those in the blood.[36,40–42] The estimated dose likely to be ingested by the infant is less than 2 mg/kg/day. Neither the drug nor its metabolite was detected in the infant's plasma in any but very low concentration,[41] and no adverse effects have been reported. The Committee on Drugs of the American Academy of Pediatrics considers the use of disopyramide compatible with breast feeding.[23]

CLASS IB ANTIARRHYTHMIC DRUGS

Lidocaine

The prototype of class Ib antiarrhythmic agents, lidocaine is very effective in suppressing ventricular ectopy and ventricular tachyarrhythmias. Onset of action is immediate following bolus intravenous administration. The effect lasts 10–20 minutes, but half-life is about 100 minutes. The drug is 70% bound to proteins, predominantly to α_1-acid glycoprotein.[43]

Lidocaine undergoes liver metabolism (90%), which depends mainly on hepatic blood flow. Currently lidocaine is the treatment of choice for ventricular arrhythmias, including emergent conditions.

Lidocaine's use as an antiarrhythmic agent during pregnancy has rarely been reported. Most of the information available is obtained from its extensive use as a local anesthetic during labor and delivery.[44–64] Stokes et al[65] described the use of lidocaine in a woman who suffered an acute myocardial infarction and underwent successful rescucitation after a cardiac arrest at 18 weeks of gestation. A male infant low in birth weight but otherwise normal, was delivered at 38 weeks. At 17 months of age his neurologic condition was normal, but growth was below the 10th percentile. Menon et al[66] reported a 15-year-old girl at late pregnancy presented with Bell's palsy and runs of sustained ventricular tachycardia. The arrhythmia was effectively controlled with lidocaine, labor was induced, and the delivery was uneventful. Juneja et al[67] used a continuous epidural infusion at term in a 20-year-old pregnant woman who presented with multiple ventricular premature beats and runs of nonsustained ventricular tachycardia in two successive pregnancies. The arrhythmia was controlled, and both infants were normal. Delivery was vaginal at the first pregnancy and cesarian section at the second one, owing to lack of progression and fetal acidosis.

Lidocaine crosses the placenta fairly rapidly after intravenous or epidural administration, and could even be detected in the umbilical cord within 2 minutes of administration.[68] The fetal/maternal serum concentration ratio is 0.5 to 0.7.[44–48,67,69,70] The lower fetal levels may be attributable to lower α_1-acid glycoprotein blood concentrations in the fetus, which are one third of that of the mother.[43] Lidocaine is a weak base and may be trapped in the slightly acidic environment of amniotic fluid. In addition, several reports have described a rise in fetal drug levels during fetal acidosis.[49,50,70] Acidosis may increase the unbound fraction of lidocaine, facilitating further fetal trapping.[51] The elimination half-life of lidocaine in a neonate acquiring the medication in utero is prolonged (180 min, vs. 100 min in adults).[45]

Scanlon et al[52] reported that offspring of mothers treated with continuous epidural blocks had significantly lower scores on tests of muscle strength and tone than did controls.

Several reports described lack of deleterious neurobehavioral effects; as in adults, however, lidocaine may produce side effects in the fetus.[53–56,69] In a study of 57 pregnant women given lidocaine for caudal, epidural, paracervical, or pudendal block, 4 out of 8 infants with drug levels above 2.5 μg/mL had Apgar scores of 6 or less.[69] Of 5 infants with central nervous system depression at birth, 3 had lidocaine levels greater than 3 μg/mL. Since fetal plasma levels are 50–70% of maternal levels, to avoid fetal toxicity, the maternal plasma levels should not exceed 4 μg/mL. Kim et al[53] reported a case in which accidental lidocaine injection to the fetus's scalp during local anesthesia for episiotomy induced severe toxicity in the newborn, producing blood levels of 14 μg/mL and manifesting as apnea, hypotonia, seizures, and fixed dilated pupils. The neonate recovered completely with normal neurologic function and behavior after 3 days and at a second evaluation 7 months later. Bozynski et al[54] described a neonate with severe lidocaine toxicity delivered 20 minutes after administration of 200 mg lidocaine to the mother for pudendal block. The neonate developed apnea and bradycardia soon after birth, requiring mechanical ventilation and intensive supportive therapy. Fetal lidocaine level was 2–3 μg/mL. The infant recovered completely within a few days, and at 2 months follow-up, his physical examination was normal. Van Dorsten and Miller[56] described fetal heart decelerations immediately after inadvertent intrauterine injection of lidocaine. The fetal bradycardia persisted 14 minutes and was accompanied with transient fetal acidosis. The delivery proceeded normally and the infant had Apgar scores 5 at 1 minute, owing to lack of respiration and hypotonia, and 9 at 5 minutes.

In the Collaborative Perinatal Project,[57] which monitored 50,282 mother–child pairs, 293 women were exposed to lidocaine during their first trimester. There was no evidence of teratogenicity, but there was greater than expected incidence of respiratory tract anomalies (three cases), tumors (two cases), and inguinal hernias (eight cases). It is not known whether these findings are related to maternal comorbidity or lidocaine, or are incidental. For the whole pregnancy duration, 947 exposures were recorded, again without evidence of teratogenicity. In other reports, no neurobehavioral abnormalities were demonstrated in infants born to mothers treated with lidocaine during their pregnancies.[55,58,59]

It thus appears that use of lidocaine in pregnancy is safe as long as the fetal acid–base status is normal and maternal blood levels are kept within mid- to-low therapeutic range. Particular attention should be given to maternal lidocaine levels in preeclamptic women, in whom due to prolonged total body clearance of epidural lidocaine administration of the drug may result in higher blood levels than in normotensive patients.[60]

Currently the FDA pregnancy risk category of lidocaine is B.[22] However, since lidocaine undergoes primarily hepatic metabolism, pregnant women with diminished hepatic blood flow, such as in congestive heart failure, should receive reduced dosage. Additionally, lidocaine should preferably be avoided when labor is prolonged or in fetal distress, conditions that are associated with fetal acidosis.

Zeister et al[61] reported a 37-year-old lactating woman with mitral valve prolapse who was treated with intravenous lidocaine for acute onset of ventricular arrhythmias. Her serum level was 2 μg/mL, and the milk concentration 2 hours later, after discontinuation of lidocaine, was 0.8 μg/mL. The infant was not allowed to nurse during the administration of lidocaine to his mother or immediately afterward. No further reports are available.

The Committee on Drugs of the American Academy of Pediatrics considers the use of lidocaine compatible with breast feeding.[23]

Mexiletine

Mexiletine, a local anesthetic structurally similar to lidocaine, is approved by the FDA for oral treatment of symptomatic ventricular tachycardia.

Unlike lidocaine, bioavailability following oral administration is about 90%, and 10% undergoes first-pass hepatic metabolism. Peak plasma mexiletine concentration is reached with 2–4 hours, and 75% is protein-bound. Elimination half-life is 7.5–10 hours.[62] Common adverse effects are gastrointestinal (nausea, vomiting), neurological (diplopia, dizziness, tremor, paresthesia), and fever and rash.

The experience with mexiletine in pregnancy is quite limited.[63,64,71–73] Timmis et al[63] successfully treated ventricular tachycardia by administering mexiletine 600 (mg/day) in combination with propanolol (120 mg/day) to a woman in her 31st gestational week. Therapy was continued, and during spontaneous delivery at the 39th gestational week the fetal/maternal mexiletine concentration ratio was 1.0. The infant was normal at birth, but a transient bradycardia of 90 beats per minute was noted for 6 hours. The infant was breast-fed while the mother continued treatment with mexiletine, resulting in mexiletine/breast milk concentrations of 0.6–0.8 mg/L. The drug could not be detected in the infant's serum, and no adverse effects were noted.

In another report,[64] mexiletine and propranolol were used to suppress ventricular tachycardia resistant to procainamide in a woman who was 14 weeks pregnant. The patient gave birth to a healthy boy, and no side effects were noted. Lownes and Ives[71] described a 26-year-old woman with a history of mitral valve prolapse, ventricular ectopy, and ventricular tachycardia who was treated with mexiletine 750 (mg/day) and atenolol (50 mg/day) throughout her conception, pregnancy, and postnatal course. During prenatal evaluations, the fetus was thought to be small for gestational age. At 39 weeks, the patient delivered vaginally a healthy male infant weighing 2600 g with an Apgar score of 9/10 at 1 and 5 minutes, respectively. Serum mexiletine levels of the mother on admission and of the child 9 hours postpartum were <0.2 and 0.4 μg/mL, respectively. During the immediate postpartum period, the infant had failure to feed and at 8 months was reevaluated for seizurelike episodes. The results of his neurologic examination and electroencephalogram showed normal development, he was found to have gastroesophageal reflux, and subsequently he developed normally. Gregg and Tomich[72] described another patient with mitral valve prolapse and symptomatic premature ventricular contractions treated with mexiletine prior to conception and throughout pregnancy. The dose of mexiletine was increased throughout the pregnancy from 30 mg/day at the time of conception to 800 mg/day at delivery. During cesarean section delivery (at 38 weeks of gestation), lidocaine was added to control ventricular ectopy. A male infant weighing 3750 g with an Apgar score of 4/9 was delivered. Subsequently, hypoglycemia in the newborn period was noted and corrected. At delivery, the maternal and cord blood mexiletine levels were 0.6 and 0.4 μg/mL, respectively.

In summary, mexiletine appears to freely cross the placenta, and fetomaternal ratio ranges from 0.7 to 1.[62,63] Although the use of mexiletine during pregnancy was initially thought to be safe,[62,63] reported fetal bradycardia, small size for gestational age,[71] low Apgar score, and neonatal hypoglycemia[72] are bothersome. Despite these concerns, no teratogenic or long-term adverse consequences have been reported.

Currently the FDA pregnancy risk category of mexiletine is C.[22] Mexiletine is secreted in breast milk. Both Timmis et al[63] and Lewis[64] found higher concentrations of mexiletine in the breast milk than in mothers' plasma; the milk/plasma ratio varied between 0.78 and 1.89.[63] However, the calculated daily quantity ingested by the infant appears to be well below therapeutic range,[64] and mexiletine levels were undetectable in the infant blood.[63]

The Committee on Drugs of the American Academy of Pediatrics considers the use of mexiletine compatible with breast feeding.[23]

Tocainide

Tocainide, an additional oral analog of lidocaine, is indicated for treatment of ventricular arrhythmias. In addition it has been used in the treatment of myotonic dystrophy and trigeminal neuralgia.

Bioavailability of tocainide is nearly 100%. Following oral ingestion, peak plasma tocainide concentration is reached at 0.5–2 hours; mean half-life is 10–14 hours, and tocainide is poorly protein-bound. About 40% is excreted unchanged in the urine. Adverse effects are dose dependent, including lightheadedness, paresthesia, tremors, diplopia, tinnitus, nausea, vomiting anorexia, skin rash, and sweating. Tocainide may have proarrhythmic effect or may aggravate congestive heart failure. Infrequently it may produce pulmonary fibrosis or bone marrow depression.[74–76]

No report of its usage in human pregnancy is available. Animal studies have shown conflicting results. In mice, tocainide and its metabolites cross the placenta to the fetus. No teratogenicity was observed in rats and rabbits exposed to doses up to 12 times the usual human dose. Similar doses in rats produced dystocia, delayed parturition, increased incidence of stillbirth, and reduced one-week offspring survival.

In spite of lack of human data, currently the FDA pregnancy risk category of tocainide is C.[22] No information about tocainide secretion into breast milk is available.

Phenytoin

Phenytoin is used mainly to treat seizure disorders. Its antiarrhythmic usage is limited,[77] mainly to cases of supraventricular and ventricular arrhythmias due to digitalis toxicity; infrequently it is used for refractory ventricular arrhythmias associated with general anesthesia and cardiac surgery, prolonged QT syndrome, or arrhythmias combined with epilepsy.[74,77–79]

Following oral administration, absorption of phenytoin is incomplete and delayed, varies with the brand of drug, and reaches peak plasma concentration within 8–12 hours. The drug is 90% protein-bound. Therapeutic serum concentration is 10 to 20 μg/mL and is similar for both cardiac arrhythmias and epilepsy. Over 90% of the drug undergoes hepatic metabolism, and mean elimination half-life (about 24 h) can be slowed in the presence of liver disease or concomitant administration of phenothiazines, dicumarol, chloramphenicol, phenylbutazone, and isoniazid. Adverse effects include nystagmus, ataxia, drowsiness, stupor and coma, nausea, epigastric pain, anorexia, hyperglycemia, hypocalcemia, skin rash, megaloblastic anemia, gingival hyperplasia, lymph node hyperplasia, peripheral neuropathy, and systemic lupus erythematosus.[74,77–79]

Phenytoin's use as an antiarrhythmic agent during pregnancy has not been reported. However, extensive information has been accumulated from its use during pregnancy for management of maternal epilepsy.[19,80–99]

Plasma phenytoin concentrations may decrease during pregnancy to about 40% at term. Therefore dose requirements correspondingly increase. These changes may result from altered drug absorption or increased clearance. Postpartum plasma concentrations rapidly return to prepregnancy values, calling for dose reduction.[80–87]

Phenytoin readily crosses the placenta. Neonatal and maternal serum concentrations are similar.[78–81] At therapeutic maternal levels, 72 hours is required for the elimination of phenytoin from the neonate.[89] Janz and Fuchs described in 1964 the teratogenic effects of phenytoin.[90] Since then numerous studies have reported the teratogenic effects in epileptic pregnant women taking phenytoin either alone or in combination with other anticonvulsants.[91–102] Hanson and Buehler reviewed the literature in 1982 and found an incidence of defects in treated epileptics varying from 2.2 to 26.1%.[97,98] The authors tentatively attributed the increased risk to the antiepileptic drugs, to genetic factors, or to their combination. However, in each study the teratogenic rate was higher in the treated mothers than in untreated epileptic or normal control mothers. Buehler et al[79] found that the teratogenic effects of phenytoin may be secondary to elevated levels of oxidative metabolites—epoxides. The suceptibility may be genetically determined.

A characteristic pattern of malformations, known as the fetal hydantoin syndrome (FHS), was described.[100–102] Clinical features of FSH, not necessarily apparent in ever infant, are as follows:

Craniofacial: broad nasal bridge, wide fontanel, low-set hairline, broad alveolar ridge, metoptic ridging, short neck, ocular hypertelorism, microcephaly, cleft lip/palate, abnormal or low-set ears, epicanthal folds, ptosis of eyelids, coloboma, coarse scalp hair.

Limbs: small or absent nails, hypoplasia, of distal phalanges, altered palmar crease, digital thumb, dislocated hip.

Growth retardation, both physical and mental, and congenital heart defects are also often observed. Reviewing the literature in 1982, Janz stated that all possible malformations may be observed in the offspring of mothers treated for epilepsy.[103] Briggs et al[104] in their recent extensive review support his statement.

The surveillance study of Michigan Medicaid recipients involving 229,101 completed pregnancies between 1985 and 1992, reported on 332 newborns exposed to phenytoin during the first trimester. A total of 15 (4.5%) exhibited major birth defects, including 5/3 (observed/expected) cardiovascular, 1/0 spina bifida, and 1/1 hypospadias. No anomalies were observed in three other categories (oral clefts, polydactyly, limb reduction defects) for which specific data were available.[19]

Twelve case reports describing infants' malignancy after in utero exposure to phenytoin have been located[104]: neuroblastoma, six cases; and a single case each for ganglioneuroblastoma, melanotic neuroectodermal tumor, extrarenal Wilms' tumor, mesenchymoma, lymphangioma, and ependymoma. These findings suggest that phenytoin may be a human transplacental carcinogen. Therefore children exposed in utero to phenytoin should be closely followed up for at least several years.

Phenytoin may cause early hemorrhagic disease of the newborn, which may be severe or even fatal when occurring during the first 24 hours after birth.[105] The mechanism suggested for this hemorrhagic tendency is unknown. Lane and Hathaway[106] suggested that phenytoin induction of microsomal hepatic enzymes may deplete the already low reserves of fetal vitamin K. Phenytoin-induced thrombocytopenia has also been reported as a mechanism for hemorrhage in the newborn.[107] In controlled trials, however, none of these potential mechanisms were proven.[106] In spite of that, Lane and Hathaway suggested oral vitamin K administration to phenytoin-treated pregnant women during the last 2 months of gestation (10 mg/day), with increased dosage (20 mg/day) during the last 2 weeks. At delivery they recommended immediate intramuscular administration of vitamin K to the newborn, combined with cord blood coagulation status evaluation.

Phenytoin may induce folic acid deficiency in the epileptic patient by impairing gastrointestinal absorption or by inducing hepatic enzymes and increasing folic acid metabolism. Biale and Lewenthal[107] described two populations treated with phenytoin and other anticonvulsants. Twenty-four pregnant women, studied retrospectively without folic acid supplementation, gave birth to 66 infants. Ten infants (15%) had major anomalies, and two mothers of the affected infants had markedly low red blood cell folate levels. The second group, consisting of 22 epileptic women who were given folic acid (2.5–5 mg/day), starting before conception in 26 pregnancies and within the first 40 days in 6, gave birth to 33 infants, without any defect. However, other reports did not confirm this association.[107–109] Hiilesmaa et al[109] treated 133 women with an average daily folic acid dose of 0.5 mg from the 6th to the 16th week of gestation. They found defects in 20 infants (15%), which is similar to the reported frequency in anticonvulsant-treated pregnant women without folate supplementation. It should be noted that in this study folic acid supplementation was initiated relatively late with a significantly lower dosage.

Dansky et al suggested that in animals as well as in humans there is a dose-related teratogenic effect of phenytoin.[110,111]

Currently the FDA pregnancy risk category of phenytoin is D.[23] That is, phenytoin usage during pregnancy involves a significant fetal risk, mainly congenital malformations and hemorrhage at birth. Phenytoin probably should not be used to control arrhythmias even for its special indications in non-pregnant patients, since safer therapeutic alternatives exist. When its usage is mandatory for maternal seizure control during pregnancy, close monitoring of plasma phenytoin levels is recommended to maintain adequate seizure control and to avoid excessively high plasma concentrations.

Phenytoin is excreted into breast milk. Milk/plasma ratio ranged from 0.18 to 0.54.[59,77–80] There is only one case report on methemoglobinemia, drowsiness, and decreased sucking activity.[81] None of the other reports described infantile adverse effects associated with maternal phenytoin usage during lactation.

The Committee on Drugs of the American Academy of Pediatrics considers the use of phenytoin compatible with breast feeding.[23]

Moricizine

Moricizine is a phenothiazine derivative, approved for treating ventricular arrhythmias. It is also effective in the management of supraventricular arrhythmias. It shortens Purkinje fiber action potential and, like class Ib antiarrhythmics, exerts minimal effect on cardiac performance. However, moricizine significantly decreases phase 0 sodium influx, in which action it is like class Ia antiarrhythmics.[79]

Moricizine is rapidly almost completely absorbed following oral administration, but it undergoes extensive first-pass metabolism, resulting in bioavailability of 35–40%. Peak plasma concentration is within 0.5–2 hours. Protein binding is 95%, and plasma half-life is 1.5 to 3.5 hours. The drug is usually well tolerated. Adverse effects include tremor, mood changes, headache, vertigo, nystagmus, dizziness, nausea, vomiting and diarrhea.[79,112,113] In the second Cardiac Arrhythmia Suppression Trial, (CAST-II), moricizine was ineffective and even somewhat harmful, being associated with increased mortality within 2 weeks of drug initiation.[114]

No reports of the use of moricizine in human pregnancy are currently available. Teratogenicity studies in rabbits and rats treated with five and seven times, respectively, the maximal human moricizine dose did not result in either teratogenic or fetotoxic effect.[22]

Currently the FDA pregnancy risk category of moricizine is B.[22] However, it should be noted that we lack any significant human experience with the drug during pregnancy, and it should be used with caution. The excretion of moricizine in human milk has been described in animals and in humans without reported problems to the fetuses,[22,23] but no published clinical experience is available.

CLASS IC ANTIARRHYTHMIC DRUGS

Flecainide

Flecainide acetate is a potent antiarrhythmic agent used for both ventricular and supraventricular arrhythmias. Because its high potential for proarrhythmia,[115,116] flecainide has been approved for the prevention of paroxysmal supraventricular tachycardias and paroxysmal atrial fibrillation/flutter associated with disabling symptoms in patients without structural heart disease. The drug has also been restricted to the treatment of sustained life-threatening ventricular arrhythmias. Bioavailability of oral flecainide dose is 95%, with peak plasma levels of 2–4 hours. Plasma half-life is 12–27 hours (average 14 h).[74,117] Flecainide is 50% protein-bound. About two-thirds of an oral dose undergoes hepatic metabolism into inactive metabolites. Drug interaction occurs when flecainide is combined with digoxin or propranolol, and dose adjustment may be required.[3] Side effects include blurred vision, dizziness, headache, nausea, paresthesia, tremor, fatigue, and nervousness.

Flecainide has been used during pregnancy for both maternal[118–120] and fetal[121–127] tachyarrhythmias. Palmer and Norris[118] described a case of 24-year-old women with symptomatic Wolff–Parkinson–White (WPW) syndrome who was treated with flecainide up to 300 mg/day. At 37 weeks of pregnancy the patient delivered spontaneously a healthy baby girl. The maternal and fetal cord blood levels were 0.63 and 0.44 mg/L, respectively (fetomaternal ratio of 0.69). Wagner et al[119] described a case of a 23-year-old woman who was treated with flecainide (200 mg/day) and sotalol (160 mg/day) for "bursts" of ventricular tachycardia and polymorphic premature ventricular contractions. While on treatment, the patient became pregnant, and the therapy was continued at the same dosage throughout the pregnancy. A normal baby was delivered by cesarian section 3 weeks before full term. At delivery, the fetomaternal flecainide level ratio was 0.86. The follow-up of the infant after one year revealed no abnormalities. Doig et al[120] reported failure of oral flecainide (300 mg daily) as well as a subsequent attempt with amiodarone to cardiovert incessant atrial tachycardia late in the course of a twin pregnancy in a 24-year-old woman. The patient cardioverted spontaneously at 31 weeks of gestation during the first stage of labor. Two healthy infants were delivered vaginally by forceps.

Flecainide has been used successfully for cardioversion of fetal supraventricular tachyarrhythmias.[121–127] Allan et al[121] treated 14 cases of fetal supraventricular tachycardias associated with intrauterine heart failure with flecainide (300 mg/day), and 12 of the 14 fetuses responded by cardioversion to sinus rhythm. In the remaining two fetuses, the tachycardias were treated successfully with digoxin. One of the fetuses treated with flecainide died after maternal treatment for 3 days. This event occurred after the fetal arrhythmia had been cardioverted to sinus rhythm and within 24 hours from cordocentesis. The authors attributed the death either to cordocentesis or to proarrhythmia induced by flecainide. The mean time for cardioversion for the series was 48 hours, and the mean age of delivery was 35 weeks. Comparison of cord and maternal blood flecainide concentrations indicated a placental transfer of approximately 80% of the drug. The data above compared favorably with the authors' earlier experience with 12 hydropic fetuses treated with digoxin and verapamil, in which there were two deaths and high rates of postnatal complications in the remaining 10 fetuses, with a mean time to cardioversion of 2–3 weeks.[123]

Perry et al.[124] described another two cases of fetal supraventricular tachycardia refractory to digoxin, alone and in combination with verapamil, that responded to the combination of digoxin and flecainide (maternal dose, 300 mg/day). The fetomaternal ratio of flecainide was 0.7–0.83 at the time of delivery, and the calculated fetal elimination half time was 29 hours. Kohl et al[125] successfully cardioverted incessant fetal tachycardia by intraumbilical administration of adenosine at the 28th week of gestation. They continued with the following maternal daily regimen: 1.2 mg β-methyl digoxin intravenously and 300 mg flecainide orally. The fetus died at the end of the 29th week, probably as a result of the proarrhythmic effect of the combination therapy.

Currently the FDA pregnancy risk category of flecainide is C.[23]

The foregoing data and other reports[124–128] suggest that flecainide is a very effective drug for cardioversion of fetal supraventricular tachycardia and is devoid of teratogenic effects. Caution is advisable because of the death of two fetuses,[118,126] however, even though neither death could be attributed with certainty to flecainide.

Flecainide is secreted in breast milk. Wagner et al[119] measured the breast milk/maternal plasma ratio, which varied between 1.57 and 2.18. McQuinn et al[129] measured breast milk and plasma flecainide concentrations in 11 healthy volunteers treated with flecainide (100 mg every 12 h for 5.5 days). Milk/plasma ratios ranged from 2.6 to 3.7. The authors estimated that the maximal daily amount ingested by the infant could be 1.07 mg, which is unlikely to cause adverse effects. The babies were not breast fed in either study.

The Committee on Drugs of the American Academy of Pediatrics considers the use of flecainide compatible with breast feeding.[23]

Propafenone

Propafenone is effective in treating supraventricular as well as ventricular arrhythmias.[130–133] However, recent studies have shown lack of efficacy or even proarrhythmic effects in treating ventricular arrhythmia (ESVEM)[134] or cardiac arrest survivors (CASH).[135] In recent years propafenone has been widely used mainly for supraventricular arrhythmias.[130,133] Although propafenone has structured features similar to those of propranolol and its β-adrenergic blocking activities are demonstrable in vitro, only mild and inconsistent beta blockade occurs in vivo.[130–132]

Following oral ingestion of propafenone, more than 95% is absorbed; there is extensive first-pass hepatic metabolism that is saturable at low doses. Therefore propafenone exhibits a dose-dependent bioavailability, which increases from 5–12% after a single dose of 150–300 mg to 40–50% with 450 mg. Peak plasma concentration is achieved within 2–3 hours. Similarly the relationship between dosage and steady state concentration is nonlinear. Increasing the dosage three-fold (from 300 to 900 mg/day) causes a 10-fold increase in steady state mean plasma concentration. Plasma half-life ranges from 2 to 10 (mean 6) hours, and the drug is 95% protein-bound.[130,131]

Propafenone is almost entirely metabolized, with less than 1% excreted unchanged in the urine. It is metabolized in vivo to 5-hydroxypropafenone of equal antiarrhythmic potency and to N-desalkylpropafenone of less potency. In approximately 7% of the population of the United States, a genetic deficiency in the hepatic cytochrome isoenzyme P-450 dbl causes the metabolism to 5-hydroxypropafenone to be impaired, with the result that in these individuals plasma half-life may be as long as 32 hours and propafenone levels may reach toxic levels at therapeutic doses.[130]

Minor adverse effects occur in about 15% of patients, and these are mainly neurological (dizziness, taste disturbance, blurred vision, headaches, parasthesias) and gastrointestinal (nausea, vomiting, anorexia, constipation). Less common adverse effects are abnormal liver function tests, ophthalmic disturbances, arthritis, arthralgia, leukopenia, and rash. Infrequently there are reports of exacerbation of asthma or shortness of breath.[79,128–130]

During pregnancy, propafenone has been used during the second and third trimester for both maternal[136,137] and fetal indications.[138,139] Brunozzi et al[136] reported the clinical case of a 22-year-old pregnant patient with valvular disease treated with propafenone for complex ventricular arrhythmia. Therapy was started during her 19th week of gestation, initially with 450 mg/day and later with 900 mg/day. The patient underwent cesarian section at 36 weeks of pregnancy and delivered a 2.450 kg neonate with Apgar score of 8/10 at 1 and 5 minutes, respectively. At birth, the fetomaternal propafenone and 5-hydroxypropafenone blood concentration level ratio was 0.29 and 0.45, respectively. There were no adverse fetal or teratogenic effects. Santinelli et al[137] treated with propafenone a 28-year-old pregnant woman with WPW syndrome. Their patient experienced an episode of ventricular fibrillation due to atrial fibrillation with fast ventricular rates, but no information is given in regard to pregnancy outcome. Gembruch et al[138,139] used propafenone in conjunction with β-methyldigoxin and/or other antiarrhythmics via direct intrauterine administration in fetuses when transplacental passage of antiarrhythmic drugs was not effective. Among fetuses with nonimmune fetal hydrops, there were four deaths. However, because of the severity of these cases and use of multiple drugs both transplacentally and direct intraperitoneally, it is not clear what was responsible for fetal death: propafenone or the arrhythmia and hydrops fetalis themselves. Libardoni et al[140] treated a 37-year-old woman for nonsustained ventricular tachycardia and paroxysmal supraventricular tachycardia with propafenone (450 mg/day initially, 900 mg/day afterward) starting at her 25th week of gestation. She gave birth to a normal child spontaneously at the 36th week. The cord/maternal ratio was 0.42 for the metabolite 5-hydroxypropafenone, and 0.14 for the parent drug. This difference can be explained by different maternal protein bindings of the two compounds (75 and 95%, respectively).

Currently the manufacturer's definition of the pregnancy risk category of propafenone is C. In spite of the widespread usage of propafenone in nonpregnant patients, the limited data available during pregnancy and the adverse outcomes described above[138,139] indicate that propafenone should be used during pregnancy only with great caution.

Libardoni and al[140] also measured ratio of breast milk to plasma and found 0.50 for 5-hydroxypropafenone, and 0.20 for propafenone. Since the infant in their report was bottle-fed, they could only calculate. Assuming a daily milk intake of 150 mL/kg, the estimated ingested amount of both the parent drug and its metabolite was about 0.03% of the maternal dose.

Lorcainide

Lorcainide is a relatively new class Ic antiarrhythmic medication. Following oral dose administration, absorption ranges to 65%. Absorption is probably dose related, and it increases with chronic therapy. About 70% is protein-bound, and its half-life is about 9 hours. Lorcainide undergoes hepatic metabolism, and less than 3% is excreted unchanged in urine. Its metabolite norlorcainide is active and its plasma concentrations are higher than the parent compound. The half-life of norlorcainide is almost three times longer than that of lorcainide.[141,142]

There is no evidence of effect on fertility, embryotoxicity, or dysmorphogenicity among rats and rabbits treated with long-term oral or parenteral lorcainide.[144]

Currently the FDA pregnancy risk category of lorcainide is C.[23]

Lorcainide is secreted in breast milk of both animals and humans. No adverse effects associated with maternal lorcainide administration and breast feeding have been currently reported.

Encainide

Encainide has been approved by the FDA for treatment of life-threatening ventricular arrhythmias.[79] Following oral ingestion there is variable absorption, ranging from 7 to 80%, with peak plasma concentration within 0.5–2 hours. Plasma half-life is 3–4 hours for encainide but may reach 12 hours for its metabolites, which are more active than the parent drug. Encainide and metabolites are more than 75% protein-bound, and the drug is excreted renally. Adverse effects include dizziness, diplopia, vertigo, paresthesia, leg cramps, and metallic taste in the mouth. Sinus arrest or atrioventricular block may occur, and proarrhythmia has been reported, especially in patients with a history of sustained ventricular tachycardia, structural heart disease, or congestive heart failure.[79,143]

There are only two reports concerning the use of encainide in human pregnancy.[144,145] Encainide and its two active metabolites o-demethylencainide and 3-methoxydemethylencainide cross the placenta. Concentrations of encainide and its metabolites in fetal plasma ranged from 30 to 300% of simultaneously collected maternal levels. Amniotic fluid levels of the three compounds were two to three times greater than the fetal plasma.[144] Strasburger et al[145] described encainide administration at the 26th week of gestation for resistant fetal tachycardia and continued throughout pregnancy and during infancy. The authors did not specify the patient's outcome. However, summarizing the outcome of 41 children treated for supraventricular tachycardia with oral encainide alone or in combination with other antiarrhythmic medication, they found efficacy of about 60%. They concluded that children younger than 6 months required higher dose for arrhythmia control and had higher incidence of adverse events. Quart[144] used an encainide maternal dose of 200 mg/day to successfully treat fetal arrhythmia. The gestational age of the fetus was not given, nor the length of therapy. Encainide could not be detected in the fetal plasma, and the concentrations of the two metabolites were less than 100 ng/mL. However, very high concentrations of the metabolites were measured in the first newborn's urine samples.

Currently the pregnancy risk category of encainide defined by the manufacturer is B.

Quart[144] also measured milk levels of encainide and one metabolite, *o*-demethylencainide, and found 200–400 and 100–20 ng/mL, respectively. These levels were comparable to maternal peak plasma levels. The second metabolite, 3-methoxy-*o*-demethylencainide, was not produced by the mother and could not be detected in her plasma nor in her milk. In animals, however, Quart found milk secretion also of this metabolite.

CLASS III ANTIARRHYTHMIC DRUGS

Amiodarone

Amiodarone, a benzofuran derivative containing two iodine molecules, is a very potent and effective class III antiarrhythmic. Introduced in the late 1960s as an antianginal drug, its peculiar antiarrhythmic properties soon became evident and, since then, it has been extensively used to treat both supraventricular and ventricular arrhythmias. The drug is very effective against atrial fibrillation and flutter, paroxysmal supraventricular tachycardia, ectopic atrial tachycardia, and supraventricular arrhythmia related to preexcitation syndromes. Amiodarone is currently probably also the most effective medication for ventricular tachyarrhythmias. In addition to its direct antiarrhytmic effects, amiodarone has noncompetitive β- and α-adrenergic-blocking properties, as well as some calcium channel blocking activity, exerting coronary and systemic vasodilatation. It also has anti-ischemic and antiadrenergic properties.[146–148]

Following oral ingestion, amiodarione is slowly, variably, and incompletely absorbed. Bioavailability is 35–65%, and peak plasma concentration is 3–7 hours. There is only minimal first-pass hepatic extraction. Onset of action after oral administration is within a few days, while intravenous administration is usually effective within a few hours. Amiodarone undergoes extensive hepatic metabolism, predominantly to desethylamiodarone. Both compounds accumulate extensively in liver, lung, fat, and skin. Myocardial concentration of amiodarone is 10–50 times that found in the plasma. Plasma protein binding is 96%. Amiodarone clearance is very slow, mainly by hepatic excretion into bile, with some enterohepatic recirculation. After cessation of drug ingestion, plasma concentration declines to 50% reduction within 3–10 days, followed by a final half-life ranging from 26 to 107 (mean 53) days.[79,146,148]

Unfortunately, amiodarone's toxicity parallels its remarkable antiarrhythmic efficacy. Pulmonary, hyper- or hypothy-roidism, neuromuscular, gastrointestinal, ocular, hepatic, and cutaneous side effects may require discontinuation of therapy.[74,146–148]

Amiodarone may interact with several drugs. Amiodarone potentiates the effect of warfarin and increases the serum levels of digoxin, quinidine, procainamide, phenytoin, and diltiazem. Dosage adjustment of these medications is frequently required when they are coadministered with amiodarone.[146–148]

There are several reports of amiodarone use during pregnancy for either the mother or the fetus.[138,139,149–165] Amiodarone and its metabolite desethylamiodarone (DEA) cross the placenta to the fetus. In 10 infants described, cord plasma concentrations of amiodarone and DEA were 0.05–0.35 and 0.05–0.55 µg/mL, respectively.[139,149–156] Cord/maternal ratios for amiodarone were 0.10–0.28 in nine cases[150–155] and 0.6 in one case,[156] and for DEA about 0.25.[149–156] Gembruch et al,[122,139] who infused amiodarone via repeated umbilical punctures, found a smaller fetomaternal ratio that probably was due to the severity of hydrops fetalis. The expected fetal concentrations were not achieved until substantial improvement of fetal heart failure had occurred.

Maternal indications for amiodarone therapy were both supraventricular (atrial fibrillation in patients with Wolff–Parkinson–White syndrome, atrial tachycardia, and fibrillation) and ventricular tachyarrhythmias.[149–154,156,157] Fetal indications were tachyarrhythmias and tachyarrhythmia-induced congestive heart failure.[158–161]

Candelpergher et al[149] treated two pregnant women for refractory atrial tachycardia. Both newborns were healthy. McKenna et al[150] treated a woman in her 34th gestational week who had paroxysms of atrial flutter/fibrillation associated with Wolff–Parkinson–White syndrome and was resistant to quinidine. A loading dose of 800 mg/day for one week was followed by a maintenance dose of 400 mg daily. At 41 weeks, the patient delivered a normal child that was slightly bradycardic (104–120 beats/min) for 48 hours. Pitcher et al[151] reported a successful treatment with amiodarone of atrial tachycardia resistant to propranolol, digoxin, and verapamil during the last 3 weeks of pregnancy. Neither the mother nor the child had untoward effects. Penn et al[152] reported a 32-year-old woman treated with amiodarone from her 16th week of gestation. Initially she received 800 mg daily for one week and later 200 mg/day. At 39 weeks of gestation she gave birth to a normal baby, but his QT interval was prolonged for an additional 7 weeks.

Robson et al[153] described two cases in which amiodarone was administrated during pregnancy for longer periods. In the first case, the patient became pregnant while on daily maintenance dose of 200 mg of amiodarone to control atrial fibrillation associated with mitral stenosis, and the drug was continued throughout the pregnancy. At 37 weeks, she delivered a healthy baby. In the second case, amiodarone (400 mg/day) was given in addition to metoprolol (50 mg/day) to control atrial tachycardia in a patient in her 22nd week; at 39 weeks, she delivered a healthy child. Strunge et al[154] described a woman who received 200–400 mg of amiodarone throughout her pregnancy. She gave birth to a healthy child. Plomp et al[155] described five pregnancies in four women treated with amiodarone. Four infants, exposed to amiodarone throughout gestation, were healthy at birth and during follow-up from 8 months to 5 years. The fifth infant, who was exposed to metoprolol throughout pregnancy and to amiodarone during the last six weeks, was born at 40 weeks with low birth weight. At 5 years of age, he reportedly continued to show abnormalities (impaired speech and delayed motor development). Rey et al[156] reported a 19-year-old pregnant patient treated with propranolol (80 mg/day) and amiodarone (400 mg/day) 4 days a week for recurrent ventricular tachycardia. Throughout the pregnancy, the patient developed diffuse thyroid enlargement, but she was clinically euthyroid and her thyroid function tests were normal. The patient gave birth to a healthy 2670 g baby with no signs of amiodarone toxicity. At delivery, maternal and fetal thyroid function tests were normal. Foster and Love[157] described a patient treated with amiodarone (400 mg/day) for ventricular ectopy and nonsustained ventricular tachycardia in her 32nd gestational week. A healthy neonate was delivered at 37 weeks by cesarean section. Postdelivery, the infant's heart rate varied from 40 to 163 beats per minute during the following 4 days, and the corrected QT interval was 0.58 second. Amiodarone and DEA levels in the fetal cord blood were 0.1 and 0.2 mg/L, respectively.

Although these initial reports showing no fetal adverse effects were encouraging, other authors reported a less favorable neonatal outcome.[158–160] DeWolf et al[158] reported a severe case of congenital hypothyroidism with goiter, associated with maternal ingestion of 200 mg daily from the 13th week of pregnancy. The baby also had persistent hypotonia and bradycardia, large anterior and posterior fontanels, and macroglossia. Cord blood levels of thyrotropin exceeded 100 mU/L (normal range, 10–20 mU/L), T_4 was 35.9 μg/L (normal range, 60–170 μg/L), and antithyroid antibodies were absent. Iodine content in the fetal urine was 144 μg/dL (normal value, <15 μg/dL). Amiodarone and DEA levels, drawn on the fifth day postdelivery, were 0.65 and 0.45 μg/mL, respectively. Bone maturation was 28 weeks. The infant required substitution therapy with levothyroxine until 20 months of age. At that time, the results of his thyroid function tests were normal, but his psychomotor development revealed 4 months retardation and a bone age of 12 months. Laurent et al[159] reported another case of neonatal hypothyroidism following maternal treatment with digoxin (0.5 mg/day) and amiodarone 1200 (mg/day) for 3 days and afterward 600 mg/day for 3 weeks, for control of fetal supraventricular tachycardia and congestive heart failure. At 35 weeks, a 2960 g infant was delivered. The infant had a heart rate of 200 beats per minute, mild heart failure, and

goiter. Thyroid function tests revealed hypothyroidism, and thyroxine replacement was started. At 3 months of age the infant recovered completely.

The use of amiodarone for the treatment of fetal supraventricular tachycardia was attempted in several cases.[160–162] Arnoux et al[160] described a case of fetal supraventricular tachycardia and congestive heart failure resistant to digoxin alone or in combination with either sotalol or verapamil that was successfully treated with digoxin and amiodarone. Amiodarone was started at 31 weeks of pregnancy and continued until term (38 weeks). A normal infant was delivered with an amiodarone cord/maternal ratio of 0.127. The comparison of doses and fetomaternal levels showed a linear concentration–dosage relation. Therefore, the authors suggested that maternal levels may be used as an indicator for fetal levels. Rey et al[161] described a case of fetal supraventricular tachycardia resistant to digoxin alone and in combination with propranolol that was successfully treated with verapamil and amiodarone. At 33 weeks of gestation, the patient delivered spontaneously a male infant weighing 2700 g with an Apgar score of 8/9 at 1 and 5 minutes, respectively. No drug levels were obtained.

Maternal amiodarone toxicity is similar to that in nonpregnant patients. Potential problems may arise, however, if epidural or general anesthesia is required during cesarean or vaginal delivery.[163] General anesthesia in patients receiving amiodarone has been associated with increased morbidity and mortality. Interaction between amiodarone and anesthetics has been observed during anesthesia for both cardiac and noncardiac surgery. Sinus arrest, junctional rhythms, heart block, atropine-resistant bradycardias, persistent hypotension, and a blunted response to phenylephrine are some of the complications reported. Epidural anesthesia is safer, but precautions should be taken to avoid any alteration of the patient's hemodynamics.

A review[164] of 34 pregnancies in which maternal amiodarone treatment was administered found that 53% of the neonates had no adverse effects and 15% had minor side effects such as bradycardia and prolonged QT interval. In a substantial percentage of neonates, however, more serious adverse effects were seen: small for gestational age (21%), prematurity (12%), and prenatal hypothyroidism (9%). The incidence of neonatal hypothyroidism seen in this series is similar to that observed in the adult population treated with amiodarone.

In summary, amiodarone is a very effective but also a potentially toxic drug for the mother and in particularly for the fetus. In particular, neonatal hypothyroidism, small size for gestational age, and prematurity may have serious consequences with regard to fetal well-being. Use of amiodarone during pregnancy should be reserved for treatment of drug-refractory, symptomatic, and/or potentially lethal tachyarrhythmias. As for adults, the risk for the fetus and the mother probably can be reduced by administration of the minimal effective amiodarone dosage (frequently 200 mg/day or less). A fetal weight below the tenth percentile increases the risk of perinatal mortality, and early delivery should be considered. Therefore particular attention should be given to the fetal intrauterine growth curve and the size of the thyroid gland. In neonates with abnormal thyrotropin levels, a complete thyroid biochemical profile should be obtained at birth, and hormonal substitution therapy should be immediately started in infants with hypothyroidism. During pregnancy, indices of maternal thyroid function should be followed closely.

Currently the FDA pregnancy risk category of amiodarone is D.[22]

The levels of the amiodarone and DEA are higher in breast milk than in maternal serum and can be detected in infant blood, but with wide circadian variation.[150,151,154,165] While desethylamiodarone crosses the placenta in greater concentration than amiodarone, higher levels of amiodarone than of DEA are found in breast milk. McKenna et al[150] measured milk/plasma ratio and found 2.31–9.21 for amiodarone and 0.8–3.8 for its metabolite at 9 weeks postdelivery in a woman being treated with 400 mg/day. They calculated that the infant is exposed to about 1.4 mg/kg/day, equivalent to adult daily dose of 100 mg. Strunge et al[154] measured high amiodarone levels (1.06–3.65 μg/mL) in an 18-year old-woman receiving 200 mg/day. Amiodarone level in the newborn serum were only 0.1 μg/mL or less in repeated measurements, and no adverse effects were noted in the nursing infant. Pitcher et al[151] measure amiodarone levels of 0.5–1.8 μg/mL in breast milk, without adverse effects to the infant. An additional three nursing mothers receiving amiodarone (200 mg/day) had milk/plasma concentration ratios that varied from 0.4 to 13.0, depending on timing of dose to sample interval. Two infants had serum amiodarone levels of 0.01–0.03 μg/mL.

Although no adverse effects were observed in the breast-fed infants, the available data are insufficient. Although elimination of amiodarone in the pediatric age group may be faster, it should be remembered that amiodarone's half-life is still several weeks. Therefore we recommend that until further information has established the infants' safety, breast feeding should be discouraged in a mother who is treated with amiodarone.

Bretylium

Bretylium, a quaternary ammonium compound, is an adrenergic blocker with class III antiarrhythmic properties. It is approved by the FDA for parenteral administration only and is used for life-threatening ventricular arrhythmias that are resistant to lidocaine and probably not amenable to intravenous amiodarone.

Bretylium is effective orally as well as parenterally, although its absorption from the gastrointestinal tract is poor and erratic with bioavailability less than 50%. Following in-

travenous administration, bretylium is widely distributed to various tissues. Its half-life ranges from 5 to 10 hours, and it is eliminated unchanged through the kidneys.[74,79]

The main adverse event is hypotension, occurring in about 50% of the treated patients. Nausea and vomiting may also occur, following rapid intravenous administration.

There is only one report of bretylium use during pregnancy in humans. Gutgesell et al[166] described a 39-year-old woman with long QT interval syndrome, who received chronic oral bretylium tosylate during pregnancy and subsequent breast feeding. The pregnancy and delivery were uncomplicated, and no side effects have been observed in the infant.

In spite of lack of information, currently the FDA pregnancy risk category definition of bretylium is C.[22] However, the high incidence of hypotension associated with bretylium administration, which may compromise uterine blood flow and consequently cause fetal hypoxia, should restrict its usage to resistant and life-threatening ventricular arrhythmias.

Gutgesell described uncomplicated breast feeding in the patient who receive chronic oral bretylium treatment,[166] but there are no additional data available about secretion of bretylium in breast milk of animals or humans, especially when this agent is administered intravenously.

Adenosine

Adenosine, a natural purine nucleoside, is very effective in the management of paroxysmal supraventricular tachycardias. Adenosine is rapidly cleared from circulation by the endothelium and blood cells; its half-life is about 7 seconds. Side effects, which are therefore very short, include headache, flushing, excess inhibition of the sinus or atrioventricular nodes, and anginal pain. Bronchoconstriction may be precipitated, mainly in asthmatic patients, that may persist for 30 minutes.[74,79]

Being a natural substance with a very short half-life, adenosine is particularly attractive for use during pregnancy.[167–172]

Podolsky and Varon[167] reported that a 40-year-old woman, at her 39th week of pregnancy, experienced a recurrent narrow-complex supraventricular tachycardia accompanied by hypotension (systolic blood pressure 80 mmHg). A similar episode had occurred 6 months earlier, and the patient was still being treated with atenolol (50 mg/day). An initial bolus of 6 mg of adenosine showed no response; but a second dose of 12 mg cardioverted her to sinus rhythm within 15 seconds. A healthy infant was born 2 weeks later. Leung et al[168] treated a 27-year old, hypotensive (systolic blood pressure 80 mmHg) women who presented to the emergency room in the 31st week of pregnancy with paroxysmal supraventricular tachycardia. Three boluses of 4, 6, and 8 mg were given at 5-minute intervals; following the third bolus, the patient cardioverted to sinus rhythm. Harrison et al[169] successfully cardioverted a 19-year-old patient who developed her tachycardia during labor in the 38th week of her pregnancy. No effect was noted on fetal heart rate or uterine contraction. Cesarian section was undertaken on failure of labor progression. Mason et al[170] reported a 34-year-old woman with paroxysmal supraventricular tachycardia at her 30th week of gestation. A single 6 mg bolus of adenosine cardioverted her to normal sinus rhythm. The authors did not observe any changes in fetal heart rate. A normal infant was delivered vaginally at term. Afridi et al[171] successfully treated reciprocating tachycardia in a 26-year-old pregnant woman with Wolff–Parkinson–White syndrome with 6 mg adenosine. Subsequently she was treated with atenolol. Her tachycardia recurred during labor, and intravenous boluses 6 and 12 mg of adenosine converted her to sinus rhythm. Fetal distress, noted during the mother's arrhythmia, resolved on return to sinus rhythm. A third recurrence of the reciprocating tachycardia was terminated with 12 mg of adenosine. A male infant was delivered by a cesarian section with Apgar scores 1/5 at 1 and 5 minutes, respectively. Adverse fetal or neonatal effects were not noted in either case.

Kohl et al[125] successfully interrupted incessant tachycardia leading to hydrops fetalis in a 28-week-old fetus by direct administration of adenosine into the umbilical vein. The adenosine abruptly terminated the arrhythmia within seconds, and digoxin and flecainide were added intraumbilically to maintain sinus rhythm. The fetus was found dead in utero at 29 weeks, presumably as a result of recurrence of tachycardia or untoward effects of the medications, probably digoxin and flecainide.

In summary, adenosine is a promising therapy during pregnancy because it is a natural endogenous substance and because of the positive reports of experience with its use in pregnancy to date.[168,172] Adverse or teratogenic effects were noted in only one case, and even then, the fatal fetal outcome is probably related not to adenosine but to the arrhythmia or to other medications. Anyhow further data are needed to establish its safety during usage pregnancy.

Currently the FDA pregnancy risk category of adenosine is C.[22]

No reports about adenosine in breast milk are available. Since its half-life is only a few seconds, adenosine is not expected to be secreted; however this assumption needs confirmation.

CONCLUSION

Many clinical situations in pregnancy require the use of cardiovascular medications. It is hard to evaluate drugs during pregnancy, so the safety experiences with many medications are limited, but certain drugs (digoxin, quinidine, β-adrenergic blockers, α-methyldopa, hydralazine) have been used with relative safety to both mother and fetus. It always is best to avoid medications in pregnancy but, when necessary, and the risk/benefit ratio is favorable, drugs for cardiovascular disease may be used.

REFERENCES

1. Meyer J, Lackner JE, Schochet SS. Paroxysmal tachycardia in pregnancy. *JAMA* 94:1901;1930.

2. Spinnato JA, Shaver DC, Flinn GS, Sibai BM, Watson DL, Marin-Garcia J. Fetal supraventricular tachycardia: in utero therapy with digoxin and quinidine. *Obstet Gynecol* 1984;64: 730–735.

3. Hill LM, Malkasian GD. The use of quinidine sulfate throughout pregnancy. *Obstet Gynecol* 1979;54:366.

4. Colin A, Lambotte R. Influence tératogène des medicaments administrés à la femme enceinte. *Rev Med Liege* 1972;27:39.

5. Guntheroth WG, Cyr DR, Mack LA, Benedetti T, Lenke RR, Petty CN. Hydrops from reciprocating atrioventricular tachycardia in a 27-week fetus requiring quinidine for conversion. *Obstet Gynecol* 1985;66(suppl):29S–33S.

6. Johnson WH, Dunnigan A, Fehr P, Benson WD. Association of atrial flutter with orthodromic reciprocating fetal tachycardia. *Am J Cardiol* 1987;59:374–375.

7. Killeen AA, Bowers LD. Fetal supraventricular tachycardia treated with high dose quinidine: toxicity associated with marked elevation of the metabolites 3(s)-3-hydroxyquinidine. *Obstet Gynecol* 1987;70:445–449.

8. Wong RD, Murthy AR, Mathisen GE, Glover N, Thornton PJ. Treatment of severe falciparum malaria during pregnancy with quinidine and exchange transfusion. *Am J Med* 1992;92: 561–562.

9. Sherer DM, Sadovsky E, Menashe M, Mordel N, Rein AJ. Fetal ventricular tachycardia associated with nonimmunologic hydrops fetalis. *J Reprod Med* 1990;35:292–294.

10. Braverman AC, Broely BS, Rutherford JD. New onset ventricular tachycardia during pregnancy. *Int J Cardiol* 1991;33: 409–412.

11. Szekely P, Snaith L. *Heart Disease and Pregnancy.* Edinburgh: Churchill-Livingstone; 1974.

12. Bellett S. *Essentials of Cardiac Arrhythmias: Diagnosis and Management.* Philadelphia: WB Saunders; 1973.

13. Merx W. Herzrhythmusstorungen in der Schwangershaft. *Dtsch Med Wochenschr* 1972;97:1987.

14. Mauer AM, Devaux LO, Lahey ME. Neonatal and maternal thrombocytopenic purpura due to quinine. *Pediatrics* 1957; 19:84.

15. Mendelson CL. Disorders of heart beat during pregnancy. *Am J Obstet Gynecol* 1956;72:1268.

16. Kambam JR, Franks JJ, Smith BE. Inhibitory effect of quinidine on plasma pseudocholinesterase activity in pregnant women. *Am J Obstet Gynecol* 1987;157:897.

17. Miller RD, Walter LW, Katzning BG. The potentiation of neuromuscular blocking agents by quinidine. *Anesthesiology* 1967;26:1036.

18. Foldes FF, Foldes VM, Smith JC, Zsigmond EK. The relation between plasma cholinesterase and prolonged apnea caused by succinylcholine. *Anesthesiology* 1963;24:208.

19. Rosa F. Personal communication. FDA; 1993. In: Briggs GG, Freeman RK, Yaffe SJ, eds. *Drugs in Pregnancy and Lactation. A Reference Guide to Fetal and Neonatal Risk.* 4th ed. Baltimore: Williams & Wilkins; 1994;284,693,759.

20. Coplen SE, Antman EM, Berlin JA, Hewitt P, Chalmers TC. Efficacy and safety of quinidine therapy for maintenance of sinus rhythm after cardioversion. A meta-analysis of randomized control trials. *Circulation* 1990;82:1106–1116.

21. Morganroth J, Goin SE. Quinidine-related mortality in the short-to-medium-term treatment of ventricular arrhythmias. A meta-analysis. *Circulation* 1991;84:1977–1983.

22. United States Pharmacopoeial Convention. *Drug Information for the Health Care Professional, IA, IB.* 15th ed. Rockville MD: USP DI; 1995.

23. American Academy of Pediatrics, Committee on Drugs. *Pediatrics* 1994;93:137–150.

24. Connolly SJ, Kates RE. Clinical pharmacokinetics of *N*-acetylprocainamide. *Clin Pharmacokinet* 1982;7:206–220.

25. Dumesic DA, Silverman NH, Tobias S, Golbus MS. Transplacental cardioversion of fetal supraventricular tachycardia with procainamide. *N Engl J Med* 1982;307:1128.

26. Given BD, Phillippe M, Sanders SP, Dzau V. Procainamide cardioversion of fetal supraventricular tachyarrhythmia. *Am J Cardiol* 1984;53:1460.

27. Lima JJ, Kuritzky PM, Schentag JJ, Jusko WJ. Fetal uptake and neonatal disposition of procainamide and its acetylated metabolite: a case report. *Pediatrics* 1978;61:491–492.

28. Heinonen OP, Slone D, Shapiro S. *Birth Defects and Drugs in Pregnancy.* Littleton, MA: Publishing Sciences Group; 1977;358.

29. Merx W, Effert S, Heinrich KW. Heart disease in pregnancy, intra- and postpartum. *Z Geburtshilfe Perinatol* 1974;178:317.

30. Allen NM, Page RL. Procainamide administration during pregnancy. *Clin Pharmacol* 1993;12:58–60.

31. Pittard III WB, Glazier H. Procainamide excretion in human milk. *J Pediatr* 1983;102(4):631–633.

32. Karim A, Cook C, Campion J. Placental and milk transfer of disopyramide and its metabolites in rats. *Drug Metab Dispos* 1978;6:346–348.

33. Jequier R, Deraedt R, Plongerm R, Vamier B. Pharmacology and toxicology of disopyramide. *Minerva Med* 1970;61 (suppl 71):3689.

34. Shaxted EJ, Milton PJ. Disopyramide in pregnancy: a case report. *Curr Opin Med Res* 1979;6:70–72.

35. Echizen H, Nakura M, Saotome T, Minoura S, Ishizaki T. Plasma protein binding of disopyramide in pregnant and postpartum women, and neonates and their mothers. *Br J Clin Pharmacol* 1990;29:423–430.

36. Ellsworth AJ, Horn JR, Raisys VA, Miyagawa LA, Bell JL. Disopyramide and *N*-monodesalkyldisopyramide in serum and breast milk. *Drug Intell Clin Pharm* 1989;23:56–57.

37. Leonard RF, Braun TE, Levy AM. Initiation of uterine contractions by disopyramide during pregnancy. *N Engl J Med* 1978;299:84–85.

38. Tadmor OP, Keren A, Rosenhak D, Gal M, Shaia M, Hornstein E, Yaffe H, Graff E, Stern S, Diamant YZ. The effect of disopyramide on uterine contractions during pregnancy. *Am J Obstet Gynecol* 1990;162:482–486.

39. Ward R. Maternal drug therapy for fetal disorders. *Semin Perinatol* 1992;16:12–20.

40. Barnett DB, Hudson SA, McBurney A. Disopyramide and its *N*-monodesalkyl metabolite in breast milk. *Br J Clin Pharmacol* 1982;14:310–312.

41. Mackintosh D, Buchanan N. Excretion of disopyramide in human breast milk. *Br J Clin Pharmacol* 1985;19:856.

42. Hoppu K, Neuvonen PJ, Korte T. Disopyramide and breast feedings. *Br J Clin Pharmacol* 1986;21:553. Letter.

43. Mitani GM, Steinberg I, Lien E, Harrison EC, Elkayam U. The pharmacokinetics of antiarrhythmic agents in pregnancy and lactation. *Clin Pharmacokinet* 1987;12:253–291.

44. Zador G, Lindmark G, Nilsson BA. Pudendal block in normal vaginal deliveries. *Acta Obstet Gynecol Scand* 1974;34 (suppl):51–64.

45. Brown WU Jr, Bell GC, Lurie AO, Weiss JB, Scanion JW, Alper MH. Newborn blood levels of lidocaine and mepivacaine in the first postnatal day following maternal epidural anesthesia. *Anesthesiology* 1975;42:698–707.

46. Kuhnert BR, Knapp DR, Kuhnert PM, Prochaska AL. Maternal, fetal, and neonatal metabolism of lidocaine. *Clin Pharmacol Ther* 1979;26:213–220.

47. Philipson EH, Kuhnert BR, Syracuse CD. Maternal, fetal, and neonatal lidocaine levels following perineal infiltration. *Am J Obstet Gynecol* 1984;149:403–407.

48. Liston WA, Adjepon-Yomoah KK, Scott DB. Foetal and maternal lignocaine levels after paracervical block. *Br J Anaesth* 1973;45:750–754.

49. Brown WU, Bell GC, Alper MH. Acidosis, local anesthetics and the newborn. *Obstet Gynecol* 1976;48:27.

50. Petrie RH, Paul WL, Miller FC, Arce JJ, Paul RH, Nakmura RM, Hon EH. Placental transfer of lidocaine following paracervical block. *Am J Obstet Gynecol* 1974;120:791.

51. Burney RG, DiFazio CA, Foster JH. Effects of pH on protein binding of lidocaine. *Anesth Analg* 1978;57:478.

52. Scanion JW, Brown WU Jr, Weiss JB, Alper MH. Neurobehavioral responses of newborn infants after maternal epidural anesthesia. *Anesthesiology* 1974;40:121–128.

53. Kim WY, Pomerance JJ, Miller AA. Lidocaine intoxication in a newborn following local anesthesia for episiotomy. *Pediatrics* 1979;64:643.

54. Bozynski ME, Rubarth LB, Patel JA. Lidocaine toxicity after maternal prudential anesthesia in a term infant with fetal distress. *Am J Perinatol* 1987;4:164–166.

55. De Praeter C, Vanhaesebrouck P, De Praeter N, Govaert P, Bogaert M, Leroy J. Episiotomy and neonatal lidocaine intoxication. *Eur J Pediatr* 1991;150:685–686. Letter.

56. Van Dorsten JP, Miller FC. Fetal heart rate changes after accidental intrauterine lidocaine. *Obstet Gynecol* 1981;57:257–260.

57. Heinonen OP, Slone D, Shapiro S. *Birth Defects and Drugs in Pregnancy.* Littleton, MA: Publishing Sciences Group; 1977.

58. Chestnut DH, Bates JN, Choi WW. Continuous infusion epidural analgesia with lidocaine: efficacy and influence during the second stage of labor. *Obstet Gynecol* 1987;69:323–327.

59. Kileff MB, James FM III, Dewan D, Floyd H, DiFazio C. Neonatal neurobehavioral responses after epidural anesthesia for cesarean section with lidocaine and bupivacaine. *Anesthesiology* 1982;57:A403. Abstract.

60. Ramanathan J, Bottorff M, Seter JN, Khalil M, Sibai BM. The pharmacokinetics and maternal and neonatal effects of epidural lidocaine in preeclampsia. *Anesth Analg* 1986;65:120–126.

61. Zeister JA, Gaarder TD, De Mesquita SA. Lidocaine excretion in breast milk. *Drug Intell Clin Pharm* 1986;20:691–693.

62. Monk JP, Brogden RN. Mexiletine: a review of its pharmacodynamic and pharmacokinetic properties, and therapeutic use in the treatment of arrhytmias. *Drugs* 1990;40:374–411.

63. Timmis AD, Jackson G, Holt DW. Mexiletine for control of ventricular disarrhythmias in pregnancy. *Lancet* 1980;2:647–648.

64. Lewis AM, Patel L, Johnston A, Turner P. Mexiletine in human blood and breast milk. *Postgrad Med J* 1981;57:546–547.

65. Stokes IM, Evans J, Stone M. Myocardial infarction and cardiac arrest in the second trimester followed by assisted vaginal delivery under epidural analgesia at 38 weeks gestation. Case report. *Br J Obstet Gynaecol* 1983;91:197–198.

66. Menon KP, Mahpatra RK. Paroxysmal ventricular tachycardia associated with Bell's palsy in a teenager in late pregnancy. *Angiology* 1984;35:534–536.

67. Juneja MM, Ackerman WE, Kaczorowski DM, Sollo DG, Gunzenhauser LF. Continuous epidural lidocaine infusion in the parturient with paroxysmal ventricular tachycardia. *Anesthesiology* 1989;71:305–308.

68. Tucker GT, Boyes RN, Bridenbaugh PO, Moore DC. Binding of anilide-type local anesthetics in human plasma. *Anesthesiology* 1970;33:304–314.

69. Shnider SM, Way EL. The kinetics of transfer of lidocaine across the human placenta. *Anesthesiology* 1968;29:944.

70. Biehl D, Shnider SM, Levinson G, Callender K. Placental transfer of lidocaine: effects of fetal acidosis. *Anesthesiology* 1978;48:409–412.

71. Lownes HE, Ives TJ. Mexiletine use during pregnancy and lactation. *Am J Obstet Gynecol* 1987;157:446–447.

72. Gregg AR, Tomich PG. Mexiletine use in pregnancy. *J Perinatol* 1988;8:33–35.

74. Marcus FL, Opie LH. Antiarrhythmic drugs. In: Opie LH, ed. *Drugs for the Heart.* 4th ed. Philadelphia: WB Saunders; 1995;207–247.

75. Holmes B, Brogden RN, Heel RC, Spiegel TM, Avery GS. Tocainide: a review of its pharmacological properties and therapeutic efficacy.; *Drugs* 1983;26:93–123.

76. Roden DM, Woosley RL. Tocainide. *N Engl J Med* 1986;315:36–41.

77. Atkinson AJ Jr, Davidson R. Diphenylhydantoin as an antiarrhythmic drug. *Annu Rev Med* 1974;25:99–113.

78. Wit AL, Rosen MR, Hoffman BF. Electrophysiology and pharmacology of cardiac arrhythmias: VIII. Cardiac effects of diphenylhydantoin. *Am Heart J* 1975;90:397–404.

79. Zipes DP. Management of cardiac arrhythmias: pharmacological, electrical, and surgical techniques. In: Braunwald E, ed. *Heart Disease: A Textbook of Cardiovascular Medicine.* 4th ed. Philadelphia: WB Saunders; 1992;628–666.

80. Lander CM, Edwards VE, Eadie MJ, Tyrer JH. Plasma anticonvulsant concentrations during pregnancy. *Neurology* 1977;27:128–131.

81. Landon MJ, Kirkley M. Metabolism of diphenylhydantoin (phenytoin) during pregnancy. *Br J OIbstet Gynaecol* 1979;86:125–132.

82. Ramsay RE, Straus RG, Wilder BJ, Willmore LJ. Status epilepticus in pregnancy: effect of phenytoin malabsorption on seizure control. *Neurology* 1978;28:85–89.

83. Dam M, Christiansen J, Munck O, Mygind KI. Antiepileptic drugs: metabolism in pregnancy. *Clin Pharmacokinet* 1979;4:53–62.

84. Lander CM, Smith MT, Chalk JB, de Wytt C, Symoniw P, Livingstone I, Eadie MJ. Bioavailability and pharmacokinetics of phenytoin during pregnancy. *Eur J Clin Pharmacol* 1984;27:105–110.

85. Nau H, Kuhnz W, Egger HJ, Rating D, Helge H. Anticonvulsants during pregnancy and lactation: transplacental, maternal and neonatal pharamcokinetics. *Clin Pharmacokinet* 1982;7:508–543.

86. Chen SS, Perucca E, Lee JN, Richens A. A serum protein binding and free concentrations of phenytoin and phenobarbitone in pregnancy. *Br J Clin Pharmacol* 1982;13:547–552.

87. Van der Klight E, Schobben F, Bree TB. Clinical pharamcokinetics of antiepileptic drugs. *Drug Intell Clin Pharm* 1980;14:674–685.

88. Shapiro S, Hartz SC, Siskind V, Mitchell AA, Slone D, Rosenberg L, Monson RR, Heinonen OP. Anticonvulsants and parenteral epilepsy in the development of birth defects. *Lancet* 1976;1:272–275.

89. Mellin GW. Drugs in the first trimester of pregnancy and the fetal life of *Homo sapiens. Am J Obstet Gynecol* 1964;80:1169–1180.

90. Janz D, Fuchs V. Are anti-epileptic drugs harmful when given during pregnancy? *German Med Monogr* 1964;9:20–23.

91. Hill RB. Teratogenesis and antiepileptic drugs. *N Engl J Med* 1973;289:1089–1990.

92. Janz D. The teratogenic risk of antiepileptic drugs. *Epilepsia* 1975;16:159–169.

93. Bodendorfer TW. Fetal effects of anticonvulsant drugs and seizure disorders. *Drug Intell Clin Pharm* 1978;12:14–21.

94. American Academy of Pediatrics, Committee on Drugs. Anticonvulsants and pregnancy. *Pediatrics* 1977;63:331–333.

95. Nakane Y, Okuma T, Takahashi R, Sato Y, Wada T, Sato T,

Fukushima Y, Kumashiro H, Ono T, Takahshi T, Aoki M, Tanimura T, Hazam H, Kawahara R, Otsuki S, Hosokawa K, Inanaga K, Nakazaw Y, Yamamoto K. Multi-institutional study of the teratogenic and fetal toxicity of antiepileptic drugs: a report of a collaborative study group in Japan. *Epilepsia* 1980;21:663–680.

96. Andermann E, Dansky L, Andermann F, Loughnan PM, Gibbons J. Minor congenital malformations and dermatoglyphic alterations in the offspring of epileptic women: a clinical investigation of the teratogenic effects of anticonvulsant medication. In *Epilepsy, Pregnancy and the Child. Proceedings of a Workshop in Berlin, September 1980.* New York: Raven Press; 1981.

97. Dansky L, Andermann E, Andermann F. Major congenital malformations in the offspring of epileptic patients. In: *Epilepsy, Pregnancy and the Child. Proceedings of a Workshop in Berlin, September 1980.* New York: Raven Press; 1981.

98. Hanson JW, Buehler BA. Fetal hydantoin syndrome: current status. *J Pediatr* 1982;101:816–818.

99. Buehler BA, Delimont D, Van Waes M, Finnell RH. Prenatal prediction of risk of the fetal hydantoin syndrome. *N Engl J Med* 1990;332:1567–1572.

100. Meadow SR. Anticonvulsant drugs and congenital abnormalities. *Lancet* 1968;2:1296.

101. Loughnan PM, Gold H, Vance JC, Phenytoin teratogenicity in man. *Lancet* 1973;1:70–72.

102. Hill RM, Horning MG, Horning EC. Antiepileptic drugs and fetal well-being. In: Boreus L, ed. *Fetal Pharmacology.* New York: Raven Press; 1973;375–379.

103. Janz D. Antiepileptic drugs and pregnancy: altered utilization patterns and teratogenesis. *Epilepsia* 1982;23(suppl 1):S53–S63.

104. Briggs GG, Freeman RK, Yaffe SJ, eds. *Drugs in Pregnancy and Lactation. A Reference Guide to Fetal and Neonatal Risk.* 4th ed. Baltimore: Williams & Wilkins; 1994.

105. Page TE, Hoyme HE, Markarian M, Jones KL. Neonatal hemorrhage secondary to thrombocytopenia: an occasional effect of prenatal hydantoin exposure. *Birth Defects* 1982;18:47–50.

106. Lane PA, Hathaway WE. Vitamin K in infancy. *J Pediatr* 1985;106:351–359.

107. Biale Y, Lewenthal H. Effect of folic acid supplementation on congenital malformations due to anticonvulsant drugs. *Eur J Obstet Reprod Biol* 1984;18:211–216.

108. Pritchard JA, Scott DE, Whalley PJ. Maternal folate deficiency and pregnancy wastage. IV. Effects of folic acid supplements, anticonvulsants, and oral contraceptives. *Am J Obstet Gynecol* 1971;109:341–346.

109. Hiilesmaa VK, Teramo K, Granstrom ML, Bardy AH. Serum folate concentrations during pregnancy in women with epilepsy: relation to antiepileptic drug concentrations, number of seizures, and fetal outcome. *Br Med J* 1983;287:577–579.

110. Dansky L, Andermann E, Sherwin AL, Andermann F. Plasma levels of phenytoin during pregnancy and the puerperium. In *Epilepsy, Pregnancy and the Child. Proceedings of a Workshop in Berlin, September 1980.* New York: Raven Press; 1981.

111. Dansky L, Andemann E, Andermann F, Sherwin AL, Kinch RA. Maternal epilepsy and congenital malformation: correlation with maternal anticonvulsant levels during pregnancy. In *Epilepsy, Pregnancy and the Child. Proceedings of a Workshop in Berlin, September 1980.* New York: Raven Press; 1981.

112. Filton A, Buckley MMT. Moricizine: a review of its pharmacological properties, and therapeutic efficacy in cardiac arrhythmias. *Drugs* 1990;40:138–167.

113. Clyne CA, Estes NAM III, Wang PJ. Moricizine. *N Engl J Med* 1992;327:255–260.

114. The Cardiac Arrhythmia Suppression Trial II (CAST-II) Investigators. Effect of the antiarrhythmic drug moricizine on survival after myocardial infarction. *N Engl J Med* 1992;327:227.

115. The Cardiac Arrhythmia Suppression Trial (CAST) Investigators. Preliminary report: effect of encainide and flecainide on mortality in randomized trial of arrhythmia suppression after myocardial infarction. *N Engl J Med* 1989;321:406.

116. Herre JM, Titus C, Oeff M, Eldar M, Franz MR, Griffin JC, Scheinman MM. Inefficacy and proarrhythmic effects of flecainide and encainide for sustained ventricular tachycardia and ventricular fibrillation. *Ann Intern Med* 1990;113:671–676.

117. Bauman JL. Cardiac drugs. In: Knoben JE, Anderson PO, eds. *Handbook of Clinical Drug Data.* 6th ed. Hamilton, IL: Drug Intelligence Publications; 1988;469–496.

118. Palmer CM, Norris MC. Placental transfer of flecainide. *Am J Dis Child* 1990;144:144. Letter.

119. Wagner X, Jonglard J, Monlin M, Miller A, Petitjean J, Pisapia A. Coadministration of flecainide acetate and sotalol during pregnancy: lack of teratogenic effects, passage across the placenta and excretion in human breast milk. *Am Heart J* 1990;119:700–702.

120. Doig JC, McComb JM, Reid DS. Incessant atrial tachycardia accelerated by pregnancy. *Br Heart J* 1992;67:266–268.

121. Allan LP, Chito SK, Shorland GK, Maxwell DJ, Priestley K. Flecainide in the treatment of fetal tachycardia. *Br Heart J* 1991;65:46–48.

122. Gembruch U, Hansman M, P edel DA, Bald R. Intrauterine therapy of fetal tachyarrhythmias: intraperitoneal administration of antiarrhythmic drugs to the fetus in fetal tachyarrhythmias with severe hydrops fetalis. *J Perinatol Med* 1988;16:39–44.

123. Maxwell DJ, Crawford DC, Curry PVM, Tynan MJ, Alan LD. Obstetric importance, diagnosis and management of fetal tachycardias. *Br Med J* 1988;297:107–110.

124. Perry JC, Ayres NA, Carpenter RJ. Fetal supraventricular tachycardia treated with flecainide acetate. *J Pediatr* 1991;118:303–305.

125. Kohl T, Tercanli S, Kececioglu D, Holzgreve W. Direct fetal administration of adenosine the termination of incessant supraventricular tachycardia. *Obstet Gynecol* 1995;85:873–874.

126. Macphail S, Walkinshaw SA. Fetal supraventricular tachycardia: detection by routine auscultation on successful in utero

management. Case report. *Br J Obstet Gynaecol* 1988;95: 1073–1076.

127. Wren C, Hunter S. Maternal administration of flecainide to terminate and suppress fetal tachycardia. *Br Med J* 1988;296:249.

128. Kofinas AD, Simon NV, Sagel H, Lyttle E, Smith N, King K. Treatment of fetal supraventricular tachycardia with flecainide acetate after digoxin failure. *Am J Obstet Gynecol* 1991;165:630–631.

129. McQuinn RL, Pisani A, Wafa S, Chang SF, Miller AM, Frappel JM, Chamberlain GVP, Camm AJ. Flecainide excretion in human breast milk. *Clin Pharmacol Ther* 1990;48:262–267.

130. Capucci A, Boriana G. Propafenone in the treatment of cardiac arrhythmias. *Drug Saf* 1995;12:55–72.

131. Funck-Brentano C, Kroemer HK, Lee JT, Roden DM. Propafenone. *N Engl J Med* 1990;322:518–525.

132. Bryson HM, Palmer KJ, Langtry HD, Fitton A. Propafenon: a reappraisal of its pharmacology, pharamcokinetics and therapeutic use in cardiac arrhythmias. *Drugs* 1993;45:85–130.

133. Kishore AGR, Camm AJ. Guidelines for the use of propafenone in treating supraventricular arrhythmias. *Drugs* 1995;50:250–262.

134. Mason JW. A comparison of seven antiarrhythmic drugs in patients with ventricular tachyarrhythmias. *N Engl J Med* 1993;329:452–458.

135. Siebels J, Capapato R, Ruppel R, Schneider MA, Kuck KH. ICD versus drugs in cardiac arrest survivors: preliminary results of the Cardiac Arrest Study Hamburg. *PACE* 1993;16:552–558.

136. Brunozzi LT, Meniconi L, Chiscchi P, Liberati R, Zuaretti G, Latini R. Propafenone in the treatment of chronic ventricular arrhythmias in a pregnant patient. *Br J Clin Pharmacol* 1988;26:489–490.

137. Santinelli V, DePaola M, Turco P, Smimmo D, Chiariello M, Condorelli M. Wolff–Parkinson–White at risk and propafenone. *J Am College Cardiol* 1988;11:1138.

138. Gembruch U, Hansmann M, Bald R. Direct intrauterine fetal treatment of fetal tachyarrhythmia with severe hydrops fetalis by antiarrhythmic drugs. *Fetal Ther* 1988;3:210–215.

139. Gembruch U, Manz M, Bald R, Rüddel H, Redel DA, Schlebusch H, Nitsch J, Hansmann M. Repeated intravascular treatment with amiodarone in a fetus with refractory supraventricular tachycardia and hydrops fetalis. *Am Heart J* 1989;118: 1335–1338.

140. Libardoni M, Piovan D, Busato E, Padrini R. Transfer of propafenone and 5-OH-propafenone to foetal plasma and maternal milk. *Br J Clin Pharmacol* 1991;32:527–528.

141. Keefe DL. Pharmacology of lorcainide. *Am J Cardiol* 1984; 54:1B–21B.

142. Eriksson CE, Brogden RN. Lorcainide: a preliminary review of its pharmacologic properties and therapeutic efficacy. *Drugs* 1984;27:279–300.

143. Brogden RN, Todd PA. Encainide: a review of its pharmacological properties and therapeutic efficacy. *Drugs* 1987;34: 519–538.

144. Quart BD. Personal communication. Bristol-Myers Company, 1988. In: Briggs GG, Freeman RK, Yaffe SJ, eds. *Drugs in Pregnancy and Lactation. A Reference Guide to Fetal and Neonatal Risk.* 4th ed. Baltimore: Williams & Wilkins; 1994;324–325.

145. Strasburger JF, Smith RT Jr, Moak JP, Gothing C, Garson A Jr. Encainide for resistant supraventricular tachycardia in children: follow-up report. *Am J Cardiol* 1988;62:50L–54L.

146. Gill J, Heel RC, Fitton A. Amiodarone: an overview of its pharmacological properties and review of its therapeutic use in cardiac arrhythmias. *Drugs* 1992;43:69–110.

147. Podrid PJ. Amiodarone: reevaluation of an old drug. *Ann Intern Med* 1995;122:689–700.

148. Rosenbaum MB, Chiale MD. Amiodarone. In: Messereli FH, ed. *Cardiovascular Drug Therapy.* Philadelphia: WB Saunders; 1990;1236–1256.

149. Candelpergher G, Buchberger R, Suzzi GL, Padrini R. Transplacental passage of amiodarone: electrocardiographic and pharmacological evidence in a newborn infant. *G Ital Cardiol* 1982;12:7982.

150. McKenna WJ, Harris L, Rowland E, Whitelaw A, Sotrey G, Holt D. Amiodarone therapy during pregnancy. *Am J Cardiol* 1983;51:1231–1233.

151. Pitcher D, Leather HM, Storey GCA, Holt DW. Amiodarone in pregnancy. *Lancet* 1983;1:597–598.

152. Penn IM, Barrett PA, Pannikote V, Barnaby PF, Campbell JB, Lyons NR. Amiodarone in pregnancy. *Am J Cardiol* 1985;56: 196–197.

153. Robson D, Jeeva Raj MV, Storey GCA, Holt DW. Use of amiodarone during pregnancy. *Postgrad Med J* 1985;61:75–77.

154. Strunge P, Frandsen J, Andreasen F. Amiodarone during pregnancy. *Eur Heart J* 1988;9:106–109.

155. Plomp TA, Vulsma T, De Vijlder JJM. Use of amiodarone during pregnancy. *Eur J Obstet Gynecol Reprod Biol* 1992;43:201–207.

156. Rey E, Bachrach LK, Buttow GN. Effects of amiodarone during pregnancy. *Can Med Assoc J* 1987;136:959–960.

157. Foster CJ, Love HG. Amiodarone in pregnancy: case report and review of literature. *Int J Cardiol* 1988;20:307–316.

158. De Wolf D, De Schepper J, Verhaaren H, Deneyer M, Smitz J, Sacre-Smits L. Congenital hypothyroid goiter and amiodarone. *Acta Paediatr Scand* 1988;77:616–618.

159. Laurent M, Betremieux P, Biron Y, Lellelloco A. Neonatal hypothyroidism after treatment by amiodarone during pregnancy. *Am J Cardiol* 1987;60:142.

160. Arnoux P, Seyral P, Llurens M, Djiani P, Ptier A, Unal D, Cano JP, Sirradimigni A, Rouault F. Amiodarone and digoxin for refractory fetal tachycardia. *Am J Cardiol* 1987;59:166–167.

161. Rey E, Duperron L, Gauthier R, Lemsy M, Grignon A, LeLorier J. Transplacental treatment of tachycardia-induced fetal heart failure with verapamil and amiodarone. *Am J Obstet Gynecol* 1985;153:311–312.

162. Wladimiroff JW, Steward PA. Treatment of fetal cardiac arrhythmias. *Br J Hosp Med* 1985;34:134–140.

163. Koblin DD, Romanoff ME, Martin DE, Hensley FA, Larach DR, Stauffer RA, Luck JC. Anesthetic management of the parturient receiving amiodarone. *Anesthesiology* 1987;66:551–553.

164. Widerhorn J, Bhandari AK, Bughi S, Rahimtoola SH, Elkayam U. Fetal and neonatal adverse effects profile of amio-

darone treatment during pregnancy. *Am Heart J* 1991;122:1162–1166.

165. Hill DA, Reasor MJ. Effects of amiodarone administration during lactation in Fischer-344 rats. *Toxicol Let* 1992;62:119–125.

166. Gutgesell M, Overholt E, Boyler R. Oral bretylium tosylate use during pregnancy and subsequent breast feeding: a case report. *Am J Perinatol* 1990;7:144–145.

167. Podolsky SM, Varon J. Adenosine use during pregnancy. *Ann Emergency Med* 1991;29:1027–1028.

168. Elkayam U, Goodwin TM. Adenosine therapy for supraventricular tachycardia during pregnancy. *Am J Cardiol* 1995;75:521–523.

169. Harrison JK, Greenfield RA, Wharton JM. Acute termination of supraventricular tachycardia by adenosine during pregnancy. *Am Heart J* 1992;123:1386–1388.

170. Mason BA, Ricci-Goodman J, Koos BJ. Adenosine in the treatment of maternal paroxysmal supraventricular tachycardia. *Obstet Gynecol* 1992;80:478–480.

171. Afridi I, Moise KJ Jr, Rokey R. Termination of supraventricular tachycardia with intravenous adenosine in a pregnant woman with Wolff–Parkinson–White syndrome. *Obstet Gynecol* 1992;80:481–483.

172. Hagley MT, Cole PL. Adenosine use in pregnant women with supraventricular tachycardia. *Ann Pharmacother* 1994;28:1241–1242.

31

USE OF VASODILATORS DURING PREGNANCY

STEVEN E. CALVIN, MD

INTRODUCTION

Though pregnancy is normally a state of relative vasodilation, pharmacologic relaxation of the vascular system is necessary in a number of clinical situations. Though a variety of vasodilating agents may be indicated for the gravid patient, use of these agents in pregnancy requires a careful review of mechanisms of action, indications, and published experience in pregnancy.

Pregnancy is characterized by changes in the vascular system designed to maintain flow to the uteroplacental bed. Nitric oxide (NO) has been shown to be the endothelial-derived relaxing factor and may be useful in cardiovascular therapeutics.[1] It has been shown that estrogen induces the enzyme NO sythetase and that the natural NO-dependent vascular relaxation of pregnancy is impaired in toxemia.[2]

Vasodilating agents act by various mechanisms to cause vascular relaxation. Either arterial or venous effects predominate, although some agents have mixed effects. Vascular responses to vasodilating agents are individual: varying by vessel type and size.[3] In pregnant guinea pigs, vessel reactivity varies with location of the vascular bed.[4] Vasodilator effects on arteries isolated from human myometrium and fetal villi show significant variation.[5] Unfortunately the uteroplacental circulation cannot compensate for drastic reductions in perfusion pressure.

Hemodynamic subsets of hypertensive women have been recognized in studies utilizing both echocardiography and pulmonary artery catheters.[6] Differences in the response to vasodilating agents of these patient subsets are important in deciding which patients should be treated and which may benefit from volume expansion prior to treatment.

A number of cardiovascular problems in pregnant women benefit from vasodilator therapy. The most frequent indication is the short- or long-term treatment of hypertension. Short-term use generally involves the control of extreme blood pressure elevation associated with pregnancy toxemia. Nonpregnant patients have been divided into those with hypertensive emergency (i.e., diastolic pressures >120 mmHg) and those with hypertensive urgency (i.e., smaller but significant elevations).[7] These distinctions may not be valid in pregnancy; most clinicians treat diastolic pressures greater than 110 mmHg. It is important to avoid excessive and rapid reductions in pressure because hypoperfusion of the uteroplacental unit may result.

Patients with chronic hypertension may be treated throughout pregnancy with vasodilators alone or in combination with other antihypertensive agents. Because the relative maternal age in pregnancy is increasing, there is an increase in the number of pregnant women who have ischemic cardiovascular disease. Some will require therapy for angina during pregnancy. A patient with primary pulmonary hypertension may choose to be pregnant and may require vasodilator therapy.

Published experience with vasodilators in pregnancy is limited. Most pharmaceutical manufacturers report animal studies evaluating fertility and teratogenic effects. These investigations often involve doses many times those used in pregnant women. Most pertinent literature is in the form of case reports of adverse reactions or observational studies in groups treated for hypertension.

The understanding of the pathogenesis of toxemia is in rapid flux. The endothelial cell is important in the maintenance of normal vascular tone. The central role played by

Cardiac Problems in Pregnancy, Third Edition
Edited by Uri Elkayam, MD, and Norbert Gleicher, MD
Copyright © 1998 by Wiley-Liss, Inc. ISBN 0-471-16358-9

these cells in the pathogenesis of preeclampsia has been described.[8] Patients with chronic hypertension are at a substantially increased risk for this reversible problem peculiar to pregnancy.

The sections that follow review individual vasodilating agents and their use in pregnancy.

HYDRALAZINE

Mechanism

Hydralazine directly reduces systemic vascular resistance. The effect is more pronounced on the arterioles than on the veins, and diastolic pressure is reduced more than systolic pressure. Renal blood flow is preserved. In studies done on isolated human placental lobules, hydralazine appears to activate guanylate cyclase, leading to increased cyclic guanosine monophosphate and relaxation of vascular smooth muscle. No evidence was found for an effect on nitric oxide production or release.[9] In pregnant ewes in which hypertension is induced by means of angiotensin II, intravenous hydralazine is an effective dilator of the uteroplacental vascular bed.[10] A similar effect is not seen when hypertension is induced by cocaine.[11]

There is no direct cardiac effect of hydralazine, but the drug stimulates the sympathetic nervous system, producing a compensatory increase in cardiac output. Most pregnant women are able to maintain and tolerate the increased cardiac output without difficulty. Because sodium retention occurs in conjunction with the increased cardiac output, hydralazine is rarely used as a first-line agent in prolonged antihypertensive therapy.

Hydralazine is available in oral and parenteral forms. Oral hydralazine is occasionally used in pregnancy. With intravenous injection, the onset of action is gradual, with a peak at 20 minutes. The half-life is 3 hours. Fetal blood levels are comparable to maternal levels, and hydralazine is present in breast milk.[12] There is no contraindication to breast feeding in patients on this medication. The most frequent side effects of hydralazine are headache and flushing related to reflex sympathetic activity. A dose-dependent lupuslike reaction also occurs in some patients. This reaction has occurred in pregnancy, with severe maternal and neonatal effects.[13] Prolonged high dose use is therefore not advisable.

Indications

The most common use of hydralazine in pregnancy is for the acute reduction of blood pressure. The usual dose is 5 mg every 20 minutes, intravenously. The goal is a diastolic pressure of less than 100 mmHg. The dose can be increased to 10 mg, but the total dose should not exceed 30 mg in 4 hours. For oral therapy, the usual starting dose is 25 mg twice daily with a maximum daily dose of 200 mg day.

Experience in Pregnancy

Hydralazine is a commonly used oral antihypertensive agent in Sweden and England. In the United States, hydralazine is most commonly given intravenously during the peripartum period. With intravenous use there is a risk of inducing hypotension and associated abnormalities in fetal heart rate tracing.[14] However when used in recommended doses for treating severe hypertension, it is effective and safe for both the mother and baby.[15] Hydralzine should not be used in combination with other vasodilating agents such as diazoxide because of the risk of severe, life-threatening hypotension.[16]

Phalangeal defects have been reported in rabbits given hydralazine and other vasodilators in early pregnancy.[17] These defects were attributed to the pharmacological effect of hypotension rather than to a direct effect on fetal chondrogenesis. On the other hand, when pregnant rats were given hydralazine in nontoxic doses, there were no teratogenic or fetopathic effects.[18] Human studies are limited. Eight mother–child pairs with first-trimester exposure to hydralazine were identified in the Collaborative Perinatal Project; no congenital malformations occurred.[19]

Doppler studies of the uterine and umbilical arteries have been performed in severely hypertensive pregnant women treated with hydralazine. There were no significant changes in blood flow characteristics after administration of hydralazine.[20]

Comparative studies have been done evaluating hydralazine and labetalol. There was a tendency to lower 5-minute Apgar scores in the hydralazine-treated group.[21] The same investigators found no negative effect on neonatal adaptation between the treatment groups.[22] A prospective, randomized clinical trial using parenteral and sublingual nifedipine also showed lower Apgar scores in babies of hydralazine-treated mothers, but both agents were felt to be safe for use with severe preeclampsia.[23]

Most preeclamptic patients are relatively hypovolemic. Some authors have recommended definition of patient subsets and volume expansion prior to the use of hydralazine.[6] In a study utilizing Swan–Ganz catheter monitoring information, it was shown that preeclamptic patients with low pulmonary capillary wedge pressure (PCWP), low cardiac index, and high systemic vascular resistance benefited from volume expansion prior to hydralazine treatment.[24] Most patients do not require invasive hemodynamic monitoring, but the use of noninvasive methods may make it easier to identify patients who would benefit from volume expansion.

At one point the original manufacturer of hydralazine discontinued production of the injectable form of the drug. It soon became clear that there was substantial demand for this drug in pregnancy, and production was resumed. Injectable hydralazine is now available from the original manufacturer and as a generic preparation.

DIAZOXIDE

Mechanism

Diaxozide, administered intravenously, dilates resistance vessels with little effect on venous capacitance. Its effects are similar to those of hydralazine. It is chemically related to the thiazide diuretics. Use of this drug can lead to profound hypotension, and prolonged use causes hyperglycemia that may necessitate insulin treatment.

Indications

Diazoxide is a very powerful vasodilator, originally used as a second-line agent in patients who failed to respond to hydralazine. Rather than using a standard nonpregnant dose, in pregnancy a minibolus regimen has been recommended.[25] Only 30 mg is given intravenously every 1–2 minutes until the desired effect has been achieved. The maximum total dose is 150 mg. Diazoxide is rarely used today because of the availability of agents with wider margins of safety.

Experience in Pregnancy

Though there are no controlled human studies on early pregnancy use, there is evidence of teratogenic and embryopathic effects in rats and rabbits exposed to diazoxide. Because of smooth muscle relaxation, diazoxide inhibits uterine contractions.[26] As a result, augmentation of labor may be necessary. The use of diazoxide poses a significant risk of hyperglycemia. This condition is probably related to suppression of insulin secretion, and diazoxide has been used orally to treat familial neonatal hyperinsulinemia.[27]

The combination of diazoxide with other vasodilating agents had the potential to cause fatal maternal hypotension.[16] In the last decade, comparative studies showed that diazoxide has significant maternal/fetal risks and side effects more often than alternative agents.[28] For this reason it should not be used in pregnant women unless the risks clearly outweigh the benefits.

MINOXIDIL

Mechanism

Minoxidil is an oral agent with a direct vasodilating effect mediated by modulation of potassium channels in vascular smooth muscle. Both diastolic and systolic pressures are reduced. The compensatory response to the decreased pressure leads to increased cardiac output and fluid retention. A major side effect of this drug is hypertrichosis, a generalized increase in the growth and pigmentation of body hair.

Indications

Minoxidil is useful for the treatment of hypertensive patients with renal insufficiency. To minimize compensatory responses, minoxidil is usually used in combination with a diuretic and an adrenergic blocking agent.

Experience in Pregnancy

Minoxidil use in pregnancy is only described in case reports. There is no clear evidence that the drug is teratogenic, although hypertrichosis was noted in newborns.[29] There is no contradindication to the use of minoxidil while breast feeding.[30]

CALCIUM CHANNEL BLOCKERS

Mechanism

Calcium channel blockers are chemically and pharmacologically diverse. The vascular relaxation caused by these agents is due to interference with the slow membrane calcium channels, leading to a reduction in intracellular calcium. Vascular smooth muscle tone is therefore reduced, and blood pressure falls.

The mechanisms of vascular response to these agents have been studied. Pregnant patients in the early third trimester who were at risk for hypertension by hyperresponse to angiotensin II showed blunted responses when pretreated with nifedipine.[31] The initial plasma renin activity in hypertensive pregnant women predicted the blood pressure lowering effect of nifedipine.[32] Elevated atrial natriuretic peptide levels have also been shown to predict the response to nifedipine by hypertensive pregnant women.[33]

Urinary prostacyclin metabolites (but not those of thromboxane) are increased in the urine of nifedipine-treated hypertensive pregnant women.[34] Such a result suggests that nifedipine may increase the vascular production of this important endogenous vasodilating substance.

Indications

Nifedipine is used for the acute treatment of severe hypertension in the peripartum period. If an immediate response is desired, the liquid-filled capsule can be bitten and swallowed. The usual oral dose is 10 mg. A subsequent 10 mg dose can be given in 20–30 minutes if the response is inadequate. The total daily dose should not exceed 120 mg. For long-term treatment, an extended-release tablet (30 or 60 mg) is given once daily.

Though both nifedipine and nicardipine are efficient antihypertensive agents, nicardipine is available as an intravenous preparation. Its safe use has been reported in pregnancy.[35] Advantages reported include a more selective effect with fewer side effects. The intravenous nicardipine dose is 1 μg/kg/min (generally 4–7 mg/h).

Experience in Pregnancy

The use of nifedipine in pregnancy has been extensively reviewed.[36] At currently recommended doses, the safety and efficacy of this agent have been demonstrated. A study evaluating the potential teratogenic effects of various types of vasodilating agents given to rabbits at doses higher than those administered in humans, showed that all the tested drugs, including nifedipine, were associated with phalangeal defects.[17] The digital effects were likely related to decreased flow during development, and not due to a specific effect on fetal chondrogenesis. A retrospective study on 37 newborns exposed to nifedipine in the first trimester showed no increase in major malformations.[29]

Studies in pregnant ewes showed a decrease in arterial pressure due to intravenous nifedipine, but there was no significant effect on resistance in the uterine artery.[37] Studies in pregnant women showed that uteroplacental blood flow was not adversely affected, despite reduction in arterial blood pressure.[38]

Doppler flow characteristics have been studied in maternal and fetal arteries after administration of calcium channel blocking agents. Despite a significant decrease in maternal blood pressure after 5 mg of nifedipine, there were no changes in umbilical cord blood flow characteristics in fetuses with normal pretreatment profiles.[39] Nifedipine has no adverse effect on uterine artery flow and may increase the umbilical blood flow in the fetus.[40] Reassuring Doppler findings were also obtained when nicardipine was studied.[41] Fetal heart rate monitoring is a common method of assessing fetal health. The effect of sublingual nifedipine on fetal heart rate patterns was evaluated in 51 patients with severe pregnancy-induced hypertension. No abnormalities in heart rate tracings were identified.[42]

A comparative study of nifedipine and α-methyldopa in pregnancy-induced hypertension showed equivalent responses and no significant difference in maternal or neonatal outcomes.[43] Oral nicardipine favorably compares to metoprolol in the treatment of chronic hypertension in pregnancy. There was no difference in neonatal outcome.[44]

Breast feeding is not contraindicated in women taking nifedipine.[30]

Recently intravenous calcium channel blockers have become available in the United States. For example, nicardipine, a dihydropyridine agent similar to nifedipine, has been used intravenously to treat hypertension in severe preeclampsia.[35] Diastolic blood pressure decreased to less than 90 mmHg in all 20 patients. Nine of these patients complained of headache after infusion was begun. There were no adverse neonatal outcomes. This agent also can be used orally.

Most of the available evidence suggests that calcium channel blockers are safe in pregnant patients when used in the usual therapeutic doses. However severe hypotension and fetal distress have been reported in patients with preeclampsia.[45] The definition of various hemodynamic subsets of preeclampsia has shown that hypovolemia is a common feature of this disorder. The potential for severe hypotension exists when these patients are treated with vasodilating agents. Some have advocated volume expansion prior to treatment.[6] The initiation of a slow-release form of nifedipine in newly diagnosed preeclamptic patients showed no demonstrable benefit.[46]

Since magnesium sulfate is given to many hypertensive pregnant patients, there is significant concern about potential synergistic vasodilating and neuromuscular blockade effects of calcium channel blockers, and indeed such paired reactions have been reported.[47,48] Although the combined use of these agents without adverse effects has been reported,[49] it is important to recognize the potential for adverse effects.

SODIUM NITROPRUSSIDE

Mechanism

Sodium nitroprusside, a potent vasodilator, is a light-sensitive, inorganic complex that exerts its hypotensive effect by direct action on the vascular smooth muscle. The mechanism involves release of NO. Arterial pressure effects predominate, but venous dilatation also occurs. The hypotensive effects are more dramatic in hypertensive than in normotensive patients. Rapid metabolism is a beneficial property of sodium nitroprusside, and severe hypotensive reactions will generally resolve in less than 10 minutes. There is no direct effect on cardiac performance.

The major factor limiting the use of this agent is the potential for accumulation of cyanogen (cyanide radical). The cyanogen produced is converted to thiocyanate in the liver, but if this mechanism and the buffering capacity of methemoglobin are overwhelmed, cyanogen toxicity can occur. Toxicity is rare unless use exceeds 2–3 hours.

Indications

Sodium nitroprusside is useful in the temporary treatment of severe hypertension unresponsive to intravenous hydralazine or calcium channel blockers. This agent is frequently used during anesthetic management because dose can be titrated, but it should not be used in patients who are hypovolemic. Some authors recommend pulmonary catheterization if nitroprusside is used in pregnant women.[6] The initial dose in pregnancy should be 0.25 μg/kg/min. If necessary, the dose may be increased in increments of 0.25 μg/kg/min to a maximum dose of 2 μg/kg/min. Cyanide toxicity is rare with the temporary use of nitroprusside, but affected patients will have laboratory evidence of metabolic acidosis.

Experience in Pregnancy

There is no evidence suggesting that nitroprusside is teratogenic, though very few pregnant women have received this agent in the first trimester. The use of nitroprusside has been reported in the predelivery period.[6]

DIPYRIDAMOLE

Mechanism

Dipyridamole is a nonnitrate oral drug that causes coronary vasodilation and decreases platelet aggregation. The effect on small resistance vessels is probably mediated by inhibition of adenosine deaminase. The adenosine that accumulates is a potent vasodilator. Because of the platelet antiaggregant effect, dipyridamole has been used for thromboembolism prophylaxis.

Indications

Dipyridamole is most commonly used in patients at risk for thromboembolic disease. Because of coronary vasodilation, this drug may be used in patients with angina. The usual dose is 50–75 mg orally, four times per day.

Experience in Pregnancy

Patients given dipyridamole as possible prophylaxis for preeclampsia did not show any adverse maternal or fetal effects.[50] One recent study has reported the use of dipyradamole in pregnancy. Though nifedipine was also used, a possibly beneficial effect was noted on blood flow in the umbilical artery.[40]

PRAZOSIN AND TERAZOSIN

Mechanism

Prazosin and terazosin are oral α_1-adrenergic blocking agents used in the treatment of hypertension. Because of compensatory effects on heart rate and sodium retention, these agents are usually used in combination with β-adrenergic blockers and diuretics.

Indications

Prazosin can be used in the treatment of hypertension associated with high plasma renin levels. The usual starting dose of prazosin is 1 mg orally twice a day.

Experience in Pregnancy

Prazosin use without adverse effects has been reported in pregnancy.[51] When pheochromocytoma complicated the third trimester of pregnancy, prazosin was used until the tumor could be resected postpartum.[52]

NITROGLYCERIN

Mechanism

The release of nitric oxide causes smooth muscle relaxation.

Indications

Nitroglycerin may be used when pregnancy is complicated by myocardial infarction or when pulmonary edema is associated with severe preeclampsia. Administration can be by the oral or intravenous route.

Experience in Pregnancy

Nitroglycerin has been used without adverse effect in the treatment of myocardial infarction in pregnancy.[53,54] In severe preeclampsia, complicated by hydrostatic pulmonary edema, intravenous nitroglycerin has been used to decrease preload and pulmonary hydrostatic pressure.[55] The usual dose is 10 μg/kg/min. Severe hypotension may result if this agent is administered to a hypovolemic patient.

SUMMARY

Vasodilating agents are most commonly used to treat the acute elevations of blood pressure seen with preeclampsia. In certain additional medical and surgical situations, dilatation of the arterial or venous vessels is indicated as well.

Pregnancy is a temporary state of decreased systemic vascular resistance; the fetus is dependent on the maintenance of uteroplacental flow. It is important to avoid large or precipitous reductions in arterial pressure. For this reason vasodilating agents must be used with caution. Prior to induction of epidural anesthesia, pregnant patients are volume-loaded to avoid sharp reductions in blood pressure. Since the vascular response to vasodilating agents is analogous to epidural blockade, it is reasonable to consider the patient's volume status prior to the intravenous use of these drugs. Some patients may require volume loading prior to treatment with vasodilating agents.[6]

Until recently, hydralazine was the most common vasodilating agent used for acute blood pressure control. At one time continued availability of the parenteral form was in question. However a generic preparation is now available. Because of the temporary difficulty in obtaining hydralazine, alternative agents were considered. The most common alternative is nifedipine, although its use is restricted to the oral route. The intravenous alternatives to hydralazine include the adrenergic blocking agent labetalol (see Chapter 29) and nicardipine, a newly available calcium channel blocker that is similar to nifedipine.

Over the last several years a fairly broad experience with nifedipine has been reported. Some centers use it for its tocolytic properties and others for its antihypertensive effects. Both nifedipine and nicardipine are reasonable alternatives to hydralazine in the acute treatment of hypertension. Sustained-release nifedipine can also be used in the treatment of chronic hypertension during pregnancy.

When hydralazine and calcium channel blockers fail to control severe hypertension, either diazoxide or sodium nitroprusside may be used. These agents should only be used for brief periods in an intensive care setting. Invasive hemodynamic monitoring should be considered.

REFERENCES

1. Warren JB, Pons F, Brady AJ. Nitric oxide biology: implications for cardiovascular therapeutics. *Cardiovasc Res* 1994; 28(1):25–30.

2. Choo V. Views on vasoactive substances. *Lancet* 1994;343: 845–846.

3. O'Rourke MF. Arterial mechanics and wave reflection with antihypertensive therapy. *J Hypertension* 1992;10(suppl)(5): S43–S49.

4. Kim TH, Weiner CP, Thompson LP. Effect of pregnancy on contraction and endothelium-mediated relaxation of renal and mesenteric arteries. *Am J Physiol* 1994;267(1 pt 2):H41–H47.

5. Allen J, Skajaa K, Maigaard S, Forman A. Effects of vasodilators on isolated human uteroplacental arteries. *Obstet Gynecol* 1991;77(5):765–771.

6. Wasserstrum N, Cotton D. Volume expansion and antihypertensive therapy in severe preeclampsia. In: Clark S, Phelan J, Cotton D, eds: *Critical Care Obstetrics.* Oradell, NJ: Medical Economics; 1987:208–229.

7. Ferguson RK, Vlasses PH. Hypertensive emergencies and urgencies. *JAMA* 1986;255(12):1607–1613.

8. Roberts JM, Taylor RN, Musci TJ, Rodgers GM, Hubel CA, McLaughlin MK. Preeclampsia: an endothelia cell disorder. *Am J Obstet Gynecol* 1989;161:1200–1204.

9. Leitch IM, Read MA, Boura AL, Walters WA. Effect of inhibition of nitric oxide synthase and guanylate cyclase on hydralazine-induced vasodilatation of the human fetal placental circulation. *Clin Exp Pharmacol Physiol* 1994;21(8):615–622.

10. Pedron SL, Reid DL, Barnard JM, Henry JB. Differential effects of intravenous hydralazine on myoendometrial and placental blood flow in hypertensive pregnant ewes. *Am J Obstet Gynecol* 1992;167(6):1672–1678.

11. Vertommen JD, Hughes SC, Rosen MA, Shnider SM. Hydralazine does not restore uterine blood flow during cocaine-induced hypertension in the pregnant ewe. *Anesthesiology* 1992;76(4):580–587.

12. Liedholm H, Wahlin-Boll E, Ingemarsson I, Melander A. Transplacental passage and breast milk concentrations of hydralazine. *Eur J Clin Pharmacol* 1982;21:417–419.

13. Yemini M, Shosham (Schwartz) Z, Dgani R, Lancet M, Mogilner BM, Nissim F, Bar-Khayim Y. Lupus-like syndrome in a mother and newborn following administration of hydralazine: a case report. *Eur J Obstet Gynecol Reprod Biol* 1989;30:193–197.

14. Vink GJ, Moodley J, Philpott RH. Effect of dihydralazine on the fetus in the treatment of maternal hypertension. *Obstet Gynecol* 1980;55:519–522.

15. Paterson-Brown S, Robson SC, Redfern N, Walkinshaw SA, de Swiet M. Hydralazine boluses for the treatment of severe hypertension in preeclampsia. *Br J Obstet Gynaecol* 1994;101(5): 409–413.

16. Henrich WL, Cronin R, Miller P, Anderson RJ. Hypotensive sequelae of diazoxide and hydralazine therapy. *JAMA* 1977; 237(3):264–265.

17. Danielsson BR, Reiland S, Rundqvist E, Danielson M. Digital defects induced by vasodilating agents: relationship to reduction in uteroplacental blood flow. *Teratology* 1989;40(4):351–358.

18. Pryde PG, Abel EI, Hannigan J, Evans MI, Cotton DB. Effects of hydralazine on pregnant rats and their fetuses. *Am J Obstet Gynecol* 1993;169(4):1027–1231.

19. Heinonen OP, Slone D, Shapiro S. *Birth Defects and Drugs in Pregnancy.* Littleton, MA: Publishing Sciences Group; 1977.

20. Duggan PM, McCowan LM, Stewart AW. Antihypertensive drug effects on placental flow velocity waveforms in pregnant women with severe hypertension. *Aust N Z J Obstet Gynaecol* 1992;32(4):335–338.

21. Hjertberg R, Faxelius G, Lagercrantz H. Neonatal adaptation in hypertensive pregnancy—a study of labetalol vs. hydralazine treatment. *J Perinat Med* 1993;21(1):69–75.

22. Hjertberg R, Faxelius G, Belfrage P. Comparison of outcome of labetalol or hydralazine therapy during hypertension in pregnancy in very low birth weight infants. *Acta Obstet Gynecol Scand* 1993;72(8):611–615.

23. Walss-Rodriguez RJ, Flores-Padilla LM. Management of severe preeclampsia/eclampsia. Comparison between nifedipine and hydralazine as antihypertensive agents. *Ginecol Obstet Mex* 1993;61:76–79.

24. Belfort M, Uys P, Dommisse J, Davey DA. Haemodynamic changes in gestation proteinuric hypertension: the effects of rapid volume expansion and vasodilator therapy. *Br J Obstet Gynaecol* 1989;96(6):634–641.

25. Dudley DK. Minibolus diazoxide in the management of severe hypertension in pregnancy. *Am J Obstet Gynecol* 1985;151(2): 196–200.

26. Landesman R, Adeodato de Souza FJ, Countinho EM, Wilson KH, Bomfim de Sousa FM. The inhibitory effect of diazoxide in normal term labor. *Am J Obstet Gynecol* 1969;103:430–433.

27. Aparicio L, Carpenter MW, Schwartz R, Gruppuso PA. Prenatal diagnosis of familial neonatal hyperinsulinemia. *Acta Paediatr* 1993;82(8):683–686.

28. Michael CA. Intravenous labetalol and intravenous diazoxide

in severe hypertension complicating pregnancy. *Aust N Z J Obstet Gynaecol* 1986;26(1):26–29.

29. Briggs G, Freeman R, Yaffe S. *Drugs in Pregnancy and Lactation.* 4th ed. Baltimore: Williams & Wilkins; 1994;621–622.

30. Committee on Drugs, American Academy of Pediatrics. The transfer of drugs and other chemicals into human milk. *Pediatrics* 1994;93:137–150.

31. Tranquilli A, Conti C, Rezai B, Garzetti G, Romanini C. Nifedipine reduces pressor responsiveness to angiotensin II in pregnant women. *Clin Exp Obstet Gynecol* 1994;21(1):45–48.

32. Manninen A, Tuimala R, Vapaatalo H. Blood pressure, plasma renin activity and calcium metabolism in hypertensive pregnancy: the effect of nifedipine. *Int J Clin Pharmacol Res* 1990;10(6):331–337.

33. Manninen A, Vuorinen P, Laippala P, Tuimala R, Vapaatalo H. Atrial natriuretic peptide and cyclic guanosine-3'5'-monophosphate in hypertensive pregnancy and during nifedipine treatment. *Pharmacol Toxicol* 1994;74(3):153–157.

34. Manninen A, Metsa-Ketela T, Tuimala R, Vapaatalo H. Nifedipine increases urinary excretion of prostacyclin metabolite in hypertensive pregnancy. *Pharmacol Toxicol* 1991;69(1):60–63.

35. Carbonne B, Jannet D, Touboul C, Khelifati Y, Milliez J. Nicardipine treatment of hypertension during pregnancy. *Obstet Gynecol* 1993;81:908–914.

36. Childress C, Katz V. Nifedipine and its indications in obstetrics and gynecology. *Obstet Gynecol* 1994;83(4):616–624.

37. Harake B, Gilbert R, Ashwal S, Power G. Nifedipine: effects on fetal and maternal hemodynamics in pregnant sheep. *Am J Obstet Gynecol* 1987;157:1003–1008.

38. Walters B, Redman C. Treatment of severe pregnancy-associated hypertension with the calcium antagonist nifedipine. *Br J Obstet Gynaecol* 1984;91:330–336.

39. Puzey MS, Ackovic KL, Lindow SW, Gonin R. The effect of nifedipine on fetal umbilical artery Doppler waveforms in pregnancies complicated by hypertension. *S Afr Med J* 1991;79(4):192–194.

40. Hirose S, Yamada A, Kasugai M, Ishizuka T, Tomoda Y. The effect of nifedipine and dipyridamole on the Doppler blood flow waveforms of umbilical and uterine arteries in hypertensive pregnant women. *Asia Oceania J Obstet Gynaecol* 1992;18(2):187–193.

41. Walker JJ, Mathers A, Bjornsson S, Cameron AD, Fairlie FM. The effect of acute and chronic antihypertensive therapy on maternal and fetoplacental Doppler velocimetry. *Eur J Obstet Gynecol Reprod Biol* 1992;43(3):193–199.

42. Lurie S, Fenakel K, Friedman A. Effect of nifedipine on fetal heart rate in the treatment of severe pregnancy-induced hypertension. *Am J Perinatol* 1990;7(3):285–286.

43. Jayawardana J, Lekamge N. A comparison of nifedipine with methyldopa in pregnancy induced hypertension. *Ceylon Med J* 1994;39(2):87–90.

44. Jannet D, Carbonne B, Sebban E, Milliez J. Nicardipine versus metoprolol in the treatment of hypertension during pregnancy: a randomized comparative trial. *Obstet Gynecol* 1994;84(3):354–358.

45. Impey L. Severe hypotension and fetal distress following sublingual administration of nifedipine to a patient with severe pregnancy induced hypertension at 33 weeks. *Br J Obstet Gynaecol* 1993;100(10):959–961.

46. Caruso A, Ferrazzani S, De-Carolis S, Romano D, Mancinelli S, De-Carolis MP. The use of nifedipine as first-line hypotensive therapy in gestational hypertension. *Minerva Ginecologica* 1994;46:279–284.

47. Waisman GD, Mayorga LM, Camera MI, Vignolo CA, Martinotti A. Magnesium plus nifedipine: potentiation of hypotensive effect in preeclampsia? *Am J Obstet Gynecol* 1988;159:308–309.

48. Ben-Ami M, Giladi Y, Shalev E. The combination of magnesium sulfate and nifedipine: a cause of neuromuscular blockade. *Br J Obstet Gynaecol* 1994;101(3):262–263.

49. Fenakel K, Fenakel G, Appelman Z, Lurie S, Katz Z, Shoham Z. Nifedipine in the treatment of severe preeclampsia. *Obstet Gynecol* 1991;77:331–337.

50. Beaufils M, Uzan S, Donsimoni R, Colau JC. Prevention of preeclampsia by early antiplatelet therapy. *Lancet* 1985;1:840–842.

51. Lubbe WF, Hodge JV. Combined α- and β-adrenoceptor antagonism with prazosin and oxprenolol in control of severe hypertension in pregnancy. *N Z Med J* 1981;94:169–172.

52. Venuto R, Burstein P, Schneider R. Pheochromocytoma: antepartum diagnosis and management with tumor resection in the puerperium. *Am J Obstet Gynecol* 1984;150:431–432.

53. Hands ME, Johnson MD, Saltzman DH, Rutherford JD. The cardiac, obstetric, and anesthetic management of pregnancy complicated by acute myocardial infarction. *J Clin Anesth* 1990;2(4):258–268.

54. Ottman EH, Gall SA. Myocardial infarction in the third trimester of pregnancy secondary to an aortic valve thrombus. *Obstet Gynecol* 1993;81(5)pt2:804–805.

55. Cotton DB, Jones MM, Longmire S, Dorman KF, Tessem J, Joyce TH III. Role of intravenous nitroglycerin in the treatment of severe pregnancy-induced hypertension complicated by pulmonary edema. *Am J Obstet Gynecol* 1986;154:91–93.

32

ANGIOTENSIN-CONVERTING ENZYME INHIBITORS AND PREGNANCY

AVRAHAM SHOTAN, MD, JOSEF WIDERHORN, MD, AGNETA K. HURST, PHARMD, AND URI ELKAYAM, MD

INTRODUCTION

Angiotensin II (A-II) levels are elevated during pregnancy; however, the normal pregnant woman develops vascular refractoriness to its pressor effects, mainly as a consequence of decreased vascular smooth muscle responsiveness.[1] Women who develop pregnancy-induced hypertension begin losing their A-II refractoriness as early as the 23rd week of gestation, several weeks before hypertension develops.[2] Angiotensin-converting enzyme inhibitors (ACE-I) competitively block the conversion of angiotensin I to A-II and thus decrease the production of A-II and aldosterone. ACE inhibition as a treatment for pregnancy-induced hypertension, therefore, seemed to make good clinical sense, and such drugs as captopril and enalapril have been used in pregnant women for more than a decade.[3–7] Numerous reports, however, have been published since 1980, indicating the association of ACE-I therapy with severe fetal and neonatal morbidity and even mortality both in animals and in humans.[8]

This chapter reviews the available experimental and clinical data related to the use of ACE-I in pregnancy in an attempt to establish a clear-cut recommendation for the use of these drugs during gestation.

EXPERIMENTAL DATA

As early as 1980, Broughton-Pipkin et al[9] reported in a letter to the *Lancet* some alarming animal data related to the use of ACE-I during pregnancy. These investigators administered a single dose of captopril, analogous to that given in human patients, to five pregnant ewes at their third trimester. The ewes went into spontaneous delivery 4–23 days later, resulting in stillbirths in four cases and severe weakness in the fifth. In another study, the same investigators treated five New Zealand White rabbits with a daily dose of captopril at the third trimester and compared pregnancy outcome with those of five control rabbits.[9] The control group gave birth to 94% live-born young (81 out of total 86 babies), whereas the captopril group gave birth to 63% live-born young (47 out of 75). The difference was statistically significant. Similar results were reported by Keith et al,[10] who administered captopril or placebo to rabbits from midpregnancy to term. Among 20 captopril-treated mothers, fetal death was 86% (145 out of 169), compared to 1% (1 of 81) in the 12 rabbits treated with placebo. Similarly, high fetal mortality was found by Ferris and Weir,[11] who treated pregnant rabbits with chronic captopril in doses of either 2.5 or 5.0 mg/kg/day from the 15th day of pregnancy. These investigators reported 80% fetal mortality at the lower and 92% at the higher dose of the drug.

Minsker et al[12] described maternal toxicity (markedly increased blood urea nitrogen levels, and even maternal death) in rabbits after chronic oral administration of enalapril at dosages 1–30 mg/kg/day and showed that this result could be prevented by saline supplementation. The period of sensitivity of fetuses to the toxic effects of enalapril was found to be limited to middle to late gestation. A high single oral dose (30 mg/kg) given late in pregnancy resulted in 100% fetal deaths.

In addition to their initial studies with captopril,[9] Broughton-Pipkin and Wallace[14] studied the effects of 1–2 mg/kg of enalapril in nine chronically cannulated pregnant ewes. Although no hormonal effect could be noted in the fetuses, there was blood pressure reduction with the higher dose and one fetal death in an apparently normal full-term

Cardiac Problems in Pregnancy, Third Edition
Edited by Uri Elkayam, MD, and Norbert Gleicher, MD

lamb. (Two additional fetuses died; however, they had been abnormal prior to the study.) Grove et al.[13] studied the effect of tosimopril in the pregnant rats and found an indication that both fosinopril and its active metabolite fosinopulat do cross the placental barrier and inhibit fetal ACE.

A number of other studies have demonstrated the effect of ACE inhibition on systolic blood pressure and renal and uterine blood flow, and this work may provide an explanation of the poor fetal outcome associated with the administration of these drugs during gestation. Olsson et al,[15] who studied the effects of intravenous captopril in goats during the last months of pregnancy and lactation, reported a more pronounced fall in arterial blood pressure and a larger increase in plasma renin activity during pregnancy compared with the lactating period or with the nonpregnant state. Mabie et al[16] investigated the effects on maternal hemodynamics and organ perfusion in two groups of 10 rats each of chronic intraperitoneal administration of captopril (10 mg/kg/day) or placebo given from the 7th day of gestation. On day 21 (1 day before delivery), mean maternal arterial pressure was 23% lower in the captopril-treated group, as a result of a 29% decrease in total peripheral resistance. The decrease in total peripheral resistance was due primarily to a decline in splanchnic and skin vascular resistances.

Ferris and Weir[11] demonstrated a significant reduction in uterine blood flow (<33%) associated with a reduction in maternal blood pressure (18%) in pregnant rabbits treated with captopril. The hemodynamic changes were associated with a significant fall in uterine venous prostaglandin levels (PGE), which may have suggested the importance of PGE synthesis in maintaining uterine blood flow and the dependency of this substance on A-II. Since these investigators found an exceedingly high fetal mortality, they suggested an important role for uterine A-II and PGE synthesis during pregnancy in the maintenance of uterine blood flow and fetal survival during pregnancy. De Moura and Vale[17] infused bradykinin in vitro through fetal vessels in six full-term, isolated, perfused human placentas before and during captopril administration. Bradykinin activity was completely abolished after passage through the fetal placental circulation, and this inactivation was blocked by captopril.

The aforementioned experimental data demonstrate that the administration of ACE-I during the second and third trimesters of pregnancy caused high fetal and perinatal mortality. This unfavorable outcome may be related to a reduction in systemic blood pressure and uterine blood flow secondary to the significant vasodilatory effect, possibly caused by a decrease in A-II production and reduced degradation of bradykinin and prostaglandins mediated by these agents.[11]

HUMAN DATA

There is evidence in humans that both captopril and enalapril cross the placenta, as indicated by similar plasma levels of captopril found in the maternal and umbilical cord venous blood at delivery,[18–21] by reduction of ACE activity in both maternal and umbilical venous blood in comparison to normal maternal and umbilical cord blood levels,[18,19] and by a significantly elevated plasma renin activity in the newborn.[21]

Oligohydramnios

Several cases of oligohydramnios have been reported in pregnancies associated with exposure to ACE-I during pregnancy.[18,19,23–28] Whether these findings suggest a role of the renin–angiotensin system in the secretion of amniotic fluid is unclear. Reduction of amniotic fluid after 30–32 weeks of gestation as reported in some cases[19,22,23] may suggest an ACE-I mediated decrease in fetal renal function and urine output as cause for oligohydramnios. This mechanism may be supported by a frequent association between oligohydramnios and neonatal anuria.[3]

Renal Failure

Broughton-Pipkin et al[29] described in 1982 the case of a patient treated with captopril at the 28th week of gestation. Although maternal blood pressure response was favorable, the infant experienced severe hypotension and renal failure and died at the age of 8 days. An autopsy examination revealed grossly normal kidneys. Since long-lasting hypotension and renal failure are rare complications in the newborn in the presence of normal kidneys, it seemed highly likely that these effects were captopril related.[30]

Rothberg and Lorenz[23] reported renal failure in a newborn born in the 35th gestational week to a patient whose captopril therapy was started prior to pregnancy. In addition, the newborn, who died on day 30 postpartum, had hypoplastic skull bones and wide sutures, limb contractures, lung hypoplasia and pneumothorax, and hypotension.

Schubiger et al[22] described a 34-year-old pregnant woman whose antihypertensive treatment with methyldopa (1500 mg/day) and verapamil (360 mg/day) was ineffective. At the 32nd week of gestation, methyldopa was replaced with enalapril (20 mg/day) and was followed by elective cesarian section delivery 17 days later. The baby was anuric but otherwise healthy. Ultrasound examination disclosed normal kidneys without urine excretion, and a cystourethrogram showed no obstruction. A renal biopsy revealed hyperplasia of the juxtaglomerular apparatus. The baby needed peritoneal dialysis from the 3rd to the 10th postpartum days. The ACE activity was completely suppressed, and plasma A-II concentration was only 5% of normal neonatal level at the 3rd day postpartum. Plasma enalaprilat concentration fell from 28 ng/mL before dialysis to less than 0.16 ng/mL after dialysis and was associated with partial recovery of ACE activity and A-II concentration. At the age of 3 months, the baby's kidney function was normal.

Rose et al[31] described seven cases of prolonged hypotension, renal failure, and anuria associated with maternal use of ACE-I during the last trimester. All these cases were reported to the Food and Drug Administration and three had been published earlier.[19,22,24] Oligohydramnios, possibly as a result of intrauterine renal failure, was observed in five of the cases. Peak serum creatinine levels in the newborns were in the range of 3.6–20 mg/dL. Two of the newborns died, whereas the other five infants recovered after peritoneal dialysis 3–10 days postpartum.

In an additional publication, Broughton-Pipkin et al[18] reported the case of a 24-year-old woman with familial hypophosphatemic rickets and malignant hypertension. She presented in her 15th week of gestation with controlled blood pressure and was treated with enalapril (10 mg/day) and furosemide (40 mg/day). Ultrasound scan disclosed a normal fetal size and amniotic fluid amount. Repeated ultrasound scans revealed reduced liquid volume, followed by complete disappearance at the 20th week of gestation and associated with slowing of fetal growth. At the 21st week, furosemide and enalapril were discontinued and replaced with labetalol (600 mg daily). There was steady improvement in amniotic fluid volume, which was actually normal at the 27th week of gestation. However, a few days later, the patient presented with a placental abruption and blood pressure of 200/130 mmHg, necessitating immediate cesarean section. After delivery, anuria was not a problem. The infant was small for date, however, and died 6 days later from respiratory distress syndrome and hypotension. The recovery of the amniotic fluid volume on discontinuation of enalapril and furosemide may be a causative proof for the relation between ACE-I and oligohydramnios during pregnancy.

Cunniff et al[32] reported the case of a 22-year-old woman with systemic lupus erythematosus and severe chronic hypertension who was treated throughout her pregnancy with enalapril 20 (mg/day), propranolol 40 (mg/day), and hydrochlorothiazide (50 mg/day). During the pregnancy, there was no evidence of active lupus disease. An ultrasound examination showed a normal amniotic fluid volume at 16 weeks, but severe oligohydramnios at 27 weeks. An amniocentesis performed to determine lung maturity showed thick meconium. The infant, delivered by emergency cesarean section at 34 weeks of gestation, had striking features: The posterior fontanel was enlarged, with decreased skull ossification, and there was a glabellar crease, a deviation of the nasal septum, and a horizontal chin crease. In addition, the chest was bell shaped, there were positional deformities of both hands, and the knees and elbows exhibited contractures. The infant had prolonged hypotension, requiring resuscitation with intravenous fluid and inotropic support, as well as respiratory failure, requiring ventilatory support, and anuria. The infant died 25 hours postpartum. At autopsy, the lungs were hypoplastic with evidence of hyaline membrane, and the kidneys were enlarged, but appeared grossly normal.

However, microscopic examination disclosed poorly demarcated corticomedullary junctions, decreased number of glomerular lobulations, paucity of tubules, and increased medullary mesenchymal tissue. The authors mentioned the similarity between the renal findings in this infant and a genetically described autosomal recessive renal tubular dysgenesis defect,[33] suggesting that the mechanism in both conditions is failure to produce glomerular filtrate or lack of blood flow from the efferent arteriole into the kidney interstitium.

Pryde et al[28] described a 30-year-old patient who was treated with enalapril from the beginning of her pregnancy. The infant was delivered by cesarean section at week 32 because of fetal distress. The newborn developed respiratory failure and profound hypertension in spite of therapy with dopamine, dobutamine, and epinephrine. Hypotension and anuria persisted until initiation of peritoneal dialysis on day 5. On day 8, ischemic jejunum was resected, and on day 9, the newborn died. At autopsy, the kidneys were large and microscopic examination showed tubular dysplasia.

Although renal biopsy reveals normal kidneys in some cases of infants with anuria,[3,23,27] Guignard et al[24] reported hemorrhagic foci in the renal cortex and medulla in a newborn to a patient with pregnancy-induced hypertension who was treated with captopril during her pregnancy. Rothberg and Lorenz[23] reported anuria in a premature dysmorphic baby born to a patient whose renovascular hypotension was treated with captopril, aldomet, and thiosemide. The treatment with captopril was initiated before pregnancy, and the newborn died 1 month after delivery. Scott and Purohit[34] reported anuria and mortality in a newborn to a patient whose renovascular hypertension was treated with enalapril. The time of starting enalapril therapy was not reported.

Neonatal Hypotension

Neonatal hypotension was evidenced in approximately 10% of reported pregnancies associated with the use of ACE-I.[18,19,23–25,28,31,34] The majority of these cases were associated with anuria.

Teratogenic Effect

Although animal experimentations suggested no teratogenic malformations with the use of ACE-I during pregnancy, such an effect cannot be excluded in humans. There have been several cases of unique bony deformity, especially skull ossification defect, after gestational exposure to these medications. As previously mentioned, Cunniff et al[32] described an infant born at 34 week of gestation to a woman with systemic lupus erythematosus and severe chronic hypertension, which had been treated during gestation with enalapril, propranolol, and hydrochlorothiazide. Physical examination revealed an enlarged posterior fontanel with decreased skull ossification. There was a glabellar crease, a deviation of the nasal septum, and a horizontal chin crease. There were marked positional deformities of both hands and contractures of the knees and elbows, and the feet were held in calcaneovalgocavus position. Duminy and Burger[35] reported a case of a 30-year-old woman with renovascular hypertension treated with captopril, propranolol, and amiloride throughout her pregnancy. She gave birth to a malformed fetus with the left leg ending in midthigh and a defective skull formation of the vault.

Mehta and Modi[25] described a 27-year-old renal transplant recipient who conceived while receiving treatment with enalapril, azathioprine, atenolol, and prednisolone. She continued taking her medications throughout pregnancy. At the 32nd week of gestation, ultrasound scan showed anhydramnios and asymmetrical growth retardation, and the patient was urgently delivered by cesarean section. The male newborn was small for date, and the occipital skull, extending anteriorly to the ears and superiorly to become confluent with the anterior fontanelle, lacked ossification. He also had squashed facies and contractures of the knees, ankles, and elbows. The infant required ventilation from birth and was hypotensive (systolic blood pressure 25 mmHg) and anuric. Ultrasound showed normal size kidneys and normal urinary tract system. The infant died subsequently on the 10th day postpartum, and necropsy revealed hypoplastic lungs, extensive intracranial hemorrhage, and normal size kidneys. There

were histologic findings of congested glomeruli and hypertrophied renal arterioles, however, and the kidneys had cortical mottling. No chromosomal abnormality was detected.

Barr and Cohen[36] reported two cases of fetal renal tubular dysgenesis and severely underdeveloped calvarial bone (Figs. 32.1 and 32.2). One patient, a 26-year-old woman with systemic lupus erythematosus with nephrogenic hypertension, was chronically treated with prednisolone, atenolol, furosemide, and captopril. Serial ultrasound examiantions showed unrelieved oligohydramnios from 20 weeks of gestation. At 33 weeks, the patient gave birth to an anuric, hypoxic, acidemic, small-for-date female infant who died 14 hours later. At autopsy, the kidneys were found to be large, and microscopic examination showed renal tubular dysgenesis. The calvarial bones were very small, leaving the top third of the head unprotected by bone. Histologically, the bone was remarkably thin, without adequate trabeculation or marrow development. In the second case, an 18-year-old hypertensive mother had conceived while being treated with lisinopril. The pregnancy was uneventful, but the infant was delivered prematurely by cesarean section at the 32nd week of gestation. For 2 weeks, there was persistent anuria, necessitating peritoneal dialysis. The infant's skull plates were small and his fontanels wide open. During the next 15 months, considerable expansion of the calvarial bones was

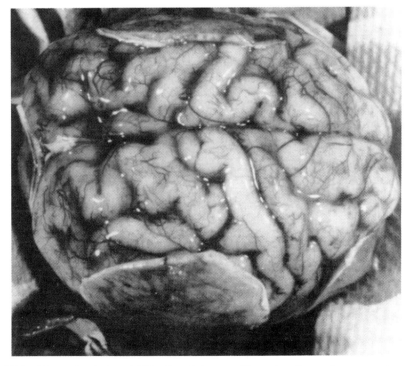

Figure 32.1 Hypocalvaria in a 1440 g female born at 33 weeks of gestation to a patient with hypertension treated with captopril during pregnancy. The skull is viewed from above, with the fibrous tissue of the fontanels and sutures removed to emphasize the diminutive size of the bones. (Reprinted with permission from Barr and Cohen.[36])

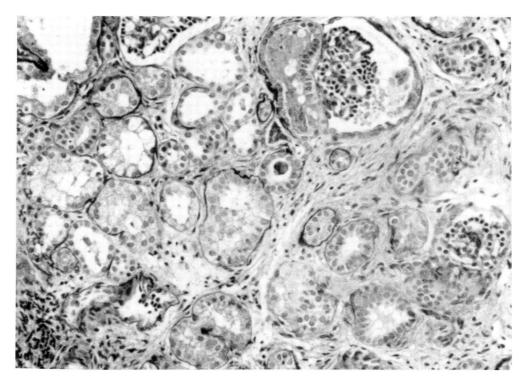

Figure 32.2   ACE inhibitor exposed kidney showing dilated Bowman's spaces and tubules, old tubular necrosis, lack of differentiation between proximal and distal convoluted tubules, and increased mesenchyme. (Reprinted with permission from Pryde et al.[28])

evident with gradual closing of the fontanels. However, he continued to be dependent on peritoneal dialysis while awaiting renal transplantation. The authors found possible links between calvarial underdevelopment, especially the membranous skull bones, and renal tubular dysgenesis. They suggested that this "kidney–skull connection" due to ACE inhibition may have been caused by intrauterine hypotension and/or chronic hypoxia.

Rothberg and Lorentz[23] reported hypoplastic skull bones and wide sutures in a newborn following gestational exposure to captopril, and Kaler et al[37] found a depressed nasal bridge, low-set ears, and micrognathia in an infant born to a patient treated with captopril, minoxide, and propranolol throughout pregnancy. In addition, the infant had clinodactyly, omphalocele, undescended testis, unusual fat distribution, hypertrichosis, and ventricular septal defect.

Patent Ductus Arteriosus

Hurault de Ligney and associated[20] reported on the initiation of captopril (75 mg/day) for preeclampsia at the 32nd week of gestation, after unsuccessful treatment with labetalol in combination with dihydralazine. Ultrasound scan disclosed intrauterine growth retardation 4 weeks prior to captopril initiation. At the 35th week, after α-methyldopa was added, a

small-for-date girl was delivered by a cesarean section. On the 11th day postpartum, a large ductus arteriosus was diagnosed and surgically corrected. Another case of persistent ductus arteriosus was reported by the same authors[19] in a 22-year-old mother whose nephrotic syndrome, complicated by hypertension, had been treated with captopril (100 mg daily) and diuretics. Once pregnancy was diagnosed, diuretics were stopped and acebutolol was added. Hypertension was controlled only until the 19th week of gestation. Intrauterine growth retardation was diagnosed, and finally oligohydramnios. At the 34th week, a small-for-date boy was delivered by cesarean section. The newborn stopped breathing at 15 minutes, needed artificial ventilation for 24 hours, and had hypotension for 10 days. A patent ductus arteriosus was diagnosed on the 3rd day postpartum and was surgically treated at 14 months.

Kreft-Jais et al[38] reported two cases of patent ductus arteriosus out of 31 pregnancies in women treated with ACE-I during gestation. Both infants were born prematurely to women given captopril until delivery. One of these infants required surgical repair after failure of attempted closure with indomethacin.

It is certainly possible that the persistent ductus arteriosus found in these four cases was related to prematurity and not necessarily to maternal captopril therapy.[3] However, the relation between persistent patency of ductus arteriosus and ACE-I-mediated potentiation of bradykinin and prostaglandins cannot be ruled out.[38]

Respiratory Complications

Respiratory complications, found in 14% of newborns[3] whose mothers were treated with ACE-I during pregnancy, included respiratory distress syndrome,[20,24,28,34,38,39] lung hypoplasia,[9,23,25] and apnea.[3,19] The incidence of respiratory distress syndrome in newborns who were born alive before 34 weeks of gestation was determined by Hanssens et al[3] to be 28%. A strong association was seen between lung hypoplasia and oligohydramnios, and this condition resulted in death in all cases.[9,23,25]

Fetal and Neonatal Mortality

In a summary of 85 reported pregnancies associated with fetal exposure to ACE-I, Hanssens et al[3] reported perinatal mortality in 11 cases, or 13%. Six of the 11 deaths occurred prepartum and presented as stillbirths; the remaining deaths occurred within the first 30 days postpartum. Perinatal death seemed to be related to severe maternal proteinuric hypertension,[38] oligohydramnios, and fetal renal and respiratory failure.[28]

Prematurity and Small Size for Date

Increased incidences of preterm delivery, cesarean section delivery, and newborns found to be small for gestational age have been reported in pregnancy associated with ACE-I therapy.[21,23,25,28,38] Kreft-Jais and associates[38] reported preterm delivery by cesarean section in 12 of 26 women who had live birth.

Breast Milk

Huttunen et al[40] measured enalaprilat concentration and ACE activity in the breast milk of three nursing mothers 4 hours after oral administration of enalapril (5–10 mg), 3–45 days postdelivery. Although serum enalaprilat levels rose markedly in the maternal serum, the drug was not detected in the breast milk, and milk ACE activity was normal compared with milk from healthy lactating women.

SUMMARY AND RECOMMENDATIONS

Numerous reports in both animals and humans have been published in the last decade describing the high degree of morbidity and even mortality in fetuses or newborns of mothers treated with ACE-I during pregnancy. Unfavorable outcomes included oligohydramnios, intrauterine growth retardation, premature labor, fetal and neonatal renal failure, bony malformations, limb contractures, persistent patent ductus arteriosus, pulmonary hypoplasia, respiratory distress syndrome, prolonged hypotension, and neonatal death.

The direct effects of ACE-I on the fetus are difficult to determine because these drugs are usually administered to women presenting with high risk pregnancies. Gestational hypertension by itself can be associated with neonatal complications, such as oligohydramnios, fetal anoxia, intrauterine growth retardation, low birth weight, and respiratory distress.[41] Therefore, in this selected group of high risk pregnancies, severity of maternal disease or consequent obstetrical decision (e.g., preterm delivery, cesarean section), as well as ACE-I, could account for some of the reported complications. However, prolonged anuria associated with renal failure and hypotension in the newborn and the unique skull ossification defect in neonates have not been commonly associated with maternal hypertension or its treatment and are very likely to be related to maternal exposure to ACE-I during gestation.

ACE inhibitors are currently a first-line treatment of hypertension and heart failure in nonpregnant patients. Because of the frequency and consistency of the reported complications associated with fetal exposure to these agents, their use should be avoided during gestation. Women in the childbearing age who are treated with ACE-I should be informed regarding the risks of continuous ACE-I treatment during pregnancy and the need to discontinue this form of therapy and replace it with an alternative treatment after conception.

In 1992 the FDA officially warned against the use of ACE-I in the second and third trimesters but not in the first trimester of pregnancy.[8] Brent and Beckman,[4] in their published information for clinical teratology counselors, did not regard exposure to ACE-I during early pregnancy as a reason for pregnancy interruption and stated that animal studies and available clinical data suggested that the deleterious effect of ACE-I was due not to the teratogenic effect but to the deleterious effect on fetal development that occurred later in gestation. However, most reported cases describing bony malformations, limb contractures, facial abnormalities, and lung hypoplasia have been associated with exposure to ACE-I throughout pregnancy. These data suggest, therefore, that complete safety of exposure to ACE-I during the first gestational trimester cannot be guaranteed, and they emphasize the need for physician and patient education regarding the risk of ACE-I during pregnancy, to avoid a dilemma associated with fetal exposure to this group of drugs during the first trimester. The great majority of available data related to the use of ACE-I in pregnancy is limited to captopril and enalapril, which seem to cause similar fetal and neonatal complications.[3,38] The safety of all other ACE-I agents currently used for the treatment of hypertension is not known and may not be known in the future. Because of the similar mechanism of action of all these agents, it seems reasonable at the present time to extend the warning related to the gestational use of captopril and enalapril to all other ACE-I drugs.

ACKNOWLEDGMENT

This chapter was reproduced with modifications with permission from Shotan et al (*Am J Med* 1994;96:451–456).

REFERENCES

1. Fleischman AR, Oakes GK, Epstein MF, Catt KJ, Chez RA. Plasma renin activity during ovine pregnancy. *Am J Physiol* 1975;228:901–904.

2. Gant NF, Worley RJ, Everett RB, MacDonald PC. Control of vascular responsiveness during human pregnancy. *Kidney Int* 1980;18:253–258.

3. Hanssens M, Keirse MJNC, Vankelecom F, Van Assche FA. Fetal and neonatal effects of treatment with angiotensin-converting enzyme inhibitors in pregnancy. *Obstet Gynecol* 1991;78:128–135.

4. Brent RL, Beckman DA. Angiotensin-converting enzyme inhibitors, an embryopathic class of drugs with unique properties: information for clinical teratology counselors. *Teratology* 1991;43:543–546.

5. Lindheimer MD, Katz A. Hypertension in pregnancy. *N Engl J Med* 1985;313:675–680. Current Concepts.

6. Lindheimer MD, Barron WM. Enalapril and pregnancy-induced hypertension. *Ann Intern Med* 1988;108:911. Letter.

7. Mochizuke M, Maruo T, Motoyama S. Treatment of hypertension in pregnancy by a combined drug regimen including captopril. *Clin Exp Hypertension Pregnancy* 1986;B5:69–78.

8. Nightingale SL. Warnings on the use of ACE inhibitors in second and third trimester of pregnancy. *JAMA* 1992;267:2445.

9. Broughton-Pipkin F, Turner SR, Symonds EM. Possible risk with captopril in pregnancy: some animal data. *Lancet* 1980;1:1256. Letter.

10. Keith IM, Will JA, Weir EK. Captopril: association with fetal death and pulmonary vascular changes in the rabbit. *Proc Soc Exp Biol Med* 1982;170:378–383.

11. Ferris TF, Weir EK. Effect of captopril on uterine blood flow and prostaglandin E synthesis in the pregnant rabbit. *J Clin Invest* 1983;71:809–815.

12. Minsker DA, Bagdon WJ, MacDonald JS, Robertson RT, Bokelman DL. Maternotoxicity and ferotoxicity of an angiotensin-converting enzyme inhibitor, enalapril, in rabbits. *Fundam Appl Toxicol* 1990;14:461–470.

13. Grove KL, Mayo RJ, Forsyth CS, Frank AA, Speth RC. Fosinopril treatment of pregnant rats: developmental toxicity, fetal angiotensin-converting enzyme inhibition, and fetal angiotensin II receptor regulation. *Toxicol Lett* 1995;80:85–95.

14. Broughton-Pipkin F, Wallace CP. The effect of enalapril (MK421), an angiotensin converting enzyme inhibitor, on conscious pregnant ewe and her foetus. *Br J Pharmacol* 1986;87:533–542.

15. Olsson K, Fyhrquist F, Benlamlih S, Dahlborn K. Effects of captopril on arterial blood pressure, plasma renin activity and vasopressin concentration in sodium-repleted and sodium-deficient goats: a serial study during pregnancy, lactation and anestrus. *Acta Physiol Scand* 1984;121:73–80.

16. Mabie WC, Ahokas RA, Sibai BM. Maternal and uteroplacental hemodynamic effects of chronic captopril in the hypertensive, term-pregnant rat. *Am J Obstet Gynecol* 1990;163:1861–1867.

17. DeMoura RS, Vale NS. Effect of captopril on bradykinin inactivation by human foetal placental circulation. *Br J Clin Pharmacol* 1986;21:143–148.

18. Broughton-Pipkin F, Baker PN, Symonds EM. ACE inhibitors in pregnancy. *Lancet* 1989;2:96–97. Letter.

19. Boutroy MJ, Vert P, Hurault de Ligny B, Miton A. Captopril administration in pregnancy impairs fetal angiotensin converting enzyme activity and neonatal adaptation. *Lancet* 1984;2:935–936. Letter.

20. Hurault de Ligny B, Ryckelynck JP, Mintz P, Levy G, Muller G. Captopril therapy in preeclampsia. 1987;46:329–330. Letter.

21. Fiocchi R, Lijnen P, Staessen J, Van Assche F, Fagard R, Amery A, Spitz B, Rademaker M. Captopril during pregnancy. *Lancet* 1984;2:1153. Letter.

22. Schubiger G, Flury G, Nussberger J. Enalapril for pregnancy-induced hypertension: acute renal failure in a neonate. *Ann Intern Med* 1988;108:215–216.

23. Rothberg AD, Lorentz R. Can captopril cause fetal and neonatal renal failure? *Pediatr Pharmacol* 1984;4:189–192.

24. Guignard JP, Burgener F, Calame A. Persistent anuria in neonate: a side effect of captopril. *Int J Pediatr Nephrol* 1981;2:133. Abstract.

25. Mehta N, Modi N. ACE inhibitors in pregnancy. *Lancet* 1989;2:96. Letter.

26. Plouin PF, Tchoboutsky C. Inhibition of angiotensin converting enzyme in human pregnancy: 15 cases. *Presse Med* 1985;14:2175–2178.

27. Knott PD, Thorpe SS, Lamont CA. Congenital renal dysgenesis possibly due to captopril. *Lancet* 1989;1:451. Letter.

28. Pryde PG, Sedman AB, Nugent CE, Barr M. Angiotensin-converting enzyme inhibitor fetopathy. *J Am Soc Nephrol* 1993;3:1575–1582.

29. Broughton-Pipkin F, Symonds EM, Turner SR. The effects of captopril (SQ14,225) upon mother and fetus in the chronically cannulated ewe and in the pregnant rabbit. *J Physiol* 1982;323:415–422.

30. Lubbe WF. The use of captopril in pregnancy. *N Z Med J* 1983;96:1029–1030. Letter.

31. Rosa FW, Bosco LA, Graham CF, Milstein JB, Dreis M, Creamer J. Neonatal anuria with maternal angiotensin-converting enzyme inhibition. *Obstet Gynecol* 1989;74:371–374.

32. Cunniff C, Jones KL, Phillipson J, Benirschke K, Short S, Wujek J. Oligohydramnios sequence and renal tubular malforma-

tion associated with maternal enalapril use. *Am J Obstet Gynecol* 1990;162:187–189.

33. Swinford AE, Bernstein J, Toriello HV, Higgins JV. Renal tubular dysgenesis: delayed onset of oligohydramnios. *Am J Med Genet* 1989;32:127–132.

34. Scott AA, Purohit DM. Neonatal renal failure: a complication of maternal antihypertensive therapy. *Am J Obstet Gynecol* 1989;160:1223–1224.

35. Duminy PC, Burger PD. Fetal abnormalities associated with the use of captopril during pregnancy. *S Afr Med J* 1981;60:805. Letter.

36. Barr M, Cohen MM. ACE inhibitor fetopathy and hypocalvaria: the kidney–skull connection. *Teratology* 1991;44:485–495.

37. Kaler SG, Patrinos ME, Lambert GH, Myers TF, Karlman R, Anderson CL. Hypertrichosis and congenital anomalies associated with maternal use of minoxidil. *Pediatrics* 1987;79: 434–436.

38. Kreft-Jais C, Plouin PF, Tchoboutsky C, Boutroy MJ. Angiotensin-converting enzyme inhibitors during pregnancy: a survey of 22 patients given captopril and nine given enalapril. *Br J Obstet Gynaecol* 1988;95:420–422.

39. Millar JA, Wilson PD, Morrison M. Management of severe hypertension in pregnancy by a combined drug regimen including captopril: case report. *N Z Med J* 1983;96:796–798.

40. Huttunen K, Gronhagen-Riska C, Fyhrquist F. Enalapril treatment of a nursing with slightly impaired renal function. *Clin Nephrol* 1989;31:278. Letter.

41. Mayden KL, Elrad H, Grylia RV, Gleicher N. Obstetric ultrasound in the management of pregnancy complicated by maternal and fetal disease. In Gleicher N, ed. *Principles of Medical Therapy in Pregnancy.* New York: Plenum; 1985;64–77.

33

ANTICOAGULATION IN PREGNANCY

WILLIAM MCGEHEE, MD

INTRODUCTION

Anticoagulant therapy is an essential component in the management of a variety of clinical events that may occur during pregnancy. While there is a general consensus that therapy is beneficial for women with venous thromboembolism and several cardiac disorders, there are other circumstances in which the role of anticoagulants is either uncertain or controversial. This chapter summarizes current standards of therapy based on clinical trials and the personal experience of the author. New information that may alter current practices is reviewed.

INDICATIONS FOR ANTICOAGULANT THERAPY

Venous Thromboembolism

The most common indication for anticoagulant therapy during pregnancy is venous thrombosis, along with its complications. The incidence of documented venous thromboembolism in the general population has been estimated to be 1 in 1000,[1] and retrospective studies (Table 33.1) have reported approximately the same incidence in pregnant women.[2,3] However, our recent experience suggests that the true incidence may indeed be substantially higher. In the period from 1992 to 1995, our anticoagulant clinic cared for 42 women with either deep vein thrombosis (DVT) or pulmonary embolism occurring during pregnancy or the immediate postpartum period. Whatever the true incidence, pulmonary embolism remains an important cause of maternal mortality (Table 33.2), ranking second only to death due to trauma.[4]

Cardiac Disease

A prosthetic heart valve is the most common cardiac indication for anticoagulant therapy. With advances in cardiac diagnosis and increased safety of valve replacement, the number of patients with prosthetic heart valves continues to increase. Long-term oral anticoagulant therapy reduces the incidence of thromboembolic complications,[5] but until recent years the incidence of thromboembolism in this heterogeneous population has been difficult to define. The risk of thromboembolism has been thought to depend on several interacting factors: the severity of the underlying cardiac disease, the design and position of the prosthesis, the presence of arrhythmia, and the age of the patient. The intensity of oral anticoagulant therapy is also important, but early clinical trials reported different risks of bleeding and thromboembolic complications. Part of this variation was due to poor standardization of the tests used in the measurement of anticoagulant intensity. It became apparent that there were large differences in the sensitivity of prothrombin time reagents.[6] With the introduction of the international normalized ratio (INR), large patient groups could be compared. With standardization of the prothrombin time, recent clinical trials have provided a clearer picture of relative risks and definition of optimal therapy. In 1995 a study of patients on long-term, well-controlled oral anticoagulant therapy defined the incidence of thromboembolism in patients with mechanical heart valves.[7] This risk was lowest in patients less than 50 years of age: 0.1/100 patient-years, with a bleeding risk of 2.5/100 patient-years. The same study confirmed that thromboembolism depends on the position and the design of the prosthesis and on the severity of the underlying heart disease.

Cardiac Problems in Pregnancy, Third Edition
Edited by Uri Elkayam, MD, and Norbert Gleicher, MD
Copyright © 1998 by Wiley-Liss, Inc. ISBN 0-471-16358-9

TABLE 33.1 Venous Thromboembolic Disease During Pregnancy Documented by Objective Test

Source of Data and Period Covered	Deliveries	Incidence (%)
De Sweit et al, 1970–1980	35,000	0.09
LAC-USC MC, 1985	16,811	0.08
LAC-USC MC, 1986	17,145	0.09
LAC-USC MC, 1987[a]	16,490	0.09

[a]One case of fatal pulmonary embolism 2 days postpartum after an apparent uncomplicated vaginal delivery.

Source: DeSweit et al[2] and author's unpublished data[3] from the Los Angeles County University of Southern California Medical Center (LAC-USC MC).

TABLE 33.2 Specific Causes of Maternal Mortality

Cause	Deaths per 100,000 Live Births
All causes	10
Trauma	1.9
Pulmonary embolism	1.2
Toxemia of pregnancy	0.9
Intracranial hemorrhage	0.9
Infection	0.6
Amniotic fluid embolism	0.6

Source: Sachs et al, *N Engl J Med* 1987; 316:667–672.

Valves of older design (caged ball or caged disk) had a substantial greater thrombotic risk (2.5/100 patient-years) than the newer tilting or bileaflet prostheses (0.7/100 patient-years). The authors of this report and the accompanying editorial[8] concluded that optimal antithrombotic therapy must be individualized depending on these risk factors. During pregnancy, the risk mandates the continuation of anticoagulant therapy, but, because there is concern about the potential risk to the fetus from coumarin drugs, oral anticoagulants are often replaced by heparin. The incidence of treatment failure associated with this alternate therapy has not been clearly defined.[9]

Other cardiac conditions that may require anticoagulant therapy during pregnancy include valvular disease, cardiomyopathy, congenital heart disease, and atrial fibrillation. The benefit of long-term oral anticoagulant therapy for isolated nonvalvular atrial fibrillation has been most apparent in patients past the childbearing age.[10] Thus, the need for anticoagulant therapy in patients with controlled nonrheumatic isolated atrial fibrillation during pregnancy is questionable. However, there is little disagreement that anticoagulants are indicated for patients with atrial fibrillation associated with rheumatic mitral valve disease, left atrial enlargement, or a history of systemic embolism.[11]

PATIENTS AT PRESUMED RISK FOR THROMBOSIS

Anticoagulant therapy has been advocated for a pregnant woman with presumed increased risk of thrombosis, usually suspected when there is a history of a previous thromboembolic event.[9] For the clinician, the definition of risk and the need to prophylactically treat such patients is problematic and controversial. Pregnancy is associated with consistent alteration in the levels of coagulation factors,[12] which tend to shorten in vitro clotting tests; but the value of these changes to predict a thrombotic event in the individual patient has never been documented. Nevertheless, new information has convincingly demonstrated that the rate of thrombin generation is increased during pregnancy. Assessment of the rate of

thrombin generation has been derived from measurement of "activation peptides," small fragments of the coagulation factors cleaved from precursor proteins during in vivo coagulation.[13] One peptide is a product of the conversion of prothrombin to thrombin (fragment 1.2, or F1.2). The plasma concentration provides an indirect measurement of in vivo thrombin generation. All normal individuals have measurable levels of F1.2 in their plasma. Low levels of F1.2 are evident in some patients with severe congenital bleeding disorders. Conversely, high values are seen in patients with active thrombosis and in some patients with underlying disorders that have been associated with increased risk of thrombosis (a prethrombotic state). During pregnancy, F1.2 and other markers of coagulation activity[14–16] are elevated, indicating increased activation of the coagulation system. Apparently, this physiologic increase in thrombin generation, by itself, does not directly influence the risk of thrombosis. Thus, while these observations confirm that a *potential hypercoaguable state* is present during pregnancy, they do not allow identification of the occasional patient who will have a clinically significant thrombosis. Moreover, animal studies have suggested that low concentrations of thrombin may serve an important antithrombotic function.[17]

Deep vein thrombosis is often preceded by an transient *environmental event:* infection, surgery, or pregnancy. Underlying congenital or acquired hemostatic abnormalities associated with thrombosis in the general population (Table 33.3) would also be expected to contribute to risk during pregnancy. The relevance of congenital or acquired hemostatic abnormalities will depend on two determinants: the degree of the alteration in the hemostatic system produced by the defect and the population incidence of the disorder.

Congenital antithrombin III (ATIII) deficiency is a well-recognized risk factor for venous thrombosis during pregnancy.[18,19] Antithrombin III binds to and inactivates thrombin and other serine proteases participating in thrombin generation. Thus, it is not surprising that the pregnant woman with increased thrombin generation and deficiency of ATIII is at increased risk of thrombosis. However, ATIII deficiency (type I) is uncommon and accounts for only a small number of patients who manifest thrombosis.

TABLE 33.3   Hemostatic Abnormalities Associated with Thrombosis

Abnormality	General Population Incidence
Antithrombin III deficiency (type I)	1:5000–10,000
Protein C deficiency	1:250
Protein S deficiency	Unknown[a]
Plasminogen abnormality	Very uncommon
Lupus anticoagulant	Unknown
Activated protein C resistance (APCR)	3–5%

[a]Depressed during pregnancy.

A second and more important series of underlying abnormalities involves the protein C and S "natural anticoagulant pathway." Thrombin is a procoagulant, since it clots fibrinogen, activates factor XIII, and aggregates platelets. Thrombin also activates factor V (V_a) and factor VIII (VIII_a), an essential function that allows continuing and accelerated thrombin generation.[20] Paradoxically, thrombin is also the trigger for a series of reactions that reduce the rate of thrombin generation. The essential features of this system[21] are illustrated in Figure 33.1. The key elements include an endothelial cell thrombin receptor, thrombomodulin, and two plasma vitamin-K-dependent proteins, protein C and S. Thrombomodulin-bound thrombin cleaves protein C to produce a serine protease-activated protein C (C_a). In concert with protein S, C_a dampens thrombin generation by cleaving V_a and VIII_a. Congenital deficiency of either protein C or S has been associated with an increased risk for thrombosis.[22,23] Heterozygote protein C deficiency is relatively common in the general population (1 in 250), but the great majority of protein-C-deficient patients lack a history of thrombosis.[24,25] The population incidence of congenital protein S deficiency has not been clearly defined, but all pregnant patients demonstrate an acquired decrease in the concentration of protein S.[26] It is intriguing to speculate that acquired protein S deficiency could be one reason for the increased rate of thrombin generation in pregnancy.

When retrospective measurements of these three important inhibitors were performed in patients who had venous thrombosis during pregnancy, a definite abnormality could be detected in only 5–10% of patients. However, the importance of underlying congenital abnormalities in the risk for venous thrombosis has dramatically increased since the discovery of a common autosomal defect associated with familial thrombosis.[27] In vitro, activated protein C prolongs the clotting time of normal plasma by inactivation of factors V_a and VIII_a. In contrast, the clotting times of the affected thrombophilia family members proved resistant to the usual action of activated protein C [activated protein C resistance (APCR)] despite normal concentrations and function of the constituent proteins C and S. APCR was later shown to be due to an abnormality[28] in one of the substrates—factor V Leiden. A single amino acid substitution at a major cleavage site for activated protein C was found in the great majority of patients with APCR. Presumably V_a is poorly inactivated, allowing increased thrombin generation and the development of a prethrombotic state. Population studies have demonstrated that heterozygote APCR is the most common congenital abnormality associated with a thrombotic tendency and is present in 3–5% of the general population.[29] Homozygotes are at higher risk for thrombosis. Although affected patients have increased levels of F1.2, they often do not manifest clinical thrombosis for many years. However, thrombosis may present spontaneously or, more commonly, when the patient is challenged by surgery, illness, or pregnancy.[30]

For some reason, APCR seems to be a very important risk factor for thrombosis during pregnancy. A surprisingly high incidence of APCR of 60% has been reported in patients who have had venous thrombosis during pregnancy.[31] In a related clinical setting, the risk of thrombosis due to oral contraceptives has been reported to be 30 times higher for patients with heterozygous APCR.[31–33] Patients with multiple genet-

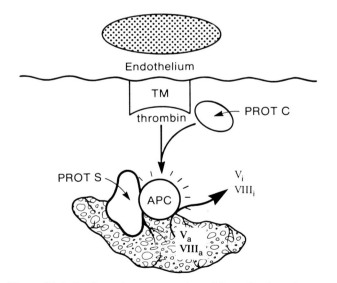

Figure 33.1 A schematic representation of the activation of protein C and its subsequent inhibition of factors VIIIa and Va. Protein S is shown as a cofactor enabling activated protein C to bind to the platelet surface. The symbols VIII_i, and V_i stand for inactivated factor VIII and factor V. TM is thrombomodulin.

ic abnormalities (APCR with protein C or S deficiency) may be at still higher risk for venous thrombosis during pregnancy.[34] This new information offers the possibility that a substantial number of patients with a true risk for venous thrombosis could be identified early in pregnancy allowing the selective application of prophylactic anticoagulant therapy. Even though APCR seems to be the most common predictor of thrombotic risk during pregnancy, some patients have had thrombosis-free pregnancies. Thus, further carefully designed, prospective clinical studies need to be performed for definition of the importance of other hemostatic abnormalities that could interact with APCR to produce clinically important thrombosis.

Antiphospholipid Autoantibodies

In 1952 Conley and Hartmen[35] reported that some patients with systemic lupus erythematous (SLE) had prolonged activated partial thromboplastin times (APPT) that were not corrected by the addition of normal plasma. Subsequently it was shown that this activity was due to the presence of an antibody.[36] The term "lupus anticoagulant" was introduced.[37] However, this label became inappropriate when similar abnormalities were noted in apparently normal individuals. Further studies have demonstrated that *lupus anticoagulants* are part of a large heterogeneous family of autoantibodies with apparent activity directed against phospholipids. Recent evidence suggests that the antigenic targets are not anionic phospholipids alone, but antigens that bind to phospholipid surfaces.[38] The best characterized antigens are β_2-glycoprotein I (β_2GPI) and several coagulation factors, including prothrombin, factor X, protein C, and protein S. The broader term, *antiphospholipid antibody syndrome,* was introduced to include patients who do not have SLE. Despite a prolonged PTT, there is usually no bleeding diathesis, but these antibodies have been associated with three important clinical conditions: thrombocytopenia, a thrombotic tendency involving either the arterial or venous circulation,[39–41] and recurrent fetal loss.[42,43]

The incidence of these antibodies in the general population is unknown, although they are more common in some ethnic groups.[44] The majority of the patients are women, and a familial association can often be demonstrated.[45] The presence of an antiphospholipid antibody is one of the more common abnormalities found in young patients with spontaneous thrombosis. Oral anticoagulants are effective in preventing recurrent thrombosis.[46] For the pregnant patient with a lupus anticoagulant, subcutaneous heparin therapy has been advocated[47] to prevent thrombosis and to improve fetal viability. When heparin is given in adequate intensity, the incidence of thrombosis is reduced but the benefit on fetal salvage has not been firmly established. Combination therapy with heparin, aspirin, and prednisone has been advocated to improve fetal viability. The true value of this strategy is currently uncer-

tain. Long-term, prospective studies of this difficult problem are under way.[48]

THERAPEUTIC OPTIONS

Heparin

Heparin is the drug of choice for management of thrombotic disorders during pregnancy.[49,50] Since it does not cross into the placenta, there is little direct risk to the fetus. The anticoagulant effect of heparin depends on interaction with plasma cofactors. Commercial or unfractionated (UF) heparin extracted from porcine intestinal mucosa or beef lung contains a mixture of heparin molecules that have varying molecular weights and different anticoagulant profiles. Many of the molecules do not interact with the plasma cofactors and, therefore, have little anticoagulant effect. When heparin forms a complex with the cofactor antithrombin III, the action of this natural inhibitor is accelerated, resulting in rapid neutralization of serine proteases generated in the coagulation cascade. Thrombin and activated factor X (X_a) are the most sensitive to the effect of heparin–antithrombin III complex. Heparin, at a higher concentration than usually used in treatment, also forms a complex with a second cofactor (heparin cofactor II), which inhibits thrombin but not X_a.

Animal studies have demonstrated that propagation of an experimentally induced venous thrombus is prevented by heparin, but a critical minimal concentration of 0.2 U/mL is required.[51] Based primarily on these studies, a therapeutic range for treatment of active venous thrombosis was defined (0.2–0.4 U/mL measured by protamine titration). When patients with venous thrombosis are given heparin in this concentration, the outcome is usually favorable.[52] Clinically, heparin concentration is estimated by prolongation of a clotting test, most commonly the activated partial thromboplastin time (APTT). However, in some situations, prolongation of the APTT may fail to accurately reflect the heparin concentration. Commercial partial thromboplastin reagents and different instruments have varying sensitivities to ex vivo samples obtained from heparin-treated patients.[53] Thus, measurement of heparin intensity by the APTT currently has the same limitations that plagued the prothrombin time before the introduction of the INR system. The result of the APTT is expressed in seconds, and a APTT ratio (subject APTT in seconds per subject baseline APTT in seconds). Commonly the patient's baseline sample (without heparin) is not available, and the mean value obtained from a population of nonpregnant control subjects is used. Normally, the APTT becomes short (to a variable degree) during pregnancy as a result of elevation of procoagulant clotting factors. Thus, for this reason alone, the reported APTT ratio may be misleading. Other conditions limit the value of the APTT for the measurement of heparin intensity. A patient with a lupus anticoagulant may have a prolonged APTT before heparin, and the addition of heparin further prolongs coagulation. Measurement of heparin concentration may require a more specific heparin assay such as the technically difficult protamine titration[50,52] or inhibition of exogenous activated factor X.[53,54] One of these specific assays should be performed whenever the interpretation of the APTT is difficult. Such tests are clearly mandated when heparin is administered to the patient with a lupus anticoagulant. In addition, periodic specific heparin assays are now recommended for all patients along with a APTT, to provide assurance that a given APTT is indicative of the desired therapeutic intensity.

Low Molecular Weight Heparin

In recent years, low molecular weight heparin (LMW heparin) or heparinoids have been prepared from UF heparin by enzymatic or chemical methods.[55] LMW heparin has now replaced UF heparin as the drug of choice for some clinical indications. Controlled trials have demonstrated effectiveness for the prophylaxis and treatment of active venous thrombosis.[56–59] The LMW anticoagulant profile differs from UF heparin[60] because the heparin molecule has a shorter chain length. LMW binds to antithrombin III and inhibits X_a but has relatively little effect on thrombin (II_a). Thus, the APTT is not a suitable assay for monitoring intensity for LMW heparin. The comparative properties of UF and LMW heparin are summarized in Table 33.4. In 1994 LMW heparin was advocated for management of venous thrombosis during pregnancy.[61,62] Like UF heparin, LMW heparin does not cross into the fetal circulation. The longer half-life of the LMW compound after subcutaneous injection might allow a single injection per day in low risk conditions, thus perhaps increasing acceptability by patients. However, no controlled clinical trials in pregnant subjects have been reported to show that only a single injection is effective. Nevertheless, when appropriate prospective studies are performed, LMW heparin will probably assume a dominant role for the treatment of venous thrombosis in pregnancy.

Oral Anticoagulants

The oral anticoagulants (coumarins or inandione derivatives) are vitamin K antagonists that interfere with posttranslational glutamic acid carboxylation of all vitamin-K-dependent proteins. Oral anticoagulants produce their anticoagulant effect by depression of prothrombin and factor X[63] but do not achieve this desired effect for several days (Table 33.5). Moreover, early depression of protein C may actually result in a prothrombotic stimulus. For the patient with active thrombosis, initial therapy without concomitant heparin[64] or premature discontinuance of heparin[65,66] before specific prothrombin becomes depressed is associated with poor therapeutic outcome. Warfarin, the drug most commonly employed in the United States, is effective for secondary prophylaxis in patients with venous thromboembolism and for cardiac patients with arrhythmias, valvular disease, or prosthetic heart valves. Large-scale studies have defined optimal intensities for patients with these indications.[67]

Oral anticoagulants cross the placenta and can adversely affect the fetus. There is clear documentation that exposure during the first 8–12 weeks of gestation is associated with a characteristic coumarin embryopathy consisting of nasal bone hypoplasia and chondrodysplasia punctata.[68] The mechanism of teratogenicity has been suggested by the description of an infant with congenital deficiency of multiple vitamin-K-dependent proteins who demonstrated characteristic "coumarin embryopathy"[69] without exposure to the drug. The authors speculated that the bleeding tendency and the fetal abnormalities were due to the observed abnormal carboxylation of vitamin-K-dependent proteins. By inference, coumarin embryopathy would be related to a pharmacologic effect of oral anticoagulants rather than to direct toxicity, and the risk would be greater with prolonged high intensity therapy.

TABLE 33.4   Comparison of Unfractionated (UF) and Low Molecular Weight (LMW) Heparin

Property	UF Heparin	LMW Heparin
Molecular weight	12,000–14,000	4000–6000
Anticoagulant action	Binds thrombin and X_a	Binds X_a
Bioavailability	30%	100%
Half-life after IV injection	45–60 min	2 h
Absorption from SQ injection	Variable	100%
Protamine		
In vitro	Good neutralization	Poor neutralization
In vivo	Good neutralization	Questionable effect
Incidence of thrombocytopenia	2.7%	0%
Monitoring test	APTT	X_a inhibition
Cost of drug	Inexpensive	Expensive
Need for monitoring	Yes	No (or infrequent)

TABLE 33.5   Vitamin-K-Dependent Proteins

Factor	Time to Depression by Oral Anticoagulants
Factor II (prothrombin)	30–80 h
Factor VII	3–5 h
Factor IX	24 h
Factor X	40 h
Protein C	3–5 h
Protein S	1–3 days

There is now general agreement that oral anticoagulants are contraindicated during the first trimester and at term because of the risk of fetal hemorrhage at delivery.[67,68] Nevertheless, because oral anticoagulants clearly reduce the thromboembolic potential for patients with mechanical heart valves, many clinicians have chosen warfarin over heparin for the intervening months. However, some data suggest that oral anticoagulants given at any time in pregnancy produce associated adverse effects, including fetal bleeding, spontaneous abortion, low birth weight, and central nervous system abnormalities.[70–75]

Most disturbing is the possibility of long-term effects that may not be apparent at birth. A single small retrospective study assessed long-term effects on children exposed to oral anticoagulants during pregnancy[76] compared to a control group of children not exposed to intrauterine warfarin. Low scores on neurological assessment and IQ tests were demonstrated. Overall, the incidence of abnormalities attributable to oral anticoagulants remains uncertain and controversial, with estimates ranging from 0 to 67%. Because of this uncertainty, oral anticoagulants should be avoided throughout pregnancy, **provided** alternate anticoagulant therapy achieves adequate protection of the mother from thrombosis.

Other Drugs

Low dose aspirin has been advocated to reduce the incidence of pregnancy-induced hypertension and appears to be safe.[77] Aspirin has also been used for two cardiac indications. Studies in nonpregnant populations with nonvalvular atrial fibrillation indicate that these regimens offer some benefit, but current information suggests that oral anticoagulants are more effective. Aspirin, given along with oral anticoagulants, has been recommended for prosthetic valve patients who have experienced thromboembolic complications despite optimal warfarin intensity.[78]

COMPLICATIONS OF ANTICOAGULANT THERAPY

The most important complication of anticoagulant therapy is bleeding. Like the risk of thrombosis, the risk of bleeding de-

pends on several interacting factors. Excessive intensity of therapy is important but is uncommon if the patient is carefully monitored by standard coagulation tests: the prothrombin time for warfarin, and the APTT for heparin. As noted above, the APTT may not accurately reflect heparin intensity, and a more specific test may be required (e.g., the X_a inhibition assay). Other conditions associated with bleeding, such as placenta previa and trauma due to accidents or assault, may complicate therapy in patients receiving anticoagulants.

Prolonged heparin therapy results in decreased bone density in some patients, but symptomatic osteoporosis or fractures are uncommon in the young pregnant woman.[79,80] The long-term effects have not been defined, but bone loss does not appear to continue after heparin is stopped. A potentially more serious complication of heparin is the appearance of an antibody that induces thrombocytopenia (heparin-induced thrombocytopenia, or HIT).[81] In some patients the HIT may be followed by a severe thrombotic syndrome (HITTS). If this complication develops, heparin must be stopped immediately, and when the indication for continued therapy is strong, an alternate anticoagulant drug must be chosen. Unfortunately, LMW heparin cannot be used because it often cross-reacts with the antibody. Warfarin, dextran, synthetic heparinoids,[82,83] or specific thrombin inhibitors[84] may be considered, depending on the individual clinical problem. The development of HIT might be expected in a small percentage of the patients on prolonged heparin therapy. However, this author has not seen reports of the HITTS in pregnant women. Monthly platelet counts could be helpful in detecting HIT, but interpretation of a fall in the platelet count may be difficult, since mild thrombocytopenia, of little consequence, is commonly seen during pregnancy.[85,86]

One rare complication of oral anticoagulant therapy deserves note. Warfarin-induced skin necrosis classically appears during the first few days of treatment. Typically, the patient develops an area of painful erythema of the skin, which rapidly progresses to hemorrhagic necrosis. Microscopic examination of the borders of such a lesion shows hemorrhage and venular thrombosis. The pathogenesis of the venular thrombosis is attributed to warfarin-induced depression of protein C or protein S, since patients with heterozygote deficiencies seem particularly sensitive to this complication.[87,88]

TREATMENT OF ACUTE VENOUS THROMBOSIS OR PULMONARY EMBOLISM

Once the diagnosis of venous thrombosis or pulmonary embolism has been reasonably established, intravenous heparin therapy is indicated. The most common approach is to administer an intravenous bolus dose of unfractionated heparin (usually 5000 units), followed by a continuous intravenous infusion. Monitoring of heparin intensity is obtained by measur-

TABLE 33.6   Adjusted-Dose Subcutaneous Heparin Therapy for High Risk Patients

Continue IV heparin for a minimum of 5 days.
Begin adjusted-dose subcutaneous heparin (ADSH) at 12-hour intervals.
Each ADSH dose is half the 24-hour dose required by IV therapy.
Overlap first ADSH dose with IV therapy.
Stop IV heparin; give second dose of ADSH.
Six hours later, obtain APTT (midinterval time).
Adjust ADSH dose to achieve targeted intensity.
Obtain specific heparin assay on this sample (X_a inhibition).
Monitor at 2-week intervals; adjust heparin dose; do platelet count monthly.
Follow at weekly intervals after 36 weeks.
Instruct patient to stop heparin at first sign of labor.
If epidural anesthesia is elected, check APTT to ensure no residual heparin.
After delivery, start IV heparin and begin oral anticoagulant therapy.
Monitor daily with prothrombin time and APTT; adjust doses appropriately.
Discharge on oral anticoagulant when INR is 2–3 (overlap for 4 days).

ing the APTT 4–6 hours later and adjusting the infusion dose to obtain a "therapeutic range." While the author advocates this method, two points of caution are worthy of consideration.

1. Bolus doses of heparin substantially larger than 5000 units produce a high plasma heparin concentration, and the clearance rate of heparin is reduced. When a APTT is obtained 3–4 hours later, the clotting time may still be prolonged from the large bolus injection. This first APTT often results in the mistaken conclusion that the infusion rate is excessive, whereupon the infusion dose of heparin is reduced. A APTT obtained several hours later may demonstrate inadequate prolongation as the heparin from the large bolus is cleared. If the initial bolus dose is limited to 5000 units, this potential error is usually avoided.

2. Treatment of active venous thrombosis with heparin is quite effective, provided a therapeutic concentration of heparin equivalent to 0.2–0.4 U/mL (defined by protamine titration or 0.35–0.67 U/mL by X_a inhibition) is rapidly achieved. Treatment failure and early recurrence of thrombosis have been convincingly linked to failure to obtain the targeted intensity during the first 24–48 hours of therapy.[89]

While measurement of heparin effect is usually assessed by measurement of the APTT, the clinician should remain aware that the APTT may not accurately reflect heparin intensity. No standardization of the APTT (similar to the INR system for the prothrombin time) has been accepted. Therefore, the APTT ratio that reflects a given heparin concentration cannot be precisely defined unless the laboratory compares the ex vivo APTT samples to a specific heparin assay, such as protamine titration or X_a inhibition.[54] While this procedure will define the relative sensitivity of the APTT system to the actual heparin concentration, individual patients may appear

either very resistant or, alternately, very sensitive to heparin (e.g., a lupus anticoagulant). Such patients require specific heparin assays to adequately determine heparin intensity.

Intravenous heparin should be continued for a minimum of 5 days. Secondary prophylaxis with adjusted dose subcutaneous heparin (ADSH) can then be initiated Table 33.6). Concentrated heparin (20,000 U/mL) and sharp small needles (disposable 1 mL insulin syringes) contribute to compliance. Some patients may develop painful areas of induration at injection sites. Changing the type of heparin (porcine to bovine) may provide some improvement, but if the problem persists, LMW heparin may be better tolerated. Our experience suggests that ADSH therapy at 12-hour intervals is well tolerated and provides effective heparin concentrations; but close follow-up is essential. The author believes that a knowledgeable and empathetic nurse plays an **indispensable** role for the optimal care of this patient population.

After delivery, heparin therapy should be continued while oral anticoagulants are introduced. Breast feeding is not contraindicated by the use of oral anticoagulant drugs.[90] The duration of secondary prophylaxis is usually 3–6 months for DVT or pulmonary embolism. This period should be extended for the patient found to have an underlying prethrombotic disorder.

PRIMARY PROPHYLAXIS FOR THE PATIENT AT PRESUMED INCREASED RISK OF VENOUS THROMBOSIS

For pregnant patients at presumed risk of thrombosis, assessment of the degree of risk should be made for each individual, since many patients will not require anticoagulant therapy. Surveillance with periodic impedance plethysmography or imaging ultrasound may be useful as an early warning of clinically important venous thrombosis in the lower extremities. Small subcutaneous doses of 5000 units at 8- to 12-hour intervals have been advocated for low risk patients. This author does not favor that approach, since such prophylactic therapy has been shown to be ineffective in patients at true risk for recurrent venous thrombosis.[91] However, higher subcutaneous "adjusted" doses of heparin provide protection equivalent to warfarin.[92] If the patient is determined to be at high risk as defined by the history, a recent thrombotic event, persistently abnormal results from a noninvasive test for venous obstruction, or a coagulation test abnormality (ATIII deficiency, APCR, lupus anticoagulant), full ADSH therapy is advised. Even with UF heparin, initial hospitalization is not required because it is not necessary to administer intravenous bolus doses. Monitoring of the ADSH intensity at midinterval time can be done in the outpatient clinic.

MANAGEMENT OF THE PATIENT WITH A PROSTHETIC HEART VALVE

The proper management of pregnant women implanted with prosthetic heart valves is the area of most significant controversy, reflecting concerns of oral anticoagulants on the fetus and the adequacy of heparin therapy in the prevention of thromboembolism in the mother (Chapter 6).

As noted above, the incidence of warfarin toxicity to the fetus has not been established. Clearly, there is some risk, particularly in the first trimester and at the time of delivery. The majority of physicians avoid warfarin during these two periods. However, there is significant controversy on the question of optimal therapy during the intervening months. Patients implanted with prosthetic valves of older design are at substantially higher risk of thrombosis than patients with "modern" prostheses.[7,93] Both groups have been treated "successfully" with oral anticoagulants during pregnancy, but at some cost in fetal morbidity and mortality. The question of whether heparin therapy would be "better" has yet to be resolved by prospective study. A comparative study of patients with prostheses of older design is progressively unlikely because of the decreasing number of women of childbearing age who have these valves. However, studies of patients with low risk modern prostheses could be designed. In 1989 a series of patients with modern prosthetic valves received treatment only with warfarin throughout pregnancy; no thrombotic events were reported, but there was a substantial rate of total fetal morbidity.[74] Fortunately, the authors reported the intensity of oral anticoagulant therapy, offering the possibility that their data could be used as a historical control for patients treated with heparin alone. Such a study should answer the question of whether heparin would be as protective as appropriately intense oral anticoagulants.

In the past, treatment with heparin has been reported to be inadequate and associated with serious thrombotic compli-

cations. Clearly, as could be predicted, subcutaneous heparin in a dose of 5000 units twice a day is inappropriate, and the clinical outcomes are disastrous.[72] Other studies also have cited thromboembolic events when heparin was employed, but the details of heparin therapy have usually not been provided. The primary concern with heparin in the treatment of any type of thrombosis is to administer the drug at an adequate intensity, which is usually defined by the APTT. As noted previously, different APTT reagents and different instruments often given conflicting results. Therefore, the sensitivity of the APTT system to be employed needs to be clearly defined,[54] a step often not provided by many clinical laboratories. For patients with prosthetic valves, particularly with the older more thrombogenic models, heparin intensity should be high, with a midinterval sample showing at least 0.3–0.4 U/mL as assessed by protamine titration or 0.55–0.8 anti-X_a U/mL. A lower intensity of 0.35–0.55 U/mL may provide adequate protection for patients with venous thrombosis. We now follow all our pregnant patients with the specific test along with a APTT and find that the APTT frequently fails to provide an accurate measure of the true heparin intensity. Previously, a APTT ratio of 1.5 was considered to reflect a therapeutic heparin concentration (obtained at midinterval time using ADSH as described earlier). We find that a ratio of 1.5 using our hospital APTT assay will not achieve even a low therapeutic intensity in 50% of patient ex vivo samples. However, a ratio of 2.0 or greater correlated with a high intensity heparin concentration (>0.55 X_a inhibition unit) in 90% of patient samples. These ratios apply to only one brand of APTT reagents and instrument. The appropriate APTT ratios will be different for other systems. However, the recommendation that the APTT ratio be at least 2–2.5 for patients with prosthetic valves is in agreement with a previously published study.[94]

High intensity heparin is mandated for the patient with a mechanical heart valve. If the appropriate therapeutic heparin intensity is achieved and close follow-up is assured, this author strongly advocates adjusted-dose subcutaneous heparin therapy throughout pregnancy. Women with prosthetic valves who desire children need to be advised prior to conception to discontinue oral anticoagulants and substitute ADSH. For the patient who becomes pregnant while still on oral anticoagulants, prompt change to heparin may decrease the risk of coumarin embryopathy. The problem of thrombosis with prosthetic heart valves should gradually decrease as the valves of newer design become less thrombogenic and our knowledge of how to administer and monitor anticoagulant therapy continues to mature.

CONCLUSION

Anticoagulants provide effective therapy for the prevention and treatment of thrombotic disorders encountered in pregnant women. While there are risks associated with anticoagulants, these can be minimized by the proper selection of patients for therapy and the application of individualized treatment plans appropriate for the underlying pathology. A favorable outcome requires close cooperation between the patient and the knowledgeable physician. In areas of remaining controversy, the author provides broad guidelines for therapy. Proper intensity of heparin therapy has been emphasized, since this appears to be the major problem in the interpretation of outcome in earlier studies. To date, we lack conclusive evidence of what constitutes optimal therapy for some patients. This can be obtained only from rigorous clinical trials. Thus, ultimate responsibility for therapeutic decisions still remains with the physician.

REFERENCES

1. Goldhaber S. Epidemiology of pulmonary embolism and deep vein thrombosis. In: Bloom AL, Forbes CD, Thomas DP, Tuddenhamm EGD, eds. *Haemostasis and Thrombosis.* 3rd ed. Edinburgh: Churchill Livingstone 1994;1327–1333.

2. De Sweit M, Fidler J, Howell R, Letsket E. In: *Advanced Medicine,* Tunbridge Wells: Pitman Medical; 1981:17;309.

3. McGehee W. Unpublished information.

4. Sachs BP, Brown DA, Driscoll SG, Shulman E, Acker D, Ransil BJ, Jewett JF. Maternal mortality in Massachusetts: trend and prevention. *N Engl J Med* 1987;316:667–672.

5. Mok CK, Boey J, Wang R, Chan TK, Cheung KL, Lee PK, Chow J, Ng RP, Tse TF. Warfarin vs dipyridamole–aspirin and pentoxylline–aspirin for the prevention of prosthetic heart thromboembolism: a prospective clinical trial. *Circulation* 1985;72:1059–1063.

6. Hirsh J, Dalen JE, Deykin D, Poller L. Oral anticoagulants: mechanism of action, clinical effectiveness and optimal therapeutic range. *Chest* 1992;102(suppl 4):312S–326S.

7. Cannegieter SC, Rosendaal FR, Wintzen AR, van der Meer FJ, Vandenbroucke JP, Briët E. Optimal oral anticoagulant therapy in patients with mechanical heart valves. *N Engl J Med* 1995;333:11–17.

8. Fihn SD. Aiming for safe anticoagulation. *N Engl J Med* 1995;333:54–55. Editorial.

9. Ginsberg JS, Hirsh J. Use of antithrombotic agents during pregnancy. *Chest* 1995;108(suppl 4):305S–310S.

10. The Boston Area Anticoagulation Trial for Atrial Fibrillation Investigators. The effect of low-dose warfarin on the risk of stroke in patients with nonrheumatic atrial fibrillation. *N Engl J Med* 1990;323:1505–1511.

11. Levine HJ, Pauker SG, Salzman EW, Eckman MH. Antithrombotic therapy in valvular heart disease. *Chest* 1992;102(suppl 4):434S–444S.

12. Todd M, Thompson J, Bowie E, Owen L. Changes in coagulation during pregnancy. *Mayo Clin Proc* 1965;40:370–383.

13. Bauer K, Rosenberg R. The pathophysiology of the prethrombotic state in humans: insights gained from studies using markers of the hemostatic system activation. *Blood* 1992;79:2039–2047.

14. Cadroy R, Grandjean H, Pichon J, Desprats R, Berrebi A, Fournie A, Boneu, B. Evaluation of six markers of hemostatic system in normal pregnancy and pregnancy complicated by hypertension or pre-eclampsia. *Br J Obstet Gynaecol* 1993;100(5):416–420.

15. Reinthaller A, Mursch-Edlmayr G, Tatra G. Thrombin–antithromnbin III complex levels in normal pregnancy with hypertensive disorders and after delivery. *Br J Obstet Gynaecol* 1990;97:506–510.

16. Bremme K, Ostlund E, Almqvist, Heinonen K, Blomback M. Enhanced thrombin generation and fibrinolytic activity in normal pregnancy and the puerperium. *Obstet Gynecol* 1992;80:132–137.

17. Hanson S, Griffin J, Harker L, Kelly A, Esmon C, Gruber A. Antithrombotic effects of thrombin-induced activation of endogenous protein C in primates. *J Clin Invest* 1993;92:2003–2012.

18. Hellgren M, Tengborn L, Abildgaard U. Pregnancy in women with antithrombin III deficiency: experience of treatment with heparin and antithrombin. *Gynecol Obstet Invest* 1982;14:127–414.

19. Leclerc JR, Geerts W, Panju A, Nguyen P, Hirsh J. Management of antithrombin III deficiency during pregnancy without administration of antithrombin III. *Thromb Res* 1986;41:567–573.

20. Rapaport SI. Blood coagulation and its alterations in hemorrhagic and thrombotic disorders. *West J Med* 1993;158:153–161.

21. Esmon CT. Protein C biochemistry, physiology and clinical implication. *Blood* 1983;62:1155.

22. Bertina RM, Broekmans AW, van der Linden IK, Mertens K. Protein C deficiency in a Dutch family with thrombotic disease. *Thromb Haemostasis* 1982;48:1–5.

23. Comp PC, Nixon RR, Cooper MR, Esmon CT. Familial protein S deficiency associated with recurrent thrombosis. *J Clin Invest* 1984;74:2082–2088.

24. Miletich J, Sherman L, Broze G. Absence of thrombosis in subjects with heterozygous protein C deficiency. *N Engl J Med* 1987;317:991–996.

25. Pabinger I, Kyrle P, Heistinger, Eichinger S, Wittmann E, Lechner K. The risk of thromboembolism in asymptomatic patients with protein C and S deficiency: a prospective cohort study. *Thromb Haemostasis* 1994;71:441–445.

26. Comp PC, Thurnau GR, Welsh J, Esmon CT. Functional and immunologic protein S levels are decreased in pregnancy. *Blood* 1986;68:881–885.

27. Dahlback B, Carlsson M, Svensson P. Familial thrombophilia due to a previously unrecognized mechanism characterized by poor anticoagulant response to activated protein C: prediction of a cofactor to activated protein C. *Proc Natl Acad Sci USA* 1993;90:1004–1008.

28. Bertina R, Koeleman B, Koster T, Rosendaal FR, Dizven RJ, de-Ronde H, van-der-Velden PA, Reitsma PH. Mutation in blood coagulation factor V associated with resistance to activated protein C. *Nature* 1994;369:64–67.

29. Dahlbäck B. Inherited thrombophilia: resistance to activated protein C as a pathogenic factor of venous thromboembolism. *Blood* 1995;85:607–614.

30. Greengard JS, Eichinger S, Griddin JH, Bauer KA. Variability of thrombois among homozygous siblings with resistance to activated protein C due to an Arg → Gln mutation in the gene for factor V. *N Engl J Med* 1994;331:1559–1562.

31. Hellgren M, Svensson P, Dahlback B. Resistance to activated protein C as a basis for venous thromboembolism associated with pregnancy and oral contraceptives. *Am J Obstet Gynecol* 1995;173:210–213.

32. Vandenbroucke J, Koster T, Briët E, Reitsma P, Bertina R, Rosendall F. Increased risk of venous thrombosis in oral-contraceptive users who are carriers of factor V Leiden mutation. *Lancet* 1994;344:1453–1457.

33. Bloomenkamp K, Rosendaal F, Helmerhost F, Buller H, Vandenbroucke J. Enhancement by factor V Leiden mutation of risk of deep-vein thrombosis associated with oral contraceptives containing third-generation progestogen. *Lancet* 1995;346:1593–1596.

34. Koeleman B, Reitsma P, Allaart C, Bertina R. Activated protein C resistance as an additional factor for thrombosis in protein C deficient families. *Blood* 1994;84:1031–1035.

35. Conley CL, Hartmenn RC. A hemorrhagic disorder caused by a circulating anticoagulant in patients with disseminated lupus erythematosus. *J Clin Invest* 1952;31:621–622.

36. Shapiro S, Thiagarajan P. Lupus anticoagulants. *Prog Hemostasis Thromb* 1982;6:263–285.

37. Feinstein D, Rapaport S. Acquired inhibitors of blood coagulation. *Prog Hemostasis Thromb* 1972;1:75.

38. Oosting J, Derksen R, Bobbink I, Hackeng T, Bouma B, de Groot P. Antiphospholipid antibodies directed against a combination of phospholipids with prothrombin, protein C or protein S: an explanation for their pathogenic mechanism? *Blood* 1993;81:2618–2625.

39. Boey M, Colaco C, Gharavi A, Elkon KB, Loizou S, Hughes GR. Thrombosis in systemic lupus erythematosus: striking association with the presence of a circulating lupus anticoagulant. *Br Med J* 1983;287:1021.

40. Mueh J, Herst K, Rapaport S. Thrombosis in patients with lupus anticoagulant. *Ann Intern Med* 1980;92:156.

41. Hart R, Miller V, Coull B, Bril V. Cerebral infarction association with lupus anticoagulants; preliminary report. *Stroke* 1984;15:114.

42. Gardlund B. The lupus inhibitor in thromboembolism and intrauterine death in the absence of systemic lupus. *Acta Med Scand* 1984;215:293.

43. Many A, Pauzner R, Carp H, Langevitz P, Martinowitz U. Treatment of patients with antiphospholipid antibodies during pregnancy. *Am J Reprod Immunol* 1992;28:216–218.

44. Stimmler M. Personal communication.

45. Exner T, Barber S, Kronemberg H, Rickard KA. Familial association of the lupus anticoagulant. *Br J Haematol* 1989;45:89.

46. Rosove M, Brewer P. Antiphospholipid thrombosis: clinical course after the first thrombotic episode in 70 patients. *Ann Intern Med* 1992;117:303–308.

47. Rosove M, Tabsh K, Wasserstrum N, Howard P, Hahn BH, Kalunian KC. Heparin therapy and prevention of pregnancy loss in women with lupus anticoagulant or anticardiolipin antibodies. *Obstet Gynecol* 1990;75:360.

48. Cowchock F, Reece E, Balaban D, Branch DW, Plouffe L. Repeated fetal losses associated with antiphospholipid antibodies: a collaborative randomized trial comparing prednisone with low-dose heparin treatment. *Am J Obstet Gynecol* 1992;166:1318–1322.

49. Hirsh J, Dalen J, Deykin D, Poller L. Heparin: mechanism of action, pharmacokinetics, dosing considerations, monitoring, efficacy and safety. *Chest* 1992;102(suppl 4):337S–351S.

50. Chiu MH, Hirsh J, Wung WL, Regoeczi E, Gent M. Relationship between the anticoagulant and antithrombotic effects of heparin in experimental venous thrombosis. *Blood* 1977;49:171–184.

51. Basu D, Gallus A, Hirsh J, Cade J. A prospective study of the value of monitoring heparin therapy with the activated partial thromboplastin time. *N Engl J Med* 1972;292:324–327.

52. Brill-Edwards P, Ginsberg JS, Johnson M, Hirsh J. Establishing a therapeutic range for heparin. *Ann Intern Med* 1993;119:104–109.

53. Levine M, Hirsh J, Gent M, Turpie A, Cruickshank M, Weitz J, Anderson D, Johnson M. A randomized trial comparing activated partial thromboplastin time with heparin assay in patients with acute venous thromboembolism requiring large daily doses of heparin. *Arch Intern Med* 1994;154:49–56.

54. van den Besselaar A, Meeuwisse-Braun J, Bertina R. Monitoring heparin therapy: relationship between the activated partial thromboplastin time and heparin assays based on ex-vivo heparin samples. *Thromb Haemostasis* 1990;63:16–23.

55. Hirsh J, Levine MN. Low molecular weight heparin. *Blood* 1992;79:1–17.

56. Hull R, Rascob GE, Pineo GF, Green D, Throwbridge AA, Elliott CG, Lerner RG, Hall J, Sparling T, Brettell HR, Norton J, Carter CJ, George R, Merli G, Ward J, Mayo W, Rosenbloom D, Brant R. Subcutaneous low-molecular weight heparin compared with continuous intravenous heparin in the treatment of proximal-vein thrombosis. *N Engl J Med* 1992;326:975–982.

57. Prandoni P, Lensing AW, Buller HR, Carta M, Cogo A, Vigo M, Casara D, Ruol A, ten-Cate JW. Comparison of subcutaneous low-molecular-weight heparin with intravenous standard heparin in the treatment of proximal-vein thrombosis. *Lancet* 1992;339:441–445.

58. Levine M, Gent M, Hirsh J, Leclerc J, Anderson D, Weitz J, Ginsberg J, Turpie AG, Demers C, Kovacs M, Geerts W, Kasis J, Desjardins L, Cusson J, Cruickshank M, Powers P, Brien W, Haley S, Willan A. A comparison of low-molecular-weight heparin administered primarily at home with unfractionated heparin administered in the hospital for proximal deep-vein thrombosis. *N Engl J Med* 1996;334:677–681.

59. Koopman M, Prandoni P, Piovella F, Ockelford P, Desiderius P, Brandjes M, et al. Treatment of venous thrombosis with intravenous unfractionated heparin administered in the hospital as compared with subcutaneous low-molecular-weight heparin administered at home. *N Engl J Med* 1996;334:682–687.

60. Barrowcliffe TW. Low molecular weight heparin(s). *Br J Haematol* 1995;90:1–7.

61. Rasmussen C, Wadt J, Jacobsen B. Thromboembolic prophylaxis with low molecular weight heparin during pregnancy. *Int J Gynaecol Obstet* 1994;47:121–125.

62. Nelson-Piercy C. Low molecular weight heparin for obstetric thromboprophylaxis. *Br J Obstet Gynaecol* 1994;101:6–8. Editorial comment.

63. Zivelin A, Rao V, Rapaport S. Mechanism of the anticoagulant effect of warfarin as evaluated in rabbits by selective depression of individual procoagulant vitamin K-dependent clotting factors. *J Clin Invest* 1993;92:2131–2140.

64. Brandjes D, Heijboer H, Buller H, de Rijk M, Jagt H, ten Cate J. Acenocoumarol and heparin compared with acenocoumarol alone in the initial treatment of proximal vein thrombosis. *N Engl J Med* 1992;327:1485–1489.

65. Wessler S, Gitel S. Warfarin: from bedside to bench. *N Engl J Med* 1984;311:645–652.

66. Hyers T, Hull R, Weg J. Antithrombotic therapy for venous thromboembolic disease. *Chest* 1992;102(suppl):409S–425S.

67. Hirsh J. Oral anticoagulant drugs. *N Engl J Med* 1991;324: 1865–1875.

68. Hall J, Pauli R, Wilson K. Maternal and fetal sequelae of anticoagulation during pregnancy. *Am J Med* 1980;68:122–140.

69. Pauli R, Lian J, Mosher D, Suttie J. Association of congenital deficiency of multiple vitamin K-dependent coagulation factors and the phenotype of the warfarin embryopathy: clues to the mechanism of teratogenicity of coumarin derivatives. *Am J Hum Genet* 1987;41:566–583.

70. Lutz D, Noller S, Spittell J, Danielson G, Fish C. Pregnancy and its complications following cardiac valve prostheses. *Am J Obstet Gynecol* 1988;131:460–466.

71. Stevenson R, Burton O, Ferianto G, Taylor H. Hazards of oral anticoagulants during pregnancy. *JAMA* 1980;243:1549–1551.

72. Iturbe-Alesio I, del Carmen Fonesca M, Mutchinik O, Santos M, Zajarias A, Salazar E. Risks of anticoagulant therapy in pregnant women with artificial heart vales. *N Engl J Med* 1986;314:1390–1393.

73. Salazar E, Zajarias A, Gutierrez N, Iturbe I. The problem of cardiac valve prostheses, anticoagulants and pregnancy. *Circulation* 1984;70(suppl 1):169–177.

74. Sareli P, England M, Berk M, Marcus R, Epstein M, Driscoll J, Meyer T, McIntyre J, Ven Geldern C. Maternal and fetal sequelae of anticoagulation during pregnancy in patients with mechanical heart valve prosthesis. *Am J Cardiol* 1989;63: 1462–1465.

75. Born D, Martinez E, Almeida A, Santos D, Carvahlo A, Moron A, Miyasaki C, Moraes S, Ambrose J. Pregnancy in patients with prosthetic heart valves: The effects of anticoagulation on mother, fetus and neonate. *Am Heart J* 1992;124:413–417.

76. Olthof E, De Vries TW, Touwen BC, Van der Veer E. Late neurological, cognitive and behavioral sequelae of prenatal exposure to coumarins: a pilot study. *Early Human Dev* 1994;38:97–109.

77. CLASP Collaborative Group. A randomized trial of low-dose aspirin for the prevention and treatment of preeclampsia among 9,364 pregnant women. *Lancet* 1994;343:619–629.

78. Stein R, Alpert J, Copeland J, Dalen J, Goldman S, Turpie A. Antithrombotic therapy in patients with mechanical and biological prosthetic heart valves. *Chest* 1992;102(suppl 4):445S–455S.

79. Deihlman T. Osteoporotic fractures and the recurrence of thromboembolism during pregnancy and the puerperium in 184 women undergoing thromboprophylaxis with heparin. *Am J Obstet Gynecol* 1993;168:1265–1270.

80. Barbour L, Kick S, Steiner J, LoVerde M, Heddleston L, Lear J, Baron A, Banton P. A prospective study of heparin-induced osteoporosis in pregnancy using bone densitometry. *Am J Obstet Gynecol* 1994;170:862–869.

81. King D, Kelton J. Heparin-associated thrombocytopenia. *Ann Intern Med* 1984;100:535.

82. Magani H. Heparin-induced thrombocytopenia (HIT); an overview of 230 patients treated with orgaron (Org 10172). *Thromb Haemostasis* 1993;70:554–561.

83. Greinacher A, Eckhardt T, Mussman J, Mueller-Eckhardt C. Pregnancy complicated by heparin associated thrombocytopenia: management by a prospectively in vitro selected heparinoid (Org 10172). *Thromb Res* 1993;71:123–126.

84. Matsuo T, Kario K, Chikahira Y, Nakao K, Yamada T. Treatment of heparin-induced thrombocytopenia by use of argatroban, a synthetic thrombin inhibitor. *Br J Haematol* 1992;82: 627–629.

85. Aster R. Gestational thrombocytopenia. A plea for conservative management. *N Engl J Med* 1990;323:264–266.

86. Ballem P. Diagnosis and management of thrombocytopenia in obstetric syndromes. In: *Obstetric Transfusion Practice.* 1993;49–76. American Association of Blood Banks.

87. Broeckmans AW, Bertina RM. Loeliger EA, Hofman V, Klingemann HG. Protein C and the development of skin necrosis during anticoagulant therapy. *Thromb Haemostasis* 1983;49:251.

88. Anderson D, Brill Edwards P, Walker I. Warfarin-induced skin necrosis in two patients with protein S deficiency; successful reinstatement of warfarin therapy. *Blood* 1989;74(suppl):409.

89. Hull R, Rascob G, Hirsh J, Jay R, Leclerc J, Geerts W, Rosenblum D, Sackett D, Anderson C, Harrison L, Gent M. Continuous intravenous heparin compared to intermittent subcutaneous heparin in the initial treatment of proximal-vein thrombosis. *N Engl J Med* 1986;315:1109–1114.

90. McKenna R, Cale E, Vasan U. Is warfarin sodium contraindicated in the lactating mother? *J Pediatr* 1983;103:325–327.

91. Hull T, Delmore T, Genton E, Hirsh J, Gent M, Sackett D, McLoughlin D, Armstrong P. Warfarin sodium versus low-dose heparin in the long-term treatment of venous thrombosis. *N Engl J Med* 1979;301:855–858.

92. Hull R, Delmore T, Carter C, Hirsh J, Genton E, Turpie G, McLaughlin D. Adjusted subcutaneous heparin versus warfarin sodium in the long-term management of venous thrombosis. *N Engl J Med* 1982;306:189–194.

93. Stein P, Alpert J, Copeland J, Dalen J, Goldman S, Turpie G. Antithrombotic therapy in patients with mechanical and biological prosthetic heart valves. *Chest* 1995;108(suppl 4):371S–379S.

94. Ginsberg J, Barron W. Pregnancy and prosthetic heart valves. *Lancet* 1994;344(8931):1170–1172.

34

DIGITALIS GLYCOSIDES IN PREGNANCY

IRVING STEINBERG, PHARMD, GLADYS MORIGUCHI MITANI, PHARMD,
EARL C. HARRISON, MD, AND URI ELKAYAM, MD

INTRODUCTION

Cardiac glycosides have been successfully used for acute and maintenance therapy of pregnant women with various cardiac disorders, with safety provided to the fetus.[1] Over the past 15 years, digitalis compounds, particularly digoxin, have been administered maternally as therapy for fetal tachyarrhythmias.[2] Thus, a thorough knowledge of digitalis preparations and their usage in pregnancy is pertinent. Before turning to the specifics of cardiac glycosides in pregnancy, a brief general review of these drugs is presented.

CLINICAL PHARMACOLOGY OF CARDIAC GLYCOSIDES

Digitalis glycosides are steroidlike compounds that produce positive inotropic effects on cardiac muscle and specific electrophysiologic effects on the conduction system. The mechanism for the positive inotropic effect is incompletely understood, but current evidence supports the concept that the cardiac glycosides increase the availability of calcium to the contractile elements during excitation/contraction coupling.[3] This action may be related to digitalis-induced, Na^+/K^+-activated ATPase inhibition in the cardiac myocyte,[4] although a positive inotropic effect without inhibiting the Na^+/K^+ pump has also been reported with therapeutic concentrations of the digitalis glycoside strophanthidin.[5] Cardiac glycosides bind avidly to the α subunit of this enzyme, which then disturbs the extracellular–intracellular electrolyte balance. The resul-

tant increase in intracellular sodium serves to enhance intracellular calcium movement (or decreased calcium extrusion), leading to enhanced contractile force.[3] Hydrogen exchange for sodium and calcium may promote further inotropic effect. Augmentation of vagal tone may also be important in the antiarrhythmic effects of digitalis. The clinically important antiarrhythmic properties of digitalis preparations result from electrophysiologic effects primarily on the atria and the atrioventricular (AV) node. Digitalis increases the refractoriness of the AV node and junctional tissue, slowing conduction, thereby controlling the ventricular rate in response to the rapid atrial rates in atrial flutter/fibrillation and supraventricular tachycardia. This effect is produced primarily by increased vagal tone, with direct effects only at high therapeutic concentrations. Enhanced vagal and sympathetic stimulus (e.g., thyrotoxicosis, fever, severe heart failure, agonist drugs) dampen digitalis control of atrial arrhythmias.[3] Digitalis may also suppress ectopic atrial pacemakers and alter propagation through reentrant pathways in the atrium.[6] Digitalis can enhance antegrade conduction through AV bypass tracts, adversely increasing ventricular response in Wolff–Parkinson–White syndrome, promoting the risk of ventricular fibrillation.

Only four of the numerous plant-derived cardiac glycoside compounds known to exist are commonly used today: digoxin, digitoxin, ouabain, and deslanoside. These pure glycoside preparations have largely replaced digitalis leaf, allowing for more accurate standardization of the active drug contents. Differences in the route of administration and the onset and duration of action often determine which preparation is used for specific clinical situations.[3]

Cardiac Problems in Pregnancy, Third Edition
Edited by Uri Elkayam, MD, and Norbert Gleicher, MD
Copyright © 1998 by Wiley-Liss, Inc. ISBN 0-471-16358-9

Digoxin

Digoxin is the most widely used digitalis preparation. Its popularity is due mainly to its intermediate duration of action and its availability in both oral and parenteral dosage forms.[7] Oral absorption of digoxin occurs primarily from the proximal small intestine. Patients with normal gastrointestinal function absorb approximately 60–75% from the tablet form, approximately 85% from the elixir, and 90–100% from the available encapsulated gel preparation.[3,7,8] Concomitant administration of cholestyramine or nonabsorbable antacids may impair the gastrointestinal absorption of digoxin. Furthermore, absorption may be diminished and erratic in patients with malabsorption syndromes. Intramuscular administration serves no advantage because it triggers the local release of muscle enzymes, and pain. Approximately 20–30% of digoxin is plasma protein bound, but because of its extensive tissue binding and high apparent volume of distribution, plasma protein binding changes are unlikely to be clinically important.

The average elimination half-life of digoxin is approximately 40 hours in adult patients with normal renal function. Excretion is primarily via the kidneys, with 60–80% excreted unchanged in the urine. Although digoxin clearance and elimination half-life have correlated well with glomerular filtration,[9] renal tubular secretion is an additional important pathway.[10] This route may be based on an ATP energy-dependent transporting P-glycoprotein expressed in renal tubular cells.[11] Quinidine and verapamil interfere with this P-glycoprotein-mediated tubular secretion, leading to increased digoxin levels when these drugs are added to therapy.[12] Biliary excretion may make up as much as 35% of digoxin clearance, and this biliary/hepatic pathway can be induced. About one-third of the body stores are lost daily in patients with normal renal function.

The average digitalizing dose is 0.5–1.0 mg (20–40 μg/kg) intravenously or 0.75–1.5 mg orally, with both routes of administration given in two to four divided doses 6–8 hours apart. The usual oral maintenance doses range between 0.125 and 0.5 mg daily. If no loading dose is given, steady state equilibrium on daily maintenance doses will be reached in approximately 5–7 days in patients with normal renal function.[7,13] Maintenance doses are adjusted according to digoxin serum levels, individual patient response, and other factors altering requirements. Usual maintenance doses must be decreased in patients with diminished renal function, and steady state conditions may take more than 2 weeks to be achieved. Concomitant administration of quinidine, amiodarone, propofenone, verapamil, or flecainide (in descending order of magnitude) may significantly increase plasma digoxin concentrations.[14]

The onset of action of digoxin occurs 15–30 minutes after intravenous administration, with peak effects reached within 1–5 hours. After oral administration, the onset of action occurs between 0.5 and 2 hours, with peak effects occurring within 6–8 hours. Since the drug adheres to a two-compartment model with a defined distribution phase, determination of therapeutic plasma concentrations should be performed at least 6–8 hours after the dose, when distribution is expected to be complete. This level corresponds to the pharmacodynamically active concentration at the myocardial effector site. Plasma concentration monitoring efficiency was emphasized in a large laboratory network review in which 24% of levels exceeding 2 ng/mL were drawn less than 6 hours after the prior dose (45% among "nonstat" outpatient assays).[15] Accepted therapeutic concentrations in adults range between 0.5 and 2.0 ng/mL.

Digitoxin

Digitoxin is the principal active ingredient in digitalis leaf and therefore has comparable pharmacokinetics. The gastrointestinal absorption following oral administration of digitoxin is 90–100% complete. Approximately 97% of the drug in plasma is bound to albumin.[16] Digitoxin is characterized by its long elimination half-life of 5–7 days; however, there is considerable interpatient variation. The drug undergoes extensive metabolism, presumably in the liver, with minor amounts of digoxin resulting as one of the cardioactive metabolites; variable degrees of enterohepatic recycling occur among patients. Some digitoxin and its metabolites are also excreted in the urine and in the feces via the bile. Because the primary excretory pathway is via the liver, the half-life of digitoxin varies little with changing renal function. This pathway is accelerated, however, by hepatic enzyme inducers. Nonhepatic routes of elimination may also increase in patients with liver disease.[17] The average digitalizing dose is 1.0 mg intravenously or 0.7–1.2 mg orally; both routes are given in two or three divided doses 4–6 hours apart. The usual oral maintenance dose is 0.1 mg daily (range of 0.05–0.3 mg/day). Steady state is reached in approximately 3–4 weeks when therapy is initiated without a loading dose. The onset of action occurs between 25 minutes to 2 hours following intravenous administration, and peak effects are reached within 4–12 hours. After oral administration, the onset of action occurs in 0.5–2 hours, with peak effects in 4–12 hours. If therapeutic plasma concentrations are to be evaluated, blood samples should be drawn no earlier than 6 hours after the dose. Therapeutic concentrations are in the range of 10–35 ng/mL.

Ouabain and Deslanoside

Ouabain and deslanoside are both poorly absorbed from the gastrointestinal tract and are available only for parenteral use. Ouabain has an onset of action within 20 minutes after intravenous administration and may be useful when rapid onset of action is required.[17] Its half-life averages 21 hours, and excretion is primarily via the kidneys, although gastrointestinal excretion can also be substantial.[17,18] Deslanoside is structurally very similar to digoxin. Its onset of action is somewhat more rapid than digoxin, but its half-life is essentially identical. Therefore, it enjoys no substantial advantage over parenteral use of digoxin. If a rapid onset of action is essential, ouabain is preferable to deslanoside.

Toxicity of Cardiac Glycosides

Unfortunately, toxicity due to digitalis preparations remains an important clinical problem. Laboratory surveys demonstrated 6.7% of 280,00 digoxin assays were in the toxic range exceeding 2 ng/mL.[15] In a prospective study, Beller et al,[19] using electrocardiographic criteria, found that 22% of digitalized hospital patients were definitely toxic and 6% were possibly toxic. It was hoped that the availability of an assay for the measurement of serum digitalis concentrations would substantially reduce this incidence of toxicity. It is now clear, however, that individual differences in sensitivity to cardiac glycosides give rise to significant overlap between toxic and nontoxic serum levels.[9]

Predisposing factors to toxicity include hypoxia, pulmonary disease, acid–base disorders, renal insufficiency, certain types and levels of severity of heart disease, concomitant drug administration (e.g., diuretics, anesthetics, calcium channel blockers, β-adrenergic blockers, amiodarone, quinidine), and serum electrolyte disorders (e.g. hypokalemia, hyperkalemia, hypomagnesemia, hypercalcemia, hyponatremia). The extracardiac signs include anorexia, nausea and vomiting, headache, fatigue, malaise, and visual disturbances such as scotomas, halos, and changes in color perception. Other neurologic symptoms, including confusion and disorientation, may also occur. Cardiotoxic signs include virtually every known rhythm disturbance. Some common arrhythmias seen with toxicity include premature ventricular complexes, ventricular tachycardia, atrial tachycardia with AV nodal block, AV junctional tachycardia, sinus arrest, first-degree block, Mobitz type I second-degree AV nodal block, and third-degree AV nodal block. Unfortunately, extracardiac toxic manifestions cannot be used reliably as premonitory signs and symptoms of impending cardiac rhythm disturbances. Cardiac toxicity may precede, or occur in the absence of, extracardiac signs.

Treatment of toxicity most importantly requires recognition of the problem and withdrawal of digitalis therapy. Potassium should be given when hypokalemia is present, but caution should be exercised in its administration because hyperkalemia may further impair AV nodal conduction. Phenytoin, lidocaine, and propranolol are often recommended to treat ectopic tachyarrhythmias due to digitalis toxicity. Occasionally, electrical cardioversion[20] or pacemaker insertion may be required. Repeated oral doses of charcoal may decrease absorption, cut off enterohepatic recirculation, and enhance nonrenal elimination of digitalis preparations.[21] Commercial digoxin-specific Fab antibody fragments (e.g., Digibind®) are available, and with careful monitoring and interpreation of follow-up levels, digoxin can be used in cases of serious toxicity and/or severely elevated blood levels.[22]

DIGITALIS GLYCOSIDES AND PREGNANCY

Digitalis preparations have been prescribed during pregnancy for many years, and digoxin remains a first-line agent in the management of cardiac arrhythmias during pregnancy.[1] Clinical experience developed over the years suggests that the use of these agents in pregnancy is relatively safe, especially considering the detrimental consequences to the mother and fetus if treatment is withheld.

Since pregnancy is associated with marked physiologic and hemodynamic changes in the maternal circulation, alterations in the pharmacodynamics and pharmacokinetics of digitalis preparations are expected. Despite the expanding number of reports and clinical studies published, clear dosing guidelines for the use of digitalis in pregnancy in maternal and fetal treatment, and the proper interpretation of plasma concentrations, are still needed. Questions remain with respect to the increasing number of reports of a digoxin-like immunoreactive substance (DLIS) that interferes with many of the commercially available digoxin radioimmunoassay kits. False-positive digoxin concentrations have been detected in the amniotic fluids and sera of pregnant women and newborn infants not exposed to digitalis.[23,24]

This section reviews studies on the pharmacokinetics of digitalis preparations in animals and humans. In addition, a review of the DLIS is included because of the significant impact it may have in interpreting the results of studies done prior to knowledge of its existence. This recent finding also brings attention to the need for proper and careful interpretation of serum digoxin concentrations in the pregnant patient population.

Animal Pharmacokinetic Studies

Before the availability of radioactive digitalis and the radioimmunoassay for measurement of serum and tissue digoxin concentrations, a placental barrier to the passage of digitalis to the fetus was thought to exist. Okita et al[25] demonstrated that digitoxin crosses the placenta of pregnant guinea pigs and that 22% of the dose appears in the fetus within an hour. The same investigators found that only 0.65% of the dose appears in rat fetuses an hour after digitoxin is given, thus demonstrating marked species difference in the placental passage of digitoxin. In three out of four guinea pigs, tissue-bound digitoxin and its metabolites were detected in the fetal heart; in one guinea pig, only the metabolite was detected. On a tissue-weight basis, higher concentrations of digitoxin were found in the fetal heart than in the maternal heart.[25] Fouron[26] studied dogs, whose metabolism of digoxin is known to be similar to that of humans.[27] They found that transplacental passage of digoxin occurred almost immediately, but fetal concentrations were lower than maternal concentrations until equilibrium was reached, at least 4 days after maternal digitalization. Significant concentrations of digoxin were also found in the amniotic fluid.[26] Hernandez et al[28] and Singh et al[29] demonstrated rapid placental passage of digoxin in pregnant ewes. A longer half-life of digoxin in the fetal serum was found than in the maternal serum following a single bolus dose of tritiated digoxin. After chronic dosing, the fetal, maternal, and amniotic fluid concentrations were essentially similar; however, the tissue binding of digoxin in all fetal lamb tissues was significantly less than that which occurred in maternal tissues. The fetomaternal tissue concentration ratio of digoxin was found to be 0.25.[28]

Human Pharmacokinetic Studies of Digoxin

Several studies have reported alterations in digoxin pharmacokinetics during pregnancy. In women receiving oral digoxin (0.25 mg daily) for rheumatic heart disease throughout their last trimester of pregnancy, Rogers et al[30] observed that average maternal serum concentrations measured 5–7 hours after the last dose increased significantly 1 month postpartum (1.1 ± 0.2 ng/mL) compared with concentrations observed at term (0.6 ± 0.1 ng/mL). This change may be due to a 50% decrease in absorption antepartum or a 50% drop in total body clearance of digoxin postpartum. The findings of Rogers et al, however, were not in agreement with a subsequent study of 15 women receiving maintenance digoxin who were studied during the third trimester and again 6–16 weeks postpartum. Luxford and Kellaway[31] observed higher digoxin renal clearance and 24-hour urine elimination of digoxin during the third trimester compared to the postpartum values. However, in 12 of 15 women, higher serum digoxin concentrations were observed during the third trimester than during the postpartum period. Increased drug bioavailability during pregnancy was suggested as an explanation for higher serum digoxin concentrations during the third trimester, while markedly reduced gastric emptying during labor was thought to be responsible for the reduction in serum digoxin concentrations at delivery.[31] Yet, these higher third-trimester levels may not suggest reduced digoxin clearance but, rather, increasing radioimmunoassay interference by digoxin-like immunoreactive substance produced increasingly through the third trimester (see further discussion on DLIS below). Many studies that have evaluated digoxin levels with respect to dose in pregnant patients have reported single-point measurements, often non–steady state, and measured after oral dosing at various stages of pregnancy, in which the influences of decreased bioavailability and/or augmented clearance cannot reliably be discriminated (see later discussion on treatment of the fetus with digoxin and table 34.1).

A more definitive description of the pharmacokinetics of digoxin was performed as part of a fetal tachyarrhythmia treatment study.[32] Six serum samples were drawn from each of 6 women (22–33.5 weeks of gestation) after an initial intravenous digoxin dose of 0.5–1 mg. Nonlinear least-squares fitting was accomplished with a two-compartment model, and any interference of digoxin-like immunoreactive substance was assessed prior to drug administration. Kinetic parameters were the following: volume of distribution = 5.7 ± 3.0 L/kg, clearance = 4.71 ± 1.99 mL/min/kg (range 1.92–7.74), half-life = 20.4 ± 12.3 hours. These parameters reflect enhanced clearance and faster half-life beyond that seen in nonpregnant subjects and indicate that the added weight of pregnancy does not represent mass that will bind digoxin beyond that observed in nongravid populations. This study using intravenous drug administration furthers the findings of Rogers et al[30] and demonstrates that the pharmacokinetic changes for digoxin in pregnancy are related primarily to increases in clearance.

Digoxin-like Immunoreactive Substance

Recent publications have established the presence of an endogenous digoxin-like immunoreactive substance (DLIS) that interferes with many of the commercially available digoxin radioimmunoassay (RIA) and fluorescence polarization immunoassay (FPIA) kits.[23,24] Apparent digoxin concentrations have been reported in sera from several patient populations not exposed to digitalis therapy. These false positive results came from women in the second and third trimesters, with and without preeclampsia,[33–35] as well as from amniotic fluid, meconium, fetal and cord blood,[36,37] serum and urine of premature and term newborns,[38–40] and sera from nonpregnant patients with hypertension,[41] renal diseases,[41,42] and liver disease.[43,44] The nature and potential biologic activity of this substance have been the subject of intense scientific scrutiny over the past decade.[45] Substances with structural similarities to digoxin (e.g., digoxin metabolites, progesterones, estrogens, cortisol, androgen precursors, spironolactone, bile salts) have been noted to cross-react with digoxin measurements using the commercial RIA and FPIA kits.[45–49] Pooled steroids have also been shown to positively react with the radioimmunoassay of digoxin, and physiologic conditions that may increase steroidogenesis could also be implicated.[24] DLIS may exhibit biologic activity, analogous to endogenous digitalis-like factors (EDLFs). However, the assumption of naturetic and vasoactive biologic activity of all DLIS compounds has been a limiting factor in the search for steroid as well as nonsteroid chemicals and peptides that are EDLFs.[45] Assays for such biologic activity of EDLFs include Na^+/K^+-ATPase inhibition and erythrocyte ^{86}Rb-uptake inhibition, and competition for cellular [^3H]oubain binding. These functional assays have shown correlation[50,51] and discordance[52,53] of DLIS with EDLF.

In pregnant women not receiving digoxin, Seccombe et al[54] detected stable DLIS concentrations in the amniotic fluid between 16 and 33 weeks of gestation, but noted an increase from 33 weeks to term. Graves et al[55] documented the presence of DLIS in the blood (range of 0.1–0.6 ng/mL of digoxin equivalents) of third-trimester pregnant women which became undetectable 24 hours postpartum. This would suggest that the DLIS of maternal origin in normal pregnancy disappears with a rapid half-life postpartum. DLIS concentrations appear to increase as gestation progresses and have been shown to be higher in preeclamptic women.[33,56] Gusdon et al,[33] who referred to the DLIS as "naturetic hormone," observed higher concentrations in preeclamptic women compared to women in the third trimester of normal pregnancy (whose levels were equal to nonpregnant controls). Additionally, Polish investigators found higher concentrations of DLIS in third-trimester pregnant women with preeclampsia (0.57 ± 0.23 vs. 0.22 ± 0.20 for normotensive) and observed a mild and scattered correlation between DLIS and a clinical scoring system assessing the severity of preeclampsia (including systolic and diastolic blood pressure, proteinuria, and edema).[35] The same authors also noted that therapy with the antihypertensive agent nitrendipine was most effective in decreasing DLIS levels, consistent with the results of others who found decreases in DLIS using nifedipine or ritodrine as tocolytic therapy.[57] Importantly, the cord and newborn levels of DLIS exceeded the maternal values in the hypertensive and normotensive groups.

Other investigators have challenged the foregoing results. Levels of DLIS were measured every 2 weeks during the third trimester in 170 women, 20 of whom developed hypertension.[34] Both normotensive and hypertensive groups showed a similar rise in DLIS levels, and there was no significant difference in these levels at each 2-week interval (although the mean levels of 0.23 and 0.17 ng/mL, respectively, were slightly less than observed in other studies). Further delineation of the impact of pregnancy-induced hypertension on DLIS levels was reported recently.[53] Nondiabetic women with preeclampsia had higher levels than their normotensive counterparts (0.35 vs. 0.22 ng/mL). Those with transient hypertension of pregnancy (without proteinuria) had intermediate values (mean = 0.28 ng/mL), and the values correlated with the diastolic blood pressure. Mirroring this pattern of results was the measurement of Na^+/K^+-ATPase inhibition. Normotensive pregnant patients with insulin-dependent diabetes mellitus (IDDM) showed DLIS and EDLF than the nondiabetic normotensive group (0.31 vs 0.22 ng/mL). However, there was no statistical increase in DLIS or EDLF in the IDDM patients with PIH or preeclampsia, triggering speculation of mechanistic differences, and possibly explaining earlier studies citing no differences between normotensive and hypertensive pregnant patients, if the populations investigated included diabetic patients. Additionally, despite similar patterns of increase for each clinical grouping, there was no correlation between DLIS and EDLF,[53] further supporting the position that other chemical entities are responsible for endogenous digitalis-like effects.

The origin of DLIS is of chemical, biologic, and clinical importance. It has been recognized through numerous studies that the levels of DLIS are at their highest in the infant and mother in the immediate perinatal period. Valdes et al[56,58] reported the presence of false positive digoxin concentrations equivalent to digoxin concentrations in the range of 0.1–1.4 ng/mL in newborn infants. In another study of 24 premature or full-term newborns not exposed to digoxin, DLIS was detected in all 24 infants in concentrations ranging from 0.6 to 5.3 ng/mL, with the highest DLIS concentrations noted in premature infants. Toronto investigators found much higher cord and maternal blood DLIS levels (average within the digoxin therapeutic range) from 31 high risk pregnancies compared with 41 uneventful ones.[59] The levels in the normal risk pregnancy in the newborns were higher than the maternal values, but the reverse was true of the high risk maternal–fetal pairs. The authors speculate that in acute maternal illness, the mother produces additional DLIS (i.e., beyond that manufactured by the fetoplacental unit), and the highly scattered and mild correlation between the cord and maternal levels in the high risk pregnancies supports this. Others contend that the source of DLIS is predominantly from the placenta or fetus. A study of fetal blood sampling at 28 ± 6 weeks demonstrated 71% of fetuses with measurable DLIS versus 34% of the women ($n = 38$). Samples at delivery showed 98% of the cord blood and 22% of the women's blood with measured DLIS ($n = 45$), and the cord blood contained higher DLIS than the fetus or mother.[37] Again, only a mild correlation ($r = 0.30$, $p < 0.05$) was noted between fetal and maternal DLIS concentrations, with no difference between full-term and preterm conceptus values. Furthermore, DLIS values of 0.4–1.6 ng/mL were measured at or before delivery in fetuses displaying cardiac pathology but without exposure to maternal digoxin, and with no maternal detection of DLIS. In contrast is the work of Schlebusch et al,[60] who found lower DLIS interference in samples from mothers and fetuses treated with digoxin for fetal tachyarrhythmias, compared with samples from those with no digoxin exposure. It may be that DLIS and digoxin bind differentially to the hydropic placenta. Fetal DLIS, with physiologic Na^+/K^+-ATPase inhibition, was evidenced in highest tissue values in the gut and adrenals and may be expressed in higher levels in stressed newborns in the perinatal period.[50,51] Finally, a single perfused placental lobule model continued to release

DLIS into the fetal side perfusate.[61] Infusion of Digibind® caused a drop in perfusion pressure and vasodilatation, illustrating the role that placental DLIS may play in fetal vascular smooth muscle tone.

There is obvious biologic impact of DLIS in fluid and electrolyte maintenance in the pregnant woman and the newborn.[45,62,63] The impact of DLIS on the therapeutic drug monitoring of digoxin in maternal and fetal therapy needs further evaluation. The pharmacokinetic parameter estimates of digoxin in mothers and newborns obviously are affected by an added "background noise" level. The assessment of response and toxicity pharmacodynamics to this drug associated with achieved levels is muddied by DLIS and the variability of assay performance.[59,63] It is incumbent on the clinician using digoxin levels to assist in monitoring maternal and fetal digoxin therapy to check with the institution's laboratory, to confirm the assay being used and its propensity to measure false positive digoxin concentrations. Efforts to reduce or eliminate DLIS via sample centrifugation and ultrafiltration,[40,60,64] sulfosalicylic acid,[65] and newer automated immunoassay techniques[64,66] should assist the clinician in monitoring the pharmacodynamic response to digoxin of the individual pregnant patient and newborn, providing, as well, further definition of the effect–concentration relationship for these patient populations.

Adverse Effects in Pregnancy

Despite the transplacental passage of digitalis, remarkably few adverse effects on the fetus have been demonstrated. Fouron[26] found digitalis effects on fetal electrocardiograms 3 hours after toxic dosages were administered to pregnant dogs. Potondi[67] reported a case of digitalis overdosage in a pregnant woman whose subsequent miscarriage was attributed to digitalis poisoning. Sherman and Locke[68] also reported a case of maternal digitalis toxicity associated with electrocardiographic changes in the newborn and subsequent death of the infant, presumably secondary to the effects of intrauterine anoxia.

Concern has been raised that digitalis may play a role in low birth weights observed occasionally in infants of mothers with heart disease. It is postulated that digitalis, by binding in the placenta, might alter the placental transport of amino acids to the fetus.[69] Another possible explanation for low birth weight may be related to an observation of Weaver and Pearson,[70] who showed that women on digitalis had earlier onset of spontaneous labor. Lower birth weights were noted in infants of these mothers. After adjusting for gestational age, the authors concluded that the weight differences were due to relative prematurity and not to growth retardation. They attributed the early onset and shorter duration of labor in digitalized patients to a direct effect of digitalis on myometrium.

Despite these isolated reports, in a large series of pregnant patients, no demonstrable clinical or electrocardiographic adverse effects were demonstrated in fetuses of mothers who consumed digitalis preparations during pregnancy.[1] This may in part be due to early gestation effects of relatively low binding of digitalis in fetal tissues, relative resistance of the fetal heart to digitalis effects, and incomplete transplacental passage.[29,71,72] This line of thought is reinforced by the overall lack of adverse clinical electrophysiologic sequelae when digoxin has been used for treatment of fetal supraventricular tachycardia and atrial flutter. Digoxin is in pregnancy risk category C of the U.S. Food and Drug Administration.

Digoxin and Breast Feeding

Digoxin is substantially released into human breast milk. Chan et al[73] obtained breast milk samples between 3 and 7 days postpartum from women taking maintenance digoxin doses. The breast milk concentrations averaged 0.64 ng/mL and were in a 0.59 ratio of the corresponding maternal blood concentrations. However, Levy et al[74] observed a closer-to-unity ratio of concentrations of digoxin in the breast milk and maternal plasma. In a woman ingesting large maintenance doses of digoxin (0.75 mg/day), Finley et al[75] found digoxin concentrations of 1.9 ng/mL in breast milk, 2.1 ng/mL in the corresponding maternal serum, and 0.2 ng/mL in the infant's serum at 7 days. In another study, digoxin was not detected in the plasmas of two nursing infants whose mothers were each taking digoxin 0.25 mg daily. The milk/plasma ratios were 0.9 and 0.8 in the first and second mother, respectively. Peak milk concentrations taken 4–6 hours after the dose were 0.96 and 0.61 ng/mL, respectively; the time-averaged concentration (using area under the concentration–time curve) were 0.78 and 0.41 ng/mL, respectively. The amount of digoxin ingested by these infants per day was estimated to be less than 0.01 of a recommended daily maintenance dose of 12.5 μg/kg/day.[76] The author suggested that digoxin could be safely taken by lactating mothers. Digoxin is also listed as one of the drugs compatible with breast feeding by the American Academy of Pediatrics.[77] However, it is prudent to always closely monitor a nursing infant for possible adverse effects.

Reinhardt et al[78] used a two-compartment model to describe the kinetics of digoxin in milk in 11 women. Following a 0.5 mg intravenous dose, rapid equilibrium, within 10–30 minutes, between maternal plasma and milk was noted. The concentrations in maternal plasma and milk declined exponentially in parallel. The ratio ranged narrowly between 0.57 and 0.67 (mean = 0.62) with no differences between foremilk and hindmilk or between intravenous and oral forms of maternal administration. Assuming a long neonatal half-life, steady state conditions, and a maternal dose of 0.5 mg/day, only 3% of therapeutic levels would be expected in the nursing infant. Therefore, breast milk from a mother who is receiving digoxin can be assumed to be safe for the nursing infant, with regular follow-up by the pediatrician.

PLACENTAL TRANSFER OF CARDIAC GLYCOSIDES

Digoxin

Digoxin appears to cross the placenta readily. Seven women were administered radioactive (tritiated) digoxin intravenously immediately before terminating pregnancy at 15–22 weeks of gestation. [^{3}H]Digoxin activity was detected in the umbilical cord within 5 minutes, and within 30 minutes fetal plasma concentrations were similar to the maternal values.[79] Fetal tissue distribution revealed the highest measured digoxin concentrations in the heart of five of the seven fetuses (second highest in the other two), with a near six-fold range per gram. The total placental digoxin exceeded any organ value by approximately 8- to 50-fold, demonstrating enhanced binding to this tissue. Digoxin was also detected in the amniotic fluid, but the concentrations were lower than from the umbilical and maternal venous samples. In another study, two 0.5 mg doses of digoxin were administered orally to 12 healthy patients 24 and 2–6 hours prior to therapeutic abortion at 12–16 weeks of gestation. In contrast to the results of Saarkoski et al,[79] measurable concentrations of digoxin could not be detected in the fetal kidney, heart, liver, skeletal muscle, and amniotic fluid; but concentrations of 5.8 ng/g wet weight were detected in the placenta, suggesting a high affinity of the placenta for digoxin binding.[80] Chan et al[73] demonstrated almost perfect correlation between placenta and maternal plasma digoxin concentrations, but an average 78-fold higher placental concentration; these values might also have been inflated by measured digoxin-like immunoreactive substance. Padeletti et al[81] noted delay in maternal–fetal equilibrium, reporting that three-quarters of cases took more than 3 hours (from maternal administration to delivery) to achieve concentration unity; delivery less than 100 minutes after digoxin administration did not produce unity. The delay in equilibrium between the two circulations was tentatively attributed to tissue and plasma protein binding of digoxin in both mother and fetus.

Further delineation of fetoplacental transport was evaluated using the single perfused human placental lobule model. Lobules from harvested healthy placentas are perfused on the maternal and fetal sides with [^{3}H]digoxin administered on the maternal side, and serial samples drawn from both sides to attempt to mimic the in vivo situation. Over a 3-hour timed experiment, Derewlany et al[82] showed measured digoxin on the fetal side at 5 minutes and transport rate equilibrium at 30 minutes; however, unity of concentrations was projected to occur only after 4 hours. The fetoplacental-to-maternal ratio was 0.36, with binding of digoxin to perfused (3.4-fold higher than maternal-side levels) and nonperfused placental tissue accounting for the remainder. This model supports the observations of Padelleti et al[81] and demonstrates avid placental binding, though not to the extent observed by Chan et al.[73]

Recently, German investigators utilized this isolated perfused placental model to demonstrate the potential impact of augmented maternal and fetal albumin concentrations on the magnitude of fetoplacental digoxin concentrations.[82a] The data suggest that higher maternal protein content reduces the fetoplacental transfer of digoxin. In another study, these investigators showed that the magnitude of digoxin transplacental transfer was also tied to the integrity of the placental perfusion.[82b] "Well-perfused" placentas showed larger fetomaternal digoxin concentration ratio than the "malperfused" placentas (mean ratio: 0.44 versus 0.30, $p < 0.05$), while the accumulation of digoxin in placental tissue showed the opposite trend. Antipyrine clearance (a flow-limited, freely diffusable, standard chemical marker of in-vitro placental passage[82c]) was used to assess placental perfusion, and the fetomaternal digoxin ratio correlated closely with the antipyrine clearance.

Serum concentrations in the cord blood at delivery were reported to be similar to the maternal serum concentrations in women receiving oral digoxin maintenance treatment.[30,83] However, Chan et al[73] observed fetal cord samples that were approximately 50% of the corresponding maternal concentrations in women receiving long-term oral therapy. Lower fetal cord concentrations compared to the maternal serum were also observed by Allonen et al[80] and were supported for short-term exposure by the data of Derewlany et al.[82] Extensive data on ratios of fetal and cord blood to maternal blood and factors influencing maternal–fetal passage of digoxin are described in studies of fetal tachyarrhythmia treatment.

Ouabain

Saarikoski[84] demonstrated rapid transplacental passage of [^{3}H]ouabain in pregnant women during the second trimester of pregnancy. The time to equilibrium between the maternal and fetal circulations was over 2 hours. The concentrations of ouabain in the fetal heart were found to be three to ten times that of fetal plasma. Thus, an uptake mechanism for ouabain in the fetal heart apparently exists by the second trimester of pregnancy. High concentrations of [^{3}H]ouabain were found in the placenta compared to the maternal and fetal values, implying a slow rate of placental transfer or a placental uptake mechanism for ouabain. Low concentrations of ouabain were also found in the amniotic fluid. Bergmans et al[85] used 0.125 mg of intravenous ouabain every 3 hours for treatment of fetal supraventricular tachycardia without success; no maternal or cord blood levels were reported.

Digitoxin

Although very little information is available regarding the use of digitoxin in pregnancy, one study demonstrated placental transfer and fetal distribution as well as evidence suggesting fetal metabolism. Okita et al[71] studied three women who terminated their pregnancies at 11–12 weeks of gestation and one woman who carried an anencephalic fetus to term. At delivery 1.7–5 hours after intravenous administration of radioactive digitoxin, less than 1% of the dose was detected in the fetuses as unchanged drug and less than 3.5% as the metabolites. In the fetus near term, concentrations of unchanged drug in the liver, gallbladder, and intestine approached the concentrations in the heart and kidneys. Concentrations of the metabolites were noted to be higher than concentrations of unchanged drug in all the tissues. Concentrations of both unchanged digitoxin and its metabolites were lower in the tissues of the fetus near term than in the fetuses at 11–12 weeks of gestation. Fetal metabolism of digitoxin was suggested by the high concentration ratios of metabolite to digitoxin observed in the liver tissues. In addition, there was evidence of biliary excretion of both unchanged and metabolized drug.

Treatment of the Fetus with Digoxin

Increased diagnostic efficiency using fetal echocardiography has promoted advanced applications of pharmacotherapy to the management of fetal arrhythmias. These techniques have realized as high as 80% success in cardioversion of fetal supraventricular tachycardia, and slightly less for atrial flutter. Management strategies have commonly instituted maternal drug administration to obtain adequate transplacental passage and fetal circulatory concentrations of effective antiarrhythmics, helping to avoid potential fetal morbidity and mortality, and to delay otherwise unavoidable early delivery. The physiochemical features of the antiarrhythmics in clinical use differ, suggesting a wide range of fetoplacental uptake. During the past 15 years, digoxin has become a mainstay in the treatment of fetal arrhythmias via maternal and direct administration (Table 34.1)[32,83,86–103b]; it is the routine drug of first choice.[103c] Additionally, digoxin has been used for its cardiotonic effects to treat fetal cardiac failure/hydrops fetalis in the absence of tachyarrhythmias.[104–106b]

Since digoxin is not ionized at blood pH (therefore no "ion trapping") and does not have known carrier- or energy-dependent transfer (i.e., no facilitated or active transport), transplacental passage of digoxin is suggested to be influenced primarily by passive diffusion. This suggestion leads to a prediction of an approximate 1:1 ratio between fetal/cord and maternal digoxin levels after maternal exposure.[30] However, this ratio has not been consistently observed in cases in which the fetus has been treated with digoxin for atrial arrhythmias, particularly when this drug has been used unsuccessfully to treat supraventricular tachycardia (Tables 34.1 and 34.2).[2,107,108] Nonimmune fetal hydrops and cardiac failure, either preceding or resulting from arrhythmia, constitute the suspected cause of incomplete passage of digoxin. The edema seen in the hydropic placenta and fetus thickens the passive diffusion barrier and reduces the transport of digoxin, contributing to a ratio of fetal/cord to maternal digoxin level lower than that found in the nonhydropic fetus. The resulting subtherapeutic fetal digoxin level represents a major factor in the more limited success of digoxin in treating supraventricular tachycardia and atrial flutter in hydropic versus nonhydropic fetuses.

Little information exists on the pharmacokinetics of digoxin in the fetus. In one case of fetal supraventricular tachycardia, Weiner and Thompson[100] first administered several drugs, including digoxin, to the mother. After a low fetal/maternal concentration ratio was demonstrated, with failure to control the arrhythmia, the fetus received a direct intramuscular injection of digoxin, with a subsequent maintenance schedule of repeated fetal administration after heart rate control. The initial schedule, based on neonatal digoxin pharmacokinetic parameters, was inadequate to provide therapeutic levels and sustained response. Two postloading dose levels obtained by cordocentesis revealed a half-life of 15.3 hours (much shorter than observed postnatally) and an enormous 97.8 L/kg volume of distribution. These parameters suggest extensive placental binding, as illustrated by the results of Saarkoski[79] and Chan et al[73] during maternal administration. The authors indicate that this shorter than expected half-life may make direct therapy impractical for prolonged rhythm control.

Data regarding fetal/cord-to-maternal concentration ratios (Table 34.1) must be interpreted with care, particularly for single-point evaluations. The time of the last dose until concentration sampling at delivery varies among studies. The length of therapy from diagnosis to delivery may have an impact on digoxin levels (particularly when given orally) as equilibration is more likely the longer the maternal course of therapy.[82] Fetal sampling during gestation may reflect differences in fetoplacental transfer compared to cord sampling at delivery; this is related to normal thinning of the placenta with advancing gestational age, and the increased surface area will promote passive diffusion of digoxin. Resolution of hydrops during therapy may increase the fetal/cord–maternal concentration ratio and can conceivably provide at delivery fetoplacental transfer data different from results seen when fetal sampling is performed earlier (Fig. 34.1).[109] Amniotic fluid samples reveal levels two- to three-fold higher than the simultaneously obtained cord blood or umbilical vein concentrations and may exceed the concomitant maternal level; this likely reflects the accumulation of digoxin in the amnion after fetal excretion.[104,109a] Finally, digoxin-like immunoreactive substance may interfere with the assay technique, altering the levels and ratios measured; this tendency has been accounted for in more recent studies.[32,110]

TABLE 34.1 Fetal Arrhythmia treatment with Digoxin: Maternal Cord-Fetal Concentrations Documented

Ref: First Author (year)	Arrhythmia	Hydrops/ Heart Failure	Gestational Age (weeks)	Dose (mg) Loading	Dose (mg) Maintenance	Maternal/ Cord-Fetal Concentration (ng/mL)	Success
Newburger[86] (1979)	SVT	Yes	36	"standard doses"		0.7/0.6	No
	SVT	No	≈35	"standard doses"		0.6/0.65	No
Kerenyi[87] (1980)	SVT	Yes	32	ND	0.25 q 6 h PO × 8	2.7/0.7	Partial
					0.25 q 12 h PO × 3		
Lingman[87] (1980)	Tach	Yes	29	0.25 IV × 2	0.25 q day PO	1.6/1.0	Yes
Harrigan[89] (1981)	SVT	Yes	26	1.5 PO in 14 h	0.25 q day PO	0.8/0.7	Yes
Belhassen[90] (1982)	AFi/WPW	No	32	ND	0.25 q 8 h PO	1.6/1.6	No
Dumesic[83] (1982)	SVT	Yes	30	ND	0.25 q 12 h PO	0.8/—	No
					0.25 q 8 h PO	1.3/—	No
					0.25 q 12 h PO	0.8/0.8	No
Allan[91] (1984)	AFl	No	34	ND	0.25 q 8 h PO	1.2/0.8	Yes
Given[92] (1984)	Atrial tach	Yes	24	1.25 PO in 16 h	0.25 q 8 h PO	1.6/0.7	Yes with procainamide
Spinnato[93] (1984)	AFl	No	33	1.5 IV in 36 h	0.25 q 12 h PO	1.2/— after LD	No at 36 h
					0.375 q day PO	1.0/0.3	Yes with quinidine
	SVT	Yes	30	0.25 PO × 2	0.5 q day PO	1.0/—	No
						2.2/— after quinidine	Yes with quinidine
	SVT	Yes	27	1.5 IV in 24 h	0.375 q day PO	1.6/0.8	Yes with quinidine
					0.5 q day PO	1.9/—	No
					0.25 q day PO	1.5/1.3 after quinidine	Yes with quinidine
King[94] (1984)	SVT	Yes	26	ND	0.125 q day PO	3.6/0.4	Rate yes, hydrops no
Nagashima[95] (1986)	AFl	Yes	30	ND	0.5 q day PO	1.0/0.62	No
	AFl	No	41	ND	0.5 q day IV	1.2/1.3	?[b]
	SVT	Yes	31	ND	0.25 q 12 h IV	1.02/—	↓ HR
					0.25 q 12 h PO	—/—	Recurrence
					0.25 q 12 h IV	1.29/—	Yes (↓ HR, ↓ hydrops; maternal toxicity)
Wiggins[96] (1986)	SVT	Yes	24	0.75–1.0 IV in 24 h	0.25 q day PO	0.30/0.36	Yes
	SVT	No	24	0.75–1.0 IV in 24 h	0.375 q day PO	0.9/0.8	Yes
Repke[97] (1986)	SVT	No	37	0.25 q 6 h PO × 4 days	0.375 q day PO	0.9/0.8	Yes
				0.25 q 3 h PO × 4 days		0.6/—	No
Mimura[97] (1987)	AF	Yes	34	ND	0.5 q day PO	1.5/0.7	No
						1.0/0.64	No
Younis[91] (1987)	SVT	Yes	ND	1.25 PO	0.425–0.5 q day PO	1.1/0.3	No

(continued)

427

TABLE 34.1 (*Continued*)

Ref: First Author (year)	Arrhythmia	Hydrops/ Heart Failure	Gestational Age (weeks)	Dose (mg) Loading	Dose (mg) Maintenance	Maternal/ Cord-Fetal Concentration (ng/mL)	Success
Weiner[100] (1988)	SVT	No	24	1.0 IV in 18 h	0.5 q day PO	0.9/—	No
				0.5 IV	0.5 q 12 h PO	1.3/—	No
				q 12 h × 2 days	0.5 q 8 h PO	1.8/0.8 (fetal)	No
					0.5 q day PO	0.7/0.9 (fetal)	No
				fetal 0.025 IM × 1			Transient
				fetal 0.070 IM in 24 h		—/1.51, 1.1	Transient
				fetal 0.200 IM in 24 h		—/1.2	Yes
				fetal 0.080 IM q 12 h			Yes
Hallak[101] (1991)	SVT	Yes	25	2.0 IV in 24 h		0.9/—	No
				fetal 0.02 IM in 24 h			partial
				1.5–2.25 PO/q day		2.5/0.5 (fetal)	Partial with hydrops
						2.3/1/1	Yes, no hydrops
Kofinas[102] (1991)	SVT	Yes	31	ND	ND	2.1/0.9	Yes with flecainide
Azancot-Benisty[32] (1992)	SVT	No	37	ND	ND	1.8/0.9	Yes
	SVT	Yes	31	ND	ND	0.8/0.6	No
	SVT	Yes	32	ND	ND	0.6/0.8	No, yes with amiodarone
	AFl	Yes	30	ND	ND	1.3/1.4	No, yes with amiodarone
	AFl	Yes	36	ND	ND	1.8/1.4	No
	SVT	Yes	25	ND[b]	ND[b]	1.6/1.2	Yes
	SVT	Yes	33	ND[b]	ND[b]	1.0/0.8	Yes
	SVT	Yes	22	ND[b]	ND[b]	1.2/1.5	Yes
	SVT	Yes	33.5	ND[b]	ND[b]	1.9/1.2	Yes
Battiste[103] (1992)	SVT	Yes	17	1.0 IV in 12 h	0.25 q 12 h PO	2.9/—	No
						1.4/0.6	Yes with Procainamide
Mozas[103a] (1995)	SVT	Yes	29	2 in 24 h PO	0.25 q in 12 h PO	0.94/1.1**	Yes
Kohl[103b] (1995)	SVT	Yes	23	1.2 IV	ND but given IV	—/—	Partial for 5 weeks with flecainide
						1.5/0.33	Yes, after adenosine

**level obtained 24 h postnatal.
[a]Second treatment before, and immediately after delivery.
[b]Maternal dose was 1–2 mg/day.

Abbreviations and symbols: AFi, atrial fibrillation; AFl, atrial flutter; HR, heart rate; IM, intramuscular; IV, intravenous; ND, none/not documented; PO, oral; SVT, supraventricular tachycardia; WPW, Wolff–Parkinson–White syndrome; ↑, increase; ↓, decrease.

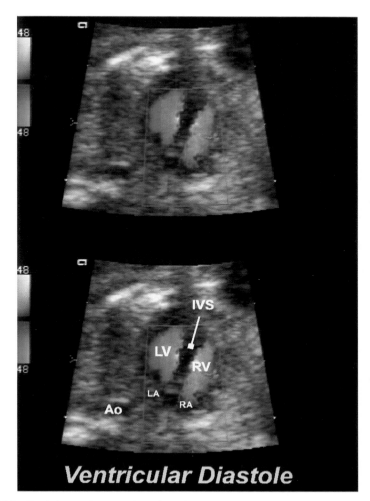

Figure 47.20 Real-time color Doppler of the four-chamber view during ventricular diastole; red represents the flow of blood into the ventricular chambers. The color enhances the identification of the interventricular septum (IVS). Ao, aorta; RV, right ventricle; LV, left ventricle; RA, right atrium; LA, left atrium.

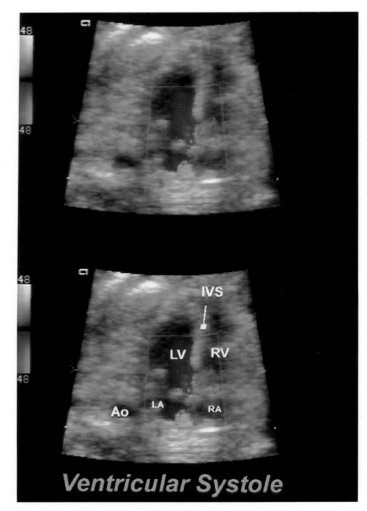

Figure 47.21 Real-time color Doppler of the four-chamber view during ventricular systole; blue represents the flow of blood along the interventricular septum of the left ventricle. In the normal heart, blood is not observed along the right interventricular septum during systole. Ao, aorta; RV, right ventricle; LV, left ventricle; RA, right atrium; LA, left atrium; IVS, interventricular septum.

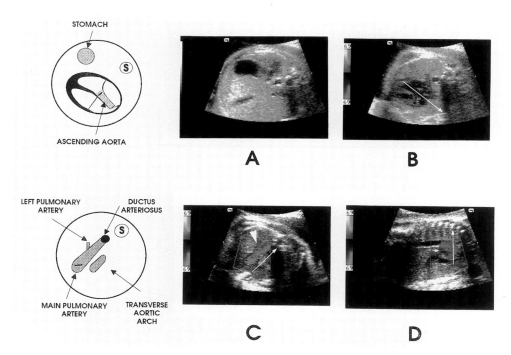

Figure 47.22 Identification of the outflow tracts. Upper schematic: the four-chamber view, with the left side of the fetus proximal to the ultrasound beam and the spine (S) at the 2 o'clock position. (*A*) Position of the fetal stomach within the left side of the abdomen. (*B*) By directing the transducer beam cephalad to the four-chamber view, the origin of the ascending aorta (small arrow) can be identified as it exits the left ventricle. Lower schematic: the orientation of the outflow tracts identified by di - recting the transducer beam in a transverse plane through the chest further cephalad to the four-chamber view. (*D*) The vessels identified are perpendicular to the ascending aorta; they include the main pulmonary artery, branching of the left pulmonary artery (arrowhead), ductus arteriosus, and transverse aortic arch (arrow). (*E*) Image of the aortic arch obtained in a left sagittal plane; arrow identifies the direction of the ascending aorta in which the transverse aortic arch is imaged perpendicular to this plane. (From DeVore.[117])

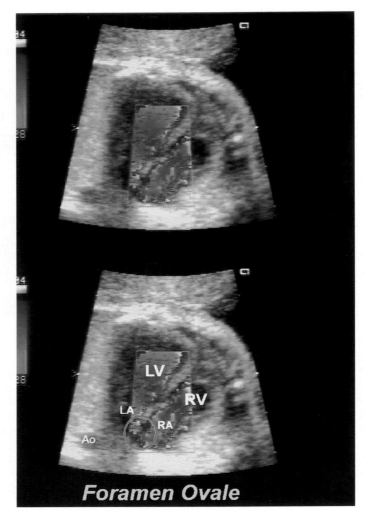

Figure 47.23 Color Doppler examination of the foramen ovale; red circle represents the flow of blood through the foramen ovale. In this image, the baseline of the color velocity was moved to the top of the velocity bar so that only one color is present in the image. This view makes it easy to see where blood is flowing but does not accurately indicate velocity. This technique is important for viewing areas of low flow, such as the foramen ovale, and for removing the aliasing effect observed in low flow states.

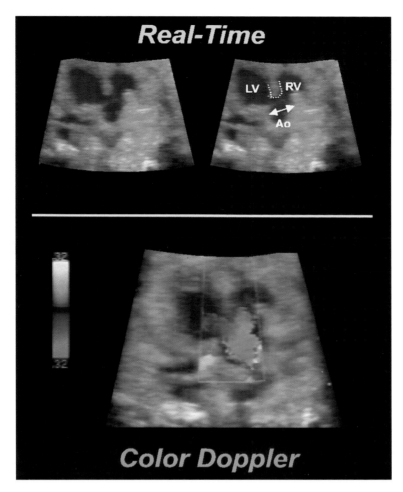

Figure 47.24 Tetralogy of Fallot. The real-time images illustrate the ventricular septal defect (dotted line), overriding the aorta. The color Doppler illustrates flow along both the right and left interventricular septum, exiting the aorta. LV, left ventricle; RV, right ventricle.

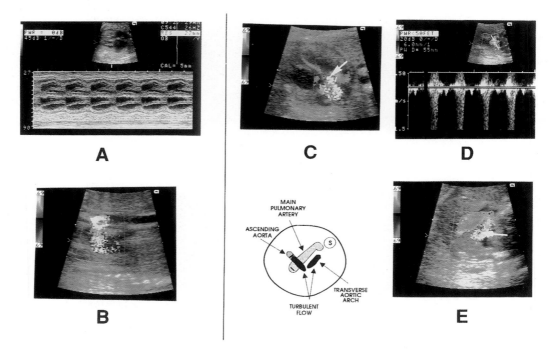

Figure 47.25 Aortic stenosis. (*A*) M-mode recording from the four-chamber view, which demonstrates normal ventricular wall contractility, with no evidence of ventricular disproportion. (*B*) The aortic arch demonstrates disturbed flow in the ascending aorta. (*C*) Blood exiting the left ventricle. The disturbed flow can be observed to originate at the aortic valve (arrow). (*D*) Pulsed Doppler of the aortic outflow tract, demonstrating increased flow across the valve. (*E*) Transverse plane in which disturbed flow is observed in the transverse aortic arch. (From DeVore.[117])

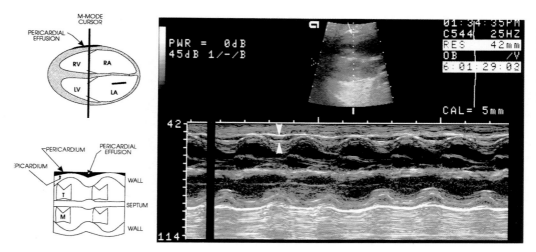

Figure 47.27 Schematic illustrates the four-chamber view from which the M-mode recording is obtained; ultrasound recording demonstrates the separation of the pericardium and the epicardium (arrowheads).

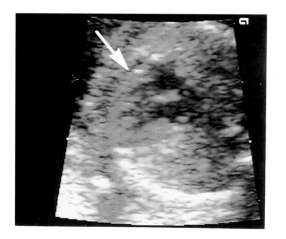
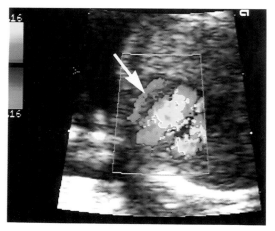
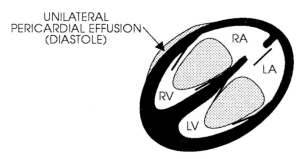

Figure 47.28 Pericardial effusion identified with real-time and color Doppler ultrasound in a 17-week fetus. The real-time image suggests separation of the pericardium from the epicardium (white arrow) along the right ventricular wall. The color Doppler image illustrates the pericardial space to be filled with color Doppler (red) (white arrow) with aliasing observed within the ventricles during diastole. RV, right ventricle; RA, right atrium; LV, left ventricle; LA, left atrium. (From DeVore and Horenstein.[121])

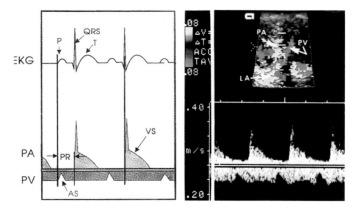

Figure 47.33 Schematic compares an electrocardiogram with the pulsed Doppler waveforms recorded from the pulmonary artery (PA) and pulmonary vein (PV) from the lung parenchyma. The real-time Doppler color image demonstrates a pulmonary vein entering the left atrium (LA) and a branch of the pulmonary artery within the lung. The left side of the fetus is at the top of the image. P, P wave of the atrial depolarization; QRS and T, electrical depolarization and repolarization of the ventricle; A, atrial systole recorded from the pulmonary veins; VS, ventricular systole recorded from the pulmonary artery; PR, interval from the onset of atrial systole to the onset of ventricular systole. (*B*) Color and pulsed Doppler recording from the lung parenchyma. (From DeVore and Horenstein.[121])

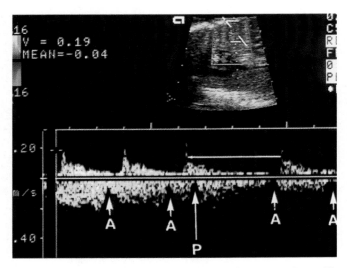

Figure 47.34 Color and pulsed Doppler recording from the lung parenchyma illustrating normal atrial contractions (A) interrupted by a premature atrial contraction (P) that is not conducted to the ventricles. This results in prolongation of ventricular systole (solid white line). (From DeVore and Horenstein.[121])

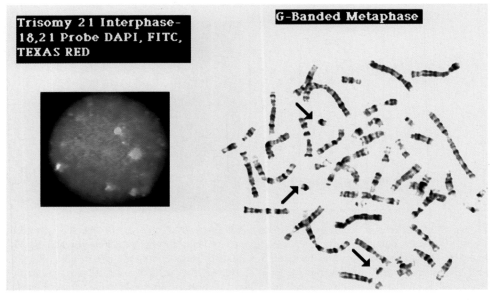

Figure 49.1 Interphase FISH analysis using probes for chromosomes 21 and 18 reveals three green (for chromonsome 21) and two red (for chromosome 18) signals (left half of the picture). This is compatible with trisomy 21 which is shown on the right half of the picture (G-banded metaphase).

TABLE 34.2   Management Success[a] in Three Studies of Fetal Arrhythmias Using Three Digoxin Regimens

Presence of Heart Failure/Hydrops	Primary Treatment		Secondary Treatment: Digoxin + Others
	Digoxin Alone	Digoxin + Verapamil	
Ito et al[2] (1994)[b]			
Yes	18/46	10/13	20/26
SVT	16/37	5/7	16/19
AFl	2/9	5/6	4/7
No	21/33	3/3	4/6
SVT	13/22	1/1	3/4
AFl	8/11	2/2	1/2
Van Engelen et al[107] (1994)[c]			
Yes	1/10		7/7
No	10/14		1/2
Gembruch et al[108] (1993)[d]			
Yes	1/9	3/7[e]	6/6
No	7/9	1/1[e]	
Frohn-Mulder et al[115b] (1995)[f]			
Yes	1/6		0/5[g]
			3/7[g,h]
No	12/22		4/4[h,i]

[a]Treatment data given as successful cardioversions/patients.
[b]Cumulated data compiled from case reports and series.
[c]Response to each regimen for specific arrhythmias not itemized; rhythm control for 88% of SVT and 66% for AFl.
[d]Only SVT among 18 fetuses studied.
[e]Verapamil used as secondary therapy after digoxin failure.
[f]35/50 patients treated; 14/50 with atrial flutter, response not itemized.
[g]Alternative treatment without digoxin.
[h]Flecainide alone.
[i]Following digoxin failure.

Abbreviations: AFl, atrial flutter; SVT, supraventricular tachycardia.

Based on the early encouraging data suggesting unity fetoplacental passage, Klein et al[111] first attempted maternal digitalization to convert supraventricular tachycardia in a fetus at 28 weeks of gestation. Despite assertive intravenous loading and oral maintenance regimens (resulting in maternal toxicity), the heart rate and hydrops did not resolve. Postnatal electrocardiogram was consistent with a Wolff–Parkinson–White pattern. No maternal or fetal/cord digoxin levels were reported. Newberger and Keane[86] gave "standard doses" of digoxin to cardiovert supraventricular tachycardia in two near-term fetuses. Short-term treatment provided no apparent success; unity transplacental passage was observed, but with low levels of 0.6–0.7 ng/mL.

The first published successes of this treatment approach followed soon after, with slightly more aggressive digoxin dosing and resultant levels of 0.7–1.0 ng/mL.[87–89] Important findings were realized from these attempts, all in preterm fetuses with some degree of heart failure or hydrops documented. Kerenyi et al[87] demonstrated only a partial response and noted the lack of unity in fetal/maternal digoxin concentration ratio (26%). Lingman et al[88] sustained lasting conversion in a fetus with a heart rate exceeding 300 beats per minute and obtained this response only one day after an intravenous loading dose of digoxin. Harrigan et al[89] observed abrupt rate conversion shortly after completion of 1.5 mg of digoxin over 14 hours. A normal heart rate was sustained, but fetal ascites and scalp edema took 19 days to resolve, with a cord blood level of 0.7 ng/mL at delivery.

The initial successes just described fostered larger series and retrospective and prospective studies to determine more precisely the rate of success with this approach and the clinical predictors of response, as well as modifications to digoxin therapy, to achieve a more reliable and long-lasting response. These alterations include more aggressive digitalizing doses

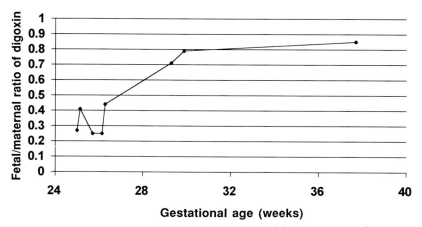

Figure 34.1 Fetal-to-maternal ratios of digoxin in a case of fetal hydrops and supraventricular tachycardia treated initially with maternal digoxin. With persistence of symptoms at 27 weeks gestation, addition of direct umbilical cord injections of amiodarone resolved the symptoms and increased the transplacental passage of digoxin. (Modified from Gembruch et al, *Am J Cardiol* 1989;118:1335.)

to the mother, fetal digoxin concentration sampling, addition of other maternal-administered drugs, and intraperitoneal, intramuscular, and umbilical cord direct delivery of digoxin and other antiarrhythmics.[2]

The initial case reports provided important findings, and replication of these results in more recent case reports and series allows us to form a better understanding of concepts of fetal treatment with digoxin:

1. In the face of fetal hydrops, the success of digoxin administered alone is diminished, largely as a result of reduced transplacental passage and lower fetal/cord blood levels. This effect has been noted by numerous authors.[32,87,92,93,97–99,101–103,111] Hansmann et al[110] found hydrops in 26 of 54 fetuses with supraventricular tachycardia and atrial flutter. Few with hydrops had rate conversion with digoxin alone, but intrauterine conversion was accomplished with the addition of other drugs and/or direct fetal administration. This group of investigators demonstrated most directly the impact of fetal hydrops on transplacental passage of digoxin via repeated fetal sampling over time (Fig. 34.1). After failure of initial maternal digitalization, the fetal-to-maternal ratio of digoxin was well below unity. With ultrasound-directed umbilical vein injections of amiodarone added to maternal digoxin, the heart rate and hydrops resolved and the fetal-to-maternal ratio of digoxin increased to near unity.[109] These data are supported by the observations of many other investigators of reduced efficacy and fetal-to-maternal ratio of digoxin (Tables 34.1 and 34.2), as well as by prolonged time until onset of sustained effect when this agent is used alone in the initial maternal treatment attempts.

Therefore, if digoxin is to be given to the mother to treat fetal arrhythmia and heart failure, it should be provided in high doses, with maternal blood levels approaching 2 ng/mL. Maternal toxicity must be closely monitored, however, because adverse effects have occurred with high plasma levels without resultant fetal cardioversion.[111] Caution is necessary when using high dose, combination conduction-depressing pharmacotherapy, since fetal demise can occur even after apparently successful rhythm conversion.[113] Van Engelen et al[107] observed that larger numbers of drugs in addition to digoxin, and longer time periods, were required to achieve control in hydropic fetuses (consistent with the early report by Harrigan et al[89]), but they were able to achieve similar high success rates in both hydropic (80%) and nonhydropic (84%) fetuses. This set of results supports earlier similar findings.[112,114] Although other authors have not found such success rates in fetal hydrops,[115] these authors did observe lower range maternal and fetal digoxin concentrations (means of 0.84 and 0.48, respectively), and congenital heart anomalies were found in the majority of the pharmacologically managed hydropic fetuses. This is not typical of fetuses undergoing digoxin treatment of tachyarrhythmias in other larger trials, where few anatomical defects are noted.[2,110] With the expected reduced fetal levels and effectiveness of digoxin when administered alone in fetuses with ultrasonigraphically demonstrated hydrops or heart failure, earlier intervention with added secondary agents and/or direct fetal therapy is suggested (Table 34.2). Resolution of hydrops may require four to six weeks after pharmacologic conversion to a normal rhythm.[111a,111b] The experience with alternative first-line agents (e.g., flecainide) instead of digoxin is limited[2,107,115a,115b], but, nonetheless, very encouraging.

2. The efficacy of digoxin alone in the treatment of atrial flutter is somewhat less than the success rate in supraventricular tachycardia[32] (Table 34.2). This is particularly noteworthy in fetuses with heart failure, as seen in the excellent compilation by Ito et al.[2] Van Engelen et al[107] reported an 88% successful rhythm control with intrauterine treatment of supraventricular tachycardia, compared with 66% with atrial flutter. The success of the single and combination digoxin and nondigoxin regimens for each of these arrhythmia groups was not itemized in their report. Additionally, in utero Wolff–Parkinson–White syndrome may worsen with exposure to digoxin, as reported by Belhassen et al,[90] similar to observations in older children and adults. Most often WPW syndrome is diagnosed only after delivery, in the neonate,[112,114] often after in utero failure of digoxin alone.[86,87,93,97,112]

3. The experience reported by Lingman et al[88] of a rapid conversion of atrial tachycardia after intravenous administration supports utilizing this route of administration for indirect digitalization of the fetus. Nagashima et al[95] treated a 31-week fetus with intravenous maternal digoxin with initial response. After the mother was switched to the same dose of oral drug, however, the fetal tachycardia recurred, only to be controlled again when therapy was switched back to the intravenous route. Breakthrough during maintenance oral digoxin therapy, followed by reestablishment of control with an additional loading dose has been reported by others.[32] This sequence demonstrates both the reduced bioavailability and delayed absorption often seen in pregnant women receiving oral medications and the need for higher oral doses.[116] More rapid cardioversion is also demonstrated using the intravenous route,[32,96] even in fetal hydrops. We recommend intravenous loading infusions of digoxin for more rapid control of fetal heart rate, and returning to intravenous administration if fetal tachyarrhythmia recurs while the mother is being maintained on high dose oral treatment. This can be done prior to, or in concurrence with, trials of other drugs or direct fetal administration.

REFERENCES

1. Cox JL, Gardner MJ. Treatment of cardiac arrhythmias during pregnancy. *Prog Cardiovasc Dis* 1993;36:137–178.

2. Ito S, Magee L, Smallhorn J. Drug therapy for fetal arrhythmias. *Clin Perinatol* 1994;21:543–572.

3. Smith TW. Digitalis: mechanisms of action and clinical use. *N Engl J Med* 1988;318:358–365.

4. Lee KS, Klaus W. The subcellular basis for the mechanism of inotropic action of cardiac glycoside. *Pharmacol Rev* 1971; 23:193–244.

5. Bernabei R, Vassalle M. The inotropic effects of strophanthidin in Purkinje fibers and the sodium pump. *Circulation* 1984;69:618–631.

6. Rosen MR, Wit AL, Hoffman BE. Electrophysiology and pharmacology of cardiac arrhythmias and toxic effects of digitalis. *Am Heart J* 1975;89:391–399.

7. Aronson JK. Clinical pharmacokinetics of digoxin. *Clin Pharmacokinet* 1980;5:137–149.

8. Doherty JE, Dalrymple GU, Murphy ML, Kane JJ, Bissett JK, de Soyza N. Pharmacokinetics of digoxin. *Fed Proc* 1977;36:2242–2246.

9. Dobbs RJ, O'Neill CJA, Deshmukh AA, Nicholson PW, Dobbs SM. Serum concentration monitoring of cardiac glycosides: how helpful is it for adjusting dosage regimens? *Clin Pharmacokinet* 1991;20:175–193.

10. Koren G. Clinical pharmacokinetic significance of the renal tubular secretion of digoxin. *Clin Pharmacokinet* 1987;13:334–343.

11. Ito S, Koren G, Harper PA, Silverman M. Energy-dependent transport of digoxin across renal tubular cell monolayers (LLC-PK1). *Can J Physiol Pharmacol* 1993;71:40.

12. Ito S, Woodland C, Harper PA, Koren G. The mechanism of the verapamil–digoxin interaction in renal tubular cells (LLC-PK1). *Life Sci* 1993;53:PL399.

13. Marcus FI, Burkhalter C, Pavlovich J, Kapadia GG. Administration of tritiated digoxin with and without a loading dose: a metabolic study. *Circulation* 1966;34:865–874.

14. Marcus FI. Pharmacokinetic interactions with digoxin and other drugs. *J Am College Cardiol* 1985;5:43A–50A.

15. Howanitz PJ, Steindel SJ. Digoxin therapeutic drug monitoring practices: a College of American Pathologists Q-probes study of 666 institutions and 18,679 toxic levels. *Arch Pathol Lab Med* 1993;117:684–690.

16. Lukas DS, DeMartino AG. Binding of digitoxin and some related cardenolides to human plasma proteins. *J Clin Invest* 1969;48:1041–1053.

17. Schneeweiss A. Digitalis glycosides. In: Schneeweiss A, ed. *Drug Therapy in Cardiovascular Disease*. Philadelphia: Lea & Febiger; 1986;723–740.

18. Selden R, Margolies MN, Smith TW. Renal and gastrointestinal excretion of ouabain in dog and man. *J Pharmacol Exp Ther* 1974;188:615–623.

19. Beller GA, Smith TW, Abelman WH, Haber E, Hud WB. Digitalis intoxication. *N Engl J Med* 1971;284:989–997.

20. Schroeder S, Harrison DC. Repeated cardioversion during pregnancy. *Am J Cardiol* 1971;27:445–446.

21. Lalonde RL, Deshpande R, Hamilton PP, McLean WM, Greenway DC. Acceleration of digoxin clearance by activated charcoal. *Clin Pharmacol Ther* 1985;37:367–371.

22. Ujhelyi MR, Robert S. Pharmacokinetic aspects of digoxin-specific Fab therapy in the management of digitalis toxicity. *Clin Pharmacokinet* 1995;28:483–493.

23. Koren G, Farine D, Maresky D, Taylor J, Heyes ART, Soldin S, MacLeod S. Significance of the endogenous digoxin-like substance in infants and mothers. *Clin Pharmacol Ther* 1984;36:759–764.

24. Hicks JM, Brett EM. Falsely increased digoxin concentrations in samples from neonates and infants. *Ther Drug Monitor* 1984;6:461–464.

25. Okita GT, Gordon RB, Geiling EML. Placental transfer of radioactive digitoxin in rats and guinea pigs. *Proc Soc Exp Biol Med* 1952;80:536–538.

26. Fouron JC. Dynamics of the placental transfer of digoxin in the dog. *Biol Neonate* 1973;23:116–123.

27. Doherty JE, Perkins WH. Tissue concentration and turnover of tritiated digoxin in dogs. *Am J Cardiol* 1966;17:47–52.

28. Hernandez A, Strauss AW, Burton RM, Goldring D. The effects of long term administration of ^{3}H-digoxin to the pregnant ewe upon the cardiovascular hemodynamics of the fetal lamb. *Am J Obstet Gynecol* 1975;121:1100–1102.

29. Singh S, Fehr PE, Mirkin BL. Elimination kinetics and placental transfer of digoxin in pregnant and nonpregnant ewes. *Res Commun Chem Pathol Pharmacol* 1978;20:31–42.

30. Rogers MC, Willerson JT, Goldblatt A, Smith TW. Serum digoxin concentrations in the human fetus, neonate, and infant. *N Engl J Med* 1972;287:1010–1013.

31. Luxford AME, Kellaway GSM. Pharmacokinetics of digoxin in pregnancy. *Eur J Clin Pharmacol* 1983;25:117–121.

32. Azancot-Benisty A, Aigrain EJ, Guirgis NM, Decrepy A, Oury JF, Blot P. Clinical and pharmacologic study of fetal supraventricular tachyarrythmias. *J Pediatr* 1992;121:608–613.

33. Gusdon JP, Vardaman M, Buckalew J, Hennessy J. A digoxin-like immunoreactive substance in preeclampsia. *Am J Obstet Gynecol* 1984;150:83–85.

34. Kerkes SA, Poston L, Wolfe CD, Quartero HW, Carabelli P, Petruckevitch A, Hilton PJ. A longitudinal study of maternal digoxin-like immunoreactive substances in normotensive pregnancy and pregnancy-induced hypertension. *Am J Obstet Gynecol* 1990;162:783–787.

35. Kaminski K, Rechberger T. Concentration of digoxin-like immunoreactive substance in patients with preeclampsia and its relation to the severity of pregnancy-induced hypertension. *Am J Obstet Gynecol* 1991;165:733–736.

36. Weiner CP, Landas S, Persoon TJ. Digoxin-like immunoreactive substance in fetuses with and without cardiac pathology. *Am J Obstet Gynecol* 1987;157:368–371.

37. Lupoglazoff JM, Jacqz-Aigrain E, Guyot B, Chappey O, Blot P. Endogenous digoxin-like immunoreactivity during pregnancy and at birth. *Br J Clin Pharmcol* 1993;35:251–254.

38. Pudek MR, Seccombe DW, Jacobson BE, Whitfield MF. Seven different immunoassay kits compared with respect to interference by a digoxin-like immunoreactive substance in serum from premature and full-term infants. *Clin Chem* 1983;29:1972–1974.

39. Ghione S, Balzan S, Decollogne S, Paci A, Pieraccini L, Montali U. Endogenous digitalis-like activity in the newborn. *J Cardiovasc Pharmacol* 1993;22(suppl 2):S25–S28.

40. Ray JE, Crisan D, Howrie DL. Digoxin-like immunoreactivity in serum from neonates and infants reduced by centrifugal ultrafiltration and fluorescence polarization immunoassay. *Clin Chem* 1991;37:94–98.

41. Deray G, Pernollet M, Devynck M, Zingraff J, Touam A, Rosenfeld J, Meyer P. Plasma digitalis-like activity in essential hypertension or end-stage renal disease. *Hypertension* 1986;8:632–638.

42. Schrader BJ, Maddux MS, Veremia SA, Mozes MF, Maturen A, Bauman JL. Digoxin-like immunoreactive substance in renal transplant patients. *J Clin Pharmacol* 1991;31:1126–1131.

43. Yang SS, Korula J, Sundheimer JE, Keyser AJ. Digoxin-like immunoreactive substances in chronic liver disease. *Hepatology* 1989;9:363–369.

44. Lucena MI, Andrade RJ, Fraile JM, Alcantara R, Gonzalez-Correa JA, Sanchez De La Cuesta F. Endogenous digoxin-like substance in liver failure. *Int J Clin Pharmacol Ther* 1994;32:567–569.

45. Goto A, Yamada K, Yagi N, Yoshioka M, Sugimoto T. Physiology and pharmacology of endogenous digitalis-like factors. *Pharmacol Rev* 1992;44:377–399.

45. Scherrman JM, Sandouk P, Guedeney X. Endogenous digoxin-like immunoreactive substances in cord serum characterized by anti-digitoxin and anti-digoxin antibodies—effect of modulated incubation conditions. *Clin Biochem* 1986;19:201–204.

46. Scherrman JM, Sandouk P, Guedeney X. Digitalis-like factors and digoxin pharmacokinetics. *Chest* 1986;89:468–469.

47. Yun WS, Ho CS, Panesar NS, Swaminathan R. The contribution of steroids to digoxin-like immunoreactivity in cord blood. *Ann Clin Biochem* 1992;29:337–342.

48. Pleasants RA, Williams DM, Porter RS, Gadsen RH Jr. Reassessment of cross-reactivity of spironolactone metabolites with four digoxin immunoassays. *Ther Drug Monitor* 1989;11:200–204.

49. Jortani SA, Valdes R Jr. Digoxim and its related endogenous factors. *Crit Rev Clin Lab Sci:* 1997; 34:225–274.

50. Seccombe DW, Pudek MR, Humphries KH, Matthewson B, Taylor GP, Jacobson BE, Whitfield MP. A study into the nature and organ source of digoxin-like immunoreactive substance(s) in the perinatal period. *Biol Neonate* 1989;56:136–146.

51. Guedeney X, Chanez C, Scherrmann JM. Existence of a digitalis-like compound in the human fetus. *Biol Neonate* 1991;59:133–138.

52. Hamlyn JM, Blaustein MP, Bova SP, DuCharme DW, Harris DW, Mandel F, Mathews WR, Ludens JH. Identification and characterization of a ouabain-like compound from human plasma. *Proc Natl Acad Sci USA* 1991;88:6259–6263.

53. Graves SW, Lincoln K, Cook SL, Seely EW. Digitalis-like factor and digoxin-like immunoreactive factor in diabetic women with preeclampsia, transient hypertension of pregnancy, and normotensive pregnancy. *Am J Hypertension* 1995;8:5–11.

54. Seccombe DW, Pudek MR, Whitfield MP, Jacobson BE, Wittmann BK, King JF. Perinatal changes in a digoxin-like immunoreactive substance. *Pediatr Res* 1984;18:1097–1099.

55. Graves SW, Valdes R, Brown BA, Knight AB, Craig R. Endogenous digoxin-like immunoreactive substance in human pregnancies. *J Clin Endocrinol Metab* 1984;58:748–751.

56. Valdes R. Endogenous digoxin-immunoreactive factor in human subjects. *Fed Proc* 1985;44:2800–2805.

57. Yapar EG, Ayhan A. The influence of tocolytic therapy on serum digoxin-like immunoreactive substance concentration. *Gynecol Obstet Invest* 1994;37:10–13.

58. Valdes R, Graves SW, Brown BA, Landt M. Endogenous substance in newborn infants causing false-positive digoxin measurements. *J Pediatr* 1983;102:947–950.

59. Koren G, Farine D, Grundmann H, Heyes J, Soldin S, Taylor J, MacLeod SM. Endogenous digoxin-like substance(s) associated with uneventful and high-risk pregnancies. *Dev Pharmacol Ther* 1988;11:82–87.

60. Schlebusch H, Mende SV, Grunn U, Gembruch U, Bald R, Hansmann M. Determination of digoxin in the blood of pregnant women, fetuses, and neonates before and during antiarrhythmic therapy, using four immunochemical methods. *Eur J Clin Chem Clin Biochem* 1991;29:57–66.

61. Di Grande A, Boura ALA, Read MA, Malatino LS, Walters WAW. Release of a substance from the human placenta having digoxin-like immunoreactivity. *Clin Exp Pharmacol Physiol* 1993;20:603–607.

62. Friedman HS, Abramowitz I, Nguyen T, Babb B, Stern M, Farrer SM, Tricomi V. Urinary digoxin-like immunoreactive substance in pregnancy: relation to urinary electrolytes. *Am J Med* 1987;83:261–264.

63. Ebara H, Suzuki S, Nagashima K, Shimano S, Kuroume T. Digoxin-like immunoreactive substances in urine and serum from preterm and term infants: relationship to renal excretion of sodium. *J Pediatr* 1986;108:760–762.

64. Fitzsimmons WE. Influence of assay methodologies and interferences on the interpretation of digoxin concentrations. *Drug Intell Clin Pharm* 1986;20:538–542.

64. Dodds HM, Norris RLG, Johnson AG, Pond SM. Evaluation and comparison of the TDxII, Stratus, and OPUS digoxin assays. *Ther Drug Monitor* 1995;17:68–74.

65. Qazzaz HM, Goudy S, Miller JJ, Valdez R Jr. Treatment of human serum with sulfosalicylic acid structurally alters digoxin and endogenous digoxin-like immunoreactive factor. *Ther Drug Monitor* 1995;17:53–59.

66. Jiang F, Wilhite TR, Smith CH, Landt M. A new digoxin immunoassay substantially free of interference by digoxin immunoreactive factor. *Ther Drug Monitor* 1995;17:184–188.

67. Potondi A. Congenital rhabdomyoma of the heart and intrauterine digitalis poisoning. *J Forensic Sci* 1967;11:81–88.

68. Sherman JL, Locke RV. Transplacental neonatal digitalis intoxication. *Am J Cardiol* 1960;6:834–837.

69. Whitsett JA, Wallick ET. [3][H]Ouabain binding and Na^+-K^+-ATPase activity in human placenta. *Am J Physiol* 1980;238:E38–E45.

70. Weaver JB, Pearson JF. Influence of digitalis on time of onset and duration of labour in women with cardiac disease. *Br Med J* 1973;3:519–520.

71. Okita GT, Plotz EJ, Davis ME. Placental transfer of radioactive digitoxin in the pregnant woman and its fetal distribution. *Circ Res* 1956;4:376–380.

72. Papp J, Nemeth M, Resch B. Foetal development of responsiveness to cardiotonic drugs in human foetus, neonate, and infant. *N Engl J Med* 1972;287:1010–1013.

73. Chan V, Tse TF, Wong V. Transfer of digoxin across the placenta and into breast milk. *Br J Obstet Gynaecol* 1978;85:605–609.

74. Levy M, Granit L, Laufer N. Excretion of drugs in human milk. *N Engl J Med* 1977;297:789.

75. Finley JP, Waxman MB, Wong PY, Lickrish GM. Drug excretion in human milk. *J Pediatr* 1979;94:339–340.

76. Loughnan PM. Digoxin excretion in human milk. *J Pediatr* 1978;92:1019–1020.

77. Committee on Drugs, American Academy of Pediatrics. Transfer of drugs and other chemicals into human milk. *Pediatrics* 1994;93:137–150.

78. Reinhardt D, Richter O, Genz T, Potthoff S. Kinetics of the translactal passage of digoxin from breast feeding mothers to their infants. *Eur J Pediatr* 1982;138:49–52.

79. Saarikoski S. Placental transfer and human fetal uptake of ^{3}H-digoxin in humans. *Br J Obstet Gynaecol* 1976;83:879–884.

80. Allonen H, Kanto J, Iisalo E. The foeto-maternal distribution of digoxin in early human pregnancy. *Acta Pharmacol Toxicol* 1976;39:477–480.

81. Padelleti L, Porclani MC, Scimone G. Placental transfer of digoxin (beta-methyldigoxin) in man. *Int J Clin Pharmacol Biopharmacol* 1979;17:82–83.

82. Derewlany LO, Leeder JS, Kumar R, Radde I, Knie B, Koren G. The transport of digoxin across the perfused human placental lobule. *J Pharmacol Exp Ther* 1991;256:1107–1111.

82a. Schmolling J, Jung S, Reinsberg J, Schlebusch H. Digoxin transfer across the isolated placenta is influenced by maternal and fetal albumin concentrations. *Reproduc Fertil Develop* 1996;8:969–974.

82b. Schmolling J, Jung S, Reinsberg J, Schlebusch H. Diffusion characteristics of placental preparations affect the passage across the isolated placental lobule. *Ther Drug Monitor* 1997;19:11–16.

82c. Bourget P, Roulot C, Fernandez H. Models for placental transfer studies of drugs. *Clin Pharmacokinet* 1995;28:161–180.

83. Dumesic DA, Silverman NH, Tobias S, Golbus MS. Transplacental cardioversion of fetal supraventricular tachycardia with procainamide. *N Engl J Med* 1982;307:1128–1132.

84. Saarikoski S. Placental transmission and foetal distribution of ^{3}H-ouabain. *Acta Pharmacol Toxicol* 1980;46:272–282.

85. Bergmans MGM, Jonker GJ, Kock HCLV. Fetal supraventricular tachycardia: review of the literature. *Obstet Gynecol Survey* 1985;40:61–68.

86. Newburger JW, Keane JF. Intrauterine supraventricular tachycardia. *J Pediatr* 1979;95:780–786.

87. Kerenyi TD, Gleicher N, Meller J, Brown E, Stienfeld L, Chitkara U, Raucher H. Transplacental cardioversion of in-

trauterine supraventricular tachycardia with digitalis. *Lancet* 1980;2:393–395.

88. Lingman G, Ohrlander S, Ohlin P. Intrauterine digoxin treatment of fetal paroxysmal tachycardia. *Br J Obstet Gynaecol* 1980;87:340–342.

89. Harrigan JT, Kangos JJ, Sikka A, Spisso KR, Natarajan N, Rosenfeld D, Leiman S, Korn D. Successful treatment of fetal congestive heart failure secondary to tachycardia. *N Engl J Med* 1981;304:1527–1529.

90. Bellhassen B, Pauzner D, Bleiden D, Sherez J, Zinger A, David M, Muhlbauer B, Laniado S. Intrauterine and postnatal atrial fibrillation in the Wolff–Parkinson–White syndrome. *Circulation* 1982;66:1124–1128.

91. Allan LD, Crawford DC, Anderson RH, Tynan M. Evaluation and treatment of fetal arrhythmias. *Clin Cardiol* 1984;7:467–473.

92. Given BD, Phillippe M, Sanders SP, Dzau VJ. Procainamide cardioversion of fetal supraventricular tachycardia. *Am J Cardiol* 1984;53:1460–1461.

93. Spinnato JA, Shaver DC, Flinn GS, Sibai BM, Watson DL, Marin-Garcia J. Fetal supraventricular tachycardia: in-utero therapy with digoxin and quinidine. *Obstet Gynecol* 1984;64:730–735.

94. King CR, Mattiloli L, Goertz KK, Snodgrass W. Successful treatment of fetal supraventricular tachycardia with maternal digoxin therapy. *Chest* 1984;85:573–575.

95. Nagashima M, Asai T, Suzuki C, Matsushima M, Ogawa A. Intrauterine supraventricular tachyarrhythmias and transplacental digitalisation. *Arch Dis Child* 1986;651:996–1000.

96. Wiggins JW, Bowes W, Clewell W, Manco-Johnson M, Manchester D, Johnson R, Appareti K, Wolfe RR. Echocardiographic diagnosis and intravenous digoxin management of fetal tachyarrhythmias and congestive heart failure. *Am J Dis Child* 1986;140:202–204.

97. Repke JT, Steinbach G. Fetal supraventricular tachycardia refractory to digoxin cardioversion: a case report. *J Reprod Med* 1986;31:195–197.

98. Mimura S, Suzuki C, Yamazaki T. Transplacental passage of digoxin in the case of nonimmune hydrops fetalis. *Clin Cardiol* 1987;10:63–65.

99. Younis JS, Granat M. Insufficient transplacental digoxin transfer in severe hydrops fetalis. *Am J Obstet Gynecol* 1987;157:1268–1269.

100. Weiner CP, Thompson MIB. Direct treatment of fetal supraventricular tachycardia after failed transplacental therapy. *Am J Obstet Gynecol* 1988;158:570–573.

101. Hallak M, Neerhof MG, Perry R, Nazir M, Huhta JC. Fetal supraventricular tachycardia and hydrops fetalis: combined intensive, direct and transplacental therapy. *Obstet Gynecol* 1991;78:523–525.

102. Kofinas AD, Simon NV, Sagel H, Lyttle E, Smith N, King K. Treatment of fetal supraventricular tachycardia with flecainide acetate after digoxin failure. *Am J Obstet Gynecol* 1991;165:630–631.

103. Battiste CE, Neff TW, Evans JF, Cline BW. In-utero conversion of supraventricular tachycardia with digoxin and pro-

cainamide at 17 weeks' gestation. *Am J Perinatol* 1992;9:302–303.

103a. Treatment of fetal supraventricular tachycardia with maternal administration of digoxin. *Int J Gynecol Obstet* 1995;50:293–294.

103b. Kohl T, Tercanli S, Kececioglu D, Holzgreve W. Direct fetal administration of adenosine for the termination of incessant supraventricular tachycardia. *Obstet Gynecol* 1995;85:873–874.

103c. Copel JA, Friedman AH, Kleinman CS. Management of fetal cardiac arrhythmias. *Obstet Gynecol Clin North Am* 1997;24:201–211.

104. De Lia J, Emery M, Sheafor S, Jennison T. Twin transfusion syndrome: successful in-utero treatment with digoxin. *Int J Gynecol Obstet* 1985;23:197–201.

104a. Kanhai HHH, van Kamp IL, Moolenaar AJ, Gravenhorst JB. Transplacental passage of digoxin in severe Rhesus immunization. *J Perinat Med* 1990;18:339–343.

105. Harris JP, Alexson CG, Manning JA, Thompson HO. Medical therapy for the hydropic fetus with congenital complete atrioventricular block. *Am J Perinatol* 1993;10:217–219.

106. Roman JD, Hare AA. Digoxin and decompression amniocentesis for treatment of feto–fetal transfusion. *Br J Obstet Gynaecol* 1995;102:421–423.

106a. Chavkin Y, Kupfersztain C, Ergaz Z, Guedj P, Finkel AR, Stark M. Successful outcome of idiopathic nonimmune hydrops fetalis treated by maternal digoxin. *Gynecol Obstet Invest* 1996;42:137–139.

106b. Anandakumar C, Biswas A, Chew SSL, Chia D, Wong YC, Ratman SS. Direct fetal therapy for hydops secondary to congenital atrioventricular heart block. *Obstet Gynecol* 1996;87:835–837.

107. Van Engelen AD, Weijtens O, Brenner JI, Kleinman CS, Copel JA, Stoutenbeek P, Meijboom EJ. Management outcome and follow-up of fetal tachycardia. *J Am College Cardiol* 1994;24:1371–1375.

108. Gembruch U, Redel DA, Bald R, Hansmann M. Longitudinal study in 18 cases of fetal supraventricular tachycardia: Doppler echocardiographic findings and pathophysiologic implications. *Am Heart J* 1993;125:1290–1301.

109. Gembruch U, Manz M, Bald R, Ruddel H, Redel DA, Schlebusch H, Nitsch J, Hansmann M. Repeated intravascular treatment with amiodarone in a fetus with refractory supraventricular tachycardia and hydrops fetalis. *Am J Cardiol* 1989;118:1335–1338.

110. Hansmann M, Gembruch U, Bald R, Manz M, Redel DA. Fetal tachyarrhythmias: transplacental and direct treatment of the fetus—a report of 60 cases. *Ultrasound Obstet Gynecol* 1991;1:162–170.

111. Klein AM, Holzman IR, Austin EM. Fetal tachycardia prior to the development of hydrops—attempted pharmacologic cardioversion: case report. *Am J Obstet Gynecol* 1979;134:347–348.

111a. Petrikovsky B, Schneider E, Ovadia M. Natural history of hydrops resolution in fetuses with tachyarrythmias diagnosed and treated in utero. *Fetal Diagn Ther* 1996;11:292–295.

111b. Parilla BV, Strasburger JF, Socol ML. Fetal supraventricular tachycardia complicated by hydrops fetalis: a role for direct fetal intramuscular therapy. *Am J Perinatol* 1996;13:483–486.

112. Kleinman CS, Copoel JA, Weinstein EM, Santulli TV, Hobbins JC. In utero diagnosis and treatment of fetal supraventricular tachycardia. *Semin Perinatol* 1985;9:113–129.

113. Owen J, Colvin EV, Davis RO. Fetal death after successful conversion of fetal supraventricular tachycardia with digoxin and verapamil. *Am J Obstet Gynecol* 1988;158:1169–1170.

114. Maxwell DJ, Crawford DC, Curry PVM, Tynan MJ, Allan LD. Obstetric importance, diagnosis, and management of fetal tachycardias. *Br Med J* 1988;297:107–110.

115. Maeda H, Koyanagi T, Nakano H. Intrauterine treatment on nonimmune hydrops fetalis. *Early Hum Dev* 1992;29:241–249.

115a. Frohn-Mulder IM, Stewart PA, Witsenburg M, Den Hollander NS, Wladmiroff JW, Hess J. The efficacy of flecainide versus digoxin in the management of fetal supraventricular tachycardia. *Prenat Diagn* 1995;15:1297–1302.

115b. Simpson JM, Milburn A, Yates RW, Maxwall DJ, Sharland GK. Outcome of intermittent tachyarrythuias in the fetus. *Pediatr Cardiol* 1997; 18: 78–82.

116. Ward RM. Pharmacologic treatment of the fetus: clinical pharmacokinetic considerations. *Clin Pharmacokinet* 1995; 28:343–350.

35

TOCOLYTIC THERAPY IN THE CARDIAC PATIENT

T. Murphy Goodwin, MD

INTRODUCTION

Preterm delivery occurs in approximately 10% of all births in the United States. In many cases no specific measures to prevent the preterm birth are possible or warranted. Nevertheless, more than 60,000 women per year are treated with intravenous tocolytics, and a much larger number receive tocolytic agents via the subcutaneous or oral route. Although the overlap between significant cardiac disease and the need for tocolysis is infrequent, the situation has the potential for serious adverse consequences for the pregnant mother. Among the questions that must be answered before initiating a plan of therapy are the following:

Have strict criteria for the diagnosis of preterm labor been applied?

What is the current neonatal outcome for a given weight and gestational age in the region?

Is the labor related to maternal compromise (e.g., hypoxemia)?

Is the labor related to fetal compromise?

What are the benefits of pharmacologic tocolytic therapy?

Are there specific harmful effects of pharmacologic tocolytic therapy and/or adjunctive therapy directed at fetal maturation?

Let us address these in order.

The current approach to preterm labor varies widely in the United States, with some advocating abandonment of pharmacologic tocolytic therapy entirely,[1] while others routinely advocate multiagent tocolytic therapy.[2] Between these extremes, it is common practice at present to accept frequent uterine contractions as sufficient justification for tocolytic therapy, even though it has been clearly shown that most patients who have only uterine contractions without evidence of cervical change will not progress in labor even without specific treatment.[3] While the confusion caused by such overtreatment is considerable, the potential for injury to the otherwise healthy patient is limited. This does not apply in the case of the pregnant cardiac patient, for whom pharmacologic tocolytic therapy may present a significant risk.

The diagnosis of preterm labor in the pregnant cardiac patient, therefore, must be based on the presence of regular uterine contractions associated with clear evidence of cervical change. Commonly accepted specific criteria have been outlined by Creasy.[4] Importantly, awaiting evidence of cervical change does not appear to reduce the efficacy of tocolysis.[5]

Any risk to the mother in attempting to arrest labor must be weighed against the benefit to the fetus of delaying delivery. While this may appear self-evident, the data for the risk/benefit equation are constantly changing. The addition of surfactant, antenatal and postnatal steroids, and high frequency ventilation have changed neonatal morbidity and mortality figures considerably since the last edition of this book. Treating physicians should rely on the outcome statistics from their own centers, updated at least annually, to be able to make informed decisions about the comparative risks and benefits of tocolytic therapy in the pregnant cardiac patient. Current neonatal outcome data for the Los Angeles County/University of Southern California Medical Center (LAC-USC) and affiliated centers is shown in Tables 35.1 and 35.2. Similar numbers would apply at many tertiary level nurseries in the United States.

Cardiac Problems in Pregnancy, Third Edition
Edited by Uri Elkayam, MD, and Norbert Gleicher, MD
Copyright © 1998 by Wiley-Liss, Inc. ISBN 0-471-16358-9

TABLE 35.1 Approximate Neonatal Survival to Discharge of Preterm Infants Born in LAC-USC and Affiliated Facilities

Gestational Age (weeks)	Birth Weight (g)	Survivors (%)
24–25	500–750	55
26–27	751–1000	80
28–29	1001–1250	93
30–31	1251–1500	96
32–33	1501–1750	98
≥34	1751–2000	99+

Currently used tocolytic regimens include β-mimetic agents, magnesium sulfate, calcium channel blockers (nifedipine), and prostaglandin synthetase inhibitors (usually indomethacin). The largest randomized experience has been accumulated with the β-mimetic ritodrine, and it is reasonable to extrapolate from what is known about this agent to other β-mimetics. In addition, because of the amount of data accumulated with regard to efficacy and safety, ritodrine has become the standard for comparison with other tocolytic regimens, in particular with regard to efficacy.

The meta-analysis of King et al,[3] together with the results of the Canadian collaborative study,[6] established that the only undisputed beneficial effect of β-mimetic therapy is a delay in delivery of 48 hours. All other tocolytic regimens have compared themselves to this standard, and none has been studied on a scale that would be necessary to demonstrate more comprehensive benefits.

Another important consideration is the relation, if any, of the stimulus for uterine activity to maternal compromise. Maternal hypoxemia can be a potent stimulus to uterine contractions, perhaps mediated through release of fetal vasopressin.[7] In any patient who presents with a change in cardiac symptoms and evidence of uterine contractions, the contractions should be presumed secondary to the deterioration in cardiac status until the patient's condition is stabilized.

Fetal compromise or growth restriction in utero may also be associated with preterm labor.[8] In this setting the fetus may signal the need for its own delivery from a hostile environment. In our experience, evidence of fetal compromise (diminished amniotic fluid, fetal growth delay, or abnormal fetal heart rate testing) is the most common reason for preterm delivery among cardiac patients, although not all these deliveries are associated with preterm labor. The mother with congenital cardiac disease is at increased risk for cardiac malformations in the fetus.[9] Such malformations may be a cause of preterm uterine activity, especially when associated with fetal hydrops.

Can the medical regimen required by the cardiac disease lead to preterm labor or complicate therapy? The principal concern in this regard is the usage of β-adrenergic antagonists. There have been a number of reports of these agents leading to increased uterine activity, in particular those that block β_1- and β_2-adrenergic receptors equally, such as propranolol.[10] In practice, however, there is no discernible effect of the more commonly used beta blockers on uterine activity. In our experience with atenolol and metoprolol, intrapartum and antepartum, we have observed no effect on uterine activity, baseline tone, or the general progress of labor.

Type II calcium blockers (nifedipine, nicardipine, nitrendipine) have their major action on smooth muscle and are used in the treatment of hypertension and angina. Such agents are potent inhibitors of uterine activity as will be discussed below.

CARDIOVASCULAR EFFECTS OF TOCOLYTIC AGENTS

Although intravenous β-mimetics have been used as the gold standard in most studies of tocolytic therapy, in the United States subcutaneous terbutaline and magnesium are gaining in popularity. A recent survey of centers around the country[11] revealed that more than 50% used intravenous magnesium as first-line therapy. The remainder used a β-mimetic, but this was often subcutaneous terbutaline. Failure of subcutaneous terbutaline to arrest labor was often followed by intravenous magnesium even in some of these centers. Intravenous ritodrine or terbutaline was used as first-line therapy in only 20%

TABLE 35.2 Approximate Neonatal Morbidity Rates (%) by Gestational Age at Birth in LAC-USC and Affiliated Facilities

Pathological Condition	Gestational Age (weeks)						
	24–25	26–27	28–29	30–31	32–33	34	35
RDS	85	81	65	30	30	20	3
PDA	80	50	50	21	17	8	
Sepsis	25	25	20	10	7	5	5
NEC	8	6	5	5	3		
IVH, grades III and IV	20	9	7	5	3		

Abbreviations: RDS, respiratory distress syndrome; PDA, patient ductus arteriosus; NEC, necrotizing enterocolitis; IVH, intraventricular hemorrhage (Papille's classification).

of centers. Less than 5% of practitioners used indomethacin or nifedipine for tocolysis, but usage of the latter agent appears to be increasing considerably in some regions.

Concern about the adverse effects of indomethacin on the fetus appears to have markedly limited use of this agent in the last several years. Several reports of increased neonatal morbidity, in particular intracranial hemorrhage and necrotizing enterocolitis, have appeared.[12,13] For this reason, the discussion of specific tocolytic drugs in women with cardiac disease will focus on β-mimetics, magnesium, and nifedipine.

Cardiac Effects of β-Mimetics

All the β-mimetics used for tocolysis are designed to be selective for β_2. Nevertheless, both because of intrinsic properties of the drugs and because of tissue distribution of β_1 and β_2 receptors, all have some β_1 effects. The majority of the undesirable side effects stem from this.

In dosages commonly required for intravenous tocolysis, a decline in peripheral vascular resistance is seen, manifesting as lowered diastolic pressure.[14] The mean arterial pressure is only slightly lowered, however, because β_1-mediated chronotropic and inotropic effects result in increased cardiac output.[15] The principal concerns for the otherwise healthy-appearing patient who receives β-mimetic therapy are pulmonary edema, myocardial injury due to ischemia, and unmasking of latent cardiac disease.

Patients on β-mimetic agents frequently demonstrate ECG changes including ST depression, T-wave flattening or inversion, and prolongation of the QT interval. The significance of these findings is debated. While Michalak et al[16] attributed these changes to ischemia, Hendricks and others noted that the changes resolve within 24 hours in 90% of patients despite continued therapy.[17] These authors postulated that the transient ECG changes are related to the temporally coincident hypokalemia induced by β-mimetics.

Several studies have shown no changes in cardiac enzymes during either short- or long-term β-mimetic therapy.[18,19] It appears unlikely that β-mimetic therapy in the otherwise healthy gravida results in ischemic injury. Despite these reassuring data, however, complaints of chest pain during therapy should usually prompt discontinuation of the medication, in particular because of the possibility of underlying undiagnosed cardiac disease. Myocardial infarction during ritodrine infusion in a previously healthy woman has been reported.[20]

The most consistently identified serious complication of β-mimetic therapy in otherwise healthy gravidas is pulmonary edema, with a reported incidence of 1–5%. It has been observed principally in the first 3 days of therapy, when the β-mimetic-mediated water retention is strongest. Most cases have been associated with excessive fluid intake and concomitant use of other medications (e.g., glucocorticoids,

prostaglandin antagonists, calcium channel blockers). Pulmonary edema is more likely to occur when certain conditions of pregnancy are present—twins, hydramnios, preeclampsia.[21]

There is no evidence of impaired cardiac function as a contributing factor in the vast majority of reported cases. Pulmonary capillary pressure assessed by central catheterization was not changed during β-mimetic infusion.[22,23] Noninvasive estimates of central hemodynamics have shown a rise in estimated pulmonary capillary pressure during ritodrine infusion but normal left ventricular function,[24,25] giving support to earlier studies that showed no change in left ventricular function in patients who developed pulmonary edema while on β-mimetic therapy. Awareness of the risk factors for pulmonary edema has apparently led to a marked reduction in this complication in recent years. The largest single trial of a β-mimetic therapy (ritodrine), reported in 1991, noted only one case of pulmonary edema among the 352 patients in the ritodrine arm of the study.[6]

Less frequently reported but serious cardiovascular consequences of β-mimetic use for preterm labor include persistent sinus bradycardia after ritodrine withdrawal[26] and Mobitz type I atrioventricular block during ritodrine infusion.[27] A variety of cardiac dysrhythmias were noted in 30 patients on Holter monitoring during terbutaline therapy.[28] Even in patients who were asymptomatic, frequent premature ventricular contractions and sustained tachycardia with T-wave inversion were noted. A case of maternal death after one week of subcutaneous terbutaline pump therapy was attributed to arrhythmia.[29] Severe hypotension following β-mimetic infusion remains a major problem in conjunction with regional anesthesia. Ephedrine is the drug of choice for reversing this effect.[30]

Several patients have been described whose initial manifestation of cardiomyopathy occurred after prolonged ritodrine or terbutaline therapy.[31,32] Although some authors have attributed this to unmasking of underlying disease, each of the four cases of peripartum cardiomyopathy associated with terbutaline use reported by Lampert experienced total recovery of cardiac function.

It is important to note that new onset arrythmias, pulmonary edema, and maternal death have been reported in association with oral and subcutaneous terbutaline pump therapy.[29,33,34] These modes of β-mimetic administration have gained in popularity in recent years, while intravenous use in hospitals has declined. The adverse cardiovascular consequences of the subcutaneous terbutaline pump, in particular, have been insufficiently characterized. Despite the widespread use of this device over the last 6 years, there have been no randomized trials and fewer than 50 patients have been described in two case series.[35,36]

Other metabolic perturbations with β-mimetic usage include hyperglycemia, ketoacidosis, hypokalemia, and lactic acidosis. While the acute hypokalemia may be marked, no cardiac effects or ECG changes have been found to result from these changes.

Should β-mimetic agents ever be used in the gravida with cardiac disease? It has been suggested that since the majority of the adverse effects of β-mimetics are mediated by their β_1 properties, these effects can be avoided by simultaneous treatment with a selective β_1 blocker or a calcium channel blocker such as verapamil. Grospietsch and Kuhn[37] reported that the practice of combining verapamil and β-mimetic therapy for a presumed cardioprotective effect has been applied widely in Europe. Grospietsch and others have shown, however, that while metoprolol does blunt the hemodynamic changes seen with β-mimetics, verapamil, in the commonly prescribed dosages, has no such effect.[38] There has been one case reported of a woman with Wolff–Parkinson–White syndrome treated simultaneously with the β-mimetic fenoterol and metoprolol.[39] Nevertheless, given the wide range of cardiac effects associated with the use of these agents even in healthy subjects, and the ready availability of safer alternatives of apparently equal efficacy (see below), β-mimetic use of tocolysis in the cardiac patient may constitute an unnecessary risk.

If β-mimetics are favored for tocolysis in the pregnant cardiac patient, their use remains contraindicated in cases of pulmonary hypertension with right-to-left shunting, aortic, mitral, or pulmonary stenosis, hypertrophic cardiomyopathy, and coarctation. In addition, β-mimetics should be avoided in any condition in which their arrhythmogenic effect would pose a risk.

Cardiac Effects of Magnesium Sulfate

The hemodynamic effects of bolus infusion of magnesium sulfate on normotensive subjects is negligible. In a study of 70 subjects in preterm labor, Thiagarajah found no significant change in pulse rate or in systolic or diastolic blood pressure.[40] A clinically insignificant drop in systolic blood pressure of 6.8% by 12 hours of infusion was the only effect noted. In Rhesus monkeys, uterine blood flow was unchanged or increased with magnesium, while it was decreased with ritodrine.[40]

Profound hypotension with infusion of magnesium has been reported rarely, but the majority of such cases have occurred under special circumstances: in previously hypertensive subjects,[41] with much larger boluses of magnesium than are currently used,[42] or in combination with other medications such as ritodrine[43] or nifedipine.[44] The combination of nifedipine and magnesium may have other adverse effects, as described below.

Direct cardiac effects of magnesium include lengthening of the PR and QRS intervals with concentrations above 10 mEq/L (normal target range for tocolysis = 4–6 mEq/L). Increased T-wave amplitude has been described at therapeutic concentrations,[45] with virtual disappearance as toxic concentrations are approached.[46] Cardiac arrest is the ultimate consequence of profound magnesium toxicity. It is preceded in sequence by neuromuscular blockade, progressing clinically from generalized weakness to paralysis. Potentiation of this neuromuscular blockade has been described with the combination of nifedipine, as discussed below.

Pulmonary edema may occur with magnesium therapy but appears to be much less common than with β-mimetics. Elliot found that pulmonary edema occurred in 1% of patients on magnesium for preterm labor[47] and was usually associated with other risk factors. Yeast et al[48] found no cases of pulmonary edema in 193 patients treated with magnesium for preterm labor but noted a 3.2% incidence (4/124) in patients treated with magnesium for preeclampsia. Pulmonary edema in preeclampsia was strongly associated with low colloid osmotic pressure, a finding not associated with preterm labor.

Other less common cardiovascular problems with magnesium usage have been reported. An association between spontaneous desaturation ($SaO_2 < 91\%$), and magnesium usage in labor has been reported; but the association was stronger for magnesium usage for preeclampsia than for preterm labor.[49] Two cases of atrial fibrillation apparently related to magnesium infusion have been reported[34,50]: one in a preeclamptic patient and one in a woman in preterm labor who had been previously treated with terbutaline. The latter case required short-term digitalization. In both cases the heart was otherwise normal.

Chest pain is occasionally reported with magnesium alone. A recent report describes a woman treated with magnesium for preterm labor who developed chest pain and inverted T waves.[51] This presumptive evidence of subendocardial ischemia resolved with decreasing rate of infusion of magnesium. The mechanism of this effect is not clear.

Two patients with unexplained hyperkalemia following magnesium infusion (one for preeclampsia, one for preterm labor) have been described.[52] Electrocardiographic changes were not described, but the potassium level reached 7.1 and 7.2 mEq/L, respectively. The hyperkalemia resolved with discontinuation of the magnesium. Both patients had a history of intravenous cocaine use.

The use of magnesium for tocolysis in patients with cardiac disease has been described in several recent reports.[53–55] Pulmonary hypertension with shunting, in which even a modest decrease in systemic resistance may be catastrophic, is one of the few cardiac contraindications to magnesium use.

Calcium Channel Blockers

Type II calcium blockers or dihydropyridines (e.g., nifedipine, nicardipine) are used for their relaxing effect on smooth muscle. Type I calcium antagonists (verapamil, diltiazem) are used for their effect on myocardial contractility and conduction but have been found to have little effect on smooth muscle in general including the myometrium.[56,57] Type II calcium blockers have minimal effect on the cardiac conducting system, and their use results in significant diminution in uterine activity. Of these agents, only nifedipine has been used widely in humans for its tocolytic effect.

The principal hemodynamic effect of nifedipine is a reduction in systemic and pulmonary vascular resistance. As a result, there is a fall in diastolic and mean arterial pressures of approximately 20% associated with a reflex tachycardia.[58] This effect is more prominent in hypertensive than normotensive subjects. There is minimal effect on the venous vessels.[59,60] Hypotension can be reduced by avoiding the sublingual route of administration, which offers little benefit—significant tocolytic action of oral nifedipine is seen in less than 20 minutes.

The combination of nifedipine and magnesium with a goal of increasing tocolytic efficacy has been described. Potentiation of the toxic effects of magnesium has occurred with this regimen, however.[44,61,62] A similar effect has been demonstrated in rats.[63] Nevertheless, extensive experience with magnesium added to chronic nifedipine therapy in hypertensive gravidas suggests that this effect is uncommon.[64] As yet, no adverse cardiovascular effects of isolated nifedipine use for tocolysis have been described. There is no reported experience with the use of nifedipine for tocolysis in the cardiac patient.

A number of oxytocin antagonists with potential for clinical tocolysis have been developed. Atosiban, the only oxytocin antagonist tested in humans, has been shown to lack any significant hemodynamic effects despite its similarity to antidiuretic hormone.[65,66] Such agents may be of value in the treatment of cardiac patients in preterm labor in the future.

EFFECT OF ADJUVANT THERAPIES FOR PRETERM LABOR ON CARDIAC DISEASE

The use of long-acting steroids (betamethasone or dexamethasone) to enhance fetal maturity is now recommended for most patients at risk for preterm delivery,[67] and women with cardiac disease may receive these safely. Although these agents have been associated with the development of pulmonary edema when used in conjunction with β-mimetics, this does not appear to be a significant risk when fluid intake is carefully monitored. They are devoid of mineralocorticoid effect. Yeast reported that there was no effect of steroids on colloid osmotic pressure.[48]

Thyrotropin-releasing hormone (TRH) is being studied for its purported beneficial effect on fetal maturation. Although this benefit is not established at present, some clinicians, encouraged by preliminary favorable reports,[68,69] have begun to use it. In the dosages normally advocated for a fetal effect, the only undesirable effects reported were maternal nausea, vomiting, and flushing. The most recent, and largest report, however, shows no fetal benefit and a transient hypertension more common in the treatment group.[70]

Antenatal vitamin K for patients in preterm labor has been advocated by some authors as a means of reducing neonatal intracranial hemorrhage.[71] Although recent reports have not confirmed a benefit to the fetus,[72] many centers have adopted the use of vitamin K. This practice may pose a problem in institutions where patients with mechanical valve prostheses are managed with Coumadin in the third trimester.[73]

CLINICAL APPROACH

The initial evaluation of the pregnant patient with cardiac disease in preterm labor should not differ from the assessment of other patients except with respect to the common practice of vigorous hydration, which should be avoided in some patients with cardiac disease. Bed rest in the left lateral position and sedation are permitted. If there is any evidence of cardiac deterioration, and other known causes of preterm labor have been ruled out, the cardiac disease should be presumed to be the cause of the preterm uterine activity. Efforts directed at understanding the cause of the deterioration and at stabilizing the patient are more appropriate than specific tocolytic therapy. A complete ultrasound should be performed to be certain that the preterm labor is not related to fetal growth delay or anomaly.

At the present time in our own institution, cardiac patients between 23 and 32 weeks of gestation who display regular uterine contractions, clear evidence of cervical change, no evidence of fetal growth delay, and no other cause for preterm labor are candidates for tocolysis with magnesium sulfate. This form of tocolysis, especially when initiated without bolus, should be tolerated even by most patients with severe disease, including those in whom β-mimetic therapy would be absolutely contraindicated.

From 32 to 35 weeks of gestation, patients with severe cardiac disease and premature labor will generally be managed with bed rest and steroids for pulmonary maturity. Pharmacologic tocolytic therapy is rarely employed, and then only after evidence of pulmonary immaturity had been documented by amniocentesis. Patients with moderate disease may be candidates for tocolysis in this gestational age range after evidence of pulmonary immaturity has been documented.

Second-line therapy for tocolysis is rarely employed under these circumstances. Our preferences would be nifedipine or, in rare circumstances, a short course of indomethacin. Steroids for fetal maturation are employed without consideration to the maternal cardiac status.

REFERENCES

1. Leveno KJ, Cunningham FG. β-Adrenergic agonists for preterm labor. *N Engl J Med* 1992;327:349–351.

2. Kosasa TS, Busse R, Wahl N, Hirata G, Nakamura RT, Hale RW. Long term tocolysis with combined intravenous terbutaline and magnesium sulfate. *Obstet Gynecol* 1994;84:369–373.

3. King JF, Grant A, Kierse MJNC, Chalmers I. Betamimetics in preterm labor: an overview of the randomized controlled trials. *Br J Obstet Gynaecol* 1988;95:211.

4. Creasy R. Preterm labor and delivery. In: Creasy R, Resnick R, eds. *Maternal Fetal Medicine: Principles and Practice*. 3rd ed. Philadelphia: WB Saunders; 1995;503.

5. Utter GO, Dooley SL, Tamura RK, Socol ML. Awaiting cervical change for the diagnosis of preterm labor does not compromise the efficacy of ritodrine tocolysis. *Am J Obstet Gynecol* 1990;163:882.

6. Canadian Preterm Labor Investigators Group. Treatment of preterm labor with the β-adrenergic agonist ritodrine. *N Engl J Med* 1992;327:308.

7. Stark RI, Wardlaw SL, Daniel SS, Husain MK, Sanocka UM, James LS, Vande-Wiele RL. Vasopressin secretion induced by hypoxia in sheep: developmental changes and relationship to β-endorphin release. *Am J Obstet Gynecol* 1982; 143:204.

8. Frederick J, Anderson ABM. Factors associated with spontaneous preterm birth. *Br J Obstet Gynaecol* 1976;83:342–350.

9. Whittemore R, Wells JA, Castellsague X. A second-generation study of 427 probands with congenital heart defects and their 837 children. *J Am College Cardiol* 1994;23:1468–1471.

10. Estrada E, Gonzalez JL, de la Vega A, Adamsons K. Treatment of dysfunctional labor with propranolol. Society for Gynecologic Investigation 38th Annual Meeting; San Antonio, TX: 1991. Abstract 227.

11. Ortho Pharmaceutical market research data; 1994.

12. Norton ME, Merrill J, Cooper BAB, Kuller JA, Clyman RI. Neonatal complications after the administration of indomethacin for preterm labor. *N Engl J Med* 1993; 329:1602–1607.

13. Major CA, Lewis DF, Harding JA, Porto MA, Garite TJ. Tocolysis with indomethacin increases the incidence of necrotizing enterocolitis in the low-birthweight neonate. *Am J Obstet Gynecol* 1994;170: 102–106.

14. Ferguson JE, Dyson DC, Holbrook RH, Schutz TH, Stevenson DK. Cardiovascular and metabolic effects associated with nifedipine and ritodrine tocolysis. *Am J Obstet Gynecol* 1989; 161:788.

15. Wagner JM, Morton MJ, Johnson KA, O'Grady JP, Speroff L. Terbutaline and maternal cardiac function. *JAMA* 1981;246: 2697.

16. Michalak D, Klein V, Marquette GP. Myocardial ischemia: a complication of ritodrine tocolysis. *Am J Obstet Gynecol* 1983;146:861–862.

17. Hendricks SK, Keroes, J, Katz M. Electrocardiographic changes associated with ritodrine-induced maternal tachycardia and hypokalemia. *Am J Obstet Gynecol* 1986;154:921–923.

18. Gerris J, Bracke M, Thiery M, Maele GV. Cardiotoxicity of ritodrine: assessment based on serum creatinine kinase activity. *Z Geburtshilfe Perinatol* 1980;184:25.

19. Hadi HA, Albazzaz SJ. Cardiac isoenzymes and electrocardiographic changes during ritodrine tocolysis. *Am J Obstet Gynecol* 1989;161:318.

20. Donnelly S, McGing P, Sugrue D. Myocardial infarction during pregnancy. *Br J Obstet Gynaecol* 1993;100:781–782.

21. Hankins GDV. Complications of β-sympathomimetic tocolytic agents. In: Clark SL, Cotton DB, Hankins GDV, Phelan JP, eds. *Critical Care Obstetrics*. 2nd ed. Boston: Blackwell Scientific; 1991;231–244.

22. Benedetti TJ, Hargrove JC, Rosene KA. Maternal pulmonary edema during premature labor inhibition. *Obstet Gynecol* 1982;59:33S–37S.

23. Philipsen T, Ericksen PS, Lyngard P. Pulmonary edema following ritodrine–saline infusion in premature labor. *Obstet Gynecol* 1981;58:304–308.

24. Hadi HA, Abdulla AM, Fadel NE, Stefadouros MA, Methen WP. Cardiovascular effects of ritodrine tocolysis: a new noninvasive method to measure pulmonary capillary pressure during pregnancy. *Obstet Gynecol* 1987;70:608–612.

25. Hadi HA, Albazzaz SJ. Measurement of pulmonary capillary pressure during ritodrine tocolysis in twin pregnancies: a new noninvasive technique. *Am J Perinatol* 1993;10:351–353.

26. Dean H, Berliner S, Garfinkel D, Shoenfeld A, Ovadia J, Pinkhas J. Sinus bradycardia following ritodrine withdrawal. *JAMA* 1982;247:1810.

27. Sherer DM, Nawrocki MN, Thompson HO, Woods JR. Type I second-degree AV block (Mobitz type I, Wenckebach AV block) during ritodrine therapy for preterm labor. *Am J Perinatol* 1991;8:150–152.

28. Schneider EP, Jonas E, Tejani N. Detection of cardiac events by continuous electrocardiogram monitoring during ritodrine infusion. *Obstet Gynecol* 1988;71:361–364.

29. Hudgens DR, Conradi SE. Sudden death associated with terbutaline sulfate administration. *Am J Obstet Gynecol* 1993;169: 120–121.

30. McGrath JM, Chestnut DH, Vincent RD, Craig SD, Atkins BL, Poduska DJ, Chaterjee P. Ephedrine remains the vasopressor of choice for treatment of hypotension during ritodrine infusion and epidural anesthesia. *Anesthesiology* 1994;80:1073–1081.

31. Blickstein I, Zalel Y, Katz Z, Lancet M. Ritodrine-induced pulmonary edema unmasking underlying peripartum cardiomyopathy. *Am J Obstet Gynecol* 1988;159:332.

32. Lampert MB, Hibbard J, Weinert L, Briller J, Lindheimer M, Lang RM. Peripartum heart failure associated with prolonged tocolytic therapy. *Am J Obstet Gynecol* 1993;168:493–495.

33. Bloss JD, Hankins GD, Gilstrap LC, Hauth JC. Pulmonary edema as a delayed complication of ritodrine therapy. *J Reprod Med* 1987;32:469–471.

34. Levy DL. Morbidity caused by terbutaline infusion pump therapy. *Am J Obstet Gynecol* 1993;169:1385. Letter.

35. Lam F, Gill P, Smith M, Kitzmiller JL, Katz M. Use of the subcutaneous terbutaline pump for long-term tocolysis. *Obstet Gynecol* 1988;72:810–813.

36. Sala DJ, Moise KJ. The treatment of preterm labor using a portable subcutaneous terbutaline pump. *J Obstet Gynecol Neonat Nurs* 1990;1:108–115.

37. Grospietsch G, Kuhn W. Effects of β mimetics on maternal physiology. In: Fuchs AR, Fuchs F, Stubblefield PG, eds. *Preterm Birth: Causes, Prevention and Management*. (2nd ed.). New York: McGraw Hill; 1993;297–298.

38. Grospietch G. Zusatz btz. Begleittherapie. In: Grospietch G, Kuhn W, eds. *Tokolyse mit Betastimulatoren.* Stuttgart, New York: Thieme; 1983;182.

39. Trolp R, Irmer M. Tocolyse mit einem Betamimetikum bei Wolff–Parkinson–White Syndrom. *Geburtshilfe Frauenheidkd* 1980;40:688.

40. Thiagarajah S, Harbert GM, Bourgeois FJ. Magnesium sulfate and ritodrine hydrochloride: systemic and uterine hemodynamic effects. *Am J Obstet Gynecol* 1985;153:666–674.

41. Bourgeois FJ, Thiagarajah S, Harbert GM, DiFazio C. Profound hypotension complicating magnesium therapy. *Am J Obstet Gynecol* 1986;154:919–920.

42. Winkler AW, Smith PK, Hoff HE. Intravenous magnesium sulfate in the treatment of nephritic convulsions in adults. *J Clin Invest* 1942;21:207–216.

43. Frolich EP. Efficacy of combined administration of magnesium sulfate and ritodrine in the treatment of premature labor. *Obstet Gynecol* 1988;71:283. Letter.

44. Waisman GD, Mayorga LM, Camera MI, Vignolo CA, Martinotti A. Magnesium plus nifedipine: potentiation of hypotensive effect in preeclampsia? *Am J Obstet Gynecol* 1988; 59:308–309.

45. Caritis SN, Edelstone DI, Meuller-Heubach E. Pharmacologic inhibition of preterm labor. *Am J Obstet Gynecol* 1979; 33:557–558.

46. Somjen G, Hilmy M, Stephen CR. Failure to anesthetize human subjects by intravenous administration of magnesium sulfate. *J Pharmacol Exp Ther* 1966;154:652–659.

47. Elliot JP, O'Keefe DF, Greenberg P, Freeman RK. Pulmonary edema associated with magnesium sulfate and betamethasone administration. *Am J Obstet Gynecol* 1979;134:717–719.

48. Yeast, JD, Halberstadt C, Meyer BA, Cohen GR, Thorp JA. The risk of pulmonary edema and colloid osmotic pressure changes during magnesium sulfate infusion. *Am J Obstet Gynecol* 1993;169:1566–1571.

49. Porter KB, O'Brien WF, Kiefert V, Knuppel RA. Evaluation of oxygen desaturation events in singleton pregnancies. *J Perinatol* 1992;12:103–106.

50. Oettinger M, Perlitz Y. Asymptomatic paroxysmal atrial fibrillation during intravenous magnesium sulfate treatment in preeclampsia. *Gynecol Obstet Invest* 1993;36:244–246.

51. Sherer DM, Cialone PR, Abramowicz JS, Woods JR. Transient symptomatic subendocardial ischemia during intravenous magnesium tocolytic therapy. *Am J Obstet Gynecol* 1992;166: 33–35.

52. Spital A, Greenwell R. Severe hyperkalemia during magnesium sulfate therapy in two pregnant drug abusers. *South Med J* 1991;84:919–921.

53. Hess DB, Hess LW, Heath BJ, Lehan PH, McColgin SW, Martin JN Jr. Morrison JC. Pregnancy after Fontan repair of tricuspid atresia. *South Med J* 1991;84: 532–534.

54. Megarian G, Bell JG, Huhta JC, Bottalico JN, Weiner S. Pregnancy outcome following Mustard procedure for transposition of the great arteries: a report of five cases and review of the literature. *Obstet Gynecol* 1994;83:516.

55. Ottman EH, Gall SA. Myocardial infarction in the third trimester of pregnancy secondary to an aortic valve thrombus. *Obstet Gynecol* 1993;81:804–805.

56. Henry P. Comparative pharmacology of calcium antagonists: nifedipine, verapamil, and diltiazem. *Am J Cardiol* 1980;46: 1047–1058.

57. Matsuyama E, Okazaki H. Comparative effects of three calcium antagonists, diltiazem, verapamil and nifedipine on the sinoatrial and atrioventricular nodes: experimental and clinical studies. *Circulation* 1981;63:1035–1042.

58. Schwab MC, Singh BN. Nifedipine: pharmacologic properties and clinical use. *Hosp Forum* 1985;20:85–99.

59. Pirhhonen JP, Erkkola RU, Ekblad UU, Nyman L. Single dose of nifedipine in normotensive pregnancy: nifedipine concentrations, hemodynamic responses, and uterine and fetal flow velocity waveform. *Obstet Gynecol* 1990;76:807–811.

60. Walters BNJ, Redman CWG. Treatment of severe pregnancy-associated hypertension with the calcium antagonist nifedipine. *Br J Obstet Gynaecol* 1984;91:330–336.

61. Ghoneim MM, Long JP. The interaction between magnesium and other neuromuscular blocking agents. *Anesthesiology* 1970;32:33.

62. Snyder SW, Cardwell MD. Neuromuscular blockade with magnesium sulfate and nifedipine. *Am J Obstet Gynecol* 1989;169: 35–36.

63. Thorp JM, Spielman FJ, Valea FA, Payne FG, Meuller RA, Cefalo RC. Nifedipine enhances the cardiotoxicity of magnesium sulfate in the isolated perfused Sprague-Dawley rat heart. *Am J Obstet Gynecol* 1990;163:655–666.

64. Sibai BM, Barton JR, Akl S, Sarinoglu C, Mercer BM. A randomized prospective comparison of nifedipine and bed rest versus bed rest alone in the management of preeclampsia remote from term. *Am J Obstet Gynecol* 1992;167:879–884.

65. Goodwin TM, Paul RH, Silver H, Spellacy W, Parsons M, Chez R, Hayashir R, Valenzuela G, Creasy GW, Merriman R. The effect of the oxytocin antagonist atosiban on preterm uterine activity in the human. *Am J Obstet Gynecol* 1994;170:474–478.

66. Goodwin TM, Millar LM, Abrams LS, Weiglein RC, Holland ML. Pharmacokinetics of atosiban in pregnant women with preterm labor. *Am J Obstet Gynecol* 1995;179:913–917.

67. NIH Consensus Conference. Effect of corticosteroids for fetal maturation on perinatal outcomes. *JAMA* 1995;273:413–417.

68. Ballard RA, Ballard PL, Creasy RK, Padbury J, Polk DH, Bracken M, Moya FR, Gross I. Respiratory disease in very-low-birthweight infants after prenatal thyrotropin-releasing hormone and glucocorticoid. *Lancet* 1992;339:510–515.

69. Knight DB, Liggins GC, Wealthal SR. A randomized, controlled trial of antepartum thyrotropin-releasing hormone and betamethasone in the prevention of respiratory disease in preterm infants. *Am J Obstet Gynecol* 1994;171:11–16.

70. ACTOBAT Study Group. Australian collaborative trial of antenatal thyrotropin-releasing hormone (ACTOBAT) for prevention of neonatal respiratory disease. *Lancet* 1995;345:877–882.

71. Pomerance JJ, Teal JG, Gogolok JF, Browns S, Stewart ME. Maternally administered antenatal vitamin K1: effect on neonatal prothrombin activity, partial thromboplastin time, and intraventricular hemorrhage. *Obstet Gynecol* 1987;70: 235–241.

72. Thorp JA, Ferrete-Smith D, Gaston LA, Johnson J,Yeast JD, Meyer B. Combined antenatal vitamin K and phenobarbital therapy for preventing intracranial hemorrhage in newborns less than 34 weeks' gestation. *Obstet Gynecol* 1995;86:1–8.

73. Iturbe-Alessio I, Fonseca MD, Mutchinik O, Santos MA, Zajarias , Salazar E. Risks of anticoagulant therapy in pregnant women with artificial heart valves. *N Engl J Med* 1986;315:1390–1393.

36

LIPID-LOWERING DRUGS IN PREGNANCY AND LACTATION

JAFNA L. COX, MD, FRCPC

INTRODUCTION

The epidemiological links between plasma cholesterol levels, coronary artery disease, and cardiovascular mortality have been conclusively established in a series of landmark studies over the past four decades.[1–3] Subsequent trials of lipid modification, now too numerous to list, have shown that pharmacological and other interventions can lower lipid levels with corresponding improvements in outcome. Two large and well-publicized trials employing statin drugs for primary[4] and secondary[5] prevention of coronary artery disease are among the most recent of the drug intervention studies. These investigations are particularly impressive in terms of showing significant treatment-related reductions in a variety of adverse cardiovascular end points, including mortality. The prevalence of hyperlipidemia in western society is high. Depending on the lipid level cut-off, as many as 60 million Americans may require educational, dietary, or pharmacological intervention.[6] Accordingly, and in view of the now proven benefit obtainable with lipid reduction, it is anticipated that expanding numbers of patients will be started on lipid lowering drug therapy. Some of these will be women of childbearing potential. This chapter summarizes the available data regarding the use of lipid-lowering drugs in pregnancy and lactation.

BILE ACID SEQUESTRANTS

Cholestyramine and colestipol are insoluble compounds that bind bile acids. As a result, enterohepatic recirculation is in-

terrupted and hepatic receptors of low density Lipoproteins (LDLs) are up-regulated, thereby increasing clearance of LDL–cholesterol.[7,8] Cholestyramine, for instance, results in a 7–25% fall in cholesterol and an 11–36% lowering of LDL-cholesterol,[7,8] and the drug was shown to reduce substantially the incidence of coronary heart disease in the Lipid Research Clinics Coronary Primary Prevention Trial.[9,10] On the other hand, treatment with cholestyramine may be associated with a slight increase in triglycerides by as much as 5% from baseline.[7]

Sequestrants are available as powders to be mixed with liquid or food. Their major side effects are limited to the gastrointestinal tract and include epigastric distress, abdominal bloating, flatulence, and constipation.[7,8] These side effects can be minimized by gradually increasing the dose of drug and by coprescribing a stool softener.[8]

Animal and human studies of cholestyramine in pregnancy have not been performed, largely because the drug is almost totally unabsorbed following oral ingestion.[11] Cholestyramine has been used to treat cholestasis during pregnancy.[12–14] No adverse maternal or fetal effects were noted, and in one study[12] treatment with 9 g daily continued for 12 weeks. There are no animal or human studies of colestipol in pregnancy, and there have been no published reports describing the use of colestipol during pregnancy.[11] However, colestipol has been observed to cross the rat placenta in measurable quantities.[15] Published experience with bile acid sequestrants during lactation is lacking.[11]

The National Cholesterol Education Program guidelines for adults[16] note that bile acid sequestrants may be suitable for treating women considering pregnancy because the agents

Cardiac Problems in Pregnancy, Third Edition
Edited by Uri Elkayam, MD, and Norbert Gleicher, MD
Copyright © 1998 by Wiley-Liss, Inc. ISBN 0-471-16358-9

are not absorbed and lack systemic toxicity. However, Appendix II, "Special Patient and Population Groups," recommends that drug therapy with lipid-lowering agents be discontinued during pregnancy because their effects on the fetus have not been well studied. Furthermore, because fat-soluble vitamins are also bound by the drug, long-term use has the potential of leading to deficiencies in the mother or fetus.[17] Both cholestyramine and colestipol are in the U.S. Food and Drug Administration's pregnancy risk category C.[11,17]

NICOTINIC ACID (NIACIN)

Nicotinic acid works by inhibiting hepatic secretion of lipoproteins. This results in a reduction of cholesterol bound to LDLs and very low density lipoproteins (VLDLs) and an increase in the levels of cholesterol bound to high density lipoproteins (HDLs).[7,8] Although effective and inexpensive, nicotinic acid has numerous subjective side effects that limit its tolerability. Prostaglandin-mediated symptoms include flushing, palpitations, and dizziness. Impaired glucose tolerance, increased blood urate, and hepatotoxicity (especially with extended-release preparations) have been reported, as have gastritis, acanthosis nigricans, and atrial arrhythmias.[7,8] Symptoms may be more pronounced in women.

Animal and human studies of nicotinic acid in pregnancy have not been carried out,[11] and published experience with the drug in human gestation could not be located. According to the product monograph,[18] safety in pregnancy has not been established, although fetal abnormalities have not been reported with its use. High doses are required to achieve lipid lowering, and the appropriate animal reproduction or teratology studies have not been reported. Niacin is distributed in the breast milk, but its effects on the nursing infant have also not been documented.[11,18] The product monograph advises that "appropriate monitoring" be observed if nicotinic acid is to be used during pregnancy, especially during initiation of therapy. However, given the lack of data, and the possibility of potent maternal side effects, the drug is probably best avoided during pregnancy. Nicotinic acid is an FDA pregnancy risk category C drug.[11]

INHIBITORS OF 3-HYDROXY-3-METHYLGLUTARYL COENZYME A (HMG CoA) REDUCTASE

The HMG CoA reductase inhibitors are a class of drugs highly effective in lowering total and LDL-cholesterol, with relatively few side effects.[19] The mechanism of action involves inhibition of the enzyme 3-hydroxy-3-methylglutaryl coenzyme A reductase in the liver, resulting in up-regulation of LDL receptors on the hepatocyte and a consequent increase in clearance of LDL particles.[19,20] HMG CoA reductase inhibitors recently were shown to reduce mortality and coronary events when used for both primary[4] prevention in men and secondary prevention in men and women.[5] Total cholesterol levels are lowered by as much as 30%, with 20–40% reductions in LDL-cholesterol and 10–20% reductions in triglycerides. Levels of HDL-cholesterol may be increased by 10% above baseline.[7,8,19,20] The most commonly used drugs in this class are lovastatin, pravastatin, simvastatin, and fluvastatin.

Side effects are few, although gastrointestinal symptoms (e.g., abdominal discomfort, nausea, diarrhea, constipation, flatulence) may lead to drug withdrawal. Headaches, fatigue, insomnia, musculoskeletal pain, and rash are infrequent but documented associations. Liver damage has been reported with a 0.1–1.5% incidence that is dose dependent, and liver enzymes should therefore be followed. Myopathy is rare, occurring more frequently during cotherapy with nicotinic acid or fibrates, with cyclosporin in transplant patients, and with participation in severe exercise.[7,8,19,20]

Because products of the cholesterol biosynthesis pathway are essential to fetal development (e.g., in the synthesis of steroids and cell membranes), HMG CoA reductase inhibitors should be avoided during pregnancy. No evidence for mutagenicity was found in experimental studies assessing lovastatin, pravastatin, or simvastatin.[11,19] However, animal studies are difficult to interpret because of marked species differences in drug pharmacokinetics and sensitivities. For instance, both rabbits and dogs are extremely sensitive to the pharmacological action of these compounds.[19,20]

Lovastatin has been shown to produce skeletal malformations in mice at plasma levels 40 times the recommended maximum human exposure, and in rats at 80 times the recommended maximum dose.[21] No evidence of teratogenesis was documented in rabbits receiving up to 3 times the recommended maximum human dose.[21] In preclinical studies, pravastatin was not teratogenic in rats receiving 240 times, and rabbits 20 times, the recommended maximum human dose.[22] Simvastatin did not induce teratogenicity in rats or rabbits given 6 or 4 times, respectively, the maximum recommended daily dose in humans.[11] Tse and Labbadia[23] used a multiple oral dosing regimen of 1 mg/kg/day of fluvastatin in pregnant rabbits, beginning on the sixth day following conception. Steady state drug concentrations were achieved in the mothers after 5 days, at which time the amount of fluvastatin detectable in the reproductive organs was 25–50% of maternal blood levels. The fetus/placenta and amniotic fluid/placenta concentration ratios declined from 0.92 and 0.97, respectively, on the tenth day postconception to 0.10 and 0.04, respectively, only 8 days later. These results suggest that at least in the rabbit, transplacental transfer of fluvastatin and its metabolites is limited at later stages of pregnancy. No tissue retention of drug was documented. Hrab et al[24] administered fluvastatin orally to mated rats from day 15 of gestation through weaning. In three separate studies, using doses of 12 and 24 mg/kg/day, the authors noted unanticipated maternal mortality, apparently due to cardiomyopathy, at the time of parturition and during lactation. An increase in stillborn pups and neonatal mortality was also documented. All adverse effects, including mortality, were completely blocked following supplementation with mevalonic acid, suggesting that the adverse maternal effects resulted from exaggerated pharmacological activity at the dose levels administered.

The single published report describing the use of lovastatin in a human pregnancy[25] involved a woman who took lovastatin (10 mg/day) and dextroamphetamine sulfate during the first trimester of pregnancy. Therapy had been started approximately 6 weeks from her last menstrual period for progressive weight gain and hypercholesterolemia, and was continued until pregnancy was diagnosed at 11 weeks of gestation. A female infant was delivered by cesarean section at 39 weeks with a constellation of abnormalities known as the VATER association (**v**ertebral anomalies, **a**nal atresia, **t**racheoesophageal fistula, and **r**enal and radial dysplasia). Chromosome analysis was normal, the family history noncontributory, and the cause of the defects otherwise unknown, although the possibility of drug-induced teratogenesis must be considered.

Unpublished information is available from the Health Protection Branch in Ottawa, Canada, regarding four pregnancies involving exposure to lovastatin that proceeded to a natural outcome (E. Pregent, personal communication, Merck Frosst Canada, 1995). Six other pregnancies have been reported during which lovastatin was taken by the mother, but all were terminated for a variety of reasons.

A 37-year-old female with diabetes mellitus was treated with lovastatin (20 mg daily) for hypercholesterolemia. Concomitant medication included methyldopa, gemfibrozil, captopril, ferrous sulfate, hydrocodone, cephalexin, ibuprofen (both Nuprin and Advil), phenylephrin HCl–chloropheniramine maleate–acetaminophen (Dristan), acetaminophen, and hydralalzine hydrochloride. The patient conceived while on therapy, and the lovastatin was discontinued when she was at least 7 weeks pregnant. The patient spontaneously aborted 4 weeks later.

A 41-year-old female was placed on lovastatin (20 mg daily) for the treatment of diet-resistant hypercholesterolemia. Concomitant medications included fluoxetine (Prozac), levothyroxine sodium, propranolol, and clonidine. The patient had been receiving lovastatin for 7 months when a positive pregnancy test led to the stoppage of the drug. Labor was induced at 9 months because of maternal hypertension, and a normal female infant was delivered by cesarean section.

A 42-year-old woman was placed on lovastatin (dosage and duration not reported) prior to conception. She subsequently delivered a stillborn baby. Death was due to fetal asphyxia subsequent to strangulation by the umbilical cord.

Tests confirmed the absence of genetic abnormalities.

In the final case, a 22-year-old woman with hirsutism was receiving lovastatin (40 mg daily). She conceived while on treatment, but the drug was discontinued at the fifth week of pregnancy. The patient delivered a newborn who initially did well (Apgar scores, 8/9; birth weight, 3400 g), although signs of heart failure manifested at 2 days postpartum. Investigations revealed aortic hypoplasia, atrial and ventricular defects, and secondary cerebral dysfunction. The newborn subsequently developed a urinary tract infection that was treated with sulfa. Because the infant was judged to be high risk, surgery was not performed, and death occurred at 4 weeks of age. The reporting physician did not feel that the neonatal outcome was related to therapy with lovastatin; an autopsy was not performed, however.

A recent review of the Bristol-Myers Squibb worldwide safety database identified 16 cases of women exposed to pravastatin during pregnancy (R. Ouellet, personal communication, Bristol-Myers Squibb, 1995). Seven of these were exposed during the first trimester, and all delivered healthy term infants. No information was available in five women who discontinued pravastatin when pregnancy was confirmed, and no data were available for the other four women.

There are no published data on the use of simvastatin in pregnancy,[26] and no cases of inadvertent exposure to the drug during pregnancy have been reported to the manufacturer (E. Pregent, personal communication, Merck Frosst Canada Inc., 1995).

During the clinical program evaluating fluvastatin, five women receiving the drug became pregnant and were discontinued from further study.[27] Two of these women gave birth to healthy babies; one experienced an ectopic pregnancy, which was ascribed to a scarred fallopian tube, and a fourth spontaneously aborted. The outcome of the fifth is unknown.

There is no published experience regarding the use of any of the HMG CoA reductase inhibitors during human lactation. Lovastatin,[21] pravastatin,[22] and fluvastatin[27] are known to pass into breast milk. It is not known whether simvastatin crosses into the breast milk.[26] All HMG CoA reductase inhibitors are assigned an FDA category X risk in pregnancy,[11] and all product manufacturers specify that the drugs are contraindicated in pregnancy and lactation.

THE FIBRATES

Fibrates reduce blood cholesterol less effectively than either nicotinic acid or the HMG CoA reductase inhibitors.[7,8,28] In the Helsinki Heart Study, gemfibrozil occasioned an 11% decrease in LDL-cholesterol levels and an 11% increase in HDL-cholesterol levels.[29] However, fibrates are very effective in managing type III lipidemia and are front-line therapy in reducing the risk of pancreatitis in patients with very high plasma triglyceride levels.[7,8] These drugs exert their effect largely by stimulating lipoprotein lipase, the enzyme responsible for the catabolism of triglyceride-rich particles. Nonsplanchnic clearance of VLDL from plasma is accelerated. Because fibrates increase cholesterol secretion into bile, there is a resultant increase in bile lithogenicity that enhances the risk of gallbladder disease.[8] Clofibrate was associated with an increased noncardiovascular mortality in a study conducted by the World Health Organization,[30] whereas in the Helsinki Heart Study,[29] gemfibrozil resulted in a 34% reduction in cardiovascular events, though without effect on overall mortality. As a consequence, gemfibrozil is the preferred agent.

Side effects are predominantly gastrointestinal and include nausea, abdominal discomfort, cholelithiasis, and cholecystitis. In addition, weight gain, myositis, drowsiness, decreased libido, and ventricular arrhythmia have all been reported.[7,8] Because the fibrates displace warfarin from albumin, warfarin dose may need to be readjusted.

Gemfibrozil has been associated with adverse effects in rats and rabbits at doses ranging between 0.5 and 3 times the maximum recommended human dose, but no developmental toxicity or teratogenicity was observed among the offspring of either species.[31] Rats exposed to 0.6 and 2 times the maximum recommended human dose before and throughout gestation experienced a dose-related reduction in conception rate and, at the higher dose, an increase in stillborns and a reduction in pup weight during lactation.[31] A dose-related increase in the incidence of skeletal variations among the offspring was also noted, including anophthalmia. Rats exposed to 0.6–2 times the maximum recommended human dose from gestation day 15 through weaning experienced dose-related decreases in birth weights and suppression of pup growth during lactation.[31] Rabbits receiving 1–3 times the maximum recommended human dose during organogenesis had a dose-related decrease in litter size and, at the high dose, an increased incidence of parietal bone variations.[31]

Studies of gemfibrozil in humans are lacking, but three unpublished cases of gemfibrozil use in pregnancy were submitted to the Parke-Davis Worldwide Adverse Experience Report Service between 1982 and 1995 (P. Suleman, Parke-Davis Canada, 1995). The first report involved a 36-year-old woman who was taking gemfibrozil (amount not specified) 6 months prior to conception and continued taking the drug for the first 2 months of pregnancy. She was being treated concurrently with clomiphene. The patient went into premature labor (time of gestation unspecified) and delivered an infant with Pierre Robin syndrome (micrognathia and abnormal smallness of the tongue, often with cleft palate, and often with bilateral eye defects including high myopia, congenital glaucoma, and retinal detachment) and patent ductus arteriosus. The child's father also had suffered Pierre Robin syndrome at birth. A second patient (no age given) inadvertently took 1200 mg of gemfibrozil for one day during her pregnancy (timing not stated), and the outcome was unknown. The third patient (no age given) took gemfibrozil (amount not stated) for an unspecified period before conception and into early pregnancy (duration not given). A healthy baby was delivered (length of gestation and birth weight not available).

It is not known whether gemfibrozil crosses into breast milk. Since, however, gemfibrozil has been shown to have tumorigenic potential in animal studies,[11] its use should be avoided by nursing mothers. Gemfibrozil is an FDA pregnancy risk category C drug.[11]

SUMMARY

Because cholesterol is a fundamental constituent of hormones and cell membranes, theoretical concerns have been raised regarding the sequelae to the developing fetus of altering cholesterol synthesis in the mother. Drugs such as the HMG CoA reductase inhibitors and the fibrates should be avoided during gestation on this basis alone. The lack of experience with these compounds during pregnancy and lactation, and the potential for adverse effects as suggested by the case reports described above, are further compelling reasons not to use them. Nicotinic acid should similarly be avoided. In general, these lipid-lowering agents should not be administered to women of childbearing age unless they are highly unlikely to conceive. In the event that a woman becomes pregnant while taking these drugs, therapy should cease immediately, and the patient should be apprised of the potential risks to the fetus. The bile acid sequestrants are not absorbed and so would not be expected to affect the fetus or nursing neonate. Nevertheless, because the effect on the fetus of lipid lowering in general during gestation has not been adequately studied, and the specific effects of these pharmacological agents in this setting are largely unknown, they should preferentially be discontinued during pregnancy as well. The potential for bile acid sequestrants to produce deficiencies in fat-soluble vitamins in both the mother and her fetus provides a further argument against their use.

Most experts recommend dietary measures as opposed to drugs for the management of lipid abnormalities in pregnant women. Indeed, because atherosclerosis is a chronic process, discontinuation of lipid-lowering drugs during pregnancy should have little impact on the outcome of long-term therapy of primary hypercholesterolemia in most instances.

REFERENCES

1. Keys A. *Seven Countries: A Multivariate Analysis of Death and Coronary Heart Disease.* Cambridge, MA: Harvard University Press; 1980.

2. Castelli WP, Garrison RJ, Wilson PWF, Abbott RD, Kalousdian S, Kannel WB. Incidence of coronary heart disease and lipoprotein cholesterol levels: the Framingham study. *JAMA* 1986;256:2835–2838.

3. Martin MJ, Hulley SB, Browner WS, Kuller LH, Wentworth D. Serum cholesterol, blood pressure, and mortality: implications from a cohort of 361,662 men. *Lancet* 1986;ii:933–936.

4. Shepherd J, Cobbe SM, Ford I, Isles CG, Lorimer AR, MacFarlane PW, McKillop JH, Packard CJ. Prevention of coronary heart disease with pravastatin in men with hypercholesterolemia. *N Engl J Med* 1995;333:1301–1307.

5. Scandinavian Simvastatin Survival Study Group. Randomised trial of cholesterol lowering in 4444 patients with coronary heart disease: the Scandinavian Simvastatin Survival Study (4S). *Lancet* 1994;344:1383–1389.

6. Sempos C, Fulwood R, Haines C, Carroll M, Anda R, Williamson DF, Remington P, Cleeman J. The prevalence of high blood cholesterol levels among adults in the United States. *JAMA* 1989;262:45–52.

7. Opie LH, Frishman WH. Lipid-lowering and antiatherosclerotic drugs. In Opie LH, ed. *Drugs for the Heart.* 4th ed. Philadelphia: WB Saunders; 1995;288–307.

8. Blum CB, Levy RI. Current therapy for hypercholesterolemia. *JAMA* 1989;261:3582–3587.

9. Lipid Research Clinics Program. The Lipid Research Clinics Coronary Primary Prevention Trial Results. I. Reduction in incidence of coronary heart disease. *JAMA* 1984;251:351–364.

10. Lipid Research Clinics Program. The Lipid Research Clinics Coronary Primary Prevention Trial Results. II. The relationship of reduction in incidence of coronary heart disease to cholesterol lowering. *JAMA* 1984;251:365–374.

11. U.S. Pharmacopoeial Convention. *Drug Information for the Health Care Professional, 1A, 1B.* 15th ed. Rockville, MD: USP DI; 1995.

12. Lutz EE, Margolis AJ. Obstetric hepatosis: treatment with cholestyramine and interim response to steroids. *Obstet Gynecol* 1969;33:64–71.

13. Heikkinen J, Maentausta, O, Ylostalo P, Janne O. Serum bile acid levels in intrahepatic cholestasis of pregnancy during treatment with phenobarbital or cholestyramine. *Eur J Obstet Gynecol Reprod Biol* 1982;14:153–162.

14. Shaw D, Frohlich J, Wittman BAK, Willms M. A prospective study of 18 patients with cholestasis of pregnancy. *Am J Obstet Gynecol* 1982;142(6 Pt 1):621–625.

15. Chabra S, Kurup CKR. Maternal transport of chlorophenoxyisobutyrate at the foetal and neonatal stages of development. *Biochem Pharmacol* 1978;27:2063–2065.

16. The Expert Panel. Report of the National Cholesterol Education Program Expert Panel on Detection, Evaluation, and Treatment of High Blood Cholesterol in Adults. *Arch Intern Med* 1988;148:36–69.

17. Briggs GG, Freeman RK, Yaffe SJ. *Drugs in Pregnancy and Lactation.* 4th ed. Baltimore, MD: William & Wilkins; 1994.

18. Krogh CME, ed. *CPS. Compendium of Pharmaceuticals and Specialties.* 30th ed. Ottawa: Canadian Pharmaceutical Association; 1995;886–887.

19. Davignon J, Montigny M, Dufour R. HMG-CoA reductase inhibitors: a look back and a look ahead. *Can J Cardiol* 1992;8: 843–864.

20. Slater EE, MacDonald JS. Mechanism of action and biological profile of HMG CoA reductase inhibitors: a new therapeutic alternative. *Drugs* 1988;36(suppl 3):72–82.

21. Mevacor. Product monograph. Merck Frosst Canada Inc.; 1995.

22. Pravachol. Product monograph. Bristol-Myers Squibb Canada; 1995.

23. Tse FLS, Labbadia D. Absorption and disposition of fluvastatin, an inhibitor of HMG-CoA reductase, in the rabbit. *Biopharm Drug Disposition* 1992;13:285–294.

24. Hrab RV, Hartman HA, Cox RH Jr. Prevention of fluvastatin-induced toxicity, mortality, and cardiac myopathy in pregnant rats by mevalonic acid supplementation. *Teratology* 1994;50: 19–26.

25. Ghidini A, Sichere S, Willner J. Congenital abnormalities (VATER) in baby born to mother using lovastatin. *Lancet* 1992;339:1416–1417.

26. Zocor. Product monograph. Merck Frosst Canada Inc.; 1995.

27. Lescol. Product monograph. Sandoz Canada Inc.; 1995.

28. Lupien PJ, Brun D, Gagné C, Moorjani S, Bielman P, Julien P. Gemfibrozil therapy in primary type II hyperlipoproteinemia: effects on lipids, lipoproteins and apolipoproteins. *Can J Cardiol* 1991;7:27–33.

29. Frick MH, Elo O, Haapa K, Heinonen OP, Heinsalmi P, Helo P, Huttunen JK, Kaitaniemi P, Koskinen P, Manninen V, Maenpaa H, Malkonen M, Manttari M, Norola S, Pasternack A, Pikkarainen J, Romo M, Sjoblom T, Nikkila EA. Helsinki Heart Study: primary-prevention trial with gemfibrozil in middle-aged men with dyslipidemia. *N Engl J Med* 1987;317:1237–1245.

30. Committee of Principal Investigators. WHO Cooperative Trial on Primary Prevention of Ischemic Heart Disease with Clofibrate to Lower Serum Cholesterol: Final Mortality Follow-Up. *Lancet* 1984;2:600–604.

31. Lopid. Product monograph. Parke-Davis; 1995.

PART VII

PREGNANCY PREVENTION IN THE CARDIAC PATIENT

37

FERTILITY CONTROL IN THE CARDIAC PATIENT

SIRI LINDA KJOS, MD

INTRODUCTION

While atherosclerotic heart disease is the leading cause of death in women, it remains relatively uncommon during the reproductive years. Rheumatic heart disease has declined with advent of penicillin, while children with congenital heart disease have matured into adulthood as a result of new techniques in cardiac surgery. These advances have changed the composition of the population of cardiac patients facing reproductive decisions, shifting it from those with acquired to those with congenital disease. Currently, over 70% of individuals with congenital heart disease survive into the third decade of life.[1] Not uncommonly, young women with congenital heart disease must face difficult reproductive choices, often with sparse solid information and many misconceptions. Often they are denied any effective contraceptive method secondary to a perceived increased risk of infectious, thromboembolic, or vascular complications attributable to the use of the contraceptive. Although research and educational efforts in this area have been limited, current evidence suggests that women with cardiac lesions may have several options for contraception. Paradoxically, pregnancy often carries a definitive risk of both maternal and infant mortality. Furthermore, planning a pregnancy to coincide with a period of optimum cardiac function and patient health should be a goal of the patient and her medical team. It is a goal that can be accomplished only by employing effective contraception.

Advances in contraceptive technology offer the woman with congenital or acquired cardiac disease many options. Contraceptive morbidity has been reduced: Low dose combination and progestin-only oral contraceptives have decreased the risk of thrombosis and embolism; the copper-medicated intrauterine devices have reduced failure rates and infection; and metabolic side effects have been decreased by the development of new long-acting progestin subdermal implants, the less androgenic "new progestins," and the lower dose oral contraceptives. Although more prospective contraceptive studies in women with cardiac disease are needed, the practitioner can be reassured that for most cardiac patients an effective and acceptable contraception can be prescribed. The goal of this chapter is to address these issues, enabling the physician to develop individually tailored contraceptive programs to meet the changing needs and demands during the reproductive epoch of a woman with cardiac disease.

COUNSELING: PLANNING AND PREVENTING PREGNANCY

Honest and open discussions regarding pregnancy planning and prevention should begin as a young woman with cardiac disease enters the menarche or, if already in this epoch, as soon as her cardiac condition becomes apparent. In a study of youth with congenital heart disease, the majority had questions about their reproductive potential and their risk of having a child with congenital heart disease.[2] Another survey of young adults with congenital heart disease revealed that 60% had little or no information about their ability to conceive, bear children, or use contraception. Several respondents noted their physicians' reluctance to prescribe oral contraceptives, and others believed they should never get pregnant.[3]

Preconception counseling should be an ongoing discussion between the patient and her physicians. Current factual data should be presented to address her pregnancy risk, including her risk of mortality, serious morbidity, and the pos-

Cardiac Problems in Pregnancy, Third Edition
Edited by Uri Elkayam, MD, and Norbert Gleicher, MD
Copyright © 1998 by Wiley-Liss, Inc. ISBN 0-471-16358-9

sibility of prolonged hospitalization. Discussion of neonatal risk should include any teratogenic or adverse effects of medicinal therapy, the risk of prematurity or fetal loss, and the risk of congenital heart disease of the newborn. The optimal timing of a pregnancy planned on the basis of social and medical reasons should be discussed. Serious questions must be openly addressed with facts and options. Would reparative surgery be best performed prior to pregnancy? Would a worsening prognosis of a woman's cardiac status limit her functional reproductive life span? Medically speaking, when would the optimal time for pregnancy be? Does this time coincide with the patient's personal life with respect to her partner, education, and goals? Ideally, the pregnancy should be timed for the patient to be at her cardiac optimum, controlled by medications that can be safely continued through pregnancy. To achieve this timing, an effective contraception regimen that poses the least risk should be chosen. Our role as physicians is to present the best possible factual data concerning a patient's pregnancy prognosis and contraceptive options, to enable her and her family to make an informed decision about childbearing. Seeking consultation with specialists experienced in caring for cardiac disease during pregnancy should be encouraged to provide a current and accurate risk assessment.

CONTRACEPTIVE OPTIONS

Coital-Dependent Methods

Periodic Abstinence (Rhythm) Method. Religious or personal beliefs may permit only rhythm or periodic abstinence, where intercourse is avoided around the period of ovulation. Success requires regular and predictable cycles, patient understanding and recognition of the ovulatory period, and, most importantly, a motivated couple committed to periods of abstinence. When periodic abstinence is the only acceptable contraceptive method, a patient's choice should be supported with proper education and encouragement. Methods such as daily recording of basal body temperature, change in quality of cervical mucus, or the results of urine hormonal testing should be used to identify and avoid intercourse during the ovulatory period.[4] The lowest reported first-year failure rates range from 10.5 to 14.4%,[5] making this a less desirable method for women who may be placed at considerable medical risk by an unwanted pregnancy.

Barrier Methods. Barrier methods, which create mechanical and/or chemical barriers to fertilization, include diaphragms, male and female condoms, spermicidal jelly or foam, contraceptive sponges (no longer marketed in the United States), and cervical caps. None of these methods produce metabolic alterations; thus no contraindications to their use in cardiac patients exist. All these methods are user dependent, requiring correct application or insertion before coitus.

This property accounts for their high first-year failure rates with actual use, 12–28%.[5] With experience and motivation, these failure rates can be substantially reduced (2–6%), but they remain well above that of experienced users of oral contraceptives (0.1–0.5%), long-acting progestins (0.04–0.4%), and intrauterine devices (0.8–2.0%).[5] Proper and explicit education detailing the use of barrier methods is required to reduce the failure rate. Condoms should be used in conjunction with spermicide to reduce the failure rate. Patient and partner behavior and their sexual behavior may need to be modified to comfortably integrate the use of barrier methods.

Although barrier methods and periodic abstinence do not require refills and medical supervision, the physician must continue to inquire at each visit whether the patient is compliant and satisfied with her method. Because these methods have a higher failure rate, the symptoms of pregnancy should be reviewed. If the patient misses a period, she should be instructed to seek immediate medical care. Prompt care becomes of paramount importance in cases of the patients who require therapy with possibly teratogenic medication such as warfarin. Warfarin embryopathy occurs in 29% of infants exposed between the 6th and 12th weeks of gestation.[6]

Hormonal Contraception

Hormonal contraceptives contain a synthetic formulation of a progestin alone or in combination with an estrogen, the latter being found only in oral contraceptives. Progestin-only contraceptives are delivered via many routes: orally or intramuscularly, subcutaneously (as an implant), or directly into the uterine cavity (via an intrauterine device). The metabolic impact is influenced not only by the delivery route but also by the dosage and hormonal potency of the various formulations. Metabolic effects of synthetic steroids are characterized as estrogenic, androgenic, or progestogenic, with combination oral contraceptives often counterbalancing estrogenic and androgenic effects. Understanding of these metabolic effects allows the proper selection to meet the specific needs with respect to a patient's cardiac status and to her lifestyle.

Oral Contraceptives (OCs)

Estrogen in OCs   During the last 30 years, the estrogen and progestin dosage in combination oral contraceptives has been reduced 5– and 25–fold, respectively, reducing the morbidity and side effects while retaining the pregnancy protection. The term "low dose" generally refers to the estrogen component in combination formulations, which contain less than 0.050 mg of ethinyl estradiol (EE_2) or its methylated derivative, mestranol. Higher dose estrogen OCs (0.050 mg or higher) are inappropriate for prescription in most patients and should be prescribed only when a higher estrogen dose is indicated. Progestin-only OCs have very low progestin dose and are referred to as "minipills." Metabolic effects from

OCs that if improperly selected and poorly monitored could adversely effect cardiac disease include thromboembolism, hypertension, fluid and water retention, and hyperlipidemia. Since these effects are dose and potency dependent, special consideration should be given to the individual patient's specific cardiac lesion. In general, the first question to be addressed is whether there are contraindications to an estrogen-containing OC preparation, which has the advantage of a lower failure rate compared with progestin-only OCs (0.1 vs 0.5% failure rate per year with perfect use).[5]

Progestins in OCs   The formulations of progestin contained in combination OCs are 19-nortestosterone derivatives, and they vary widely in their dosage and androgenic and progestational potency. Norethindrone (NET) and its two derivatives, ethynodiol diacetate (ED) and norethindrone acetate, which are metabolized to northindrone, have equivalent biological effects per dose. Levonorgestrel (LNG) is 10–20 times more potent and more androgenic than the norethindrones and is marketed in a lower dose.[7] The new "third-generation" progestins are derivatives of LNG and are widely used in Europe. Two of these, norgestimate and desogestrel, have recently become available in the United States; both are metabolized to LNG. The third, gestodene, has yet to reach the United States market and is active in its original form. The new progestins offer the advantage of a higher reported progestin activity and decreased androgenic activity.[8,9] The low dose NET preparation (≤0.50 mg), the least androgenic of the "old" progestins, exhibits minimal androgenic effects.[10] While the "third-generation" progestins look promising, further study is necessary comparing their efficacy with the existing progestins using low progestin dose formulations.

Progestin-Only OCs   The progestin-only "minipill" provides an invaluable option for women who have contraindications (e.g., hypertension, thrombosis) to the estrogen component of OCs. The minipill can also be prescribed to nursing women. The two preparations available, one with NET (0.35 mg/day) and the other with LNG (0.075 mg/day) have a lower mean daily dose of progestin than is found in any of the combination OCs.

Hormonal methods act primarily to inhibit the midcycle gonadotrophin surge, preventing ovulation. Additionally, they retard conception by alterations in the composition of the cervical mucus, in the motility of the uterus and oviduct, and in the endometrial lining, which together results in decreased sperm penetration, fertilization, and implantation.

Metabolic Effects of Oral Contraceptives

HYPERCOAGULABILITY   In older preparations, a higher estrogen dosage was found to be associated with increased venous and arterial thromboembolic complications, including myocardial infarction, cerebrovascular accidents, deep venous thrombosis, and pulmonary embolism.[11,12] The increased risk for embolic complications has been attributed to the estrogen component of OCs, which produces a dose-dependent increase in hepatic globulin production of factors VII and X. Recent large prospective population studies, using current low dose estrogen preparations, demonstrated no increased risk of myocardial infarction, pulmonary embolism, or cerebral vascular accident.[13–15]

HYPERTENSION   Another hepatic globulin elevated in dose-dependent fashion by estrogen is angiotensinogen. Even a mild, but not usually clinically significant rise in blood pressure is seen with the low dose EE_2 preparations (0.030–0.040 mg).[16] No hypertensive effect was seen in the women using the two progestin-only preparations (NET 0.35 mg, LNG 0.075 mg) during the 2-year study. In women with cardiac disease, selecting a combination OC containing estrogen over a progestin-only method should take into consideration the increase in blood pressure and coagulability.

CARBOHYDRATE METABOLISM   Synthetic estrogens are neutral with respect to their effect on glucose tolerance. A 10-fold increase in dose of ethinyl estradiol does not affect glucose tolerance.[17] Conversely, progestins decrease glucose tolerance, by promoting increased insulin resistance and secretion in a dose-dependent fashion.[18] A large prospective study found a proportional increase in serum glucose levels with increased doses of progestins: each 1 mg increase in NET, NET acetate, or ED dose was associated with a 5–10 mg/dL increase in 1- and 2-hour serum glucose levels of a glucose tolerance test (OGTT), while each 1 mg increase in NG and LNG dose was associated with an 18–35 mg/dL increase.[19] In muscle and adipose cells, progestins exert a contrainsulin effect, increasing peripheral insulin resistance, while in the liver they appear to promote glycogen storage, an insulin-like effect. Estrogens, in turn oppose the peripheral action of progesterone and increase insulin sensitivity in muscle and adipose cells. When prescribed in combination, the net effect on carbohydrate metabolism appears to depend on the molar concentration ratio of estrogen to progestin.[20] Today's low dose combination OCs, whether containing the new progestins or the older preparations in lower dosages, tend to be estrogen dominant in their metabolic effect. They have been shown to have minimal effect on glucose tolerance, serum insulin, or glucagon levels in healthy women.[8,18,21–25]

LIPID METABOLISM   Estrogen exerts favorable changes on serum lipids, increasing high density lipoprotein cholesterol (HDL-C) and decreasing low-density lipoprotein cholesterol (LDL-C).[26] It also increases serum total triglycerides, an effect of uncertain cardiovascular risk in women. Conversely, progestins exhibit an adverse dose-dependent effect on serum lipid levels, increasing LDL-C and decreasing HDL-

C.[26] Adverse lipid changes have been associated with increased cardiovascular risk and atherosclerosis, a factor of critical importance in women with atherosclerotic cardiac disease. In combination OCs, estrogen counterbalances this effect by favorably altering the lipid levels. Whether today's combination OCs, whether containing low progestin doses (<1.0 mg NET or <0.100 mg LNG mean daily dose) or less androgenic new progestins, the current low dose estrogen/progestin formulation, they are largely estrogen dominant in their metabolic effect. Recent prospective studies in healthy women using these formulations have not found adverse changes in HDL-C or LDL-C, or ratios of total cholesterol to HDL-cholesterol. Only the more androgenic progestin, LNG in a triphasic preparation, has been shown to lower HDL_2 compared with the norethindrone, gestodene, or desogestrel formulations.[9,27,28] These findings have been confirmed in a large cross-sectional study examining women using seven different low estrogen dose (0.030–0.040 mg EE_2) formulations, but with varying progestin doses and types, in contrast to women using no hormonal contraception.[10] Women using combination OCs with the two least potent, lower dose progestins, NET (0.5 mg) and desogestrel, respectively, had a 12 and 14% reduction in LDL-C levels and a 10 and 12% increase in HDL-C levels compared to controls. In contrast, women using the more potent, higher dose LNG combinations of 0.150 and 0.250, had a 5 and 16% decrease in HDL-C levels, as a result of a 29% and 43% reduction in the HDL_2 subclass. Finally, women using progestin-only "minipills" (0.35 mg) also demonstrated no adverse lipid changes.

CARDIOVASCULAR DISEASE   The possibility of exacerbating any existing risk of cardiovascular disease is a major concern for physicians contemplating the prescription of OCs to women with heart disease. The increased risk of myocardial infarction, which was reported in older studies using high estrogen dose OCs, was demonstrated to be related to increased venous and arterial thrombosis.[29,30] Accelerated atherosclerosis with OC use has never been demonstrated in either primate[31] or human studies, nor has any increased risk of myocardial infarction been shown in former OC users.[32] In large prospective cohort studies of healthy OC users, no increased risk of cardiovascular disease in current[33,34] or prior[35] oral contraceptive use has been demonstrated.

Long-Acting Progestins   Two preparations, depo-medroxy-progesterone acetate (DMPA) and Norplant are currently available in the United States. Their sustained release of a progestin inhibits ovulation. Thus their contraceptive mechanism is similar to that of OCs with the advantage of not requiring daily administration.

Injectables   Since injectable contraceptives became available in the 1960s, they have been used widely throughout the world. Only recently, after the lack of association between

DMPA and breast cancer[36] was clearly demonstrated, was DMPA approved for use in the United States. Norethisterone enanthate, another widely prescribed injectable progestin, is not available in the United States. DMPA is administered every 3 months in a 150 mg dose and has one of the lowest contraceptive failure rates (0.3%).[5] Its contraceptive effect generally lasts up toward 4 months, providing a safety window for the patient tardy in keeping her 3-month appointment. After discontinuation of usage, there may be a prolonged delay in return of menses and fertility, making DMPA a less desirable method in women planning to conceive in the near future. Weight gain and irregular menses, from intermenstrual spotting to amenorrhea, are common side effects. More commonly, amenorrhea develops after prolonged use. Patients should be counseled prior to prescription and reassured that DMPA-associated menstrual irregularities are not harmful.

METABOLIC EFFECTS OF DMPA   Since it does not contain estrogen, DMPA does not increase liver globulin production, and thus clotting factors or angiotensinogen do not increase. Nor has this agent been associated with increased blood pressure,[37,38] thromboembolism, or clotting factors.[39] Healthy women using DMPA do exhibit a deterioration in glucose tolerance that is statistically significant, but not clinically significant (i.e., the OGTT values remained well within the normal range).[38,39] The effect of DMPA on serum lipids appears to be relatively minor,[40] with some investigators reporting lowered HDL-C levels but not LDL-C levels,[40,41] and others reporting increased LDL-C.[39] As used for contraception, DMPA is a relatively high dose progestin.

Implants   Currently, only one implantable progestin, Norplant, is available. In the near future, new implants not requiring surgical removal should be available. Current studies are under way testing a biodegradable, 1-year implant of a LNG preparation. Norplant, a subcutaneous implant of six Silastic capsules containing LNG, provides excellent pregnancy protection for up to 5 years by the sustained release of low levels of LNG.[42] Its yearly failure rate is 0.04%.[5] Again, as is the case with progestin-only methods, irregular bleeding, from amenorrhea to frequent or prolonged bleeding, is a common but not harmful side effect occurring in approximately three-quarters of users during the first year.[43] Afterward, irregularities tend to resolve, with bleeding patterns returning to a cyclic menstrual pattern.

METABOLIC EFFECTS OF NORPLANT   As with DMPA, a statistically but not clinically significant increase in glucose and insulin levels during glucose tolerance testing was reported in healthy Norplant users.[44] In two long-term studies examining lipid metabolism, fasting serum triglyceride, total cholesterol, and LDL-cholesterol and HDL-cholesterol were found to have significantly decreased at 2 and at 5 years.[45,46]

Hormonal Contraception in Women with Cardiac Disease

Existing Studies No prospective studies exist examining hormonal contraceptive use in cardiac patients. In the one cross-sectional study examining contraceptive choices in 330 women with prior cardiac surgery, 7 women were identified who had used oral contraceptives for a mean of 26.2 ± 3.1 months.[47] Although the formulation was unspecified, no pregnancies or adverse outcomes were reported. Six of these women had undergone a mitral comissurotomy, and the remaining one had had a congenital lesion repaired. Aside from this study, one case report documents an embolic stroke in a 21-year-female smoker, who "was 3 months postpartum and had used oral contraceptives since delivery."[48] The formulation and estrogen dose were unspecified, nor was it specified whether there was a standard delay of 3–6 weeks in the initiation of a combination OC after delivery. After diagnosis of an embolic occlusion, physical examination revealed a midsystolic click and an echocardiogram with thickened, redundant mitral leaflets with marked prolapse and posterior mitral leaflet thrombus. Another study, examining coagulation states in former OC users who had experienced cerebrovascular insufficiency, found evidence of hypercoagulability, decreased plasma antithrombin II activity, increased platelet coagulant activity, and elevated β-thromboglobulin levels, compared with controls.[49] These changes were not felt to be secondary to OCs, which had been discontinued 4 months to 14 years earlier, but were related to the severity of the mitral valve prolapse (MVP). Increased platelet coagulant activities have been documented in mitral valve prolapse patients compared with control patients.[50] The severity of the platelet coagulant hyperactivity increased with progressively symptomatic MVP disease, being present in 100% of those who had experienced a thromboembolic event. Similarly, shortened platelet survival time has been documented in patients with rheumatic mitral valve disease and mitral valve prolapse with histories of thromboembolism.[51] Although MVP may be relatively common to younger women (up to 17% in women in their 20s),[52] usually it is asymptomatic and follows a benign course. In a follow-up study of 237 minimally symptomatic or asymptomatic patients with MVP, a subset of patients who were at risk for sudden death, infective endocarditis, or cerebral embolic events were identified by echocardiography to have redundant valve leaflets.[53] In patients with nonredundant valves, complications occurred in less than 1% compared to 10% in those with redundant valves.

Chronically anticoagulated patients with prosthetic valves present an exception to the use of estrogen-containing oral contraceptives. With ovulation, these women are at high risk of developing hemorrhagic corpus luteum cysts, secondary to the normal disruption of the ovarian capsule. Intraperitoneal bleeding, when present, usually occurs between days 20 and 26 of the menstrual cycle, and these women have a high propensity for recurrent bleeding.[54] This may lead to catastrophic bleeding requiring emergency surgery. In these women the consistent inhibition of ovulation and imposition of cycle control provided by a combination OC makes it an excellent contraceptive choice for these women.[55] The progestin-only OCs provide less consistent protection from ovulation,[56] making them a less desirable choice. DMPA also regularly inhibits ovulation, however the irregular bleeding that also is characteristic may pose a problem in the anticoagulated patient.

Recommendations for Hormonal Prescription in Women with Cardiac Disease In view of the paucity of data examining the effects of oral contraceptives, DMPA, or Norplant prescription in women with cardiac disease, the physician must rely on a large body of reassuring data in healthy women. The most prudent choice of hormonal contraception would be a progestin-only method, whether the minipill OC or DMPA or Norplant in women with valvular heart disease, with prosthetic heart valves not requiring anticoagulation, and with most forms of congenital heart disease. Studies have shown that the progestin-only methods do not affect blood pressure and coagulation factors, both important in cardiac patients. These methods also have been demonstrated to have a minimal metabolic effect on lipids and carbohydrates. Estrogen-containing oral contraceptives are contraindicated in any cardiac patient at risk for thromboembolism. With caution, low dose combination OCs may be used in women with asymptomatic MVP that has been confirmed by echocardiography to have no regurgitation or redundancy,[57] with prosthetic valve replacements requiring chronic anticoagulation and with repaired cardiac lesions and subsequent stable cardiac function. Although mild fluid retention (3–4 lb) is a more common side effect of estrogen-containing OCs,[56] all patients using hormonal methods must be routinely monitored for signs and symptoms of fluid retention, which could place them at risk for congestive heart failure. As with all cardiac patients, changes in medication, such as the prescription of a hormonal contraceptive, require supervision for side effects or interactions with other medications.

Selection among the progestin-only methods depends more on the lifestyle and compliance of the individual patient. In a patient for whom daily compliance poses a problem, such as a sexually active teenager with a cardiac lesion, a highly efficacious method such as Norplant or DMPA should be considered. If the patient has no history of hormonal contraception use, it is prudent to begin with a trial of the progestin-only minipills. Should any problems arise, the drug can easily and immediately be discontinued. If no adverse effects are noted, consideration may be given to either of the long-acting progestins. When prescribing any hormonal method in women with cardiac disease, frequent examinations to monitor for possible increased blood pressure and fluid retention should be scheduled. Equally important is discussing individual compliance and the patient's satisfaction with her method of contraception.

Intrauterine Devices

Medical Risks Associated with Intrauterine Device (IUD) Use The litigation and controversy linking the use of the intrauterine device and pelvic inflammatory disease (PID) has made many physicians reluctant to prescribe the IUD. Studies have shown that this association was attributable to only one type of IUD, the Dalkon Shield,[58,59] which is no longer marketed. This device uniquely increased the relative risk of PID in its users ($RR = 8.3$) compared with all other IUDs. That finding led to an abrupt drop in usage and availability of all IUDs in the 1980s. Recent studies have clarified the risk factors associated with the use of IUDs and reestablished their safety in appropriately selected patients. Two IUDs are currently on the United States market, the Progestasert (Progesterone T) and Paraguard (Copper T 380A). The Progestasert continuously releases low doses of progesterone locally into the endometrial cavity, decreasing menstrual blood loss. This device, which must be replaced annually, has an annual failure rate of 2.0%: higher than that of the Paraguard (0.8%), which was approved for 10 years of use in 1990.[5]

It is important to clarify the risk of pelvic inflammatory disease when considering the prescription of IUDs in women with cardiac disease who are at risk for subacute bacterial endocarditis. When the Dalkon Shield is excluded, the greatest risk of pelvic inflammatory disease associated with IUD use occurs during the first 4 months after insertion.[58] Postinsertion infections result from the introduction of bacteria into the sterile endometrial cavity during the insertion procedure. Studies have demonstrated that by 30 days after IUD insertion, the endometrial cavity becomes sterile.[65] The strongest support for the safety of the intrauterine device comes from a recent meta-analysis of data from 13 prospective randomized trials, conducted by the World Health Organization, involving almost 23,000 IUD insertions with over 58,000 woman-years of use.[61] Combination of these studies found the overall incidence of PID in IUD users to be 1.6 per 1000 woman-years of use, and this risk was not increased over time. There was, however, a sixfold increase in risk of developing PID during the first 20 days postinsertion compared to afterward. The presence of sexually transmitted diseases also was found to be positively associated with PID risk in IUD users. Other investigators have demonstrated no increase in risk of PID beyond the first 4 months after insertion (RR, 1.0–1.3, excluding Dalkon Shield) compared to controls using no method of contraception.[58] Secondly, the development of PID and subsequent tubal infertility in prior IUD users was also related to exposure risk to sexually transmitted diseases, specifically being increased in women with multiple sexual partners, a history of PID or nulliparous women under the age of 25.[58,59,62] When these factors were

adjusted for, IUD use was not a risk factor. Accordingly, the use of IUDs should be restricted to women at low risk of exposure to sexually transmitted disease: monogamous, parous women without a history of recent sexually transmitted disease.

Intrauterine Device and Cardiac Disease A large study examining contraceptive use in 330 women after cardiac surgery (250 with mitral comissurotomy, 77 with valve replacement and 3 with repair of congenital heart disease) was reported in 1985.[63] The majority, 170 women (52%), had used a copper-medicated IUD, either the Copper T380A or Copper T200 for a mean of 31 ± 6 months. All underwent antibiotic prophylaxis (parenteral gentamicin, 80 mg, and ampicillin, 1 g, administered 30 min prior to insertion and two subsequent doses administered at 8 h intervals afterward), and all were prescribed supplementary iron daily. Although menorrhagia was reported more frequently in the IUD users compared to women who chose other contraceptive methods (29% vs. 12% in those with mitral comissurotomy and 59% vs. 39% in those with valve replacement receiving warfarin anticoagulant therapy), there were no significant differences in mean hemoglobin levels between the IUD users and cardiac patients using other contraceptives with or without anticoagulant therapy. Only one patient discontinued the IUD secondary because of severe bleeding. Of significant importance, none of the IUD users developed bacterial endocarditis, developed congestive heart failure associated with menorrhagia, or became pregnant.

Recommendations for IUD Prescription in Cardiac Patients The IUD offers one of the most effective methods of reversible, long-acting contraception, without any metabolic disturbance. Unless special indications for the Progestasert IUD exist, the Copper T380A is recommended, since it offers 10 years of protection with only one insertion, decreasing the risk of repeated postinsertion infections. The metabolic neutrality of the IUD makes it an especially attractive choice for cardiac patients with associated vascular disease. Care should be taken to select appropriate candidates at low risk for sexually transmitted disease: monogamous women in a stable relationship who also are multiparous and have no history of active, recent, or recurrent pelvic infection. Until the new recommendations were released in 1997,[64a] the American Heart Association has always recommended antibiotic prophylaxis for subacute bacterial endocarditis at time of insertion or removal in cardiac patients with valvular heart disease, prosthetic heart valves, most congenital heart disease, idiopathic hypertrophic subaortic stenosis, mitral valve prolapse with regurgitation, history of endocarditis, or previous rheumatic fever on continuous oral penicillin.[64b] Parenteral prophylaxis, either intramuscular or intravenous, was recommended[65] and is supported by the preceding study by Abdalla et al.,[64] where ampicillin (2 g) plus gentamicin

(1.5 mg/kg) is given 30 minutes prior to insertion and two subsequent doses at 8-hour intervals afterward. In penicillin-allergic patients, vancomycin (1 g) given slowly intravenous over one hour should be substituted.[64] When the risk of endocarditis is decreased, either the postinsertion doses may be eliminated or oral prophylaxis (amoxicillin, 3 g, given 1 h prior to insertion followed by 1.5 g 6 h later) may be substituted. In cardiac patients not at risk specifically for endocarditis, the physician should consider prophylaxis to reduce postinsertion infection.[66] Recommended antibiotics include doxycycline (200 mg prior to insertion and 100 mg 12 h later), erythromycin (500 mg prior to insertion and again 6 h later),[15] or azithromycin (500 mg prior to insertion). Prior to insertion, both cervical culture for *Neiserria gonorrhea* and a *Chlamydia trachomatis* screen must be negative. Likewise, careful aseptic technique must be followed during insertion. The procedure should be delayed if bacterial vaginitis/cervicitis or pelvic tenderness is detected until an etiology is established and the symptoms resolved. A 4- to 6-week postinsertion examination allows the detection of infection and identifies expulsions. Prescription of supplemental iron intake and annual hemoglobin measurements is recommended, since menstrual blood loss generally is doubled with copper-medicated IUD use compared to control cycles.

Prescription of IUDs in nulliparous women is a relative contraindication, prohibited primarily from the medical-legal risk of subsequent infertility in a patient with unproven fertility. Successful, long-term use of copper-medicated IUDs in women with type I diabetes, 78% of whom were nulliparous, has been reported.[67] This group of patients are similar to cardiac patients in that they are at risk for serious sequelae secondary to infection. Generally nulliparous women tend to be younger and unmarried, both factors that place them at increased risk of sexually transmitted diseases and pelvic inflammatory disease. Nulliparous women are also at increased risk of vasovagal symptoms and postinsertion pain.[66] In a study of 87 healthy women undergoing IUD insertions without anesthesia, 12% demonstrated tachycardia, 11% bradycardias, and 1% premature ventricular contractions.[68] These episodes were associated with a high degree of anxiety and pain. All episodes were self-limiting. The authors' motivation for their study was an initial case of cardiac arrest with successful resuscitation after a painful IUD insertion in a patient with a history of syncopal episodes coincidental with injections. Although not documented in the literature, an arrhythmia may present an increased risk to the cardiac patient. Care must be taken with IUD insertion in these patients. A paracervical block using 10–20 ml of 1% lidocaine is particularly beneficial in decreasing pain during insertion or removal.[66] Gentleness, reassurance, and a careful explanation also help alleviate a patient's anxiety and pain.

Education of IUD users is important and should include an explanation of the progression of pelvic inflammatory disease from an untreated sexually transmitted disease such as chlamydial or gonococcal cervicitis. Patients should be taught to watch for the early signs of PID: increased and abnormal vaginal discharge, dyspareunia, heavy and painful menses, lower abdominal pain, and fever. These symptoms demand a prompt physical exam, cultures, and microscopic wet mount and Gram stain examination. Bacterial vaginitis or cervicitis should be treated with oral antibiotic therapy (clindamycin or metronidazole) without IUD removal. Clinical pelvic infections or positive venereal cultures mandate IUD removal and aggressive antibiotic therapy. Close follow-up for resolution of symptoms is a must. Additionally, gonococcal and chlamydial cultures should be obtained during each patient's annual gynecological examination. These general principles of good gynecological care are of paramount importance when the IUD is prescribed for women with cardiac disease.

Permanent Sterilization

Sterilization in the Female Cardiac Patient Permanent sterilization is the most effective form of contraception in women who no longer desire or are able to conceive. Although the operative risk may seem substantial, when it is amortized over the remaining reproductive lifespan of the cardiac patient with the assurance of pregnancy prevention, the benefits generally outweigh the risks. Careful preoperative planning should further minimize these risks. Bilateral tubal ligation can be performed via many operative variations of technique, all of which ligate and excise or fulgurate a portion of both fallopian tubes. This procedure may be performed either postpartum or unrelated to parturition.

When bilateral tubal ligation is performed related to delivery, it is a very simple, cost-efficient procedure. During a cesarean delivery, it is generally easily performed and requires minimal extra operating time. After a vaginal delivery, a small infraumbical incision is generally made in the delivery room immediately after delivery, to provide access for ligation. Blood loss is generally less than 20 ml. Most commonly regional anesthesia is employed, often using the epidural placed during labor. However, the procedure also may be performed under local anesthesia and conscious intravenous sedation. This surgery is ideally suited for the cardiac patient. Because the risk of the delivery far exceeds the operative risk associated with postpartum sterilization, the preparations effected for delivery can be used for the postpartum surgery. In women with severe cardiac compromise, central hemodynamic monitoring has generally been placed for the preceding labor and delivery. The timing of the tubal ligation may be delayed for 24–48 hours if necessary. Epidural anesthesia also may be continued, reactivated, or placed in the operating/delivery room. An equally satisfactory anesthesia, which should not be overlooked in cardiac patients, is the use of local infiltration with conscious intravenous sedation. Plans for postpartum sterilization should be incorporated into the overall discussion of route of delivery, type of anesthesia, and cardiac monitoring. Only in rare circumstances should postpartum sterilization be canceled in these patients, since the one-time risk can generally be managed to provide a lifetime protection from pregnancy.

Similarly, with planning and hemodynamic monitoring if needed, the risk of interval tubal sterilization can be minimized to make this an option for the woman with severe cardiac disease, particularly if she has completed her childbearing or if a pregnancy would place her at an unacceptably high risk. Again, anesthesia options range from general to epidural to local infiltration with intravenous sedation. Interval sterilization may be performed either via exploratory laparotomy or laparoscopic route (with minimal or no insufflation of the abdominal cavity). The technique of local anesthesia and laparoscopic sterilization has been used in healthy patients for years, requiring an average of 10 minutes of operating time.[69–71] Its successful use in cyanotic heart patients, with hemodynamic monitoring, was reported in 1983.[72] The authors used direct trocar entry, physically tented the abdominal wall to minimize the pneumoperitoneum, and used nitrous oxide to minimize serum pH disturbances. Most importantly, the use of local infiltration and sedation avoids the vasodilatory effect of general anesthesia and any increase in left-to-right shunt. Additionally, selection of optimal laparoscopy candidates without prior laparotomies, obesity, or known pelvic pathology, as well as experience on the part of the surgeon, contribute to operative success under local anesthesia.[73] The "minilaparotomy" tubal ligation utilizing a 3–5 cm suprapubic incision is the most frequent method of interval sterilization and is performed worldwide.[74] It lends itself very well to local anesthesia.[75] A uterine manipulator is useful in both laparoscopy and minilaparotomy and mandates parenteral antibiotic prophylaxis, as do all procedures involving the urogenital tract. An additional suprapubic probe during laparoscopy may also be used to lift the uterus, avoiding a uterine manipulator.

In summary, close collaboration and thorough preoperative evaluation by a team consisting of the gynecological surgeon, the anesthesiologist, and the cardiologist can reduce morbidity in these patients. Anticoagulation, if used, must be discontinued prior to surgery. Continuous hemodynamic monitoring and bacterial endocarditis prophylaxis should be used. Strong consideration should be given to local anesthesia with intravenous sedation in cases of cyanotic heart disease.[72]

Male Sterilization Another option, not to be overlooked in cardiac patients who are in stable, married relationships, is permanent sterilization for the spouse. Vasectomy should always be considered when the issue of permanent sterilization of the female cardiac patient is being addressed. Discussion must include the possibility of remarriage, since the patient's partner may realistically anticipate becoming a widower at a relatively young age. He must be also sure in his desire for no more children.

THE UNPLANNED PREGNANCY

Counseling and Medical Indications for Abortion in Cardiac Patients

The role of the physician in counseling any woman with an unplanned pregnancy is first to listen to and respect her desires. The cardiac patient who wants her pregnancy but is unsure of the safety of continuing deserves in-depth counseling very similar to that provided for women planning to conceive. An open dialogue, in language comprehensible to the patient and her family, should include a presentation of the anticipated course of pregnancy based on the best available information. What is the patient's current cardiac status? How will pregnancy alter it? Will she require prolonged bed rest or hospitalization? What will delivery be like? What are the risks of serious complications and possible death? What are the risks to the fetus with respect to normal intrauterine development and any teratogenic exposures? If the patient has a congenital lesion, what are the risks of her passing the condition on to her child? What treatments or actions can be done to reduce the patient's risk? Does she have a support system, both social and financial to help her during pregnancy? Conversely, what are the risks of pregnancy termination? Will termination improve either the short-term or the long-term maternal morbidity or mortality? Could termination with subsequent corrective cardiac surgery substantially improve the next pregnancy outcome to mother and child? After counseling, a patient must make her own final decision. For some, any serious increase in mortality risk may be unacceptable, while for others, under no circumstance will terminating the pregnancy be acceptable.

Today, with specialized care provided by a team including a cardiologist, a perinatologist, and an anesthesiologist, a therapeutic abortion is rarely indicated because of heart disease.[76,77] A general consensus can be found for recommendation for therapeutic abortion when maternal mortality with pregnancy exceeds 25–50%: congestive heart failure in early pregnancy, pulmonary hypertension, Eisenmenger's syndrome, uncorrected cyanotic congenital malformations, cardiomyopathy, and the Marfan syndrome with aortic involvement.[76–80] In cases of Eisenmenger's syndrome, the risk of a first- or second-trimester abortion has been shown to be significantly lower than delivery in the third trimester.[81] With the remaining cardiac lesions, which comprise over 90% of cases, it should be possible to anticipate a successful outcome for both mother and child. In these cases, a cardiologist experienced in pregnancy should evaluate the patient.

Abortion in Cardiac Patients: Surgical Considerations

As is in the case in tubal ligation, a careful evaluation must be done before abortion is performed. Prophylaxis for bacterial endocarditis should be given when indicated.[64a] A preoperative anesthesia assessment should determine the level of hemodynamic monitoring required and the best anesthesia choice. During the first trimester, prior to 14 weeks of gestation, terminations can be easily and most safely performed via dilatation and suction curettage under local anesthesia, using a paracervical block augmented with intravenous sedation administered by the anesthesiologist. The risk of termination beyond this point increases with increasing second-trimester gestational age.

Medically induced abortions, employing prostaglandin E_2 or hypertonic saline, are generally contraindicated in cardiac patients secondary to their cardiovascular effects. Thus second-trimester terminations in these patients require surgical dilatation and evacuation. Several anesthesia options exist. Most second-trimester terminations can usually be accomplished under local block with conscious sedation. If more complete anesthesia is necessary, epidural anesthesia, following the guidelines similar to those used for pregnant cardiac patients, may be used to avoid general anesthesia.[82] Surgical procedures are usually preceded by the placement of cervical laminara or osmotic dilators. Prior to their placement, antibiotic prophylaxis should be instituted. Because of the increased risk, a second-trimester abortion should be performed by a surgeon experienced in this procedure in a hospital setting. Care must be taken in the use of uterine contracting agents secondary to their side effects: fluid retention (oxytocin), vasoconstriction and hypertension (ergotrates, vasopressin) and hypotension and tachycardia (prostaglandins).[66] As with all surgery on cardiac patients, careful preoperative evaluation and planning will minimize and control most risk factors.

An in-depth discussion of future contraceptive method and future pregnancy plans must be part of the discussion surrounding the patient's decision to terminate. An unwanted or unplanned pregnancy is a failure of medical care. Contraceptive counseling and pregnancy planning must be a routine part of cardiac and gynecological care. It must begin early, as each patient reaches her menarche.

SUMMARY

Just as advances in surgical and medical care have made successful pregnancy outcomes in women with cardiac disease a reality, advances in contraceptive therapy have made fertility control for these women possible. Although a great deal of work remains to be done to document the safety of contraception in cardiac patients, much can be extrapolated from the large body of contraceptive experience in healthy women. As more women with congenital lesions survive to bear children, this information will become available. With the exception of estrogen-containing oral contraceptives, women with cardiac disease generally may be prescribed most forms of contraception. The method of contraceptive choice should be individually tailored to the demands of a patient's specific cardiac lesion as well as her lifestyle and future pregnancy plans. A more frequent schedule of follow-up not only allows assessment of potential problems, but should promote an increased dialogue on pregnancy planning. This responsibility should be shared by the patient's cardiologist and gynecologist. By being able to offer efficacious contraceptive methods for these women, the goal of planned pregnancy, when cardiac status is at its optimum, can truly become a reality.

REFERENCES

1. Moller J, Anderson R. 1000 Consecutive children with cardiac malformation with 26- to 37-year follow-up. *Am J Cardiol* 1992;70:661–667.
2. Wright M, Jarvis S, Wannamaker E, Cook D. Congenital heart disease: functional abilities in young adults. *Archi Physiol Med Rehab* 1995;66:289–293.
3. Gantt LT. Growing up heartsick: the experiences of young women with congenital heart disease. *Health Care Women Int* 1992;13:241–248.
4. Brown JB, Blackwell LF, Billings JJ, et al. Natural family planning. *Am J Obstet Gynecol* 1987;157:1082–1089.
5. Trussel J, Hatcher RA, Cates W, Stewart F, Kost K. Contraceptive failure in the United States: an update. *Stud Fam Plann* 1990;21:51–54.
6. Iturbe-Alessio I, del Carmen Fonseca M, Mutchinik O, Santos MA, Zajarias A, Salazar E. Risks of anticoagulant therapy in pregnant women with artificial heart valves. *N Engl J Med* 1986;315:1390–1393.
7. Dorflinger LJ. Relative potency of progestins used in oral contraceptives. *Contraception* 1985;31:557–570.
8. Bringer J. Norgestimate. A clinical overview of a new progestin. *Am J Obstet Gynecol* 1992;166:1969–1977.
9. Kjaer K, Lebech A-M, Borggaard B, Refn H, Pedersen LR, Schierup L, Bremmelgaard A. Lipid metabolism and coagulation of two contraceptives: correlation to serum concentrations of levonorgestrel and gestodene. *Contraception* 1989;40:665–673.
10. Gosland IF, Crook D, Simpson R, Proudler T, Felton C, Lees B, Anyaor U. Devenport M. Wynn V. The effects of different formulations of oral contraceptive agents on lipid and carbohydrate metabolism. *N Engl J Med* 1990;323:1375.
11. Layde PM, Feral V. Further analysis of mortality in oral contraceptive users: Royal College of General Practitioners' oral contraception study. *Lancet* 1981;1:541–546.

12. Stampfer MJ, Willet WC, Colditz GA,Speizer FE, Hennekens CH. A prospective study of past use of oral contraceptive agents and risk of cardiovascular diseases. *N Engl J Med* 1988;319:1313.

13. Porter JB, Hunter JR, Jick H, Stergachis A. Oral contraceptives and nonfatal vascular disease. *Obstet Gynecol* 1985;66:1.

14. Porter JB, Jick H, Walker AM. Mortality among oral contraceptive users. *Obstet Gynecol* 1987;70:29.

15. Rosenberg L, Palmer JR, Lesko SM, Shapiro S. Oral contraceptive use and the risk of myocardial infarction. *Am J Epidemiol* 1990;131:1009.

16. Wilson ES, Cruickshank J, McMaster M, Weir RJ. A prospective controlled study of the effect on blood pressure of contraceptive preparations containing different types of dosages and progestogen. *Br J Obstet Gynaecol* 1984;91:1254.

17. Spellacy WN, Buhl WC, Birk SA. The effect of estrogens on carbohydrate metabolism: glucose, insulin and growth hormone studies on one hundred seventy-one women ingesting premarin, mestranol and ethinyl estradiol for six months. *Am J Obstet Gynecol* 1971;114:388–392.

18. Spellacy W. Carbohydrate metabolism during treatment with estrogen, progestogen and low-dose oral contraceptive preparations on carbohydrate metabolism. *Am J Obstet Gynecol* 1982;142:732.

19. Perlman JA, Russell-Briefel R, Ezzati T, Lieberknecht G. Oral glucose tolerance and the potency of contraceptive progestins. *J Chronic Dis* 1985;38(10):857–864.

20. Kalkhoff RK. Metabolic effects of progesterone. *Am J Obstet Gynecol* 1982;142:735.

21. Loke DFM, Ng CSA, Samsioe G, Holck S, Ratnam SS. A comparative study of the effects of a monophasic and a triphasic oral contraceptive containing ethinyl estradiol and levonorgestrel on lipid and lipoprotein metabolism. *Contraception* 1990;42:535–554.

22. Petersen KR, Souby SO, Pederson RG. Desogestrel and gestodene in oral contraceptives: 12 months' assessment of carbohydrate and lipoprotein metabolism. *Obstet Gynecol* 1991;78:666–672.

23. Runnebaum B, Grunwald K, Rabe T. The efficacy and tolerability of norgestimate/ethinyl estradiol (250 μg of norgestimate/35 μg of ethinyl estradiol): results of open, multicenter study of 59,701 women. *Am J Obstet Gynecol* 1992;166:1963–1968.

24. Spellacy WN, Buhi WC, Birk SA. Carbohydrate metabolism prospectively studied in women using a low estrogen oral contraceptive for six months. *Contraception* 1979;20:137–148.

25. Van der Vage N, Kloosterboer HJ, Haspels AA. Effect of seven low-dose combined oral contraceptive preparations on carbohydrate metabolism. *Am J Obstet Gynecol* 1987;156:918–922.

26. Wahl P, Walden C, Knopp R, Hoover J, Wallace R, Heiss G, Rifkind B. Effect of estrogen/progestin potency on lipid/lipoprotein cholesterol. *N Engl J Med* 1981;308:862.

27. Kloosterboer HJ, van Wayjen RG, van del Ende A. Comparative effects of monophasic desogestrel plus ethinyl estradiol and triphasic levonorgestrel plus ethinyl estradiol on lipid metabolism. *Contraception* 1986;34:125.

28. Percival-Smith RK, Morrison BJ, Sizto R, Abercrombie B. The effect of triphasic and biphasic oral contraceptive preparations on HDL-cholesterol and LDL-cholesterol in young women. *Contraception* 1987;35:179.

29. Layde PM, Feral V. Further analysis of mortality in oral contraceptive users: Royal College of General Practitioners' oral contraception study. *Lancet* 1981;1:541–546.

30. Mann JI, Inman WHW. Oral contraceptives and death from myocardial infarction. *Br Med J* 1975;2:245–248.

31. Clarkson TB, Shively CA, Morgan TM, Koritnik DR, Adams MR, Kaplan JR. Oral contraceptives and coronary artery atherosclerosis of cynomolgus monkeys. *Obstet Gynecol* 1990;75:217–222.

32. Carr BR, Ory H. Estrogen and progestin components of oral contraceptives: Relationship to vascular disease. *Contraception* 1997;55:267–272.

33. Porter JB, Hunter JR, Jick H, Stergachis A. Oral contraceptives and nonfatal vascular disease. *Obstet Gynecol* 1985;66:1.

34. Porter JB, Jick H, Walker AM. Mortality among oral contraceptive users. *Obstet Gynecol* 1987;70:29.

35. Rosenberg L, Palmer JR, Lesko SM, Shapiro S. Oral contraceptive use and the risk of myocardial infarction. *Am J Epidemiol* 1990;131:1009.

36. WHO Collaborative Study of Neoplasia and Steroid Contraceptives. Breast cancer and depo-medroxyprogesterone acetate: a multinational study. *Lancet* 1991;338:833–888.

37. Toppozada HK, Koetswang S, Almakhu VE, Khan T, Darovec AP, Chatterjee TK, Molitor Peffer MP, Apelo R, Linchtenberg R, Crosignani PG, deSouza JC, Huidubro MG, Haspels AA. World Health Organization Expanded Programme of Research, Development and Research Training in Human Reproduction, Task Force on Long-Acting Systemic Agents for the Regulation of Fertility. Multinational comparative clinical evaluation of two long-acting injectable contraceptive steroids: northisterone enanthate and medroxyprogesterone acetate: final report. *Contraception* 1983;28:1–20.

38. Liew DFM, Ng CSA, Yong YM, Ratnam SS. Long-term effects of depo-provera on carbohydrate and lipid metabolism. *Contraception* 1985;31:51–64.

39. Fahmy K, Khairy M, Allam G, Gobran F, Alloush M. Effect of depo-medroxyprogesterone acetate on coagulation factors and serum lipids in Egyptian women. *Contraception* 1991;44:431–444.

40. Garza-Flores J, De la Cruz DL, Valles de Bourges V, Sanchez-Nuncio R ,Martinez M, Fusiwara JL, Perez-Palacios G. Long-term effect of depo-medroxyprogesterone acetate on lipoprotein metabolism. *Contraception* 1991;44:61–71.

41. Deslypere JP, Thiery M, Vermeulen A. Effect of long-term hormonal contraception on plasma lipids. *Contraception* 1985;31:633–642.

42. Diaz S, Pavez M, Miranda P, et al. Long-term follow-up of women treated with Norplant® use. *Contraception* 1987;35:551.

43. Darney PD, Atkinson E, Tanner S, MacPherson S, Hellerstein S, Alvardo A. Acceptance and perceptions of Norplant® among users in San Francisco USA. *Stud Fam Plann* 1990;21:152.

44. Konje JC, Otolorin EO, Ladipo AO. The effect of continuous subdermal levonorgestrel (Norplant) on carbohydrate metabolism. *Am J Obstet Gynecol* 1992;166 (1 Pt 1):9.

45. Singh K, Viegas OAC, Liew D, Singh P, Ratnam SS. Two-year follow-up of changes in clinical chemistry in Singaporean Norplant®-2rod acceptors: Metabolic changes. *Contraception* 1989;39:147–154.

46. Singh K, Viegas OAC, Loke D, Ratnam SS. Effect of Norplant® implants on liver, lipid and carbohydrate metabolism. *Contraception* 1992;45:141–153.

47. Abdalla MY, El Din Mostafa E. Contraception after Heart Surgery. *Contraception* 1992;45:73–80.

48. Busch EH, Synder DW, Barron RE. Embolic stroke in a woman with mitral valve prolapse who used oral contraceptives. *Chest* 1986;90:454–455.

49. Elam MB, Viar MJ, Ratts TE, Chesney CM. Mitral valve prolapse in women with oral contraceptive-related cerebrovascular insufficiency. Associated persistent hypercoagulable state. *Arch Intern Med* 1986;146:73–77.

50. Walsh PN, Kansu TA, Corbett JJ, Savion PJ, Goldburgh WP, Schaiz NJ. Platelets, thromboembolism and mitral valve prolapse. *Circulation* 1981;63:552–559.

51. Steele P, Weily H, Rainwater J, Vogel R. Platelet survival time and thromboembolism in patients with mitral valve prolapse. *Circulation* 1979;80:43–45.

52. Savage DD, Garrison RJ, Devereux RB, Castell WP, Anderson SJ, Levy D, McNamara PM, Stokes J3d, Kannel NB, Feinleib M. Mitral valve prolapse in the general population. Epidemiologic features: the Framingham Study. *Am Heart J* 1983;106:571–576.

53. Nishimura RA, McGoon MD, Shub C, Miller FA, Ilstrup DM, Tajik AJ. Echocardiographically documented mitral-valve prolapse. Long-term follow-up of 237 patients. *N Engl J Med* 1985;313:1305–1309.

54. Peters WA, Thiagarajah S, Thorton WN. Ovarian hemorrage in patients receiving anti-coagulant therapy. *J Reprod Med* 1979;22:82.

55. Droegemuller W. Benign gynecoloic lesions. In: Droegemueller WM, Herbst AL, Mishell DR Jr, Stenchever MA, eds. *Comprehensive Gynecology.* St. Louis: CV Mosby; 1987;440–492.

56. Mishell DR Jr. Contraception, sterilization, pregnancy termination. In: Droegemueller WM, Herbst AL, Mishell DR Jr, Stenchever MA, eds. *Comprehensive Gynecology.* St. Louis: CV Mosby; 1987;269–318.

57. Sullivan JM, Lobo RA. Considerations for contraception in women with cardiovascular disorders. *Am J Obstet Gynecol* 1993;168:2006–2011.

58. Lee NC, Rubin GL, Ory HW, Burkman RT. Type of intrauterine device and the risk of pelvic inflammatory disease. *Obstet Gynecol* 1983;62:1.

59. Lee NC, Rubin GL. The intrauterine device and pelvic inflammatory disease revisited: new results from the Women's Health Study. *Obstet Gynecol* 1988;72:1.

60. Mischell DR Jr. Intrauterine devices. In: Lobo RA, Mishell DR Jr., Paulson RJ, Shoupe D, eds. *Infertility, Contraception, and Reproductive Endocrinology,* 4th Edition. Massachusetts: Blackwell Scientific; 1997;851–862.

61. Mishell DR Jr, Bell JH, Good RG, Moyer DL. The intrauterine device: a bacteriologic study of the endometrial cavity. *Am J Obstet Gynecol* 1966;96:119.

62. Farley TMM, Rosenberg MJ, Rowe PJ, Chen J-H, Meirek O. Intrauterine devices and pelvic inflammatory disease: an international perspective. *Lancet* 1992;339:785–788.

63. Cramer DW, Schiff I, Schoenbaum SC, Gibson M, Belisle S, Albrecht B, Stillman RJ, Berger MJ, Wilson E, Stadel BV. Tubal infertility and the intrauterine device. *N Engl J Med* 1985;312:941.

64. Abdalla MY, El Din Mostafa E. Contraception after heart surgery. *Contraception* 1992;45:73–80.

64a. Dajani AS, Taubert KA, Wilson W, Bolger AF, Bayer A, Ferrieri P, Gewitz MH, Shulman ST, Nouri S, Newburger JW, Hutto C, Pallasch TJ, Gage TW, Levison ME, Peter G, Zuccaro G Jr. Prevention of bacterial endocarditis: Recommendations of the American Heart Association. JAMA 1997;277: 1794–1801.

64b. Dajani AS, Bisno AL, Chung KJ, Durack DT, Freed M, Gerber MA, Karchmer AW, Millard HD,, Rahimatoola S, Shulman ST, Watanakunakorn C, Taubert KA . Prevention of bacterial endocarditis: Recommendations of the American Heart Association. JAMA 1990;264:2919–2922.

65. Prevention of bacterial endocarditis. *Med Let* 1987;29:109–110.

66. Barbara AJS, David TD. Infective endocarditis in obstetrics and gynaecologic practice. *Obstet Gynecol* 1986;154:180–188.

67. Hatcher RA, Trussel J, Stewart F,Stewart GK, Kowald D, Guest F, Cates W, Policar M. *Contraceptive Technology.* 16th ed. New York: Irvington; 1994;347–377.

68. Kimmerle R, Berger M, Weiss R, Kurz K-H. Effectiveness, safety and acceptability of a copper intrauterine device (CU Safe 300) in type I diabetic women. *Diabetes Care* 1993;16:1227–1230.

69. Acker D, Boehm FH, Askew DE, Rothman H. Electrocardiogram changes with intrauterine contraceptive device insertion. *Am J Obstet Gynecol* 1973;115:458–461.

70. Wheeless CR. Anesthesia for diagnostic and operative laparoscopy. *Fertil Steril* 1971;22:690–694.

71. Poindexter AN, Abdul-Malak A, Fast J. Laparoscopic tubal sterilization under local anesthesia. *Obstet Gynecol* 1990;75: 5–8.

72. Peterson HB, Hulka F, Spelman FJ, Lee S, Marchbanks PA. Local versus general anesthesia for laparoscopic sterilization: a randomized study. *Obstet Gynecol* 1983;90:203–209.

73. Snabes MC, Poindexter AN. Laparoscopic tubal sterilization under local anesthesia in women with cyanotic heart disease. *Obstet Gynecol* 1991;78:437–440.

74. Bruhat M-A, et al., translated by Duvivier R, Vancaillie TG. *Operative Laparoscopy.* MEDSI/McGraw-Hill, Paris, France, 1989; p. 169–176.

75. Speroff L, Darney PD. *A Clinical Guide for Contraception.* Williams and Wilkins, Baltimore, MD, 1992; p. 265–306.

76. McCann M. Laparoscopy and minilaparotomy: Two major advances in female sterilization. *Stud Fam Plann* 1980;11:119.

77. Elkayam U, Gleicher N. Cardiac problems in pregnancy. I. Maternal aspects. *JAMA* 1984;251:2837–2838.

78. Clark SL. Structural cardiac disease in pregnancy. In: *Critical Care Obstetrics,* 2nd Ed. Clark SL, Cotton DB, Hankins GDV, Phelan JP (Eds.) Blackwell Scientific Publications, Boston, MA, 1991; p. 114–135.

79. Shabetai R. Cardiac diseases. In: *Maternal-Fetal Medicine: Principles and Practice.* 3rd Ed. WB Saunders, Philadelphia, PA, 1994; p. 768.

80. Goodwin TM, Greenspoon JS. Heart disease in pregnancy. In: *Management of Common Problems in Obstetrics and Gynecology,* 3rd Ed. Blackwell Scientific Publications, Boston, MA, 1994; p. 3–11.

81. Shabetai R. Congenital or acquired heart disease. In: *Medical Counseling Before Pregnancy.* Hollingsworth DR, Resnik R. (Eds.). Churchill Livingstone, New York, NY, 1988; p. 445–473.

82. Gleicher N, Midwall J, Hochgerger D, et al. Eisenmenger's syndrome in pregnancy. *Obstet Gynecol Surv* 1979;34:721–741.

83. Jones MM, Joyse TH. Anesthesia for the patient with pregnancy-induced hypertension and the pregnant cardiac patient. In: Clark SL, Cotton DB, Hankins GDV, Phelan JP, (eds.) *Critical Care Obstetrics,* 2nd ed. Blackwell Scientific Publications, 1991;559–578.

FETAL SECTION

38

EMBRYOLOGY OF THE HEART

Enid Gilbert-Barness, MD, Diane Debich-Spicer, BS, and Orestes Borrego, MD

INTRODUCTION

After fertilization, the embryo undergoes a period of rapid mitotic divisions called cleavage. During this process it becomes a solid sphere of cells, the morula, and then a hollow sphere with an internal cluster of cells at one pole, the blastocyst. Diffusion is adequate for a short while after growth and implantation have been achieved. Eventually the size of the embryo exceeds the efficiency of diffusion.

EMBRYOLOGY OF THE HEART

The first stage of cardiac development is the formation of vascular plexuses on either side of the developing head fold (Table 38.1). These fuse in the midline to form a straight cardiac tube with a series of dilatations representing the primitive chambers. The wall of the tube consists of three layers: endocardium, cardiac jelly, and epimyocardium.

Two components of the splanchnic mesoderm are separated by a layer of embryonic connective tissue known as cardiac jelly. The outer layer gives rise to the epicardium and myocardium and is called the epimyocardial mantle. The endothelial component gives rise to the definitive endocardium.

Between the 19th and 20th days, the heart bulges ventrally into the pericardial space and consists of a single midline structure composed of an endocardial tube surrounded by cardiac jelly and the epimyocardial mantle.

Localized expansion produces four dilated regions in the developing heart tube: bulbus cordis, ventricle, atrium, and sinus venosus. Even though the more caudal portions of the tube have not yet fused, paired atria and horns of the sinus venosus can be discerned embedded in the septum transver-

sum (Fig. 38.1).[1] Branches of the paired dorsal aortae loop ventrally around the foregut as the first pharyngeal arch arteries, joining the cephalic end of the bulbus. At their caudal ends, the endocardial tubes connect with vitelline, umbilical, and cardinal veins. Early in the 4th week, the dorsal mesocardium breaks down, allowing continuity between both sides of the pericardial space. This passage dorsal to the heart, between its attached arterial and venous ends, persists as the transverse sinus of the pericardium. This primitive heart tube undergoes a looping, assuming an S-shaped configuration within the pericardium.

During its continued growth the heart tube loops in two dimensions. A loop is formed by the ventral projection of the bulbus and ventricle. Simultaneously, a counterclockwise rotation (as viewed ventrally) takes place, bringing the atrium out of the septum transversum and placing it dorsal to the left ventricle. As a result, the apex of the bulboventricular loop is displaced toward the right (Fig. 38.2).[2] With continued growth, the lateral extremities of the atrium progressively envelop the distal portion of the bulbus cordis, persisting as the right and left atria.

Movements produce a groove between the left ventricle and the bulbus cordis that is known as the bulboventricular or conoventricular sulcus. A corresponding ridge in the interior of the heart tube is called the bulboventricular flange. The ends of the tube diverge laterally as the left and right horns of the sinus venosus, retaining communication with the veins entering the heart.

Expansion occurs in the bulbus and ventricle, but at their junction the lumen remains narrow, forming the primary interventricular foramen. These chambers extend caudally by growth of the epimyocardium and cavitation of its internal surface. The irregular nature of the process produces the tra-

Cardiac Problems in Pregnancy, Third Edition
Edited by Uri Elkayam, MD, and Norbert Gleicher, MD
Copyright © 1998 by Wiley-Liss, Inc. ISBN 0-471-16358-9

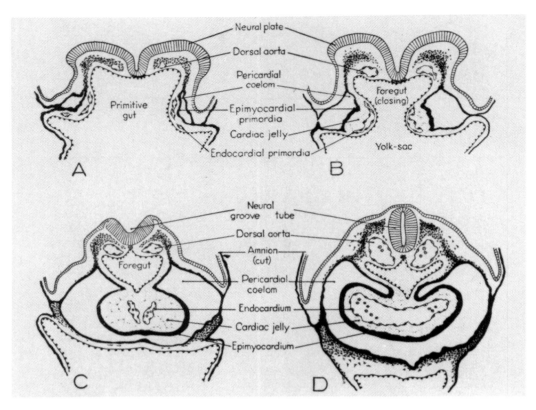

Figure 38.1 Cross sections of embryos at various stages of cardiac development showing formation: (A) approximation; (B) and fushion; (C,D) of endothelial heart tubes (endocardium) of each side to form the midline heart. Note the thickening of the splanchnic mesoderm to form the epimyocardial mantle, its separation from the endocardium by the cardiac jelly, and the attachment of the heart to the foregut by the forming dorsal mesocardium (unlabeled). (From Corliss,[1] with permission.)

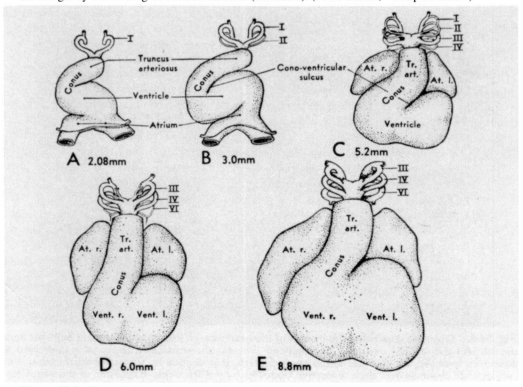

Figure 38.2 Ventral views of reconstructions of hearts from embryos of various stages, showing the formation of the bulboventricular (conoventricular) loop and sulcus, as well as the reduction in the latter and shift in position of the truncus toward the midline with age. Note the regions of the bulbus cordis: right ventricle, conus cordis, and truncus arteriosus. (From Kramer.[2])

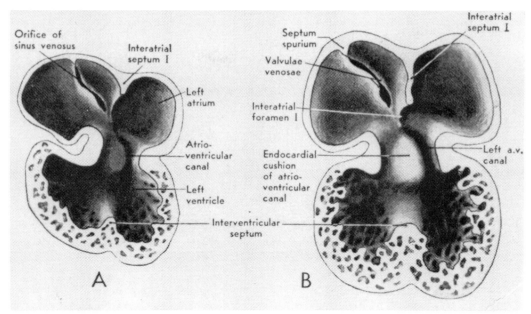

Figure 38.3 Diagrams illustrating the interior of the heart as seen in a frontal section in embryos during the fifth (A) and sixth (B) weeks of development. Whereas the atrioventricular canal is undivided and positioned over the left ventricle at the younger stage, it is divided by the endocardial cushions into two separate channels over their respective ventricles by the sixth week. Expansion of the ventricles at their apices leaves a muscular ridge between them, the muscular portion of the interventricular septum. As this region is incorporated into the atrium, the borders of the sinus venosus protrude as the right and left venous valves (valvulae venosae). The septum primum (interatrial septum I) grows caudally toward the endocardial cushions, its free edge forming the boundary of the ostium primum (interatrial foramen I). (From Corliss,[1] with permission.)

beculated appearance of the future ventricles. Since this extension does not take place at the junction of the two chambers, a ridge of muscular tissue persists between them, forming the muscular portion of the interventricular septum (Fig. 38.3).[1]

There are three regions of the bulbus cordis. The most proximal becomes trabeculated and will give rise to the right ventricle; the conus cordis becomes the outflow tract for both ventricles; and the most distal is the truncus arteriosus, which becomes the ascending aorta and pulmonary trunk. With expansion of the ventricles, the apex of the heart shifts toward the left with the extension of the atrium to the right atrioventricular canal that is positioned over the muscular interventricular septum.

During development, venous drainage to the heart changes from a bilateral pattern to one in which most of the blood returns to the right side. Whereas the right horn of the sinus venosus becomes enlarged, the left horn and midportion remain small, persisting in the adult as the coronary sinus of the atrium. The left horn of the sinus venosus is separated from the left side of the atrium by a crescent-shaped groove that forms between them. This invagination extends past the midline to the right atrium. As a result, the left horn

and midportion of the sinus venosus empty into the right side of the atrial chamber.

During this period the heart has developed from a straight tube with linearly arranged compartments to an intermediate arrangement in which the left and right sides each consist of an atrium and a ventricle. However, the heart remains essentially a tube, albeit tortuous, the two sides not yet separated from each other.

Separation of the Atria and Ventricles

Partitioning of the atrium occurs by progressive wrapping of the expanding atrium around the truncus and aortic sac. A crescent-shaped indentation or ridge is produced in its cephalic wall. The free concave edge of this ridge faces anteroinferiorly, toward the endocardial cushions. Although this structure, the septum primum, appears as a reduplication of the atrial wall, it continues to grow actively until its free edge reaches the endocardial cushions. While it exists, the space between the edge of the septum primum and the cushions is known as the ostium primum. Eventually this space is closed by fusion of the septum with the cushions. Preparato-

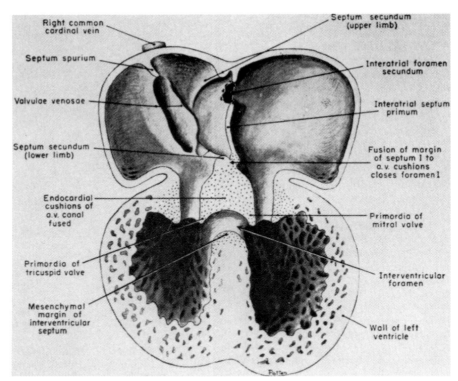

Figure 38.4 Atrial and ventricular septation: **I.**

Figures 38.4–38.6 Series of diagrams showing the changes occurring in the interior of the heart during atrial and ventricular septation. Note the orientation of the venous valves, their regression, the fusion of remnants of the left one with the septum secundum, and the derivation of the valves of the coronary sinus and inferior vena cava from the caudal portion of the right one. Also illustrated is the formation of the septum secundum and its relationship to the ostium secundum (interatrial foramen II) and the septum primum establishing the foramen ovale. The path of blood entering the right atrium is indicated by the white arrows in Figure 38.6. The formation of the left and right atrioventricular valves from endocardial cushions is shown also. (From Patten,[3] with permission.)

ry to closure of the ostium primum, perforations appear in the cephalic portion of the septum primum and coalesce to form a single opening, the ostium secundum. In this manner communication between the two atria is maintained after closure of the ostium primum (Figs. 38.4–38.6).[3,4]

The crescent-shaped septum secundum grows down, with its free edge overlapping the ostium secundum on its right side, and forms the boundary of an oval opening. The former is the limbus foramen ovalis, and the latter is the foramen ovale. Since septum secundum does not fuse with septum primum, a channel between the foramen ovale and the ostium secundum allows passage of the blood from right to left atrium. The overlapping of these septa acts as a valve preventing reversal of the blood flow. The position of the limbus foramen ovalis is such that a portion of the blood entering the right atrium from the inferior vena cava is directed into the foramen ovale. The septum primum fuses with the septum secundum after birth, sealing this channel.

Shortly after the formation of the septum primum, a vein from the venous plexus of the developing lung buds can be found opening into the atrium to the left of the interatrial septum. By this means, vascular drainage of the pulmonary structures is effected via the left atrium. As the atrium expands, the primitive pulmonary vein is incorporated into its wall up to the secondary branches. As a result, four separate pulmonary veins open into the left atrium.

A muscular ridge grows up from the base of the ventricle, dividing the right and left sides of the ventricle to form the interventricular septum. Endocardial cushion tissue forms the membranous septum, thus closing the ventricular septum.

Development of Endocardial Cushion Tissue

With the formation and fusion of the endocardial cushions, a substantial amount of connective tissue is brought to a central location between the resultant atrioventricular orifices.

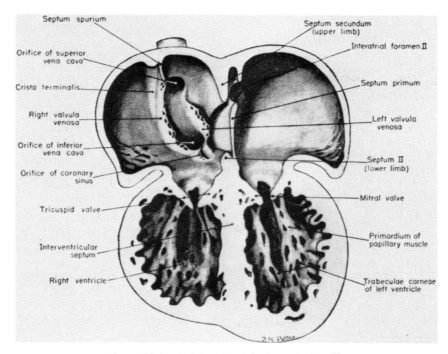

Figure 38.5   Atrial and ventricular septation: **II.**

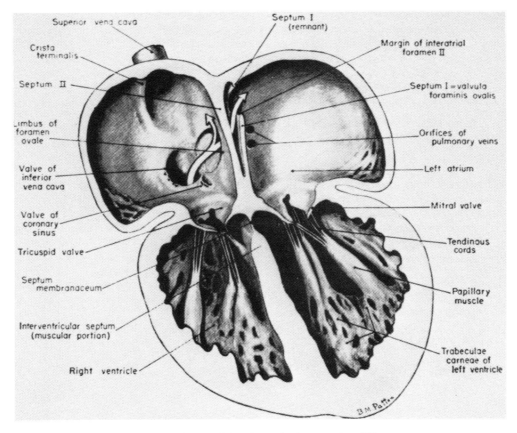

Figure 38.6   Atrial and ventricular septation: **III.**

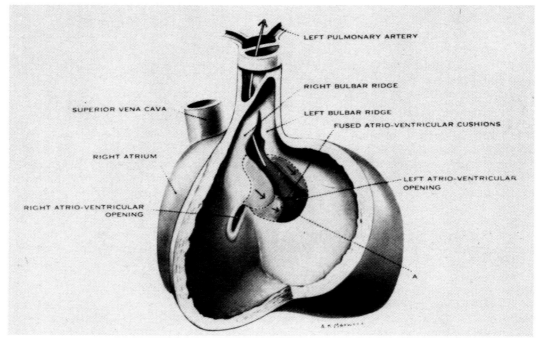

Figure 38.7 Closure of the interventricular foramen: **I.**

Figures 38.7–38.9 Series of diagrams illustrating the spiral disposition of the truncoconal septum and the closure of the interventricular foramen by merger of proliferations from the endocardial cushions (A) and the conus (bulbar) ridges. (From Hamilton and Moss,[5] with permission of Williams & Wilkins Co.)

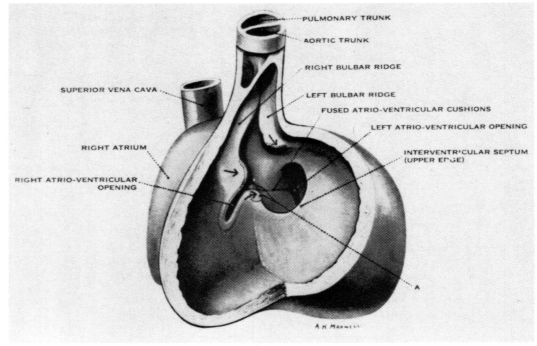

Figure 38.8 Closure of the intraventricular foramen: **II.**

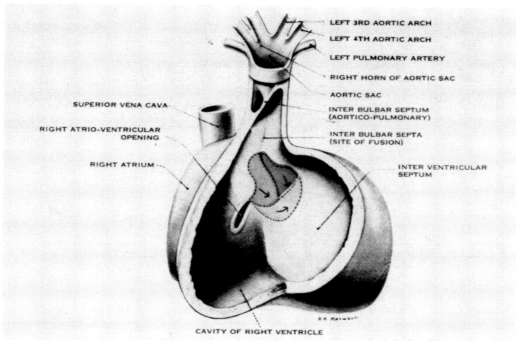

Figure 38.9   Closure of the intraventricular foramen: **III.**

This process is accompanied by an invagination of the epicardium in the atrioventricular sulcus. It eventually meets the endocardium, effectively separating the musculature of the atrium from that of the ventricle. Some cardiac muscle fibers remain, bridging from the floor of the right atrium to the dorsal extension of the muscular interventricular septum. There the fibers branch, with some continuing into each ventricle. This array will become the bundle of His and its main branches. Simultaneously a more differentiated connective tissue develops in the valvular projections as they become flattened out to form the definitive cusps. The cusps become elongated by an undercutting mechanisms that also frees some of the trabeculae from the ventricular wall. Replacement of some of the muscle with connective tissue in the latter structures produces the chordae tendineae anchored to the still muscular papillary muscles.

Septation and Spiraling of the Truncus Arteriosus

The formation of a spiral septum divides the conus and truncus into the systemic and pulmonary outflow tracts. In addition, the proximal edge of the septum effects the closure of the interventricular foramen by fusing with the superior margin of the muscular interventricular septum, the endocardial cushions, and their tubercles.

At the 5–6 mm (crown–rump) fetal stage, accumulations of mesenchymal tissue form two ridges that are distributed along the conus and truncus in a spiral manner. Although the tissue is continuous throughout those regions, it develops to a greater degree at three locations: between the ventral roots

of aortic arches 4 and 6; in the truncus arteriosus at the level of formation of the semilunar valves; and, more proximally, in the conus. The ridges progressively protrude into the respective lumina, eventually meeting and fusing to form a septum. The most distal ridges divide the aortic sac frontally so that the sixth arch (and the pulmonary trunk arising from it) occupies a dorsal position and the fourth arch (which will form the aorta) is ventrally placed. This aorticopulmonary septum spirals as it approximates the conus (Figs. 38.7–38.9).[5]

Completed Development of the Heart

The heart assumes its definitive structure by the 8th week (days 45–57) of development, summarized in Table 38.1.

Early in fetal life, the inner surfaces of both ventricles show prominent trabeculae (Fig. 38.10). These largely disappear from the left ventricle (LV) before birth, giving it the smooth unbroken surface that distinguishes it from the right ventricle (RV). The right border of the heart is formed by the right atrium (RA); the inferior border and most of the anterior surface by the RV. The left border of the heart is formed by a narrow strip of the anterior surface of the LV. Because of their important role in intrauterine circulation, the RA and the auricular appendage are large and prominent. Both the left atrium (LA) and the auricular appendage are small in the fetus and newborn.[6,7]

Circulation of Blood Before Birth (Fig. 38.11)

Before birth, oxygenated blood from the placenta normally passes through the umbilical vein to the umbilicus and enters

Blood pressure in the umbilical arteries at the time of birth normally averages about 80 mmHg systolic and 45 mmHg diastolic. It is usually about 10 mm higher in the first 24 hours, and by 10–14 days after birth the systolic pressure is 90–100 mmHg.[6]

Closure of the Temporary Fetal Vessels

Six structures present during fetal life disappear after birth. Four of these—the umbilical vein, the ductus venosus and the paired umbilical arteries—make possible the flow of blood between the placenta and the fetus during intrauterine life. The other two—the FO and DA—are designed to adjust the circulation through the right and left sides of the heart before birth and to obviate passage of part of the blood through the lungs.

These six structures become nonfunctioning soon after birth. The umbilical arteries and vein contract and constrict, and the small lumen remaining after contraction is obliterated by proliferation of the intima. Fibrous cords persist as permanent evidence of the earlier existence of these vessels. The portion of the umbilical vein extending between the umbilicus and the liver becomes the ligamentum venosum. The proximal portions of the umbilical arteries persist as the internal iliac arteries and the more distal obliterated portions become the lateral umbilical ligaments.[6]

The FO is an oval foramen near the center of the interatrial septum that measures about 8 mm in diameter at term. During intrauterine life blood flows through it because the pressure of the blood entering the RA from the placenta pushes the septum aside and permits early passage into the LA.

After birth the volume of blood entering the RA is proportionately reduced and the pressure is no longer higher on the right side. When the pressure on the two sides is equalized, or is higher in the LA than in the right, the septum primum is held in place and covers the FO in the septum secundum (Fig. 38.12). Blood normally ceases flowing through the FO as soon as the umbilical cord is cut, and the septa thereafter are in juxtaposition.

Increases in oxygen tension in the RA will lead to contraction of the DA, but anoxic states such as the respiratory distress syndrome may cause the DA to remain open after birth.

At autopsy it is impossible to tell from the appearance of the DA whether an infant was stillborn or lived for several or more hours. The DA in a term infant is 8–10 mm long and slightly less in diameter.

When a continuous longitudinal incision is made through the PA, DA, and descending aorta, the region of the DA is visible grossly as a circumscribed area in which the wall is thinner and more translucent than that of the permanent vessels (Fig. 38.13) and which, when unstretched, often forms fine wrinkles, a condition that is not found in the aorta or PA. Microscopic examination reveals definite differences in the walls of the permanent vessels and the wall of the DA. The cells of the latter are much less compact and have fewer elastic fibers, slightly more muscle cells, and considerably more interstitial fluid.

A cross section of the DA from a stillborn infant or one who dies during the first or second day of life shows a lumen about the size of the aorta and PA. The wall is composed of loosely arranged muscle cells and elastic tissue. The internal elastic lamina is a dense compact layer except for occasional areas in which gaps are associated with beginning intimal proliferation and mounds of the inner media protrude into the lumen. Proliferation of the intima may begin before birth, resembling that ordinarily found 1–2 days after birth. Any contraction that occurs immediately after birth must be in the nature of a spasm that disappears after death, since it is impossible to differentiate the DA of an infant several hours or more old from that of a stillborn fetus in which such functional changes could not be expected to have occurred.

In infants who survive for a longer time after birth, the DA shows a gradually increasing density of the media caused by contraction of the muscle and elastic fibers and disappearance of the intervening spaces. This change is responsible for most of the reduction in the size of the vessel, accompanied by increased collagen in mounds of proliferating intima or media with final obliteration of the lumen. The changes do not proceed uniformly in all parts of the DA, and some areas may be completely closed while others retain an appreciable lumen for many weeks. Even if the DA becomes functionally closed immediately after birth because of the cessation of placental circulation and establishment of respiration, the anatomic closure is only gradual, and for at least a week or 10 days a grossly visible opening can be demonstrated in the vessel. For several months a smaller opening may be identified on microscopic examination.[6] Figure 38.14 demonstrates the pressure and oxygen saturation of various chambers of the heart after closure of the DA.

MOLECULAR BASIS OF CARDIAC DEVELOPMENT

Temporal and Spatial Regulation of Cardiomorphogenesis

Temporal and spatial sequences of cardiac morphogenesis are highly regulated processes involving cell proliferation, migration, differentiation, and sorting at specific time periods and location in embryogenesis. Therefore, even partial failure of these highly coordinated processes can lead to disruption of normal cardiac development.[10]

Extracellular Matrix

Extracellular matrix (ECM) is a highly elaborated structure involving regulated, intimate associations of proteins, pro-

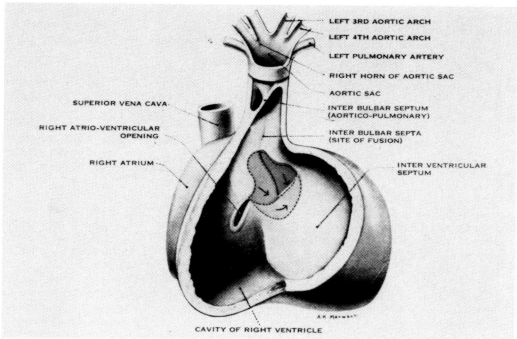

LEFT 3RD AORTIC ARCH
LEFT 4TH AORTIC ARCH
LEFT PULMONARY ARTERY
RIGHT HORN OF AORTIC SAC
AORTIC SAC
INTER BULBAR SEPTUM (AORTICO-PULMONARY)
INTER BULBAR SEPTA (SITE OF FUSION)
INTER VENTRICULAR SEPTUM

SUPERIOR VENA CAVA
RIGHT ATRIO-VENTRICULAR OPENING
RIGHT ATRIUM

CAVITY OF RIGHT VENTRICLE

Figure 38.9 Closure of the intraventricular foramen: **III.**

This process is accompanied by an invagination of the epicardium in the atrioventricular sulcus. It eventually meets the endocardium, effectively separating the musculature of the atrium from that of the ventricle. Some cardiac muscle fibers remain, bridging from the floor of the right atrium to the dorsal extension of the muscular interventricular septum. There the fibers branch, with some continuing into each ventricle. This array will become the bundle of His and its main branches. Simultaneously a more differentiated connective tissue develops in the valvular projections as they become flattened out to form the definitive cusps. The cusps become elongated by an undercutting mechanisms that also frees some of the trabeculae from the ventricular wall. Replacement of some of the muscle with connective tissue in the latter structures produces the chordae tendineae anchored to the still muscular papillary muscles.

Septation and Spiraling of the Truncus Arteriosus

The formation of a spiral septum divides the conus and truncus into the systemic and pulmonary outflow tracts. In addition, the proximal edge of the septum effects the closure of the interventricular foramen by fusing with the superior margin of the muscular interventricular septum, the endocardial cushions, and their tubercles.

At the 5–6 mm (crown–rump) fetal stage, accumulations of mesenchymal tissue form two ridges that are distributed along the conus and truncus in a spiral manner. Although the tissue is continuous throughout those regions, it develops to a greater degree at three locations: between the ventral roots

of aortic arches 4 and 6; in the truncus arteriosus at the level of formation of the semilunar valves; and, more proximally, in the conus. The ridges progressively protrude into the respective lumina, eventually meeting and fusing to form a septum. The most distal ridges divide the aortic sac frontally so that the sixth arch (and the pulmonary trunk arising from it) occupies a dorsal position and the fourth arch (which will form the aorta) is ventrally placed. This aorticopulmonary septum spirals as it approximates the conus (Figs. 38.7–38.9).[5]

Completed Development of the Heart

The heart assumes its definitive structure by the 8th week (days 45–57) of development, summarized in Table 38.1.

Early in fetal life, the inner surfaces of both ventricles show prominent trabeculae (Fig. 38.10). These largely disappear from the left ventricle (LV) before birth, giving it the smooth unbroken surface that distinguishes it from the right ventricle (RV). The right border of the heart is formed by the right atrium (RA); the inferior border and most of the anterior surface by the RV. The left border of the heart is formed by a narrow strip of the anterior surface of the LV. Because of their important role in intrauterine circulation, the RA and the auricular appendage are large and prominent. Both the left atrium (LA) and the auricular appendage are small in the fetus and newborn.[6,7]

Circulation of Blood Before Birth (Fig. 38.11)

Before birth, oxygenated blood from the placenta normally passes through the umbilical vein to the umbilicus and enters

TABLE 38.1   Summary of the Development of the Heart

Age (days)	Size	Event
18	Presomite	Angiogenic tissue appears; reversal of cardiogenic plate
19–20	1–2 somites	Appearance of endothelial heart tubes
21	4 somites	Fusion of endothelial heart tubes
21–22	6 somites	Differentiation of atria, ventricle, and bulbus cordis; first beats of heart
25	14–16 somites	Fusion of primitive atria, regression of dorsal mesocardium, formation of bulboventricular loop
26–27	20 somites to 10 mm	Circulation of blood established
32	5 mm	Septum primum appears
33	6 mm	Interventricular septum appears
35	8 mm	Foramen secundum present
36–37	0–10 mm	Atrial cushions fused
43	15 mm	Bulbar ridges fused
46	17 mm	Interventricular foramen closed, coronary arteries formed
47	18 mm	Septum secundum appears

Source: Modified from WJ Hamilton, HW Mossman, B Hamilton, *Mossman's Human Embryology.* Baltimore: Williams & Wilkins; 1972.

the fetal liver as a continuation of the same vessel. It moves through the liver via the ductus venosus. As the ductus venosus emerges from the liver it is joined by the hepatic veins, and together they enter the inferior vena cava (IVC). Blood entering the RA through the IVC is a mixture of freshly oxygenated blood from the placenta and venous blood from the abdominal organs and lower extremities. It is joined in the RA by blood from the superior vena cava (SVC). The greater part of the blood from the IVC is shunted in an isolated stream directly through the foramen ovale (FO) into the LA. The head and upper extremities receive blood somewhat more highly saturated with oxygen than the rest of the body. A large amount of the blood entering the RA passes through the FO into the LA and from there to the LV, the aorta and the general circulation.

The remainder of the blood from the RA passes into the RV and then through the pulmonary artery (PA). About 10–15% of the blood from the RV enters the lung through the PA, which divides into right and left branches and continues as the ductus arteriosus (DA), joining the aorta immediately distal to the origin of the left subclavian artery; it then enters into the peripheral circulation, having thus bypassed the lungs. Consequently, only part of the blood entering the PA enters the lungs and returns through the pulmonary veins to the LA.[8]

The fetal pulmonary arteries develop a thickened medial layer in response to high pressure and to hypoxia-induced constriction. Pulmonary vascular resistance drops in the first 2–3 days of life, accompanying constriction of the DA, and reaches adult levels at about 2 weeks.[5,9]

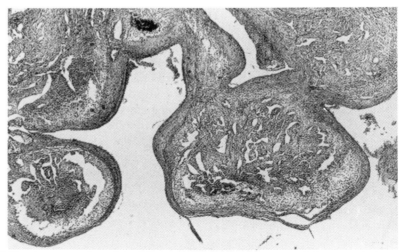

Figure 38.10   A cross section of the left ventricle of a small premature infant reveals deep trabeculation in the ventricular wall. This feature disappears as the heart grows.

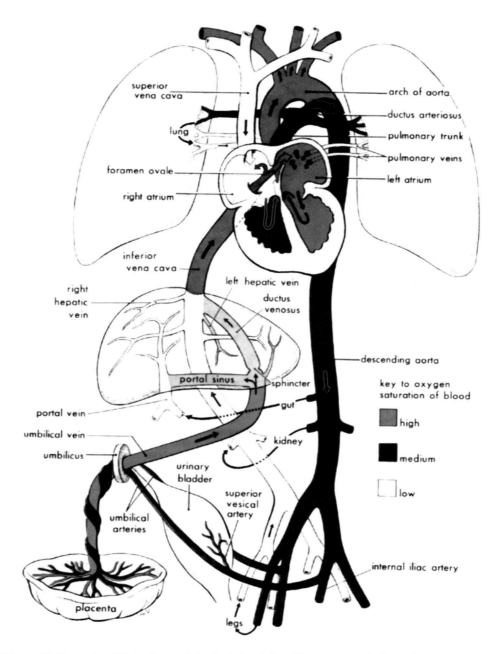

Figure 38.11 A simplified scheme of the fetal circulation. The gray tones indicate the oxygen saturation of the blood, and the arrows show the course of the fetal circulation. The organs are not drawn to scale. Three shunts permit most of the blood to bypass the liver and the lungs: the ductus venosus, the foramen ovale, and the ductus arteriosus. (From Moore.[8])

The blood in the LA is derived from the RA through the FO and to a lesser extent from the pulmonary veins. It flows through the LV into the ascending aorta and is distributed to the head, neck, and arms through branches arising from the arch. Immediately distal to the subclavian artery it is joined by the DA with blood from the RV; this mixture enters the descending aorta.

Blood returns to the placenta through the two umbilical arteries, which arise as branches of the right and left internal iliac arteries.

Blood pressure in the umbilical arteries at the time of birth normally averages about 80 mmHg systolic and 45 mmHg diastolic. It is usually about 10 mm higher in the first 24 hours, and by 10–14 days after birth the systolic pressure is 90–100 mmHg.[6]

Closure of the Temporary Fetal Vessels

Six structures present during fetal life disappear after birth. Four of these—the umbilical vein, the ductus venosus and the paired umbilical arteries—make possible the flow of blood between the placenta and the fetus during intrauterine life. The other two—the FO and DA—are designed to adjust the circulation through the right and left sides of the heart before birth and to obviate passage of part of the blood through the lungs.

These six structures become nonfunctioning soon after birth. The umbilical arteries and vein contract and constrict, and the small lumen remaining after contraction is obliterated by proliferation of the intima. Fibrous cords persist as permanent evidence of the earlier existence of these vessels. The portion of the umbilical vein extending between the umbilicus and the liver becomes the ligamentum venosum. The proximal portions of the umbilical arteries persist as the internal iliac arteries and the more distal obliterated portions become the lateral umbilical ligaments.[6]

The FO is an oval foramen near the center of the interatrial septum that measures about 8 mm in diameter at term. During intrauterine life blood flows through it because the pressure of the blood entering the RA from the placenta pushes the septum aside and permits early passage into the LA.

After birth the volume of blood entering the RA is proportionally reduced and the pressure is no longer higher on the right side. When the pressure on the two sides is equalized, or is higher in the LA than in the right, the septum primum is held in place and covers the FO in the septum secundum (Fig. 38.12). Blood normally ceases flowing through the FO as soon as the umbilical cord is cut, and the septa thereafter are in juxtaposition.

Increases in oxygen tension in the RA will lead to contraction of the DA, but anoxic states such as the respiratory distress syndrome may cause the DA to remain open after birth.

At autopsy it is impossible to tell from the appearance of the DA whether an infant was stillborn or lived for several or more hours. The DA in a term infant is 8–10 mm long and slightly less in diameter.

When a continuous longitudinal incision is made through the PA, DA, and descending aorta, the region of the DA is visible grossly as a circumscribed area in which the wall is thinner and more translucent than that of the permanent vessels (Fig. 38.13) and which, when unstretched, often forms fine wrinkles, a condition that is not found in the aorta or PA. Microscopic examination reveals definite differences in the walls of the permanent vessels and the wall of the DA. The cells of the latter are much less compact and have fewer elastic fibers, slightly more muscle cells, and considerably more interstitial fluid.

A cross section of the DA from a stillborn infant or one who dies during the first or second day of life shows a lumen about the size of the aorta and PA. The wall is composed of loosely arranged muscle cells and elastic tissue. The internal elastic lamina is a dense compact layer except for occasional areas in which gaps are associated with beginning intimal proliferation and mounds of the inner media protrude into the lumen. Proliferation of the intima may begin before birth, resembling that ordinarily found 1–2 days after birth. Any contraction that occurs immediately after birth must be in the nature of a spasm that disappears after death, since it is impossible to differentiate the DA of an infant several hours or more old from that of a stillborn fetus in which such functional changes could not be expected to have occurred.

In infants who survive for a longer time after birth, the DA shows a gradually increasing density of the media caused by contraction of the muscle and elastic fibers and disappearance of the intervening spaces. This change is responsible for most of the reduction in the size of the vessel, accompanied by increased collagen in mounds of proliferating intima or media with final obliteration of the lumen. The changes do not proceed uniformly in all parts of the DA, and some areas may be completely closed while others retain an appreciable lumen for many weeks. Even if the DA becomes functionally closed immediately after birth because of the cessation of placental circulation and establishment of respiration, the anatomic closure is only gradual, and for at least a week or 10 days a grossly visible opening can be demonstrated in the vessel. For several months a smaller opening may be identified on microscopic examination.[6] Figure 38.14 demonstrates the pressure and oxygen saturation of various chambers of the heart after closure of the DA.

MOLECULAR BASIS OF CARDIAC DEVELOPMENT

Temporal and Spatial Regulation of Cardiomorphogenesis

Temporal and spatial sequences of cardiac morphogenesis are highly regulated processes involving cell proliferation, migration, differentiation, and sorting at specific time periods and location in embryogenesis. Therefore, even partial failure of these highly coordinated processes can lead to disruption of normal cardiac development.[10]

Extracellular Matrix

Extracellular matrix (ECM) is a highly elaborated structure involving regulated, intimate associations of proteins, pro-

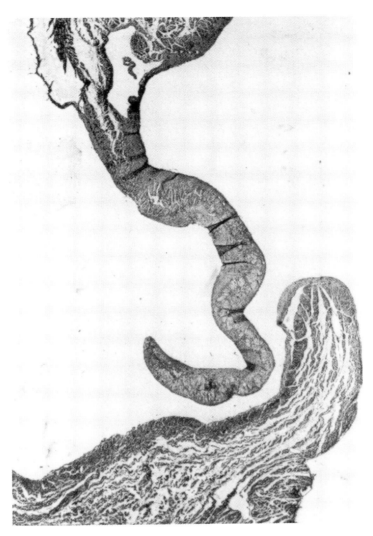

Figure 38.12   Foramen ovale from infant 4 days old. Although anatomically patent, it was functionally closed. (From Gilbert-Barness E[6])

teoglycans, and glycosaminoglycans. Each of these morphoregulatory molecules has a specialized function in fulfilling the ECM's multiple purposes. The main purpose, however, is serving the cell as a substrate for growth and providing a stable milieu around them. In addition, the ECM provides a suitable scaffold for functioning among the cells in a given milieu. The circulatory system evolves within and along with the ECM in cardiogenesis and angiogenesis.[11,12]

Fibronectin

Fibronectin is a glycoprotein belonging to a group of adhesion molecules with diverse molecular structures whose major property is their ability to bind with other ECM components and to specific integral cell membrane proteins. Fibronectin is a large multifunctional glycoprotein consisting of two chains held together by disulfide bonds.[13] Fibronectin is produced by fibroblasts, monocytes, endothelial cells, and cells of other types. It binds to other ECM components including collagen, fibrin, heparin, and proteoglycans via specific domains and to cells via integrin receptors. Integrins are transmembrane glycoproteins made up of α and β chains whose intracellular domains interact, in areas of focal adhesion, with elements of the cytoskeleton, to signal cell attachment, locomotion, or differentiation.[14] Fibronectin is thought to be directly involved in the attachment, spreading, and migration of cells. It also serves to enhance the sensitivity of certain cells, such as capillary endothelial cells, to the proliferative effects of growth factors.

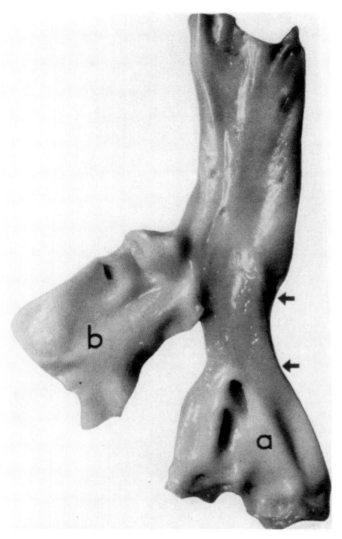

Figure 38.13   Main pulmonary artery (a) gives off branches to right and left lungs and continues as the ductus arteriosus (between arrows) and enters aorta immediately to arch (b). Note difference in opacity of ductus arteriosus and other vessels. Before removal from the body, the ductus arteriosus appeared to be of the same caliber as pulmonary artery and aorta. Infant aged 10 hours. (From Gilbert-Barness E[6])

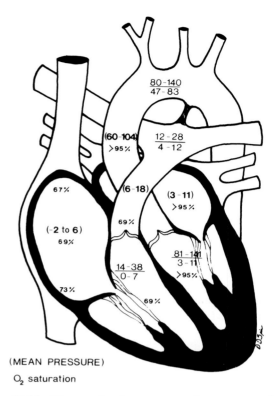

(MEAN PRESSURE)

O₂ saturation

Figure 38.14   Diagram showing pressure and oxygen saturation of the various chambers of the heart established after closure of the DA.

Collagen

Collagen is the most common protein found in the body and the major product of the fibroblast. It provides the tensile strength and the framework for the embryo to develop and evolve.

Various types of collagen are associated with the cardiac development. The interstitial collagens form the major structural as well as functional components during development and in the adult.[10] These collagens are principally types 1 and 3. Transient expression of type 2 has also been reported. Collagen types 5, 6, and 8 are also present in small quantity dur-

ing development, being evident in the neonatal periods when the expression and deposition of collagen is critical to the formation of different regions of the heart. Early expression of collagen seems to be predominantly type 1 with less type 3; however, this ratio changes with later development when type 3 becomes predominant. This expression of interstitial collagens appears to be coordinated with the expression of specific receptors (integrins) and may be associated with increased heart rate and/or increases in pressure. The formation of the basic arrangement of collagen in the endomysium and perimysium is established in the neonate or earlier. The network of collagens is essential for attaching the cellular components of the developing heart in a three-dimensional manner. The attachment of collagen is at precise regions on the myocyte at or near the Z bands. However, attachment to capillaries and fibroblasts does not appear to be at precise sites.[10,15–17]

GROWTH FACTORS

Molecular Markers

Growth factors are a group of molecules that regulate the complex process of cell growth and differentiation. Some of these factors act on a variety of cell types, whereas others have relatively specific targets. Growth factors may act by endocrine, paracrine, or autocrine signaling, with paracrine being the most common mode of operation. Many cells have specific receptors for specific factors produced either by themselves or by other cell types.

Transforming Growth Factor β (TGF-β)

TGF-β stimulates fibroblast chemotaxis and the production of collagen and fibronectin by cells and inhibits collagen degradation by decreasing proteases and increasing protease inhibitors. Within the endocardial cushion, TGF-β and a specific isoform of the fibroblast growth factor (FGF) receptor are coexpressed. In addition, recent studies have documented the expression of the negative helix–loop–helix relation in the developing endocardial cushion. Existing evidence suggests a critical role for TGF-β in heart development and heart malformation. Basic FGF (b-FGF) is present in the extracts of many organs and is elaborated by activated macrophages, whereas acidic FGF (a-FGF) is confined to neural tissue.[18,19]

Growth Factors

Growth factors such as transforming growth factor β, fibroblast growth factors, and platelet-derived growth factors (PDGFs) appear to play significant roles in cardiac development.[18]

Integrins

Integrins of the β_1 family are expressed in a precise temporospatial manner during embryogenesis of several systems, including heart, lung, kidneys, and integument. β_1 Integrin mRNA and protein are expressed most abundantly in regions of the heart undergoing elaborate morphogenetic remolding, especially developing trabeculae and endocardial cushions.

Neural Crest

During early embryonic development, the neural crest provides ectomesenchymal cells to the heart and aortic arch arteries, which are essential for the normal development of these structures. Ectomesenchymal cells derived from the cardiac neural crest form the walls (excluding endothelium) of all the persisting aortic arch arteries and they support their development. Neural crest cells in the third, fourth, and sixth arches migrate to the outflow tract of the heart, where they participate in outflow septation.[20,21]

REFERENCES

1. Corliss CE. *Patten's Human Embryology: Elements of Clinical Development.* New York: McGraw-Hill; 1976.

2. Kramer TC. The partitioning of the truncus and conus and the formation of the membranous portion of the interventricular septum in the human heart. *Am J Anat* 1942;71:343–370.

3. Patten BM. Persistent interatrial foramen primum. *Am J Anat* 1960;107:271–280.

4. Patten BM. *Foundations of Embryology.* 2nd ed. New York: McGraw-Hill; 1964.

5. Hamilton WJ, Mossman HW. *Boyd and Mossman's Human Embryology.* Baltimore: Williams & Wilkins; 1972.

6. Gilbert-Barness E, Debich-Spicer D. Cardiovascular system, pt I, chap 18. In *Potter's Pathology of the Fetus and Infant.* Gilbert-Barness E, ed. Philadelphia: Mosby-Year Book; 1997.

7. Moore KL. *Essential of Human Embryology.* Philadelphia: BC Decker; 1988;127–135.

8. Moore KL. *Before We Are Born: Basic Embryology and Birth Defects.* 3rd ed. Philadelphia: WB Saunders; 1989;202–225.

9. Rudolph AM, Heymann, MA. Coarctation of the aorta in the fetal and neonatal periods. *Birth Defects; orig art ser* 1972;8:19.

10. Clark EG, Markwald RR, Takao A, eds. *Developmental Mechanisms of Heart Disease.* New York: Futura Publishing; 1995.

11. Borg TK, Burgess ML. Holding it all together: organization and function(s) of the extracellular matrix in the heart. *Heart Fail* 1993;8:230–238.

12. Streuli CH, Bissell MJ. Mammary epithelial cells, extracellular matrix and gene expression. *Cancer Treat Res* 1991;53:365–381.

13. Carver W, Price RL, Raso DS, Terracio L, Borg TK. Distribution of β_1 integrin in the developing rat heart. *J Histochem Cytochem* 1994;42:167–175.

14. Hynes RO. Integrins: versatility, modulation and signaling in cell adhesion. *Cell* 1992;69:11–25.

15. Bashey RI, Hernandez AM, Jimenez SA. Isolation, characterization and location of cardiac collagen type VI. *Circ Res* 1992;70:1006–1016.

16. Carver W, Terracio L, Borg TK. Expression and accumulation of collagen in the neonatal heart. *Anat Rec* 1993;236:511–520.

17. Swiderski RE, Daniels KJ, Jensen KL, Solursh M. Type II collagen is transiently expressed during avian cardiac valve morphogenesis. *Dev Dyn* 1994;200:294–304.

18. Enenstein J, Waleh NS, Kramer RH. Basic FGF and TGF-β differentially modulate integrin expression of human microvascular endothelial cells. *Exp Cell Res* 1992;203:499–503.

19. Chien KR. Overview: molecular analysis of cardiac developmental phenotypes: problems, progress, and prospects. In: Clark EG, Markwald RR, Takao A, eds. *Developmental Mechanisms of Heart Disease.* New York: Futura Publishing; 1995;3–28.

20. Kirby ML. Cellular and molecular contributions of the cardiac neural crest to cardiovascular development. *Trends Cardiovasc Med* 1993;3:18–23.

21. Kirby ML. A preview of the molecular basis of neural crest contribution of heart development. In: Clark EG, Markwald RR, Takao A, eds. *Developmental Mechanisms of Heart Disease.* New York: Futura Publishing; 1995;221–225.

39

BIOPHYSICS OF THE DEVELOPING HEART

PAGE A. W. ANDERSON, MD

INTRODUCTION

This chapter describes cardiac function in the fetus and in the neonate, emphasizing the changes that occur with development and birth. The information is presented in a manner that distinguishes primary changes in myocardial contractility from changes related to secondary factors such as ventricular volume (preload), ventricular interaction, and arterial pressure (afterload). The effects of all these factors are important in the support of the fetal and neonatal circulation and the adaptation of the heart to the changes in circulation with birth.

In the following sections, which provide an understanding of how the fetal heart functions and its ability is modulated, we focus on results from the intact animal. We also draw on results from isolated cardiac muscle. (In the isolated preparation, force and length can be controlled precisely, whereas in the intact heart, where ventricular volume changes from one cardiac cycle to another, such control is difficult at best, hindering an appreciation of alterations in cell function or contractility.) Our focus on the intact animal is based on the concept that only by exploring in the intact fetal heart the ways in which the various factors that determine cardiac function interact can we grasp how heart function is modulated during development and in response to birth and to pathophysiologic states.

We will consider the overall mechanical function of the heart to depend on four factors, which have been classically treated as independent variables: (1) muscle length or ventricular diastolic volume (i.e., the preload imposed on the myocardium just prior to contraction, e.g., ventricular end-diastolic volume); (2) inotropy, the intrinsic ability of the myocardium to contract, which is modulated by changes in the sensitivity of the cardiac myofilaments to calcium and cytosolic calcium concentration, through such agents as cardiac glycosides, β-adrenergic agonists, and the physiological variables heart rate and postextrasystolic potentiation; (3) afterload, or the load imposed on the myocardium following activation and during the cardiac contraction (e.g., the arterial pressure the ventricle must exceed to generate a stroke volume); and (4) the interaction of the right and left ventricle (e.g., the effect of right ventricular end-diastolic volume on left ventricular systolic and diastolic function). Although this separation of factors that affect heart function may be somewhat artificial at the basic level of cell function, the approach allows the description of the dependence of in vivo fetal cardiac performance on heart rate, ventricular volume (preload), arterial pressure (afterload), and inotropic state. We will explore the ways in which these dependencies alter cardiac output.

An understanding of these dependencies and their interaction is essential in explaining how the fetal heart responds to different forms of stress and adapts with birth. Knowing what mechanisms are available to alter the function of the fetal heart will allow us to treat pathophysiologic states with therapeutic modalities that exploit these dependencies or make use of these mechanisms. Our need to understand how fetal cardiac function can be modulated is further driven by our present ability to perform *in utero* surgery on the human fetus (e.g., *in utero* diaphragmatic hernia repair) and by our present and hoped-for future abilities to palliate or correct congenital defects in utero.[1-4] With these therapeutic possibilities in mind, we outline how specific physiological and hormonal variables alter the function of the fetal heart and fetal cardiac output.

Cardiac Problems in Pregnancy, Third Edition
Edited by Uri Elkayam, MD, and Norbert Gleicher, MD

FUNCTION OF THE FETAL HEART AND ITS MODULATION

Ventricular Filling and Ejection

Diastole Fetal ventricular volume increases during diastole from its end-systolic volume to its end-diastolic volume. The components of diastole that result in the end-diastolic volume of the fetal ventricle are similar to those of the adult heart. An appreciation of these components is important in applying Doppler and echocardiographic techniques to the interrrogation of diastolic filling in the fetal heart. These components of fetal ventricular diastolic filling have been well characterized in the adult heart. Opening of the tricuspid and mitral valves, which occurs when atrial pressure exceeds that in the ventricle, begins the period of rapid ventricular filling (Fig. 39.1). In the nonstressed fetus, the normal variability in heart rate reveals the presence during low heart rates of slow ventricular filling during the middle of diastole (Fig. 39.1). The end of diastole is marked by atrial systole. This increase in atrial pressure further increases ventricular volume to its end-diastolic level. Atrial systole also contributes to the effectiveness of the subsequent ventricular contraction through the appropriate temporal relation of atrial systole to ventricular systole, inducing what has been termed stretch-activation.

When heart rate is increased, the duration of diastole is decreased, and the period of slow ventricular filling disappears, as in the adult heart. The components of rapid ventricular filling and atrial systole become summed into a monotonic increase in ventricular volume. Figures 39.1 and 39.2 illustrate that the characteristics of this diastolic filling waveform coupled to the ventricular rearrangement that occurs during early systole at small end-diastolic volumes make it difficult to determine the contribution of atrial systole to end-diastolic volume at rapid fetal heart rates. The volumetric change that accompanies a change in a minor axis measurement of a ventricle may also be difficult to deduce because of the geometric relation. For example, a large change in a ventricular dimension when the ventricle is filling from a relatively small volume will reflect a smaller increment in ventricular volume than a small increase in that dimension when the ventricle is filling from a larger end-systolic volume. These observations follow from the nonlinear (in some dimensions almost cubic) effect of a ventricular dimension on ventricular volume. Figures 39.1 and 39.2 illustrate the differences in the contributions of different components of diastolic filling to ventricular volume when the duration of diastole is altered.

The relative contributions of rapid and slow filling and atrial systole to end-diastolic volume appear to change with development. Doppler interrogation of diastolic flow across the atrioventricular valves *in utero* has led to the conclusion that atrial systole is the major contributor to the increase in ventricular volume during embryonic life. In the late gestation fetal lamb, sonomicrometric measurements of ventricu-

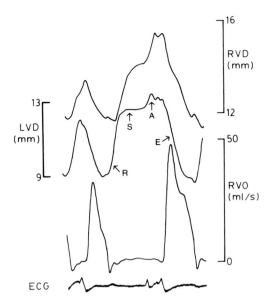

Figure 39.1 Right and left ventricular dimension, pulmonary artery flow, and electrocardiographic waveforms obtained from an *in utero* fetal lamb that had undergone the surgical introduction of the physiological instrumentation 5 days earlier. A sonomicrometric dimension transducer was implanted in the interventricular septum, and two dimension transducers were placed on the endocardial surface of the right and left ventricular free wall.[9] Rapid filling (R) of both ventricles occurs during early diastole. When diastole is longer, a period of slow ventricular filling (S) occurs during mid-diastole. The end of diastole is marked by a further increment in ventricular filling (A), a result of atrial systole. Systole or the ejection phase is lettered E. These data illustrate the presence in the late gestation fetus of the components of diastolic filling described in the adult heart. The fetal differences in right and left ventricular end-diastolic volume are illustrated by these data: The right ventricular end-diastolic dimension is much larger than that of the left ventricle (see also Fig. 39.23). The waveforms (top to bottom) are as follows: right ventricular dimension (RVD), left ventricular dimension (LVD), pulmonary artery flow (RVO), and electrocardiogram (ECG).

lar volume suggest that rapid and slow filling phases are the most important contributors to ventricular filling, as they are in the adult heart.

The maturational decrease in myocardial compliance[5,6] has been used to explain why in the immature heart, atrial systole, compared to the earlier filling phases, has the greatest effect on end-diastolic volume (see below). However, at all ages the contribution of atrial systole to ventricular end-diastolic volume and stroke volume (see below) has its greatest effect when the normal temporal coupling relationship between atrial and ventricular systole is maintained. The changes in the relative timing of atrial and ventricular systole that occur during a fetal supraventricular or ventricular tachycardia or when the atrial pacemaker site is changed can have profound negative effects on fetal right and left ven-

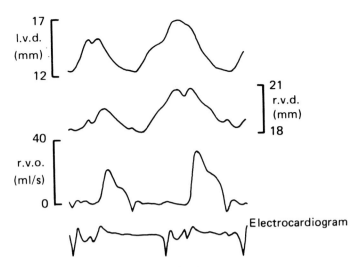

Figure 39.2   Waveforms illustrating the effect of differences in ventricular end-diastolic volume on the dimension waveform during early systole. The right and left ventricular dimension and pulmonary flow waveforms were obtained during right atrial pacing of an *in utero* lamb that had undergone cardiovascular instrumentation 4 days earlier. The waveforms on the left, were obtained at a pacing rate of 280 beats/per minute, and those on the right after introduction of a longer paced interval to allow right and left ventricular filling to larger end-diastolic volumes. The pulmonary flow waveform denotes the onset of ventricular ejection. Marked systolic rearrangement occurs at the smaller end-diastolic volumes (the waveforms on the left). The systolic rearrangement is identified by the increase in right ventricular dimension during early systole. Note that at the larger end-diastolic volume on the right the systolic rearrangement in the left ventricle is not evident at all and is much decreased in the right ventricle. The waveforms (top to bottom) are as follows: septum to left ventricular free wall dimension (l.v.d.); septum to right ventricular free wall dimension (r.v.d.); pulmonary artery flow or right ventricular output (r.v.o.); and the electrocardiogram. (From Anderson et al, *J Physiol* 1987;387:297–316, with permission.)

tricular output (Figs. 39.3–39.5). As discussed below, such tachycardias markedly shorten diastolic filling time, decrease ventricular end-diastolic volume, and so decrease stroke volume. The decreased myocardial compliance of the immature heart compounds the negative effect on end-diastolic volume of shortened diastolic filling time. Consequently, when diastolic filling time is shortened, venous pressure must be increased to achieve end-diastolic volumes necessary to maintain fetal stroke volume and cardiac output. The clinical manifestations of this increased venous pressure in the fetus with supraventricular tachycardia are ascites and pleural and pericardial effusions.

Systole   The components of ventricular systole are the same as those seen in the adult heart (Figs. 39.6 and 39.7). The onset of ventricular contraction increases ventricular pressure and closes the tricuspid and mitral valves. The following period of ventricular systole, which precedes aortic and pulmonic valve opening, is called isovolumic because volume remains constant.

The isovolumic portion of systole is accompanied by a change in ventricular shape. The smaller the end-diastolic

volume, the greater is the increase in the ventricular minor axis dimension and the decrease in the major axis (or length) of the ventricle. At small end-diastolic volumes this systolic rearrangement complicates the accurate assessment of end-diastolic volume by means of a single ventricular dimension or plane (e.g., see Figs. 39.2 and 39.3). Consequently, when such an approach is used, the extent to which end-diastolic volume is compromised by a fast rate or decreased blood volume cannot be fully appreciated.

The next component of ventricular systole is the ejection phase. When ventricular pressure exceeds arterial pressure, the semilunar valves open and the ventricles eject their stroke volume. With ventricular relaxation and fall in ventricular systolic pressure, aortic and pulmonic valve closure occurs. Similar to the adult heart, ventricular pressure appears to reach zero or even a negative value at end-systole, and as a result, the ventricle acts like a suction pump during the onset of diastolic filling when the tricuspid and mitral valves open.

The sections that follow use the waveforms of ventricular pressure, dimension, and stroke volume to characterize how heart rate, ventricular volume, arterial pressure (afterload), and inotropy affect the function of the fetal heart. The mea-

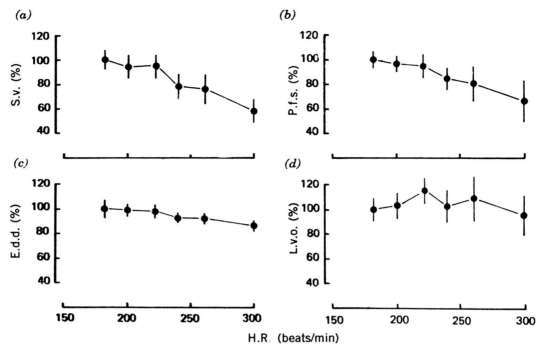

Figure 39.3 Effects of right atrial pacing on left ventricular end-diastolic volume, stroke volume, and output in a group of fetal lambs that had undergone cardiovascular instrumentation 4–12 days prior to the study. Values are expressed as a percentage of the value obtained at the slowest rate, the latter being considered as 100%, paced rates, 182–300 beats/per minute. (*A*) Percentage change in left ventricular stroke volume (S.v.). (*B*) Percentage change in percent fractional shortening (P.f.s.). (*C*) Percentage change in end-diastolic dimension (E.d.d.). (*D*) Percentage change in left ventricular output (L.V.O.). Vertical bars represent 2 standard deviations of the mean. (Reprinted from Anderson et al, *J Physiol* 1986;372:557–573, with permission.)

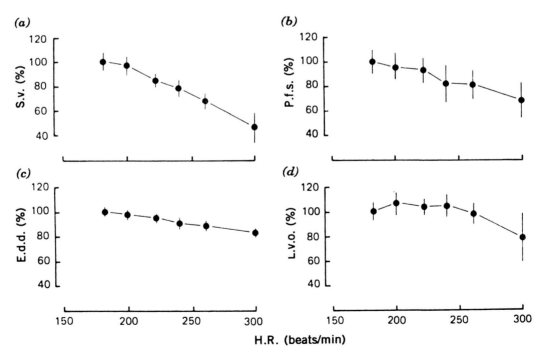

Figure 39.4 Effects of left atrial pacing on left ventricular end-diastolic volume, stroke volume, and output in the same group of fetal lambs described in Figure 39.3. See legend to Figure 39.3 for conditions and variables. (Reprinted from Anderson et al, *J Physiol* 1996;372:557–573, with permission.)

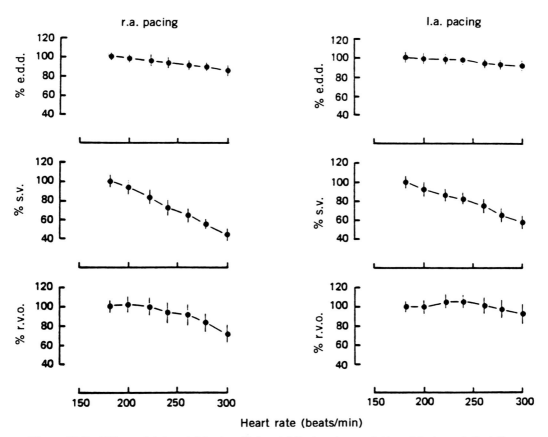

Figure 39.5   Effects of right atrial (r.a.) and left atrial (l.a.) pacing on right ventricular end-diastolic volume, stroke volume, and output in a group of *in utero* fetal lambs that had undergone cardiovascular instrumentation 4–17 days prior to the study. *In vitro* calibration of the right ventricular dimension waveform has demonstrated that these changes in end-diastolic dimension are an accurate measure of changes in right ventricular end-diastolic volume. Values are normalized and expressed as percentages; 100% represents the slowest values. Percentage change in right ventricular end-diastolic dimension, % e.d.d.; percentage change in right ventricular stroke volume, % s.v.; percentage change in right ventricular output, % r.v.o.; paced rates, 182–300 beats/per minute. Vertical bars represent 2 standard deviations about the mean. (Reprinted from Anderson et al, *J Physiol* 1987;387:297–316, with permission.)

sures of systolic and of diastolic function that can be directly determined from these waveforms include the maximum rate of ventricular systolic pressure development (the maximum first derivative of pressure, $dP/dt_{max}, P_{max}$: e.g., see Fig. 39.7), which is a measure of inotropy sensitive to preload and afterload that occurs at or just prior to semilunar valve opening.[7,8] The maximum rate of fall of ventricular pressure (maximum negative first derivative of ventricular pressure) provides a measure of ventricular diastolic relaxation and marks end-systole. These measures have been commonly used to describe adult heart function.

The end-systolic and end-diastolic volumes of the fetal right and left ventricles, which reflect the effects of venous return and atrial pressure on ventricular filling and the effects of ventricular volume, inotropy, and afterload on systolic function, are assessed using ventricular dimensions mea-

sured just prior to the onset of rapid ventricular filling in early diastole and following atrial systole. In general, the largest end-diastolic diameter provides the best approximation of end-diastolic volume. As noted above, however, if the largest value is used during rapid heart rates and hypovolumic states, end-diastolic volume may be overestimated. The usefulness of ventricular dimension waveforms for describing right and left ventricular end-diastolic volume has been validated in the fetal lamb heart (Fig. 39.8).[9,10]

The Frank–Starling Relation

Ventricular volume's effect on the ability of the adult heart to develop pressure and eject blood was described in the late nineteenth and early twentieth centuries by Frank[11] and Starling.[12] Frank demonstrated that when end-diastolic volume

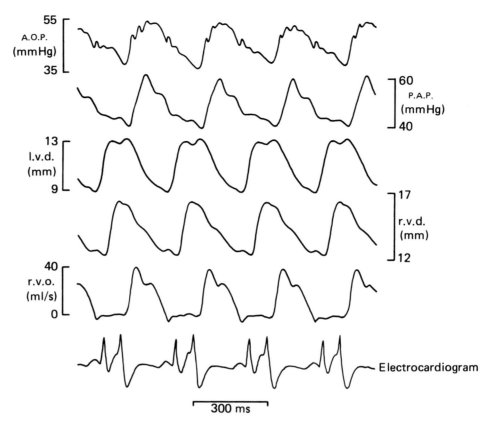

Figure 39.6   Data obtained during a period of spontaneous rhythm from an *in utero* lamb at 131 days of gestation and 6 days after cardiovascular instrumentation. The waveforms (top to bottom) are as follows: bracheocephalic arterial pressure, AOP; pulmonary artery pressure, PAP; septum to left ventricular free wall dimension, LVD; septum to right ventricular free wall dimension, RVD; pulmonary artery flow (i.e. right ventricular output), RVO; and the electrocardiogram. (From Anderson et al; *J Physiol* 1987;387:297–316, with permission.)

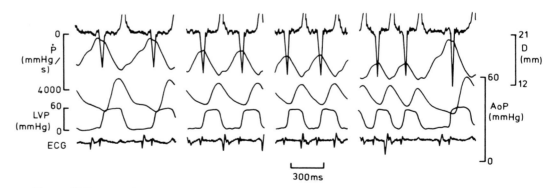

Figure 39.7   The effect of increasing heart rate on left ventricular pressure development (first derivative of left ventricular pressure, P_{max}) and left ventricular end-diastolic volume (left ventricular end-diastolic dimension) in an *in utero* fetal lamb (138 days of gestation). Although end-diastolic volume and end-diastolic pressure fall with increasing heart rate, the ability of the heart to develop pressure, as described by P_{max}, is enhanced. When end-diastolic volume is allowed to return to or exceed the control value (data on far left), the positive inotropic effect of heart rate on P_{max} is further revealed. Traces (top to bottom) are as follows: first derivative of left ventricular pressure (a positive deflection is in a downward direction); left ventricular dimension, D; aortic pressure, AoP; left ventricular pressure, LVP; and electrocardiograms, ECG. (Reprinted from Anderson et al, *Am J Obstet Gynecol* 1980;138:33–43, with permission.)

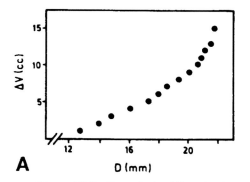 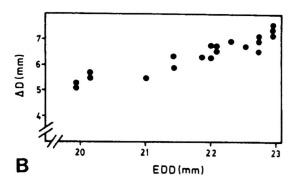

Figure 39.8 Data obtained from *in vitro* calibration of left ventricular dimensions and *in vivo* measurements of left ventricular end-systolic and end-diastolic dimensions illustrating the presence of the Frank–Starling relation in the *in utero* fetal lamb, late in gestation. (*A*) In vitro study of the relationship between minor axis dimension (D) and increments in ventricular volume (V) in a lamb heart from a day-old animal (instrumented at 115 days of gestation; see also Fig. 39.11). (*B*) The in vivo relationship between end-diastolic dimension (EDD) and the amount of systolic shortening of this dimension (D = EDD − end-systolic dimension) from the same lamb, studied the day prior to delivery, 144 days of gestation. (From the laboratory of P.A.W. Anderson.)

is increased, the isolated heart is able to generate a higher maximum systolic pressure and a higher maximum rate of rise of pressure (P_{max}). Starling demonstrated that stroke volume increases in response to an increase in venous return.

The cellular basis of the Frank–Starling mechanism arises in part from the sarcomere. Changing sarcomere length modulates (1) the number of myosin heads that interact with actin and (2) the sensitivity of the myofilaments to calcium (i.e., how many actin–myosin interactions occur at a given cell calcium concentration). Based on the length of the myosin-containing thick filaments and that of the actin-containing thin filaments, the optimum sarcomere length for actin–myosin interaction is 2.0–2.2 μm. At longer sarcomere lengths, the extent of overlap of the thick and thin filaments decreases, reducing the number of potential cross-bridge interactions. At shorter sarcomere lengths, the interdigitation of the thin filaments through the M line interferes with cross-bridge attachments. Sarcomere length also affects the sensitivity of the monofilaments to calcium, as described by force or myofibrillar ATPase activity as a function of calcium concentration (Fig. 39.9). Increasing sarcomere length beyond the optimal thick/thin filament overlap increases the sensitivity of the myofilaments to calcium, shifting the force–pCa relation and the half-maximal activation of force or ATPase activity to lower calcium concentrations.

The Frank–Starling relation also appears to have a basis in the cardiac cell's membranes. Stretching or distorting the sarcolemma can alter membrane current: for example, by increasing a calcium current. Regardless of the cellular basis of the Frank–Starling mechanism, fetal and embryonic cardiac muscle manifests the presence of this relation when end-diastolic volume and muscle length are increased (Fig. 39.10). The physiological manifestations include a higher systolic

pressure, a greater stroke volume, and an increase in P_{max} (Figs. 39.11 and 39.12).[7,9–13]

These findings aside, a controversy has existed over the importance of this relation in the function of the intact fetal heart.[14,15] The following numbered paragraphs review findings that support contrasting viewpoints about the effects of fetal ventricular volume on cardiac function as measured by stroke volume and cardiac output. In our opinion, the reader will conclude that modulating end-diastolic volume is an important factor in altering stroke volume and cardiac output in the fetal heart. These paragraphs are included, however, because of the apparently extreme positions put forward earlier about the presence and the role of the Frank–Starling relation in the fetal heart.

1. *In vivo* studies of right ventricular output in the fetal lamb by Heymann and Rudolph[14] found that large increases in end-diastolic pressure, in response to a volume infusion, produced only a small increase in cardiac output. These results generated the concept that the Frank–Starling mechanism is not operative in the fetal heart and that the stroke volume of the fetal heart is somehow fixed.

2. In a subsequent study of the neonatal lamb,[6] Klopfenstein and Rudolph found evidence for a developmental acquisition of the ability of the heart to respond to a change in ventricular volume: A volume infusion increased left ventricular output in the lamb during the first neonatal week by a smaller percentage than in the 6-week-old lambs. It must be noted that the measured increase in cardiac output of the 1-week-old lamb was actually *greater* than that of the older animal. The percentage increase in the output of the younger lamb was

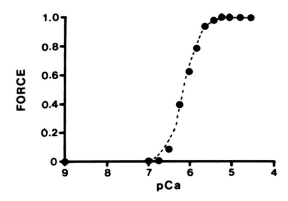

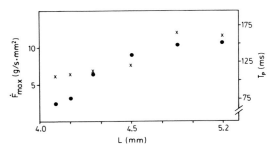

Figure 39.10 Illustration of the Frank–Starling relation in cardiac muscle isolated from a fetal lamb heart: the maximum rate of rise of force–cross-sectional area (F_{max}; circles) obtained from a fetal lamb's trabeculae carneae (126 days of gestation) over a range of muscle lengths (L). The time to maximum tension (T_p) for these contractions is plotted as a cross.

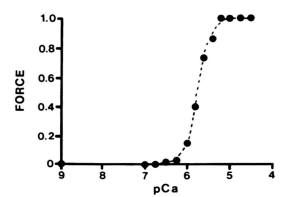

Figure 39.9 The sensitivity of cardiac myofilaments to calcium is described by the relation between force and the negative log of calcium concentration (pCa). The cardiac preparations were chemically skinned to remove all the cell membranes, to permit control of the calcium concentration in the solution bathing the myofibrils. At low calcium concentrations, no force is generated ,and then at a calcium concentration of approximately 1 μM, a large increase in force development for small increases in calcium concentration is observed. The pCa at which half-maximal force is generated is used to characterize the sensitivity of the myofilaments to calcium. The force–pCa relation in the lower panel is shifted to the right relative to the relation in the top panel. This indicates that the preparation, which provided the data in the lower panel, has a lower sensitivity to calcium. The differences in the relative amounts of the isoforms of cardiac troponin T, the thin filament regulatory protein, contained in these preparations correlate with the differences in myofilament sensitivity to calcium. (From Nassar et al, *Circ Res* 1991;69:1470–1475, with permission.)

lower because its control value, corrected for body weight, was higher than that of the 6-week-old. The relatively higher control output in the younger lamb may be the result of an increased level of inotropy in the newborn.

3. Gilbert[17] and Thornburg et al[15,18] concluded that the functional reserves of the fetal right and left ventricles,

measured by an increase in stroke volume or output in response to an increase in end-diastolic volume, are smaller than those of more mature animals. Their results were interpreted as supporting the concept that the fetal and neonatal hearts are operating at or near the maximum effect of the Frank–Starling relation on cardiac output (Fig. 39.13). However, these data clearly demonstrate the presence of a Frank–Starling relation in the fetus. The ventricular function curves illustrate a large increase in stroke volume when atrial pressure is increased from 1 mmHg to 5 mmHg.

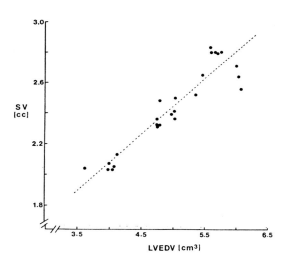

Figure 39.11 The Frank–Starling relation, characterized by the effect of end-diastolic volume on stroke volume, in an *in utero* fetal lamb that had undergone cardiovascular instrumentation 7 days earlier. A range of left ventricular end-diastolic volumes was obtained by altering the pacing interval. Left ventricular end-diastolic volume was computed by measuring three left ventricular dimensions and using an ellipsoid model and *in vitro* calibration. LVEDV, left ventricular end-diastolic volume; SV, stroke volume. (From the laboratory of P.A.W. Anderson.)

VOLUME   INFUSION

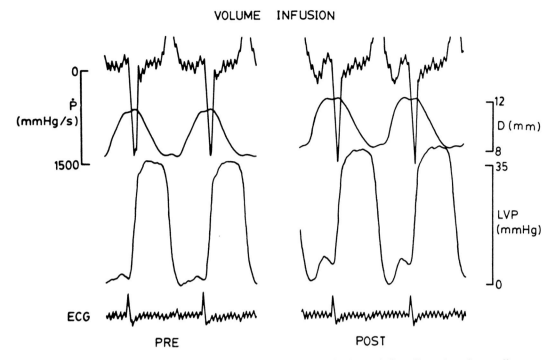

Figure 39.12   The effect of a volume infusion on left ventricular end-diastolic and peak systolic pressure, left ventricular end-diastolic and end-systolic dimensions, and peak first derivative of left ventricular pressure in a fetal lamb (138 days of gestation) that had undergone cardiovascular instrumentation 6 days earlier. The increase in circulating blood volume has a positive effect on end-diastolic volume, peak systolic pressure, and peak first derivative of pressure. The increase in systolic pressure is consistent with the exaggerated response to an increase in blood volume seen in the fetal lamb compared to the adult animal. The increase in end-diastolic volume is accompanied by an increase in systolic shortening consistent with an increase in stroke volume, the result of the Frank–Starling relation (see also Fig. 39.11). Tracings (top to bottom) are as follows: first derivatives of left ventricular pressure, P; left ventricular pressure, LVP; and electrocardiogram, ECG; pre; prior to infusion: post; following infusion. (From the laboratory of P.A.W. Anderson.)

4. Kirkpatrick et al[13] concluded that the Frank–Starling relation is important in the fetal heart when they found that increasing ventricular end-diastolic volume increases stroke volume.

5. In further support of this conclusion, in our fetal studies, increases or decreases in right and left ventricular end-diastolic volume were associated with significant increases or decreases in stroke volume (Fig. 39.11), respectively.[7,9,10]

The explanations for the apparently conflicting results from these fetal studies and the consequently differing conclusions are several. They include the sensitivity of the different methods used (e.g., the ability to measure whether and to what extent end-diastolic volume is changed by a specific intervention) and the sensitivity of the method used to measure beat-to-beat changes in stroke volume.

For example, in the studies of Heymann and Rudolph,[14] Gilbert,[17] and Thornburg et al,[15,18] end-diastolic volume and the effects of circulating blood volume on this variable were estimated by measuring atrial mean pressure and ventricular end-diastolic pressure. These measures are especially unreliable for assessing a change in ventricular end-diastolic volume at high end-diastolic pressures, because of the fetal myocardium's low compliance[5,6] (see Fig. 39.14 and later sections: Ventricular Interaction and Myocardial Compliance). Over the normal range of fetal end-diastolic pressures, a small increase in ventricular filling pressure produces a large increase in end-diastolic volume, while at high filling pressures, a large increase in filling pressure results in a very small increase in end-diastolic volume.[5]

Another explanation for the apparently conflicting results is the effect of increasing circulating blood volume on arterial pressure and the effects of increased arterial pressure on ventricular stroke volume (see later section: Afterload). Rudolph and associates found that when afterload was controlled, increasing left ventricular end-diastolic volume increased stroke volume.[19,20] Consequently, the failure to

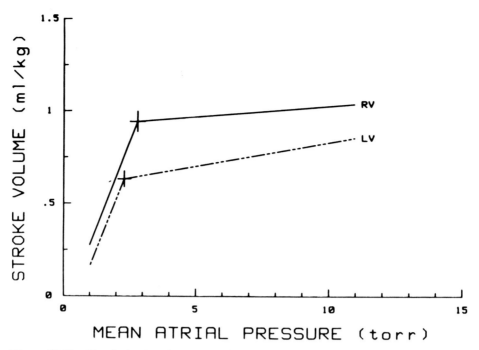

Figure 39.13   Ventricular function curves (right and left ventricular stroke volume as a function of mean atrial pressure) obtained from a group of fetal lambs. The ascending limb of the right ventricular function curve was steeper than that of the left. At all the filling pressures, right ventricular stroke volume exceeded that of the left ventricle. Although little increase in stroke volume is achieved at atrial pressures in excess of 5 torr (=5 mmHg), the presence of a Frank–Starling relation is clearly demonstrated in these fetal lambs over the range of physiologically normal atrial pressures. (From Reller et al, *Pediatr Res* 1987;22:621–626, with permission.)

demonstrate an increase in fetal cardiac output or stroke volume at high and often nonphysiological filling pressures does not test whether an increase in fetal end-diastolic volume increases stroke volume.

In contrast, ventricular dimension transducers can accurately monitor changes in end-diastolic volume. This technique, based on sonomicrometry, was first applied to the fetal left ventricle by Kirkpatrick et al[21] and shown to monitor accurately changes in end-diastolic volume. This approach was further developed to monitor fetal right ventricular dimensions[9] and, by means of multiple ventricular dimension transducers, to measure fetal left ventricular end-diastolic volume and so describe the relation between end-diastolic volume and stroke volume (Figs. 39.8 and 39.11).

Fetal ventricular stroke volume has been estimated by means of several techniques, including electromagnetic flow probe,[9,10,14] indicator dilution techniques, and systolic change in a ventricular dimension.[13] Although the systolic change in ventricular dimension can be useful in assessing whether end-diastolic volume affects systolic shortening or stroke volume (Fig. 39.8), *in vitro* calibration of the dimension signal is required to obtain an accurate estimate of stroke volume. The output of an electromagnetic flow probe is easily and accurately calibrated, allowing stroke volume to be monitored from beat to beat while physiological interventions are carried out. Transient changes in ventricular output are more accurately assessed with this approach than with indicator dilution techniques, which provide an average output over many systoles. Unfortunately, flow probes, which encircle the vessel, ultimately compromise the vessel lumen and increase ventricular afterload, or the resistance against which the ventricle ejects blood (see below). From a pragmatic viewpoint, this narrowing is rarely of significance during the first 7–10 days following instrumentation, and its presence can be identified by measuring ventricular and arterial pressures. In the studies described below, when a narrowing of the vessel was identified, the physiological data obtained from that lamb were rejected.

The importance of the Frank–Starling mechanism in the fetus is easily demonstrated by combining the techniques of sonomicrometry to measure ventricular dimensions and electromagnetic flow transducers to measure pulmonary artery and aortic flow, providing an excellent approach for examining the relationship between fetal ventricular end-diastolic

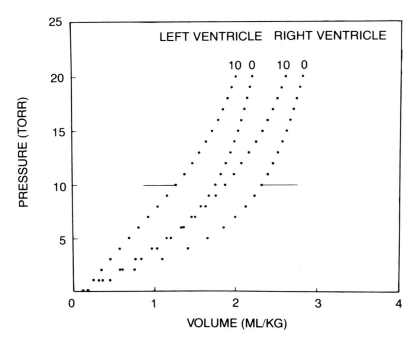

Figure 39.14   The effect of changing pressure in the contralateral ventricle on the passive pressure–volume relations of fetal lamb ventricles *in vitro*. The pressure–volume curves of the fetal right and left ventricles were obtained with the contralateral ventricles being filled at two different pressures, 0 and 10 torr. The standard error bars at 10 torr are provided by the horizontal lines. When the pressure in the contralateral ventricle is increased, the ipsilateral passive pressure–volume relation is shifted to the left (i.e., the higher the right ventricular end-diastolic pressure, the less the left ventricle will fill for a given left atrial pressure). Right ventricular filling is affected by left ventricular end-diastolic pressure or volume in a similar manner. These relations demonstrate that experiments in which fetal ventricular end-diastolic pressure is raised to pathologically elevated levels (>8 or 10 torr) will achieve little increase in end-diastolic volume and so will not be useful in testing the presence of the Frank–Starling relation in the fetal animal. (From Pinson et al, *J Dev Physiol* 1987;9:253–269, with permission.)

volume and stroke volume. Importantly, this relationship can be examined over a physiologic range of filling pressures by controlling diastolic filling time and heart rate through altering the atrial electronic pacing pattern. This approach provides a wide range of end-diastolic volumes (e.g., Figs. 39.7, 39.8, and 39.15).[9,10] Using this approach, the fetal right and left ventricle demonstrate a significant and positive relationship between end-diastolic volume and stroke volume. An increase in end-diastolic dimension is associated with an increase in stroke volume (Fig. 39.8). Moreover, when fetal left ventricular end-diastolic volume is measured *in vivo* using three left ventricular dimensions, an excellent linear correlation is found between end-diastolic volume and stroke volume (Fig. 39.11). P_{max} and other measures of ventricular performance also demonstrate the positive effect of end-diastolic volume on ventricular function (Fig. 39.16).[7,22,23]

Importantly, the Frank–Starling relation is physiologically important in moment-to-moment changes in cardiovascular state. In the chronically instrumented fetal lamb, large changes in end-diastolic and end-systolic volume can occur from one beat to the next.[7,9,10,13,22,23] These changes in volume may occur with maternal movements; for example, when the ewe lies on her abdomen, a sudden precipitous decrease in fetal left ventricular end-diastolic volume can occur, followed by a return to a volume equal to or exceeding that observed when the ewe was standing. These large beat-to-beat and minute-to-minute changes in fetal stroke volume that occur in late gestation (Fig. 39.11) demonstrate the dynamic ability of the fetal right and left ventricles to modulate cardiac output in response to varying hemodynamic states and changes in venous return.

The presence of the Frank–Starling mechanism in the fetal heart has special significance when one is considering the effects of birth on the left ventricle. Left ventricular stroke volume increases with birth (Fig. 39.17B; see Effects of Birth, below).[8,16,24–26] For example, left ventricular stroke volume has been shown to increase from 1.1 mL/kg to 2.0 mL/kg and output from 180 mL/kg/min[24] to 400–425

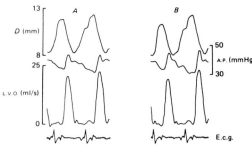

Figure 39.15 The dynamic effects of altering heart rate and so the duration of diastolic filling on left ventricular filling and stroke volume: data from an in utero fetal lamb that had undergone cardiovascular instrumentation to permit study of the affects of introducing a longer paced interval into the paced rate. (*A*) First systole in response to a paced rate of 240 beats per minute (pacing interval, 250 ms); second systole follows a paced interval of 400 ms. (*B*) First systole in response to a paced interval of 280 beats per minute (paced interval, 215 ms), and the second systole again follows a paced interval of 400 ms. Note that at the faster rate the end-diastolic dimension and stroke volume are smallest. Following the 400 ms interval, stroke volume is larger following the faster paced rate. The right atrium is being paced. Tracings (top to bottom) are as follows: left ventricular minor axis dimension, D; aortic pressure, A.P.; ascending aortic flow, L.V.O.; and electrocardiogram, e.c.g. (Reprinted from Anderson et al, *J Physiol* 1986;372:557–573, with permission.)

mL/kg/min.[16,25–27] Studies that monitor left ventricular end-diastolic dimensions in the lamb prior to and following delivery demonstrate that an increase in left ventricular end-diastolic volume is a significant contributor to the enhanced function of the neonatal heart.[8,21,23] Thus, the Frank–Starling mechanism is a contributor to the left ventricle's ability to markedly increase its stroke volume and output with birth.

Although these findings demonstrate that the Frank–Starling relation is operational in the *in vivo* fetal right and left ventricle, these studies do not address the following questions: Why is the output of the fetal heart unaffected by increasing end-diastolic pressure over a range that in the neonate results in a significant increase in output[15,17,18,28] (see Fig. 39.18)? A potentially important contributor is the extracardiac constraint that is lost with birth.[29] Another is the effect of birth on ventricular interaction that follows, for example, from the marked fall in pulmonary artery pressure and resistance during the first minutes of neonatal life, the marked increase in pulmonary venous return, and the increase in left ventricular end-diastolic volume (see below).

Ventricular Interaction

Ventricular interaction characterizes how the diastolic volume and pressure and systolic pressure in one ventricle alter diastolic filling and systolic function in the contralateral ventricle. Although this interaction has been well described in the adult heart, the effect of ventricular loading on the function of the contralateral ventricle has yet to be fully characterized in the fetus.

In the adult heart the effects of ventricular filling and pressure development of, for example, the left ventricle on those of the right have been studied extensively. In the adult heart the right ventricle has little effect on left ventricular function unless, as a consequence of cardiac disease or pulmonary hypertension, the right ventricle is enlarged and hypertrophied. In the presence of the normal thin-walled adult right ventricle, the effects of ventricular interaction are dominated by the effects of the left ventricle on right ventricular function. The greater the filling of the left ventricle and the higher its end-diastolic pressure, the less the right ventricle is filled by a giv-

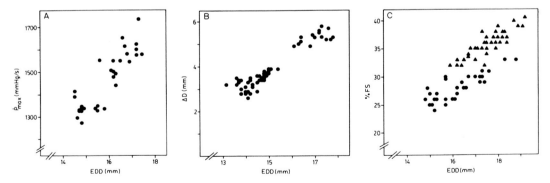

Figure 39.16 Characterization of the Frank–Starling relation in the left ventricle of the *in utero* fetal lamb: (*A*) effect of end-diastolic dimension (EDD) on the maximum rate of rise of left ventricular pressure, P_{max}, (*B*) systolic shortening (end-diastolic dimension − end-systolic dimension, ESD), and (*C*) percent fractional shortening [100(EDD − ESD/EDD)]. Data obtained at two infusion rates of isoproterenol 0.006 μg/kg/min, (circles) and 0.024 μg/kg/min (triangles). (Reprinted from Ref. 7, with permission.)

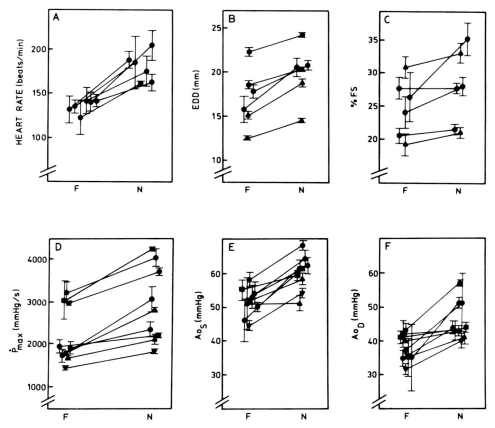

Figure 39.17   The effects of birth on cardiovascular hemodynamics in six lambs that had undergone cardiovascular instrumentation at least 4 days prior to birth: the change from fetal (F) to neonatal (N) life (the mean and 2 standard deviations) of (A) heart rate; (B) ventricular end-diastolic dimension, EDD; (C) percent fractional shortening, %FS; (D) maximum rate of rise of left ventricular pressure, $\dot{P}_{max}$; (E) aortic systolic pressure, Ao$_S$; and (F) diastolic aortic pressure Ao$_D$. Connected values in (B)–(F) were obtained at the same heart rates (squares, paced intervals of 250 ms; circles, 300 ms; upright triangles, 350 ms; inverted triangles, 400 ms). (Reprinted from Anderson et al, *Am J Physiol* 1984;247:H371–H379, with permission.)

en venous pressure. Similarly, alterations in the development of left ventricular pressure and left ventricular contraction can compromise right ventricular systolic function.

The developmental changes in ventricular interaction are a consequence of differences in ventricular mass and shape (see Fig. 39.19). These differences follow, in part, from the lower pulmonary artery pressure of the adult. In contrast, fetal right and left ventricular systolic pressures are similar (Fig. 39.6), while the end-diastolic volume of the fetal right ventricle is greater than that of the left. As a consequence, the fetal right ventricular mass is similar to or greater than that of the left ventricle, in contrast to the adult heart, where right ventricular mass is much less than in the left ventricle (Fig. 39.19). Not surprisingly, *in vitro* studies of the fetal and neonatal heart demonstrate that changes in right ventricular volume significantly affect the extent to which the left ventricle is distended by a given filling pressure,[5] while in the

adult heart, the effects of right ventricular volume have very modest effects on left ventricular function (Fig. 39.20).

Romero et al,[5] using hearts obtained from fetal, newborn, and adult sheep, assessed whether developmental changes in the right and left ventricles modulate the effects of right and left ventricular volume on the filling of the contralateral chamber (Fig. 39.20). When right ventricular distending pressure exceeds 5 mmHg, left ventricular filling is compromised. The extent of the compromise is greatest in the fetal heart and least in the adult heart. When right ventricular filling pressure is increased to pathological levels (e.g., 15 mmHg), the fetal left ventricular volume is decreased by 30% while that of the adult heart is decreased by only 10%. Similarly, left ventricular diastolic pressure limited right ventricular filling at all ages. Thus, in the normal newborn the neonatal fall in right ventricular end-diastolic volume may through ventricular interaction have a powerful effect on the

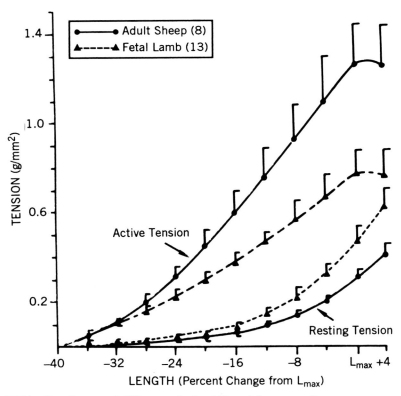

Figure 39.21 Developmental differences in the ability of the myocardium to contract and develop pressure and myocardial passive characteristics or compliance, illustrated in data obtained from preparations isolated from 8 adult (*circles*) and 13 fetal (*triangles*) sheep. The immature myocardium is less compliant (stiffer) than that of the adult. On the other hand, the adult myocardium is able to develop a much greater force per cross-sectional area than is the immature myocardium. Each point in the vertical bars represents the mean ± SEM. (From Friedman, *Prog Cardiovasc Dis* 1972;15:87–111, with permission.)

will result in relatively larger end-diastolic volumes in the adult heart, compared to the fetus and the newborn. When left ventricular passive pressure–volume data for hearts from different stages of development are mathematically modeled, the fetal left ventricular data generate a significantly larger slope than those of the newborn and adult left ventricles, reflecting the developmental fall in myocardial stiffness (Fig. 39.22). Myocardium from the right ventricle of the late gestation fetus and the newborn are similar, but for both these stages of development the immature right ventricle is stiffer than that of the adult. Thus, compared to the adult heart, the greater stiffness of the immature right and left ventricles will result in relatively smaller increases in ventricular end-diastolic volume in response to the same venous filling pressure.

Another factor that contributes to the effects of development on ventricular filling is chamber size. The developmental changes in ventricular shape and mass[31,32] (see Figs. 39.19 and 39.23) in fetal, newborn, and adult hearts affect wall tension as a function of change in internal radius.[5] The tension–radius relations of both fetal ventricles demonstrate

the greatest increase in wall tension for comparable increases in chamber dimension (Fig. 39.24). These developmental differences in ventricular wall tension–radius relations appear to exceed the effects of differences in myocardial compliance.[5]

The foregoing analyses of *in vitro* ventricular volume–wall tension and passive pressure–volume relations are instructive in explaining why ventricular-function curves (stroke volume or output as a function of atrial filling pressure) of the *in vivo* fetal heart demonstrate such small increases in stroke volume when end-diastolic pressures are increased beyond the physiological range. A consequence of the decreased distensibility of the fetal ventricles beyond the physiological range of filling pressures is the minimal effect of increasing pressure to these pathologic levels on stroke volume. In summary, the apparent absence of the Frank–Starling relation in the fetal heart at high filling pressures is, in part, a consequence of the relatively decreased fetal myocardial compliance of the fetal heart and the decreased distensibility of the fetal right and left ventricle.

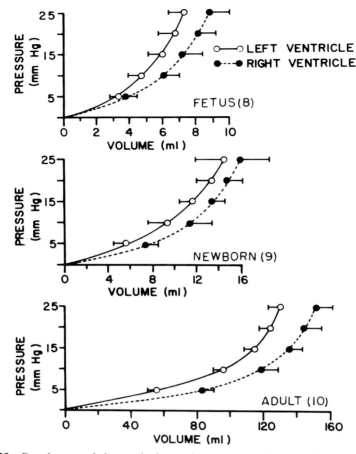

Figure 39.22   Developmental changes in the passive pressure–volume relations of the heart, illustrated by data obtained from hearts from 8 fetal, 9 newborn, and 10 adult sheep. The data further illustrate the developmental increase in myocardial compliance. Each point in the horizontal bars represents mean, ± SEM. No significant differences were observed between the passive pressure–volume relations of the fetal right and left ventricles. In the newborn heart, the passive pressure–volume relation of the left ventricle was shifted significantly to the left of the right ventricular curve. (From Romero et al, *Am J Physiol* 1972;222:1285–1290, with permission.)

Afterload

The term "afterload" is derived from the concept that if the end-diastolic volume is a load applied to the ventricle before contraction (i.e., preload), then afterload is the load or pressure the heart must eject against after systole has begun. In isolated muscle, the greater the afterload, the slower the contraction velocity and the smaller the amount of muscle shortening (Fig. 39.25). Increasing afterload in vivo has a similarly negative effect on ventricular function, regardless of the stage of development. Although afterload is made up of several components, the major *in vivo* component is arterial pressure. The higher the arterial pressure, the higher the afterload. A consequence of a higher afterload is a greater myocardial oxygen consumption: When ejecting from the same end-diastolic volume against a higher systolic pressure, the

ventricle must develop a higher wall tension to eject blood and so consume a greater amount of oxygen.

The fetal heart is not able to eject against arterial pressures that are well tolerated by the adult heart; this is because the adult left ventricular wall is thicker and the adult myocardium contains a relatively greater number of myofibrils. For example, the adult human heart easily sustains a normal cardiac output in the presence of mean systemic arterial pressures of 100 mmHg. In contrast, the preterm infant's heart fails in the face of such pressures—sometimes acutely, while at other times more slowly—and the infant acquires the signs and symptoms of a congested circulation and ultimately metabolic acidosis.

The effect of afterload on fetal ventricular stroke volume is clearly evident over the normal range of fetal arterial pressures.[15,18] This effect is exemplified in Figure 39.26, where

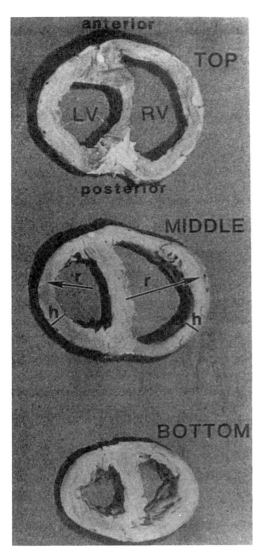

Figure 39.23 Transverse, cross-sectional slices of fetal lamb ventricles one-quarter (*top*), half (*middle*), and three-quarters (*bottom*) of the distance from the atrioventricular valves to the ventricular apex, illustrating why changes in right ventricular end-diastolic volume are going to have a greater effect on right ventricular wall stress than similar changes in left ventricular end-diastolic volume on left ventricular wall stress. Specifically, the right ventricular cavity is relatively larger and has a greater radius of curvature. Considering the LaPlace relation for similar pressures, right ventricular wall stress must be higher. LV = left ventricle, RV = right ventricle, r = radius, h = wall thickness. (From Pinson et al, *J Dev Physiol* 1987;9:253–269, with permission.)

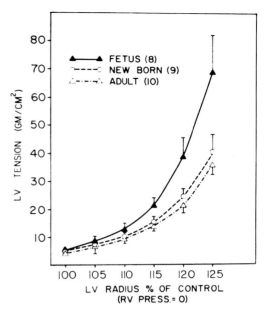

Figure 39.24 Developmental changes in the left ventricular wall tension–radius relation. At any radius, left ventricular wall tension was significantly greater in the fetal heart than in that from the newborn or adult. No significant differences were observed between the newborn and the adult. The control left ventricular radius (100%) corresponded to the radius at a calculated wall tension of 5 g/cm². Numbers in parentheses are the number of hearts studied. (From Romero et al, *Am J Physiol* 1972;222:1285–1290, with permission.)

increasing arterial pressure decreases fetal ventricular stroke volume and output. Of note, the fetal left ventricle is better able to maintain its stroke volume than is the right ventricle (Fig. 39.27). The greater sensitivity of the fetal right ventricle to an increase in overload in comparison to that of the left

probably has to do with fetal ventricular end-diastolic volume, wall tension, and stroke volume, given that these values are larger for the right ventricle than for the left ventricle (consider Fig. 39.23).

This sensitivity of the fetal heart to afterload is important in considerations of the hemodynamic effects of *in utero* hypoxemia. Fetal cardiovascular function is profoundly affected by hypoxemia. The effects include a decrease in cardiac output and heart rate, an increase in arterial pressure, and a redistribution of cardiac output. The contributions of the hypoxemia-induced increase in arterial pressure to these pathophysiological effects have been examined.[33,34] The depressed right ventricular function curves that result from hypoxemia (Fig. 39.28) vanish when nitroprusside is used to eliminate the systemic hypertension even when hypoxemia is allowed to persist: in the presence of nitroprusside and hypoxemia, the right ventricular function curve becomes similar to the control.

The negative effect of an increase in arterial pressure on fetal ventricular stroke volume is also revealed when the fetus receives an infusion of saline solution or blood. Mean arterial pressure is elevated in response to such an infusion out of proportion to the response observed in the adult heart. This negative effect of afterload on ventricular stroke volume contributes to the finding that increasing fetal circulating blood

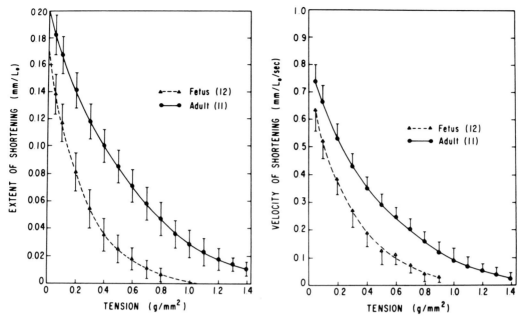

Figure 39.25 The ability of the ventricle to shorten against a given load increases with development. These data illustrate the myocardial basis of this increase. For any given tension, the adult myocardium is able to shorten a greater amount and at a higher velocity. Numbers in parentheses are the numbers of lamb and sheep from which heart muscle was isolated. Each point in the vertical bars represents the mean ± SEM. (From Friedman, *Prog Cardiovasc Dis* 1972;15:87–111, with permission.)

volume and so ventricular end-diastolic volume may not increase ventricular stroke volume.

This interaction among circulating blood volume, arterial pressure, and ventricular output has a broader significance than simply its usefulness in interpreting the results of experiments that assess the presence of the Frank–Starling relation in the fetal heart. Consider the successful *in utero* repair of diaphragmatic hernias and the proposed use of cardiac surgery and cardiac bypass technology to treat congenital heart defects *in utero*. The application of such procedures and techniques to the fetus, with their effects on ventricular volume and circulating blood volume, requires a full understanding of the mechanisms that modulate fetal ventricular function and how they may be affected by these invasive procedures.

Inotropy (Contractility)

Effects of β-Adrenoreceptor Stimulation   The outputs of the fetal right and left ventricles are often characterized as being near maximal in the intact *in utero* fetus. The apparent resistance of the fetal heart to perturbations that might be expected to increase ventricular output, including catecholamine stimulation,[35] is surprising in the light of observations resulting from other developmental studies. One is the striking ability of the immature heart to increase its output with

birth. Another is the catecholamine enhancement of force development in isolated fetal myocardium.[6,7,36]

We have used isoproterenol, a β-adrenoreceptor agonist, to address whether inotropy of the *in vivo* fetal ventricle can be enhanced.[37] The markers for an increase in ventricular inotropy were the maximum rate of rise of the ventricular pressure, stroke volume, and cardiac output (Fig. 39.29).

Infusions of isoproterenol produce twofold or greater increases in P_{max} and are associated with an enhancement of ventricular systolic function (Fig. 39.16). When stroke volume and left ventricular output are examined, left ventricular output is increased by 50% or more with infusion rates that would be considered small or modest if used in a patient (Fig. 39.30). Left ventricular end-diastolic volume falls with the associated isoproterenol-induced increase in heart rate. Despite the fall in preload, stroke volume does not fall. When the effects of heart rate on ventricular filling are controlled, stroke volume increases by 40–50% (Fig. 39.31). These results clearly demonstrated the positive effects of catecholamine stimulation on *in vivo* fetal ventricular function. Positive inotropic interventions increase the ability of the ventricle to develop pressure and to eject blood. These findings are of importance in the light of presently performed and potential future invasive procedures to treat or palliate congenital malformations in the human fetus.[1–4] A complete understanding of the effects of inotropic interactions on the im-

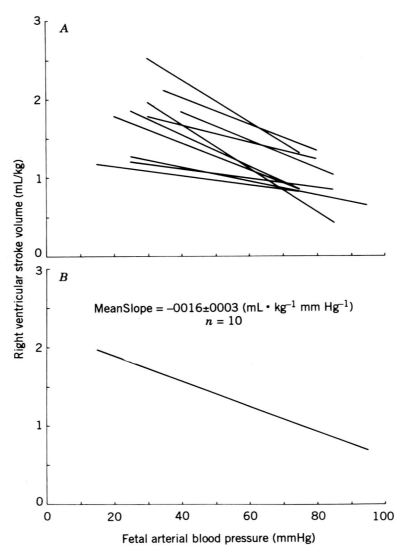

Figure 39.26   The effects of pulmonary artery pressure on fetal right ventricular stroke volume. These data illustrate the sensitivity of the right ventricle to an increase in afterload or arterial pressure: The higher the fetal blood pressure, the lower the right ventricular stroke volume. (*A*) Stroke volume–arterial pressure coordinates from ventricular function curves obtained at normal, reduced, and elevated arterial pressures. Each line represents the regression for an individual experiment. (*B*) Mean slope of the regression lines in (*A*). In the mature fetal lamb, the arterial pressure is approximately 40–50 torr and has an average stroke volume of approximately 1.4 mL/kg. This regression yields the same relation between arterial pressure and stroke volume. By the end of the first postnatal week, pulmonary arterial pressure is approximately 20 torr and stroke volume has increased to about 2 mL/kg. Based on this regression analysis, the postnatal decrease in arterial pressure would be expected to increase right ventricular stroke volume to about 2 mL/kg. (From Thornburg, Morton, *J Physiol* 1983;244:H656, with permission.)

mature heart will permit sound therapeutic decisions in the care of the sick fetus and neonate.

Effects of Heart Rate on Ventricular Function   The effects of heart rate on fetal ventricular function depend on the variable being monitored and the experimental design. The fol-

lowing subsection aims to separate the different effects of heart rate on ventricular function, considering them in the context of the Frank–Starling relation (ventricular end-diastolic volume), inotropy (contractility), and afterload (arterial pressure).

Because of the complex interaction of the effects of heart

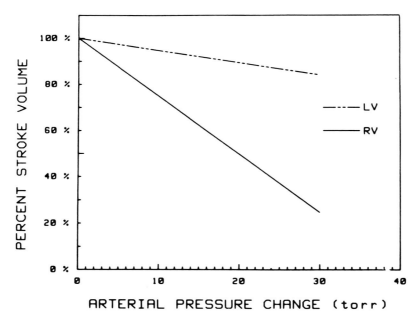

Figure 39.27   Relation between afterload and fetal right and left stroke volume, illustrated by average responses obtained from group of fetal lambs. Stroke volume is expressed as a percentage of the control and arterial pressure as the increment above control. Consistent with the geometric differences between the fetal right and left ventricle (see Fig. 39.23), an increase in afterload or arterial pressure has a greater effect on fetal right ventricular stroke volume than that of the left ventricle. (From Reller et al, *Pediatr Res* 1987;22:621–626, with permission.)

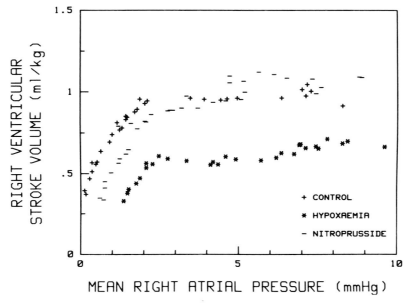

Figure 39.28   The effect of fetal hypoxemia on the relation between right ventricular stroke volume and right atrial pressure (stars) is eliminated by treating the hypoxemia-induced hypertension with nitroprusside (dashes). The control relation prior to inducing hypoxemia is illustrated with plus signs. (From Reller et al, *J Dev Physiol* 1989;11:263–269, with permission.)

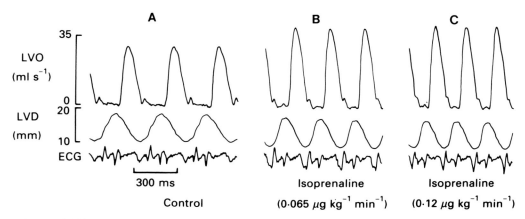

Figure 39.29   The positive effect on left ventricular stroke volume and output that follows from the chronotropic and inotropic effects of isoproterenol in the fetal lamb. Isoproterenol was infused at two different rates in this fetal lamb that had undergone instrumentation 5 days earlier (gestational age 126 days). (*A*) Control. (*B*) 0.065 μg/kg/min. (*C*) 0.12 μg/kg/min. Tracings (top to bottom) are as follows: ascending aortic blood flow, LVO; left ventricular anterior–posterior axis dimension, LVD; and the electrocardiogram, ECG. The time base is the same in all three panels. (From Anderson et al, *J Physiol* 1990;430:441–452, with permission.)

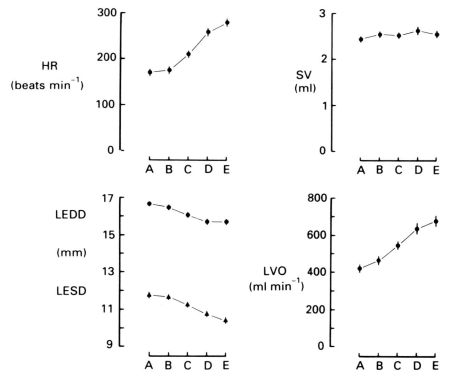

Figure 39.30   Effects of isoproterenol on mean spontaneous heart rate (HR) and left ventricular stroke volume (SV), end-diastolic (LEDD) and end-systolic (LESD) dimensions, and output (LVO) (*n* = 7) for controls (*A*) and during isoproterenol infusions at the following rates (μg/kg/min): (*B*) 0.0063, (*C*) 0.024, (*D*) 0.071, and (*E*) 0.241. Tracings (top to bottom) are as follows: Points and bars are least-square means ± SEM. Average SEM, expressed as a percentage of the means for each group of measurements: HR = 4.0%, LEDD = 0.9%, LESD = 1.5%, SV = 2.9%, and LVO = 5.0%. (From Anderson et al, *J Physiol* 1990;430:441–452, with permission.)

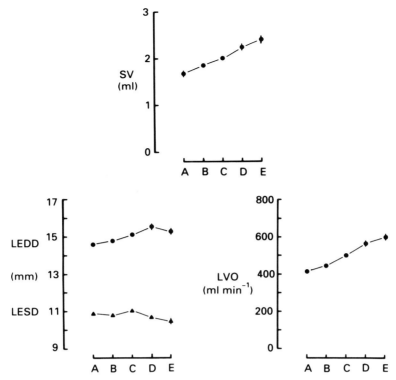

Figure 39.31 Effects of isoproterenol on mean left ventricular stroke volume (SV), end-diastolic (LEDD) and end-systolic (LESD) dimensions, and output (LVO) when heart rate was controlled using atrial pacing ($n = 6$) for controls (*A*) and during isoproterenol infusions at the following rates (μg/kg/min): (*B*) 0.0063, (*C*) 0.024, (*D*) 0.071, and (*E*) 0.241. Points and bars are least-square means ± SEM. Average SEM, expressed as a percentage of the means for each group of measurements: SV = 2.9%, LEDD = 0.9%, and LVO = 2.8%. (From Anderson et al, *J Physiol* 1990;430:441–452, with permission.)

rate on variables that control fetal ventricular function, essentially diametrically opposite viewpoints have been reached as to how and whether heart rate modulates fetal ventricular function, for example, as measured by cardiac output. Because some viewpoints have been accepted dogma, it is valuable to review the findings that support these different conclusions.[38–45]

Heart Rate and Inotropy (In Vivo)   Considering here only increases in heart rate brought about by atrial pacing, it is noted that an increase in heart rate has a positive inotropic effect on the *in vivo* fetal heart's ability to develop systolic pressure.[22,23,38] When rate is increased, the heart shows an increased ability to generate pressure (e.g., P_{max} increases despite a fall in left ventricular end-diastolic volume: Fig. 39.7). When end-diastolic volume is allowed to return to its low rate value or when it does so spontaneously (Figs. 39.7 and 39.16), P_{max} is even further accentuated at the faster rate. This increase in the rate of pressure development occurs when atrial pacing is used to increase heart rate, and sponta-

neous increases in heart rate, bring about even greater developmental rates.

An increase in rate also enhances the ability of the ventricle to eject blood.[9,10,23,44] As described below next, however, this positive effect of rate on stroke volume requires that end-diastolic volume not fall with the rate increase and the shortened diastolic filling time. If these conditions are fulfilled, ejection phase measures of ventricular function are consistently enhanced when heart rate is increased. Examples of this positive effect include increases in the rate of ejection, systolic shortening of ventricular dimensions, and stroke volume (Figs. 39.16 and 39.32).

Thus, the positive inotropic effect of heart rate is most clearly revealed *in vivo* when end-diastolic volume is held constant. On the other hand, when end-diastolic volume falls with the rate increase, the positive effect of heart rate on inotropy can be obscured (see below, and Figs. 39.3–39.5 and 39.32). The complex interaction of diastolic filling time and enhancement of inotropy provides an explanation for the range of findings observed when the effect of heart rate on

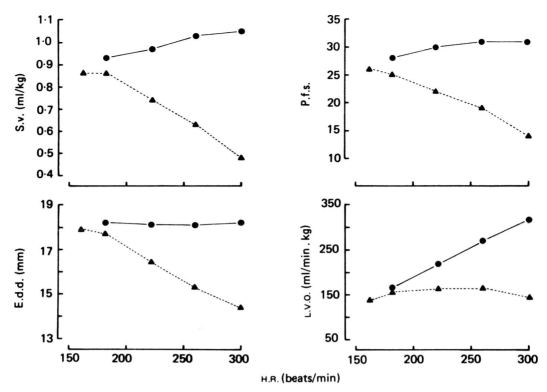

H.R. (beats/min)

Figure 39.32   Effects of atrial pacing on fetal left ventricular end-diastolic volume, stroke volume and output, and stroke volume and output when end-diastolic volume is kept constant. A comparison of left ventricular filling and ejection during right atrial pacing for systoles during pacing rates of 150–300 beats per minute (*triangles*) and the subsequent systoles (*circles*) that follow the introduction of a longer paced interval (400 ms; e.g., see Fig. 39.2). Left ventricular end-diastolic dimensions (EDD) following the longer paced intervals were within 0.1 mm, while the dimensions during continuous pacing at a constant rate became progressively smaller with each increase in rate. For the systoles with comparable end-diastolic dimensions (*circles*), stroke volume (SV, corrected for body weight), percent fractional shortening (PFS), and left ventricular output (LVO, corrected for body weight) were larger, the faster the preceding paced rate. Data were obtained from a fetal lamb 10 days after surgery. (From Anderson et al, *J Physiol* 1986;372:557–573, with permission.)

fetal cardiac output is examined (see below, Heart Rate and Cardiac Output).

Heart Rate and End-Diastolic Volume   When atrial pacing is used to increase heart rate, end-diastolic volume decreases in both the right and left ventricle. The same phenomenon occurs in the adult heart. The decrease in end-diastolic volume results in a decrease in stroke volume (Figs. 39.3–39.5).

The rate-induced fall in end-diastolic volume can be circumvented by infrequently interpolating among the shorter paced intervals a longer paced interval. The longer diastolic-filling time allows the ventricles to eject from the same end-diastolic volume (preload) at different overall rates. The stroke volumes of these systoles are significantly greater than those that begin from smaller end-diastolic volumes (Figs. 39.15 and 39.32).[9,10] The aortic diastolic pressure that precedes ventricular ejection is similar for these systoles, re-

moving as a confounding effect on stroke volume variations in afterload.

The increase in stroke volume at faster rates, observed using this mechanism for keeping end-diastolic volume constant, demonstrates the positive inotropic effect of heart rate (see Fig. 39.32 and preceding subsection, Heart Rate and Inotropy). The faster the paced rate, the larger the stroke volume. Thus, in the fetus, a large increase in output occurs with an increase in heart rate when the fall in end-diastolic volume is circumvented. The response of the fetal heart is quite similar to the response of the adult heart when heart rate is increased and an arteriovenous fistula is used to increase venous return.[39,40]

Heart Rate and Site of Atrial Pacing   The relationship between heart rate, end-diastolic volume, and stroke volume is complicated in the fetus by atrial pacing site and the fetal circulation. The foramen ovale, an essential fetal connection, allows blood returning from the placenta to flow from the right to the left atrium. Consequently, flow into the fetal right atrium from the inferior vena cava contributes to both left and right ventricular filling. If the phasic relation of the right and left atrial pressure waveforms is altered, the flow patterns through the foramen ovale will be affected, hence the right and left ventricular end-diastolic volumes. Consequently, when the site of atrial pacing alters the normal sequence of right and left atrial contraction, fetal right and left ventricular outputs can be differentially affected.[9,10]

An increase in heart rate through right atrial pacing decreases right ventricular end-diastolic volume and stroke volume more than left atrial pacing at the same rate (Fig. 39.5).[9] The left ventricle is affected in the opposite manner by the site of atrial pacing[10]: Increasing heart rate with left atrial pacing produces a greater fall in left ventricular end-diastolic volume and stroke volume than does right atrial pacing (Figs. 39.3 and 39.4). This approach for varying the end-diastolic volumes of the two ventricles may prove to be of value in exploring the *in vivo* effects of the relatively noncompliant immature right ventricle on left ventricular function.

In summary, the effects of atrial pacing site on right and left ventricular output are as follows: When right atrial pacing is used to increase heart rate, a significant decrease in right ventricular output occurs, while increasing heart rate with right atrial pacing results in no significant change in left ventricular output. Conversely, increasing heart rate through left atrial pacing results in a decrease in left ventricular output, but right ventricular output is unchanged.

These results and those discussed earlier demonstrate that in the fetus, heart rate, end-diastolic volume, arterial pressure, and inotropy are important variables in determining stroke volume, and therefore the cardiac output of the fetus. The identification of these relationships in the fetus demonstrate that they are in place prior to birth and will be useful in the adaptation of the neonate to the increased metabolic needs and the changes in right and left ventricular workload that occur with birth. Indeed, increases in heart rate, left ventricular end-diastolic volume, and inotropy do occur with birth (see Effects of Birth, below).

Heart Rate and Cardiac Output   The effects of heart rate on fetal cardiac output result from the interaction of rate-induced changes in ventricular end-diastolic volume and inotropy. These effects are similar to those observed in the heart of the adult. In both adult and fetus, when heart rate is increased by atrial pacing, end-diastolic volume falls, stroke volume falls, and cardiac output remains unchanged over a broad range of rates.[39–43] Thus, in both the fetus and the adult the extents to which ventricular end-diastolic volume decreases and stroke volume decreases strongly affect whether heart rate increases cardiac output.

A spontaneous increase in heart rate in the fetus usually results in an increase in ventricular output (Fig. 39.33), just as an exercise-induced increase in heart rate in the adult serves to increase cardiac output. The similarity of the responses of the adult and the fetal cardiac output to heart rate changes supports the conclusion that preload and inotropy, the hemodynamic modulators of ventricular function, are present over a broad range of development. Importantly, they modulate stroke volume. Consequently, all the variables in the following equation are important in the fetal, neonatal, and adult heart:

$$\text{ventricular output} = \text{stroke volume} \times \text{heart rate}$$

These effects of rate, inotropy, end-diastolic volume, and pacing site can be imagined easily to interact in a manner so complicated that different conclusions about the effect of heart rate on fetal cardiac output can be reached (e.g., see Figs. 39.32 and 39.33).

Rudolph and Heymann[44] observed in the chronically instrumented fetus that, in general, an increase in total (biventricular) cardiac output occurs when heart rate is increased over a broad range of rate and that beyond this range, output falls with further increases in rate. To obtain slow fetal heart rates, acetylcholine, a negative inotropic agent, was admin-

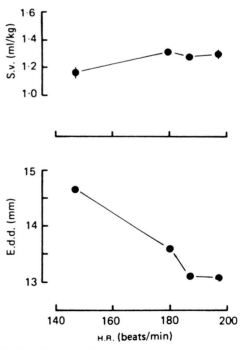

Figure 39.33   When fetal heart rate increases spontaneously, ventricular output usually increases. In this sample, end-diastolic dimension (EDD) fell with an increase in rate while stroke volume (SV, corrected for body weight) increased. The increase in stroke volume and rate resulted in a marked increase in left ventricular output. (From Anderson et al, *J Physiol* 1986;372:557–573, with permission.)

istered to the fetus (consequently, some of the decrease in cardiac output at low heart rates can be attributed to an acetylcholine-induced decrease in contractility). These observations, coupled with these authors' earlier finding that an increase in cardiac output does not occur when right ventricular end-diastolic pressure is increased markedly resulted in the following conclusion: Stroke volume is relatively fixed in the fetus; consequently, the stressed fetus must have only one mechanism through which cardiac output can be increased—namely, an increase in heart rate.

A conclusion diametrically opposite to that of Rudolph and Heymann was reached by Kirkpatrick et al,[38] who believe that an increase in heart rate does not increase fetal ventricular output. On monitoring left ventricular volume by means of ventricular dimension transducers (see Fig. 39.2), they found no increase in left ventricular output with an increase in heart rate. This appeared to be a consequence of the heart rate induced decrease in end-diastolic volume (see Figs. 39.3–39.5 and 39.32).

Spontaneous or Atrial Pacing-Induced Increase in Rate
When we monitored stroke volume of the right and the left ventricle in the chronically instrumented fetal lamb using electromagnetic flow transducers,[9,10] we found that the most important consideration is whether the heart rate change occurs spontaneously or through atrial pacing. When atrial pacing is used in assessing the effects of rate on output free of the concomitant effects associated with spontaneous changes in heart rate, an increase in heart rate does not increase right or left ventricular output. The inotropic effect of the greater heart rate and the increased number of beats per minute is offset by the decrease in stroke volume that follows from the fall in end-diastolic volume.

Rudolph and Heymann[44] found that a spontaneous increase in rate was always associated with an increase in output, and Kirkpatrick et al[38] found no increase in output. In our assessment of the effects of spontaneous changes in heart rate on ventricular output in the fetal lamb,[9,10] a spontaneous increase in rate was associated usually with an increase in right and left ventricular output, occasionally with no increase in output, and rarely with a fall in output.

An explanation of these various findings is provided by the following. The effects of a spontaneous change in heart rate on ventricular output must be a consequence of how the underlying stimuli, which induce the rate change, affect inotropy, venous return, and arterial pressure, and therefore stroke volume. Through the use of ventricular dimension transducers, venous return can be shown to increase during some spontaneous increases in heart rate as end-diastolic volume is maintained despite a decrease in diastolic filling time. On other occasions, inotropy can be shown to be enhanced (e.g., stroke volume is increased despite a fall in end-diastolic volume: the opposite to what occurs when an increase in rate is induced by atrial pacing; contrast Figs. 39.32 and 39.33).

Furthermore, concomitant variations in ventricular afterload can modify ventricular ejection and so modulate the effects of a spontaneous rate change on stroke volume[15,18,45] (and see above: Effects of Afterload).

The Force–Interval Relationship

The presence of the relationship, described above, between heart rate and ventricular performance must be considered in a more general way than simply: Does ventricular output vary with a change in heart rate? Broader questions are suggested: (1) How does the heart, having undergone activation and contraction, return itself to a state of readiness to generate tension or eject blood by the next beat? (2) Does this process change qualitatively and quantitatively with development? These questions are relevant to the modulation of cytosolic calcium concentration, essential for cardiac contraction and to the issue of whether the control of cytosolic calcium concentration is affected by development.

The general relationship between the pattern of stimulation and force of contraction, which has been studied extensively in the adult heart (e.g., as postextrasystolic potentiation, the positive staircase that follows a change in rate, or the response to paired pacing), where it has been termed the force–frequency, interval–strength, or force–interval relationship.[22] In adult myocardium these changes in the force of contraction are the result of changes in the cytosolic calcium concentration during systole (Fig. 39.34; see also Fig.

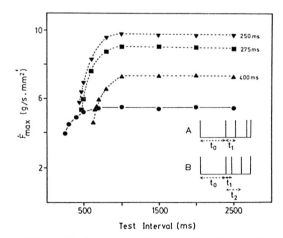

Figure 39.34   The force–interval curves, F_{max} (the maximum rate of rise of force) described as a function of the test interval (t_1 or t_2) from an isolated fetal *trabeculae carneae cordis* (132 days of gestation): basic interval $t_0 = 3000$ ms; first-stage curve has varying t_1 (circles). Three second-stage curves as follows: fixed t_1 (= 250 ms) and varying t_2 (inverted triangles), $t_1 = 275$ ms (squares), and $t_1 = 400$ ms (upright triangles). *Inset:* Schematic representation of the pacing sequence of the two-stage experiment (stages A and B). (From Anderson et al, *Am J Obstet Gynecol* 1980;138:44–54, with permission.)

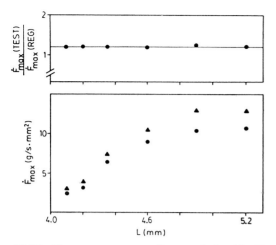

Figure 39.35 Top = postextrasystolic potentiation (the F_{max}–interval ratio, F_{max} of the potentiated test contraction, $t_2 = 2500$ ms, following an extrasystole, $t_1 = 300$ ms, divided by F_{max} of the preceding regular contraction) as a function of muscle length for an isolated *trabeculae carneae* from a fetal lamb (126 days of gestation). Bottom = Values of F_{max} for the test contractions (*triangles*) and the preceding regular contractions (*circles*). (From Anderson et al, *Am J Obstet Gynecol* 1980;138:44–54, with permission.)

39.35).[46] A developmental difference in the relation between the pattern of stimulation and the force of contraction indicates a developmental change in the control of activator calcium and the systems that modulate cytosolic calcium.

If ontogeny recapitulates phylogeny, the following phylogenetic difference in a force–interval relation might be found in the developing heart. In adult mammalian myocardium, an extrasystole elicits a weaker contraction than the preceding contraction at the basic rate, whereas in amphibian myocardium the maximum tension of the extrasystole is greater than that of the preceding steady state contraction.[47] Such differences between the two phyla in the myocardial response to an extrasystole suggest a corollary: Amphibian myocardium is thought to depend primarily on extracellular calcium for the source of activator calcium, and immature mammalian myocardium is thought to have a greater dependence on extracellular calcium than that of the adult heart.[48–50] Consequently, the maximum tension of the extrasystolic contraction of the fetal myocardium could be anticipated to be greater than the maximum tension of the contraction at the basic rate. However, this potential developmental difference does not occur; in both adult and fetal mammalian myocardium, that is, extrasystoles elicit weaker contractions.

Mammalian myocardia of the fetus, neonate, and adult never demonstrate the properties of the amphibian force–interval relationship.[47] Thus, even though the contraction of the amphibian myocardium and that of the immature mammal are more dependent on extracellular calcium concentration, the qualitative properties of the mammalian force–interval relationship do not recapitulate phylogenetic ones, or if they do, the changes must occur prior to the fetal stage of development.[22]

It is sometimes asked whether a quantitative difference in this descriptor of contractility, the force–interval relationship, exists among the different stages of development. Postextrasystolic potentiation has been shown to be less in the human neonate than in the older infant.[51] Similarly, paired pacing produces less enhancement in contractility in isolated fetal myocardium than in that of the adult.[38] Unfortunately, these points in development were studied using different pacing patterns, preventing a direct comparison from one age to another. The same heart rate and timing of the extrasystole must be used at the different ages; for example, the more prematurely an extrasystole is introduced in the basic pacing cycle, the greater is the postextrasystolic potentiation.[22] Additional concerns about using these data to understand how development affects the control of myocardial cytosolic calcium concentration include the possibility that quantitative differences between patient populations may reflect differences in the state of the patient, and that inotropy and disease states, rather than differences in the patients' ages, alter the force–interval relationship.[52,53]

Conceptually experimental approaches based on describing the force–interval relationship are useful in testing for the presence of alterations in cytosolic calcium concentration with development and birth. The following discussion will provide an understanding of how this approach can be applied to describing developmental changes in contractility and will confirm the usefulness of this approach by demonstrating that this relation is unaffected by muscle length and is altered by changes in inotropy.

Evaluations of the force–interval relationship can be carried out using an unlimited number of pacing patterns, since any variation in the stimulus pattern reveals to some extent the characteristics of this relationship. In other words, included in each response of the heart to a variation in the pattern of pacing or heart rate is a partial description of how contractility (a working definition being a change in cytosolic calcium concentration during contraction or a change in the sensitivity of the myofilaments response to calcium) is modulated and what the basic level of contractility is at the time of study.

Restitution of Contractility Following a Contraction   The restitution of contractility following a contraction (see Fig. 39.34) and the alteration of this process by the introduction of an extrasystole can be described by the following experiment. This approach has been used to examine the force–interval relationship in isolated muscle, and a modification of it has been used to study this relation in the *in vivo* heart. The *in vitro* muscle is paced at a constant rate (basic interval = t_0), and infrequently but regularly an extra stimulus is interpolated at various coupling intervals following the previous regular stimulus (the extrasystolic interval, t_1). The shorter t_1, the more premature the extrasystole (Fig. 39.34). In adult myocardium, as the extrasystolic interval t_1 is increased, contractility (described by the maximum rate of rise of force of an isometric contraction, F_{max}) in the extrasystole rises monotonically from its smallest value at the shortest t_1 to equal that of the preceding contraction at the basic pacing rate when t_1 approaches the basic pacing interval, t_0. Stated in another manner, these experiments demonstrate that the myocardium requires time following a contraction to regain its full ability to contract.

The monotonic time course of this increase in contractility from one contraction to the next (i.e., the restitution of contractility) is qualitatively the same *throughout* mammalian development. However, quantitative differences do exist. The increase in contractility is far more rapid during early development in some mammals (e.g., in neonatal kitten myocardium and rabbit cardiac myocytes vs. cells from the adults).[54,55] Of interest, in the sheep, an animal that is more advanced in development at birth, the restitution of contractility in myocardium from the midgestation fetus appears to be similar to that of the adult.[22]

The presence of developmental differences in the restitution of contractility can be explained by changes in the dependency of the cell on extracellular sources of calcium and by the developmental increase in the intracellular stores of calcium, more specifically, the sarcoplasmic reticulum (SR). When the cell is stimulated to contract, the junctional and corbular components of the SR (containing calsequestrin, a calcium-binding protein, and the SR calcium release channel) release calcium into the cytosol. The longitudinal SR (containing an SR calcium ATPase, SERCA2) removes calcium from the cytosol,[48,54–57] allowing the cell and so the myocardium to relax. This organization of the SR components appears to provide the functional basis for the restitution of contractility. When the SR storage and release of calcium is disabled with ryanodine, restitution is markedly blunted. In that with development, the SR increases in amount and its differentiation,[55,58] a developmental change in the restitution of contractility could follow from alterations in this membrane system (e.g., in the time required for movement of calcium within the SR or for recovery of the system's ability to release calcium).

Postextrasystolic Potentiation   Potentiation in the forcefulness of the contraction that occurs after an extrasystole reflects the ability of the cell to modulate cytosolic calcium concentration and provides a quantitative measure of how contractility is altered by development, pathophysiological states, and inotropic interventions.

The effects of an extrasystole on the subsequent postextrasystole (described *in vitro* by the ratio of F_{max} of the potentiated beat to F_{max} of the preceding contraction at the basic rate) can be described using the following pacing pattern.

Two stimuli are interpolated infrequently into the basic pacing sequence (see Fig. 39.34 and earlier subsection: Method for Examining *In Vivo* Force–Interval Relationship). The first of the two stimuli is the stimulus to elicit the extrasystole. It is introduced at an interval t_1 following the preceding regular contraction. The second stimulus that elicits the postextrasystole is applied at various longer intervals (postextrasystolic interval, t_2). The effects of the extrasystoles on the restitution of contractility can be described by varying the timing of the extrasystole or the timing of the postextrasystole, generating different restitution curves. Although such restitution curves are qualitatively similar (Fig. 39.34), they differ quantitatively. The postextrasystolic constitution of contractility rises to a plateau value that is greater than F_{max} of the contraction at the regular rate.

The level of the plateau and slope of the postextrasystolic restitution of contractility depend on the prematurity of the extrasystole: The more premature the extrasystole (the shorter the t_1), the steeper the slope of the restitution of contractility, and the greater the amount of postextrasystolic potentiation (Fig. 39.34). Postextrasystolic potentiation is also dependent on heart rate (i.e., the basic pacing interval). For example, postextrasystolic potentiation is increased when the basic rate is slowed, and the prematurity of the extrasystole, t_1, is held constant. These characteristic dependencies of the force–interval relationship are found in all mammalian myocardia, both adult and fetal.[22,47,52,59] Thus, the quantitative characteristic of postextrasystolic potentiation depend on the basic pacing interval (i.e., the heart rate) and the timing of the extrasystole following the contraction at the basis rate (t_1, Fig. 39.34). Consequently, the same rate and pattern of stimulation (i.e., pacing patterns) must be used to compare postextrasystolic potentiation in hearts of different stages of development. Changes in potentiation are the result of developmental changes in cytosolic calcium concentration.

The basis of using quantitative changes in postextrasystolic potentiation for examining developmental changes in myocardial function or contractility is supported by the finding that changes in maximum cytosolic calcium concentration underlie alterations in force.[46] In adult myocardium, postextrasystolic potentiation appears to result from an enhanced release of calcium from the SR. This conclusion is supported by the abolition of postextrasystolic potentiation of force and of cytosolic calcium concentration by ryanodine, just as this agent blunts the restitution of contractility.[46]

The Force–Interval Relationship: In Vivo

Postextrasystolic Potentiation   *In vivo* postextrasystolic potentiation can be described by the ratio of the maximum rate of rise of ventricular pressure (P_{max}) in the postextrasystole divided by P_{max} of the preceding contraction at the basic heart rate. This ratio has been used to reveal quantitative changes in inotropic state (e.g., the effect of inotropic agents, disease states, and development).[8,52,53] The findings that inotropic stimulation and disease alter the force–interval relationship support the use of this relationship for assessing developmental changes in myocardial contractility.

The general characteristics of the force–interval relationship *in vivo* in the chronically instrumented animal and in the patient are the same as those observed *in vitro*.[8,22,52,60] No differences in the qualitative characteristics are found among the fetus, neonate, and adult,[8,22,61] including the child and adult human.[53,60]

Method for Examining In Vivo Force–Interval Relationship
The approach used to examine the force–interval relationship *in vivo* was modified from the *in vitro* one. The new design (Fig. 39.36) takes into consideration the intrinsic heart rate, the physiological properties of the atrioventricular conduction system, and the variations in ventricular end-diastolic volume (see Frank–Starling relation) produced by the timing of the extrasystole and the postextrasystole:

1. The basic pacing rate t_0 must be faster than that used in the isolated muscle experiments because of the intrinsic heart rate *in vivo*. Indeed, the changes in resting heart rates during gestation and neonatal life necessitate the use of a range of pacing rates during each *in vivo* study in which comparisons are to be made. For example, the increase in heart rate that follows birth prevents the use of a pacing rate that easily controls fetal heart rate the day prior to birth.[23]

2. The refractory periods and conduction times of the atrioventricular conduction system vary with development, making it impossible to use the same range of extrasystolic intervals t_1 for a given pacing rate or pacing cycle length, t_0, at all stages of development. In general, the later in gestation or the older the lamb, the longer the refractory period and the slower the conduction velocity of the atrioventricular conduction system.[8,22] For example, an extrasystole can be obtained easily at a coupling interval (t_1) of 200 ms in the lamb on the 135th day of gestation, but not at all in the lamb 120 days following birth. Similarly, the heart of the 120-day-old neonate cannot be paced continuously at a cycle interval of 300 ms (200 beats/min) without the Wenckebach phenomenon. Sympathetic tone also affects atrioventricular conduction. For example, during a fetal isoproterenol infusion, an extrasystole with a t_1 as short as 160 ms can be obtained, while in the absence of isoproterenol, an extrasystole can never be elicited at this interval. The increases in circulating catecholamine levels at birth and their subsequent fall[62,63] may explain the decrease in refractory period and conduction times that occurs in the first few hours following delivery and the gradual return of these values to prenatal levels over the subsequent neonatal days.

3. The same general relationship between the basic pacing rate and the prematurity of the extrasystole exists at all the ages studied; in essence, the faster the heart rate, the earlier the extrasystole can be successfully

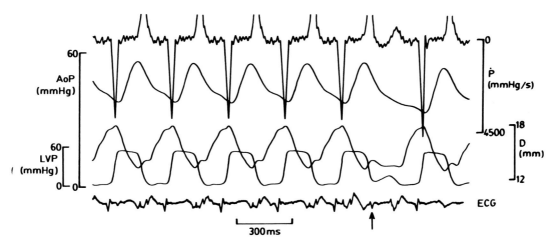

Figure 39.36 Postextrasystolic potentiation in the left ventricle of the fetal lamb, demonstrated by introducing an extrasystole during the performance of a force–interval experiment in an *in utero* lamb (134 days of gestation, 15 days after cardiovascular instrumentation): basic cycle interval $t_0 = 300$ ms; first test interval $t_1 = 195$ ms. The potentiation is illustrated by the increase in the maximum first derivative of left ventricular pressure P_{max}. The positive first derivative is in a downward direction. The arrow denotes the QRS of the first test systole. Traces (top to bottom) are as follows: P, the first derivative of left ventricular pressure; AoP, aortic pressure; D, left ventricular minor axis dimension; LVP, left ventricular pressure; ECG, electrocardiogram. (From Anderson et al, *Am J Obstet Gynecol* 1980;138:33–43).

elicited. This observation can be explained in two ways: (a) there is a developmental decrease in heart rate, and a simultaneous increase in the refractory time of the atrioventricular (AV) node, and (b) the heart rate and the AV node refractory time reflect sympathetic tone (e.g., the higher the sympathetic tone, the faster the heart rate and the shorter the refractory time). Thus, coupling the heart rate and the length of the extrasystolic interval follows from the balance of parasympathetic and sympathetic tone and the developmental changes in the electrophysiological properties of the heart.

4. With regard to the *in vivo* effects of the pacing pattern on ventricular end-diastolic volume, the pacing rates and patterns often alter diastolic filling time[7,22,23] and so end-diastolic volume. The faster the rate, and the more prematurely the extrasystole is introduced, the smaller the end-diastolic volume of the extrasystole is likely to be (e.g., see Figs. 39.7 and 39.33). The timing of the postextrasystole also affects the end-diastolic volume preceding the potentiated contraction. Consequently, if the effects of the force–interval relationship are to be evaluated *in vivo* and the confounding effects of the Frank–Starling relation on P_{max} are to be circumvented, end-diastolic volume must be monitored to ensure that systoles with the same end-diastolic volumes are being compared (Figs. 39.36 and 39.37).

Description of the In Vivo *Force–Interval Relation*   Alteration of the rate and pattern of stimulation in the fetus and neonate produces a complex interaction of hemodynamic variables. Importantly, these interactions are the same as those seen in the adult heart. Figure 39.36 illustrates the changes brought about by the introduction of an extrasystole. The rise in ventricular pressure induced by the extrasystole prevents the rapid diastolic filling that normally occurs immediately following the regular systole. Following the extrasystole, ventricular diastolic filling is more rapid than that following systoles at the basic rate, a result of higher atrial pressure (due to the extrasystole interfering with atrial emptying). In this example, the maximum extrasystolic pressure does not reach the aortic pressure, yet the minor axis dimension decreases. This may be due in part to fiber rearrangement during this isovolumic systole, but often the effect is associated with a prominent V wave in the left atrial pressure waveform, suggestive of mitral regurgitation. In terms of the effect of afterload, when the extrasystolic pressure is not sufficient to open the aortic valve, aortic pressure continues to fall. Consequently, the aortic diastolic pressure preceding the postextrasystolic systole may be lower than at the regular rate, as discussed in the following paragraph (see also earlier section, Afterload).

In the example provided (Fig. 39.36) P_{max} of the postextrasystole is greater than that of the regular systole, while

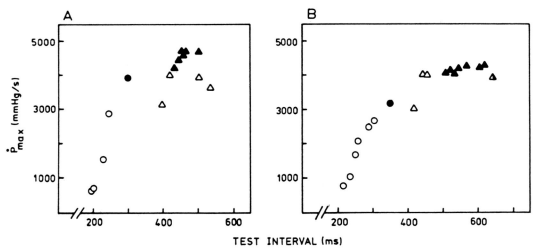

Figure 39.37   (A) First-stage (circles) and second-stage (triangles) curves of P_{max} versus interval for an *in utero* fetal lamb (136 days of gestation, 14 days postoperation) at a basic interval of $t_0 = 205$ ms. Solid symbols denote systoles preceded by the same left ventricular end-diastolic dimension (EDD); open symbols, test systoles with an EDD less than that of the preceding regular systole (solid circle). (B) First-stage (circles) and second-stage (triangles) P_{max}–interval curves for the same fetal lamb, studied on the same day, at a slower basic cycle interval, $t_0 = 350$ ms; the second-stage experiment had the same fixed first test interval, $t_1 = 205$ ms, as in (A). Solid symbols indicate systoles with equal EDD; open symbols represent an EDD less than that of the preceding regular systole (solid circle); and the half-solid triangle is P_{max} of a systole preceded by an EDD greater than that of the preceding regular systole but P_{max} was obtained after left ventricular ejection had begun. (From Anderson et al, *Am J Obstet Gynecol* 1980;138:33–43.)

P_{max} of the extrasystole is smaller than that of the regular systole (the effect of variation in end-diastolic volume on P_{max} is considered below). The ejection phase characteristics of the postextrasystolic contraction are enhanced: The amount and rate of ejection (minor axis shortening) are greater than those of the regular systole. This enhancement of systolic properties may be related, in part, to the lower aortic diastolic pressure and the heart's ability to eject more effectively against a lower afterload.[18,15,45,64] However, when the aortic diastolic pressures preceding the postextrasystolic contraction and the preceding systole at the basic rate are equal, postextrasystolic potentiation of the ejection phase characteristics is still found. The arterial pulse width for the potentiated systole is, as expected, larger than that for the systole at the basic rate.

The relationship between the extrasystolic coupling interval (t_1) and the heart's ability to develop pressure P_{max} (Fig. 39.37) is similar to the F_{max}–interval relationship of the isolated muscle: The earlier the extrasystole is introduced (i.e., the shorter t_1) the smaller P_{max} of the extrasystole. As t_1 increases, P_{max} of the extrasystole increases monotonically to equal P_{max} of the preceding systole at the basic heart rate. When a second systole is introduced following the extrasystole, pressure development in this postextrasystole (P_{max}) is affected in a similar manner to F_{max} of the postextrasystole in vitro (Fig. 39.37). That is, at the shortest t_2, P_{max} has its smallest value; and as t_2 is increased, P_{max} rises to a value that exceeds P_{max} of the preceding systole at the basic rate, demonstrating postextrasystolic potentiation.

The Frank–Starling mechanism affects the quantitative characteristics of the in vivo force–interval relation: The pacing and coupling intervals affect diastolic filling time, end-diastolic volume, P_{max}, and so the shapes of P_{max}–interval curves. For example, the end-diastolic volume preceding an extrasystole is (usually) smaller than the end-diastolic volume of extrasystoles preceded by a longer extrasystolic interval (Fig. 39.36). In addition, changing the basic heart rate is also likely to change end-diastolic volume (Fig. 39.7). For example, faster heart rates usually result in smaller end-diastolic volumes. Consequently, although the shapes of the force–interval curves are similar in vitro and in vivo, the responses of the in vivo heart are being modulated by changes in end-diastolic volume (Fig. 39.37) while in vitro muscle length is unaffected by the pacing patterns, and sarcomere length is constant.

Although end-diastolic volume falls with an increase in rate, P_{max} is usually greater at the faster rate (Figs. 39.7 and 39.37). At times the fetal results mimic those obtained in the intact adult animal by Kavaler et al[65] and Noble et al[66]: P_{max} is changed little by a change in rate. However, in general, the fetal heart response is similar to that of the adult, described by Mahler et al[42]: When a pause is introduced to allow the end-diastolic volume to return to that at the lower rate, P_{max} is enhanced markedly at the faster rate (Fig. 39.7).

When the end-diastolic volume preceding the postextrasystole is the same as that for the preceding systole at the basic rate, the general characteristics of the in vivo relationship are the same as those found in vitro:

1. When end-diastolic volume is serendipitously constant for postextrasystoles enlisted at different t_2, P_{max} increases as t_2 increases, revealing the increase in contractility (restitution of contractility) observed in vitro. The importance of end-diastolic volume is illustrated in Figure 39.37A: the fall in P_{max} at the longest t_2 is a consequence of a decrease in end-diastolic volume.

2. Postextrasystolic potentiation of P_{max} depends on the prematurity of the preceding extrasystole: The more prematurely the extrasystole is elicited (the shorter t_1), the greater the amount of postextrasystolic potentiation.

3. For a constant extrasystolic interval (t_1), the slower the heart rate, the greater the amount of postextrasystolic potentiation

The effect of afterload (i.e., aortic diastolic pressure, on P_{max}) is illustrated in Figure 39.37B: P_{max} of the postextrasystole at the longest t_2 has fallen. This is a consequence of aortic diastolic pressure falling to a level that allows left ventricular ejection to begin before the first derivative of left ventricular pressure has reached its maximum value. (This blunting of P_{max} is most likely to happen when the extrasystole is mechanically ineffective and t_2 exceeds the sum of t_0 and t_1.) This effect of diastolic pressure on P_{max} has also been demonstrated in the adult heart.[67–69]

A wide variety of heart rates and the extrasystolic coupling intervals (t_1) can be used for the in vivo evaluation of postextrasystolic potentiation. The complex interaction of rate and extrasystolic coupling interval on postextrasystolic potentiation demands that the same pacing parameters be used if, for example, hearts are to be compared from one point in development to another or if the effects of cardiovascular disease are to be assessed. This is especially important if quantitative measures, based on postextrasystolic potentiation, are to be compared at different stages of development.

In conclusion, careful attention to the interaction of the hemodynamic variables of preload and afterload and the effects of altering the pacing pattern on the quantitative characteristics of the force–interval relationship (e.g., postextrasystolic potentiation) allows the force–interval relation to be used successfully to assess changes in contractility from day to day in the same heart, as well as differences in contractility among hearts.

Effects of Length on the Force–Interval Relationship   Importantly, preload must be shown not to affect postextrasystolic potentiation if it is to be used as a quantitative measure for characterizing the effects on the heart of development, stress, and birth. The finding that a change in inotropy alters the ratio of P_{max} of the postextrasystole to P_{max} of the preceding systole at the basic heart rate (both systoles being preceded by the same end-diastolic volume) demonstrates that this measure fulfills an essential requirement for its use in assessing inotropy or contractility. If the measure is preload dependent, for example, the increases in left ventricular end-diastolic volume that occur with birth[8,23] would preclude the use of postextrasystolic potentiation to determine whether birth alters inotropy. Restated, if end-diastolic volume affects postextrasystolic potentiation, this measure cannot be used for the *in vivo* assessment of developmental changes in myocardial contractility. (Consider the confounding effects of afterload on the end-systolic pressure–volume relation in the neonate.[70])

To test whether the force–interval relationship, as described by postextrasystolic potentiation, can be used to describe changes in contractility in the developing heart, we carried out a series of *in vitro* and *in vivo* experiments to test whether postextrasystolic potentiation is independent of muscle length. The following subsections describe these experimental results and demonstrate that postextrasystolic potentiation provides a measure that is unaffected by muscle length. Consequently, these results support the use of the force–interval relationship in assessing changes in contractility.

IN VITRO.   When the length of isolated fetal muscle is changed, the force developed in a contraction changes. However, the qualitative characteristics of the force–interval relationship remain the same (see Fig. 39.35). Importantly, such a length change does not affect either the force–interval ratio or the shapes of the force–interval curves that describe the dynamic beat-to-beat changes in contractility (Fig. 39.38). Stated differently, these results are comparable with the following relationship:

$$F_{max} = F(R,P)F(L) \qquad (39.1)$$

The results support the assumption that $F(R,P)$, the function that describes how contractility changes from beat-to-beat, as manifested by altering the rate and pattern of stimulation, is the same at all muscle lengths. In Equation 39.1, the effect of length is described by $F(L)$. The results of force–interval relation experiments performed on isolated myocardium of fetal sheep and of the adult rabbit, dog, and cat[52,59,61,71] and the isolated heart of the adult dog[68,69,72] are described by the relation in this equation. The effect of introducing an extrasystole (i.e., postextrasystolic potentiation) at a given muscle length *l* can be described as follows: where F_{maxpot} is the response of the potentiated contraction; F_{maxreg} the response of the regular contraction, $F(R,P)_{pot}$ the solution of $F(R,P)$ for the potentiated contraction, $F(R,P)_{reg}$

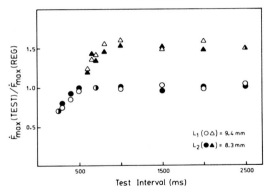

Figure 39.38   Effect of muscle length on the normalized force–interval curves: F_{max} of the test contraction divided by F_{max} of the preceding regular contraction, described as a function of the test interval, t_1 or t_2, for an isolated moderator muscle bundle from a fetal lamb of 136 days of gestation. First-stage results are circles, and second-stage results are triangles. The curves were obtained at a longer muscle length L_1 (open symbols) and a shorter length L_2 (solid symbols). Basic pacing interval t_0 was 3000 ms; for the second-stage curve, the fixed first test interval t_1 was 275 ms. (Data from Anderson et al.[22])

the solution of $F(R,P)$ for the preceding contraction at the basic rate, and $F(L)_l$ the solution of $F(L)$ for a given length *l*. Thus, the function that describes the Frank–Starling relation, $F(L)$, can be separated from the function that describes the effects of a change in rate and pattern of stimulation or inotropic state, $F(R,P)$, by making the F_{max}–interval ratio. By making the ratio, it is possible to eliminate the Frank–Starling effect (Figs. 39.35 and 39.39).

IN VIVO.   The variations in end-diastolic volume from one beat to the next can make it difficult to test for the dependence of the force–interval relationship on ventricular volume. Fortunately, over a wide range of t_2 (see description of *in vivo* force–interval experiment above), the end-diastolic volumes of potentiated systoles are equal to the end-diastolic volume of the preceding systole at the basic paced heart rate. These systoles allow us to examine whether the effects of the Frank–Starling relation can be separated from the effects of altering inotropy. When left ventricular volume is increased by a volume infusion, P_{max}, aortic pressure, and end-diastolic pressure are increased (see Figs. 39.12 and 39.39). Although P_{max} of the potentiated contraction and that at the basic rate increase after a volume infusion, the ratio of P_{max} of the potentiated systole to P_{max} of the preceding regular systole (P_{max}–interval ratio) remains constant (the end-diastolic volumes of the regular and potentiated systoles being equal, Fig. 39.39). Thus, in the *in vivo* developing heart, the effects of the force–interval relationship on ventricular function can be separated from the effects of the Frank–Starling mechanism.

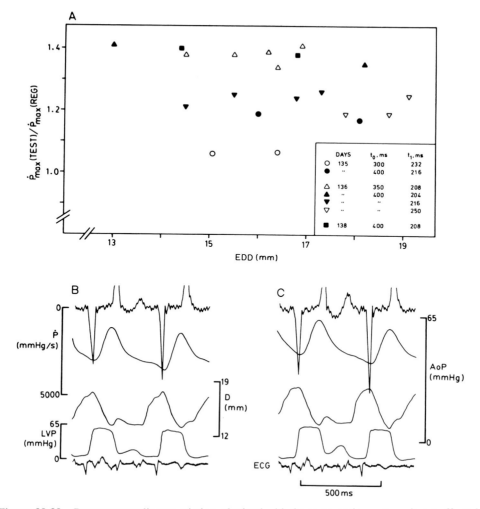

Figure 39.39 Postextrasystolic potentiation, obtained with the same pacing pattern, is not affected in the *in utero* lamb by left ventricular end-diastolic dimension (EDD). (*A*) Potentiation described by the P_{max}–interval ratio (P_{max} of the second test contraction divided by P_{max} of the preceding regular contraction; both systoles preceded by the same EDD). The ratios obtained at several EDD, for each pacing interval are compared for a fetal lamb instrumented at 132 days of gestation. The symbols indicate the day of gestation, the basic pacing interval (t_0), and the timing of the fixed first test interval (t_1). The effect of end-diastolic dimension on postextrasystolic potentiation ($t_0 = 300$ ms, $t_1 = 205$ ms) in a fetal lamb (at 138 days of gestation, instrumented 16 days earlier) is shown (*B*) before and (*C*) after a left atrial volume infusion. Tracings (top to bottom) are as follows: P_{max}, first derivative of pressure; AoP, aortic pressure, D, left ventricular minor axis dimension; and ECG, electrocardiogram. (Data from Anderson et al.[7])

Effect of Inotropy on the Force–Interval Relationship In the classical definition, an inotropic intervention is a maneuver that changes contractile strength in the absence of a change in muscle length (or ventricular volume). We have adopted here an elaboration of this definition of inotropy, based on the force–interval relationship. This definition provides the framework for classifying the effects of inotropic agents and the inotropic state of the myocardium. The rationale and justification for this definition have been reviewed

elsewhere.[73] For our present purposes, we focus on the inotropic action of sympathomimetic agents (e.g., isoproterenol), since myocardial innervation and catecholamine content increase with development while α and β-adrenoreceptor number and ratio change. Thus, understanding how sympathomimetic agents affect the force–interval relationship may be useful in interpreting how this measure of contractility is affected by developmental changes in α and β-adrenoreceptors, cardiac sympathetic innervation, and the transition from *in utero* to postnatal life (see below, The Effects of Birth).[36,74–85]

IN VITRO.   Unlike the effect of a change in muscle length, an inotropic intervention alters the shape of the force–interval curves and the amount of potentiation. For example, isoproterenol increases the slope of restitution curves and brings the plateaus of the curves closer together, resulting in a decrease in postextrasystolic potentiation (Fig. 39.40).[86] At higher concentrations of isoproterenol, the curves become biphasic and, ultimately, the second-stage curves can "droop" below the first-stage curves, producing "postextrasystolic depression" (Fig. 39.40). These effects are blocked competitively by practalol or propranolol.[86] From these results it follows that the function describing the relationship between the rate and pattern of stimulation (a solution of which produces these curves) must contain (i.e., depend on) inotropy.

The effects of an inotropic agent on the force–interval relationship have clear developmental implications: If during the control state (i.e., responses obtained at a constant rate), no developmental differences in the relationship are revealed, inotropic agents may, and probably will, reveal developmental differences in the way myocardial performance can be modulated by inotropic agents.

If the force–interval relationship is considered (see above) to be comparable to a description of contractility, inotropic agents do expose developmental differences in contractility. When isolated myocardium from the puppy is exposed to isoproterenol or norepinephrine, the change in postextrasystolic potentiation depends on age.[87] For example, in Figure 39.41, at the youngest age, norepinephrine is shown to induce an increase in postextrasystolic potentiation, while at older ages, postextrasystolic potentiation is decreased, and by 2 months of age postextrasystolic depression is induced by the same dose. The developmental differences in the response to norepinephrine are reminiscent of the different effects of α and β-adrenoreceptor stimulation of the adult myocardium: α-stimulation enhances postextrasystolic potentiation while β-stimulation induces postextrasystolic depression.[86] The developmental differences in the effects of norepinephrine on the force–interval relationship occurred despite the absence of a change in the dose–response relation at a constant pacing rate.[87]

The effects of inotropic agents on the shapes of the F_{max}–interval curves at different ages further reveal developmental changes in myocardial contractility. The force–interval curves of fetal lambs and neonatal puppy myocardium remain monotonic in concentrations of isoproterenol or nor-

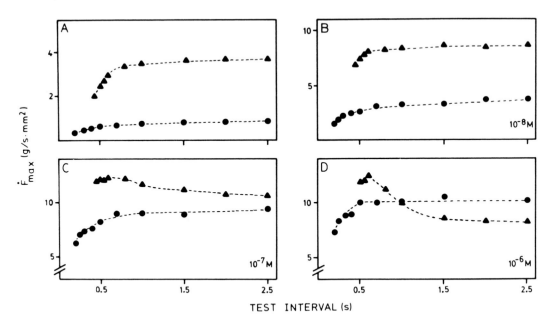

Figure 39.40   Effects of isoproterenol on the force–interval relationship of an adult rabbit papillary muscle: Results from the first-stage (circles) and second-stage (triangles; t_1 = 200 ms) experiments before (*A*) and during exposure to isoproterenol at various concentrations: (*B*) 10^{-8} M, (*C*) 10^{-7} M, and (*D*) 10^{-6} M. During exposure to 10^{-7} M and 10^{-6} M isoproterenol the second-stage curves were biphasic (i.e., they "drooped"). This characteristic effect of β-adrenoreceptor stimulation of adult myocardium is not seen in the rabbit in the first 3 weeks of life. (From the laboratory of P.A.W. Anderson.)

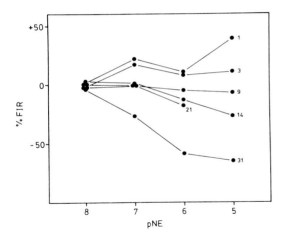

Figure 39.41 Norephinephrine (NE) dose–response curves, expressed as a percent change in the force–interval ratio from control (FIR), obtained from a litter of puppies. Numbers to the right of the curves are the puppies' ages in days.

epinephrine much higher than those that induce biphasic force–interval curves in myocardium for older animals. (These biphasic changes are inhibited competitively by a β-adrenoreceptor antagonist, see above; Fig. 39.40.)

The presence of different sympathomimetic effects on contractility at different developmental periods provides a tool that can be used to explore how and when during development the myocardium achieves adultlike properties. This information can also be used to examine the underlying mechanisms that produce these differences. The finding, for example, that the number of α-adrenoreceptors is highest in the newborn lamb myocardium and falls with time following birth may be related to the developmental differences in the force–interval responses to catecholamine stimulation.

Developmental differences in the effects of various inotropic agents on the force–interval relation may be relevant to the treatment of low cardiac output in the sick premature or full-term infant. When should a sympathomimetic agent be used, which one, and at what dose? Furthermore, these developmental changes reveal the power of the force–interval relationship as a tool in dissecting developmental changes in contractility and their basis. Coupling changes in the physiological responses to the various developmental changes in cell systems, such as how altered expression of the guanine-binding proteins affects the adenylate cyclase system, will lead to a better understanding of how these processes alter contractility.

IN VIVO.   Enhancement of the *in vivo* fetal heart's inotropic state, as measured by an increase in ventricular output, has proven difficult to demonstrate.[35,45] An isoproterenol infusion may have complex effects on the fetal circulation, ultimately appearing to alter the distribution of cardiac output

and decreasing placental flow.[37] However, the initial effect of isoproterenol is a significant increase in fetal ventricular output (Figs. 39.30 and 39.31).

The positive effects of isoproterenol on inotropy are further revealed by means of the force–interval relation: Postextrasystolic potentiation falls, as it does in isolated fetal myocardium (Fig. 39.42).[7] Isoproterenol (e.g., 0.05 μg/kg/min) abolishes postextrasystolic potentiation of P_{max} and ventricular ejection characteristics (Fig. 39.42). These *in vivo* effects are similar to those of isoproterenol *in vitro*. Importantly, these effects of isoproterenol on postextrasystolic potentiation are not altered by end-diastolic volume.

Effects of Congenital Cardiac Defects   The relationship, as described by the P_{max}–interval ratio, has been used successfully in the child[53] to demonstrate differences in contractility between normal, hypertrophied, and failing ventricular myocardium. Although at a constant rate, other descriptors of ventricular function were unable to demonstrate a difference, the hearts of children with left ventricular hypertrophy were found to have a significantly greater amount of postextrasystolic potentiation. Furthermore, the shape of the P_{max}–interval curves of hearts with stable hypertrophy or no hypertrophy were qualitatively different from those of the child in heart failure.[53] Children with congestive heart failure had strikingly different force–interval curves: They were biphasic, resulting in postextrasystolic depression in some patients, reminiscent of the effects of β-sympathomimetic stimulation on the force–interval relation of isolated myocardium (consider Refs. 53 and 86).

Thus, as in isolated muscle, the force–interval relationship of the *in vivo* heart satisfies two major criteria for an index of contractility: The amount of potentiation for a given rate and pattern of stimulation is not altered by a change in ventricular volume, whereas exposure to an inotropic agent does alter the amount of potentiation. The insensitivity of the force–interval relationship to a change in ventricular volume is of special importance because of the large and acute increases in left ventricular volume that occur with birth (Fig. 39.17). The preload independence of this measure ensures that changes in postextrasystolic potentiation with birth are due to a change in contractility, not to an increase in left ventricular end-diastolic volume.

EFFECTS OF DEVELOPMENT ON CONTRACTILITY

It is assumed frequently that contractility or inotropic state is enhanced by development. Certainly, in view of the developmental changes in other myocardial properties, it seems highly likely that changes in contractility occur. With development, cellular organization and amount of myofibrils, sarcoplasmic reticulum, and mitochondria increase, while

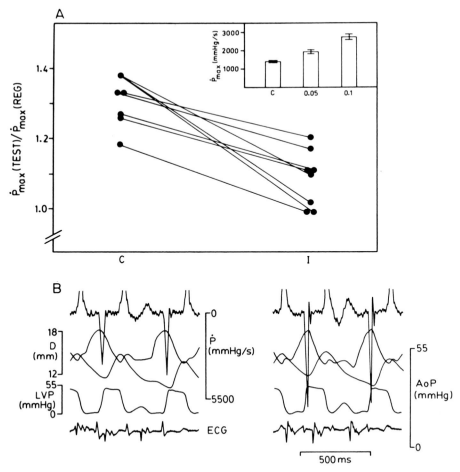

Figure 39.42   The inotropic agent isoproterenol affects postextrasystolic potentiation. Thus, altering inotropy alters this measure of contractility while a change in end-diastolic volume does not (see Fig. 39.36). (*A*) The effect of isoproterenol on the P_{max}–interval ratio for six fetal lambs: data points above C were obtained in the absence of isoproterenol; those in the presence of isoproterenol are above the I. The three lines drawn from the top data point indicate the responses of one lamb to three different doses of isoproterenol. The higher the infusion dose, the lower the ratio (i.e., the smaller the amount of postextrasystolic potentiation). (*B*) The response to an extrasystole ($t_0 = 300$ ms, $t_1 = 210$ ms) for a fetal lamb (139 days of gestation, instrumented 17 days earlier) during the control state and in response to an infusion of isoproterenol (0.02 μg/kg/min) on the same day. Tracings (top to bottom) are as follows: P, first derivative of pressure; D, left ventricular minor axis dimension; AoP, aortic pressure; LVP, left ventricular pressure; and ECG, electrocardiogram. (Data from Anderson et al, *Am J Obstet Gynecol* 1980;138: 44–54).

contractile protein isoform expression changes.[55,88–90] Furthermore, consistent with an increase in contractility with development, the cytosolic calcium concentration transient during a contraction increases during postnatal life.[91]

Despite all these effects of development, a change in the force per cross-sectional area (corrected for differences in the amount of contractile material per cross section among preparation from the fetal and adult sheep) has sometimes not been found.[92] (However, consider Fig. 39.21). Glycerinated muscles from the adult and the fetal sheep generated the same

tensions at equal sarcomere lengths.[92] Furthermore, in this species, the estimated maximal velocity of sarcomere shortening did not appear to undergo any developmental change. In contrast to these findings, studies of other species have demonstrated developmental increases in the ability of the myocardium to generate tension and to shorten that, interestingly, appear to be unrelated to changes in the relative amount of contractile material.[93–95]

The apparent absence of developmental differences in contractility observed in sheep myocardium is reminiscent of

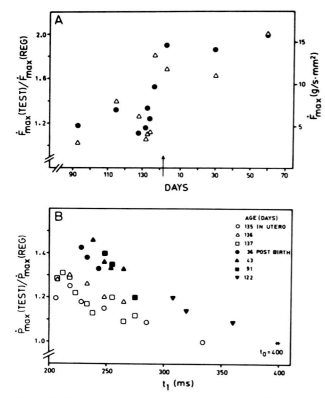

Figure 39.43 (A) F_{max}–interval ratios (circles) and F_{max} (triangles, the maximum rate of rise of force) obtained from isolated ventricular trabeculae from sheep hearts as a function of gestational age (left of arrow) and age following birth (right of arrow). F_{max}–interval ratio is F_{max} of the postextrasystolic contraction divided by F_{max} of the preceding regular contraction, the extrasystolic interval being the same for each ratio. (B) The P_{max}–interval ratios (FIR) obtained from a lamb instrumented *in utero* at 124 days of gestation as a function of the extrasystolic interval, t_1. The older the animal, the greater the P_{max}–interval ratio for any given t_1. The ratios obtained in the first days following birth (not plotted) fell initially below those obtained at gestational ages of 135, 136, and 137 days (open symbols), then gradually returned to the fetal level by 7–15 days of life, and then rose above the fetal values (solid symbols). (Data from Anderson et al.[8])

comparisons of normal and hypertrophied myocardium. These studies demonstrated no difference in force-generating ability.[59,96] However, when the force–interval relationship was used, significant differences between normal and hypertrophied myocardium were found to exist; postextrasystolic potentiation was increased in hypertrophied myocardium.[59]

Comparable to the positive effect of hypertrophy on postextrasystolic potentiation is the positive effect of development on the same characteristic (Fig. 39.43).[8,87] In sheep in the last 2 weeks of gestation, there is a sudden large increase in the amount of postextrasystolic potentiation (Fig. 39.43). *In vitro,* potentiation increases somewhat further in the first days of neonatal life and remains constant thereafter. Other studies, which did not control for rate and pattern and stimu-

lation, have also demonstrated a change in the force–interval relation with development.[38,51] The most straightforward interpretation of these changes is that the range over which cytosolic calcium concentration is modulated is increased with development. Teleologically, this developmental change, which describes a greater availability of activator calcium during the postextrasystole, indicates that the myocardial reserves in contractility are increasing in the days just prior to birth.

In the intact chronically instrumented fetal lamb, postextrasystolic potentiation also increases during gestation, similar to the increase in potentiation observed in isolated myocardium. However, as discussed below, postextrasystolic potentiation *in vivo* changes dynamically around the time of birth: Postextrasystolic potentiation begins to fall by 2 hours prior to delivery and continues to fall in the hours and days that follow delivery, then rising over the following days and weeks to reach and exceed the amount of postextrasystolic potentiation observed in the same lambs prior to delivery (Fig. 39.44).

These findings support the concept that the growth of the heart with development and the accompanying hypertrophy of the cardiac cells are modulated by the same mechanisms used in the adult heart to respond to a pathologic state.[59] Thus, just as cell size is increased by growth and by hypertrophy, contractility, as characterized by postextrasystolic potentiation, is induced to change with development in the same manner as with some forms of hypertrophy in the heart of the child and the adult.

EFFECTS OF BIRTH

The physiologic transformation the fetus undergoes when it becomes a neonate is a subject that is fascinating to all who are interested in growth and development. The effect of birth on the left ventricle provides an example of how the developing heart alters ventricular volume, heart rate, and inotropic state to adapt to a change in work load. Large changes in ventricular dynamics must occur to accommodate the large increase in left ventricular output and the smaller increase in right ventricular output that accompany birth and the transition from the fetal to the postnatal circulation.[8,16,24–26,28] Few studies have described how the fetal left ventricle adapts to birth in the absence of the acute effects produced by the extensive instrumentation required to examine the effects of birth. The acquisition of data from the heart that has recovered from surgery presents a difficult problem because it requires that the animals undergo cardiovascular instrumentation days before birth. This prenatal recovery is essential in that the fetal response to surgery includes the use of three mechanisms that may be brought into play to bring about the neonatal increase in ventricular output: heart rate, the Frank–Starling relation, and inotropy.

for volume challenges at this stage of development, in the presence of a normal blood volume, resulting in little increase in stroke volume and cardiac output. The neonatal displacement of ventricular filling to the steeper part of the passive pressure–volume relation is transient. The day after birth the end-diastolic volume is larger, but the end-diastolic pressures have fallen to fetal levels.

The neonatal increase in left ventricular end-diastolic volume, evidenced by the increase in end-diastolic pressure and dimensions, may result from several aspects of the neonatal rearrangement of the circulation. One experimental approach used to mimic the effects of postnatal respiration of air is *in utero* ventilation with oxygen. Those experiments demonstrate that in response to the increase in arterial oxygen content, placental blood flow decreases, and flow in the ductus arteriosus reverses in direction to go predominantly from the aorta to the pulmonary artery. The change in direction of flow reflects the marked fall in pulmonary vascular resistance that accompanied gaseous ventilation of the lungs and increase in blood oxygenation. This fall in resistance also causes the right ventricular output to go through the pulmonary vascular bed to the left atrium and ventricle. In the response to the increase in pulmonary blood flow from these two sources (left-to-right ductal shunting and right ventricular output), left ventricular output and stroke volume increase.[98,99] These findings suggest that with birth, the fall in pulmonary vascular resistance and the increase in pulmonary venous return are important contributors to the neonatal increase in left ventricular end-diastolic volume, and so left ventricular output.

The neonatal fall in pulmonary artery pressure could also enhance left ventricular output through altering the interaction between the right and left ventricle: The decrease in right ventricular afterload enhances right ventricular ejection and results in a smaller right ventricular end-systolic and end-diastolic volume. (Echocardiography has demonstrated a fall in the human right ventricular size with birth.[30]) This decrease in right ventricular volume permits greater filling of the left ventricle, even if there is no neonatal change in left atrial pressure. This effect of ventricular volume interaction is amplified by the neonatal increase in left atrial pressure.

When left ventricular dimensions are monitored on the day prior to and on the day of delivery,[8,23] a wide range of fetal and neonatal end-diastolic dimensions can be observed in the same animal. Indeed, some lambs exhibit fetal and neonatal systoles with the same end-diastolic dimension, suggesting that at times the postnatal increase in ventricular work can be achieved without the use of the Frank–Starling relation.[23] Although such systoles are uncommon, they demonstrate an increase in inotropy with birth: When fetal and neonatal systoles at the same heart rate and end-diastolic volume are compared, a neonatal increase in P_{max} and, to a lesser extent, percentage of fractional shortening is found to occur[23], consistent with a neonatal increase in inotropic state separate from the effects of heart rate. Recalling that in-

creases in aortic pressure decrease the ability of the ventricle to eject blood,[15,18,64] we see that the relatively smaller increase of the ejection phase descriptors with birth, relative to P_{max}, may be a consequence of the associated neonatal increase in aortic pressure and so afterload.

The force–interval relationship also changes with birth; postextrasystolic potentiation falls markedly following birth (Fig. 39.43), supporting the presence of an increase in inotropic state through sympathetic stimulation. The fall begins 3–4 hours prior to birth, but the greatest portion of the fall occurs following delivery. The fall in potentiation and the rise in P_{max} are the same as those produced by a fetal isoproterenol infusion (Fig. 39.42). The enhanced left ventricular stroke volume at comparable filling pressures, observed with *in utero* ventilation, is also consistent with an increase in inotropy. Interestingly, the *in utero* ventilation observations were acquired in the presence of β-adrenergic sympathetic blockage and are augmented by isoproterenol.[98,99] However, the prenatal decrease in postextrasystolic potentiation appears to correlate with the increase in circulating levels of catecholamines that begins prior to birth, suggesting that the increases in inotropy and plasma catecholamine concentration are coupled.

In the days and weeks that follow birth, postextrasystolic potentiation gradually returns to or exceeds the fetal level of potentiation, while P_{max} decreases to the level found in the fetus and that of the child and the adult. These maturational changes suggest that the heart is reacquiring the functional reserves that are used to cope with the increased cardiac work of neonatal life. This postnatal reacquisition of myocardial reserves is an important process, enabling the infant to respond to stress and to the hemodynamic loads imposed in later infancy by congenital cardiac defects.

SUMMARY

The function of the fetal right and left ventricles are modulated by changes in heart rate, ventricular end-diastolic volume, inotropy, and afterload. Fetal heart uses the first three of these mechanisms to adapt to neonatal life. Although the heart of the normal neonate is capable of further increases in rate, inotropic state, and left ventricular end-diastolic volume, the extensive use of these mechanisms with birth temporarily compromises the ability of the neonatal heart to respond to additional neonatal stresses.

ACKNOWLEDGMENTS

This work was supported in part by grants HL 20749, HL 33680, and HL 42250 from the National Heart, Lung, and Blood Institute, and by a grant-in-aid from the American Heart Association, with funds contributed in part by the Association's North Carolina affiliate. The author thanks Mrs. Annette Oakeley, Miss Nancy Halpern, and Ms. Elizabeth Fair, for without their assistance the contents of this chapter would have been markedly reduced. The author also thanks Mrs. Roberta Parker for her secretarial assistance and Mr. Peter Solet for his secretarial and editorial assistance.

REFERENCES

1. Bical O, Gallix P, Toussaint M, Landais P, Gaillard D, Karam J, Neveux JY. Intrauterine versus postnatal repair of created pulmonary artery stenosis in the lamb. *J Thorac Cardiovasc Surg* 1990;99:686–690.

2. Harrison MR, Adzick NS, Longaker MT, Goldberg JD, Rosen MA, Filly RA, Evans MI, Golbus MS. Successful repair *in utero* of a fetal diaphragmatic hernia after removal of herniated viscera from the left thorax. *N Engl J Med* 1990;322:1581–1584.

3. Sandhu SK, Heckman JL, Balsara R, Russo PA, Dunn JM. Chronic alterations in cardiac mechanics after fetal closed heart operation. *Ann Thorac Surg* 1994;57:1409–1415.

4. Schmidt KG, Sliverman NH, Harrison MR, Callen PW. High-output cardiac failure in fetuses with large sacrococcygeal teratoma: diagnosis by echocardiography and Doppler ultrasound. *J Pediatr* 1989;114:1023–1028.

5. Romero T, Covell JW, Friedman WF. A comparison of pressure–volume relations of the fetal, newborn and adult heart. *Am J Physiol* 1972;222:1285–1290.

6. Friedman WF. The intrinsic physiologic properties of the developing heart. *Prog Cardiovasc Dis* 1972;15:87–111.

7. Anderson PAW, Manring A, Crenshaw C Jr. Biophysics of the developing heart. II. The interaction of the force–interval relationship with inotropic state and muscle length (preload). *Am J Obstet Gynecol* 1980;138:44–54.

8. Anderson PAW, Glick KL, Manring A, Crenshaw C Jr. Developmental changes in cardiac contractility in fetal and postnatal sheep: *in vitro* and *in vivo. Am J Physiol* 1984;247:H371–H379.

9. Anderson PAW, Killam AP, Mainwaring RD, Oakeley AE. *In utero* right ventricular output in the fetal lamb: the effect of heart rate. *J Physiol* 1987;387:297–316.

10. Anderson PAW, Glick KL, Killam AP, Mainwaring RD. The effect of heart rate on *in utero* left ventricular output in the fetal sheep. *J Physiol* 1986;372:557–573.

11. Frank O. Zur Dynamik des Herzmuskels. *Z Biol* 1895;32:370–447.

12. Starling EH. *The Linacre Lecture on the Law of the Heart* (Cambridge; 1915; monograph). London: Longmans, Green; 1918.

13. Kirkpatrick SE, Pitlick PT, Naliboff J, Friedman WF. Frank–Starling relationship as an important determinant of fetal cardiac output. *Am J Physiol* 1976;231:495–500.

14. Heymann MA, Rudolph AM. Effects of increasing preload on right ventricular output in fetal lambs *in utero. Circulation* 1973;48(suppl IV):37.

15. Thornburg KL, Morton MJ. Filling and arterial pressures as determinants of left ventricular stroke volume in fetal lambs. *Am J Physiol* 1986;251:H961–H968.

16. Klopfenstein HS, Rudolph AM. Post-natal changes in the circulation and responses to volume loading in sheep. *Circ Res* 1978;42:839–845.

17. Gilbert RD. Venous return and control of fetal cardiac output. In: Longo LD, Reneau DD, eds. *Circulation in the Fetus and Newborn.* New York: Garland Publishing; 1978;Volume 1 299–316.

18. Thornburg KL, Morton MJ. Filling and arterial pressures as determinants of RV stroke volume in the sheep fetus. *Am J Physiol* 1983;244:H656–H663.

19. Hawkins J, Van Hare GF, Schmidt KG, Rudolph AM. Effects of increasing afterload on left ventricular output in fetal lambs. *Circ Res* 1989;65:127–134.

20. Van Hare GF, Hawkins JA, Schmidt KG, Rudolph AM. The effects of increasing mean arterial pressure on left ventricular output in newborn lambs. *Circ Res* 1990;67:78–83.

21. Kirkpatrick SE, Covell JW, Friedman WF. A new technique for the continuous assessment of fetal and neonatal cardiac performance. *Am J Obstet Gynecol* 1973;116:963–972.

22. Anderson PAW, Manring A, Crenshaw C Jr. Biophysics of the developing heart. I. The force–interval relationship. *Am J Obstet Gynecol* 1980;138:33–43.

23. Anderson PAW, Manring A, Glick KL, Crenshaw C Jr. Biophysics of the developing heart. III. A comparison of the left ventricular dynamics of the fetal and neonatal lamb heart. *Am J Obstet Gynecol* 1982;143:195–203.

24. Rudolph AM, Heymann MA. Fetal and neonatal circulation and respiration. *Annu Rev Physiol* 1974;36:187–207.

25. Berman W Jr, Musselman J. Myocardial performance in the newborn lamb. *Am J Physiol* 1979;237:H66–H70.

26. Breall JA, Rudolph AM, Heymann MA. Role of thyroid hormone in postnatal circulatory and metabolic adjustments. *J Clin Invest* 1984;73:1418–1424.

27. Lister G, Walter TK, Versmold HT, Dallman PR, Rudolph AM. Oxygen delivery in lambs, cardiovascular and hematologic development. *Am J Physiol* 1979;237:H668–H675.

28. Downing SE, Talner N, Gardner TH. Ventricular function in the newborn lamb. *Am J Physiol* 1965;208:931–937.

29. Grant DA, Kondo CS, Maloney JE, Walker AM, Tyberg JV. Changes in pericardial pressure during the perinatal period. *Circulation* 1992;86:1615–1621.

30. Sahn DJ, Lange LW, Allen HD, Goldberg SJ, Anderson C, Giles H, Haber K. Quantitative real-time cross-sectional echocardiography in the developing normal human fetus and newborn. *Circulation* 1980;62:588–597.

31. Pinson CW, Morton MJ, Thornburg KL. An anatomic basis for fetal right ventricular dominance and arterial pressure sensitivity. *J Dev Physiol* 1987;9:253–269.

32. Versprille A, Janse J, Harinck E, van Nie C, Neef K. Functional interaction of both ventricles at birth and the changes during the neonatal period in relation to the changes of geometry. In: Longo LD, Reneau DD, eds. *Fetal and Newborn Cardiovascular Physiology.* New York: Garland STMP Press; 1978;Volume 1 pp 399–413.

33. Reller MD, Morton MJ, Thornburg KL. Right ventricular function in the hypoxaemic fetal sheep. *J Dev Physiol* 1986;8:159–166.

34. Reller MD, Morton MJ, Giraud GD, Reid DL, Thornburg KL. The effect of acute hypoxaemia on ventricular function during beta-adrenergic and cholinergic blockade in the fetal sheep. *J Dev Physiol* 1989;11:263–269.

35. Lorijn RHW, Longo LD. Norepinephrine elevation in the fetal lamb: oxygen consumption and cardiac output. *Am J Physiol* 1980;239:R115–R122.

36. Artman M. Developmental changes in myocardial contractile responses to inotropic agents. *Cardiovasc Res* 1992;26:3–13.

37. Anderson PAW, Fair EC, Killam AP, Nassar R, Mainwaring RD, Rosemond RL, Whyte LM. The *in utero* left ventricle of the fetal sheep: the effects of isoprenaline. *J Physiol* 1990;430: 441–452.

38. Kirkpatrick SE, Naliboff J, Pitlick PT, Friedman WF. The influence of poststimulation potentiation and heart rate on the fetal lamb heart. *Am J Physiol* 1975;229:318–323.

39. Sugimoto T, Sagawa K, Guyton AC. Effect of tachycardia on cardiac output during normal and increased venous return. *Am J Physiol* 1966;211:288–292.

40. Cowley AW, Guyton AC. Heart rate as a determinant of cardiac output in dogs with arteriovenous fistula. *Am J Cardiol* 1971;28:321–325.

41. Guyton AC. *Textbook of Medical Physiology.* Philadelphia: WB Saunders; 1971.

42. Mahler F, Yoran C, Ross J Jr. Inotropic effect of tachycardia and poststimulation potentiation in the conscious dog. *Am J Physiol* 1974;227:569–575.

43. Ross J Jr, Linhart JW, Braunwald E. Effects of changing heart rate in man by electrical stimulation of the right atrium: studies at rest, during exercise, and with isoproterenol. *Circulation* 1965;32:549–558.

44. Rudolph AM, Heymann MA. Cardiac output in the fetal lamb: the effects of spontaneous and induced changes of heart rate on right and left ventricular output. *Am J Obstet Gynecol* 1976;124:183–192.

45. Gilbert RD. Effects of afterload and baroreceptors on cardiac function in fetal sheep. *J Dev Physiol* 1982;4:299–309.

46. Weir WG, Yue DT. Intracellular calcium transients underlying the short-term force–interval relationship in ferret ventricular myocardium. *J Physiol* 1986;376:507–530.

47. Anderson PAW, Manring A, Sommer JR, Johnson EA. Cardiac muscle: an attempt to relate structure to function. *J Mol Cell Cardiol* 1976;8:123–143.

48. Martonosi A. Membrane transport during development in animals. *Biochim Biophys Acta* 1975;415:311–333.

49. Chin TK, Friedman WF, Klitzner TS. Developmental changes in cardiac myocyte calcium regulation. *Circ Res* 1990;67: 574–579.

50. Artman M, Graham TP Jr, Boucek RJ Jr. Effects of postnatal maturation on myocardial contractile responses to calcium antagonists and changes in contraction frequency. *J Cardiovasc Pharmacol* 1985;7:850–855.

51. Arcilla RA, Lind J, Zetterqvist P, Oh W, Gessner IH. Hemodynamic features of extrasystoles in newborn and older infants. *Am J Cardiol* 1966;18:191–199.

52. Anderson PAW, Manring A, Johnson EA. The force of contraction of isolated papillary muscle: a study of the interaction of its determining factors. *J Mol Cell Cardiol* 1977;9:131–150.

53. Anderson PAW, Manring A, Serwer GA, Benson DW, Edwards SB, Armstrong BE, Sterba RJ, Floyd RD IV. The force–interval relationship of the left ventricle. *Circulation* 1979;60:334–348.

54. Maylie JG. Excitation–contraction coupling in neonatal and adult myocardium of cat. *Am J Physiol* 1982;242:H834–H843.

55. Nassar R, Reedy MC, Anderson PAW. Developmental changes in the ultrastructure and sarcomere shortening of the isolated rabbit ventricular myocyte. *Circ Res* 1987;61:465–483.

56. Meissner G. Ryanodine activation and inhibition of the Ca^{2+} release channel of sarcoplasmic reticulum. *J Biol Chem* 1986; 261:6300–6306.

57. Martonosi AN. Mechanisms of Ca^{2+} release from sarcoplasmic reticulum of skeletal muscle. *Physiol Rev* 1984;64:1240–1320.

58. Nayler WG, Fassold E. Calcium accumulating and ATPase activity of cardiac sarcoplasmic reticulum before and after birth. *Cardiovasc Res* 1977;11:231–237.

59. Anderson PAW, Manring A, Arentzen CE, Rankin JS, Johnson EA. Pressure-induced hypertrophy of cat right ventricle: an evaluation with the force–interval relationship. *Circ Res* 1977;41:582–588.

60. Sink JD, Anderson PA, Wechsler AS. Postoperative left ventricular contractility in the cardiac surgical patient: an evaluation of the force–interval relationship. *Ann Thorac Surg* 1985;40:475–482.

61. Anderson PAW, Rankin JS, Arentzen CE, Anderson RW, Johnson EA. Evaluation of the force–frequency relationship as a descriptor of the inotropic state of canine left ventricular myocardium. *Circ Res* 1976;39:832–839.

62. Eliot RF, Lam R, Leake RD, Hobel CJ, Fisher DA. Plasma catecholamine concentrations in infants at birth and during the first 48 hours of life. *J Pediatr* 1980;96:311–315.

63. Geis WP, Tatooles CJ, Priola DV, Friedman WF. Factors influencing neurohumoral control of the heart in the newborn dog. *Am J Physiol* 1975;228:1685–1689.

64. Mahler F, Ross J Jr, O'Rourke RA, Covell JW. Effects of changes in preload, afterload and inotropic state on ejection and isovolumic phase measures of contractility in the conscious dog. *Am J Cardiol* 1975;35:626–634.

65. Kavaler F, Harris RS, Lee RJ, Fisher VJ. Frequency–force behavior of *in situ* ventricular myocardium in the dog. *Circ Res* 1971;28:533–544.

66. Noble MIM, Wyler J, Milne ENC, Trenchard D, Guz A. Effect of changes in heart rate on left ventricular performance in conscious dogs. *Circ Res* 1969;24:285–295.

67. Wallace AG, Skinner NS Jr, Mitchell JH. Hemodynamic determinants of the maximal rate of rise of left ventricular pressure. *Am J Physiol* 1963;205:30–36.

68. Burkhoff D, Yue DT, Franz MR, Hunter WC, Sunagawa K, Maughan WL, Sagawa K. Quantitative comparison of the force–interval relationships of the canine right and left ventricles. *Circ Res* 1984;54:468–473.

69. Burkhoff D, Yue DT, Franz MR, Hunter WC, Sagawa K. Mechanical restitution of isolated perfused canine left ventricles. *Am J Physiol* 1984;246:H8–H16.

70. Klautz RJ, Teitel DF, Steendijk P, van Bel F, Baan J. Interaction between afterload and contractility in the newborn heart: evidence of homeometric autoregulation in the intact circulation. *J Am College Cardiol* 1995;25:1428–1435.

71. Anderson PAW, Manring A, Johnson EA. Force–frequency relationship: a basis for a new index of cardiac contractility? *Circ Res* 1973;33:665–671.

72. Yue DT, Burkhoff D, Franz MR, Hunter WC, Sagawa K. Postextrasystolic potentiation of the isolated canine left ventricle relationship to mechanical restitution. *Circ Res* 1985;56:340–350.

73. Manring A, Anderson PAW. The contractility of cardiac muscle. *CRC Crit Rev Bioeng* 1980;4:165–201.

74. Baker SP, Potter LT. Cardiac β-adrenoceptors during normal growth of male and female rats. *Br J Pharmacol* 1980;68:65–70.

75. Chen F-CM, Yamamura HI, Roeske WR. Ontogeny of mammalian myocardial β-adrenergic receptors. *Eur J Pharmacol* 1979;58:255–264.

76. Cheng JB, Cornett LE, Goldfein A, Roberts JM. α-Adrenergic receptor is present in fetal but not adult sheep myocardium. *Fed Proc* 1980;39:399.

77. DeChamplain J, Malmfors T, Olson L, Sachs C. Ontogenesis of peripheral adrenergic neurons in the rat: pre- and postnatal observations. *Acta Physiol Scand* 1970;80:276–288.

78. Felder RA, Calcagno PL, Eisner GM, Jose PA. Ontogeny of myocardial adrenoceptors. II. Alpha adrenoceptors. *Pediatr Res* 1982;16:340–342.

79. Friedman WF. Neuropharmacologic studies of perinatal myocardium. *Cardiovasc Clin* 1972;4:43–57.

80. Hoar RM, Hall JL. The early pattern of cardiac innervation in the fetal guinea-pig. *Am J Anat* 1970;128:499–508.

81. Schumacher W, Mirkin BL, Sheppard JR. Biological maturation and β-adrenergic effectors: development of β-adrenergic receptors in rabbit heart. *Mol Cell Biochem* 1984;58:173–181.

82. Schumacher WA, Sheppard JR, Mirkin BL. Biological maturation and beta-adrenergic effectors: pre- and postnatal development of the adenylate cyclase system in the rabbit heart. *J Pharmacol Exp Ther* 1982;223:587–593.

83. Whitsett JA, Darovec-Beckerman C. Developmental aspects of β-adrenergic receptors and catecholamine-sensitive adenylate cyclase in rat myocardium. *Pediatr Res* 1981;15:1363–1369.

84. Yamada S, Yamamura HI, Roeske WR. Ontogeny of mammalian cardiac α_1-adrenergic receptors. *Eur J Pharmacol* 1980;68:217–221.

85. Assali NS, Brinkman CR III, Woods JR Jr, Nuwayhid BS, Dandavino A. Ontogenesis of the autonomic control of cardiovascular functions in the sheep. In: Longo LD, Reneau DD, eds. *Fetal and Newborn Cardiovascular Physiology.* Volume 1 New York: Garland STMP Press; 1978;pp:47–92.

86. Manring A, Anderson PAW, Nassar R, Howe WR. Can sympathomimetic agents be classified by their action on the force–interval relationship? *Life Sci* 1983;32:329–336.

87. Anderson PAW, Manring A, Nassar R. Developmental changes in cardiac contractility. *Pediatr Res* 1979;13:339.

88. Hunkeler NM, Kullman J, Murphy AM. Troponin I isoform expression in human heart. *Circ Res* 1991;69:1409–1414.

89. Anderson PAW, Greig A, Mark TM, Malouf NN, Oakeley AE, Ungerleider RM, Allen PD, Kay BK. Molecular basis of human cardiac troponin T isoforms expressed in the developing, adult, and failing heart. *Circ Res* 1995;76:681–686.

90. Boheler KR, Carrier L, de la Bastie D, Allen PD, Komajda M, Mercadier JJ, Schwartz K. Skeletal actin mRNA increases in the human heart during ontogenic development and is the major isoform of control and failing adult hearts. *J Clin Invest* 1991;88:323–330.

91. Anderson PAW, Henderson PM, Nassar R. The calcium transient in cardiac myocytes increases with development. *Circulation* 1993;88:1–436.

92. McPherson RA, Kramer MF, Covell JW, Friedman WF. A comparison of the active stiffness of fetal and adult cardiac muscle. *Pediatr Res* 1976;10:660–664.

93. Sheridan DJ, Cullen MJ, Tynan MJ. Qualitative and quantitative observations on ultrastructural changes during postnatal development in the cat myocardium. *J Mol Cell Cardiol* 1979;11:1173–1181.

94. Urthaler F, Walker AA, Kawamura K, Hefner LL, James TN. Canine atrial and ventricular muscle mechanics studied as a function of age. *Circ Res* 1978;42:703–713.

95. Davies P, Dewar J, Tynan M, Ward R. Post-natal developmental changes in the length–tension relationship of cat papillary muscles. *J Physiol* 1975;253:95–102.

96. Spann JF Jr, Buccino RA, Sonnenblick EH, Braunwald E. Contractile state of cardiac muscle obtained from cats with experimentally produced ventricular hypertrophy and heart failure. *Circ Res* 1967;21:341–354.

97. Comline RS, Silver M. The composition of fetal and maternal blood during parturition in the ewe. *J Physiol* 222:233–256.

98. Morton MJ, Pinson CW, Thornburg KL. *In utero* ventilation with oxygen augments left ventricular stroke volume in lambs. *J Physiol* 1987;383:413–424.

99. Teitel DF, Dalinghaus M, Cassidy SC, Payne BD, Rudolph AM. *In utero* ventilation augments the left ventricular response to isoproterenol and volume loading in fetal sheep. *Pediatr Res* 1991;29:466–472.

40

AUTONOMIC CONTROL OF FETAL CARDIAC ACTIVITY

Claudio Giorlandino, md, and Giovanni Gambuzza, md

INTRODUCTION

The fetal circulation is different from that of the adult. This difference is particularly evident because of the anatomical communication of the left and right heart at the level of the atria and because of the presence of the ductus arteriosus, which shifts approximately 60% of the blood of the right ventricle to the aorta distal to the ductus.[1] The consequence is a different distribution of oxygenated blood in the fetal circulation: The left ventricle perfuses mainly the myocardium and the central nervous system (CNS), whereas the right ventricle through the ductus arteriosus perfuses the descending aorta and the districts distal to the ductus.

The fetal heart rate is also very different from that of an adult. To maintain a relatively high cardiac output, the fetal heart rate is higher. A statistically significant difference in the slope of regression lines has been demonstrated for heart rate observations before and after the 14th week of gestation (Fig. 40.1).[2] This has led to different hypotheses concerning the mechanisms that control the fetal heart rate during the various phases of gestation.

The partial pressure of fetal blood oxygen is regulated mainly through chemoreceptors, with the most important ones being found at the level of the aorta. These aortic chemoreceptors are extremely sensitive to variations in oxygen levels, and they initiate the regulatory mechanisms in response to hypoxia. The initial response to hypoxia is tachycardia and a blood pressure increase, mediated by catecholamines, corticotropin, and vasopressin.[3] When hypoxia decreases to a partial oxygen pressure below 16 mmHg, a shift to bradycardia occurs,[4] probably through a vagal response mediated by aortic chemoreceptors.

The fetus responds to hypoxia with a redistribution of blood flow. The afterload on the right ventricle is increased by catecholamine secretion. Consequently, both right and left atrial diastolic blood residues accumulate, and the diastolic atrial pressure increases. The left ventricular preload is increased and perfusion to critical areas, such as myocardium and brain, is in turn increased. Hypoxia determines a decrease in vascular resistance at the level of the brain, which further facilitates redistribution of blood flow to vital areas of the body.

The umbilical circulation absorbs more than 40% of fetal cardiac output.[5] Recently, it has become possible to evaluate resistance in uterine, placental, and umbilical vessels throughout gestation. Doppler velocimetry studies have shown that vascular resistance decreases progressively during the course of gestation.[6] Concomitantly, in the uterine arteries there is a progressive increase in the diastolic component of the velocimetry curve. By the end of gestation the resistance in uterine arteries is low, and systolic and diastolic velocities to be appear similar.[7] Flow velocity in the fetal aorta, however, does not change in parallel in normal pregnancy.[8]

Obviously, the mechanisms described above do not operate independently, but are closely linked in a complex relationship not yet fully understood. For a more detailed discussion on the anatomy, hemodynamics, and other physiologic parameters of the fetal heart, see Chapters 39, 41, and 43.

Cardiac Problems in Pregnancy, Third Edition
Edited by Uri Elkayam, MD, and Norbert Gleicher, MD
Copyright © 1998 by Wiley-Liss, Inc. ISBN 0-471-16358-9

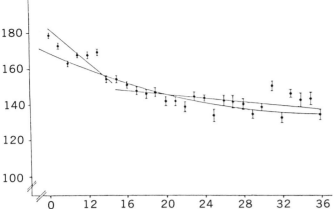

Figure 40.1   Fetal heart rate during the course of pregnancy: curve shows general trend; two regression lines are calculated for experimental values before and after the 14th week. The difference between the slopes of the two regression lines is significant.[2]

AUTONOMIC SYSTEM

The fetal heart beat originates, as in the adult heart, in the sinoatrial node. Following spontaneous depolarization of pacemaker cells, the electrical impulse travels through the right and left atria (beginning of *atrial systole*) along a specialized tract of the atrioventricular (AV) node, and from there to the branches of the bundle of His and the Purkinje fibers (*ventricular systole*).

The chronotropic activity of the sinoatrial node is under the influence of the autonomic nervous system. The rate of the impulses from the sinoatrial node decreases when the parasympathetic impulse prevails and increases when the sympathetic impulse prevails. In the pacemaker cells, acetylcholine increases the cellular membrane permeability to potassium ions, leading to an increased K^+ flow to the extracellular space, with a consequent increase in the resting potential. Catecholamine, on the other hand, reduces the K^+ flow to the extracellular space, therefore decreasing the resting potential of the cell and increasing the rate of depolarization.

The parasympathetic innervation of the heart originates from the cardiac branches of the vagus nerve, which originate from the recurrent laryngeal nerves and the thoracic vagi immediately distal to them. These nerves are interconnected with the heart nerves of the sympathetic innervation, forming dorsal and ventral cardiopulmonary plexuses in the mediastinum at the base of the heart. The dorsal plexus is located dorsal to the aortic arch and pulmonary artery; the smaller ventral plexus is located anterior to the aorta and pulmonary artery. The dorsal and ventral plexuses are the origin of the right and left coronary cardiac nerves and left lateral cardiac nerve which, together with other small nerves originating from the plexuses and the thoracic vagi, innervate the heart.[9]

The sympathetic innervation of the human heart origi-

nates from the stellate ganglia and the caudal halves of the cervical sympathetic trunks below the level of the cricoid cartilage. As mentioned above, these nerves link up with the parasympathetic nerves at the level of the ventral and dorsal cardiopulmonary plexuses, located anterior and posterior to the pulmonary artery from which the heart nerves originate.[9]

Development of the Parasympathetic and Sympathetic Systems

Studies on the ontogenetic development of both the parasympathetic and sympathetic innervation of the heart are mainly derived from the chick embryo model, since the chick heart and the human heart have similar characteristics during the early stages of development.[10]

In the human embryo, development of vagal innervation starts in the early days of the 8th week of gestation.[11] At approximately 10 weeks, nerve fibers from the right vagosympathetic trunk colonize the heart, the veins, and the pulmonary artery.[12] Vagal innervation of the heart is complete by the 12th week in the atria and by the 13th week in the ventricles.[11] The first ganglia cells appear at 8 weeks between the aorta and the pulmonary artery. At the 13th week, the gangliar structures are concentrated in five main groups: in the regions of the upper rear of the atria, the interatrial sulcus, and the atrioventricular sulcus, and in the tunica adventitia of the roots of the aorta and the pulmonary artery.[11] Irregular cells with the morphological features of mature ganglia cells can be first seen in the 120 mm fetus.[13] The process of expansion of the ganglia continues up to about the 34th week of gestation.[14]

The origin and development of the functional activity of the parasympathetic nervous system have been studied with field stimulation at the gestational ages of 12 and 20 weeks.[15] This method involves the release of neurotransmitters by myocardial autonomic structures. Their effects can be measured by changes in tension of the myocardial tissue: The release of acetylcholine provokes a decrease in tension (*negative inotropic effect*). Before the 13th week of gestation, no response to stimulation is observed, thus suggesting immaturity of the autonomic nervous system. After that period, a response can be observed, which is more frequently of the cholinergic rather than the adrenergic type. The inhibitory effect produced by acetylcholine appears even before the autonomic innervation of the heart has developed. The negative chronotropic effect on the sinoatrial node can be observed as early as the 7th week of gestation.[15,16] In contrast, nicotine does not seem to exert any inhibitory effect,[15] thus suggesting the absence of gangliar nicotine receptors up to the 20th week. Since ganglia may be functionally immature up to 20 weeks of gestation, vagal transmission to the heart may not take place. An increase in vagal tone on fetal heart rate with the progression of gestation has been demonstrated in vivo by Schifferti and Caldero-Garcia,[17] who administered atropine to pregnant women between 15 and 40 weeks of gestation. This measure blocked vagal control, in turn determining an increase in fetal heart rate more pronounced as pregnancy progresses, from an increase of 5 beats per minute at 15 weeks to 20 beats per minute at 40 weeks. These data suggest that the progressive decrease in fetal heart rate from the 4th month of pregnancy on may be the result of a progressive increase in vagal tone.

Studies on the ontogenesis of the sympathetic innervation have been primarily based on the identification of catecholamine by histochemical fluorescent methods.[18] Data on the presence of fluorescent nerve trunks up to the 13th week of pregnancy are inconsistent: One study reports the presence of low level of fluorescence as early as the 10th week,[19] whereas other researchers demonstrate the absence of fluorescence in these early stages and up to the 18th week.[20] Between 13 and 23 weeks, fluorescent nerve structures can be demonstrated uniformly, and they appear denser in the atria than in the ventricles.[21]

In contrast to this late appearance of innervation, the human fetal heart is able to synthesize norepinephrine from the 13th week of gestation.[16] Based on the evidence that sympathetic nerve terminals are absent and only small cellular fluorescent formations are present, a humoral rather than adrenergic nerve mechanism of sympathetic control has been suggested for the early stages of development.[19,20]

The presence of β-adrenergic receptors in the human heart between 12 and 22 weeks has been demonstrated by the higher sensitivity of the atrial tissue to isoproterenol than to norepinephrine.[22] Studies on field stimulation of atrial tissue at 12–20 weeks have been conducted to study the functional development of adrenergic transmission.[15] A positive inotropic effect has been demonstrated with this method from weeks 13–14 on. The positive inotropic effect is increased by phenoxybenzamine, which blocks neuronal uptake of norepinephrine, and decreased by propranolol, which blocks β-adrenergic receptors. The involvement of norepinephrine in the positive inotropic response produced by field stimulation appears therefore likely.[15]

The greater frequency and earlier presence of cholinergic responses in the experiments just described suggest that the functional activation of the parasympathetic system occurs slightly ahead of the sympathetic system. High doses of nicotine determine an excitatory effect that is blocked by propranolol. This effect is presumably due to the release of norepinephrine. Since nicotine determines the release of norepinephrine from both the sympathetic neurons and the chromaffin tissue, and since an excitatory response has been observed at 8 weeks,[15] it has been suggested that in the early stages of development, even before sympathetic transmission is established, the chromaffin tissue may be the principal site for the release of norepinephrine.

SYMPATHETIC AND PARASYMPATHETIC CONTROL OF THE FETAL HEART AND CIRCULATION

The facilitory influence of sympathetic activity on the heart is counterbalanced by the inhibitory effect of vagal activity. Differing results have been obtained in research on animals, specifically on chronically instrumented fetal sheep. Assalie et al[23] reported that atropine blockage of the cholinergic receptors resulted in a significant increase (10%) in heart rate in fetuses at term. In premature and immature fetuses, the increase was less significant (2 and 4%, respectively). In contrast, propanolol blocking of β-adrenergic receptors produced a more evident effect, decreasing the heart rate by 10% in immature fetus, 12% in premature fetuses, and 14% in fetuses at term. These data show that the sympathetic system predominates in the control of the heart rate in the sheep fetus.

The parasympathetic system does not begin to play an important role until the near-term period. This role becomes even more marked in the neonatal period. Simultaneous blocking of cholinergic and β-adrenergic receptors decreases fetal heart rate and thus confirms the predominance of the sympathetic system in the control of the fetal heart rate. In the neonatal stage, the situation is reversed. The same dual blockage causes a marked increase in heart rate, as would be expected from a predominance of the parasympathetic system.

Since the two components of the autonomic nervous system are totally active, the opposite effects of the sympathetic and parasympathetic systems do not add up algebraically, and this discrepancy must be accounted for. In animal studies, in particular, it has been reported that the response of the heart rate to a given level of vagal stimulation varies substantially according to the prevalence of sympathetic activity.[24,25] This exaggerated vagal inhibitory response to the increase of sympathetic tone has been defined as *accentuated antagonism*. At the sinoatrial node level, the effect of sympathetic activity is progressively attenuated as the level of vagal activity rises. This occurs through the inhibitory effect of acetylcoline, liberated by the vagal fibers, on the release of norepinephrine via contiguous sympathetic terminals.[25] How this interaction between the sympathetic and parasympathetic system takes place is still to be determined.

As to the control of the circulation by the autonomic nervous system, it appears that a progressive increase in neurohumoral control over the peripheral circulation occurs with advancing gestation. This turns out to be exerted to a markedly greater degree by the α-adrenergic system than by gangliar structures.[27,28] The neurohumoral control reaches a peak at term and then decreases progressively during the neonatal period.[23] In contrast, it is the parasympathetic system that plays a markedly dominating role in the control of the pulmonary circulation and of the blood flow through the ductus arteriosus.[29]

RECEPTOR SYSTEM

Baroreceptor Reflex

The literature offers contradictory data on the increase of the baroreceptor response during the course of pregnancy. Such an increase has been reported by some authors[30] and denied by others.[31,32] The part played by the autonomic nervous system in baroreceptor control has been studied in chronic fetal sheep preparations by Ismay et al[32] When phenylephrine was used to induce a sharp increase in arterial pressure, it was observed that the baroreceptor reflex was abolished by atropine and increased by propanolol. This pair of results shows that the activity of the baroreceptor response depends on parasympathetic control and is inhibited by the sympathetic system. An increase in the sensitivity of the baroreceptors has been observed in adult rabbits when α-adrenergic receptors are blocked.[33] It seems, however, that chemoreceptor systems, which are extremely sensitive to changes in the partial oxygen pressure, exert predominant control over fetal hemodynamics, rather than the baroreceptor systems. In the condition of fetal stress, the release of catecholamines into the bloodstream and their action on α-adrenergic vessel receptors appear to represent the main stimulus for the selective redistribution of blood flow, which is observed in hypoxia (vasodilatation in the coronary, cerebral, and umbilical circulations and vasoconstriction in the visceral, lung, muscle, and cutaneous zones).[34]

Chemoreceptor Reflex

Walker et al[35] demonstrated that the response to hypoxia in chronic fetal sheep preparations depends on gestational age. In fetuses before 0.8 of term gestation, hypoxia produces a modest increase in blood pressure but does not cause significant changes in heart rate. In the fetus after 0.8 of term gestation, one observes bradycardia and an increase in blood pressure. The roles of the parasympathetic and sympathetic systems in these responses were also evaluated.

Before 0.8 of term gestation, it was observed that hypoxia gave rise to a balanced increase in sympathetic and parasympathetic activities before any significant effect on the fetal heart rate occurred. After 0.8 of term gestation, there was a predominant increase in parasympathetic activity, superimposed on a concomitant but less effective sympathetic activity, with bradycardia appearing as a result.

The chemoreceptor response to changes in fetal homeostasis also was analyzed in a number of studies on fetal sheep preparation in which changes in fetal P_{O_2}, P_{CO_2}, and pH occurred. In these investigations, maternal inspiratory gas tension was altered by administering mixtures of varying composition, whereupon occlusions of the maternal internal iliac artery were provoked, followed by provocation of compression of the umbilical cord in toto, or either umbilical veins or arteries separately.

Initially, in the presence of a modest decrease in P_{O_2} and an increase in P_{CO_2}, one observes a bradycardia that can be considered to be of chemoreceptor origin and appears to be mediated by the vagus. When a significant increase in blood pressure occurs, bradycardia persists but seems to be caused by simultaneous chemo- and baroreceptor stimulation in response to the increase in afterload, provoked by the peripheral vasoconstriction and mediated by the adrenergic nervous system. When hypoxia and acidosis persist, the initial bradycardial response may be followed by an increase in fetal heart rate, provoked by an increase in myocardial contractility that is due to increased release of adrenal catecholamines. When hypoxia and acidosis exceed a critical level, however, a predominant vagal activity is imposed on the increased sympathetic tone. This results in the appearance of bradycardia aimed at saving glycogen reserves, especially those of the myocardium, in an attempt to keep the fetus alive.

HEMODYNAMIC CONTROL

Changes in cardiac output may be caused by changes in heart rate (*chronotropic effect*) or in the force of the contractions (*inotropic effect*) through the control exerted on the heart by its sympathetic and parasympathetic innervation. The energy of contraction is also proportional to the length of the myocardial fibers in the preload, diastolic phase (*Frank–Starling relation*). The fetal heart, however, behaves differently from the heart of an adult. The autonomic nervous system plays a fundamental role in the maintenance of physiologic cardiocirculatory conditions and in the reactions of the fetal cardiocirculatory apparatus to conditions of fetal stress.

The fetal lamb was used successfully by Dalton et al[36] to demonstrate the interaction of the β-sympathetic (*cardioacceleratory*) and parasympathetic (*cardioinhibitory*) systems under known physiologic conditions. These investigators used drugs with blocking actions on the two systems, administering the minimum doses needed to obtain complete blocking. The response was evaluated, measuring mean heart rate and heart rate variability, measured as the mean beat-to-beat difference (MABB) for the highest frequencies and as the root mean square deviation (2MSD) of R-R intervals for lower frequencies. Atropine, which blocks the action of acetylcholine, liberated by postganglionic parasympathetic nerves, was used as a blocker. The heart rate increased rapidly, but the MABB fell. No differences dependent on gestational age were observed. No changes in either blood gases, hematocrit, or blood pressure were noted. There was, however, some reduction in respiratory movements, probably in response to the central action of atropine, which causes a prolonged episode of high voltage electrocortical activity[37] and reduces respiratory activity.

Atropine reduces the MABB much more significantly than the 2 MDS, suggesting that high frequency variability is more influenced by the parasympathetic system. Use of the selective blocking agent propanolol rapidly reduced the heart rate, but did not influence either MABB or 2MSD. No significant change occurred in blood gases, hematocrit, blood pressure, or breathing activity. If atropine is added to propanolol, variability is greatly reduced, clearly demonstrating that variability is the result of a push–pull relationship between the two components of the autonomic nervous system. Phentolamine, a sympathetic blocking agent, caused a slow rise in the heart rate, and MABB and 2MSD increased significantly. This event was accompanied by a small fall in arterial pressure.

To establish which CNS structures are responsible for normal beat-to-beat variability, one has to refer to animal studies. In fetal lambs, if the brain is destroyed but the spinal cord is left intact up to and through the cervical region, the heart rate tracing becomes "flat." If, however, the brain stem is transected on its upper parts, heart rate variability remains normal.[37]

The effect of adrenergic and catecholamine stimulation on fetal heart rate have already been discussed. At this point it should be added that circulating catecholamines, and in particular adrenaline, can also produce effects that are mediated not by nerves but by endocrine action. Although noradrenaline seems to be the predominant catecholamine in fetal life,[38] all circulating catecholamines may be liberated under different stimuli, consequently becoming able to influence fetal heart rate.[39] The medulla of the fetal adrenal gland seems to be able to react to anoxia independently of the CNS.[40]

Jones and Robinson[39] showed that in the catheterized lamb, fetal hypoxia is followed by an increase in adrenaline and noradrenaline in the circulation. The first consequence was an increase in arterial pressure, followed by a reduction in heart rate which, however, soon returned to normal levels. When hypoxia was induced by acute maternal hemorrhage,[40] bradycardia again appeared, together with hypertension and a rise in the differential pressure. The heart rate soon returned to normal. This response is similar to the response toward baroreceptor stimulation. These studies suffer from the "impurity" of any response to catecholamines that is obtained through anoxia. Vapaavouri et al[27] established that the fetal heart differs from that of the adult in its response to adrenergic stimulation. The tachycardial response is less evident in the fetus than in the adult.[41] It is also probable that there are differences in the concentrations and interactions of adrenergic receptors.

In evaluating the activity of the fetal adrenal system and

the resulting control over the fetal heart, one faces the problem of differentiation between the production of catecholamine by the mother and/or the fetus. For a long time it was thought that the fetal and maternal systems were separate, with no transplacental transfer occurring.[39] Chen et al,[42] however, suggested the existence of a catecholamethyltransferase, which denatures catecholamines on passage across the placenta. Other studies[43–45] conclude that transfer of maternal catecholamines to the fetus takes place to a limited extent only and does not exceed 20% of the original maternal concentration. If we accept the validity of these observations, we must conclude that the maternal sympathetic system exerts great influence on the fetal adrenal sympathetic system and its cardiocirculatory activity.

During the course of fetal life there is a continuous change in the response to adrenergic stimuli.[27,41] It has also been demonstrated that the response to catecholamines is modified by thyroid hormones.[46,47] These observations suggest that thyroid hormones exert a permissive action on the β-adrenergic activity of receptors in the fetal heart. Dipak[48] demonstrated that thyroid activity is mediated through an increase in the number of β-adrenergic receptor binding sites.

The opioid peptides are produced by the fetal hypophysis, predominantly by the intermediate lobe.[49] This portion of the hypophysis is particularly prominent in the fetus. In the adult, opioids produce hypertension and bradycardia by decreasing sympathetic while increasing vagal tone at the autonomic nuclei of the brain stem.[50] An increase in opioid levels in plasma[51] and amniotic fluid[52] has been noted in association with fetal distress, abnormal heart rate patterns, and acidosis. To demonstrate a depressive action of opioids on fetal heart activity, a specific antagonist (naloxone) has been administered to fetuses, resulting in improvement in beat-to-beat variability.[53] Maternal and fetal opioid levels have recently been correlated through the secretion of cortisol, a hormone that passes freely through the placental barrier and acts as an inhibitor for the synthesis of proopiomelanocortine.[54]

The mechanism that regulates changes in fetal behavioral states is still unknown. Walker et al[55] suggested that such changes could be related to diurnal variations of uterine blood flow. Nathanielsz et al[56] proposed entrainment of a periodicity of fetal behavior by a sensory pathway that develops in response to the pressure of uterine contractions of the fetal body. We have hypothesized that fetal behavior may be influenced by maternal plasma cortisol levels. Visser et al[57] also noticed that the fetal heart rate resembles the pattern of maternal plasma cortisol variations.

One of the most interesting aspects of fetal heart rate activity relates to the action of prostaglandins, since they are involved in the control of the ductus arteriosus.[58] Because of its relaxing action on the pulmonary circulation,[59] PGE-2 has been used in an attempt to treat pulmonary hypertension in neonates.[60]

REFERENCES

1. Rudolph AM. Distribution and regulation of blood flow in the fetal and neonatal lamb. *Circ Res* 1985;57:811–821.

2. Romanini C, Arduini D, Marchetti P, Pasetto A, Mancuso S. Osservazioni sulla frequenza cardiaca fetale in epoca precoce di gravidanza. *Ann Ostet Ginecol Med Perinatale* 1980;101: 49–55.

3. Boddy K, Jones CT, Mamtel L, Ratcliffe J, Robinson JS. Changes in plasma ACTH and corticosteroid of the maternal and fetal sheep during hypoxia. *Endocrinology* 1974;94: 588–592.

4. Saling E. Fetal blood gas and acid base status during normal labour. In: Saling E, ed. *Foetal and Neonatal Hypoxia.* Baltimore: Williams & Wilkins; 1968;32–41.

5. Cameron JM, Renean DD, Guilbeau EJ. Multicomponent analysis of the fetal system. In: Longo LD, Reneau D, eds. *Fetal and Newborn Cardiovascular Physiology.* New York: Garland STPM Press; 1978;437–550.

6. Trudinger BJ, Cook CM, Collins J, Bombardieri J, Gles WB. Fetal umbilical artery velocity waveforms and placental resistance: clinical significance. *Br J Obstet Gynaecol* 1985;92: 23–30.

7. Campbell S, Griffin DR, Pearce JM, Diaz-Recanses J, Cohen-Overbeek TE, Wilson K. New Doppler technique for assessing uteroplacental blood flow. *Lancet* 1983;1:675–683.

8. Griffin D, Bilardo K, Masini L, Diaz Recanses J, Pearce JM, Wilson K, Campbell S. Doppler blood flow waveforms in the descending thoracic aorta of the human fetus. *Br J Obstet Gynaecol* 1984;91:997–1006.

9. James RD, Brands CH, Hopkins DA, Johnston DE, Murphy DA, Armour JA. Anatomy of human extrinsic cardiac nerves and ganglia. *Am J Cardiol* 1986;57:299–309.

10. Pappano AJ. Ontogenetic development of autonomic neuroeffector transmission and transmitter reactivity in embryonic and fetal hearts. *Pharmacol Rev* 1977;84:429–496.

11. Smith RB. The development of the intrinsic innervation of the human heart between 10 mm and 70 mm stages. *J Anat* 1070;107:271–279.

12. Gardner E, O'Rhahilly R. The nerve supply and conducting system of the human heart at the end of the embryonic period proper. *J Anat* 1976;121:571–587.

13. Smith RB. Intrinsic innervation of the human heart fetus between 70 mm and 420 mm CRL. *Acta Anat* 1971;78:200–209.

14. Smith RB. The development of automatic neurons in the human heart. *Anat Anz* 1971;129:70–76.

15. Walker D. Functional development of the automatic innervation of the human fetal heart. *Biol Neonat* 1975;25:31–43.

16. Gennser G. Response to adrenaline, acetylcholine and change of contraction frequency in early human fetal hearts. *Experientia* 1970;26:1105r–1107r.

17. Schifferti PY, Caldero-Gardia R. Effects of atropine and beta-adrenergic drugs on the heart rate of the human fetus. In: Boreus L, ed. *Fetal Pharmacology.* New York: Raven Press; 1973; 259–279.

18. Enermar A, Flick B, Hakanson R. Observation on the appearance of norepinephrine in the sympathetic nervous system of the chick embryo. *Dev Biol* 1965;11:283–286.

19. Patanen S, Korkala D. Catecholamines in human fetal heart. *Experientia* 1974;30:798–799.

20. Dail WG, Palmer GC. Localization and correlation of catecholamine containing cells with adenylcyclase and phosphodiesterase activities in human fetal heart. *Anat Rec* 1973;177: 265–288.

21. Gennser G, Studnitz W. Noradrenaline synthesis in human fetal heart. *Experientia* 1975;31:1422–1424.

22. Coltart DJ, Spilker BA. Development of human fetal inotropic response to catecholamines. *Experientia* 1972;28:525–526.

23. Assalie NS, Brinkman CR, Woods R, Dandauino A, Muwayhid B. Ontogenesis of the automatic control of cardiovascular functions in the sheep. In: Longo LD, Reneau DD, eds. *Fetal and Newborn Cardiovascular Physiology.* New York: Garland STPM Press; 1978;47–91.

24. Levy MN, Zieske H. Autonomic control of caridac pacemaker activity and atrioventricular transmission. *J Appl Physiol* 1969;27:465–470.

25. Levy MN. Sympathetic–parasympathetic interaction. *Fed Proc* 1984;43:2598–2602.

26. Levy MN. Sympathetic–parasympathetic interaction in the heart. *Circ Res* 1971;29:437–445.

27. Vapaavouri EK, Shinebourne EA, Williams RK, Heymann MA, Rudolph AM. Development of cardiovascular responses to autonomic blockade in intact fetal and newborn lambs. *Biol Neonatorum* 1973;22:177–178.

28. Van Patten GR, Harris WH, Mears GJ. Development of fetal cardiovascular responses to alpha-adrenergic agonists. In: Longo LD, Reneau DD, eds. *Fetal and Newborn Cardiovascular Physiology.* New York: Garland STPM Press; 1978;92–123.

29. Rudolph AM, Heymann MA. Control of the fetal circulation. In: *Fetal and Neonatal Physiology.* London: Cambridge University Press, 1973;89–111.

30. Shinebourne EA, Vapaavouri EK, Williams EK, Heymann MA, Rudolph AM. Development of baroreflex activity in an anaesthetized fetal and neonatal lamb. *Circ Res* 1972;31:710–718.

31. Maloney JE, Cannata J, Dowling MH, Else W, Ritchie B. Baroreflex activity in conscious fetal and newborn lambs. *Biol Neonat* 1977;31:340–350.

32. Ismay MJA, Lumbers ER, Stevens AD. The action of angiotensin II on the baroreflex response on the conscious ewe and the conscious fetus. *J Physiol* 1979:288:467–469.

33. Aars H. Effects of altered smooth muscle tone on aortic diameter and aortic baroreceptor activity in anaesthetized rabbits. *Circ Res* 1971;28:254–260.

34. Boddy K. Fetal circulation and breathing movements. In: Beard RW, Nathaliensz PW, eds. *Fetal Physiology and Medicine.* Philadelphia: WB Saunders; 1976;303–308.

35. Walker AM, Cannata JP, Dowling MH, Ritchie BC, Maloney JE. Age dependent patterns of autonomic heart rate control during hypoxia in fetal and newborn lambs. *Biol Neonatorum* 1979;34:198–208.

36. Dalton KJ, Phil MB, Dawes GS, Patrick JE. The autonomic nervous system and fetal heart rate variability. *Am J Obstet Gynecol* 1983;146:456–462.

37. Dawes GS. The central control of fetal breathing and skeletal muscle movements. A review. *J Physiol* 1984;346;1–18.

38. Greenberg RE, Lind J. Catecholamines in tissue of the human fetus. *Pediatrics* 1961;27:904–911.

39. Jones CT, Robinson RO. Plasma catecholamines in the fetal and adult sheep. *J Physiol* 1975;248:15–33.

40. Artal R, Glatz TH, Lam R, Nathanielsz PW, Nobel CJ. The effect of acute maternal hemorrhage on the release of catecholamines in the pregnant ewe and fetus. *Am J Obstet Gynecol* 1979;135:818–822.

41. Friedman WF. The intrinsic physiologic properties of the developing heart. In: Friedman WF, Lesch M, Sonnenblick EH, eds. *Neonatal Heart Disease*. New York: Grune & Stratton; 1973;21–49.

42. Chen CH, Klein DC, Robinson JC. COMT in rat placenta, human placenta, choriocarcinoma grown in culture. *J Reprod Fertil* 1974;39:407–410.

43. Condorelli S, Cosmi E. Passaggio placentare di alcune amine adrenergiche. *Acta Anaesthesiol Ital* 1970;21:539.

44. Cosmi E, Condorelli S. Passaggio transplacentare di catecolamine nella pecora. *Acta Anaesthesiol Ital* 1973;24:43–55.

45. Morgan CD, Sandler M, Panigel M. Placental transfer of catecholamines in vitro and in vivo. *Am J Obstet Gynecol* 1972;112:1068–1075.

46. Goswami A, Rosenberg IN. Thyroid hormone modulation of epinephrine induced lipolysis in rat adipocytes: a possible role of calcium. *Endocrinology* 1978;2223–2233.

47. Tse J, Wren RW, Kud JF. Thyroxine-induced receptors and adenosine 3-5-monophosphate system in the heart may be related to reputed catecholamine supersensitivity in hyperthyroidism. *Endocrinology* 1980;107:6–16.

48. Dipak K (Das Dibendu Bandyopadhhyay-Suschitra Bandyopadhyay). Thyroid hormone regulation of beta-adrenergic receptors and catecholamine sensitive adenylate cyclase in fetal heart. *Acta Endocrinol* 1984;106:569–576.

49. Stark RI, Frantz AG. The ACTH P-endorphin in pregnancy. In: *Neonatologia Clinica ed Ostetrica*. Rome: Pensiero Scientifico; 1984.

50. Lagamma MD, Edmund F. *Endogenous Opiates and Cardiopulmonary Function*. Chicago: Year-Book Medical Publishing; 1984;1–41.

51. Shabaan MM, Hung TT, Hoffman DI. Beta-endorphin and beta-lipotropin concentrations in umbilical cord blood. *Am J Obstet Gynecol* 1982;144:560–568.

52. Riss PA, Bieglmayer C. Immunoreactive endorphin peptides in amniotic fluid during labour. *Br J Obstet Gynaecol* 1983;90:49–50.

53. Goodlin RC. Naloxone and its possible relationship to fetal endorphin levels and fetal distress. *Am J Obstet Gynecol* 1983;90:49–50.

54. Giorlandino C, Vizzone A, Gentili P, Arduini D. Maternal endocrine situation and fetal behavior: possible correlation mechanisms. *New Trends* 1986;3:303–308.

55. Walker AM, Oakes GK, McLaughlin MK, Ehrenkranz LA, Alling DW, Chez RA. 24 hour rhythms in uterine and umbilical flows of conscious pregnant sheep. *Gynecol Invest* 1977;8:288–294.

56. Nathanielsz PW, Bailey A, Poore AR, Thorburn GD, Harding R. The relationship between myometrial activity and sleep state and breathing in fetal sheep during the last third of pregnancy. *SAm J Obstet Gynecol* 1980;653–657.

57. Visser GHA, Goodman JDS, Levine DH, Dawes GS. Diurnal and other cyclic variations in human fetal heart rate at term. *Am J Obstet Gynecol* 1982;142:535–544.

58. Coceani F, Olley PM. The response of the ductus arteriosus to prostaglandins. *Can J Physiol Pharmacol* 1973;51:220–225.

59. Lock JE, Olley PM, Coceani F. Direct pulmonary vascular responses to prostaglandins in the conscious newborn lamb. *Am J Physiol* 1980;H631:–H638.

60. Lock JE, Coceani F, Olley PM, Sawyer PR, Rowe RD. Use of prostacyclin in persistent fetal circulation. *Lancet* 1979;1:1343.

41

THE CARDIAC FUNCTION IN THE FETUS

Giuseppe Rizzo, MD, Alessandra Capponi, MD, and Carlo Romanini, MD

INTRODUCTION

In the past, the intrauterine environment has limited the possibility of studying circulation in the human fetus. Much of our understanding and present knowledge of fetal hemodynamics are therefore derived from animal studies.[1,2] During the last few years technological advances in ultrasound have, however, made the study of the human fetal heart possible. In particular, the advent of pulsed and color Doppler techniques has allowed us to examine noninvasively fetal cardiovascular pathophysiology, thus enabling hemodynamic studies of fetuses under normal and abnormal conditions.

This chapter outlines the principles of Doppler ultrasonography and its practical uses in the study of fetal cardiac function, and discusses the current and possible future applications of this investigative technology.

THE STUDY OF CARDIAC FUNCTION

General Principles

The parameters used to describe fetal cardiac velocity waveforms differ from those used in fetal peripheral vessels. In the latter situation, indices such as the pulsatility index, the resistance index or the systolic/diastolic (S/D) ratio are used. These indices are derived from relative ratios between systolic, diastolic, and mean velocity and are therefore independent of the absolute velocity values and of the angle of insonation between the Doppler beam and the direction of the blood flow.[3]

At the cardiac level, all measurements represent absolute values. Measurements of absolute flow velocities, therefore,

require knowledge about the angle of insonation, which may be difficult to obtain with accuracy. The error in the estimation of the absolute velocity, resulting from the uncertainty of angle measurement, is strongly dependent on the magnitude of the angle itself. For angles of less than about 20°, the error will be practically of no significance. For larger angles, the cosine term in the Doppler equation,

$$fd = \frac{(2FT \cos \alpha)V}{c}$$

where fd is the Doppler shift, FT the frequency transducer transmission, α the angel of insonation, V the velocity of blood flow, and c the velocity of ultrasound in tissue, changes the small uncertainty in the measurement of the angle into a large error in velocity computation.[3] As a consequence, it is always necessary to keep the Doppler beam as parallel as possible to the bloodstream when obtaining recordings, and all recordings with an estimated angle greater than 20° should be rejected.

Color Doppler may solve many of these problems by showing in real time the flow direction, thus allowing the investigator to align the Doppler beam properly in the direction of the blood flow. To record velocity waveforms, the pulsed Doppler is generally preferred to the continuous wave Doppler because of the range resolution of the former. During recordings the sample volume is placed immediately distal to the locations to be investigated (e.g., distal to the aortic semilunar valves to record the left ventricle outflow). However, in conditions of particularly high velocities (e.g., in the ductus arteriosis) the continuous Doppler may be useful because it avoids the aliasing effect.

Cardiac Problems in Pregnancy, Third Edition
Edited by Uri Elkayam, MD, and Norbert Gleicher, MD
Copyright © 1998 by Wiley-Liss, Inc. ISBN 0-471-16358-9

Parameters Measured

The parameters most commonly used to describe the cardiac velocity waveforms are the following:

peak velocity (PV), expressed as the maximum velocity at a given moment (e.g., systole, diastole) on the Doppler spectrum

time to peak velocity (TPV), or acceleration time, expressed by the time interval between the onset of the waveform and its peak

time velocity integral (TVI), calculated by planimetering the area underneath the Doppler spectrum

It is possible also to calculate *absolute cardiac flow* from both atrioventricular valve and outflow tracts by multiplying TVI times valve area times fetal heart rate (HR). These measurements are particularly prone to errors, mainly due to inaccuracies in valve area.

The valve area is derived from the valve diameter, which is near the limits of ultrasound resolution and is then halved and squared in its calculation, thus amplifying potential errors. However, they can be used properly in longitudinal studies over short time intervals in which the valve dimensions are assumed to remain constant. Furthermore, it is also possible to accurately calculate the relative ratio between the right and left cardiac output (RCO/LCO), thus avoiding the measurements of the cardiac valve, since the relative dimensions of aorta and pulmonary valves remain constant through gestation in absence of cardiac structural diseases.[4]

The evaluation of the *ventricular ejection force* (VEF) has recently also been used to assess fetal cardiac function.[5,6] VEF, a Doppler index based on Newton's law, estimates the ratio of energy transferred from right and left ventricular myocardial shortening to work done by accelerating blood into the pulmonary and systemic circulation, respectively.[7] This index appears to be less influenced by changes in preload and afterload than other Doppler indices[7] and thus may be more accurate than other Doppler variables, such as peak velocities for the assessment of ventricular function in adults with chronic congestive heart failure.

VEF is calculated according to Newton's second law of motion. Indeed, the force developed by ventricular contraction accelerates a column of blood into the aorta or pulmonary artery, respectively, and represents a transfer of the energy of myocardial shortening to the work done in the pulmonary and systemic circulation. Newton's second law defines the force as the product of mass and acceleration. The mass component in this model is the mass of blood accelerated into the outflow tract over a time interval. It can be calculated as the product of the density of blood (1.055), the valve area, and the flow velocity integral during acceleration time (FVI$_{AT}$), which is the area under the Doppler spectrum envelope up to the time of peak velocity. The acceleration

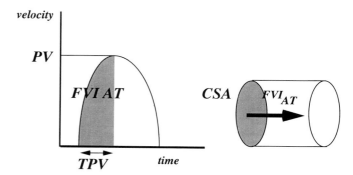

Figure 41.1   Schematic representation of a velocity waveform recorded at the level of outflow tract and cross-sectional area (*CSA*) of the vessel. The shaded area inside the velocity waveforms represents the flow velocity integral during the acceleration time (FVI$_{AT}$). During the time interval to peak velocity (TPV), a mass of blood passes through the cross-sectional areas. This mass (M) can be presented by a small cylinder of fluid of base area CSA and length to FVI$_{AT}$. The mass undergoes a mean acceleration equal to the ratio of PV to TPV. The product of mass (corrected for blood density) and acceleration yields the force developed by the ventricle. (Reprinted with permission from Rizzo et al, *Ultrasound Obstet Gynecol* 1995;5:247–255.)

component of the equation is estimated as the peak velocity (PV) divided by the time interval to peak velocity (TVP), as represented in Fig. 41.1. Thus, VEF can be calculated using the following equation:[7]

$$VEF = (1.055 \times valve\ area \times FVI_{AT}) \times \frac{PV}{TPV}$$

Recordings, Velocity Waveform Characteristics, and Their Significance

Blood flow velocity waveforms can be recorded at all cardiac levels in the human fetus, including venous return, foramen ovale, atrioventricular valves, outflow tracts, pulmonary arteries, and ductus arteriosis. Various factors affect the morphology of the velocity waveforms from different areas. Among these are preload,[8] afterload,[8–10] myocardial contractility,[11] ventricular compliance,[12] and fetal heart rate.[13] The impossibility of obtaining simultaneous recordings of pressure and volume prevents the full differentiation of these factors in the human fetus. Since, however, each parameter and site recording is more specifically affected by one of these factors, it is possible to indirectly elucidate the underlying pathophysiology by performing measurements at various cardiac levels.

Venous Circulation   Blood flow velocity waveforms may be recorded from the superior and inferior vena cava, the ductus venosus, the hepatic veins, and the pulmonary veins, as well as from the umbilical vein. The vascular area most intensively studied is the inferior vena cava (IVC). The IVC ve-

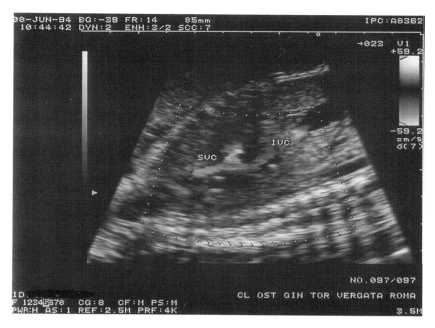

Figure 41.2   Parasigittal view of the fetal trunk showing the inferior vena cava (IVC) and superior vena cava (SVC) entering in the right atrium. (See color plates.)

locity waveforms, recorded from the segment of the vessel just distal to the entrance of the ductus venosus (Figs. 41.2 and 41.3),[14] are characterized by a triphasic profile. A first forward wave occurs concomitant with ventricular systole, a second forward wave of smaller dimensions occurs with ear-ly diastole, and a third wave with reverse flow during atrial contraction.[15] Several indices have been suggested to ana-lyze the IVC waveforms, but the most frequently used is the percentage of reverse flow, quantified as the percentage of TVI during atrial contraction (reverse flow) with respect to

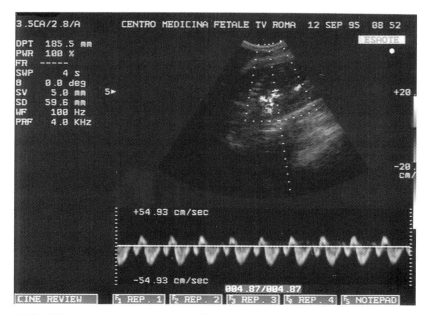

Figure 41.3   Velocity waveforms from the inferior vena cava in a normal fetus at 34 weeks of gesta-tion. Note the small amount of reverse flow during atrial contraction (upper panel). (See color plates.)

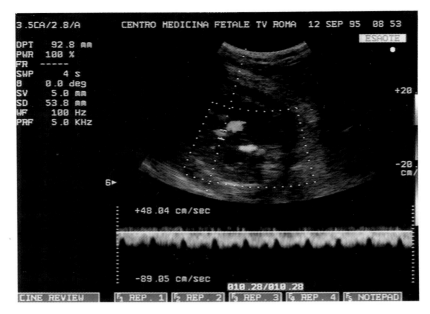

Figure 41.4   Velocity waveforms from the ductus venosus in a normal fetus at 36 weeks of gestation. Note the presence of forward flow during atrial contraction. (See color plates.)

total forward TVI (first and second wave).[15] This index is considered to be related to the pressure gradient present between the right atrium and the right ventricle during end diastole, which is a function of both ventricular compliance and ventricular end-diastolic pressure.[16]

The ductus venosus (DV) can be seen in a transverse section of the upper fetal abdomen at the level of its origin from the umbilical vein. Color is then superimposed, and the pulsed Doppler sample volume is placed just above its inlet (close to the umbilical vein) at the point of maximum flow velocity, as expressed by color brightness. DV flow velocity waveforms exhibit a biphasic pattern, with a first peak concomitant with systole (S), a second peak concomitant with diastole (D), and a nadir during atrial contraction (A) (Fig. 41.4). Among the indices suggested to quantify velocity waveforms from DV, the ratio of S peak velocity to A peak velocity (S/A) has been proven to be an angle-independent parameter that efficiently describes DV hemodynamics.[17]

The morphology of the velocity waveforms from hepatic veins is similar to that of IVC. There is a scarcity of reports on the use of these vessels in the human fetus. From data available, however, it may be argued that the analysis of these vessels may have significance similar to that of the analysis of IVC.[15]

Pulmonary vein velocity waveforms may be recorded at the level of their entrance into the right atrium (Fig. 41.5). Their morphology is similar to that of the DV and is characterized by positive velocities during atrial contraction (Fig. 41.6). The striking variations in the velocity waveform morphology between IVC and pulmonary vein is of interest and

reflects the different hemodynamic conditions occurring in systemic and pulmonary venous circulations during intrauterine life.

Umbilical venous blood flow is usually continuous (Fig. 41.7). However, in the presence of a relevant amount of reverse flow during atrial contraction in the inferior vena cava, the umbilical venous flow pulses with heart rate. In normal pregnancies these pulsations occur only before the 12th week of gestation. They are secondary to the stiffness of the ventricles at this gestational age, which causes a high degree of reverse flow into the inferior vena cava.[18] Later in gestation, the presence of such pulsations in the umbilical vein represents a finding of severe cardiac compromise (Fig. 41.8).[18]

Atrioventricular Valves   Flow velocity waveforms at the level of the mitral and tricuspid valves are recorded from the apical four-chamber view of the fetal heart (Fig. 41.9) and are characterized by two diastolic peaks, corresponding to early ventricular filling (E wave) and to active ventricular filling during atrial contraction (A wave) (Fig. 41.10). The ratio between E and A waves (E/A) is a widely accepted index of ventricular diastolic function, and it is an expression of both cardiac compliance and preload conditions.[8,19]

Outflow Tracts   Flow velocity waveforms from the aorta and pulmonary artery, respectively, are recorded from the five-chamber (Fig. 41.11) and short-axis views of the fetal heart (Fig. 41.12). PV and TPV are the most commonly used indices. The former is influenced by several factors, includ-

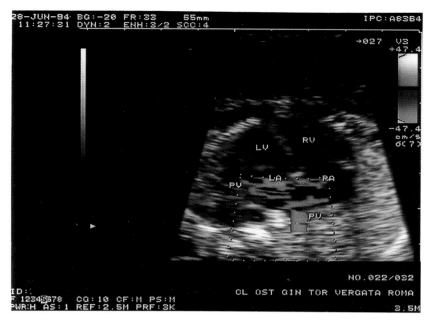

Figure 41.5 Cross-sectional section of the fetal chest showing the pulmonary veins (PV) entering in the left atrium (LA): RA, right atrium; LV, left ventricle, RV, right ventricle. (See color plates.)

ing valve size, myocardial contractility, and afterload,[9] while the latter is believed to represent the mean arterial pressure.[20]

Ductus Arteriosis Ductal velocity waveforms are recorded from a short axis, showing the ductal arch, and are characterized by a continuous forward flow through the entire cardiac cycle.[21] The parameter most commonly analyzed is the PV during systole or, similarly to peripheral vessels, the pulsatility index, PI[21,22]:

$$PI = \frac{\text{systolic velocity} - \text{diastolic velocity}}{\text{mean velocity}}$$

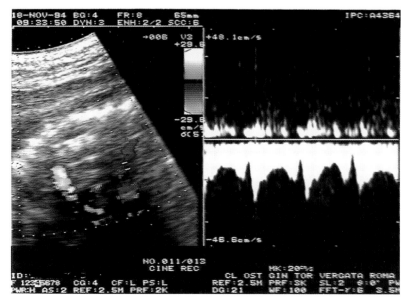

Figure 41.6 Velocity waveforms from the left pulmonary vein in a normal fetus at 36 weeks of gestation. Note the presence of forward flow during atrial contraction. (See color plates.)

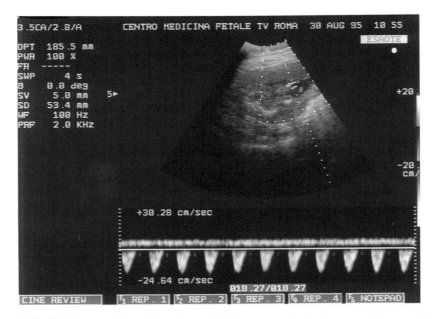

Figure 41.7   Velocity waveforms from the umbilical artery and vein in a normal fetus at 14 weeks of gestation. Note the presence of continuous flow in the umbilical vein. (See color plates.)

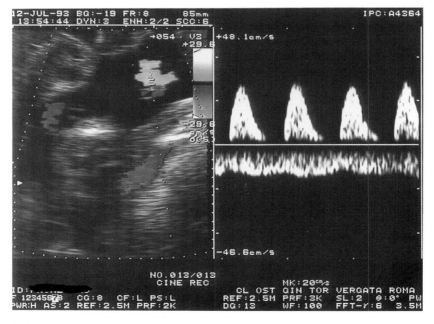

Figure 41.8   Velocity waveforms from the umbilical artery and vein in a severely growth-retarded fetus at 28 weeks of gestation. Note the absence of end-diastolic velocity in umbilical artery and presence of end-diastolic pulsations in the umbilical vein. (See color plates.)

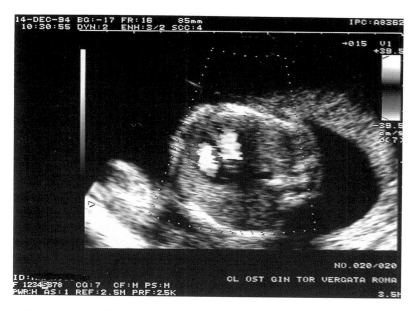

Figure 41.9   Apical four-chamber view of the fetal heart during diastole, showing the ventricular filling. (See color plates.)

Reproducibility

A major concern in obtaining absolute measurements of velocities or flow is reproducibility. To obtain reliable and reproducible recordings it is, as noted before, particularly important to minimize the angle of insonation, to verify in real time and color flow imaging the correct position of the sample volume before and after each Doppler recording, and to limit the recordings to periods of fetal rest and apnea, since behavioral states greatly influence the recordings.[23] In these conditions it is necessary to select a series of consecutive velocity waveforms (in our center, 10) characterized by uniform morphology

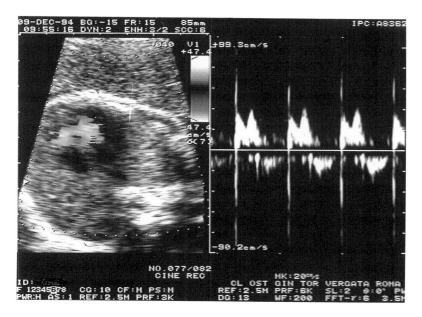

Figure 41.10   Velocity waveforms from the mitral valve in a normal fetus at 38 weeks of gestation. The E/A ratio is 0.81. (See color plates.)

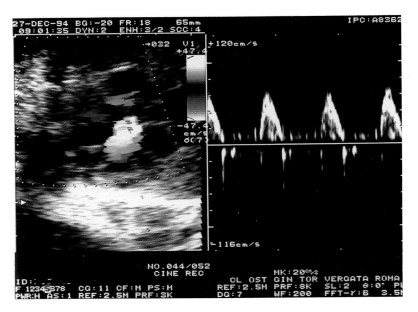

Figure 41.11 Five-chamber view of the fetal heart during systole, showing the left ventricular ejection into aorta and the corresponding velocity waveforms. (See color plates.)

and high signal-to-noise ratio, before performing the measurements. Using this technique of recording and analysis, we managed to obtain a coefficient of variation below 10% for all the echocardiographic indices except those requiring the measurement of valve dimensions. Our results are also in agreement with those reported by other centers (Groenenberg et al,[24] coefficient of variation < 7%; Al-Ghazali et al,[25] coefficient of variation < 7.6%; Reed et al,[26] maximal variation < 10%).

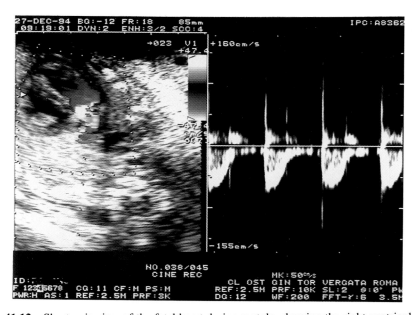

Figure 41.12 Short-axis view of the fetal heart during systole, showing the right ventricular ejection into the pulmonary artery and the corresponding velocity waveforms. (See color plates.)

NORMAL RANGES OF CARDIAC DOPPLER INDICES

The advent of equipment that can provide transvaginal color Doppler images has allowed us to record flow velocity waveforms from 11 weeks of gestation onward.[27] The following changes occur at all cardiac levels from this gestational age or up to 20 weeks: The percentage reverse flow of IVC significantly decreases,[27,28] the E/A ratio at both atrioventricular levels dramatically increases,[27,28] and PV and TVI values in outflow tracts increase, with this being particularly evident at the level of pulmonary valve.[27] These changes suggest a rapid development of ventricular compliance (which may explain the decrease of IVC reverse flow and the increase of E/A) and a shift of cardiac output toward the right ventricle (probably secondary to a decrease in right ventricle afterload due to the fall of placental resistance).

After 20 weeks of gestation there is a further, but less evident, decrease of IVC reverse flow[14] associated with a significant decrease of the S/A ratio from DV.[29]

At the level of atrioventricular valves, the E/A ratios increase,[30,31] while PV values linearly increase at the level of both pulmonary and aortic valves.[32] Small changes are also present in TPV values during gestation.[33] TPV values at the level of the pulmonary valve are lower than at the aortic level, suggesting a slightly higher blood pressure in the pulmonary artery than in the ascending aorta.[34] Quantitative measurements have shown that the right cardiac output (RCO) is higher than the left cardiac output (LCO) and that from 20 weeks onward the RCO/LCO ratio remains constant with a mean value of 1.3.[35,36] This value is lower than that reported in the fetal sheep (RCO/LCO) = 1.8), and the difference may be explained by the higher brain weight in humans, which increases the left cardiac output.[37]

In normal fetuses VEF exponentially increases with advancing gestation both at the level of right and left ventricles. No significant differences are present between right and left VEF values, and the ratio between right and left VEF values remains stable during gestation (mean value = 1.09).

Ductal PV increases linearly with gestation, and its values represents the highest velocity in the fetal circulation occurring under normal conditions.[21,22] Values of systolic velocity above 140 cm/s in conjunction with a diastolic velocity exceeding 30 cm/s are considered characteristic of ductal constriction.[21]

CARDIAC DOPPLER FINDINGS IN ABNORMAL GESTATIONS

Fetuses with Delayed Growth

Intrauterine growth-retarded (IUGR) fetuses, secondary to uteroplacental insufficiency, are characterized by selective changes of peripheral vascular resistance (i.e., the so-called brain-sparing effect) that influence cardiac hemodynamics.[38,39] Secondary to the brain-sparing effect, selective modifications occur in cardiac afterload, with decreased left ventricle afterload due to the cerebral vasodilatation and increased right ventricle afterload due to the systemic vasoconstriction. Furthermore, hypoxemia can impair myocardial contractility, while the usually present polycythemia may alter blood viscosity and therefore preload.

As a consequence, IUGR fetuses show impaired ventricular filling, with a lower E/A ratio at the level of the atrioventricular valves,[31] lower PV in aorta and pulmonary arteries (Fig. 41.13),[40] increased aortic and decreased pulmonary TPV,[33] and a relative increase of LCO, associated with decreased RCO.[25] These hemodynamic intracardiac changes are compatible with a preferential shift of cardiac output in favor of the left ventricle, leading to improved perfusion of the brain. Thus, in the early stages of compromise, the supply of substrates and oxygen can be maintained at near-normal levels despite an absolute reduction in placental transfer.

Longitudinal studies of progressively deteriorating IUGR fetuses have allowed the elucidation of the natural history of hemodynamic modifications during uteroplacental insufficiency.[18,40] Such studies have shown that TPV in aorta and pulmonary arteries and the ratios between right and left ventricular outputs remain stable during serial recordings. These findings are consistent with the absence of other significant changes in outflow resistances (a parameter inversely related to TPV values) and with cardiac output redistribution after the establishment of the brain sparing mechanism.[40] PV and cardiac output gradually decline in deteriorating IUGR fetuses, however, suggesting a progressive deterioration of cardiac function. As a consequence, cardiac filling is also impaired. Studies in the fetal venous circulation[41] have demonstrated that an increase of IVC reverses flow during atrial contraction (Fig. 41.14) and occurs with progressive fetal deterioration, suggesting a higher pressure gradient in the right atrium. The next step of fetal compromise lies in the extension of abnormal reversal of blood velocities in the IVC to the ductus venous, inducing an increase in the S/A ratio, mainly due to a reduction of the A component of the velocity waveforms[17] (Fig. 41.15). Finally, the high venous pressure induces a reduction of velocity at end of diastole in the umbilical vein, causing typical end-diastolic pulsations (Fig. 41.8).[42] The development of these pulsations is close to the onset of fetal heart rate anomalies and is frequently associated with acidemia at birth.[42,43]

The pathophysiological basis of these phenomena is still poorly understood. It is thus unknown whether these changes are due to a direct impairment of intrinsic cardiac contractility or secondary to extrinsic factors, such as peripheral resistances, preload, or afterload.

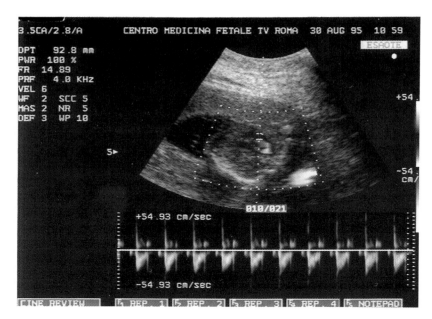

Figure 41.13   Velocity waveforms in a severely growth-retarded fetus at 28 weeks of gestation from pulmonary artery velocity waveforms. The PV is 34 cm/s (normal mean for gestation, 62 cm/s) and the TPV is 14 ms (normal mean for gestation 34.7 ms). (See color plates.)

Studies of VEF in IUGR have demonstrated that it is significantly and symmetrically decreased at the level of both ventricles (Fig.41.16).[6] The presence of a symmetrical decrease of VEF from both ventricles, despite the dramatically different hemodynamic conditions in ejection of the two ventricles (i.e., reduced cerebral resistances for the left ventricle and increased splanchnic and placental resistances for the right ventricle), supports a pivotal role of the intrinsic myo-

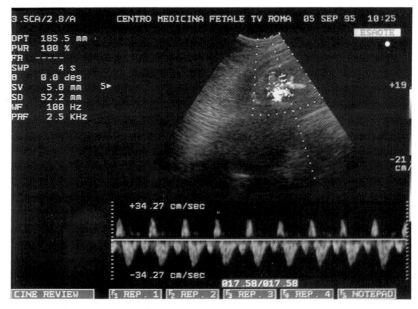

Figure 41.14   Velocity waveforms in a severely growth-retarded fetus at 30 weeks of gestation from inferior vena cava. The percentage reverse flow during atrial contraction is 29% (normal mean for gestation, 12%). (See color plates.)

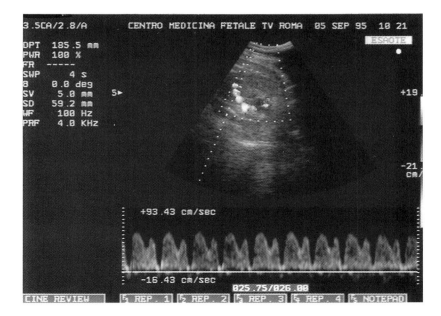

Figure 41.15 Velocity waveforms in a severely growth-retarded fetus at 32 weeks of gestation from the ductus venosus. The S/A is 9 (normal mena for gestation, 1.8). (See color plates.)

cardial function in the compensatory mechanism of the IUGR fetus following the establishment of the brain-sparing effect. Indeed, it was demonstrated in fetuses, followed longitudinally until either intrauterine death or the onset of abnormal fetal heart rate patterns requiring early delivery, that VEF dramatically decreases in a short time interval (one week), thus showing a severe impairment of ventricular force (Fig. 41.17).[6] Furthermore, a significant relationship between the severity of fetal acidosis at cordocentesis and VEF

values validates the association between this index and the severity of fetal compromise.[6]

Fetuses of Diabetic Mothers (see also Chapter 51)

Infants of diabetic mothers have long been recognized to be at risk of developing hypertrophic cardiomyopathy.[44] This disease is characterized by a thickening of the interventricular septum and ventricular walls and by systolic and diastolic

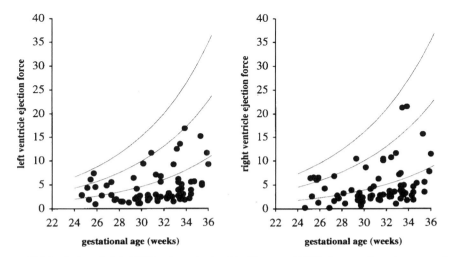

Figure 41.16 Left and right VEF values obtained in 72 severe IUGR fetuses plotted on normal reference limits for gestation. (Reprinted with permission from Rizzo et al, *Ultrasound Obstet Gynecol,* 1995;5:247–255.)

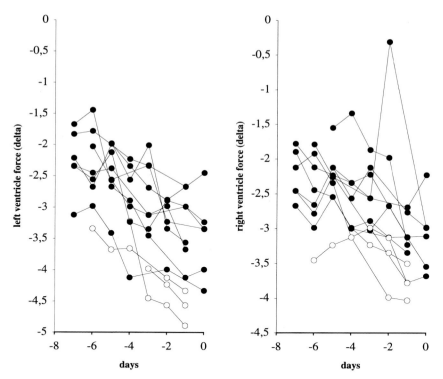

Figure 41.17   Serial changes in left and right VEF values in 12 IUGR fetuses followed longitudinally until the onset of antepartum fetal heart rate late decelerations (closed points) or until intrauterine death (open points). (Reprinted with permission from Rizzo et al, *Ultrasound Obstet Gynecol,*
1995;5:247–255.)

dysfunction of the neonatal heart, which may result in congestive heart failure in the immediate postnatal period.[45]
Echocardiography studies of the fetal heart have allowed
demonstration of the prenatal presence of hypertrophic cardiomyopathy and its progressive development with fetal
growth.

M-mode studies in fetuses of insulin-dependent diabetic
mothers have shown an increased thickness of ventricular
walls that is particularly evident at the level of the interventricular septum.[46–48] The increased cardiac size does
not merely reflect the larger size of the fetuses of diabetic
mothers (i.e., macrosomia), but represents a selective or-
ganomegaly. Indeed, the control of cardiac sizes for two biometric parameters closely related to fetal weight, fetal abdominal circumference and biparietal diameter, showed
increased wall thickness in fetuses of diabetic mothers irrespective of fetal size.[46,49]

Longitudinal echocardiographic studies have allowed elucidation of the natural history of the development of fetal
hypertrophic cardiomyopathy. Fetuses of diabetic mothers
showed an accelerated increase of cardiac size, and the
growth curves differ from those of normal fetuses.[49] Although the cardiac walls are already thicker than in normal
fetuses at 20 weeks of gestation, the accelerated increase of

cardiac size is mainly evident during the late second
trimester.[49] The cause for the increased growth rate of cardiac size during the late second trimester is unclear. Because
no association and/or correlation with the metabolic control
has been demonstrated, it has been speculated that a different degree of sensitivity of fetal myocardium to factors accelerating its growth exists at different gestational stages.
This hypothesis is supported by data of Thorsson and Hinz,[50]
showing a reduction from fetus to adult in the number and
affinity of insulin receptors.

Echocardiographic studies[46,49] have shown that the increase of cardiac wall thickness influences fetal cardiac function. At the level of both atrioventricular valves, fetuses of
diabetic mothers showed lower E/A ratios than normal fetuses.[49] Longitudinal studies have shown that these changes are
already present in early gestation and that development of diastolic function is delayed, with a slower rate of change of
E/A ratios during gestation.[49] Transvaginal echocardiography has allowed us to demonstrate differences in cardiac
functional development as early as at 12 weeks gestation, and
these anomalies seem to be particularly evident in the presence of poorer metabolic control.[51]

The low E/A values might be explained by an impaired
development of ventricular compliance in fetuses of diabet-

ic mothers secondary to cardiac will thickening. Such an effect would be consistent with the significant relationship existing between both interventricular septum and lateral ventricular wall thickness and the severity of the impairment of E/A values.[46] Moreover, as reported above, the E/A ratio is also influenced by the preload. Polycythemia is frequently present at birth in infants of diabetic mothers.[52] This condition increases blood viscosity, which may reduce preload, and thus also potentially affect the E/A ratio during intrauterine life. This hypothesis is supported by recent data showing a significant relationship between fetal hematocrit and the E/A values. This relationship, which was developed after steps had been taken to control for cardiac thickness and fetal heart rate,[53] suggests a significant impact of fetal blood viscosity on cardiac diastolic function.

Peak velocities at the level of aortic and pulmonary outflow tracts are significantly higher in fetuses of diabetic mothers than in normal fetuses.[46] Increased peak velocities could be secondary to reduced outflow tract dimensions, decreased afterload, increased cardiac contractility, or increased flow volume. These factors are difficult to differentiate in the human fetus. An obstruction of the left ventricle outflow tract, due to the hypertrophy of the septal musculature resulting in an increase of aortic peak velocities, has been described in infants of diabetic mothers.[54] However, in this condition the obstruction is usually limited to the left ventricular outflow tract and does not affect the right ventricular. Thus, the presence of a bilateral increase of pulmonary peak velocities remains unexplained. Similarly, a decrease in afterload seems unlikely on the basis of the lack of differences between control fetuses and fetuses of diabetic mothers in time to peak values. An increased contractility is, however, compatible with postnatal studies, showing a systolic ventricular contractile function above normal in infants of diabetic mothers.[55] Finally, the higher values of peak velocities may be explained on the basis of an increased intracardiac flow volume secondary to the relative larger size of such fetuses, considering the cardiac output as a function of fetal weight.

These abnormalities in cardiac hemodynamics also impair the venous circulation. We have demonstrated that the percentage reverse flow in IVC is increased in fetuses of diabetic mothers. Furthermore, fetuses with more marked hemodynamic anomalies showed a lower pH in the umbilical artery at birth, an increased hematocrit, and a higher morbidity.[29] No variations were, however, evident in fetal peripheral vessels.

We therefore speculated that the mechanisms of fetal distress are different in fetuses of diabetic mothers and those with IUGR. In the former group the development of hypertrophic cardiomyopathy plays a pivotal role in the genesis of fetal distress, while in the latter group the changes in cardiac function are secondary to a modification in peripheral resistance.

After birth the hypertrophic changes of the myocardium

regress to normal over a period of several months and usually have disappeared by 1 year of age.[55,56] It is, however, unknown whether these perinatal modifications affect cardiac function during adult life. Moreover, significant changes occur during the transitional circulation. In normal fetuses the E/A ratios at the level of both atrioventricular valves significantly increase during the first days of life, and the E wave is usually higher than the A wave, resulting in an E/A higher than 1.[56] No changes in E/A ratio occur, during the first 5 days of life in newborns of diabetic mothers, however, and E/A remains lower than 1.[56] These anomalies might explain the relatively high incidence immediately after birth of transitory tachypnea and pulmonary edema in infants of diabetic mothers.[19]

Fetal Anemia

Red cell isommunization can result in a progressive destruction of fetal red cells, leading to fetal anemia. Intravascular fetal blood transfusion by cordocentesis represents a standard treatment of fetal anemia, and this procedure leads to rapid injection of a large amount of blood with respect to overall fetoplacental volume.

Doppler echocardiography has made it possible to elucidate the hemodynamic response of the human fetus to anemia and its rapid correction.[57,58]

Before transfusion (in a condition of anemia), the left and right cardiac outputs are significantly higher than normal, and a significant relationship is present between the severity of fetal anemia and cardiac output.[57,58] As a consequence of the high volume flow, the PVs at the outflow tracts are increased.[55] Furthermore, the E/A at both atrioventricular valves is increased (Fig. 41.18).[58] Venous flow is similarly affected with an increase of peak velocities in DV.[59]

The fetal cardiac output is increased, presumably to maintain adequate oxygen delivery to organs. Although the mechanisms causing the increase of cardiac output are still unclear, two main factors have been suggested: (1) decreased blood viscosity leading to increased venous return and cardiac preload, and (2) peripheral vasodilatation due to a fall in blood oxygen content and therefore reduced cardiac afterload.[60] The first mechanism is supported by the high E/A values from atrioventricular valves seen in anemic fetuses.

There is, however, no evidence for the redistribution of cardiac output in this clinical situation similar to that described in hypoxic IUGR fetuses (brain-sparing effect), since the RCO/LCO ratio is normal in anemic fetuses.[58] This clinical picture is also in agreement with the normal PI values in fetal peripheral vessels of anemic fetuses.[61] These findings suggest that in red cell isoimmunization, the changes in fetal cardiac function are mainly related to the low blood viscosity, which in turn leads to a hyperdynamic cardiac state.

After intravascular transfusion, there is a significant temporary fall in right and left cardiac output,[57] associated with

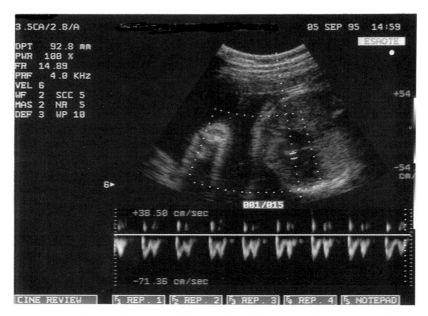

Figure 41.18 Velocity waveforms from the tricuspid valve at 30 weeks of gestation in a pregnancy complicated by rhesus isoimmunization 30 minutes after intravascular transfusion. The E/A is 1.4 (normal mean for gestation, 0.74). (See color plates.)

increased E/A ratios.[58] The latter changes may be related to the increased preload secondary to the relatively large amount of blood transfused.

The decrease of cardiac output may be secondary to four different factors (heart rate, preload, myocardial, contractility or afterload). The first factor may be excluded, since cardiac output also decreases in the absence of any significant changes in fetal heart rate.[57] Preload should be decreased to support the decrease of cardiac output, but the high E/A values suggest an increase or preload rather than a decrease.[58] Similarly, an impaired myocardial contractility seems unlikely on the basis of the velocity waveforms in aorta and pulmonary artery.[58] Therefore, an increase in cardiac afterload seems to offer the best explanation for the decrease in cardiac output.[58] This hypothesis is consistent with experimental animal studies showing a posttransfusion increase of mean arterial pressure and therefore of cardiac afterload.[62]

It is noteworthy that the fall of cardiac output in the human fetus is significantly reduced to the amount of expansion of the fetoplacental volume.[58] Moreover, within 2 hours of transfusion, all echocardiographic parameters return to normal ranges, suggesting a possibility of rapid recovery of the fetal circulation in response to volume expansion.[58]

Discordant Twins

Twin pregnancies have a high rate of perinatal complications which are particularly evident in pairs with discordant growth.[63] Studies limited to umbilical arteries have provided conflicting results about whether discordant sizes are associated with discordant Doppler indices.[64–67] These discrepancies may be explained on the basis of different classification criteria.

In a study reported in 1994, we carefully selected two groups of twin pregnancies with discordant growth, all classified by rigid criteria.[68] In the first group, the etiology was malnutrition of one twin due to placental insufficiency limited to one placenta. A criterion of inclusion was the presence of dichorionic placentas, thus virtually excluding the possibility of blood shunts between fetuses. Other criteria were the absence of either chromosomal or structural anomalies, since these intrinsic causes of the growth defects indicate delivery on the basis of presence of late decelerations, suggestive of fetal hypoxemia of the smaller twin. Serial recordings in the larger twin showed no difference in comparison to normal singleton pregnancies in all the vessels investigated, thus suggesting normal placental and fetal hemodynamics. The smaller twin showed, however, progressive changes of Doppler indices similar to those described above in singleton growth-retarded fetuses secondary to placental insufficiency. As a consequence of these hemodynamic changes, the absolute values of the Doppler indices in the smaller twin or the delta values between the smaller and the larger twin can be used as tools of fetal surveillance or prediction of fetal distress similarly to singleton pregnancies. This study also confirmed other work showing how a high delta value in the umbilical artery can predict low birth weight and adverse perinatal outcome in twin pregnancies.[64,67] The combined study of several vascular districts may further improve the diagnostic efficacy of Doppler ultrasonography.

A second group of twin pregnancies studied had been affected by the twin-to-twin transfusion syndrome. The classic pathophysiologic background of this syndrome is a shift of blood volume from one twin, the donor, to the recipient twin.[69] As a result of the transfusion, the donor twin becomes anemic, decreases in growth rate, and develops oligohydramnios as a consequence of oliguria, while the recipient twin becomes polycythemic and plethoric and, as a consequence of the volume overload, may develop polyhydramnios, cardiomegaly, cardiac insufficiency, and hydrops.[69] This concept, however, has recently been questioned by data obtained at cordocentesis showing small differences in cord hemoglobin between fetuses with classical sign of twin-to-twin transfusion syndrome.[70] These observations suggest that the mechanisms generating this syndrome are more complex than mere shifts of blood volume that probably become massive only at a late stage. In most cases, in fact, serial recordings obtained in this second group of twin fetuses demonstrated changes of Doppler indices only at the time of the last recording, close to the delivery due to fetal distress. These changes are present at the cardiac and venous levels and are consistent with a condition of anemia (increased PV at outflow tract and decreased percentage reverse flow in IVC) in the smaller twin and of massive blood transfusion (decreased PV at outflow tract, increased percentage reverse flow in IVC, and umbilical vein pulsations) in the larger twin. Indeed, these Doppler patterns are similar to those described before and immediately after intravascular blood transfusion. The absence of differences in PI values from fetal vessels even close to delivery should not be surprising, inasmuch as these indices are only minimally affected by fetal anemia or polycythemia[61] and confirm earlier reports limited to the umbilical artery.[65] The absence of obvious changes in cardiac and venous Doppler indices in the weeks preceding delivery, despite growth discordance between twins and the presence of oligohydramnios and polyhydramnios, suggests a different pathophysiological mechanism at an early stage of the syndrome. It has, in fact, been suggested that the twin-to-twin transfusion syndrome may develop first as a consequence of the placental insufficiency affecting the donor twin.[70] According to this hypothesis, placental insufficiency increases vascular resistance in the donor twin, resulting in a preferential shunt, at a later stage of the disease, toward the recipient twin. Our data do not support this theory because we were unable to document in serial recordings any Doppler changes suggestive of placental insufficiency.

POSSIBLE TREATMENTS

Since cardiac decompensation plays a pivotal role in the final steps of fetal distress secondary to different etiologies, pharmacological treatment aimed at improving cardiac function may prove useful, particularly in fetuses in which gesta-

tional age and/or fetal weight do not allow delivery. To this end we recently investigated the effects on cardiac function of normal and IUGR fetuses, of thyrotropin-releasing hormone (TRH), administer via the mother, to induce fetal lung maturation.[71] TRH administration showed a rapid effect on the circulation of both appropriately grown and IUGR fetuses. In IUGR fetuses, maternal TRH dramatically increases outflow tract PV (Fig. 41.19) and cardiac output, while decreasing the percentage reversal flow in the inferior vena cava during atrial contraction (Fig. 41.20). In normally grown fetuses these changes are limited to the level of the outflow tracts, resulting in increased peak velocity and cardiac output. No significant effects were found in any fetuses in either the ratio between left and right cardiac output, fetal heart rate, or pulsatility index of the fetal middle cerebral artery, descending aorta, and umbilical. A concomitant increase of peak velocity and cardiac output may reflect changes in either afterload or preload, or intrinsic cardiac contractility. The absence of a significant change in Doppler-measured peripheral resistance argues against a modification in afterload as a possible etiology. Similarly, the absence of a change of reverse blood flow during atrial contraction in the inferior vena cava in normal fetuses, despite an increase in cardiac output, makes it unlikely that the increase results from an altered preload. This leaves the third possibility (i.e., intrinsic cardiac contractility) as the most likely explanation.

An increased cardiac contractility is compatible with the action of thyroid hormones and may explain the reduction in IUGR fetuses of percentage reverse flow in the inferior vena cava. The improvement in cardiac contractility of IUGR fetuses may decrease the atrioventricular pressure gradient, resulting in an enhanced venous return of blood from the placenta, thus reducing the reverse flow during atrial contraction. On the other hand, in appropriately grown fetuses the improvement in cardiac contractility may not significantly affect the already low reverse flow in the inferior vena cava. Furthermore, in a group of IUGR fetuses, serially followed, we noted that the hemodynamic effects induced by TRH remain constant for at least 8 hours after administration. It is noteworthy that a second administration of TRH induces further improvement in contractility, thus suggesting a possible potentiating effect (Fig. 41.21).

It is not possible to establish with certainty whether this treatment is in fact beneficial to IUGR fetuses or whether it causes harm by increasing oxygen and nutrient consumption. However, a negative effect seems unlikely based on data demonstrating that TRH administration improves fetal heart variability, an index directly related to fetal oxygenation.[17] Similarly, the absence of modifications in PI values in peripheral vessels does not support the occurrence of changes in fetal oxygenation during the period of observation. Furthermore, thyroid hormones have been shown to have cardioprotective actions in the ischemic animal hearts[18] and in the rescue of human myocardial function after cardiac

into normal and abnormal cardiac physiology. *Circulation* 1990:81:498–505.

16. Appleton CP, Hatle LK, Popp RL. Superior vena cava and hepatic vein Doppler echocardiography in healthy adults. *J Am College Cardiol* 1987;10:1032–1039.

17. Rizzo G, Capponi A, Arduini D, Romanini C. Ductus venosus velocity waveforms in appropriate and small for gestational age fetuses. *Early Hum Dev* 1994;39:15–26.

18. Rizzo G, Arduini D, Romanini C. Pulsations in umbilical vein: a physiological finding in early pregnancy. *Am J Obstet Gynecol* 1992;167:675–677.

19. Laboritz AJ, Pearson C. Evaluation of left diastolic function: clinical relevance and recent Doppler echocardiographic insights. *Am Heart J* 1987;114:836–851.

20. Kitabatake A, Inouse M, Asao M, Masuyama T, Tanouchi J, Morita T, Mishima M, Uematsu M, Shimazu T, Hori M, Abe H. Noninvasive evaluation of pulmonary hypertension by a pulsed Doppler technique. *Circulation* 1983;68:302–309.

21. Huhta JC, Moise KJ, Fisher DJ, Shariff DF, Wasserstrum N, Martin C. Detection and quantitation of constriction of the fetal ductus arteriousus by Doppler echocardiography. *Circulation* 1987;75:406–412.

22. Van de Mooren K, Barendregt LG, Waladimiroff J. Interventricular septal thickness in fetuses of diabetic mothers. *Obstet Gynecol* 1992;79:51–54.

23. Rizzo G, Arduini D, Valensise H, Romanini C. Effects of behavioral states on cardiac output in the healthy human fetus at 36–38 weeks gestation. *Early Hum Dev* 1990;23:109–115.

24. Groenenberg IAL, Hop WCJ, Wladimiroff JW. Doppler flow velocity waveforms in the fetal cardiac outflow tract; reproducibility of waveform recording and analysis. *Ultrasound Med Biol* 1991;17:583–587.

25. Al-Ghazali W, Chita SK, Chapman MG, Allan LD. Evidence of redistribution of cardiac output in asymmetrical growth retardation. *Br J Obstet Gynaecol* 1989;96:697–704.

26. Reed KL, Sahn DJ, Scagnelli S, Anderson CF, Shenker L. Doppler echocardiographic studies of diastolic function in the human fetal heart: changes during gestation. *J Am College Cardiol* 1986;8:391–395.

27. Rizzo G, Arduini D, Romanini C. Fetal cardiac and extracardiac circulation in early gestation. *J Maternal-Fetal Invest* 1991;1:73–78.

28. Wladimiroff JW, Huisman TWA, Stewart PA, Stijnen T. Normal fetal Doppler inferior vena cava, transtricuspid and umbilical artery flow velocity waveforms between 11 and 16 weeks' gestation. *Am J Obstet Gynecol* 1992;166:46–49.

29. Rizzo G, Capponi A, Rinaldo D, Arduini D, Romanini C. Inferior cava velocity waveforms predict neonatal complications in fetuses of insulin dependent diabetic mothers. *J Maternal Fetal Invest* 1994;4:13.

30. Reed KL, Meijboom EJ, Sahn DJ, Scagnelli SA, Valdes-Cruz LM, Skenker L. Cardiac Doppler flow velocities in human fetuses. *Circulation* 1986;73:41–56.

31. Rizzo G, Arduini D, Romanini C, Mancuso S. Doppler echocardiographic assessment of atrioventricular velocity waveforms

in normal and small for gestational age fetuses. *Br J Obstet Gynaecol* 1988;95:65–69.

32. Kenny JF, Plappert T, Saltzman DH, Cartire M, Zollars L, Leatherman GF, St. John Sutton MG. Changes in intracardiac blood flow velocities and right and left ventricular stroke volumes with gestational age in the normal human fetus: a prospective Doppler echocardiographic study. *Circulation* 1986;74:1208–1216.

33. Rizzo G, Arduini D, Romanini C, Mancuso S. Doppler echocardiographic evaluation of time to peak velocity in the aorta and pulmonary artery of small for gestational age fetuses. *Br J Obstet Gynaecol* 1990;97:603–607.

34. Machado MVL, Chita SC, Allan LD. Acceleration time in the aorta and pulmonary artery measured by Doppler echocardiography in the midtrimester normal human fetus. *Br Heart J* 1987;58:15–18.

35. Allan LD, Chita SK, Al-Ghazali W, Crawford DC, Tynan M. Doppler echocardiographic evaluation of the normal human fetal heart. *Br Heart J* 1987;57:528–533.

36. De Smedt MCH, Visser GHA, Meijboom EJ. Fetal cardiac output estimated by Doppler echocardiography during mid- and late gestation. *Am J Cardiol* 1987;60:338–342.

37. Rizzo G, Arduini D. Cardiac output in anencephalic fetuses. *Gynecol Obstet Invest* 1991;32:33–35.

38. Peeters LLH, Sheldon RF, Jones, MD, Makowsky EI, Meschia G. Blood flow to fetal organ as a function of arterial oxygen content. *Am J Obstet Gynecol* 1979;135:637–646.

39. De Vore GR. Examination of the fetal heart in the fetus with intrauterine growth retardation using M-mode echocardiography. *Semin Perinatol* 1988;12:66–79.

40. Rizzo G, Arduini D. Fetal cardiac function in intrauterine growth retardation. *Am J Obstet Gynecol* 1991;165:876–882.

41. Rizzo G, Arduini D, Romanini C. Inferior vena cava flow velocity waveforms in appropriate and small for gestational age fetuses. *Am J Obstet Gynecol* 1992;166:1271–1280.

42. Arduini D, Rizzo G, Romanini C. The development of abnormal heart rate patterns after absent end diastolic velocity in umbilical artery: analysis of risk factors. *Am J Obstet Gynecol* 1993;168:43–49.

43. Indick JH, Chen V, Reed KL. Association of umbilical venous with inferior vena cava blood flow velocities. *Obstet Gynecol* 1991;77:551–557.

44. Gutgesell HP, Speer ME, Rosenberg HS. Characterization of the cardiomyopathy in infants in diabetic mothers. *Circulation* 1980;61:441–450.

45. Reller MD, Kaplan S. Hypertrophic cardiomyopathy in infants of diabetic mothers: an update. *Am J Perinatol* 1988;5:353–358.

46. Weber HS, Copel JA, Reece A, Green J, Kleinman CS. Cardiac growth in fetuses of diabetic mothers with good metabolic control. *J Pediatr* 1991;118:103–107.

47. Rizzo, G, Arduini D, Romanini C. Cardiac function in fetuses of type I diabetic mothers. *Am J Obstet Gynecol* 1991;164:837–843.

48. Vielle JC, Sivekoff M, Hanson R, Fanaroff AA. Interventricular septal thickness in fetuses of diabetic mothers. *Obstet Gynecol* 1992;79:51–54.

49. Rizzo, G, Arduini D, Romanini C. Accelerated cardiac growth and abnormal cardiac flows in fetuses of type I diabetic mothers. *Obstet Gynecol* 1992;80:369–376.

50. Thorsson AV, Hintz RL. Insulin receptors in the newborn: increase in receptor affinity and number. *N Engl J Med* 1977;297:908–912.

51. Rizzo, G, Capponi A, Rinaldo D, Arduini D, Romanini C. Effects of thyrotropin releasing hormone on cardiac and extracardiac fetal flows in appropriately grown and growth retarded fetuses. *Ultrasound Obstet Gynecol* 1995;6:8–14.

52. Widness J, Susa J, Garcia J. Increased erythropoiesis and elevated erythropoietin levels in infants born to diabetic mothers and in hyperinsulinemic rhesus fetuses. *J Clin Invest* 1981;67:637–641.

53. Rizzo G, Pietropolli A, Capponi A, Cacciatore C, Arduini D, Romanini C. Analysis of factors affecting ventricular filling in fetuses of type I diabetic mothers. *J Perinatal Med* 1994;22:125–132.

54. Gutgesell HP, Mullins CE, Gillette PC, Speer M, Rudolph AJ, McNamara DG. Transient hypertrophic subaortic stenosis in infants of diabetic mothers. *J Pediatr* 1976;89:120–125.

55. Mace S, Hirschfeld SS, Riggs T, Faranoff AA, Mecketz JR. Echocardiographic abnormalities in infants of diabetic mothers. *J Pediatr* 1979;95:1013–1019.

56. Condoluci C, Rizzo G, Arduini D, Romanini C. Transitional circulation in infants of diabetic mothers In: *6th Fetal Cardiology Symposium*. 1991. Abstract 23.

57. Moise KJ, Mari G, Fisher DJ, Hutha JC, Cano LE, Carpenter RJ. Acute fetal hemodynamic alterations after intrauterine transfusion for treatment of severe red blood cell alloimmunization. *Am J Obstet Gynecol* 1990;163:776–784.

58. Rizzo G, Nicolaides KH, Arduini D, Campbell S. Effects of intravascular fetal blood transfusion on fetal intracardiac Doppler velocity waveforms. *Am J Obstet Gynecol* 1990;163:1231–1238.

59. Oepkes D, Vandenbussche FP, Van Bel F, Kanhai HHH. Fetal ductus venosus blood flow velocities before and after transfusion in red-cell alloimmunized pregnancies. *Obstet Gynecol* 1993;82:237–241.

60. Fumia FD, Edelstone DI, Holzman IR. Blood flow and oxygen delivery as functions of fetal hematocrit. *Am J Obstet Gynecol* 1984;150:274–282.

61. Bilardo CM, Nicolaides KH, Campbell S. Doppler studies in red cell isoimmunization. *Clin Obstet Gynecol* 1989;32:719–727.

62. Chestnut DH, Pollack KL, Weiner CP, Robillard JE, Thompson CS, DeBruyn CS. Does furosemide alter the hemodynamic response to rapid intravascular transfusion of the anemic lamb fetus? *Am J Obstet Gynecol* 1989;161:1571–1575.

63. Ho SK, Wu PK. Perinatal factors and neonatal morbidity in twin pregnancy. *Am J Obstet Gynecol* 1980;122:979–987.

64. Framakides G, Schulman H, Saldana LR, Bracero LA, Fleisher A, Rochelson B. Surveillance of twin pregnancies with umbilical artery velocity waveforms. *Am J Obstet Gynecol* 1986;153:789–792.

65. Giles WB, Trudinger BJ, Cook CM. Fetal umbilical artery velocity waveforms in twin pregnancies. *Br J Obstet Gynaecol* 1985;92:490–497.

66. Pretorius DH, Machester D, Barkin S, Parker S, Nelson TR. Doppler ultrasound of twin–twin transfusion syndrome. *J Ultrasound Med* 1988;7:117–124.

67. Giles WB, Trudinger BJ, Cook CM, Connelly AJ. Doppler umbilical artery Doppler studies in the twin–twin transfusion syndrome. *Obstet Gynecol* 1990;76:1097–1099.

68. Rizzo G, Arduini D, Romanini C. Cardiac and extra-cardiac flows in discordant twins. *Am J Obstet Gynecol* 1994;170:1321–1327.

69. Blickstein I. The twin–twin transfusion syndrome. *Obstet Gynecol* 1990;76:714–721.

70. Saunders NJ, Snijders RJM, Nicolaides KH. Twin–twin transfusion syndrome during the 2nd trimester is associated with small intertwin hemoglobin differences. *Fetal Diagn Ther* 1991;6:34–36.

71. Rizzo G, Arduini D, Capponi A, Romanini C. Cardiac and venous flow in early gestation in fetuses of insulin dependent diabetic mothers. *Am J Obstet Gynecol* 1995;79:1226–1236.

42

THE NORMAL AND ABNORMAL FETAL HEART RATE

William Cusick, MD, Louis Buttino, Jr., MD, and Norbert Gleicher, MD

INTRODUCTION

Auscultation of a normal fetal heart rate can provide reassurance to the parents and physician throughout pregnancy. During the first trimester, initiation of the embryonic heart beat represents a significant developmental milestone. The ultrasound detection of this embryonic heart activity provides prognostic information for the pregnancy. Beginning in the early second trimester and continuing until term, the auscultation of fetal heart sounds at routine prenatal examinations verifies fetal life. In the third trimester, assessment of the fetal heart rate tracing in the form of a nonstress test can provide information regarding the fetal well-being. Finally, in the intrapartum period monitoring of the fetal heart rate can provide information on the fetal status during labor and may afford the trained clinician the opportunity to intervene before the development of significant fetal hypoxia and/or acidemia.

Fetal heart rate monitoring is simply a tool at the clinician's disposal. The quantity and quality of information provided by continuous fetal heart rate monitoring is highly dependent on the expertise of the individual utilizing this modality. Abnormalities of the fetal heart rate tracing and their significance can be determined only by one who has acquired a sound understanding of the normal fetal heart rate. This chapter reviews the principal elements and control mechanisms of a normal fetal heart rate. In addition, the characteristics and significance of the most common heart rate patterns are discussed. Finally, we discuss the influence of fetal hypoxia, neurological injury, structural cardiac disease, and cardiac arrhythmias on the interpretation of the continuous fetal heart tracing.

INSTRUMENTATION

Two techniques are available for monitoring the continuous fetal heart rate. External fetal heart rate monitoring (EFM) involves the use of a small Doppler transducer contained within a small plastic disk, which is secured to the maternal abdomen. Movement of the fetal heart structures (atrioventricular valves) induces a Doppler shift of the signal, which is subsequently translated by a microprocessor into a heart rate. The noninvasive nature of this technique allows for the use of EFM in any patient regardless of cervical dilation or membrane status. Unfortunately, the dependence on Doppler technology subjects EFM to signal loss due to fetal/maternal movement, maternal obesity, and particularly, with maternal expulsive efforts during the third stage of labor. Furthermore, the specific cardiac event used to determine heart rate may vary from one beat to the next. This sampling variability, although minimized by the use of monitors with autocorrelation, results in an exaggeration of the true heart rate variability. Thus, true beat-to-beat variability cannot be determined using EFM.

Internal fetal heart rate monitoring (IFM) utilizes a small spiral electrode that is attached to the presenting fetal part (scalp, breech). It is a minimally invasive technique that offers two distinct advantages over EFM: first, the instantaneous fetal heart rate, based on measurement of the R-R interval in the fetal cardiac cycle, is a true representation of the actual heart rate and therefore eliminates any false variability. Second, with the electrode attached directly to the fetus, signal loss is minimized. Before the electrode can be placed, however, the cervix must be dilated and the membranes ruptured. The fetal eyes, fontanels, and scrotum should be avoid-

Cardiac Problems in Pregnancy, Third Edition
Edited by Uri Elkayam, MD, and Norbert Gleicher, MD
Copyright © 1998 by Wiley-Liss, Inc. ISBN 0-471-16358-9

ed during electrode placement. Rare complications of scalp infection and bleeding have been associated with the use of scalp electrodes.[1]

SIGNIFICANCE OF COMMON FETAL HEART RATE PATTERNS

Fetal heart rate monitoring is typically employed in an effort to track fetal status, particularly during labor. We now turn to a description of the most commonly observed fetal heart rate changes and review their clinical significance.

Baseline Changes

The presence of normal fetal heart rate baseline characteristics (heart rate variability) with spontaneous or induced accelerations is indicative of fetal well-being.[2] The absence of such characteristics, however, does not necessarily imply the opposite (i.e., fetal hypoxia and/or acidemia). Various alterations at the level of the fetal cardiac muscle, cardiac conduction system, and/or central nervous system may influence the baseline characteristics of the fetal heart rate tracing in the absence of fetal hypoxia and/or acidemia. A clinical differentiation of baseline changes is therefore potentially important.

Rate A baseline fetal heart rate between 110 and 160 beats per minute is considered normal. The normal baseline fetal heart rate in early pregnancy is slightly higher than at term, and it declines progressively throughout gestation.[3] The reduction in baseline heart rate has been attributed to increasing vagal (parasympathetic) tone in the fetus with advancing gestational age.[3] Sympathetic influences are also important in fetal heart rate control.[4] Changes in the fetal heart rate secondary to fetal movement, uterine contractions, and other external stimuli are manifested through alterations in the relative contribution of parasympathetic and sympathetic influences.[5-8] It is the sum total of sympathetic and parasympathetic influences that determines the fetal heart rate at any time. For more detail see Chapter 41.

Fetal tachycardia is a sustained heart rate above 160 beats per minute. The causes of fetal tachycardia are varied and include fetal arrhythmias, maternal/fetal infections, drugs, and hyperthyroidism. The highest fetal heart rates are typically seen in the presence of supraventricular fetal arrhythmias (supraventricular tachycardia, atrial flutter, and atrial fibrillation). Rates above 200–300 beats per minute are common. Some fetal heart monitors are unable to interpret such high rates and will instead display a heart rate that may represent only half the true rate. Real-time ultrasound is therefore essential for confirming the actual heart rate and defining the underlying rhythm disturbance. As an isolated finding, fetal tachycardia is not associated with fetal acidosis.[2]

Bradycardia is defined as a baseline heart rate less than 120 beats per minute. Brief periods of sinus bradycardia may be seen in the healthy fetus. Rates of 100–120 beats per minute are frequently seen at night and appear to be related to fetal circadian cycles.[9] Sustained heart rates below 80 beats per minute are, however, suggestive of fetal heart block and may be the first sign of an underlying structural cardiac defect. Detailed fetal echocardiography is required to define a bradycardial dysrhythmia and to allow for a thorough assessment of cardiac structure. Isolated bradycardia is not associated with fetal hypoxia. In fact, the nonhypoxic fetus with sinus bradycardia may exhibit normal variability and spontaneous accelerations during continuous fetal heart rate monitoring (Fig. 42.1).

Variability Inspection of the normal fetal heart rate tracing between uterine contractions will yield an appreciation of short- and long-term fluctuations in the baseline heart rate. These fluctuations, referred to as short- and long-term variability, provide visible evidence of the active, dynamic control of fetal heart rate by the sympathetic and parasympathetic nervous systems. Short-term variability refers to the change in heart rate from one beat to the next and can be assessed using IFM.[10] Short-term variability is typically described as present or absent and appears to be influenced most by the parasympathetic nervous system.[6] Conversely, long-term variability is more dependent on sympathetic influences.[6] These slow oscillations of the fetal heart rate above and below the prevailing baseline have an average amplitude of 10–25 beats per minute and a frequency of 3 or more cycles per minute. Long-term variability can be assessed using either IFM or EFM.

Variability of the fetal heart rate is under central nervous system (CNS) control. Consequently, any factors that interfere with the normal functioning of the CNS will affect fetal heart rate variability. This relationship is best illustrated in the fetus with a neurological injury, where the fetal heart rate tracing exhibits minimal or absent short- and long-term variability.[11-13] Likewise, drugs that depress the CNS, such as β-adrenergic blocking agents and narcotics, may also result in diminished fetal heart rate variability. Most commonly, decreased fetal heart rate variability is seen in the preterm fetus where, because of relative CNS immaturity, amplitude is variable (lower) compared to older fetuses.[14] Short periods of decreased heart rate variability may, however, also be seen in a healthy fetus during labor.[15]

Clinically the biggest concern is that diminished fetal heart rate variability may also be a manifestation of fetal hypoxia/acidemia.[2,6,16,17] In most such instances, other abnormalities of the fetal heart rate pattern (e.g., variable or late decelerations) accompany or precede the onset of diminished variability.

Accelerations Baseline accelerations/decelerations are short-term increases/decreases in the fetal heart rate not as-

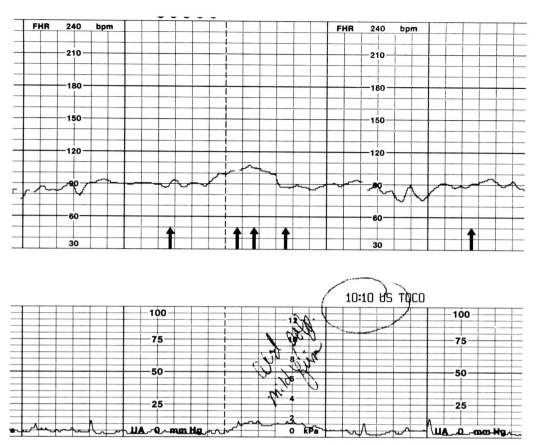

Figure 42.1 Fetal heart rate tracing of a fetus with a large atrio-ventricular canal defect and sinus bradycardia; long-term variability and spontaneous heart accelerations are evident.

sociated with uterine contractions. Short-term accelerations of the fetal heart rate are commonly seen in association with fetal movement.[18,19] Accelerations of the fetal heart rate, like long-term variability, are mediated through an increase in sympathetic discharge. The decrease in baseline fetal heart rate and the increasing amplitude of both accelerations and long-term variability seen with advancing gestational age reflect the functional maturation of the fetal central nervous system.

Accelerations of the fetal heart rate typically occur in response to fetal movement. Accordingly, they are most frequently seen during fetal wake cycles. As is the case with fetal heart rate variability, baseline accelerations are of lesser amplitude in the preterm compared to the term infant.[20] The *nonstress test (NST)* is a noninvasive method of evaluating fetal status. In the nonhypoxic fetus, a *reactive NST* is defined as a fetal heart rate tracing with normal baseline characteristics and repetitive fetal accelerations (spontaneous or induced) of sufficient amplitude and duration. It is considered a reassuring sign of fetal well-being. In contrast, the *nonreactive NST* tends to be nonreassuring, though it does not necessarily indicate the presence of fetal compromise.

Periodic Changes

Periodic changes refer to the increases (accelerations) and decreases (decelerations) in fetal heart rate that occur in association with uterine contractions. Fetal heart rate accelerations were described earlier; decelerations in the fetal heart rate, which are further classified based on their configuration and temporal relationship with uterine contractions, are classified as early, variable, or late decelerations.

Early Decelerations   Early decelerations are so named because they start with the onset of uterine contraction. This deceleration pattern is characterized by a shallow, symmetrical heart rate decrease of minimal amplitude (< 5–10 beats/min), which returns to baseline with resolution of the contraction. The drop in heart rate is mediated through an increase in vagal (parasympathetic) tone produced in response to elevated fetal intracranial pressure that accompanies uterine contractions.[7]

Early decelerations represent a reflex slowing of the fetal heart rate, produced in response to increased intracranial pressure. This benign heart rate pattern is frequently seen during labor, particularly at cervical dilations of 4–8 cm.[21] It is not associated with fetal hypoxia and/or acidemia.[2,22–24]

Variable Decelerations   As the name would suggest, variable decelerations are decreases in the fetal heart rate that show variability in onset, duration, amplitude, and appearance from contraction to contraction. They are the most common deceleration pattern seen during labor, when uterine contractions lead to intermittent umbilical cord compression. In the nonhypoxic fetus, fetal hypertension secondary to umbilical artery occlusion causes a reflex increase in parasympathetic tone, leading to an instantaneous decrease in heart rate. With resolution of arterial occlusion, the fetal hypertension resolves and the heart rate returns to baseline.[25] Occasionally, small accelerations of the fetal heart may be seen immediately preceding and following the heart rate deceleration. These *shoulders* associated with the variable deceleration are thought to be in response to fetal hypovolemia secondary to selective umbilical vein occlusion.[18] The presence of variable decelerations of the fetal heart rate may, however, also be reflective of hypoxia. In such a setting, the decrease in fetal heart rate is independent of vagal control and is the result of direct fetal myocardial depression.[25] The difference in potential clinical significance of these two causes for variable deceleration will be obvious.

Variable decelerations are the most common deceleration seen during labor and may be classified on the basis of duration and magnitude as mild, moderate, or severe.[22] Nonrepetitive variable decelerations, particularly if mild and without associated baseline heart rate changes, are not indicative of fetal hypoxia.[6] Because of the unpredictable nature and variable progression of this heart rate pattern, however, continued surveillance is warranted. The healthy fetus at term can tolerate such decelerations for short periods without developing significant fetal hypoxia and/or acidemia. However, the likelihood for fetal hypoxia/acidemia increases with the severity and frequency of these decelerations.[14,15,22] Concerns about hypoxia are further heightened when a sustained fetal heart rate above the baseline follows resolution of the deceleration (*overshoot*).[26] Eventually, the intermittent stress reflected by repetitive decelerations of sufficient severity will lead to sustained hypoxia/acidemia in the fetus. This result can be manifested in the loss of normal baseline characteristics of the fetal heart rate tracing in the form of fetal tachycardia and the loss of heart rate variability. When continued variable decelerations are associated with absent fetal heart rate variability or baseline tachycardia, fetal acidemia is likely.[2,6,16,17]

Late Decelerations   Symmetric, low amplitude (< 20 beats/min) decelerations that begin after the peak of the uterine contraction are called late decelerations. The timing of the deceleration and the *scooped shape* of the deceleration help to distinguish this heart rate pattern from early decelerations. The appearance of late decelerations has been attributed to transient fetal hypoxia that occurs with impairment of uteroplacental circulation during the course of uterine contractions. Two alternate mechanisms may lead to the appearance of late decelerations in the fetus. First, fetal hypertension that develops in a setting of impaired uterine blood flow and decreased oxygen delivery results in a reflex increase in vagal tone that leads to a slowing of the fetal heart rate. Alternatively, in the presence of fetal hypoxia, the decrease in heart rate is thought to occur secondary to direct myocardial depression.[27]

Late decelerations are one of the earliest signs of fetal hypoxia and, accordingly, demand prompt evaluation.[28] Any maternal (anemia, hypoxia, hypertension), placental (abruption, uteroplacental insufficiency), or fetal (anemia) factor that limits oxygen delivery to the fetus can cause fetal hypoxia and lead to the development of late decelerations on the fetal heart rate tracing. Intermittent late decelerations can be seen during the course of labor in many patients. If the decelerations are infrequent, sustained fetal hypoxia/acidemia is unlikely. This is especially true if no other periodic or baseline heart rate changes are present.[6] Nevertheless, such decelerations are reflective of intermittent fetal hypoxia. Accordingly, the clinician should attempt to alleviate the decelerations by optimizing fetal oxygen delivery. Potentially treatable causes should be addressed and corrected. Potentially beneficial interventions include change in maternal position, oxygen administration, correction of maternal hypotension, relief of uterine hypertonus, and/or correction of maternal/fetal anemia.

Late decelerations, like variable decelerations, are graded as mild, moderate, or severe, based on their duration and magnitude. All else being equal, the greater the severity of decelerations, the more significant the fetal hypoxia/acidemia.[22] Late decelerations of sufficient duration and severity may eventually exceed the fetus's ability to compensate, resulting in hypoxia and/or acidemia. The fetus with repetitive late decelerations, in the absence of normal fetal heart rate baseline characteristics, is likely to possess significant hypoxia/acidemia.[16,17]

Special Patterns

Lambda Pattern   The lambda pattern is characterized by an acceleration of the fetal heart rate immediately followed by a deceleration (Fig. 42.2). This pattern may accompany any type of deceleration and is seen in 4% of all intrapartum fetal heart rate tracings. As an isolated finding, the lambda pattern has not been associated with adverse fetal outcome.[29]

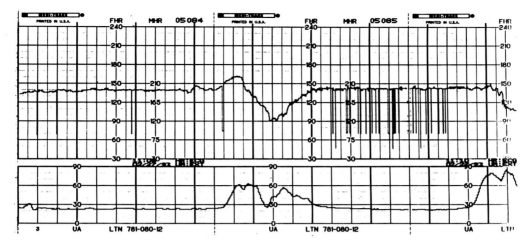

Figure 42.2   Lambda pattern in association with a variable deceleration.

Sinusoidal Pattern   The sinusoidal heart rate pattern was first described in anemic fetuses affected by severe isoimmunization.[30] Anemia from other causes may result in similar fetal heart rate changes. The characteristic features of the sinusoidal pattern are (1) stable baseline of normal rate; (2) low frequency (2–5 cycles/min), low amplitude (5–15 beats/min) oscillations of the heart rate above and below the baseline rate; and (3) absent short-term variability, with no periods of normal heart rate variability[31] (Fig. 42.3). Similar changes in the fetal heart rate have been observed after the intrapartum administration of analgesics to the mother.[32–34] Unlike the true sinusoidal pattern, the *pseudosinusoidal pattern* is not suggestive of fetal compromise. The intermittent nature of the fetal heart rate changes, and the temporal relationship to the maternal administration of analgesics (alphaprodine, butorphanol, meperidine) assists in differentiating this benign pattern from the true sinusoidal pattern. The true sinusoidal pattern should then be considered with major concern and may, in fact, be indicative of impending intrauterine fetal demise. The "pseudo" pattern does not denote such a high risk situation.

INFLUENCE OF FETAL DISEASE ON CONTINUOUS FETAL HEART TRACING

Hypoxic Fetus

Continuous fetal heart rate monitoring is frequently implemented in an effort to evaluate fetal status. When used appropriately, continuous fetal heart rate monitoring can assist the clinician in the early detection of fetal hypoxia. In the hypoxic/acidemic fetus, alterations in the baseline fetal heart rate are typically preceded by decelerations (variable or late). Such decelerations, as described above, are suggestive of intermittent fetal stress (hypoxia). This episodic stress is generally well tolerated by the healthy fetus. However, fetal hypoxia/acidemia may occur in cases of severe, persistent decelerations or in fetuses with limited reserve, for example, premature fetuses. As fetal hypoxia/acidemia progresses, baseline heart rate changes may occur. Initially, this effect can be manifested by a transient period of increased fetal heart rate variability.[6] Ultimately, this increased variability gives way to diminished long- and short-term variability.

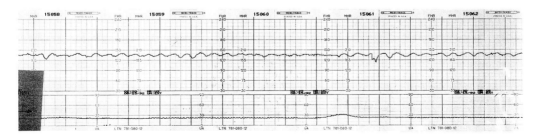

Figure 42.3   Sinusoidal fetal heart rate pattern in a fetus with severe anemia secondary to Rh isoimmunization.

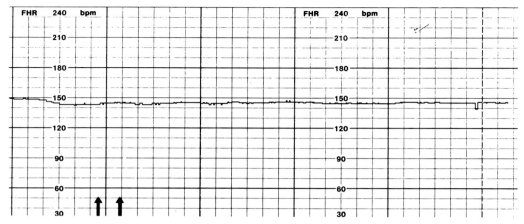

Figure 42.4 External fetal heart rate tracing in a 30-week fetus with trisomy 18. The heart rate is within the normal range and fixed; long-term variability is absent.

Baseline fetal tachycardia may develop subsequently. An ominous deceleration pattern (repetitive variable, late decelerations), combined with changes in the baseline characteristics of the continuous heart rate tracing (loss of fetal heart rate variability or tachycardia), is strongly suggestive of fetal hypoxia and requires prompt evaluation.[2,6,16,17] With continued fetal hypoxia/acidemia, the ability of the fetus to maintain a stable baseline heart rate may be lost. The resultant wandering baseline may make it difficult to recognize previously visible variable and late decelerations. Ultimately, just prior to fetal demise, profound bradycardia occurs.[35]

Neurologically Impaired Fetus

When the neurological control of the fetal heart is impaired because of preexisting or acquired damage to the CNS, alterations of the fetal heart tracing may be seen.[11–13] Fetal anencephaly, intracranial bleeding, prior anoxic injury, and CNS tumors may therefore lead to alterations of the fetal heart rate tracing in the absence of fetal hypoxia/acidemia. Similar changes may be seen in the fetus with aneuploidy.[13] Most commonly, the continuous fetal heart rate pattern in the fetus with neurological injury is flat, lacking both short-term and long-term variability. Typically, the baseline heart rate is fixed and within the normal range[11,13] (Fig. 42.4). Hypoxia and/or acidemia, manifested by repetitive decelerations and/or baseline tachycardia, may, however, also affect the neurologically impaired fetus and be superimposed upon an already existing abnormal baseline rate. The correct diagnosis through fetal monitoring of fetal hypoxia/acidemia in fetuses with preexisting neurological impairment can therefore be very difficult and/or impossible, leading to the performance of emergency cesarean sections under the false assumption of intrapartum fetal compromise.

Fetus with Isolated, Structural Cardiac Disease

The impact of associated chromosomal abnormalities or of rhythm disturbances on the heart rate tracing of the fetus with structural cardiac disease was discussed earlier. Unfortunately, little has been published regarding the influence of isolated structural cardiac disease on continuous fetal heart rate tracing. Jackson et al reported on the intrapartum course in 11 fetuses with isolated hypoplastic left ventricle. Despite the marked alteration of cardiac anatomy, the frequency of fetal heart rate abnormalities was not increased.[36] One would not expect that fetuses with less severe (e.g., atrial or ventricular septal defects, aortic coarctation, pulmonary stenosis) and valvular abnormalities would have a higher frequency of fetal heart rate abnormalities.

Fetus with Cardiac Dysrhythmia

Continuous fetal heart rate monitoring of the fetus with a cardiac dysrhythmias is inherently difficult. Moreover, as noted, the logic of many fetal heart rate monitors result in an erroneous representation of the actual heart rate in the setting of many fetal tachyarrhythmias. At such high cardiac rates, baseline accelerations and variability of the fetal heart rate are nonexistent. Although similar problems may exist in monitoring the fetus with complete heart block, some fetuses with bradyarrhythmias may exhibit reassuring accelerations and variability despite the low baseline heart rate (Fig. 42.1).

CONCLUSION

Fetal heart rate assessment can provide valuable insight into the fetal condition. To realize this benefit, a sound understanding of the normal fetal heart rate characteristics and the physiologic basis for their control is required. Adherence to a standard classification for describing normal and abnormal fetal heart rate changes will minimize confusion and facilitate communication among health care providers. Although a reactive fetal heart rate tracing can exclude significant hypoxia, an abnormal heart rate tracing does not always imply the converse. Familiarity with the common heart rate patterns and their clinical significance will facilitate accurate diagnoses and appropriate interventions in the compromised fetus.

Some recent studies have suggested that continuous fetal monitoring may result in an unneeded increase in cesarean section rates performed for falsely assumed fetal distress.[37] Since fetal heart rate monitors do not perform cesarean sections (and physicians do), these studies further emphasize the need for a proper clinical evaluation of fetal heart rate tracings. Such a proper evaluation presupposes understanding of the limitations of fetal heart rate tracing in the assessment of fetal compromise.

REFERENCES

1. Ledger WJ. Complications associated with invasive monitoring. *Semin Perinatol* 1978;2:187–194.
2. Beard RW, Filshie GM, Knight CA, et al. The significance of the changes in the continuous fetal heart rate in the first stage of labour. *J Obstet Gynaecol Br Commonw* 1971;78:865–881.
3. Schifferti P, Caldero-Garcia R. Effects of atropine and beta adrenergic drugs on the heart rate of the human fetus. In: Boreus L, ed. *Fetal Pharmacology.* New York: Raven Press; 1973;259.
4. Renou R, Newman W, Wood C. Autonomic control of fetal heart rate. *Am J Obstet Gynecol* 1969;105:949–953.
5. Itskovitz J, LaGamma EF, Rudolph AM. Heart rate and blood pressure responses to umbilical cord compression in fetal lambs with special reference to the mechanism of variable deceleration. *Am J Obstet Gynecol* 1983;147:451–457.
6. Martin CB. Physiology and clinical use of fetal heart rate variability. *Clin Perinatol* 1982;9:339–352.
7. Paul WM, Quilligan EJ, MacLaghlan T. Cardiovascular phenomenon associated with fetal head compression. *Am J Obstet Gynecol* 1964;90:824–826.
8. Yeh M-N, Morishima HO, Niemann WH, et al. Myocardial conduction defects in association with compression of the umbilical cord: experimental observations, on fetal baboons. *Am J Obstet Gynecol* 1975;121:951–956.
9. Patrick J, Campbell K, Carmichael L, et al. Influence of maternal heart rate and gross fetal body movements on the daily pattern of fetal heart rate near term. *Am J Obstet Gynecol* 1982;144:533–538.
10. Nageotte MP, Freeman RK, Freeman AG, et al. Short-term variability assessment from abdominal electrocardiogram during the antepartum period. *Am J Obstet Gynecol* 1983;145:566.
11. Phelan JP, Ahn MO. Perinatal observations in forty-eight neurologically impaired term infants. *Am J Obstet Gynecol* 1994;171:424–431.
12. Schifrin BS, Hamilton-Rubenstein T, Shields, JR. Fetal heart rate patterns and the timing of fetal injury. *J Perinatol* 1994;14:174–181.
13. Treadwell MC, Sorokin Y, Bhatia RK, Eden RD, Evans MI. Comparison of intrapartum fetal monitor tracings of karyotypically abnormal and control infants. *Fetal Diagn Ther* 1993;8:385–387.
14. Westgren M, Holmquist P, Svenningsen NW, et al. Intrapartum fetal monitoring in preterm deliveries: prospective study. *Obstet Gynecol* 1982;60:99–106.
15. Petrikovsky BM, Vintzileos AM, Nochimson DJ. Heart rate cyclicity during labor in healthy term fetuses. *Am J Perinatol* 1989;6:289–291.
16. Paul RH, Suidan AK, Yeh SY, et al. Clinical fetal monitoring. VII. The evaluation and significance of intrapartum baseline FHR variability. *Am J Obstet Gynecol* 1975;123:206–210.
17. Zanini B, Paul RH, Huey JR. Intrapartum fetal heart rate: correlation with scalp pH in the preterm fetus. *Am J Obstet Gynecol* 1980;136:43–47.
18. Lee CY, Di Loreto PC, O'Lane JM; A study of fetal heart rate acceleration patterns. *Obstet Gynecol* 1975;45:142–146.
19. Navot D, Yaffe H, Sadovsky E. The ratio of fetal heart rate accelerations to fetal movements according to gestational age. *Am J Obstet Gynecol* 1984;149:92.
20. Sorokin Y, Dierker LJ, Pillay SK, et al. The association between fetal heart rate patterns and fetal movements in pregnancies between 20 and 30 weeks gestation. *Am J Obstet Gynecol* 1982;143:243–249.
21. Hon EH. The electronic evaluation of the fetal heart rate: preliminary report. *Am J Obstet Gynecol* 1958;75:1215–1229.
22. Kubli FW, Hon EH, Khazin AF, et al. Observations on heart rate and pH in the human fetus during labor. *Am J Obstet Gynecol* 1969;104:1190–1206.
23. Tejani N, Mann LI, Bhakthavathsalan A. Correlation of fetal heart rate patterns and fetal pH with neonatal outcome. *Obstet Gynecol* 1976;48:460–463.
24. Young BK, Katz M, Klein SA. The relationship of heart rate patterns and tissue pH in the human fetus. *Am J Obstet Gynecol* 1979;143:685–690.
25. Barcroft J. *Researchers on Prenatal Life.* Oxford: Blackwell Scientific Publications; 1946.
26. Goodlin RC, Lowe EW. A functional umbilical cord occlusion heart rate pattern. *Obstet Gynecol* 1974;43:22–29.
27. Martin CB Jr, de Haan J, Van der Wilot B, et al. Mechanisms of late decelerations in the fetal heart rate. A study with autonomic blocking agents in fetal lambs. *Eur J Obstet Gynecol Reprod Biol* 1979;9:361.
28. Murata U, Martin CB, Ikenoue T, et al. Fetal heart rate accelerations and late decelerations during the course of intrauterine death in chronically catheterized rhesus monkeys. *Am J Obstet Gynecol* 1982;144:218–222.
29. Brubaker K, Garite TJ. The lambda fetal heart rate pattern: an assessment of its significance in the intrapartum period. *Obstet Gynecol* 1988;72:881–885.

30. Manseau P, Vaquier J, Chavinie P., Sureau, C. Le rythme cardiaque foetal "sinusoidal" aspect evocateur de la souffrance foetale au cours de la grossesse. *J Gynecol Obstet Biol Reprod* 1972;1:343.

31. Mondanlou HD, Freeman RK. Sinusoidal fetal heart rate pattern: its definition and clinical significance.*Am J Obstet Gynecol* 1982;142:1033–1037.

32. Gray J, Cudmore D, Lether E, et al. Sinusoidal fetal heart rate pattern associated with alphaprodine administration. *Obstet Gynecol* 1978;52:678.

33. Angel J, Knuppel R, Lake M, Sinusoidal fetal heart rate patterns associated with intravenous butorphanol administration. *Am J Obstet Gynecol* 1984;149:465.

34. Epstein H, Waxman A, Gleicher N, et al. Meperidine induced sinusoidal fetal heart rate pattern and reversal with naloxone. *Obstet Gynecol* 1982;59:225.

35. Cetrulo CL, Schifrin BS. Fetal heart rate patterns preceding death in utero. *Obstet Gynecol* 1976;48:521–527.

36. Jackson GM, Ludmir J, Castelbaum AJ, Huhta JC, Cohen AW. Intrapartum course of fetuses with isolated hypoplastic left heart syndrome. *Am J Obstet Gynecol* 1994;165:1068–1072.

37. Vintzileos AM, Nochimson OJ, Guzman ER, Knuppel RA, Lake M, Schifrin BS. Intrapartum electronic fetal heart rate monitoring versus intermittent auscultation: a meta-analysis. *Obstet Gynecol* 1995;85:149–155.

43

INTRAUTERINE ELECTROCARDIOGRAPHY AND THE SYSTOLIC TIME INTERVALS OF THE FETAL CARDIAC CYCLE

Yuji Murata, MD, Shigeharu Doi, MD, Tomoaki Ikeda, MD, Sueng-Dae Park, MD, and Toru Kanzaki, MD

INTRODUCTION

Despite inherently limited access, fetal surveillance by a variety of means has come to play a role of paramount importance in clinical perinatal medicine. Electronic monitoring of fetal heart rate (FHR) has been, by far, the most popular method used for this purpose. The clinical value of FHR monitoring, however, has been questioned. Several studies[1–4] have failed to demonstrate that such monitoring reduces perinatal mortality or improves the long-term outcome of the infants. Since perinatal mortality and morbidity are so low, and intrapartum FHR monitoring has become so routine in current clinical practice, it is practically impossible to design a study that can unequivocally demonstrate that it makes a significant contribution.

Demonstration of positive impacts on perinatal mortality and morbidity is extremely difficult for several reasons. The first is that except for mortality itself, the parameters to be used to define the quality of outcome of the infant are unclear. Second, any medical or surgical interventions taken during labor and/or at delivery may significantly alter the outcome. Last, since the incidence of perinatal morbidity, particularly that due to intrapartum injury, is very low, a great many patients would need to be recruited into a study for the results to reach statistical significance.

Many studies have been carried out on the other fetal surveillance techniques that may either replace or supplement intrapartum FHR monitoring. Using methodology similar to that for FHR monitoring, numerous researchers have inves-

tigated the fetal electrocardiogram (FECG) and the systolic time intervals (STI) of the cardiac cycle with hopes of achieving a significant clinical application. In this chapter we summarize the current body of knowledge on FECG and STI of the cardiac cycle. The past and current research literature is reviewed, and where possible, clinical correlation and application of these surveillance techniques are discussed.

FETAL ELECTROCARDIOGRAM (FECG)

Historical Overview

Cremer[5] was the first to describe FECG. The quality of the signal was so poor that its practical use was not even considered. Early in the 1960s, investigators attempted direct application of electrodes onto the fetal scalp during labor and delivery to improve signal quality.[6,7] Since then, a variety of different routes and instruments have been used, such as needle electrodes through the maternal abdomen[8] and intrauterine probe electrodes.[9] Most of these devices were investigational only and never became popular. After some modifications, fetal scalp electrodes came to provide improved signal quality and are in use today. However, they cannot be applied during labor until after rupture of the amniotic membranes, along with some cervical dilatation.

Despite their early attempts to modify the instrumentation to improve FECG signals, Hon and coworkers[10] reported rather discouraging findings of FECG as a predictor of fetal

Cardiac Problems in Pregnancy, Third Edition
Edited by Uri Elkayam, MD, and Norbert Gleicher, MD

compromise after observing dying fetuses. Hon subsequently utilized the QRS complex taken by FECG to calculate fetal heart rate.

As is true of ECG from the adult, properly processed FECG can be used for qualitative and quantitative analysis. Attempts to evaluate fetal cardiovascular performance on the basis of FECG patterns began in the early 1970s.[11] Also receiving detailed attention were FECG changes in relation to FHR patterns during labor[12] or in relation to EEG changes.[13] Later the ST waveform became a focus of FECG analysis, comparing the relative amplitude changes in T and R waves.[14]

FECG can be used by itself to obtain measurements of variables such as the duration of the P wave or the P-R interval.[15] FECG can also be combined with techniques such as the Dopplercardiogram to obtain measurements of systolic time intervals such as the preejection period.[16]

FECG Detection Methods

Abdominal FECG   The earliest FECG, described by Cremer in 1906,[5] was obtained by combined abdominal and vaginal electrodes. The difficulties in recording clear signals through the maternal abdomen were recognized by different investigators, who independently attempted to improve signal quality.[17–19]

Although abdominal FECG can be recorded noninvasively at almost any period of pregnancy, the signal amplitude is usually so small that only the QRS complex is recognizable. In addition, quality of the abdominal FECG is extremely limited as a result of poor signal-to-noise ratio and contamination by maternal ECG and electromyogram signals.

However, abdominal FECG has been improved to the degree that FHR can be counted, fetal arrhythmia can be detected, and (with the aid of averaging techniques) FECG waveform changes can be detected.[20]

Fetal Scalp ECG   Hunter[6] used clip electrodes, one directly attached to the fetal scalp (unipolar configuration) and the other on the maternal perineum. The indifferent electrode was placed on the maternal thigh. Signal quality was significantly improved by reducing maternal ECG signal amplitude, but maternal motion noise still interfered with clear recordings. Hon[7] relocated the perineal electrode to the vagina, successfully reducing maternal motion noise. This technique yielded FECG signals with an amplitude of 50–75 μV. Later, Hon and Lee[21] modified the electrodes to silver/silver chloride, which increased the FECG amplitude to 300–500 μV with significant improvement in the signal-to-noise ratio.

The electrodes currently used for FECG recordings include one attached to the fetal scalp and a second, displaced by a few millimeters, in contact with the electrically conducting amniotic fluid, cervix, or vagina. Comparisons of various FECGs obtained from fetal lambs indicated that the best FECG using the unipolar configuration was recorded with one electrode on the fetal scalp and the other on the maternal thigh.[22] FECGs so obtained are of sufficiently good quality to allow interpretation of the ECG waveform.

Lilja and coworkers, however, used a bipolar configuration with two electrodes placed on the fetal scalp. This arrangement provided lower baseline fluctuation than did the unipolar method.[23]

Scalp electrodes can be applied only after rupture of the membranes. Some cervical dilatation is also necessary to admit an applicator to pass through the cervix. Such attachment of scalp electrodes for the purpose of continuous FHR monitoring has been reported to increase scalp damage[24,25] and/or infectious morbidity in fetus.[26–28]

Rosen demonstrated FECG changes associated with an injection of a β-adrenergic agonist into a fetal lamb. The changes occurred on the ST segment and were seen on the FECG tracing obtained through a precordial lead but not through a standard lead I. Rosen concluded that a standard lead I was unsuitable for detecting the ST waveform changes (Fig. 43.1).[29]

FECG obtained through scalp electrodes is not comparable to tracings from ECG, which uses 12-lead recording including precordial leads. The configuration of FECG does, however, closely resemble lead II of the neonate ECG.[30]

Direct Fetal ECG   FECG has also been obtained directly from human fetuses undergoing antenatal fetal blood sampling or cystocentesis between 16 and 38 weeks of gestational age. A wire attached to the sampling needle was connected to the ST Analyzer (described later). Adequate quality of FECG signal was obtained with the needle in the fetal abdomen during an intrahepatic umbilical vein sampling or an aspiration of fetal urine, but not when it was in the placental cord insertion.[31]

Signal Processing and Analysis

Filters   The normal FECG consists of various components with different frequencies between 0.05 and 80 Hz, the ST segment being the slowest moving portion and the QRS complex the fastest (Fig. 43.2).[32]

Raw FECG signals, however, contain extraneous noise arising from various sources. Baseline fluctuation also makes it difficult to record consistently interpretable signals. Filters are used to eliminate or reduce electrical noise, particularly low frequency noise, which often produces apparent changes in the ST waveform.[33] On the other hand, the slow-moving part of the ST waveform appears to be vulnerable and can be distorted easily by inappropriate filters.[34] For instance, Hon[35] pointed out that FECG processed using a band pass filter (BPF) of 1.5–50 Hz loses both low and high frequency portions. Subtle changes occurring in the ST segment, therefore, may become obscured and unreliable. The other parts

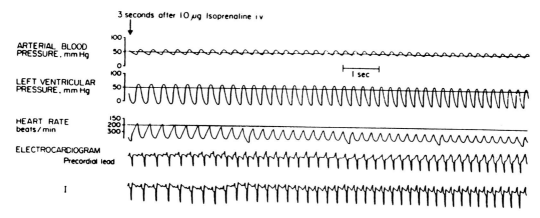

Figure 43.1 FECG changes after an intravenous injection of β-adrenergic agonist (isoprenaline, 0.4 µg/kg) into a fetal lamb. The changes occurring in the ST segment were seen only on the FECG tracing obtained through a precordial lead (second row from the bottom), not through a standard lead I (bottom row). (From Rosen.[29])

of the FECG can also be distorted, and any interpretation of the waveform becomes meaningless.

Early studies indicated rather inconsistent FECG changes during fetal distress. Mayes and his coworkers failed to demonstrate consistent changes in FECG in fetuses suffering hypoxia.[36] Hon and Lee reported inconsistent findings in 22 fetuses that died during the observation.[10] These inconsistent results may well have been produced by different instrumen-

tation and methods of signal manipulation, including the filter characteristics. It is, therefore, mandatory to include the filter characteristics in any report in which FECG waveform is studied.

Lindecrantz and coworkers[22] recommend the use of a filter having a bandwidth of 0.05–100 Hz. Table 43.1 demonstrates the ranges of band pass filters used by various investigators who reported FECG waveform analysis.

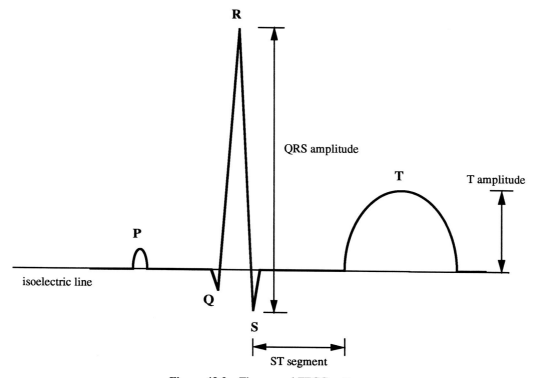

Figure 43.2 The normal FECG pattern.

TABLE 43.1 Band Pass Filter (BPF) Characteristics for FECG Waveform Analysis

Ref: First Author (Year)	BPF Frequency (Hz)
Greene[14] (1982)	200–16,000
Lilja[23] (1985)	0.1–800
Murray[15] (1989)	0.16–500 (3 dB limit)
Newbold[61] (1989)	0.1–40
Rosen[65] (1989)	0.07–100 (3 dB limit)
Thaler[37] (1988)	0.5–300
Lindecrantz[22] (1988)	0.05–100

Signal-Averaging Techniques   To prevent random noise from contaminating the FECG signal, an averaging technique has been used to superimpose successive readings of the cardiac cycle. Usually 10–20 cycles are superimposed, using the peak of R wave as a trigger point. This method, introduced by Hon and Lee,[21] can produce a significant increase in the signal-to-noise ratio, provided the trigger point in each cardiac cycle is accurate and that each component of FECG remains stable in relation to the trigger point for 10–20 cycles while they are averaged. In practice, however, noise often alters the configuration of the QRS complex and thus the accurate detection of the trigger point is difficult. Even with an optimal QRS detector, averaging may produce a false decrease in QRS amplitude, and thus create a false increase in T/QRS ratio (described later).[29]

Generally, as the number of cardiac cycles averaged increases, FECG waveform become more distorted. Rapid changes in FECG waveform may also be obscured. On the other hand, if the number of cycles is too small, one spurious cycle may affect the results significantly.

Thaler and coworkers, noting a T wave distortion that was due to the averaging technique, developed a mechanism to average the T wave separately from the other complexes of FECG.[37] The distortion that prompted this innovation appeared to have been caused by a rapid change in Q-T interval.

FECG Morphology   The characteristic pattern of an FECG obtained from a normal fetus (Fig. 43.2) includes a small P wave, a small Q wave, a large R wave, a variable-sized S wave, and an ST segment that is usually almost isoelectric.[38] The T wave is also often isoelectric.

The amplitudes of the FECG components are relative, depending on various factors such as the nature and position of the electrodes. The amplitudes also differ between different fetuses, or even within the same fetus, regardless of whether contractions are occurring at the time of reading.

Isoelectric Line   The isoelectric line is judged from the level of the P-Q interval or the pre-P portion of the FECG. An amplitude and a duration of any signal component are measured as a height (voltage) from this line or a length (time) between onset and offset from this line.

P Wave   The P wave is usually small. The mean duration of the P wave is 58.8 ms (SD, 7.6 ms). The P wave has been shown to decrease in amplitude during labor by approximately 30%.[39] The P wave sometimes becomes inverted, but the significance of this is not known. An inverted P wave was not found to be associated with uterine contractions, fetal acidosis, or hypoxia.[40] Unusually tall P waves having no diagnostic significance also have been recorded.[40]

PR Segment   Commonly this segment is depressed below the isoelectric line, especially in the presence of a QRS complex with a large amplitude. The P-R interval indicates atrioventricular node conduction time and is sensitive to vagal tone. FHR (R-R interval) is one of the factors affecting the P-R interval.

QRS Complex   The QRS complex possesses the largest amplitude, ranging from 200 to 300 μV when measured using a silver/silver chloride wire electrode.[23] The frequency of the QRS complex ranges from 20 to 40 Hz. This complex is used as a trigger to count heart rate after filtration through a high pass filter, which distorts the other lower frequency components of FECG, resulting in signals unsuitable for waveform analysis.

As described before, the amplitudes of FECG components are different in each subject. Thus comparison of absolute signal amplitudes between different fetuses is virtually meaningless. The amplitude of QRS is therefore used as a reference to observe an alteration in the amplitude of the other FECG components. For example, a ratio between the amplitudes of the T wave and QRS is calculated to quantify T-wave changes.

No QRS-complex pattern was found to be indicative of fetal condition. The following patterns were observed in a full range of fetal conditions: presence of the Q wave, notching of the R wave, presence of an S wave.[40]

ST Segment   The ST segment of FECG is usually isoelectric.[38] The ST-T segment represents ventricular repolarization of the heart and thus is thought to be related to myocardial metabolism. The absolute position of the ST segment, above or below the isoelectric line, however, does not correlate with any particular fetal condition, nor does it appear to directly correlate with myocardial hypoxia as in the adult.[40] Either an elevation or a depression of the ST segment is considered to be a pathological change.

T Wave   In normal fetuses the T wave is often isoelectric or has a positive deflection. The amplitude is less than or equal to the amplitude of the P wave.[23] T-wave amplitude that exceeds the P-wave amplitude, a tall and peaked T, and a negative T are all considered to be pathologic.

FECG And Fetal Pathophysiology

The major insults the fetus receives during intrauterine life, especially during the intrapartum period, originate from hypoxia and from acidosis as a consequence of hypoxia. In studies of FECG as an indicator of hypoxia, investigations have focused on changes in the ST segment.

The ST segment and T wave, being the period of ventricular repolarization, are particularity sensitive to metabolic events across the myocardial cell membranes, which change in response to the concentration of potassium ions and alteration of the sodium pump.[41]

The autonomic nervous system and increased circulating catecholamines induced in response to hypoxia are reported to be responsible for the changes in the ST waveform.[42] The autonomic nervous system also significantly affects these time intervals, particularly the P-R interval representing atrioventricular conduction time.

Basic Studies of FECG   In early studies using laboratory animals, changes in the ST segment and T wave were observed in association with experimentally produced hypoxia, but the results were not consistent. Pardi and coworkers[11] reported that ST-waveform changes in the exteriorized fetal lamb were demonstrable with severe hypoxemia but not with mild hypoxemia. They concluded, therefore, that FHR was a more sensitive indicator for fetal hypoxemia. Myers observed ST-T elevation in asphyxiated fetal monkeys. The changes, however, occurred late in the sequence of asphyxia, and no relationship could be identified between the FECG changes and the severity of the insult.[43] Rosen later speculated that this lack of FECG change in early stages of asphyxia was due to the standard lead I used by Myers. A standard lead I was demonstrated to be unsuitable for detecting ST-waveform changes.[29]

Increase in the amplitude of the T wave is consistently associated with hypoxia/acidosis. Since the comparison of an absolute amplitude of the T wave between different individual subjects is difficult, if not impossible, a quantitative expression of the FECG changes is made by taking a ratio between the amplitude of the T wave and that of QRS complex,-the T–QRS ratio.

Metabolic States   Rosen and colleagues demonstrated an inverse linear relationship between fetal blood pH and ST-T change, represented by T/QRS ratio, during hypoxic insults experimentally given to pregnant guinea pigs.[44] The study also reported a significant positive correlation between the fetal blood lactate concentration and T/QRS ratio (Fig. 43.3). In a separate study, Rosen and Isaksson[45] observed FHR and FECG changes, particularly those in the ST-T segment, and produced a scoring system based on alterations in the FECG. Acute fetal guinea pig preparations exposed to graded hypoxia were used in this study (Fig. 43.4; Table 43.2). They

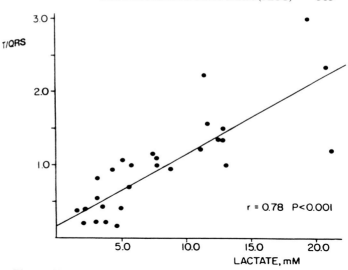

Figure 43.3   Correlation between T/QRS ratio and blood lactate concentrations observed during intrauterine asphyxia in chronically instrumented fetal lambs. (From Rosen et al.[45])

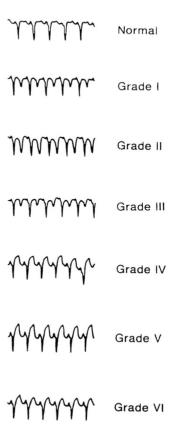

Figure 43.4   The fetal ECG scoring system established from fetal guinea pigs exposed to graded hypoxia. (From Rosen.[45])

TABLE 43.2 The Fetal ECG Scoring System Established from Fetal Guinea Pigs Exposed to Graded Hypoxia

Grade I	Appearance of negative T waves, the amplitude exceeding that of the P waves
Grade II	Maximally negative T waves
Grade III	Gradual decrease in the amplitude of the negative T waves
Grade IV	Elevation of the S-T segment and the T wave, the amplitude of the T wave being higher than that of the P waves
Grade V	Maximal increase in the amplitude of the T wave
Grade VI	Decrease in the amplitude of the T waves during continuous hypoxia

Source: Rosen.[29]

also demonstrated that the degree of ST-T alteration was closely related to a decrease in myocardial glycogen in the mature fetal guinea pig. Myocardial ATP and creatinine phosphate did not change prior to myocardial failure associated with bradycardia.[45]

The role of myocardial glycogenolysis in FECG changes was later substantiated by work using exteriorized fetal lambs. Hökegard and colleagues claimed that the physiological background to these ST-T changes is the anaerobic breakdown of myocardial glycogen stores.[46] Later they demonstrated that the extent of the FECG changes during hypoxia correlates strongly with the depletion of cardiac glycogen stores and creatine–phosphate, both of which were measured directly in the fetal sheep myocardium obtained by repeated biopsy. This decrease of glycogen is apparent even with a slight change in FECG, such as the appearance of negative T waves.[47]

Greene and his coworkers[14] observed ST-waveform changes in chronically instrumented fetal lambs. The T/QRS ratio was less than 0.30 in normal fetuses, without showing diurnal or other rhythms. Despite normal pH, persistent elevation of T/QRS ratio was seen in the animals prior to death or in those with anemia and/or hypotension. There was a strong correlation of the T/QRS ratio to the rate of rise in the lactate concentration. The data indicated that significantly raised lactate levels could precede a decrease in pH. This is why, according to Greene and coworkers, the chronically hypotensive and/or anemic lamb fetuses demonstrated elevated T/QRS ratios despite the presence of normal pH. This observation is supported by the earlier suggestion of Dawes and colleagues[48] that the major part of the increase of blood lactate during asphyxia originates from myocardial glycogenolysis. Rosen's observation during the course of labor in chronically instrumented fetal lambs with slowly developing asphyxia indicated that T-wave changes appeared approximately 10 hours prior to a drop in pH.[29]

Hökengard and coworkers demonstrated that similar changes in ST waveform observed in animal fetuses can be induced by injecting β-adrenergic agonists such as isoprenaline into a fetus. Further, they showed that the administration of β-adrenergic blockade with propanolol reversed the ST-waveform changes caused by mild and moderate hypoxia, but not severe hypoxia.[46] The relationships among catecholamines, myocardial glycogenolysis, and electrocardiographic changes have been extensively studied in adults as well as in neonates. A significant linear correlation was demonstrated between circulating adrenaline concentration and T/QRS ratio in chronically instrumented fetal lambs exposed to hypoxic insults (Fig. 43.5).[42]

Central Nervous and Cardiovascular States The changes in ST-T segment appeared in early phases of hypoxia simultaneously with changes in fetal cerebral function as measured by somatosensory-evoked electroencephalographic (EEG) responses in exteriorized lamb fetuses.[13]

Not only did ST changes occur prior to the development of fetal acidosis[14] but they also appeared in the absence of overt hypoxia.[42] Moreover, the ST-waveform changes were demonstrated before obvious changes in FHR and before evidence of cardiac failure determined by *dP/dt* in fetal lambs.[44,47] The increased amplitude of the T wave during the early phase of hypoxic insult given to the fetuses may be a result of β-adrenergic stimulation, which simultaneously raises FHR, myocardial contractility, and myocardial glycogenolysis. In this regard, Rosen suggested that the increase in T-wave amplitude could serve as an index of "myocardial energy balance." When the balance is negative, myocardial glycogen will be utilized and the ST-waveform changes will appear.[29]

Clinical Application of FECG Any technique used for intrapartum fetal surveillance, including FECG analysis, should be proven to decrease perinatal mortality and/or morbidity prior to general clinical application. Reduction in the incidence of operative deliveries, thus reducing maternal mortality and/or morbidity without worsening fetal outcome, can also be considered acceptable. For this purpose, Apgar scores, fetal scalp or umbilical blood sampling for respiratory gases and pH, and FHR monitoring have traditionally been used to determine fetal outcome. Some authors, however, say that these parameters are poor indicators for identifying the truly compromised fetus or newborn.[1,2,49–51]

To predict long-term neurological outcome of the infant, such as cerebral palsy due to ischemic encephalopathy produced during labor and delivery, the immediate performance of the newborns, as indicated by necessity for respiratory support and/or presence of seizure activities, may offer more useful information.[52,53]

Although FECG can predict fetal hypoxia, investigators have yet to demonstrate that FECG can lead to a diminution

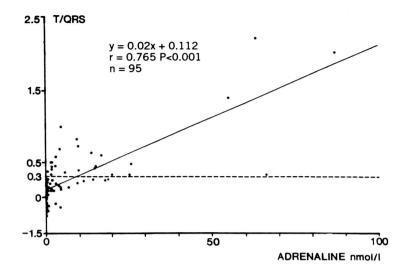

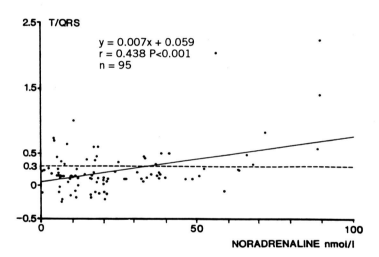

Figure 43.5   Linear correlations between T/QRS ratio and circulating adrenaline (top) and between T/QRS ratio and circulating noradrenaline (bottom) observed in chronically instrumented fetal lambs exposed to hypoxic insults. (From Rosen et al.[42])

in the rate of perinatal morbidity. In any event, this would be difficult to do because the incidence of infants damaged by intrapartum hypoxia is so low that a tremendously large population would have to be recruited into a prospective study for the results to reach statistical significance.

Past studies on human FECG as a parameter of fetal well-being are discouraging. Hon and Lee, for instance, observed 22 fetuses that died during their study and reported that FECG changes did not occur until late in the stage of fetal compromise.[10] Myers, using primate fetuses, also found that ST-T changes were a late phenomenon in the course of severe asphyxia.[43] These results tend to contradict the recent observations. Discrepancies in observation and/or interpreta-

tion are probably due to differences in the methodologies employed, including the electrodes, filters, and amplification systems that were used. It is, therefore, very difficult to compare these results of clinical studies performed by different investigators.

In a later section, we compare the results of human FECG analysis with the traditional parameters of fetal surveillance.

Signal Quality and Processing   Most data on signal quality and processing thus far published were collected in regard to human fetuses of gestational ages greater than 36 weeks. There have been no studies of FECG dealing with preterm fetuses. In the majority of studies, the fetuses exhibited cephalic presentation, and there were few descriptions of FECG obtained through electrodes placed on the fetal buttocks during breech delivery. Rosen reported the feasibility of breech electrodes for ST-waveform analysis.[29] On the other hand, Westgate and coworkers warned that a breech-presenting fetus might produce unusual-looking FECG patterns and that false negative waveforms were sometimes recorded.[54]

In regard to quality of the signals obtained from the fetuses, Murphy and coworkers reported that 35% of FECG waveforms in their study were unsuitable for analysis because of poor signal quality.[55] Lilja considered 11% to be unsuitable for analysis,[56] whereas Murray,[40] having accepted FECG with a signal-to-noise ratio of at least 6:1, rejected only 2.6% of his recordings. These differences are obviously due to the use of different electrodes, electronic systems, and analytical algorithms.

Quality of the FECG signals often deteriorates during uterine contractions, particularly in the second stage of labor. The FECG baseline usually drifts significantly as a result of uterine contraction, producing unreliable readings. Cockburn and associates, who described the difficulties in keeping acceptable FECG signals during the second stage of labor, reported that 64% of the second stage tracings had analyzable ST segments. These investigators also stated that without immediately available technical expertise, difficulties could have hampered the use of FECG monitoring by clinical obstetricians.[57]

ST Waveform and T/QRS Ratio Many studies using human fetal ECG have focused on the T/QRS ratio for quantitative analysis. In addition to measuring this ratio, however, it has been recommended that qualitative observation on the ST waveform be performed. A negative T wave and/or ST depression should be regarded as highly abnormal even in the absence of T/QRS elevation.[58]

NORMAL FETUSES As noted earlier, direct comparison of the results reported by different investigators is greatly hindered by differences in the various methodologies utilized. Currently two commercially available instruments allow investigators to analyze FECG on line during the intrapartum period. The STAN fetal monitor (ST Analyzer, Cinventa AB,

Sweden) offers a simultaneous display of both continuous FHR and T/QRS ratio. The T/QRS ratio is calculated by averaging 10 or 30 consecutive fetal ECG complexes of good signal quality. The other apparatus is the Nottingham model,[59] which employs time-coherent weighted averaging to produce a stable baseline before any measurements are made.

Newbold and her associates compared the two instruments by feeding the same FECG signals and found that the STAN monitor showed higher T/QRS ratios than did the Nottingham system. According to the investigators, this is probably because the isoelectric line in the STAN monitor had been set from the PR segment.[60]

Table 43.3 shows the T/QRS ratios observed from normal intrapartum fetuses by different groups of investigators. Here a normal fetus was defined as one with normal FHR pattern and with normal umbilical cord acid–base and lactate status at delivery. The differences seen here can be explained by the difference in the equipment used in the studies.

Using the STAN monitor, Lilja reported the highest T/QRS ratio to be 0.26 (SD 0.19) during labor with umbilical artery blood pH of 7.25 or greater.[62] Moreover, Maclachlan, using the STAN monitor, observed a range of 0.00–0.32 with a median of 0.13 (97.5th percentile = 0.28) among the fetuses in labor when no subsequent medical intervention during the neonatal period was required.[63]

Arulkumaran and his coworkers demonstrated that T/QRS ratios from antepartum fetuses between 16 and 38 weeks of gestation had no correlation with gestational age and FHR and that the values were comparable with those described in term fetuses during labor.[31]

UTERINE CONTRACTIONS Most investigators agree that uterine contractions affect FECG, particularly during the second stage of labor. Thaler and coworkers observed a significant increase in the T/QRS ratio during the first half of a uterine contraction from a mean precontraction value of 0.18 to a value of 0.26. During the second half of the contraction, the ratio fell to 0.2 and then returned to the precontraction level. The authors attributed this movement to an increase in catecholamine level during a uterine contraction.[37]

As described earlier, uterine contractions frequently not only produce noisy FECG readings but also cause a baseline

TABLE 43.3 T/QRS Ratios Observed from Normal Intrapartum Fetuses[a] **by Different Groups of Investigators**

Ref: First Author (year)	Ratio	Hardware
Lilja[56] (1988)	0.148 (SD 0.048)	ST Analyzer (STAN)
Newbold[61] (1989)	0.10 (Range 0.04–0.23)	Microcomputer
Newbold[60] (1991)	0.10 (5th–95th percentile, 0.04–0.16)	Nottingham model

[a]Normal fetuses were defined as fetuses with normal FHR pattern, normal umbilical cord acid–base, and lactate status at delivery.

drift. Newbold and her associates, however, did not observe significant changes in T/QRS ratio as labor progressed. They speculated that all changes in T/QRS ratio during labor are due to artifact from the baseline drift as well as to poor quality FECG signals.[64]

COMPARISON TO FHR PATTERNS   When FHR monitoring was considered to be the gold standard for the ascertainment of fetal well-being, the results of ST-waveform studies were compared with FHR patterns during labor. Pardi and colleagues claimed that there was a significant correlation between elevation of the T/QRS ratio and the appearance of abnormal FHR pattern represented by some variable and late decelerations.[12] This observation, however, was not confirmed by subsequent research.[55,60]

Lilja and associates, observing 46 fetuses without clinical evidence of hypoxia, demonstrated that intrapartum FHR monitoring produced a higher incidence of abnormal or suspicious patterns (74%) than did elevated (>0.25) T/QRS ratio (33%). This result may be difficult to interpret. The authors indicated that the elevation of T/QRS was sometimes transient. More importantly, differences in pattern recognition by different investigators should not be overlooked, since the incidence of abnormal or suspicious FHR patterns seems excessively high among the normal intrapartum fetuses.

Maclachlan and group demonstrated that an abnormal FHR pattern was a more sensitive indicator than an elevated T/QRS in the prediction of fetal acidosis as determined by fetal scalp blood sampling, the accuracy being 71% and 29%, respectively.[63]

Recent studies do not appear to support the relationship between abnormal FHR findings and T/QRS ratio, as suggested by Pardi in 1974.[12]

FETAL PH, GAS, AND LACTATE LEVELS   One might anticipate that the correlation between ST-waveform behavior and fetal acid/base status would also be poor. Pardi examined the changes in ST and T waves and found no direct correlation with fetal scalp pH.[12]

On the other hand, Jenkins and coworkers, on observing 4 normal and 10 acidotic fetuses at birth, determined that significantly more fetuses demonstrated a long-term increase in ST elevation and T-wave height when umbilical cord pH was less than 7.20.[38] Umbilical vein lactate level was also shown to have a significant linear correlation with T/QRS ratio obtained no more than 30 minutes before delivery (Fig. 43.6).[23] However, the same study failed to demonstrate a statistically significant relationship between T/QRS and umbilical cord pH. The relationship between T/QRS ratio and umbilical cord lactate level was not substantiated by the later study carried out by Newbold et al.[60]

A series of subsequent studies by many different investigators on the changes in the ST and T waves failed to find

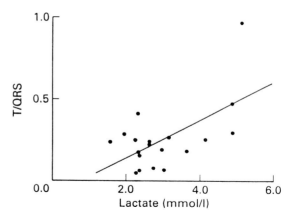

Figure 43.6   Linear correlation between T/QRS ratio obtained within 30 minutes before delivery and umbilical vein lactate level. (From Lilja et al.[23])

any significant correlation with fetal acidosis, determined by umbilical blood sample[40,55,60,65] or scalp blood sample.[63] Of interest, Rosen and colleagues studied 163 fetuses in the first stage of labor and recorded abnormal T/QRS ratios from 46 of them. Acidosis (defined by umbilical artery pH < 7.15 at birth) was seen in 7 fetuses, giving a positive predictive value of 15%.[65]

Even among the acidotic fetuses with elevated T/QRS ratio, the nature of the acidosis was not metabolic but respiratory in origin in the majority of cases.[60,63,65] Maclachlan and coworkers concluded that abnormal FHR pattern predicted 71% of fetuses subsequently showing acidosis, whereas elevated T/QRS did so in 29% of fetuses.[63]

Johanson and coworkers support the significance of T/QRS ratio in predicting fetal acidosis. They reported their experience with three fetuses that had significant acidosis confirmed by scalp blood sampling. Two of these fetuses revealed T/QRS ratios greater than 0.25, and the diagnosis of the other was equivocal due to poor quality of FECG.[66]

Arulkumaran and his coworkers reported that a standard bicarbonate value possessed better correlation with elevated T/QRS ratio than did umbilical cord pH. According to their results, a T/QRS ratio of less than 0.25 was associated with normal buffering capacity at 99.3% accuracy. Interestingly, the same authors indicated that most fetuses with a T/QRS ratio of greater than 0.25 had an abnormal ratio from the onset of labor.[67]

APGAR SCORES   No significant relationship has been demonstrated between T/QRS ratio and Apgar score at either 1 or 5 minutes.[55,60]

P-R Interval   The P-R interval represents the atrioventricular node conduction time, and normally there is a significant positive correlation with the R-R interval. Murray observed the behavior of the P-R interval in FECG of normal as well as acidotic fetuses.[40] His study indicates that all the fetuses able to maintain a positive correlation ($r > 0.3$) between the P-R and R-R intervals demonstrated umbilical artery pH of greater than 7.24 at birth.

On the other hand, fetuses showing a negative correlation between the two intervals were associated with umbilical arterial pH between 7.17 and 7.29 (mean 7.25), as documented by scalp or umbilical cord sampling. The author speculated that this inverse correlation is due to metabolically impaired myocardium, which now is unable to maintain an adequate heart rate, thus increasing the P-P interval despite an increase in sympathetic tone as indicated by a shortened P-R interval.

Furthermore, an alteration of the ST-segment height relative to the isoelectric line by greater than 5% of the QRS height together with a negative P-R/R-R correlation indicated an umbilical artery pH in the range of 6.99 to 7.26.

Prospective Clinical Studies   Westgate and associates carried out a prospective randomized study on 1200 women in labor later than 34 weeks of gestation.[54] Comparisons were made for neonatal outcome, obstetrical course, and intervention given to the patient between the control group (FHR monitoring only) and the study group (FHR monitoring plus ST-waveform analysis by STAN ST wave analyzer). The patients were treated following a strict protocol according to which every patient except for normal fetuses received fetal scalp blood sampling for the diagnosis of fetal distress. A normal T/QRS ratio was defined as between -0.10 and 0.25, an intermediate T/QRS ratio as between 0.25 and 0.50 for more than 30 minutes, and an abnormal T/QRS ratio as greater than 0.50 for more than 15 minutes. Also considered abnormal were negative T-wave components or ST depression with T elevation.

The results indicated that addition of ST-waveform monitoring to FHR monitoring significantly reduced the proportion of deliveries in fetal distress. The rates of operative delivery, incidence of asphyxia at birth, and neonatal outcome were not affected. Metabolic acidosis and low 5-minute Apgar scores were less common in the study group than in the control group but not at a level of statistical significance.

In response to this report by Westgate et al,[54] Cockburn et al reported their own study, which did not include FHR monitoring. They concluded that use of the ST-wave analyzer reduced by 10-fold the need for scalp blood sampling during labor, without altering the number of operative interventions for fetal distress and the number of babies with metabolic acidosis at delivery.[57]

Greene and Westgate,[68] having accumulated 2400 patients, noted a significant reduction in the total number of fetal blood samplings compared with the number performed on 1200 patients as presented earlier by the same group.[54]

SYSTOLIC TIME INTERVALS (STIs) OF THE FETAL CARDIAC CYCLE

Historical Overview

The first study of systolic time intervals (STIs) in a human fetus was reported by Persianinov et al.[69] These investigators performed simultaneous noninvasive recordings of fetal electrocardiograms and phonocardiograms through the maternal abdomen. Weissler and his coworkers, who first worked extensively with adult subjects, found fetal STIs, especially the preejection period (PEP) of the cardiac cycle, to be faithful indicators that reflect the functional integrity of the fetal myocardium.[70]

The majority of basic studies in the 1970s were carried out to explore pathophysiological responses of fetal STIs. These were studies of laboratory animals, usually chronically instrumented fetal sheep and monkeys. Although the potential of clinical application was repeatedly demonstrated, many technical questions remained to be answered. Even today, a large prospective, randomized study will still be necessary to statistically prove the positive impact of STIs on perinatal medicine.

Definition of STIs

Figure 43.7 depicts the electrical and mechanical events that are occurring sequentially during one cardiac cycle. The electrical events include the P wave, QRS complex, ST segment, and T wave. The onset of the Q wave is usually used as a reference point for various measurements. The important mechanical events are the cardiac valvular motions. An interval between the Q wave on ECG and any mechanical event is defined as an electromechanical STI, whereas an interval between two mechanical events is called a mechanical STI. Table 43.4 displays both electromechanical and mechanical STIs, along with the interval being measured, the physiologic implications, and methods commonly used to determine the intervals.

Electromechanical Latent Time (EMLT)   The EMLT is the interval between the onset of ventricular depolarization and the closure (Mc) of the left atrioventricular (AV) valve. This is one of the electromechanical STIs. Following the preceding cardiac cycle, the AV valves remain open until the contraction of the ventricular myocardium begins. Ventricular contraction increases the intraventricular pressure, reversing the pressure gradient from the ventricle to the atrium, promoting valve closure. The EMLT can be described, therefore, as the lag time between the electrical excitation and the onset of mechanical activity of the ventricle.

Isovolumetric Contraction Time (ICT)   The ICT is a mechanical STI that is defined as the interval between AV valve

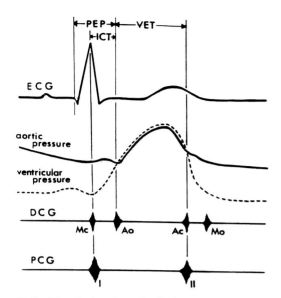

Figure 43.7 Electrical and mechanical events occurring during one cardiac cycle (top to bottom): electrocardiogram, ECG; aortic pressure tracing: intraventricular pressure tracing; ultrasound Doppler cardiogram, DCG; and phonocardiogram, PCG. Additional abbreviations: PEP, preejection period; ICT, isovolumic contraction time; VET, ventricular ejection time; Mc, Ao, Ac, and Mo on the DCG are atrioventricular (AV) valve closure, semilunar valve opening, semilunar valve closure, and AV valve opening, respectively. I and II on the PCG channel indicate the first and second sounds of the heart.

closure (Mc) and semilunar valve opening (Ao). During this period the ventricles are normally closed chambers filled with blood. When the myocardium contracts, the intraventricular pressure initially rises without changing the volume of the ventricle (isovolumetric contraction). When intraventricular pressure comes to exceed the aortic or pulmonary pressure, the semilunar valves open (Ao) and ejection of blood into the great vessels commences.

Preejection Period (PEP)   The PEP is the sum of the EMLT and ICT intervals. It is measured as the distance from the onset of the Q wave to the semilunar valve opening (Ao). It can also be described as the interval from the onset of ventricular depolarization to the beginning of ejection from the ventricle. The PEP has been the most extensively studied electromechanical STI in fetuses, infants, and adults, and it is known as a sensitive indicator of myocardial performance.

Ventricular Ejection Time (VET)   The VET is the period during which blood is ejected from the ventricles to the great vessels. At the beginning of ejection, the intraventricular pressure equals the resting (diastolic) pressure, it soon reaches its maximum (systolic) pressure, and then falls. At the point at which the intraventricular pressure becomes lower than diastolic pressure, the semilunar valve closes (Ac), and the heart enters the diastolic phase. The VET is a representative mechanical STI and has been investigated thoroughly in both infants and adults.

TABLE 43.4   Definition of Systolic Time Intervals

Systolic Time Intervals	Interval to Be Measured (refer Fig. 43.1)[a]	Physiologic Implications	Methods
Electromechanical latent time (EMLT)	Q–MC	Delay from ventricular depolarization to onset of mechanical contraction	ECG and Dopplercardiogram, ECG and M-mode, or ECG and ventricular catheter
Isovolumic contraction time (ICT)	Mc–Ao	Time required for ventricular muscle to increase intraventricular pressure until ejection starts	Doppler cardiography
Preejection period (PEP)	Q–Ao	Time between onset of ventricular depolarization and beginning of ejection	ECG and Dopplercardiogram, ECG and M-mode, or ECG and aortic catheter
Ventricular ejection time (VET)	Ao–Ac	Duration of blood ejection from ventricles to great vessels	Dopplercardiogram or M-mode
Mechanical systole	Mc–Ac or S1–S2	Total duration of ventricular muscle contraction	Dopplercardiogram or phonocardiogram
Total systole	Q–Ac or Q–S2	Total time required for heart to complete systole starting from electrical excitation	ECG and Dopplercardiogram, ECG and M-mode, or ECG and phonocardiogram, or ECG and aortic pressure

[a]The symbols Ao, Ac, Mo, and Mc are traditionally used to represent the opening and closing of the left semilunar (aortic) and the left atrioventricular (mitral) valves, respectively.

Mechanical Systole Mechanical systole is the interval from AV valve closure (Mc) to semilunar valve closure (Ac) during which the ventricular muscle continuously contracts. This phase is a mechanical STI that consists of two other mechanical STIs, the ICT and VET.

Total Systole Total systole, an electromechanical STI, is the sum of PEP and the VET. This interval is the total time required for the heart to complete the systolic phase.

Method of Determination of STIs

To be able to observe STIs, particularly electromechanical STIs such as EMLT, PEP, or total systole, an investigator must record the sequence of both electrical and mechanical events simultaneously. For recording the electrical activity of the fetal heart, either direct or indirect electrocardiogram (ECG) can be used.

Direct FECG is obtained by means of scalp electrodes attached to the fetal presenting part during delivery. This usually allows an investigator to appreciate the ECG morphology, but application is restricted to the period after the amniotic membranes have ruptured. Although the incidence of complications appears to be low, there have been some problems arising from the application of fetal scalp electrodes.[24–28,71,72]

An indirect FECG signal is obtained noninvasively by placing electrodes on the maternal abdomen. Such a signal is usually recorded with lesser quality than direct FECG. Indeed, often only the QRS complex can be identified. In one study, where the only purpose of the FECG was to time the Q wave for the measurement of STIs, abdominal FECG could be successfully performed in approximately 80% of the patients studied.[73]

Simultaneous FECG and Phonocardiogram (PCG) Some early investigations reported the use of PCG in conjunction with FECG.[69,74] As Figure 43.7 indicates, fetal PCG signals do not provide the timing of the semilunar of AV valve openings. This method, therefore, cannot determine the PEP or VET.

Simultaneous FECG and Dopplercardiogram (DCG) With appropriate filtering techniques, Doppler signals obtained from the fetal heart can be used to identify cardiac valve motions.[16] Four distinctive bursts in one cardiac cycle have been identified as the AV valve closure (Mc), the semilunar valve opening (Ao), the semilunar valve closure (Ac), and the AV valve opening (Mo).[75,76]

This method does not allow one to separately record the signals from the semilunar valve and from the AV valve. De Muylder et al[77] demonstrated consistent differences in the PEP values obtained from the right and the left ventricles via catheters in fetal lambs (Fig. 43.8). The authors emphasized the importance of obtaining the PEP from the same ventricle if the STI is to be used in evaluation of fetal myocardial function. Guided by two-dimensional real-time ultrasound, pulsed Doppler signals from the fetal aortic valve were recorded simultaneously with abdominal FECG.[78] This method allowed the authors to observe the PEP from the left ventricle.

Simultaneous FECG and Echocardiogram Fetal echocardiogram guided by real-time ultrasound was recorded together with abdominal FECG, allowing separate measurement of the right and left ventricular PEPs and VETs (Fig. 43.9).[79] The reported values of left ventricular PEP determined by echocardiogram appeared to be compatible with those observed earlier using the Dopplercardiogram.[80]

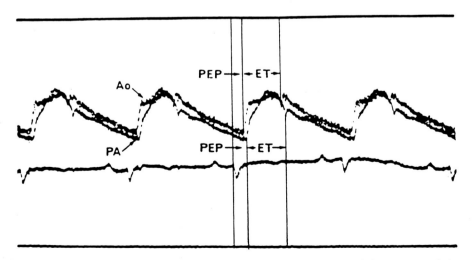

Figure 43.8 A simultaneous recording of aortic pressure, pulmonary arterial pressure, and electrocardiogram of a fetal lamb, demonstrating consistent differences in both the preejection period (PEP) and ventricular ejection time (ET) between the right and ventricles. (From De Muylder et al.[77])

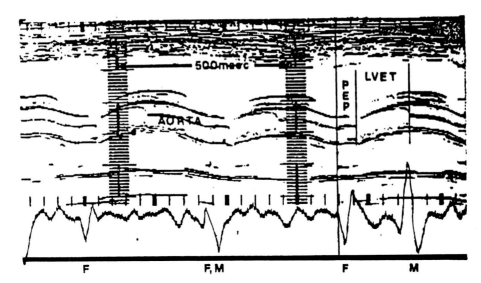

Figure 43.9   The left ventricular systolic time intervals determined by simultaneous recording of M-mode echocardiogram of aortic valve motion and abdominal fetal electrocardiogram (ECG). The preejection period (PEP) is measured from the onset of fetal QRS (F on the ECG) to aortic valve opening. The left ventricular ejection time (LVET) is measured from the aortic valve opening to closure. (From Kleinman and Donnerstein.[80])

Simultaneous FECG and Aortic or Pulmonary Blood Pressure Tracing   In an experimental setting, where a catheter can be inserted into the aorta with its tip located close to the aortic valve, the onset of aortic pressure increase indicates the timing of the aortic valve opening and allows the PEP to be determined. The right ventricular PEP can also be determined by means of a catheter inserted in the pulmonary artery. Length and compliance of the catheter may affect the measurements, but this technique has been considered to be appropriate for comparing the changes in STIs in an individual subject.[77,81] The distance between the Q wave and a dicrotic notch closely represents the total systole.

Simultaneous FECG and Ventricular Pressure Tracing
A catheter located within either the left or right ventricle can measure the ventricular pressure curve. The onset of the pressure rise corresponds to the AV valve closure, allowing the measurement of EMLT in conjunction with FECG.

STIs and Fetal Pathophysiology

Basic knowledge about normal and pathologic STIs of the fetal cardiac cycle has been developed from the results of studies using laboratory animals, especially chronically instrumented fetal lambs and primates. The results obtained using animals must be carefully interpreted: They may not be readily applicable to human fetuses because of physiological differences between species; also, differences in the anesthesia, medications, and stresses applied to the subjects may invalidate direct comparisons.

The following sections discuss physiologic factors that affect the fetal STIs, mainly two extensively investigated STIs, and PEP and VET, by comparing the results from laboratory animals and human fetuses.

Basic Studies of STIs

Physiologic Responses

GESTATIONAL AGE   Regardless of the species studied, the relationship between the PEP and gestational age of the fetus has been consistent. Human fetuses either antepartum[78,82,83] or intrapartum,[16] and monkey[84] and sheep fetuses,[81,85] revealed a lengthening of the PEP associated with advancing gestational age. Murata et al demonstrated that this physiologic lengthening of the PEP was due to a concurrent increase in the QRS duration secondary to an increase in the myocardial volume associated with advancing gestational age of monkey fetuses.[84] Organ et al[82] subsequently confirmed this finding in human fetuses.

There has been no significant relationship observed between the VET and gestational age of either the human[16,83] or the monkey fetus.[86]

FETAL HEART RATE   The relationship between the PEP and FHR has been somewhat controversial. In infants, children, and adults, reports indicate a shortening of the PEP associated with increasing heart rate, a relationships that has been reported in the fetus, as well.[87,88] Other studies, however,[16,78,84,89] failed to demonstrate a direct relationship between the PEP and FHR either in human or primate fetuses. The latter findings are consistent with the observation that heart rate changed by vagal stimulation or cardiac pacing did not alter the PEP in adult humans.[90]

Murata and coworkers demonstrated that this relationship between the PEP and FHR does not exist in fetal monkeys under physiologic conditions. The authors did, however, demonstrate this relationship when the fetus was receiving an intravenous infusion of epinephrine.[84]

Based on these findings, it appears that adrenergic stimulation, having chronotropic and inotropic stimulation at the same time, increases both FHR and myocardial contractility, thus shortening the PEP.[91]

The inverse correlation between the VET and FHR has been repeatedly demonstrated in adults, infants, and fetuses of various species. As FHR decreases from 180 beats per minute to 115 beats per minute in the human fetus,[16] and from 250 to 150 in the monkey fetus,[86] the VET lengthens in a linear fashion. No further lengthening was observed thereafter in either species.

PRELOAD   An inverse correlation between the PEP and the left ventricular end-diastolic pressure (LVEDP) was demonstrated in a monkey fetus, indicating that an increase in preload enhances myocardial contractility and thus shortens the PEP following the Frank–Starling law.[73] Continuous observation of the PEP of the human antepartum fetus with supraventricular arrhythmia revealed a shortened PEP following a long R-R interval, which prolonged a diastolic phase to increase preload. Conversely, a short R-R interval was followed by a prolonged PEP.[92,93] Similar phenomena were also seen in intrapartum human fetuses showing FHR arrhythmia.[94]

BLOOD PRESSURE   An increase in diastolic pressure lengthens the PEP by requiring more time for the intraventricular pressure to exceed intraaortic pressure before the semilunar valve opens. This relationship was not associated with any changes in the EMLT and ICT.[84]

No significant relationship has been found between the PEP and pulse pressure under physiologic conditions. An inverse correlation, however, was demonstrated in one distressed monkey fetus that exhibited a wide range of pulse pressures (Fig. 43.10).[84]

CORONARY BLOOD FLOW   An inverse correlation was found between coronary blood flow (mL/kg/beat) and the PEP under physiologic conditions in chronically instrumented fetal lambs. The radioactive microsphere technique was used to determine coronary blood flow. This relationship, however, no longer existed when the fetuses were exposed to experimental stresses that produced fetal hypoxemia or hypercapnia.[81]

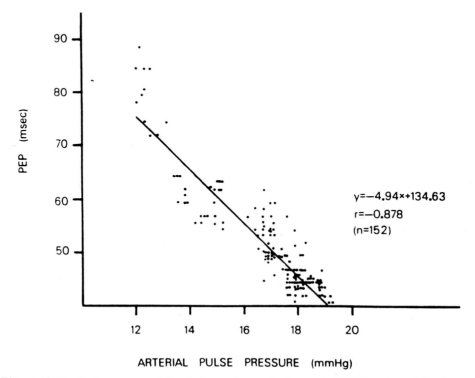

Figure 43.10   An inverse correlation between the preejection period (PEP) and arterial pulse pressure in a distressed monkey fetus. (From Murata et al.[84])

FETAL BREATHING MOVEMENTS AND DIURNAL VARIATION
No diurnal variation in the PEP or VET has been documented, but De Muylder et al[85] observed a shortening of the PEP in chronically instrumented fetal lambs, during the period of fetal breathing. Interestingly, these authors did not show any effects of fetal breathing activity per se on the PEP or VET.

Pathologic Responses

HYPOXIA   Conflicting results have been reported by different investigators on the behavior of the PEP during fetal hypoxia. Very likely the discrepancies reflect differences in the stages and/or degrees of hypoxia. Also, in some animal experiments, different conditions of the fetal preparation were used, either a stable condition without medication or an acute condition with considerable stress.

In early studies, Organ and his coworkers reported a shortening of the PEP when an exteriorized animal was exposed to an abrupt drop of P_{O_2} by making the mother breathe 100% N_2. The mother was intubated and was receiving anesthesia intravenously.[95] Subsequently, other investigators using laboratory animals[96,97] also reported a shortening of the PEP associated with fetal hypoxia. In human fetuses, although there was no consistent correlation observed between the PEP and fetal scalp blood pH or respiratory gases, Doig et al[98] observed a significantly shortened PEP in three very acidemic or hypoxic fetuses during labor.

Murata et al,[84] on the other hand, observed a further prolongation of PEP associated with combined acidemia and hypoxemia in rhesus monkey fetuses. They noted that acidemia alone produced a proportional prolongation of the PEP. Prolongation of the PEP in one antepartum fetus that did not survive was also reported by Organ and his coworkers.[82]

These observations suggest that the PEP shortens during the acute phase of hypoxia primarily as a result of the adrenal medullary secretion of catecholamines. When hypoxia becomes more severe, hypoxic depression of the myocardium overrides the catecholamine effects and thus the PEP becomes prolonged. This has been elegantly elucidated by an experiment performed by Fouron et al.[99] These investigators observed a shortening of the PEP due to changes in the ICT at the onset of hypoxemia. When acidemia was induced, the PEP slowly lengthened, initially because of a prolongation of the EMLT and later because of an increase in the already shortened ICT. This process developed slowly, and at the end of 2 hours of acidemia the PEP returned to preexperimental values. The authors concluded that STI can be normal and misleading when acidosis complicates hypoxemia.

Both hypoxemia and combined hypoxemia and acidemia shortened the VET, which was corrected for the R-R interval.[86]

ACIDEMIA   Murata et al[84] demonstrated a significant inverse correlation between the PEP and fetal arterial pH observed in chronically instrumented fetal monkeys (Fig. 43.11). The prolongation of PEP was not different whether the decrease of pH was of metabolic or respiratory origin. The prolongation of the PEP also appeared to be accompanied by the prolongation of both ICT and EMLT, indicating that two separate factors are responsible for the PEP prolongation: depression of myocardial contractility and a delay between electrical activation and the onset of mechanical contraction. Similar results were obtained from different species of laboratory animals.[81,100]

Bärtling and Klöck[101] compared the PEP with scalp blood pH from intrapartum human fetuses. They observed that normal pH (>7.3) was associated with a PEP between 65 and 80 ms. A decrease in pH in a linear fashion was accompanied by PEP values of less than 65 ms or more than 80 ms. These authors also failed to demonstrate any relationship between the PEP and base excess in fetal scalp blood.

More recently, Fouron also observed prolongation of the PEP when acidosis was experimentally induced in fetal lambs.[99] Under their experimental conditions, the STIs can be normal and misleading when acidosis complicates hypoxemia, since hypoxemia per se shortens the PEP.

Acidemia per se did not consistently affect the VET, but the combination of acidemia and hypoxemia was associated with a shortening of the VET corrected for FHR.[86]

OTHER STRESSES   A transient prolongation of the PEP and PEP/VET ratio was noted by De Muylder et al[102] during a recovery period of 2–3 days after the surgery to create the chronically instrumented fetal lambs. The prolongation of the PEP and PEP/VET was observed despite normal arterial pH of the fetus.

In another study, maternal alcohol intoxication was associated with a prolongation of both PEP And PEP/VET ratio.[100] The authors speculated that direct deleterious effects of alcohol on myocardial fibers were responsible for these changes.

In one fetus with supraventricular tachycardia, Schlotter and coworkers observed a prolonged PEP and total systole. This fetus became acidotic during delivery, but survived the perinatal period. The child, however, died from congestive heart failure at 2 years of age.[103]

Using M-mode echocardiography, Sørensen and Børlum measured the right and left VETs separately while the mothers were experiencing moderate exercise. No significant alterations in the fetal VETs due to maternal moderate exercise were demonstrated.[104]

Clinical Application of STIs

Antepartum Fetuses

NORMAL FETUSES   As described earlier, gestational age of the fetus is one of the important factors that changes the PEP. The PEP obtained from the normal antepartum fetus at term

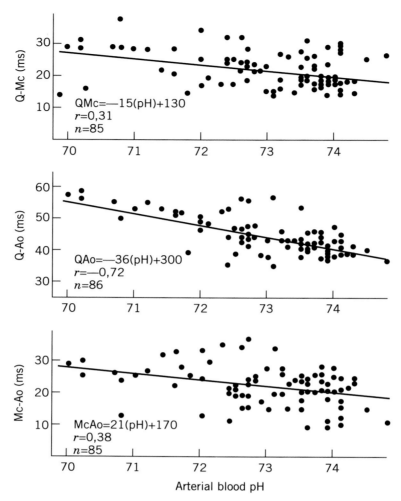

Figure 43.11 Correlation between systolic time intervals and arterial pH in rhesus monkey fetuses: electromechanical latent time (Q-Mc), preejection period (Q-Ao), and isovolumetric contraction time (Mc-Ao). (From Murata et al.[84])

ranges between 60 and 80 ms, depending on the investigators. Figure 43.12 shows the values reported by Murata et al from normal antepartum human fetuses of gestational ages 33–42 weeks. The normal range of the PEP was expressed as the 5th and 95th percentiles obtained.[73] The same investigators reported that antepartum PEP was approximately 9.5% shorter than intrapartum PEP at equivalent gestational age. Similar findings were obtained by comparing the PEP before and after contraction stress testing (CST) of the FHR. The difference was 9.1%, the PEP before the CST without significant uterine activities being shorter than that after the CST.

Organ and his associates,[82] considering the physiologic effects of FHR and gestational age on the PEP, proposed the use of the PEP140, 40 which normalizes PEP values to a standard FHR of 140 beats per minute and a gestational age of 40 weeks. The reported value of the PEP140, 40 from 95 normal antepartum fetuses was 72.9 ± 2.8 ms.

Using M-mode echocardiography, Sørensen and Børlum[104] measured the right and left VETs separately in normal antepartum fetuses between 18 and 36 weeks of gestation. Normal values of the right and left VETs were reported to be 159 ms, with a range of 142–287 ms, and 147 ms with a range of 140–169 ms, respectively.

PREDICTION OF FETAL WELL-BEING Murata et al[73] observed a significant association of abnormal outcome of an infant with prolonged PEP obtained within a week prior to delivery. A markedly prolonged PEP associated with hydrops fetalis at 27 weeks of gestation was reported by Kleinman and Donnerstein.[80]

Organ et al,[82] on the other hand, reported eight cases of shortened and four cases of normal PEP140, 40 among 13 fetuses whose subsequent perinatal courses were abnormal. One instance of a prolonged PEP140, 40 resulted in a neona-

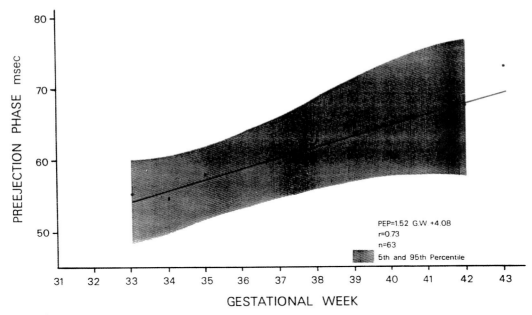

Figure 43.12   Normal range of the preejection period defined by the 5th and 95th percentiles from antepartum human fetuses between 33 and 42 weeks of gestation. (From Murata et al.[73])

tal death. Although Sampson failed to demonstrate any significant relationship between the PEP and maternal plasma unconjugated estriol level,[88] the author reported on one fetus with a shortened PEP associated with subsequent fetal asphyxia.

As discussed earlier, the definition of fetal outcome as either normal or abnormal is difficult and was not uniform among the investigators cited above. This statement applies particularly to retrospective observations in which the outcome of the fetus may have been altered or obscured by various aspects of clinical management. Abnormal PEP either shortened or prolonged, appeared to be associated with abnormal conditions of the fetus. Alteration of PEP may depend on the timing of PEP determination relative to developmental stage and/or degree of the stress the fetus is experiencing.

Thus far there are no studies published dealing with antepartum VET as a potential indicator of fetal well-being.

Intrapartum Fetuses

NORMAL FETUSES   During the intrapartum period after rupture of the amniotic membranes, FECG can be obtained by means of scalp electrodes, and the STIs can be determined. The published values of PEP determined during labor from normal term fetuses range from 70.0 to 74.0 ms among the different investigators. Table 43.5 presents the normal values of the STIs reported by different investigators.[16,98,101,105,106] Of interest, Doig et al[98] measured the PEP, ICT, and LVET during and between uterine contractions at different phases of labor: latent, active, and second stage. They demonstrated no significant differences among the values obtained during the different phases of labor or in relation to uterine contractions.

CORRELATION WITH FHR PATTERNS   In the history of perinatal medicine, the fetal heart rate pattern has been one of the

TABLE 43.5   Normal Values of Systolic Time Intervals

	Intervals (ms)		
Ref: First Author (year)	EMLT	ICT	PEP
Organ[105] (1973)			73.0 (10.0)
Murata[16] (1974)	41.3 (3.3)	29.4 (5.6)	70.0 (2.4)
Bärtling[101] (1979)			72.0 (7.9)
Doig[98] (1982)	41.6 (8.5)		76.0 (9.9)
Lewinsky[106] (1994)	44 (4.1)		73 (5.5)

most extensively studied parameters for the understanding of fetal physiology. Comparative studies of FHR patterns and STIs, therefore, have contributed significantly to understanding of the pathophysiologic changes of the systolic time intervals that appear concurrently with FHR changes of known etiology.

1. *Accelerations* Transient acceleration of the FHR was not associated with any consistent change in the PEP.[16,89] However, Hawrylyshyn and his coworkers[93] observed a prolongation of the PEP due to FHR accelerations associated with fetal movements. They attributed the prolongation of PEP to a prolongation in the ICT due to a delay in the semilunar valve opening.

2. *Early Decelerations* Organ et al[87] reported prolongation of PEP associated with early decelerations of FHR. In contrast, Hon,[107] using a similar method developed separately, demonstrated a lack of change in the PEP during early decelerations of FHR. This lack of PEP change may have been a result of limited resolution, but it could also be explained by noting that the PEP is not affected by heart rate changes caused by vagal stimulation, as demonstrated in 1967 by Harris et al.[90]

   The VET appeared to maintain its relationship with the FHR during early decelerations.[107]

3. *Variable Decelerations* Prolongation of the PEP during variable decelerations of FHR has been a consistent observation by most investigators.[95,107–108] During umbilical cord occlusion, which has been thought to be a major cause of variable deceleration of FHR, the preload decreases because the venous return through the umbilical vein has decreased, and the afterload increases because resistance of the umbilical artery has increased. Both decreased preload and increased afterload serve to prolong the PEP.

   Evers observed a two-step increase in the PEP during a variable deceleration.[97] The author attributed the first PEP prolongation, occurring at the onset of the umbilical occlusion, to the decrease in preload and the increase in afterload. The second rise in the PEP, according to Evers, may be due to fetal hypoxia caused by persistent occlusion of the cord, reflecting a chemoreceptor-induced reflex.

   Delay during umbilical cord occlusion in the closure and opening of the AV and semilunar valves, respectively, is responsible for prolonging the PEP during variable deceleration of FHR, according to Hawrylyshin et al.[93]

4. *Late Decelerations* Since the etiology of late deceleration has been considered to be hypoxia, the behavior of the PEP during late deceleration is similar to that during hypoxia as already described. Murata and Mar-

tin[16] observed prolongation of the PEP fetuses with mild to moderate late deceleration during labor. In one report, Organ et al[87] described a shortening of the PEP associated with late deceleration. Later, however, they noted two different types of PEP response, depending on whether fetal hypoxia was acute or chronic. Shortening of the PEP was seen in acute hypoxia, during which fetal myocardial contractility was enhanced by catecholamine surge. During chronic hypoxia, catecholamines became ineffective, increasing myocardial contractility and resulting in a prolongation of the PEP.[82]

PREDICTION OF FETAL OUTCOME Lewinsky[106] determined the PEP, PEP/VET ratio, and ICT on 89 intrapartum fetuses showing FHR patterns suggestive of fetal distress and subsequently being delivered by cesarean section. According to their retrospective analysis on the 89 fetuses, 25 asphyxiated fetuses, defined by umbilical artery pH less than 7.2 and/or 5-minute Apgar score less than 7, revealed significantly elevated values of the PEP, PEP/VET ratio, and ICT, on comparison with the remaining fetuses, characterized by a normal outcome. The authors concluded that PEP/VET ratio was the best parameter for the prediction of fetal outcome, with a positive predictive value of 100% and a negative predictive value of 98.4%.

SUMMARY

In the modern practice of perinatal medicine, the importance of surveillance of fetal well-being throughout pregnancy cannot be overemphasized. Electronic fetal heart rate monitoring has been mainstay of fetal surveillance. Yet the contribution of FHR monitoring, particularly that during intrapartum, is currently being questioned. FHR monitoring was not thoroughly tested prior to its widespread clinical application, and we are now forced either to reestablish its clinical value or to develop new methodology that supplements or replaces it.

As this chapter indicates, thus far a majority of the published reports appear to support the conclusion that both FECG and STI are excellent parameters, reflecting ongoing fetal cardiovascular pathophysiology. Besides the technical difficulties that remain to be overcome, both FECG and STI must undergo properly controlled, large-scale prospective studies to test their abilities to improve perinatal mortality and morbidity.

REFERENCES

1. Haverkamp A, Thompson H, McFee J, Cetrulo C. The evaluation of continuous fetal heart rate monitoring in high risk pregnancy. *Am J Obstet Gynecol* 1976;125:310–320.

2. Haverkamp A, Orleans M, Langerdoerefer S. A controlled trial of the differential effects of intrapartum fetal monitoring. *Am J Obstet Gynecol* 1979;134:399–412.

3. Wood C, Renou P, Oats J. A controlled trial of fetal heart rate monitoring in a low risk obstetric population. *Am J Obstet Gynecol* 1981;141:527–534.

4. MacDonald D, Grant A, Sheridan-Pereira M, Boylan P, Chalmers I. The Dublin randomized controlled trial of intrapartum fetal heart monitoring. *Am J Obstet Gynecol* 1985;152:524–539.

5. Cremer M. Über die direkte Ableitung der Akionstrome des menschlichen Herzens vom Oesophagus und über das Elektrokardiogramm des Fötus. *Munchener Mediz Wochensch* 1906;53:811–813.

6. Hunter C, Lansford K, Knoebel S, Braunlin R. A technique for recording fetal ECG during labour and delivery. *Obstet Gynecol* 1960;16:567–570.

7. Hon E. Instrumentation of fetal heart rate and fetal electrocardiography. II. A vaginal electrode. *Am J Obstet Gynecol* 1963;86:772–784.

8. Figueroa-Longo J, Poseiro J, Alvarez L, Caldero-Garcia R. Fetal electrocardiogram at term labor obtained with subcutaneous fetal electrodes. *Am J Obstet Gynecol* 1966;96:556–564.

9. Randall N, Steer P. Detection of the fetal ECG during labour by an intrauterine probe. *J Biomed Eng.* 1988;10:159–164.

10. Hon E, Lee S. The fetal electrocardiogram. I. The electrocardiogram of the dying fetus. *Am J Obstet Gynecol* 1963;87:804–813.

11. Pardi G, Uderzo A, Tucci E, Arata G. In: Crosignani P, Pardi, G, eds. *Fetal Evaluation During Pregnancy and Labor. Experimental and Clinical Aspects.* New York: Academic Press; 1971.

12. Pardi G, Tucci E, Uderzo A, Zanini D. Fetal electrocardiogram changes in relation to fetal heart rate patterns during labour. *Am J Obstet Gynecol* 1974;118:243–250.

13. Rosen K, Hrbek A, Karlsson K, Kjellmer I, Olsson T, Riha M. Changes in the ECG and somato-sensory evoked EEG responses (SER) during intrauterine asphyxia in the sheep. *Biol Neonate* 1976;30:95–101.

14. Greene K, Dawes G, Lilja H, Rosen K. Changes in the ST waveform of the fetal lamb electrocardiogram with hypoxaemia. *Am J Obstet Gynecol* 1982;144:950–958.

15. Murray HG. The intropartum fetal electrocardiogram—a study of time intervals. In *Fetal and Neonatal Physiology Measurements III.* (Gennser G, Marsal K, Svenningsen N, and Lindstrom K, eds.) Department of Obstetrics and Gynaecology; Malmo, Sweden, 1989; 133–138.

16. Murata Y, Martin CJ. Systolic time intervals of the fetal cardiac cycle. *Obstet Gynecol* 1974;44:224–232.

17. Maekawa M, Toyoshima J. The fetal electrocardiogram of the human subject. *Acta School Med Univ Kyoto* 1938;12:519.

18. Strassman E, Mussey R. Technic and results of routine fetal electrocardiography during pregnancy. *Am J Obstet Gynecol* 1938;36:986.

19. Ward J, Kennedy J. The recording of the fetal electrocardiogram. *Am Heart J* 1942;23:64.

20. Abboud S, Becker A. An improved detection algorithm in fetal electrocardiography. *J Electrocardiogr* 1989;22(suppl):238–242.

21. Hon E, Lee S. Noise reduction in fetal electrocardiography. II. Averaging techniques. *Am J Obstet Gynecol* 1963;87:1086–1096.

22. Lindecrantz K, Lilja H, Widmark C, Rosen K. Fetal ECG during labour: a suggested standard. *J Biomed Eng* 1988;10:351–353.

23. Lilja H, Greene, K, Karlsson K, Rosen K. ST waveform changes of the fetal electrocardiogram during labour—a clinical study. *Br J Obstet Gynaecol* 1985;92:611–619.

24. D'Souza S, Black P, MacFarlane T. Fetal scalp damage and neonatal jaundice: a risk of routine fetal scalp electrode monitoring. *J Obstet Gynecol* 1982;2:161–164.

25. Sharp D, Couriel J. Penetration of the subarachnoid space by fetal scalp electrode. *Br Med J* 1985;291:1169.

26. Jonkhof-Slok T, Weyerman M. Scalp electrode associated neonatal *Escherichia coli* meningitis—a case report. *J Perinatol Med* 1991;19:217–219.

27. Okada D, Chow A, Bruce V. Neonatal scalp abscess and fetal monitoring: factors associated with infections. *Am J Obstet Gynecol* 1977;129:185.

28. Amann S, Fagnant R, Chartrand S, Monif G. Herpes simplex infection associated with short-term use of fetal scalp electrode—A case report. *J Reprod Med* 1992;37:372–374.

29. Rosen K. Alterations in the fetal electrocardiogram as a sign of fetal asphyxia—experimental data with a clinical implementation. *J Perinatol Med* 1986;14:355–363.

30. Symonds E. Vectorcardiography and acid–base balance in the human fetus. *Br J Obstet Gynaecol* 1972;79:416–423.

31. Arulkumaran S, Nicolini U, Fisk N, Tannirandorn Y, Rosen K, Rodeck C. Direct antenatal fetal electrocardiographic waveform analysis. *Br J Obstet Gynaecol* 1991;98:829–831.

32. Greene K. The ECG waveform. *Baillieres Clin Obstet Gynaecol* 1987;1:131–155.

33. Hon E, Hess O. The clinical value of fetal electrocardiography. *Am J Obstet Gynecol* 1960;79:1012–1023.

34. Berson A, Pipberger H. The low frequency response of electrocardiographs, a frequent source of recording error. *Am Heart J* 1960;71:770–789.

35. Hon E. A fetal electrocardiographic electrode. *Yale J Biol Med* 1966;39:54–58.

36. Mayes B, Bradfield A, Smyth E. Clinical experience in foetal electrocardiography. *Med J Aust* 1963;22:905.

37. Thaler I, Timor I, Goldberg I. Interpretation of the fetal ECG during labor: the effect of uterine contractions. *J Perinatol Med* 1988;16:373–379.

38. Jenkins H, Symonds E, Kirk D, Smith P. Can fetal electrocardiography improve the prediction of intrapartum fetal acidosis? *Br J. Obstet Gynaecol* 1986;93:6–12.

39. Marvell C, Kirk D, Jenkins H, Symonds E. The normal condition of the fetal electrocardiogram during labour. *Br J Obstet Gynaecol* 1980;87:786–796.

40. Murray H. The fetal electrocardiogram: current clinical developments in Nottingham. *J Perinatol Med* 1986;14:399–404.

41. Nobel D, Cohen I. The interpretation of the T wave of the electrocardiogram. *Cardiovasc Res* 1978;12:13.

42. Rosen K. Dagbjarsson A, Henriksson B, Langercrantz H, Kjellmer I. The relationship between circulating catecholamines and ST waveform in the fetal lamb electrocardiogram during hypoxia. *Am J Obstet Gynecol* 1984;149:190–195.

43. Myers R. Two patterns of perinatal brain damage and their condition of occurrence. *Am J Obstet Gynecol* 1972;112:246.

44. Rosen K, Hökegard K, Kjellmer I. A study of the relationship between the electrocardiogram and hemodynamics in the fetal lamb during asphyxia. *Acta Physiol Scand* 1976;98:275.

45. Rosen K, Isaksson O. Alterations in fetal heart rate and ECG correlated to glycogen, creatine phosphate and ATP levels during graded hypoxia. *Biol Neonatorum* 1976;30:17–24.

46. Hökegard K, Kjellmer I, Rosen K. ECG changes in the fetal lamb during asphyxia in relation to beta-adrenoreceptor stimulation and blockade. *Acta Physiol Scand* 1979;105:195–203.

47. Hökegard K, Eriksson B, Kjellmer I, Magno R, Rosen K. Alterations in myocardial metabolism in relation to electrocardiographic changes and cardiovascular functions during graded hypoxia in fetal lamb. *Acta Physiol Scand* 1981;113:1–7.

48. Dawes G, Mott J, Shelley J. The importance of cardiac glycogen for the maintenance of life in foetal lambs and newborne animals during anoxia. *J Physiol (London)* 1959;146:516–538.

49. Dijxhoorn M, Visser G, Fidler V, Touwen B, Huisjen H. Apgar score, meconium and acidemia at birth in relation to neonatal neurological morbidity in term infants. *Br J Obstet Gynaecol* 1986;93:217–222.

50. Steer P, Eigbe F, Lissauer T, Beard R. Interrelationships among abnormal cardiotocogram in labour, meconium staining of the amniotic fluid, arterial cord blood pH, and Apgar scores. *Obstet Gynecol* 1989;74:715–721.

51. Winkler C, Hauth J, Tucker J, Owen J, Brumfield C. Neonatal complications at term as related to the degree of umbilical artery acidaemia. *Am J Obstet Gynecol* 1991;164:637–641.

52. Levene M, Sands C, Grindulis H, Moore J. Comparison of two methods of predicting outcome in perinatal asphyxia. *Lancet* 1986;ii:67–68.

53. Gilstrap L, Leveno K, Burris J, Williams M, Little B. Diagnosis of birth asphyxia on the basis of fetal pH, Apgar score and newborn cerebral dysfunction. *Am J Obstet Gynecol* 1989;161:825–830.

54. Westgate J, Harris M, Curnow J, Greene K. Randomized trial of cardiotocography alone or with ST waveform analysis for intrapartum monitoring. *Lancet* 1992;340:194–198.

55. Murphy KW, Russell VP, Johnson P, Valeute J. Clinical assessment of fetal electrocardiogram monitoring during labour. *Br J Obstet Gynaecol* 1992;99:32–37.

56. Lilja H, Aruklumaran S, Lindecrantz K, Ratnam S, Rosen K. Fetal ECG during labour: a presentation of a microprocessor system. *J Biomed Eng* 1988;10:348–350.

57. Cockburn J, Pearch J, Chamberlain C. Intrapartum fetal monitoring. *Lancet* 1992;340:610.

58. Rosen K. Model of clinical interpretation of ST waveform changes. *Fetal ECG Res News* 1990;1:27.

59. Kirk D, Smith P. Techniques for the routine on-line processing of the fetal electrocardiogram. *J Perinat Med* 1986;14:391–397.

60. Newbold S, Wheeler T, Clewlow F. Comparison of the T/QRS ratio of the fetal electrocardiogram and the fetal heart rate during labour and the relationship of these variables to condition at delivery. *Br J Obstet Gynaecol* 1991;98:173–178.

61. Newbold S, Wheeler T, Clewlow F, Soul F. Variation in the T/QRS ratio of fetal electrocardiograms recorded during labour in normal subjects. *Br J Obstet Gynaecol* 1989;96:144–150.

62. Lilja H, Karlsson K. Lindecrantz K, Rosen K. Microprocessor-based waveform analysis of the fetal electrocardiogram during labor. *J Gynecol Obstet* 1988;30:109–116.

63. Maclachlan N, Spencer J, Harding K, Arulkumaran S. Fetal acidaemia, the cardiotocograph and the T/QRS ratio of the fetal ECG in labour. *Br J Obstet Gynaecol* 1992;99:26–31.

64. Newbold S, Clewlow F, Wheeler T. The effect of uterine contractions on the T/QRS ratio of the fetal ECG. Presented at Fourth International Conference on Fetal and Neonatal Physiological Measurements. Noordwijkerhout; 1991.

65. Rosen K, Arulkumaran S, Thavarasah A. ST waveform analysis of the fetal ECG during labor—initial report of the STAN Multicenter Trial. In *Fetel and Neonatal Physiology Measurements III.* (Gennser G, Marsal K, Svenningsen N, and Linstrom K, eds) Department of Obstetrics and Gynaecology; Malmo, Sweden. 1989; 177–183.

66. Johanson R, Rice C, Shoker A. ST-waveform analysis of the fetal electrocardiogram could reduce fetal blood sampling. *Br J Obstet Gynaecol* 1992;99:167–168.

67. Arulkumaran S, Lilja H, Lindecrantz K. Fetal ECG waveform analysis should improve fetal surveillance in labour. *J Perinatol Med* 1990;18:13–22.

68. Greene K, Westgate J. Fetal ECG waveform for intrapartum monitoring. *Lancet* 1992;340:1171.

69. Persianinov L, Illyin I, Karpman V, Saveliera G. The dynamics of fetal cardiac activity. *Am J Obstet Gynecol* 1966;94:367–377.

70. Weissler A, Peeler R, Rochll WI, Durham N. Relationship between left ventricular ejection time, stroke volume and heart rate in normal individuals and patients with cardiovascular disease. *Am Heart J* 1961;62:367–371.

71. Letherman J, Parchman M, Lawler F. Infection of fetal scalp electrode monitoring sites. *Am Fam Physician* 1992;45:579–582.

72. McGregor J, McFarren T. Neonatal cranial osteomyelitis: a complication of fetal monitoring. *Obstet Gynecol* 1989;73:490–492.

73. Murata Y, Martin CJ, Ikenoue T, Lu P. Antepartum evaluation of the pre-ejection period of the fetal cardiac cycle. *Am J Obstet Gynecol* 1978;132:278–284.

74. Goodlin R, Girard J, Holman A. Systolic time intervals in the fetus and neonate. *Obstet Gynecol* 1972;39:295–301.

75. Murata Y, Takemura H, Mochizuki S, Kurachi K. The phase and frequency analysis of fetal and placental Doppler signals by ultrasound. *Med Ultrasound* 1970;8:1–16.

76. Murata Y, Takemura H, Kurachi K. Observation of fetal cardiac motion by M-mode ultrasound cardiography. *Am J Obstet Gynecol* 1972;111:287–294.

77. De Muylder X, Fouron J, Bard H, Riopel L, Urfer F. The difference between the systolic time interval of the left and right ventricles during fetal life. *Am J Obstet Gynecol* 1984;149:737–740.

78. Giorlandino C, Gentili P, Vizzone A, Rizzo G, Arduini D. A new method for the measurement of pre-ejection period in the human fetus. *Br J Obstet Gynaecol* 1986;93:307–309.

79. DeVore G, Donnerstein R, Kleinman C, Hobbins J. Real-time-directed M-mode echocardiography: a new technique for accurate and rapid quantitation of the fetal preejecton period and ventricular ejection time of the right and left ventricles. *Am J Obstet Gynecol* 1981;141:470–471.

80. Kleinman C, Donnerstein R. Ultrasonic assessment of cardiac function in the intact human fetus. *J Am College Cardiol* 1985;5:84S–94S.

81. Murata Y, Miyake K, Quilligan E. Preejection period of cardiac cycle in fetal lamb. *Am J Obstet Gynecol* 1979;133:509–514.

82. Organ LW, Bernstein A, Hawrylyshyn PA. The pre-ejection period as an antepartum indicator of fetal well-being. *Am J Obstet Gynecol* 1980;137:810–819.

83. Wolfson R, Sador I, Pillay S, Timor-Tritsch J, Herz R. Antenatal investigation of human fetal systolic time intervals. *Am J Obstet Gynecol* 1977;129:103–107.

84. Murata Y, Martin CJ, Ikenoue T, Petrie R. Cardiac systolic time intervals in fetal monkeys: pre-ejection period. *Am J Obstet Gynecol* 1978;132:285–293.

85. De Muylder X, Fouron J, Bard H, Lafond J. Physiologic modulations of the systolic time intervals in fetal lamb. *Can J Physiol Pharmacol* 1985;63:893–897.

86. Murata Y, Martin CJ, Ikenoue T, Petrie R. Cardiac systolic time intervals in fetal monkeys: ventricular ejection time. *Am J Obstet Gynecol* 1980;136:603–608.

87. Organ L, Bernstein A, and Smith K. The prejection period of the fetal heart: pattern of changes during labor. *Am J Obstet Gynecol* 1974;120:49–55.

88. Sampson M. Antepartum measurement of the preejection period in high-risk pregnancy. *Obstet Gynecol* 1980;56:289–295.

89. Robinson H, Adam A, Flemming J, Houston A. A fetal electromechanical intervals in labor. *Br J Obstet Gynaecol* 1978;85:172–716.

90. Harris W, Schoenfeld C, Wissler A. The effect of adrenergic receptor activation and blockade on the systolic pre-ejection period, heart rate and arterial pressure in man. *J Clin Invest* 1967;46:1704–1712.

91. Tally R, Meyer J, McNay J. Evaluation of the pre-ejection period as an estimate of myocardial contractility in dogs. *Am J Cardiol* 1971;27:384–391.

92. Murata Y, Pijls N, Miyake K, Schmidt P, Martin CJ, Singer J. Antepartum determination of the pre-ejection period of fetal

cardiac cycle: its relation to newborn body weight. *Am J Obstet Gynecol* 1979;133:515–518.

93. Hawrylyshyn PA, Organ LW, Bernstein A. A new computer technique for continuous measurement of the pre-ejection period in the human fetus: physiologic significance or pre-ejection period patterns. *Am J Obstet Gynecol* 1980;137:801–809.

94. Smith, GC, Fleming JE, Whitfield CR. Post-extrasystolic potentiation in a human fetus detected during measurement of systolic time intervals in labour. *Eur J Obstet Gynecol Reprod Biol* 1990;37:205–210.

95. Organ L, Milligan J, Goodwin J, Bain M. The preejection period of the fetal heart: response to stress in the term fetal lamb. *Am J Obstet Gynecol* 1973;115:377–385.

96. Morgenstern J, Czerny H, Schmidt H, Schulz J, Wernicke K. Systolic time intervals of the fetal cardiac cycle. *J Perinatol Med* 1978;6:173–196.

97. Evers JL. Cardiac pre-ejection period during prenatal life. *Gynecol Obstet Invest* 1980;11:193–213.

98. Doig J, Adam A, Flemming J, Whitfield C. Fetal cardiac electromechanical intervals during labour and effects of hypoxia and cord compression. *Br J Obstet Gynaecol* 1982;89:145–148.

99. Fouron JC, Lafond JS, Bard H. Effects of hypoxemia with and without acidemia on the isometric contraction time and the electromechanical delay of the fetal myocardium: an experimental study on the ovine fetus. *Am J Obstet Gynecol* 1990;162:262–266.

100. Lafaond J, Fouron J, Bard H, Urfer F. Changes in the systolic time intervals of the fetal heart after surgical manipulation of the fetus. *Am J Obstet Gynecol* 1983;147:285–288.

101. Bärtling T, Klöck F. Die pre-ejektion Periode des menschelichen fetalen Herzens. Bedeutung des base-line Schwankung in der pernatal Periode. *Z Geburtshilfe Perinat* 1979;183:202–211.

102. De Muylder X, Fouron JC, Bard H, Urfer FN. Changes in the systolic time intervals of the fetal heart after surgical manipulation of the fetus. *Am J Obstet Gynecol* 1983;147:285–288.

103. Schlotter CM. Antepartum noninvasive evaluation of persistent fetal cardiac arrhythmias (author's transl). *Geburtshilfe Frauenheilkd* 1981;41:32–35.

104. Sørenson K, Børlum K. Fetal heart function in response to short-term maternal exercise. *Br J Obstet Gynaecol* 1986;93:310–313.

105. Organ L, Bernstein A, Rowe I. The preejection period of the fetal heart. *Am J Obstet Gynecol* 1973;115:369–373.

106. Lewinsky RM. Cardiac systolic time intervals and other parameters of mycardial contractility as indices of fetal acid–base status. *Baillieres Clin Obstet Gynaecol* 1994;8:663–681.

107. Hon E, Murata Y, Zanini D, Martin CJ, Lewis D. Continuous microfilm display of the electromechanical intervals of the cardiac cycle. *Obstet Gynecol* 1974;43:722–728.

108. Bärtling T, Klöck F, Courtin E. Ein neues Verfahren sur online Registrerung der pre-ejektion Periode des menschenlichen fetalen Herzens parallel zum CTG. *Z Gebrutshilfe Perinat* 1978;169:182–186.

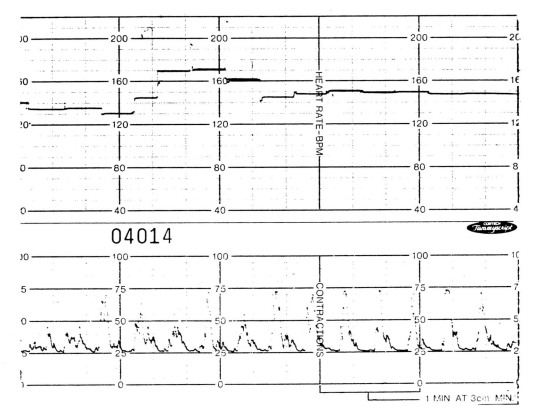

Figure 44.1 External fetal monitoring (Roche-Fetasonde): beat-to-beat variability (upper panel) and M-shaped complexes representing ultrasonic recognition of a moving fetal cardiac structure, most likely a mitral valve (lower panel).

A prerequisite for an *internal* ECG is rupture of the membranes. Consequently, a scalp electrode cannot and will not be attached to the fetus when rupture of membranes is medically contraindicated. In such instances, an abdominal ECG (not to be confused with *external* fetal monitoring based on the detection of cardiac motion by ultrasound) can be obtained. Both maternal and fetal ECGs will then be recorded on the same tracing. With appropriate axis conditions of the fetal heart, a fetal ECG tracing of adequate quality will be obtained (as a single lead) and can be differentiated from maternal ECG components. This technique, though rarely used in clinical practice, has been utilized by a number of investigators (Fig. 44.2).

The physical theory of the intrauterine ECG is discussed in detail in Chapter 2. *This* chapter, which demonstrates how a fetal ECG may be used as a tool in the diagnosis and therapy of intrauterine dysrhythmias. It also reviews the emergence of fetal echocardiography as the primary tool for the diagnosis and evaluation of fetal arrhythmias. Other noninvasive diagnostic modalities such as phonocardiography may add to the diagnosis.

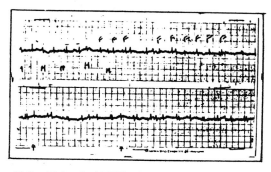

Figure 44.2 Abdominal ECG taken at 20 weeks of gestation because of irregular fetal heart rate. Upper tracing identifies the fetal complexes (M). Lower tracing indicates two premature systoles (arrows) with partial compensatory pauses. The relatively normal appearance of the QRS complex indicates a supraventricular origin. (Reproduced from Shenker,[1] with permission of Williams & Wilkins.)

The Fetal Echocardiogram

During the last decade, experience with fetal echocardiography expanded dramatically, and the procedure is now recommended in cases of suspected fetal arrhythmias. This has come about because of problems in obtaining a fetal ECG. Cameron et al[3] have suggested that the use of a fetal ECG is severely limited with current techniques and that such records are especially difficult to obtain between 28 and 34 weeks, when many arrhythmias are discovered. The authors of an earlier study felt that before the advent of fetal echocardiography, arrhythmias in the human fetus could be classified only by rhythm (*regular* or *irregular*) and rate (*bradycardia* or *tachycardia*), since only ventricular systole could be recorded, whether by electrical or mechanical means. Kleinman et al[6] stated that because transabdominal fetal electrocardiograms cannot demonstrate atrial depolarization, this technique is of "unfortunately" limited value in the analysis of cardiac rhythm disturbances. They then, however, suggested that the fetal echocardiogram may be a source of information that is useful both diagnostically and therapeutically, since it provides information on heart rate, atrial–ventricular conduction, and cardiac structure. Even investigators who are willing to accept that a fetal ECG can identify the type of arrhythmia when recordings are of good quality point out that it is often impossible to record abdominal fetal ECG signals during the second half of pregnancy.

Most authors therefore have concluded that echocardiography is superior to intrauterine electrocardiography in diagnosing intrauterine dysrhythmias, since with intrauterine electrocardiography, even in the best cases, only the fetal QRS complexes can be clearly visualized.[2,4,5,7] In contrast, echocardiography permits a noninvasive and safe sequential definition of cardiac arrythmias in utero, as well as an assessment of the hemodynamic consequences; in addition, arrhythmias occurring during administration of transplacental medication can be followed up easily.[8]

The utilization of echocardiography has allowed the differentiating of many different arrhythmias.[2–4,9–11] Cross-sectional echocardiography also allows the identification of associated structural abnormalities.[2] Simultaneous M-mode recording of aortic, mitral, or tricuspid valvular leaflet excursion and/or atrioventricular wall motion defines timing relationships between atrial and ventricular systole.[5] Finally, pulse Doppler echocardiography has been found to be valuable in the quantification of hemodynamics during arrhythmias, the characterization of cardiac rhythm, and the identification of certain anomalies.[4,8,12] In 1990 Santulli[13] described a recommended approach to fetal echocardiography. Not only are many authorities[4,5,7,13] recommending cross-sectional imaging, M-mode, and Doppler studies for the accurate interpretation of arrhythmias, but some insist that it should be mandatory.[7]

THE DIAGNOSIS OF INTRAUTERINE ARRHYTHMIAS

It appears that the detection rate of intrauterine arrhythmias varies in proportion to the interest of physicians in the detection of these anomalies. Under study conditions in our teaching department at Mount Sinai Hospital in Chicago, short bursts of either tachy- or bradyarrhythmias were reported almost weekly on a labor floor with appropriately 3000 births per year. An incidence of one dysrhythmia per 50–100 patients in labor thus appears to represent a realistic estimate. Klapholz et al[14] reported, however, that in their experience arrhythmias occur in 3–5% of all births during labor.

Dysrhythmias often last only briefly; frequently, therefore, they are considered to be artifacts or are overlooked. At times, abnormalities of the fetal heart rate are recognized; however, the necessary follow-up with a fetal echocardiogram or ECG does not always occur, either because adequate equipment is not available or because the need for further follow-up is not recognized.

When, then, should additional studies be obtained to either rule out or confirm intrauterine fetal dysrhythmia? It was noted in Chapter 42 that the normal fetal heart rate changes with gestational age. At term, a normal heart rate lies between 120 and 160 beats per minute. Heart rates of more than 180 beats per minute should be considered suspicious for tachyarrhythmias; heart rates of less than 100 beats per minute should be viewed with suspicion until a bradyarrhythmia has been ruled out. A large number of fetal arrhythmias will be identified based on such a simple screening system; some will, however, be missed, since the heart rate may be within a normal range and still be arrhythmic or dysrhythmic. Further recognition of fetal heart rate or conduction abnormalities must rely on fetal echocardiograms or ECGs or, as built into some monitoring apparatus, beat-to-beat variability recording. Specific fetal abnormalities are discussed in more detail later. They are divided into the same subgroups as in the adult. Beat-to-beat monitoring is an unusual exercise in the adult and, therefore, it deserves some additional attention at this point.

The importance of beat-to-beat variability monitoring for the detection of intrauterine arrhythmias lies in its graphic representation of heart rate patterns that are difficult to recognize in fetal ECGs. Thus, short bursts of fetal tachyarrhythmias may be lost in regular ECG tracings. The beat-to-beat monitoring capability of some monitors, which is based on the summation of the fetal heart rate during three cardiac cycles, may still be recordable. Thus, even very short bursts of tachyarrhythmias may be recognized (Fig. 44.3).

A large variety of fetal monitors is commercially available. Just as every labor floor requires adequate internal monitoring capacity, so should internal ECG monitoring capacity be geared toward the number of deliveries on the service.

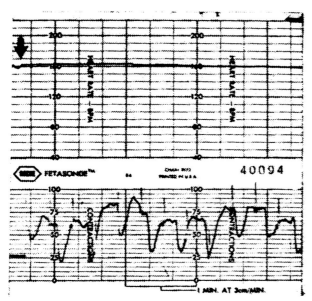

Figure 44.3 Intrapartum fetal monitoring (Roche-Fetalsonde) with scalp electrode (Corometrics) attached. Lower panel demonstrates a wandering baseline that may prevent, in certain instances, the appropriate recording of the fetal heart rate. Small QRS complexes representing the fetal ECG are demonstrable. Upper panel represents the recording of the fetal heart rate, which in this tracing is approximately 160 beats per minute (arrow). Note the straight line, which indicates no beat-to-beat variability, as otherwise a step-wise pattern would be seen.

For only minor additional costs most modern monitors with internal capability can be upgraded to give ECG output capacity. Not every internal monitor on the labor floor requires such an adjustment; however, a properly functioning monitor with ECG capability should always be available when the suspicion of a dysrhythmia arises during routine fetal heart rate monitoring. Also available should be fetal ultrasound equipment, with capability for real-time cross-sectional M-mode and Doppler scanning. Such equipment is necessary for the diagnosis of fetal arrhythmias that are undetected prior to the onset of labor. A fetal echocardiogram will also be able to define the existence of any cardiac anomalies that may be present concomitantly with a rate or rhythm disorder of the fetal heart.

SPECIFIC ARRHYTHMIAS

Brady Arrhythmias

Sinus Node Dysfunction

Sinus Bradycardia (Fig. 44.4)   In the adult, sinus bradycardia is defined as a slow but normal heart rate of less than 60 beats per minute with normal spread of the atrial excitation.

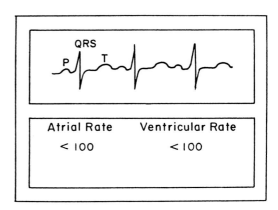

Figure 44.4   Sinus bradycardia.

With a normal fetal heart rate, defined as between 120 and 160 beats per minute, a diagnosis of sinus bradycardia is made under 100 beats per minute. This diagnosis requires, however, confirmation by means of demonstration that excitation is originating in the sinus node and is normal in its spread throughout the atrium.

As in the adult, sinus bradycardia is sometimes a sign of excellent physical fitness, as demonstrated by its frequent occurrence in athletes. In the fetus it is also a relatively benign finding. However, sinus bradycardia may reflect other pathological conditions. Therefore, fetal heart rate monitoring is used extensively for antepartum fetal evaluation. For more details, see Chapter 42.

Even in the adult, not all sinus bradycardias are benign. Sinus bradycardias may be manifestations of sinus node dysfunction, increased cerebral pressure, hypothyroidism, and hypothermia. Among known causes of sinus bradycardia in the fetus, the following have been reported in the literature: fetal head and umbilical cord compression, maternal hypotension, maternal seizures, maternal voiding, paracervical block anesthesia, and medication exposure to propranolol and reserpine.[1,15-18]

In the fetus, it is also necessary to differentiate between "short-term" fetal heart rate decelerations and "long-term" fetal bradycardia. Most clinicians classify fetal heart rate decelerations that last longer than one minute as *"bradycardia."* Since these "bradycardias" in fact, represent prolonged decelerations, they have to be differentiated from sinus bradycardias, which may last for hours and may have less ominous implications. Freeman et al,[19] however, suggested that for any fetal heart rate finding to be classified as a baseline change (i.e., tachycardia or bradycardia), it must last at least 15 minutes.

Whenever a prolonged fetal heart rate of less than 100 beats per minute is recognized by either external or internal fetal monitoring, it is important to obtain a fetal ECG and/or echocardiogram. The differential diagnosis of sinus bradycardia includes heart block and blocked atrial ectopic beats.[20] It also should always be remembered that a maternal ECG may be transmitted through the fetus (Chapter 46). Under such a circumstance, erroneous external or internal fetal monitoring can suggest persistent fetal sinus bradycardia (Fig. 47.5) when, in fact, the fetus is dead and the maternal ECG has been read as that of the fetus. A number of such instances have been reported in the literature and have, at times, presented the basis for legal action. The maternal heart rate, therefore, should be checked against the fetal heart rate when an apparent persistent fetal sinus bradycardia is recognized. Ideally, simultaneous maternal and fetal ECGs should be obtained to rule out maternal transmission through a dead fetus.

Sinoatrial Block   In this dysrhythmia, a sinus impulse is generated but neither atrial nor ventricular depolarization occurs because the sinus impulse is prevented from reaching either atrium or ventricle. In the fetus, sinoatrial block is seen most frequently in the cases of severe umbilical cord compression and also may be observed in instances of head compression. The fetal heart rate will drop significantly and may reach levels as low as 40–60 beats per minute. As a consequence of the blockage of the sinus impulse, the P-P interval of the ECG will be prolonged, most frequently to some multiple of the regular interval. If a sinoatrial *Wenckebach exit block* is present in addition, the P-P interval may be progressively and periodically shortened until a P wave is dropped. Wenckebach blocks are discussed in more detail later. Only infrequently is a sinoatrial block accompanied by an AV block.

Although ECG changes thus vary with associated conditions, a number of ECG abnormalities are found rather consistently. For example, the ECG will show either decreased amplitude of P waves or changes in the morphology of the P waves as the blockage of the sinus impulse leads to an arrest, followed by an escaped beat. The escaped beats may originate anywhere along the atrial conduction pathway, most frequently, however, they are nodal in origin. Escape beats are essential in these situations and have to be considered life-saving until normal sinus excitation resumes.[1]

The etiology of a sinoatrial block in the fetus is not completely understood. It is believed that a strong parasympathetic input at the sinus node may result in sinoatrial blockage. As in the adult, hyperkalemia has been implicated. However, the other associated etiologies in the adult, such as drug therapy with digitalis and quinidine, or acute myocardial damage, have not been reported in the fetus.[1,21]

Frequently, an intrauterine ECG will not allow unequivocal diagnosis of sinoatrial block because technical deficiencies prevent the adequate diagnosis of P-wave changes. In such cases, all that can be noted are shorter or longer fetal heart rate decelerations that require obstetric intervention. The mode of intervention remains controversial. Whenever doubt exists about the existence of fetal acidosis, a fetal scalp pH should be obtained if technically possible. If values are in the acidotic range (pH < 7.20), immediate delivery is indicated. Some investigators[16] have suggested treating such a dysrhythmia in utero with atropine, to increase fetal cardiac output, which in turn is believed to inhibit the parasympathetic input on the sinus node. Those who oppose pharmacological intervention with atropine argue that the slow rate reflects a protective reflex of the fetal heart and should not be changed.[22]

Wandering Atrial Pacemaker   In the discussion of sinoatrial block, we mentioned the occurrence of atrial escape beats. With a wandering atrial pacemaker, such escape beats occur because of an underlying sinus bradycardia. Pacemakers within the atrium and the AV junction generate such escape

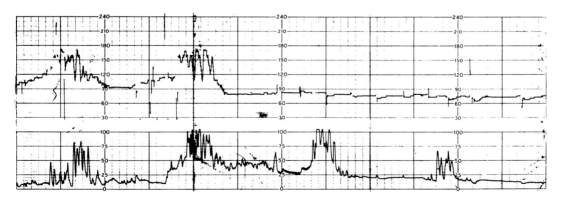

Figure 44.5   Terminal phase of fetal monitoring in a fetus with sudden loss of heart rate after an uneventful pregnancy in a 27-year-old woman (G_1, P_0) at term. The preceding labor had been normal when, after three variable decelerations, a sudden persistent "bradycardia" of approximately 80 beats per minute occurred (upper panel). The heart rate turned out to correspond to the maternal rate, and fetal death was diagnosed. Shortly thereafter, a stillborn infant with multiple congenital abnormalities, including a large omphalocele, was delivered.

beats. Consequently, the ECG will show a characteristic picture of late P waves, which have varying forms and varying PR intervals. Atrial fusion complexes may occasionally occur when QRS complexes overlap as a result of excitations in either the atria, the sinus, or the AV nodes. In some instances, the pacemaker may "wander" through the atrium, starting at the sinus node, proceeding through the atrium to the AV node and back again. In adults, this is most often considered to be a benign disorder, but it may also occur as a sign of the *sick sinus syndrome*. Only one case reported in the literature showed a neonatal ECG pattern consistent with this diagnosis.[23] Therefore, at this stage, no significant clinical importance can be attached to a wandering atrial pacemaker in the fetus. It is emphasized, however, that the escape beats, especially in association with sinoatrial block, fulfill a life-preserving function.

AV Block The PR interval in an ECG represents the time needed for the excitation to pass through the atrium, the AV node, the His bundle, and the bundle branches. In the adult, the PR interval should not exceed 0.2 second. In children, the PR interval is somewhat shortened, and in the fetus, as discussed in other chapters, it seems to vary with gestational age. Heart block, or AV block, may exist in one of three forms; *first-degree AV block, second-degree (partial) AV block,* or *third-degree (complete) AV block.*

First-Degree AV Block (Fig. 44.6) This is defined as a PR interval that exceeds the normal duration. It is essential that all atrial beats be followed by ventricular beats, thus indicating normal (even if delayed) progression of the excitation from the atria toward the ventricles. This form of AV block is usually caused by impaired conduction in the AV junction. It may be due to a *trifascicular block,* but this case is rare.

Surprisingly, no case of first-degree heart block has been reported in a fetus. Since first-degree heart blocks are recognized in the neonatal period, it must be assumed that the condition is underdiagnosed in utero.

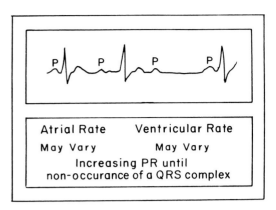

Figure 44.7 Second-degree (partial) AV block.

Second Degree (Partial) AV Block (Fig. 44.7) Second-degree AV block is characterized by atrial impulses that, intermittently, are not capable of penetrating the conduction system and therefore do not excite the ventricles. This form of AV block can appear in two forms: *Mobitz type I block (Wenckebach)* and *Mobitz type II block.*

Wenckebach block (Fig. 44.8) is defined by an increasing PR interval. Finally, an atrium-derived impulse will be completely blocked, resulting in nonoccurrence of the corresponding ventricular beat. This type of block is almost always localized to the AV node.[24] In the adult, *Wenckebach blocks* frequently appear in association with heightened vagal tone, or they may occur spontaneously. Other etiologies include drug therapy with morphine and digitalis, β-adrenergic blocking agents, and calcium antagonists. In general, a *Mobitz type I block* is considered benign if not associated with other known pathology and will be transient in the majority of cases.[24] Figure 44.9 demonstrates a *Wenckebach block* recognized in the immediate neonatal period in a viable male delivered after uneventful labor.

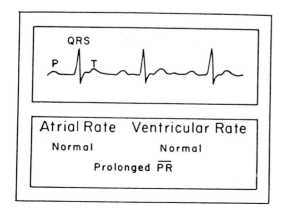

Figure 44.6 First-degree AV block.

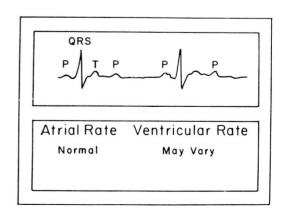

Figure 44.8 Mobitz type I (Wenckebach) block.

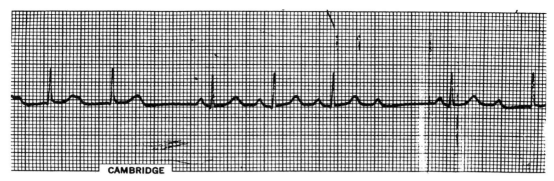

Figure 44.9 Wenckebach block, diagnosed in a male infant shortly after delivery. Maternal history was negative and labor had been uneventful.

In the adult, *Mobitz type II block* is considered a more serious disorder. In the fetal experience, this kind of second-degree AV block will be present in most fetuses with very rapid atrial rates, as may be observed in supraventricular tachycardia.[1] This form of second-degree AV block is characterized by a normal or increased PR interval, which is fixed except when beats are dropped. Unlike *Mobitz type I,* where the QRS duration is usually normal, the QRS in Mobitz type II block may be prolonged. Complexes may exhibit bizarre patterns, similar to those discussed in connection with bundle branch block. The origin of *Mobitz type II block* is usually either the His bundle or a trifascicular block.

Only a small number of second-degree blocks in utero have been reported.[25]

Third-Degree (Complete) AV Block (Fig. 44.10)   This form of AV block is the most frequently diagnosed conduction defect in the antepartum period. At the turn of the century, it had already been recognized that congenital heart blocks were commonly associated with a variety of cardiovascular anomalies. The incidence of major cardiovascular malformations in children with congenital third-degree (complete) AV block

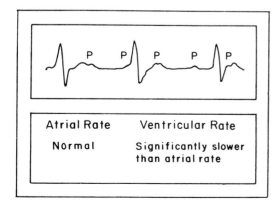

Figure 44.10 Third-degree (complete) AV block.

ranges from 25 to 50%.[9,26] Children with congenital complete heart block exhibit the same complications as adults. Follow-up studies suggest that when children with complete heart block as their only cardiac problem have a ventricular rate of more than 55 beats per minute, they generally show a satisfactory prognosis, with normal development. Children who have additional cardiac problems and/or a heart rate of less than 55 beats per minute exhibit severe complications such as Stokes–Adams attacks or syncope, congestive heart failure, and death in infancy or early childhood.[27,28] The reported incidence of complete heart block is 1 per 20,000 live births. The first diagnosis prior to birth was made by Plant and Stevens[29] in 1945. Since then, an increasing number of cases have been reported, and different methodologies have been employed in the antepartum diagnosis.

The first review of the subject was published by Teteris and associates[30] in 1968. In this report, 15 of 29 infants died with congenital heart disease. Shenker[1] reviewed that experience and added 13 cases. Among those 28 infants, 5 were found to have congenital heart disease, and 6 died either from congenital heart disease or with a pacemaker in situ.[1,31–40] The very high incidence of major cardiovascular congenital abnormalities in association with congenital heart block is confirmed by more recent studies.[41]

Increasing attention has focused on the association between congenital AV block and maternal collagen vascular disease, especially *systemic lupus erythematosus (SLE).* In 1966 Hull and associates[42] were able to show that 14 of 22 children born to 11 mothers with clinical or overt connective tissue disease exhibited congenital complete heart block. A similar association was reported in 1977 by McCue et al[43] and by Chameides and associates,[44] and in the following year by Berube and coworkers.[40]

In 1983 Scott et al[45] convincingly demonstrated a quantitative association between the antiribosomal SSA (anti-Ro) antibody in SLE mothers and congenital heart block in their offspring. While association is not causation, Litsey et al[46] were later able to strengthen this association by demonstrating these autoantibodies deposited in the area of the conduction system in a stillborn infant with the intrauterine diagnosis of complete block. Scott[47] argues against the term "*neonatal lupus syndrome*" in affected infants and recommends instead the use of "*transferred connective tissue disease.*" Why all SSA (anti-Ro)-positive females do not give birth to apparently affected children is still unknown. The incidence of neonatal disease in the presence of maternal autoantibody appears similar to that in a variety of autoimmune diseases.[48] Whether immunosuppressive therapy in SSA (anti-Ro)-positive mothers reduces the incidence of congenital heart block is still unknown. Such a reduction can be expected if the autoantibody is, in fact, causative, and if its suppression is achieved in a timely fashion. Since SS (anti-Ro) antibodies can occur with autoimmune diseases other than SLE, an investigation for the presence of the antibody is recommended in all relevant autoimmune conditions.

The importance of this association cannot be overemphasized. It allows the prospective search for congenital fetal heart block in the offspring of mothers with known connective tissue disease and, vice versa, the search for dormant connective tissue disease in mothers of infants with congenital AV block. Investigators first reported in utero diagnosis of complete AV block in a fetus from a SLE mother by means of echo and phonocardiography in 1979.[49] These noninvasive modalities are attaining increasing importance in the antepartum diagnosis of fetal heart disease. For more details, see Chapter 47.

A correct diagnosis in utero is of major clinical importance, for if the resulting fetal bradycardia is falsely interpreted as fetal distress, a cesarean section may be performed unnecessarily. Reid and associates,[50] who discussed this undesirable contingency, were also the first to document a case of fetal congenital third-degree block in a seemingly healthy mother. After extensive investigation, the patient was found to be positive in the antinuclear antibody test, showing the speckled pattern and a titer of 1:80. Mothers of infants born with congenital complete AV block should therefore be thoroughly investigated for overt autoimmune disease.

Except in cases of autoimmune disease, the pathophysiology of congenital third-degree AV block is still poorly understood. The AV node and His bundle develop separately and join early in fetal development.[51] It has been suggested that failure of the AV node and the His bundle to achieve union may explain the presence of congenital AV block in at least some cases.[52]

How, then, is the diagnosis in utero made? A high degree of suspicion should exist if the mother is known to have connective tissue disease. Otherwise, the presenting symptom will be fetal bradycardia. Again, it is important to differentiate fetal bradycardia from fetal distress. With complete AV block, none of the excitation passes from the atria into the ventricles. Rather, contraction in the ventricles is due to ex-

citations in an infranodal pacemaker, which is usually located in the His bundle. Most cases of complete heart block may be localized to the AV node or infranodally, in which case it is caused by a block in the bundle of His or bilateral bundle branch block.[24] Additionally, characteristics of the ECG include a PP interval that is shorter than the PR interval and a sometimes distorted QRS complex. The QRS complex may or may not be distorted, depending on the site from which the ventricular signal originates. According to Shenker,[1] fetal heart rates as low as 20 beats per minute have been reported; however, the majority of fetuses will exhibit heart rates in the range of 50–70 beats per minute. The in utero diagnosis of complete block will depend on the proper utilization of antepartum fetal ECG, phonocardiography, and echocardiography.[7,11,49]

The in utero treatment of congenital heart block can be considered to be experimental. In the majority of cases, congenital heart block will be tolerated in utero. Decompensation, leading to *nonimmunologic hydrops,* will only occur with extremely low ventricular rates or associated congenital cardiac defects that lead to regurgitation by either mitral or tricuspid valves. Intrauterine treatment, if indicated, usually involves drug therapy through the mother in an attempt to speed up the fetal ventricular rate (see Chapter 45 for more details). Standards drugs are betamimetic agents such as terbutaline, often in combination with digitalis and furosemide, once signs of fetal hydrops have developed. Carpenter et al[53] more recently suggested intrauterine ventricular pacing as an alternative approach in severely affected fetuses.

AV Disassociation   AV disassociation exists whenever the atria and ventricles are under the control of two separate pacemakers. While present in complete AV block, this condition can occur in the absence of a primary conduction disturbance. *AV disassociation with heart block* is caused by an excitation of a pacemaker in the AV junction of the Purkinje system, triggered when all the impulses from the sinoatrial node or the atria become blocked in the area of the AV conduction system. AV disassociation, unrelated to heart block, may occur under two circumstances. First, it may develop with an AV junctional rhythm in response to severe sinus bradycardia. When the sinus rate and the escape rate are similar and the P waves occur just before, in, or following the QRS complex, *isorhythmic dissociation* is said to be present. Second, AV disassociation can be caused by an enhanced lower (junctional or ventricular) pacemaker that competes with normal sinus rhythm and frequently exceeds it. This condition has been called *interference AV disassociation* because the rapid lower pacemaker results in bombardment of the AV node in a retrograde fashion, rendering it refractory to the normal sinus impulses. The failure of antegrade conduction is a physiologic response in that circumstance.[24]

The antepartum diagnosis of AV disassociation was made for the first time in 1979 by Platt and associates,[54] who indicated the difficulties in reaching this diagnosis in utero. In the first case, the diagnosis was made not by either abdominal or intrauterine ECG but by demonstrating a different contraction rate of atria and ventricles by means of ultrasonography. Sonography was performed because fetal bradycardia of 60–80 beats per minute was recognized in the antepartum period. This infant was delivered by cesarean section because of obstetrical indications and was found to have multiple congenital abnormalities that were incompatible with life. The pattern was considered consistent with the *polysplenia syndrome.*

In the second case, the diagnosis was also made because of fetal bradycardia of 50 beats per minute. Real-time ultrasonography suggested cardiac dynamics compatible with complete AV disassociation. At term, simultaneous maternal and fetal ECGs confirmed the diagnosis. After a normal delivery, the infant became septic on day 3 of life, went into congestive heart failure, and died. No congenital abnormalities of the heart were detected on postmortem examination. Interestingly, this fetus showed multiple ventricular ectopic beats both ante- and postpartum. Because of the associated abnormality of AV disassociation, this case was not included in our discussion of ventricular ectopic beats.

Bundle Branch Block Disorders (Fig. 44.11) Bundle branch block disorders represent impaired conduction in specific areas of the conduction system. The accurate diagnosis of either left or right bundle branch block is dependent on a complete ECG (Fig. 44.11). Since intrauterine ECGs are limited to a single lead, the diagnosis of bundle branch block disorders in utero by means of electrocardiography does not seem feasible. A widened QRS complex should be considered with suspicion and should be followed up in the neonatal period.

Tachyarrhythmias

Premature Complexes

Atrial Premature Complexes (Fig. 44.12)   This arrhythmia, which may be the most frequent in utero arrhythmia, was reported by Reed et al[55] in 76 of 86 identified intrauterine arrhythmias. Lingman et al[41] reported it in 84 of 94 supraventricular arrhythmias in a total of 113 identified arrhythmias.

Premature atrial beats originate from an abnormal focus, which may lie anywhere within the atrium. In the adult, such ectopic atrial beats are generally considered benign although they may precede more serious cardiac dysrhythmias such as atrial fibrillation, atrial flutter, and atrial tachycardia. In listening to the fetal heart, premature atrial beats may at times be confused with potentially more serious ectopic ventricular beats. In most cases it will be necessary to perform an ECG to differentiate between the two. On a purely statistical basis, in a majority of cases, premature beats will be atrial in origin. The classical sign of an atrial ectopic beat is a P wave preceding the QRS complex, which is usually normal in configuration and duration. In a majority of cases, these P waves will occur prematurely and will be followed by an incomplete compensatory pause (Fig. 44.12), thus the name "premature atrial beat." In some instances—for example, in association with "*aberrant conduction*" through the cardiac conduction system—the QRS complex may be distorted in both amplitude and configuration. The QRS complex then looks wide and in most cases is similar to that seen with right bundle branch block. It may be difficult and sometimes impossible to differentiate between ectopic atrial beats with aberrant conduction from ventricular ectopic beats without the help of a His bundle ECG. The chance for aberrant conduction increases with an increase in prematurity of the ectopic atrial beat.[24]

As already noted, these arrhythmias represent the most frequently encountered arrhythmias in the fetus. In general, the diagnosis should not be made unless confirmed by either

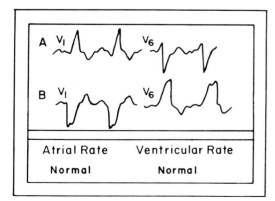

Figure 44.11 (*A*) Right bundle branch block. (*B*) Left bundle branch block.

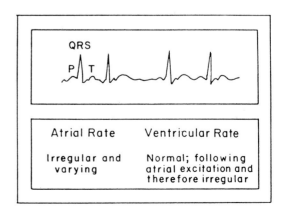

Figure 44.12 Ectopic atrial beats.

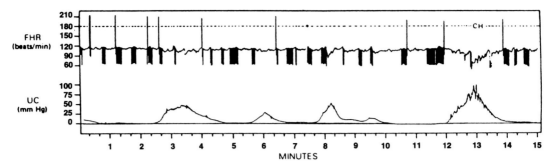

Figure 44.13   Direct fetal monitoring strip chart showing intermittent bursts of bigeminal rhythm. (Reproduced from Sugarman et al, *Obstet Gynecol* 1978;182:371–375, with permission of the American College of Obstetricians and Gynecologists.)

a fetal ECG or echocardiogram. Premature atrial beats have been described before 20 weeks of gestational age.[56] As early as 1930, investigators described fetal extrasystoles, which they identified by phonocardiographic techniques.[57] Antepartum fetal heart rate arrhythmias at that time were estimated at approximately 10% (an even higher number than in our own experience). An increasing number of cases with premature atrial beats in the antepartum period has been reported ever since,[31,55,58] although many remain undiscovered until the intrapartum period.[31,59,60] The consensus of these reports has been that premature atrial beats in the antepartum period represent a benign arrhythmia that usually disappears within the first week of life in neonates in whom extrasystoles were still detectable after birth. A number of cases have been reported in which premature atrial beats occurred in the form of either a bigeminus or trigeminus (Figs. 44.13 and 44.14).[23,61,62] The terms *"bigeminus"* and *"trigeminus"* are unfortunately used in the obstetrical literature in the context of atrial ectopic beats. This practice should not be confused with use of the same terminology in association with ventricular ectopic beats in postuterine life, where the occurrence of bigeminus and trigeminus may be of much more serious clinical significance. It is generally believed that there is no increased incidence of congenital heart disease in fetuses with premature atrial beats unless such beats occur in association with other arrhythmias or unless fetal heart murmurs are detected.[1,17] Single cases of supraventricular ectopic beats have, however, been reported in association with severe fetal decompensation and even death.[63] The recognition of premature atrial beats should therefore not be considered alarming, but should instigate a thorough reevaluation of the pregnancy. It remains unknown whether the presence of premature atrial beats in the fetus may precede the onset of sustained atrial dysrhythmias such as atrial tachycardia, flutter, or fibrillation. An erroneous diagnosis of complete heart block is possible when premature atrial beats are blocked.[19] The resulting fetal bradycardia may then falsely indicate fetal distress.[20]

Intrauterine therapy does not appear indicated.

Ventricular Premature Complexes (Fig. 44.15).   In the adult patient with structural heart disease, ventricular ectopic beats are relatively more frequent than ectopic atrial beats. In normal healthy adults, the presence of the former rarely has clinical significance unless accompanied by additional specific findings.[24] A similar statement can be made about the clinical significance of premature ventricular ectopic beats in utero. Shenker[1] summarized 16 reported cases in 1979.[31,32,59,64,65] Since then, additional cases have been reported,[23,41,55] all of which took an uneventful course and did not exhibit long-term sequelae after delivery. The only case of associated neonatal death was also associated with complete *congenital fetal heart block.*[33] Thus, in summary, ventricular beats appear to be benign in most cases.

Bigeminal Rhythm.   Bigeminal rhythm is characterized by the prematurity of every alternate beat. No ventricular case of either bigeminus or trigeminus in utero has been reported. Thus Shenker's[1] statement that ventricular premature systoles may cause bigeminy and trigeminy[1] probably means that this is a theoretical possibility. In contrast, supraventricular extrasystoles that give the ECG picture of bigeminy and trigeminy have been reported. The term *"bigeminal rhythm,"* if applied in association with ventricular ectopic beats, represents a different level of significance from that associated with atrial ectopic beats. After birth, the terms *"bigeminus"* and *"trigeminus"* are reserved for ventricular ectopy. The obstetrical literature has, however, made wide use of these terms in association with atrial ectopic beats.

Tachycardias

Sinus Tachycardia (Fig. 44.16).   Whereas in the adult, sinus tachycardia is defined as a sinus heart rate faster than 100 beats per minute, in the fetus, sinus tachycardia is defined as a sinus-initiated heart rate of more than 180 beats per minute. As in the adult, fetal sinus tachycardia must be distinguished from a number of different ectopic tachycardias. The clinical

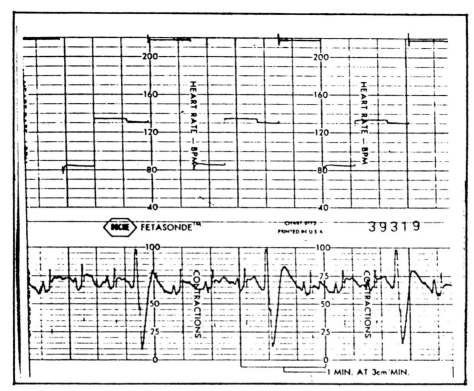

Figure 44.14   Fetal monitoring recording at 25 mm/s. Upper tracing shows the beat-to-beat fetal heart rate from the direct ECG obtained from the fetal scalp electrode during atrial trigeminy with ventricular extrasystoles. Three different heart rates are present. Lower tracing clearly shows atrial trigeminy with ventricular extrasystoles by direct ECG. (Reproduced from Young et al, *Obstet Gynecol* 1979;54:427–432, with permission of the American College of Obstetricians and Gynecologists.)

differentiation is important. Sinus tachycardia rarely exceeds 200 beats per minute and is not a primary arrhythmia; instead, it represents a physiologic response to a variety of stresses, such as fever, volume depletion, anxiety, exercise, thyrotoxicosis, hypoxemia, hypotension, or congestive heart failure.[24]

Beat-to-beat variability is almost always present in the normal fetus and remains in the range of 5–15 beats per minute.[1] Similar to sinus bradycardia, sinus tachycardia may occur either in short bursts or as a persistent state. Among causes of sinus tachycardia in the fetus, the following have been reported: cytomegalovirus disease, administration of

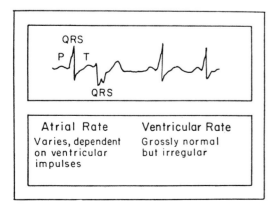

Figure 44.15   Ectopic ventricular beats.

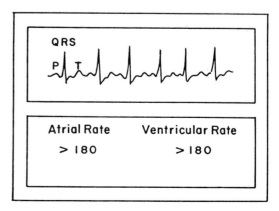

Figure 44.16   Sinus tachycardia.

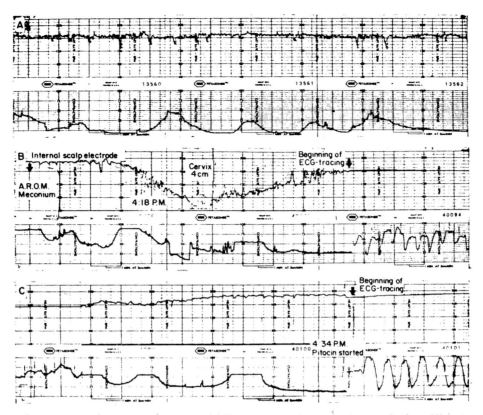

Figure 44.17 Fetal heart rate tracings indicating intrauterine meconium aspiration: (*A*) external monitor, (*B*) internal scalp electrode placed, prolonged bradycardia after amniotomy, and (*C*) internal scale electrode, slow rise of fetal heart rate to a sinus tachycardia of 180 beats per minute. In (*B*) and (*C*) the mother was positioned on her left side. Since uterine contractions were recorded by external monitor, the elevated baseline is solely an artifact; it does not represent an elevated resting pressure. (Reproduced from Gleicher et al, *Diagn Gynecol Obstet* 1980;2:151–155.)

drugs (e.g., isoxsuprin, atropine, scopolamine), maternal fever, amnionitis, early fetal hypoxia, and maternal anxiety state.[1,22,66] Additional causes that can be extrapolated from the adult experience may include severe thyrotoxicosis, profound circulatory collapse, and electrolyte imbalances. In the adult patient with severe advanced chronic airway disease, a sustained sinus tachycardia can frequently be observed. We reported the occurrence of sinus tachycardia in a fetus with the presumptive diagnosis of intrauterine meconium aspiration (Fig. 44.17).[66] It is tempting to speculate that in intrauterine meconium aspiration, pathophysiologic mechanisms similar to those in adult airway obstruction may cause fetal sinus tachycardia. The main differential diagnosis of sinus tachycardia is supraventricular tachycardia.

Whenever sinus tachycardia is observed in utero, an underlying cause must be searched for. Sinus tachycardia is often the first clinical sign of amnionitis, appearing long before fever or leukocytosis with left shift.

Atrial Fibrillation (Fig. 44.18).   This dysrhythmia is probably underrecognized in utero.[1] The contraction of the atria

is not defective. The AV node and the ventricles are, however, exposed to very rapid and very irregular stimuli from the atria. Consequently, many of these stimuli will be blocked at the AV node, while others may pass through into the lower lying conduction, resulting in rapid and irregular ventricular

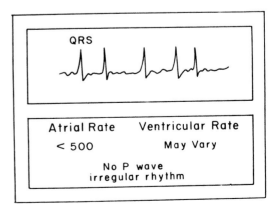

Figure 44.18 Atrial fibrillation.

contractions. The morbidity associated with atrial fibrillation is related to the ventricular response rate, the loss of the contribution of the atrial contraction to cardiac output, the proportion of ineffective ventricular beats and the occurrence of embolization.[24] The reported cases of antepartum diagnosis of atrial fibrillation are increasing.[4,10,31,55,68] One infant also showed supraventricular tachycardia but did not exhibit any congenital heart disease.[68] Another was diagnosed with Eisenmenger's syndrome and died soon after birth.[31]

The reported clinical experience with the intrapartum diagnosis of atrial fibrillation is too small to allow any significant conclusion. It remains to be determined whether a real association with congenital heart disease exists. Atrial fibrillation may occur in paroxysmal or persistent forms. It may be seen in normal subjects. It may occur in patients with heart or lung disease who develop acute hypoxia, hypercapnia, or metabolic or hemodynamic derangements. Persistent atrial fibrillation usually occurs in patients with cardiovascular disease, most commonly rheumatic heart disease, chronic lung disease, atrial septal defect, and a variety of miscellaneous cardiac abnormalities. Atrial fibrillation also occurs with thyrotoxicosis.[24]

Extrapolation to the fetal experience is impossible. However, a possible association with thyrotoxicosis or congenital mitral stenosis deserves further investigation. The diagnosis of intrauterine atrial fibrillation necessitates in all instances of fetal ECG or echocardiogram. On simple heart rate auscultation, atrial fibrillation with normal or slightly increased ventricular rate can be misdiagnosed as a sinus rhythm with numerous extrasystoles. The diagnosis is especially difficult in the fetus because a heart rate of 120 beats per minute, considered to represent tachycardia in the adult, is normal. Thus, the diagnosis should never be made unless clear documentation can be obtained.

Atrial Flutter (Fig. 44.19).   In the adult, atrial flutter is less common than atrial fibrillation. In the fetal experience, more cases of atrial flutter have been reported.[41,69–73] The small

total of reported cases suggests underreporting of this condition. In one study only half of all cases that were recognized in the neonatal period were diagnosed in the antepartum period.[74]

The underlying mechanism for this dysrhythmia is still poorly understood and highly controversial. It is believed to be a reciprocating rhythm or circus current movement. In contrast to the conditions of atrial fibrillation, the atria contract in the majority of cases at a rate of 250–350 beats per minute. An accompanying AV block is almost always present, and its ratio usually follows even numbers. Consequently, the ventricular rate will be in the range of approximately 75 to 150 beats per minute depending on whether a 4:1 or a 2:1 block is present. The ventricular rate does not necessarily follow that rule, however. On occasion, two sites of block may occur at the AV junction. For example, a high junction 2:1 and a lower 3:2 block may exist, resulting in a ventricular rate that is not a constant multiple of the atrial rate.

As in cases of atrial fibrillation, an ECG is essential for the accurate diagnosis of atrial flutter. With a variable AV block, an irregularity of the heart rate will be detectable by auscultation alone. However, with a fixed degree of block, the fetal heart rate may be regular and in the normal range for term pregnancy, and the abnormality may thus be easily overlooked.

Among the reported cases of atrial flutter diagnosed in the antepartum period, one fetus was found to have a tetralogy of Fallot.[72] Another report cited hydrops fetalis found at birth.[73] Among the survivors, most neonates required intensive therapy, which included either pharmacologic cardioversion with digitalis or electric cardioversion. One infant was found to be acidotic at birth.[70] Our own experience includes two cases with short bouts of atrial flutter that were diagnosed in the antepartum period. In both cases the infants showed prolonged periods of intermittent supraventricular tachycardia that was interrupted by very brief episodes of atrial flutter. One of the infants also exhibited flutter in the neonatal period and required digitalis therapy as well as electric cardioversion.[75]

Since the experience with atrial flutter in the antepartum period is still very limited, its clinical significance remains to be determined. Shenker[1] suggested that atrial flutter may represent a potentially serious arrhythmia. It can cause intrauterine congestive heart failure and result in fetal hydrops.[74]

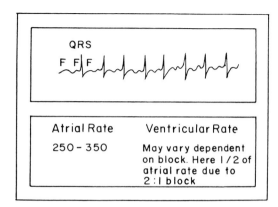

Atrial Rate	Ventricular Rate
250 - 350	May vary dependent on block. Here 1/2 of atrial rate due to 2:1 block

Figure 44.19   Atrial flutter.

Paroxysmal Supraventricular Tachycardia (Fig. 44.20). Supraventricular tachycardia represents one of the most frequently diagnosed arrhythmias in the neonate, and the number of well-documented cases of in utero supraventricular tachycardia has steadily increased.[1–3,6,9,11,23,55,63,69,75,76] Southall et al[77] reported an incidence of 4–6 per thousand pregnancies.

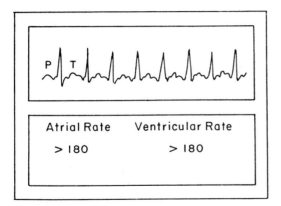

Figure 44.20 Paroxysmal supraventricular tachycardia.

To make the diagnosis, the ECG has to show a rate of at least 180 beats per minute (Figs. 44.20, 44.21), but it will frequently show a rate of significantly more than 200 beats per minute (Fig. 44.22).

Paroxysmal supraventricular tachycardia is classically called *paroxysmal atrial tachycardia,* since this dysrhythmia has been believed to be due to rapid discharges from an abnormal atrial pacemaker. More recent investigations indicate that frequently, although not in all instances, paroxysmal supraventricular tachycardia results from a reciprocating rhythm (i.e., from sustained reentry of the excitation).[24] This concept is discussed in more detail later in conjunction with *the Wolff–Parkinson–White syndrome.* The mechanisms causing supraventricular tachycardia were reviewed by Manolis and Estes.[78]

The clinical significance of intrauterine supraventricular tachycardia may vary. It is generally accepted that similar to the adult experience, the vast majority of cases will be benign. The causes of supraventricular tachycardia are seldom known, since most of the infants show no signs of organic heart disease after birth. However, a number of underlying causes should be considered, including atrial septal defects, congenital mitral valve disease, and the Wolff–Parkinson–White Syndrome.[1,79] We reported the development of intrauterine supraventricular tachycardia in two fetuses and, after birth, appearance of the Wolff–Parkinson–White syndrome.[79] Other such cases have also been reported.[69,79–81] The association between supraventricular tachycardia in the neonatal period and the Wolff–Parkinson–White syndrome had been recognized even earlier.[82] Bergmans et al[76] reported a 15% association between intrauterine supraventricular tachycardia and Wolff–Parkinson–White syndrome. Congenital heart disease appears to represent only a rare cause of supraventricular tachycardia. The importance of atrial ectopic beats in the pathogenesis of idiopathic supraventricular tachycardia remains to be determined.

What is the clinical significance of supraventricular tachycardia in utero? It appears that supraventricular tachycardia occurring in utero may be either paroxysmal and short-lived or persistent. Two factors seem most important for the eventual prognosis of the newborn. First, congenital heart disease in association with supraventricular tachycardia (reported by Shenker[1] to occur in 5–10% and by Bergmans et al[76] in 6.8% of cases) is associated with high neonatal mortality. Second, the appearance of congestive heart failure, either in utero or in the neonate, may lead to increased neonatal morbidity. Intrauterine congestive heart failure is dis-

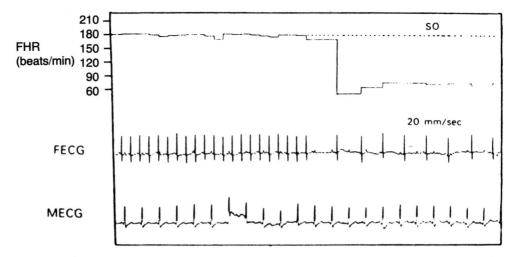

Figure 44.21 Direct fetal ECG showing spontaneous conversion from supraventricular tachycardia to sinus rhythm. (Reproduced from Sugarman et al, *Obstet Gynecol* 1978;182:371–375, with permission of the American College of Obstetricians and Gynecologists.)

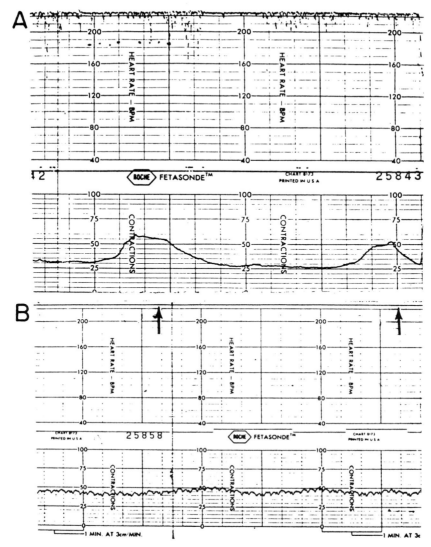

Figure 44.22 Supraventricular tachycardia in a fetus monitored with an internal scalp electrode. (*A*) A fetal heart rate of more than 220 beats per minute (upper panel) and uterine contractions (lower panel). (*B*) The same fetus, with lower panel now exhibiting the fetal ECG, indicative of supraventricular tachycardia, while the upper panel demonstrates a heart rate of more than 220 beats per minute (arrows) and an absolute lack of beat-to-beat variability.

cussed in more detail in Chapter 45. It is interesting to note, however, that among the 19 cases reviewed by Shenker,[1] 7 of 9 diagnosed in the antepartum period were found at birth to have varying degrees of congestive heart failure. In contrast, only 3 of 10 cases detected intrapartum showed signs of congestive heart failure at birth. These findings indicate that prolonged episodes of supraventricular tachycardia may predispose to intrauterine congestive heart failure. This notion is not shared by all investigators. Some have stated that supraventricular tachycardia by itself is not predictive of either the development or the severity of congestive heart failure in the newborn.[69,70]

Based on published literature and our own experience,[75] we have concluded that the duration of supraventricular tachycardia and the presence of a persistent pattern of supraventricular tachycardia determine whether congestive heart failure will or will not develop. We have speculated that the heart that is allowed to recover, with normal sinus rhythm patterns interposed between bouts of supraventricular tachycardia, is at less risk of failing than the heart that is subjected to persistent tachycardia over a prolonged period.[75] Neonates that experience this dysrhythmia in utero will exhibit an increased birth weight and heavier than normal placenta, and will diurese more significantly during the first few days of life than neonates with normal heart rate, even if apparent heart failure has not been diagnosed.[1] These findings also indicate that a minor degree of congestive heart failure may be present in a majority of cases when an intrauterine supraventricular tachycardia occurs. It has been suggested that supraventricular tachycardia is better tolerated in the fetus than in the newborn. The newborn, consequent to tachycardia, frequently develops significant heart failure as a result of the heavier load on the neonatal ventricles, which act in series and not in parallel as in the fetus.[1] Very severe fetal hydrops has, however, also been reported in association with antenatal supraventricular tachycardia.[80,83,84]

The management of the fetus with intrauterine supraventricular tachycardia depends on duration as well as persistence of dysrhythmia and the fetal condition. The latter will be evaluated by routine parameters of fetal antepartum testing, such as nonstress and stress testing, ultrasonography for signs of intrauterine congestive heart failure, intrauterine echocardiography, and fetal movement charts.

The older advice to obstetricians who recognized supraventricular tachycardia in utero had been to ignore it as a benign condition. More recently, however, a more aggressive approach has been suggested.[1,75,79] It is our opinion that all cases should be individualized. Gestational age at the time of diagnosis and fetal maturity play significant roles in the decision-making process. In the case of a term infant with proven lung maturity, delivery within a reasonably short time appears to be the correct management. This advice will be followed by most clinicians if signs of impending intrauterine congestive failure can be found. Such management will, however, be more controversial when no signs of fetal decompensation can be detected. It is still questionable whether active management in these cases is indicated. Therefore, individualization must remain the basis of management. When the fetus is not expected to exhibit mature lung function, delivery is judged against the risk of respiratory distress in the neonate. A more aggressive approach is indicated when signs of fetal decompensation and/or congestive heart failure can be found. In the absence of such signs, more conservative management should be implemented. A majority of fetuses with intrauterine supraventricular tachycardia will do well without any form of active management. The few in need of aggressive management will be detected only if each infant with supraventricular tachycardia enters a very rigorous investigational protocol.

We have proposed such a protocol,[75] which requires the following: A fetal ECG from maternal abdominal leads should be obtained if possible whenever a fetal tachycardia more than 180 beats per minute is noted. We now have moved to performing fetal echocardiography, including cross-sectional views, M-mode, and Doppler studies on all such patients. The resulting data will assist in the diagnosing of the arrhythmia, the determining of the hemodynamic effects, and the ruling out of any major congenital abnormalities (Chap-

ter 42). Serial sonographic investigations of the fetus at weekly intervals can be performed to look for early signs of congestive heart failure (e.g., presence of pericardial effusion, fetal ascites, fetal scalp edema, polyhydramnios, an enlarged edematous placenta). In addition, an attempt can be made to discern any enlargement of the fetal heart and liver. Treatment in utero is not indicated unless fetal congestive heart failure is present at a gestational age at which delivery appears contraindicated. When delivery seems feasible in the presence of congestive failure, it should be attempted by the most clinically prudent route. In some cases of severe congestive heart failure, it may be advisable to deliver the fetus by cesarean section to avoid the superimposed stress of labor on an already compromised fetus.

All infants diagnosed in the antepartum period who exhibit supraventricular tachycardia should be cared for in a tertiary care setting. Close observation of these infants in the neonatal period is essential.

The role of supraventricular tachycardia in unexplained antepartum stillbirth is still controversial.[1] In the adult experience supraventricular tachycardia rarely causes death. Extrapolating from that experience, a sudden death syndrome due to supraventricular tachycardia in utero seems highly unlikely. One investigator suggested that fetal acidosis in itself may contribute to fetal arrhythmias.[71] Utilizing Doppler flow techniques, Reed et al[55] demonstrated that the conversion of fetal tachyarrhythmias to normal sinus rhythms increases the mean velocity and cardiac index of the fetal heart.

In summary, supraventricular tachycardia in utero will, in the majority of cases, represent a benign condition. Because a few cases go on to more serious fetal decompensation, however, close supervision of all cases is indicated. Intrauterine therapy is not indicated unless signs of fetal decompensation are seen at a time when delivery is contraindicated. Intrauterine therapy may involve digoxin,[84] verapamil,[85] quinidine,[81] and other agents[79] that are usually given through the mother. Intrauterine therapy is discussed in more detail in Chapter 45.

Complex Atrial Dysrhythmias As number of additional more complex atrial dysrhythmias have been reported in adults, but not in the fetus. These include *sinus node reentry, atrial reentrant tachycardia,* and *multifocal atrial tachycardia* (MAT).[24] We noted earlier that we have seen patients who experienced varying supraventricular tachyarrhythmias in utero. It would not be surprising to see some cases of these dysrhythmias also occurring in utero.

Derangements Arising from the AV Junction These dysrhythmias refer to excitations that originate in the AV junction, which includes fibers that are close to the AV node in the lower right atrium, the AV node, and the His bundle. Dysrhythmias that may originate in this area include ectopic junctional beats and AV junctional tachycardias, which may be of three types: *nonparoxysmal junctional tachycardia (ventricular rate 70–130 beats/min), paroxysmal AV nodal reentrant tachycardia (ventricular rate 140–200 beats/min) and AV reentrant tachycardia.*[24]

Wolff–Parkinson–White Syndrome (anomalous AV excitation) (Fig. 44.23).   As in the adult, the Wolff–Parkinson–White syndrome has been recognized in neonates to be associated with a pronounced tendency for the occurrence of atrial tachyarrhythmias such as paroxysmal atrial tachycardia, atrial flutter, and atrial fibrillation. The same association now has been made for this situation in utero. We noted earlier in this chapter that some fetuses with supraventricular tachyarrhythmia displayed a Wolff–Parkinson–White syndrome pattern at birth.[75] Additional cases have been reported in the literature.[69,79,80]

The Wolff–Parkinson–White syndrome is characterized by a typical ECG appearance: P waves are normal, the PR interval is 0.11 second or less, and the QRS duration is increased and shows a slur on the initial phase of the QRS complex, which is called the delta wave.[24] From this description, it will be evident that the diagnosis in utero cannot be made with available ECG technology. The association of this syndrome with intrauterine tachyarrhythmias has been retrospectively estimated by us to occur in approximately 10% of cases[79] and by Bergmans et al[76] in approximately 15%. This estimation range requires confirmation through a larger number of reported cases. Intrauterine tachyarrhythmias should, however, always be suspected to have an underlying Wolff–Parkinson–White syndrome. Wolff–Parkinson–White syndrome may also be associated with certain congenital anomalies, the most important of which is *Ebstein's anomaly.*[24] We have suggested that in pregnancy, patients with Wolff–Parkinson–White syndrome may be predisposed to arrhythmias.[87] It is tempting to speculate that in both mother and fetus hormonal factors of pregnancy may influence and increase the incidence of symptomatic Wolff–Parkinson–White syndrome, which results in arrhythmias.

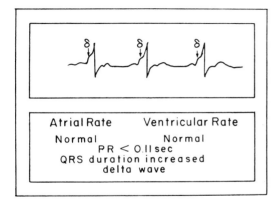

Figure 44.23   Wolff–Parkinson–White syndrome.

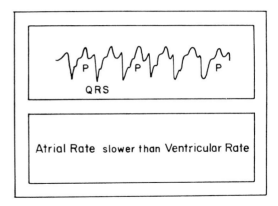

Figure 44.24   Ventricular tachycardia.

Ventricular Tachycardia (Fig. 44.24).   In the adult experience, this dysrhythmia is found less frequently than its atrial counterpart. However, if it does occur, the clinical implications are far more serious.

Ventricular tachycardia is defined as three or more consecutive ventricular premature beats. Until very recently, only one case had been reported in a fetus.[88] Shenker[1] added two more to the published experience; later additional cases were reported.[60] In one of the cases reported by Shenker, the infant died at age 12 hours with ventricular and atrial septal defects and bilateral hydronephrosis. In the other cases there was no evidence of congenital abnormalities, and the neonate improved after treatment with propranolol for ventricular premature contractions in the neonatal period.[1] Another reported case cited a completely uneventful postpartum course and no abnormalities.[60]

The experience with ventricular tachycardia in the antepartum period is too limited to allow conclusions. As with other intrauterine dysrhythmias, the principle that the occurrence of any intrauterine dysrhythmia always calls for a reevaluation of the pregnancy should be upheld. In the adult, it is important to distinguish ventricular tachycardia from supraventricular tachycardia because of the clinical implications and because the two arrhythmias are managed in completely different ways. Pharmacologic maneuvers with intravenous administration of certain medications such as verapamil or adenosine can be hazardous. It is therefore imperative to make an accurate diagnosis before instituting therapy for in utero tachycardia. The dysrhythmia by itself should not be the basis of intervention.

Ventricular Fibrillation (Fig. 44.25).   Ventricular fibrillation lasting for longer than a few seconds is synonymous with instant death. Treatment in utero therefore does not seem possible, even if the condition is recognized. To our knowledge, no case of ventricular fibrillation in a fetus has been reported. For ventricular fibrillation not to occur in utero would be

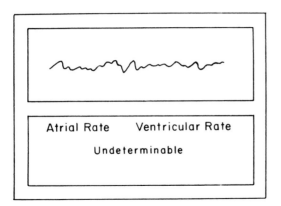

Figure 44.25 Ventricular fibrillation.

unlikely. and it is tempting to attribute some unexplained deaths in utero to this dysrhythmia.

SUMMARY

In our introduction, we outlined the theoretical difficulties in obtaining a reliable fetal ECG, either abdominally or by internal fetal scalp electrode. We also commented on the establishment of fetal echocardiography as the primary tool for diagnosing fetal arrhythmias. Shenker,[1] one of the most well-informed investigators in the field, stated in 1979 that knowledge of fetal cardiac arrhythmias diagnosed during pregnancy and labor is incomplete. Some progress has been made in this area, but there is still a need for additional information. Shenker summarized the necessity for the antepartum diagnosis of cardiac fetal arrhythmias as follows:

1. The need to distinguish fetal dysrhythmias from fetal distress.
2. The need to recognize the coexistence of congenital heart disease and varying forms of dysrhythmias.
3. The need to be able to recognize (and treat[80]) congestive heart failure, both in utero and immediately after birth.
4. The need to be able to prepare for immediate cardiac workup and treatment at time of delivery.
5. The need to recognize the relationship between maternal collagen vascular disease and congenital third-degree AV block.

Lingman et al[41] reinforced the need for closer evaluation of all fetal cardiac arrhythmias by demonstrating an increased incidence of congenital abnormalities (6.2% vs. 2.0%), fetal distress in labor (20.4% vs. 13.5%), and perinatal (3.5% vs. 0.7%) as well as neonatal mortality (1.8% vs. 0.1%) in a large study group of 113 cases.

Increasing sophistication of intrauterine electrocardiography may result in major advances in the antepartum diagnosis of cardiac abnormalities in the fetus. For example, Katz et al[89] diagnosed mitral and aortic stenosis based on a fetal ECG. The early diagnosis of congenital lesions not only will benefit the fetus immediately after birth, but also will prevent unnecessary maternal morbidity from cesarean sections performed for falsely diagnosed fetal distress. Of the available means of cardiac diagnosis, fetal echocardiography is the most accurate. Utilizing other procedures such as fetal ECG or phonocardiography may in some cases enhance the antepartum diagnosis of fetal arrhythmias.

REFERENCES

1. Shenker L. Fetal cardiac arrhythmias. *Obstet Gynecol Survey* 1979;34:561–572.
2. Allan LD, Anderson RH, Sullivan ID, Campbell S, Holt DW, Tynan M. Evaluation of fetal arrhythmias by echocardiography. *Br Heart J* 1983;50:240–245.
3. Cameron A, Nicholson S, Nimrod C, Harder J, Davies D, Fritzler M. Evaluation of fetal cardiac dysrhythmias with two-dimensional, M-mode, and pulsed Doppler ultrasonography. *Am J Obstet Gynecol* 1988;158:286–290.
4. DeVore GR, Siassi B, Platt LD. Fetal echocardiography. III. The diagnosis of cardiac arrhythmias using real-time-directed M-mode ultrasound. *Am J Obstet Gynecol* 1983;146:792–799.
5. Huhta JC, Straburger JF, Carpenter RJ, Reiter A, Abinader E. Pulsed Doppler fetal echocardiography. *J Clin Ultrasound* 1985;13:247–254.
6. Kleinman CS, Donnerstien RL, Jaffe CC, DeVore GR, Weinstein EM, Lynch DC, Talner NS, Berkowitz RL, Hobbins JC. Fetal echocardiography, a tool for evaluation of in utero cardiac arrhythmias and monitoring of in utero therapy: analysis of 71 patients. *Am J Cardiol* 1983;51:237–243.
7. Silverman NH, Enderlein MA, Stanger P, Teitel DF, Heymann MA, Golbus MS. Recognition of fetal arrhythmias by echocardiography. *J Clin Ultrasound* 1985;13:255–263.
8. Lingman G, Dahlstrom JA, Eik-Nes SH, Marshal K, Ohlin P, Ohrlander S. Haemodynamic assessment of fetal heart arrhythmias. *Br J Obstet Gynaecol* 1984;91:647–652.
9. Allan LD, Crawford DC, Anderson RH, Tynan M. Evaluation and treatment of fetal arrhythmias. *Clin Cardiol* 1984;7:467–473.
10. Crawford D, Chapman M, Allan L. The assessment of persistent bradycardia in prenatal life. *Br J Obstet Gynaecol* 1985;92:941–944.
11. Kleinman CS. Prenatal diagnosis and management of intrauterine arrhythmias. *Fetal Ther* 1986;1:92–95.
12. Strasburger JF, Huhta JC, Carpenter RJ, Garson A, McNamara DG. Doppler echocardiography in the diagnosis and management of persistent fetal arrhythmias. *J Am College Cardiol* 1986;7:1386–1391.
13. Santulli TV. Fetal echocardiography: assessment of cardiovascular anatomy and function. *Clin Perinatol* 1990;17:911–940.

14. Klapholz H, Schifrin BS, Rivo E. Paroxysmal supraventricular tachycardia in the fetus. *Obstet Gynecol* 1974;43:718–721.

15. Budnick ISS, Leikin S, Hoeck LE. Effects in the newborn infant of reserpine administered antepartum. *Am J Dis Child* 1955;90:286–289.

16. Goodlin RC, Haesslein HC. Fetal reacting bradycardia. *Am J Obstet Gynecol* 1977;129:845–856.

17. Redman TF. The significance of some unusual foetal cardiac arrhythmias. *J Obstet Gynaecol Br Emp* 1985;65:304–309.

18. Webster RD, Codmore DW, Gray J. Fetal bradycardia without fetal distress. Case presentation and review of the literature. *Obst Gynecol* 1977;50(suppl):50s–53s.

19. Freeman RK, Garite TJ, Nageotte MP. *Fetal Heart Rate Monitoring.* 2nd ed. Baltimore: Williams & Wilkins; 1991;69–71.

20. Dgani R, Borenstein R, Levavi E, Feigl A, Kauli N, Lancet M. Prenatally diagnosed blocked atrial premature beats. *Obstet Gynecol* 1978;51:507–509.

21. Ferrer PI. Arrhythmias in the neonate. In: Roberts NK, Gelband H, eds. *Cardiac Arrhythmias in the Neonate, Infant, and Child.* New York: Appleton-Century-Crofts; 1977;ch 17.

22. Queenan JT. Discussion of ref. 16. *Am J Obstet Gynecol* 1977;129:845.

23. Sugarman RG, Lawlinson KF, Schifrin BS. Fetal arrhythmias. *Obstet Gynecol* 1978;52:301–307.

24. Josephson ME, Marchlinski FE, Buxton AE. In: Isselbacher KJ, Braunwald E, Wilson JD, Martin JB, Fauci AS, Kasper DL, eds. *Harrison's Principles of Internal Medicine.* 13th ed. New York: McGraw-Hill; 1994;1011–1036.

25. Chan TS, Potter RT, Liu L. Congenital intraventricular trifascicular block. *Am J Dis Child* 1973;125:82–87.

26. Griffiths SP. Congenital complete heart block. *Circulation* 1971;43:615–617. Editorial.

27. Michaelsson M, Engl MA. Congenital complete heart block: an international study of the natural history. *Pediatr Cardiol* 1972;4:86.

28. Hochberg SH. Congenital heart block. *Am J Obstet Gynecol* 1964;88:238–241.

29. Plant RK, Stevens RA. Complete A-V block in a fetus. Case report. *Am Heart J* 1945;30:615–618.

30. Teteris NJ, Chisholm JW, Ullery JC. Antenatal diagnosis of congenital heart block. Report of a case. *Obstet Gynecol* 1968;32:851–853.

31. Komaromy B, Gaal J, Lampe L. Fetal arrhythmia during pregnancy and labour. *Br J Obstet Gynaecol* 1977;84:492–496.

32. Sorland S, Torp KH, Jenssen J. Hjerte-arytmier hos foster og nyfdt. En oversikt og omtale av 5 kasus. *Nor Laegeforen* 1963;83:1654–1659.

33. Armstrong DG, Murata Y, Martin CB Jr, Ikenoue T. Antepartum detection of congenital complete fetal heart block: a case report. *Am J Obstet Gynecol* 1976;126:291–292.

34. Smith JJ, Schwartz ED, Blatman S. Fetal bradycardia: fetal distress or cardiac abnormality? *Obstet Gynecol* 1960;15:761–764.

35. Dunn HP. Antenatal diagnosis of congenital heart block. *J Obstet Gynaecol Br Emp* 1960;67:1006–1007.

36. Sokol RJ, Hutchinson P, Krouskop RW, Brown EG, Reed G, Vasquez H. Congenital complete heart block diagnosed during intrauterine fetal monitoring. *Am J Obstet Gynecol* 1974;120:1115–1117.

37. Abdulla U, Charters DW. Congenital heart block diagnosed antenatally associated with multiple fetal abnormality. *Br Med J* 1975;4:263.

38. Altenburger KM, Jedziniak M, Roper WL, Hernandez J. Congenital complete heart block associated with hydrops fetalis. *J Pediatr* 1977;9:618–620.

39. Hamilton LA Jr, Fisher E, Horn C, DuBrow I, Vidyasagar D. A new prenatal cardiac diagnostic device for congenital heart disease. *Obstet Gynecol* 1977;50:491–494.

40. Berube S, Lister G Jr, Towes WH, Creasy RK, Heymann MA. Congenital heart block and maternal systemic lupus erythematosus. *Am J Obstet Gynecol* 1978;130:595–596.

41. Lingman G, Lustrom N-R, Marsal K, Ohrlander IS. Fetal cardiac arrhythmia: clinical outcome in 113 cases. *Acta Obstet Gynecol Scand* 1986;65:263–267.

42. Hull D, Binns BA, Joyce D. Congenital heart block and widespread fibrosis due to maternal lupus erythematosus. *Arch Dis Child* 1966;4:688–690.

43. McCue CM, Mantakas ME, JB, Ruddy S. Congenital heart block in newborns of mothers with connective tissue disease. *Circulation* 1977;56:82–90.

44. Chameides L, Truex RC, Vetter V, Raskind WJ, Galioulo FM Jr, Noonan JA. Association of maternal systemic lupus erythematosus with congenital complete heart block. *N Engl J Med* 1977;297:1204–1207.

45. Scott JS, Maddison PJ, Taylor PV, Esscher E, Scott O, Skinner RP. Connective tissue disease, antibodies to micronucleoprotein and congenital heart block. *N Engl J Med* 1983;309:209–212.

46. Litsey SE, Noonan JA, O'Conner WM, et al. Maternal connective tissue disease and congenital heart block. Demonstration of immunoglobulin in cardiac tissue. *N Engl J Med* 1985;312:98–100.

47. Scott JS. Connective tissue disease antibodies and pregnancy. *Am J Reprod Immunol* 1984;6:19–24.

48. Weinstein A, Parke AL. Pregnancy and the rheumatic diseases: the connective tissue diseases. In: Gleicher N, ed. *Principles of Medical Therapy in Pregnancy.* New York: Plenum Press; 1985;1013–1020.

49. Madison JP, Sukhum P, Williamson DP, Campion BC. Echocardiography and fetal heart sounds in the diagnosis of fetal heart block. *Am Heart J* 1979;98:505–509.

50. Reid RL, Pancham SR, Kean WF, Ford PM. Maternal and neonatal implications of congenital complete heart block in the fetus. *Obstet Gynecol* 1979;54:470–474.

51. James TN. Cardiac conduction system: fetal and postnatal development. *Am J Cardiol* 1970;25:213–226.

52. Carter JB, Blieden LC, Edwards JE. Congenital heart block: anatomic correlation and review of the literature. *Arch Pathol* 1974;97:51–57.

53. Carpenter RJ Jr, Strasburger JR, Garson A Jr, Smith R, Deter RL, Engelhardt HT Jr. Fetal ventricular pacing for hydrops sec-

ondary to complete atrioventricular block. *J Am College Cardiol* 1986;8:1434–1436.

54. Platt LD, Manning FA, Gray C, Guttenburg M, Turkel SB. Antenatal detection of fetal A-V dissociation utilizing real-time B-mode ultrasound. *Obstet Gynecol* 1979;53(suppl):59s–61s.

55. Reed KL, Sahn DJ, Marx GR, Anderson CF, Shenker L. Cardiac Doppler flow during fetal arrhythmias: physiologic consequences. *Obstet Gynecol* 1987;70:1–6.

56. Nielson JS, Moestrup JK. Fetal electrocardiographic studies of cardiac arrhythmias and the heart rate. *Acta Obstet Gynecol Scand* 1968;47:247–256.

57. Hyman AS. Irregularities of the fetal heart. Phonocardiographic study of fetal heart sounds from fifth to eighth months of pregnancy. *Am J Obstet Gynecol* 1930;20:332–347.

58. Itskovitz J, Timor-Tritsch I, Brandes JM. Intrauterine arrhythmia: atrial premature beats. *Int J Gynaecol Obstet* 1979;16: 419–421.

59. Hon EH, Huang HS. The electronic evaluation of fetal heart rate. VII. Premature and missed beats. *Obstet Gynecol* 1962; 20:81–90.

60. Young BK, Katz M, Klein SA. Intrapartum fetal cardiac arrhythmias. *Obstet Gynecol* 1979;54:427–432.

61. Harrigan JT, Acerra D, LaMagra R, Hoeveler J, Chandra N. Fetal cardiac arrhythmia during labor. *Am J Obstet Gynecol* 1977;128:693–694.

62. Schneider H, Weinstein HM, Young BK. Fetal trigeminal rhythm. *Obstet Gynecol* 1977;50(suppl):58s–61s.

63. Freistadt H. Fetal bigeminal rhythm. Report of a case. *Am J Obstet Gynecol* 1962;84:13–14.

64. Schlotter CM, Kunz S. Fegale Parasystolie—eine seltene Form fetaler Arrhythmie bei Hydramnion und Hydrops fetalis. *Z Geburtshilfe Perinatol* 1978;182:371–375.

65. Eibschitz I, Abinader EG, Klein A, Sharf M. Intrauterine diagnosis and control of fetal ventricular arrhythmia during labor. *Am J Obstet Gynecol* 1975;122:597–600.

66. Odendaal HJ, Crawford JW. Fetal tachycardia and maternal pyrexia during labor. *S Afr Med J* 1975;49:1873–1875.

67. Gleicher N, Chin JM, Brown BL, Kerenyi TD. Intrauterine meconium aspiration syndrome. *Diagn Gynecol Obstet* 1980;2: 151–155.

68. Carretti NG, Galli PA, Pellegrino P. Fetal paroxysmal supraventricular tachycardia: report of a case documented by trans-vaginal electrocardiogram during fetal distress in labour. *Acta Obstet Gynecol Scand* 1974;53:275–277.

69. Newberger JW, Keane JF. Intrauterine supraventricular tachycardia. *J Pediatr* 1979;17:581–583.

70. Levkoff AH. Perinatal outcome of paroxysmal tachycardia of the newborn with onset in utero. *Am J Obstet Gynecol* 1969; 104:73–79.

71. Symonds EM. Fetal cardiac arrhythmias and fetal acid base status. *N Z J Obstet Gynaecol* 1972;12:170–175.

72. Pearl W. Cardiac malformations presenting as congenital atrial flutter. *South Med J* 1977;70:622–624.

73. Van der Horst RL. Congenital atrial flutter and cardiac failure presenting as hydrops foetalis at birth. *S Afr Med J* 1970;44: 1037–1039.

74. Moller JH, Davachi F, Anderson RC. Atrial flutter in infancy. *J Pediatr* 1969;75:643–651.

75. Chitkara U, Gleicher N, Longhi R, Gergely LRZ, Kerenyi TD. Persistent supraventricular tachycardia in utero. *Diagn Gynecol Obstet* 1980;2:291–298.

76. Bergmans M, Jonker G, Kock H. Fetal supraventricular tachycardia: review of the literature. *Obstet Gynecol Survey* 1985;40: 61–68.

77. Southall DP, Richard J, Hardwick RA, Shinebourne EA, Gibbons GL, Thelwall-Jones H, de Swiet M, Hohnston PG. Prospective study of fetal heart rate and rhythm patterns. *Arch Dis Child* 1980;55:506–511.

78. Manolis AS, Estes NAM III. Supraventricular tachycardia: mechanisms and therapy. *Arch Intern Med* 1987;147: 1706–1716.

79. Gleicher N, Elkayam U. Cardiac problems in pregnancy. II. Fetal aspects. *JAMA* 1984;252:78–80.

80. Klein AM, Holzman IA, Austin EM. Fetal tachycardia prior to the development of hydrops. Attempted pharmacologic cardioversion. Case report. *Am J Obstet Gynecol* 1979;136: 347–348.

81. Kileen AK, Bowers LD. Fetal supraventricular tachycardia treated with high dose quinidine: toxicity associated with marked elevation of the metabolite, 3(5)-3-hydroxyquinidine. *Obstet Gynecol* 1987;70:445–448.

82. Herin P, Thoren C. Congenital arrhythmias with supraventricular tachycardia in the perinatal period. *Acta Obstet Gynecol Scand* 1973;52:381–386.

83. Silber DL, Durnin RE. Intrauterine atrial tachycardia, associated with massive edema in a newborn. *Am J Dis Child* 1969;117:722–726.

84. Kerenyi TD, Gleicher N, Meller J, Brown E, Steinfeld L, Chitkara U, Raucher H. Transplacental cardioversion of intrauterine supraventricular tachycardia with digitalis. *Lancet* 1980;2:393–394.

85. Kelin V, Repke J. Supraventricular tachycardia in pregnancy: cardioversion with verapamil. *Obstet Gynecol* 1984;63: 16s–18s.

86. Lubbers WJ, Losekoot TG, Anderson RH, Wellens HJJ. Paroxysmal supraventricular tachycardia in infancy and childhood. *Eur J Cardiol* 1974;2:91–99.

87. Gleicher N, Meller J, Sandler RZ, Sullum S, Wolff–Parkinson–White syndrome in pregnancy. *Obstet Gynecol* 1981; 58:748–752.

88. Muller-Schmidt P. Die paroxysmale Tachikardie in utero. *Geburtshilfe Frauenheilkd* 1959; 19:401–407.

89. Katz M, Vales-Cruz LM, Greco MA, Yanagawa Y, Klein SA, Mufarrij A, Young BK. Diagnosis of congenital mitral and aortic stenosis from the fetal electrocardiogram. *Obstet Gynecol* 1979;54:372–374.

45

INTRAUTERINE THERAPY OF RHYTHM AND RATE DISORDERS AND HEART FAILURE

WILLIAM CUSICK, MD, LOUIS BUTTINO, JR., MD, AND NORBERT GLEICHER, MD

INTRODUCTION

Prenatal ultrasound examinations have allowed the trained clinician to detect abnormalities of the fetal heart rate and structure prior to birth (see Chapter 42–44). As in the adult, abnormalities of the fetal heart rate and structure may result in the development of heart failure. In addition, fetal heart failure has been associated with fetal infections, chromosomal abnormalities, and anemia.[1] In its most severe form, fetal heart failure is manifested as hydrops fetalis, defined as generalized edema of fetal soft tissue. The fetus with hydrops is at increased risk for fetal death. Unfortunately for the hydropic fetus with structural cardiac disease, little can be done antepartum to correct the underlying pathology. For the fetus with hydrops due to cardiac dysrhythmia, anemia, or infection, however, therapeutic modalities exist that may allow for the reversal of hydropic changes. This chapter revews fetal heart failure, with emphasis on potential etiologies and available in utero therapies.

PHYSIOLOGY OF HEART FAILURE

Much of the relevant information about intrauterine heart failure has been extrapolated from the extrauterine experience. In extrauterine life, heart failure is defined as a pathologic state in which the heart fails to pump blood at a rate commensurate with the requirement of the metabolizing tissues, or can do so only from an abnormally elevated filling pressure, as a result of an abnormality in cardiac function.[2] Acceptance of this definition for fetal life does not necessar-

ily imply, however, that the same mechanisms lead to heart failure in the fetus and in the adult. Our understanding of the biophysics of the developing heart is still incomplete. Recent work has shed important light on the topic,[3–5] which is reviewed elsewhere in this volume (Chapter 39).

In postuterine life, a distinction is made between heart failure due to myocardial damage associated with abnormal ventricular function and congestive states due to other causes that are not usually dependent on myocardial function. Congestive heart failure is subdivided into high and low output failure, acute versus chronic, right- versus left-sided, backward versus forward, and systolic versus diastolic forms.[2] But even in the adult situation, a clear distinction between opposite terms cannot always be made. Such a differentiation, even more difficult in the fetal experience, is usually not used in published case reports. Braunwald[2] describes the foregoing terms as useful in a clinical setting but stresses that they are solely descriptive and do not signify fundamentally different disease states.

Extrapolating from the adult experience, low output cardiac failure could arise in the fetus in one of the following etiologies: myocardial disease, valvular disease, pericardial disease, obstructive cardiac or pulmonary lesions, hypertension, and coronary artery disease. High output failure can be associated with fetal anemia, hyperthyroidism, and arteriovenous (AV) shunting. Acute heart failure in the adult is usually the result of either a large myocardial infarction or valve rupture. Neither event has been reported in fetuses. Chronic heart failure in the adult is frequently due to hypertensive or valvular disease. In the fetal experience, a distinction between acute and chronic forms of heart failure has not been made.

Cardiac Problems in Pregnancy, Third Edition
Edited by Uri Elkayam, MD, and Norbert Gleicher, MD
Copyright © 1998 by Wiley-Liss, Inc. ISBN 0-471-16358-9

Neither has there been made a distinction between right- and left-sided failure of the fetal heart. Because of the obvious differences in cardiac blood flow in intra- and extrauterine life, conditions that primarily affect the right ventricle, such as valvular pulmonic stenosis or pulmonary hypertension, will play little or no role in utero. Since most of the returning blood is shifted through the foramen ovale into the left atrium and bypasses the fetal lungs, right-sided failure will not occur. However, if excessive fluid loads reach one of the ventricles for prolonged periods of time, a bilateral failure of the fetal heart may ensue. This type of failure may occur because the muscle bundles that compose both ventricles are continuous or because the ventricles share the interventricular septum. In the adult experience, a rigid differentiation between backward and forward heart failure is considered to be artificial. Both appear to operate in most patients who show signs and symptoms of chronic heart failure.[2]

The differential diagnosis of heart failure in the adult entails the "congested state"[2]: salt and water retention consequent to renal failure and/or excessive parenteral administration of fluids and electrolytes. Excessive intrauterine transfusion therapy in cases of fetal anemia could represent such a situation for the fetus.

CAUSES OF INTRAUTERINE HEART FAILURE

Some authors differentiate between underlying and precipitating causes of heart failure. Such a distinction may be important when a chronic condition does not lead to decompensation of the heart and when there must be a precipitating cause of heart failure, in addition to the underlying cause. In the fetal situation, such a distinction has not been made because long-lasting chronic conditions are uncommon. Poeschmann et al have published an excellent review of fetal hydrops and its many causes.[1] Although hydrops is a nonspecific term referring to the presence of excessive fluid in the fetus and amniotic space irrespective of cause, fetal heart failure is the most frequently recognized etiology. Table 45.1 lists causes of fetal hydrops.

Cardiac Causes

Fetal cardiac abnormalities are the most common identifiable cause for fetal hydrops. Abnormalities of both cardiac structure and rhythm have been implicated. Fortunately, cardiac causes of fetal hydrops are amenable to prenatal diagnosis with detailed ultrasonography and fetal echocardiography.

Structural Cardiac Disease Fetal hydrops has been reported in association with many of the most common structural cardiac lesions. Intracardiac neoplasms (teratoma, rhabdomyoma) have also been associated with the development of fetal hydrops. With some cardiac defects (e.g., complete

TABLE 45.1 Causes of Fetal Hydrops

Cardiovascular
    Structural heart disease
    Fetal dysrhythmia
Chromosomal
    Trisomy 21
    Monosomy XO
    Other
Fetal anemia
    Hemolytic diseases (Rh, ABO, etc.)
    Maternal–fetal hemorrhage
    Fetal blood loss
    Fetal hemoglobinopathies (α-thalassemia, G-6DP deficiency)
Placental causes
    Stuck-twin syndrome (twin–twin transfusion)
    Chorangioma
Infectious
    TORCH infections
    Parvovirus infection
Miscellaneous
    Fetal neoplasms
    Fetal intrathoracic masses
Unexplained

atrioventriicular canal defects, transposition) a concomitant arrhythmia is frequently present. With other lesions, the cardiac rhythm remains normal. Although the precise etiology of heart failure is unknown in these cases unaccompanied by cardiac dysrhythmias, low output cardiac failure due to obstruction of venous and/or arterial blood flow may be responsible.

Fetal Dysrhythmia Cardiac arrhythmia brings about heart failure in adult cardiac patients more often than any other precipitating cause.[2] The operative mechanisms vary with rhythm disorders and may be multifactorial. For example, dissociation between atrial and ventricular contraction interferes with the atrial booster pump and results in the loss of atrial contributions to ventricular filling. At the same time, it produces a rise in atrial pressure. Tachycardia can also be a contributing factor if it serves to shorten the diastolic period, thus decreasing left ventricular filling. However, heart failure can also be caused by bradyarrhythmias. A marked decrease in beats per minute will significantly affect cardiac output.

Table 45.2 summarizes some of the mechanisms of cardiac failure with various rhythm disorders based on reported adult experiences.[2] Since comparable data from the human fetus are not available, the table does not necessarily reflect fetal conditions.

Supraventricular Dysrhythmias Chapter 44 indicates that a vast majority of supraventricular dysrhythmias will not lead to cardiac decompensation of the fetus. Supraventricular

TABLE 45.2   Mechanisms of Adult Heart Failure in Association with Dysrhythmias[a]

Dysrhythmias	Mechanism of Heart Failure
Tachyarrythmias	Reduced time for ventricular filling; Myocardial ischemia
Supraventricular, ventricular arrythmias	Dissociation between atrial and ventricular contractions results in loss of atrial booster pump mechanism
Ventricular tachycardia and arrhythmias with abnormal intraventricular conduction	Further impairment of myocardial performance because synchronicity of ventricular contractions is lost
Complete AV block (with marked bradycardia)	Failure to meet requirement for large increase in stroke volume to prevent reduction in cardiac output

[a]The mechanism for heart failure in association with dysrhythmias may be multifactorial. For example, dissociation between atrial and ventricular contractions interferes with the atrial booster pump mechanism, resulting in loss of the atrial contribution to ventricular filling and at the same time producing an increase in atrial pressure. Shortness of the diastolic period due to tachycardia is also a contributing factor resulting in diminution of left ventricular filling. In cases of ventricular tachycardia and arrhythmias with abnormal intraventricular conduction, an impairment of myocardial performance may result from the loss of synchronicity of ventricular contractions. Heart failure can also be caused by bradyarrhythmias, where a marked decrease in the number of heart beats per minute may result in a significant decline in cardiac output.

Source: Modified from Braunwald.[2]

tachycardia is, however, one of the most frequent dysrhythmias precipitating congestive heart failure. It is our interpretation of published reports[6,7] as well as our own experience[8] that only prolonged episodes of supraventricular tachycardia will lead to congestive heart failure in utero. This opinion, however, is by no means unanimous.[9,10] As in postuterine life, heart failure will not occur as a sudden event. Shenker[6] very clearly demonstrated that even apparently unaffected newborns who had exhibited supraventricular tachycardia in utero were heavier at birth and diuresed more than control infants. This suggests that fetal cardiac function may be affected even before clear signs of hydrops develop. Other supraventricular dysrhythmias such as atrial fibrillation and atrial tachycardia with block are not believed to lead to congestive heart failure in utero unless associated with congenital abnormalities of the fetal heart. Atrial flutter appears to be a more serious disorder and has been associated with development of fetal hydrops[11,12] even in the absence of a cardiac lesion.

Fetal supraventricular dysrhythmias, and in particular supraventricular tachycardia, appear to be closely associated with the presence of congenital Wolff–Parkinson–White syndrome,[13,14] which is discussed in more detail under the heading of Abnormal Conduction.

Ventricular Dysrhythmias   Ventricular dysrhythmias have not been associated with the development of congestive heart failure in utero. Theoretically such a possibility may exist, however (Table 45.2).

Abnormal Conduction   Abnormal conduction can lead to fetal congestive heart failure in two principal ways. As noted in detail in Chapter 44, the Wolff–Parkinson–White syn-

drome has been closely associated with the occurrence of supraventricular tachyarrhythmias in utero. A 10–15% rate of association has been suggested by us[14] and others.[15] Supraventricular arrhythmias, in turn, may lead to congestive heart failure. This association between Wolff–Parkinson–White syndrome and supraventricular arrhythmias in utero should not come as a surprise. A similar association for the postuterine life was made a long time ago.[15]

Third-degree (complete) AV block is the conduction disorder diagnosed most frequently in utero. It is associated with a very high incidence of structural cardiac anomalies in the fetus,[16,17] subclinical autoimmune disease in the mother,[18–20] and the occurrence of intrauterine congestive heart failure if the ventricular rate of the fetal heart is exceedingly low.[21,22] For more details, the reader is referred to Chapter 44.

Chromosomal Causes

The association between fetal hydrops and aneuploidy is well established. Many fetuses with chromosomal abnormalities possess abnormalities of the cardiac and extracardiac structures, both of which may contribute to the development of heart failure. Trisomy 21 and monosomy XO are the two most common karyotypic abnormalities present in hydropic fetuses.[1] It is still not clear why some of these chromosomally abnormal fetuses become hydropic and others remain unaffected.

Fetal Anemia

Anemia is associated with a decrease in the oxygen-carrying capacity of the fetal blood. To maintain proper oxygenation

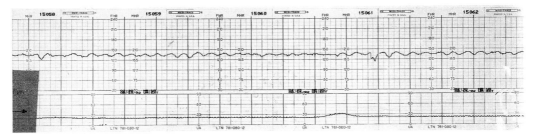

Figure 45.1 Characteristic sinusoidal fetal heart rate pattern in a 30 week fetus with anemia secondary to isoimmunization.

of the different tissues, cardiac output increases. A normal fetal heart will be able to sustain an increasing cardiac output; a compensated heart that is either overloaded or diseased may not. Anemia in the fetus may be a result of both maternal and fetal disease processes. Independent of the cause, if the anemia is severe and sustained, in utero fetal heart failure may develop, leading to the development of fetal hydrops. Severely anemic fetuses may initially be identified after demonstration of a characteristic fetal heart rate pattern. The sinusoidal pattern (Fig. 45.1), although initially described in the setting of severe isoimmunization,[23] may be seen in fetuses rendered anemic by a variety of factors.[24] More recently, a pseudo-siausoidal pattern has been associated with the intrapartum administration of maternal narcotics,[25,26] lending support to the theory that the pattern is the result of loss of autonomic control of the fetal heart rate.[23]

Hemolytic Diseases Hemolytic disease of the fetus occurs when maternal antibodies against fetal red blood cells cross the placenta.[27] Rh disease, the presence of anti-D antibodies in the mother, represents the most important maternal–fetal incompatibility. Before the administration of anti-D immunoglobulin to prevent isoimmunization became routine, 90% of all reported cases of severe hemolytic disease of the fetus were due to the interaction of D-positive fetal red blood cells and maternal anti-D alloantibodies. Since the clinical introduction of immune prophylaxis, other causes of hemolytic disease of the fetus, such as antigens other than D in the Rh system, and so-called irregular antibodies, have increased in relative importance.[27,28]

Hemolytic disease of the fetus progresses slowly. Congestive heart failure and hydrops will occur only in the most severe cases and only rarely in the first pregnancy. In subsequent pregnancies, the chance of more pronounced disease increases. If maternal antibodies capable of inducing fetal hemolytic disease are present, the pregnancy should in most cases by monitored with serial amniocenteses. Fetal hemolysis results in an elevated bilirubin content of the amniotic fluid. Spectrophotometric measurements of bilirubin in amniotic fluid provides an estimation of the severity of fetal involvement. Most institutions utilize the method developed by

Liley,[29] which is based on the evaluation of optical density of amniotic fluid at 450 μm (delta 450). Specific Liley graphs allow an accurate comparison of interlaboratory results in three levels of severity. The rise in optical density at 450 μm is proportional to the degree of severity of Rh disease in the affected fetus. Between 20 and 25% of fetuses with erythroblastosis fetalis have hemolysis so severe that they ultimately develop universal edema with ascites (immune hydrops). The mechanisms responsible for the development of fetal hydrops are complex, and their discussion would exceed the purpose of the chapter.

All hydrops fetalis was formerly attributed to fetal heart failure, caused by progressive fetal anemia. More recent evidence indicates that the causative mechanisms for hydrops are more variable.[30] Heart failure will develop in only a small percentage of hydropic fetuses and rarely, if ever, will it represent the primary cause of hydrops fetalis.[29] Once fetal involvement in the severe zone (zone 3) of the Liley graph has been determined, intervention is indicated. If the fetus is too immature for delivery, intrauterine transfusion of the fetus represents the most appropriate form of therapy. In successful cases, fetal well-being clearly improves after such therapy. Among the recorded changes is the resolution of fetal sinusoidal heart rate after intrauterine transfusions[31]; however, the opposite effect has also been reported. In at least two instances, sinusoidal fetal heart rate was noted for the first time shortly after intrauterine transfusion.[32,33]

Maternal–Fetal Hemorrhage Although small minor maternal–fetal transfusions occur in the majority of pregnancies, large hemorrhages (>30mL) occur in only 0.3–0.7% of pregnancies.[34,35] In some cases of large fetal–maternal bleeds, particularly in association with massive placental abruption, in utero fetal death may result. Alternatively, if the maternal–fetal hemorrhage is large and/or sustained, fetal anemia may develop. As is the case for anemia associated with Rh disease, such fetuses may develop overt heart failure, manifested by hydrops.

Fetal Blood Loss Acute blood loss has not been reported in association with intrauterine heart failure. However, sinusoidal fetal heart rate patterns in association with acute blood loss have been reported.[36,37] As in the adult experience, rapid loss of large amounts of blood results in shock rather than heart failure. Sinusoidal fetal heart rate then will result, not as an indication of intrauterine heart failure, but as a preterminal event.

Fetal Hemoglobinopathies Fetuses homozygous for α-thalassemia are unable to produce α-globin chains. The resultant hemoglobin H (β4) produced has a high oxygen affinity and is prone to hemolysis.[38] Similarly fetuses with G-6PD deficiency are prone to hemolysis with maternal ingestion of oxidants.[39] With severe hemolysis, fetal anemia and, subsequently, heart failure may develop. Although these disorders are not common causes for fetal hydrops, their genetic basis makes them one of the few etiologies associated with recurrent nonimmune fetal hydrops.

Placental Causes

Stuck-Twin syndrome The stuck-twin syndrome, also referred to as twin–twin transfusion, is a complication occurring almost exclusively in monochorionic twin gestations. The condition is the result of arteriovenous communications in the single chorionic plate shared by both twins. Consequently, both fetuses are at risk for heart failure; the donor (blood-losing) twin because of high output cardiac failure, and the recipient (hypertransfused) twin because of volume overload.[40]

Chorangioma Placental chorangioma may result in the development of fetal hydrops and heart failure due to increased shunting of fetal blood.

Infectious Causes

Intrauterine infections may be either bacterial or viral. Both types have been implicated in the development of in utero heart failure. The mechanism by which infection leads to failure are variable. Viral infections, particularly TORCH (**t**oxoplasmosis, **o**ther, **r**ubella virus, **c**ytomegalovirus, and **h**erpes simplex virus) infections, have been the organisms most frequently implicated as infectious causes of fetal hydrops. Recently, parvovirus B19 has received much attention for its association with fetal hydrops and death. In this instance, hydrops appears to be the result of severe fetal anemia secondary to a transient, virally induced red cell aplasia.[41]

Miscellaneous

Fetal hydrops has been described in association with a variety of extracardiac malformations of the fetus. In the case of pulmonary lesions, heart failure may be mediated through an obstruction to blood flow. In the case of certain fetal neo-plasms, such as teratomas, high output heart failure may be secondary to increased blood flow to the fetal tumor. Other times, despite an extensive evaluation, no obvious cause for fetal hydrops is identified.

CLINICAL MANIFESTATIONS

Once intrauterine congestive heart failure has become clinically evident, the diagnosis is not difficult to make. Rapid advances in sonography, and more specifically fetal echocardiography, allow the trained sonologist to diagnose abnormalities of heart structure, rhythm, and structure prenatally. Table 45.3 summarizes the most significant sonographic and Doppler findings in fetuses with intrauterine heart failure (Figs. 45.2–45.4). Many of the sonographic findings, such as polyhydramnios, placentomegaly, fetal ascites, and fetal skin edema, are nonspecific and may be present in fetuses in the absence of heart failure. The more findings present, in particular in the presence of abnormal Doppler changes, the more likely the diagnosis of fetal heart failure.

When intrauterine heart failure is suspected, the diagnosis will be established by actively searching for the findings listed in Table 45.3. Having made the diagnosis of in utero congestive heart failure, the clinician proceeds to identify the underlying cause (Table 45.1). Identifying the precise etiology for hydrops will allow for appropriate in utero therapy, when available, directed at correcting the underlying pathology.

TREATMENT OF INTRAUTERINE HEART FAILURE

The key to appropriate treatment of the fetus with in utero congestive heart failure is in defining the precipitating cause. Unfortunately, little can be offered prenatally for the hydropic fetus with an underlying chromosomal abnormality and/or structural cardiac defect. Conversely, the fetus with congenital heart failure due to fetal arrhythmia or anemia may benefit from available in utero therapies. Such therapy will be dictated, in part, by the gestational age of the fetus. In

TABLE 45.3 Sonographic/Doppler Findings in Intrauterine Congestive Heart Failure

Placentomegaly
Polyhydramnios
Pericardial/pleural effusion
Cardiomegaly
Fetal skin edema
Fetal ascites
AV valve regurgitation
Umbilical vein pulsations

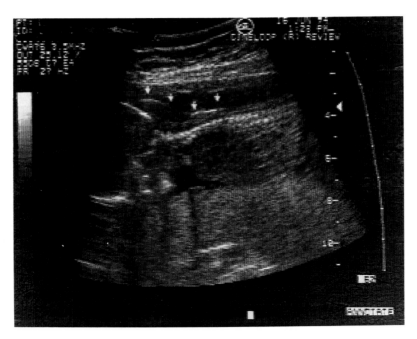

Figure 45.2   Longitudinal image of a hydropic fetus showing fetal scalp edema (arrowheads).

the setting of fetal immaturity, in utero therapy is the preferred course. With fetal maturity, prompt delivery may be effected if in utero therapy is technically cumbersome (intrauterine blood transfusion) or proves unsuccessful (persistent arrhythmia despite medication).

Fetal Dysrhythmias

Fetal dysrhythmias represent the most frequent indications for intrauterine intervention. If the fetus can be delivered safely, extrauterine therapy is probably preferable over in-

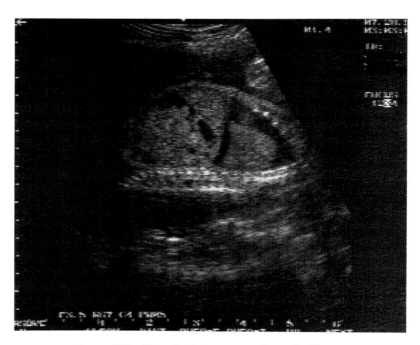

Figure 45.3   Pleural effusion surrounding a fetal lung.

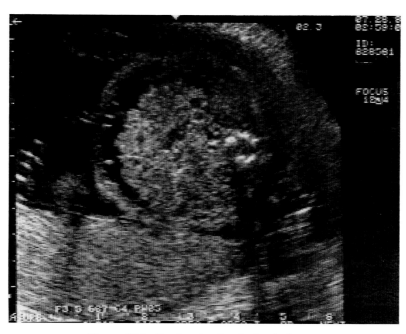

Figure 45.4   Fetal ascites in a hydropic fetus.

trauterine treatment, in accordance with principles stated earlier. Whenever an intrauterine dysrhythmia is diagnosed, the following questions need to be asked:

1. Is this a dysrhythmia that is known to lead to congestive heart failure? If the answer is yes, a search for signs of fetal heart failure should be performed (Table 45.3).

2. Is this a dysrhythmia that is known to be associated with structural cardiac defects? If the answer is yes, a careful ultrasound evaluation of the fetal heart should be performed (Chapter 46).

Supraventricular Tachycardia   Supraventricular tachycardia as a cause of intrauterine congestive heart failure was first treated pharmacologically in utero in 1980.[42] Transplacental cardioversion was first achieved by giving digitalis to the mother. Digitalis has been widely reported to cross the placenta, achieving an equilibrium in fetal and maternal sera.[43] However, such an equilibrium does not appear to occur in cases of fetal heart failure. Both we[8] and Harrigan et al[44] noted clearly lower digitalis levels in fetuses of properly digitalized mothers. Moreover, Weiner and Thompson[45] reported the cordocentesis of a fetus after failed digitalis therapy. While the maternal digitalis concentration was 1.8–2.6 μg/mL, fetal concentrations reached only 0.8 μg/mL. The difference in levels is not well understood and has been reviewed extensively.[46]

Digitalis, still the principal drug for intrauterine cardioversion of supraventricular tachycardia,[42,45,47–52] is given to the fetus through the mother by either the intravenous or oral route. To overcome the maternofetal gradient, some investigators suggest direct administration of the drug under ultrasonographic guidance into either amniotic fluid or fetal muscle.[45]

In postuterine life, drug therapy for supraventricular tachycardias varies depending on the underlying mechanisms.[53] For example, AV nodal reentrant tachycardia (AVNRT), which constitutes the majority of cases, is usually treated with verapamil hydrochloride, during acute attacks, while chronic therapy is given with either digoxin, verapamil, or propranolol hydrochloride. Among AV reciprocating supraventricular tachycardias, the second most common mechanism, the orthodromic form occurs most frequently and often is associated with the Wolff–Parkinson–White syndrome. Acute episodes can be terminated with lidocaine hydrochloride, procainamide, quinidine, or dysopyramide. Digitalis is considered to be contraindicated when a Wolff–Parkinson–White syndrome is present. Verapamil may be useful in such patients, although it is contraindicated with atrial flutter or fibrillation. The newest therapeutic approaches involve such agents as flecainide acetate and encainide hydrochloride. Antidromic AV reciprocating supraventricular tachycardia can also be associated with a Wolff–Parkinson–White syndrome. The initial therapeutic approach to such patients is usually procainamide.[53]

It is obviously impossible to establish in the fetus the underlying electrophysiologic differential diagnosis for supraventricular tachycardia. Therefore, the choice of digitalis as an initial therapeutic agent can be supported, especially since the relative fetal safety of the drug has been established.[46] Our advanced understanding of the electrophysiology of supraventricular tachyarrhythmias allows us, however, to predict that some fetuses with supraventricular tachycardia will not benefit from digitalis therapy and may, in fact, deteriorate. This speculation has already been confirmed by individual case reports.[45,54,55] Digitalis therapy for intrauterine supraventricular tachycardia should be given only under close observation of the fetus. If digitalization does not achieve cardioversion, or if the fetal status continues to deteriorate, digitalis should be withdrawn and an alternative drug regimen instituted.

Whenever drugs are utilized during pregnancy, their fetal effects are of special concern. This excludes many of the newer antiarrhythmic drugs from first-line use, since their safety in pregnancy has not yet been established. Several authors[46,56,57] have reviewed in great detail the use of antiarrhythmic drugs in pregnancy, and the reader is referred to these reviews or any comparable reference before a specific drug is chosen. Many different pharmaceutical agents have been utilized in cases of fetal supraventricular tachycardia: quinidine,[48,55,58,59] procainamide,[45,60,61] verapamil,[13,48,62,63] and propranolol.[47,59] More recently, successful fetal cardioversion has been reported with the use of flecainide,[64–67] and adenosine[68] in pregnancy. At present, many of these drugs appear to be acceptable as a second line of therapy if digitalis has failed.

All medications are to be given to the mother in standard therapeutic (pregnancy) doses, considering the expansion of plasma volume during gestation. Since the fetal effect of these drugs is dependent on the placental passage, appropriate plasma levels in the mother are essential. Published data suggest that appropriate therapeutic drug levels in fetuses with heart failure may be difficult to achieve at times. The more severely affected a fetus, the more difficult is pharmacologic cardioversion in utero. To overcome the obvious circulatory insufficiency of the severely hydropic fetus, Weiner and Thompson[45] and others[69] have recommended direct fetal treatment. Other investigators hope to improve fetal fluid overload via treatment with diuretics such as furosemide.

A variety of drug regimen are thus available for the treatment of supraventricular tachycardia in utero. While some authorities have recommended fetal treatment even in the absence of congestive heart failure,[49,50] we use this approach only if persistent supraventricular tachycardia occurs before the fetus is viable, or if (even early) signs of congestive heart failure are apparent at a time when delivery is not feasible.

Atrial Fibrillation and Flutter The association between atrial fibrillation and intrauterine congestive heart failure has not been made. Short episodes of atrial fibrillation have been recorded, however, associated with prolonged supraventricular tachycardia.[42] The risk of converting a patient with supraventricular tachycardia is especially pronounced with the antidromic AV reciprocating type[53] in the presence of the Wolff–Parkinson–White syndrome when digitalis is given for cardioversion.[70,71] Some of the reported cases of intrauterine atrial fibrillation and/or flutter were thus undoubtedly iatrogenically induced.

Atrial flutter appears to represent a more significant clinical problem in utero. Even though its incidence seems severely underreported, cases of severe fetal decompensation have appeared in the literature (Chapter 44). Because the reported experience with intrauterine atrial flutter is so limited, it is difficult to make treatment recommendations. Since congenital anomalies of the heart can be associated with this rhythm disorder, it is important to rule them out. When this has been done, it appears reasonable to follow guidelines similar to those applicable in cases of supraventricular tachycardia, where we recommend pharmacologic intervention only in cases of previability of the fetus. Standard drug treatment can be utilized.[53] with digitalis probably representing once again, the first drug of choice.

Third-Degree (Complete) AV Block In the majority of cases, complete AV block is well tolerated in utero and will not require intervention until after birth. However, with extremely low ventricular rates (< 50 beats/min) and/or associated structural lesions of the heart, which may lead to regurgitation of mitral or tricuspid valves, hydrops may develop.[72,73] Before intrauterine therapy becomes a consideration, the fetal heart should be evaluated sonographically. Moreover, because of the close association with maternal autoimmune disease, the maternal autoimmune status requires evaluation even in the absence of known or apparent clinical disease (Chapter 44).

It used to be thought that once a fetus had developed complete AV block, therapy directed at the associated autoantibody abnormality (SSA/anti-Ro) would be of no benefit. Recent case reports, however, suggest differently. Copel et al reported on five cases of congenital heart block treated with steroids between 20 and 23 weeks of gestation. Although the maternal autoantibody levels remain unchanged, the degree of heart block improved in two fetuses. In addition, fetal hydrops, present in three fetuses, resolved after the initiation of therapy.[74] Similarly, Ishimaru et al reported a single case in which a diminution in fetal heart block was noted after administration of corticosteroids to the mother.[75] Whether very early suppression of those autoantibodies decreases the incidence of complete AV block in the offspring of autoantibody-positive mothers is under investigation.

If ultrasonographic evaluation of the fetal heart excludes the presence of a major congenital heart defect, and if the ventricular rate is below 50 beats per minute, the potential exists for development of congestive heart failure in utero. Sonographic signs are the same as those listed in Table 45.3. Hydropic fetuses will die in utero if not delivered before such a terminal event takes place.

Only under previable circumstances can intrauterine pharmacological intervention be recommended. Such intervention will be directed toward an increase in ventricular rate of the fetal heart. Drugs that have been utilized for that purpose include atropine, isoproterenol, and terbutaline. Digitalis has been given to improve ventricular function.[76] To decrease fetal fluid overload, diuretics also may be used. All medications are usually given to the mother, and they achieve their fetal effects through transplacental passage. Recently, Carpenter et al[76] recommended fetal ventricular pacing for hydrops secondary to complete AV block as an alternative to pharmacological intervention or in cases of failure of drug therapy. It remains to be seen whether the application of any of these proposed treatment modalities in utero will improve the prognosis of hydropic infants, which historically has been exceedingly poor.[77–79]

Fetal Anemia

Fetal anemia, due to immune and nonimmune causes, can be treated with intrauterine blood transfusion if the fetus is too immature for delivery.[30] Other treatment modalities have proved disappointing. Whether cardiac support of the fetus with drugs such as digitalis enhances well-being has not been established. Anecdotal reports on the use of digitalis and diuretics in an attempt to enhance fluid absorption in hydropic fetuses have appeared intermittently in the literature.

Stuck-Twin Syndrome

Recently, two therapeutic modalities have been described aimed at improving the dismal prognosis for twin pairs complicated by the stuck-twin syndrome: serial, therapeutic amniocentesis[80–82] and fetoscopic laser occlusion of chorioangiopagus.[83] Therapeutic amniocentesis involves the removal of a large volume (500–10,000 mL) of amniotic fluid from around the recipient twin. Amniocentesis is repeated if polyhydramnios recurs. The goal of this therapy is to normralize the amniotic fluid volume between the twins. Initial results have been encouraging, with overall neonatal survivial rates of 44–80%.[80,81] Fetoscopic laser occlusion of chorioangiopagus was designed in an attempt to obliterate the abnormal arteriovenous communications that are felt to be responsible for the development of the syndrome. DeLia et al reported a fetal survival of 56% in 22 patients treated in the early second trimester.[83] Because of the limited experience and technical complexities of fetoscopic laser occlusion of chorioangiopagus, such an approach remains investigational at this time.

Infections

Unfortunately, effective fetal therapies for hydrops due to TORCH infection are lacking. Hydrops secondary to intrauterine infection with syphylis may be amenable to penicillin therapy.[84] As discussed earlier, fetal hydrops secondary to acute parvovirus infection is secondary to severe anemia. Treatment with intrauterine blood transfusion has proven to be highly effective.[41]

PROGNOSIS

Although heart failure in the fetus manifested by hydrops fetalis in its most severe form is an uncommon occurrence, the increasing use of diagnostic ultrasound will likely result in a higher prenatal detection rate of these affected fetuses. Potential etiologies for fetal heart failure are many and varied. The ultimate prognosis depends on the underlying etiology and the availability of effective therapies. A detailed evaluation, incorporating targeted ultrasound, fetal echocardiography, fetal karyotyping, hematologic evaluation, and assessment for intrauterine infection are essential in any attempt to diagnosis the underlying cause of fetal heart failure. Knowing the etiology of heart failure allows the clinician to individualize treatment. For the fetus with heart failure due to anemia, cardiac dysrhythmia, stuck-twin syndrome, and intrauterine infection, in utero therapies exist that may improve neonatal outcome.

REFERENCES

1. Poeschmann RP, Verheijen RHM, VanDongen PWJ. Differential diagnosis and causes of nonimmunological hydrops fetalis: a review. *Obstet Gynecol Survey* 1991;46:223–231.
2. Braunwald E. Heart failure. In: Isselbacher KJ, Braunwald E, Wilson JD, Martin JB, Fauci AS, Kasper DL, eds. *Harrison's Principles of Internal Medicine.* 13th ed. New York: McGraw-Hill; 1994;998–1009.
3. Anderson PAW, Manring A, Crenshaw C Jr. Biophysics of the developing heart. The force-interval relationship. *Am J Obstet Gynecol* 1980;138:33–43.
4. Anderson PAW, Manring A, Crenshaw C Jr. Biophysics of the developing heart. II. The interaction of the force–interval relationship with inotropic state and muscle length (preload). *Am J Obstet Gynecol* 1980;138:44–54.
5. Redman TF. The significance of some unusual fetal cardiac arrhythmias. *J Obstet Gynaecol Br Emp* 1985;65:304–309.
6. Shenker L. Fetal cardiac arrhythmias. *Obstet Gynecol Survey* 1979;34:561–572.
7. Naheed ZJ, Strasburger JF, Deal BJ, Benson DW Jr, Gisding SS. Fetal tachycardia: mechanisms and predicators of hydrops fetalis. *J Am College Cardiol* 1996;27:1736–1740.

8. Chitkara U, Gleicher N, Longhi R, et al. Persistent supraventricular tachycardia in utero. *Diagn Gynecol Obstet* 1980;2: 291–298.

9. Newberger JW, Keane JF. Intrauterine supraventricular tachycardia. *J Pediatr* 1979;95:780–786.

10. Levkoff AH. Perinatal outcome of paroxysmal tachycardia of the newborn with onset in utero. *Am J Obstet Gynecol* 1969;104:73–79.

11. Van der Horst RL. Congenital atrial flutter and cardiac failure presenting as hydrops foetalis at birth. *S Afr Med J* 1970;44: 1037–1039.

12. Moller JH, Davachi F, Anderson RC. Atrial flutter in infancy. *J Pediatr* 1969;75:643–651.

13. Berman M, Joyner G, Kock H. Fetal supraventricular tachycardia: review of the literature. *Obstet Gynecol Survey* 1985;40:61–68.

14. Gleicher N, Elkayam U. Cardiac problems in pregnancy. II. Fetal aspects. *JAMA* 1984;252:78–80.

15. Herin P, Thoren C. Congenital arrhythmias with supraventricular tachycardia in the perinatal period. *Acta Obstet Gynecol Scand* 1973;52:381–386.

16. Morquio L. Sur une maladie infantile et familiale caracterisée par des modification permanentes du pouls et des attaques syncopales et epileptiformes et la morte subite. *Arch Med Enfant* 1901;4:462–467.

17. Griffiths SP. Congenital complete heart block. *Circulation* 1971;43:615–617. Editorial.

18. Hull D, Binns BA, Joyce D. Congenital heart block and widespread fibrosis due to maternal lupus erythematosus. *Arch Dis Child* 1966;4:688–690.

19. McCue CM, Mantakas ME, Tingelstad JB, Ruddy S. Congenital heart block in newborns of mothers with connective tissue disease. *Circulation* 1977;56:82–90.

20. Altenburger KM, Jedziniak M, Roper WL, Hernandez J. Congenital complete heart block associated with hydrops fetalis. *J Pediatr* 1977;9:618–620.

21. Michaelsson M, Engl MA. Congenital complete heart block: an international study of the natural history. *Pediatr Cardiol* 1972;4:86.

22. Hochberg SH. Congenital heart block. *Am J Obstet Gynecol* 1964;88:238–241.

23. Rochard F, Schifrin BS, Goupil F, Legrand H, Blotiere J, Sureau C. Nonstressed fetal heart rate monitoring in an antepartum period. *Am J Obstet Gynecol* 1976;126:699–706.

24. Gleicher N, Runowica CD, Brown BL. Sinusoidal fetal heart rate pattern in association with amnionitis. *Obstet Gynecol* 1980;56:109–112.

25. Angel JL, Knuppel R, Lake M. Sinusoidal fetal heart rate pattern associated with intravenous butorphanol administration: a case report. *Am J Obstet Gynecol* 1984;149:465–467.

26. Epstein H, Waxman A, Gleicher N, et al. Meperidine induced sinusoidal fetal heart rate pattern and reversal with naloxone. *Obstet Gynecol* 1982;59:22S–25S.

27. Cunningham FG, MacDonald PC, Gant NF, Leveno KJ, Gilstrap LC. Hemolysis from isoimmunization. In: Cunningham FG, MacDonald PC, Gant NF, Leveno KJ, Gilstrap LC.,

eds. *Williams Obstetrics*. 19th ed. Norwalk, CT: Appleton & Lange, 1993; 1004–1013.

28. Smith BD, Haber JM, Queenan JT. Irregular antibodies in pregnant women. *Obstet Gynecol* 1967;29:118–124.

29. Liley AW. Liquor amnii analysis in the management of the pregnancy complicated by rhesus sensitization. *Am J Obstet Gynecol* 1961;83:1359–1364.

30. Bowman JM. The management of Rh-isoimmunization. *Obstet Gynecol* 1981;78:(52)1–16.

31. Hatjis CG, Mennum M, Sacks LM, Schwarz RH. Resolution of a sinusoidal fetal heart rate pattern following intrauterine transfusion. *Am J Obstet Gynecol* 1978;132:109–111.

32. Mueller-Heubach E, Cartis SN, Edelstone DI. Sinosoidal fetal heart rate pattern following intrauterine transfusion. *Obstet Gynecol* 1977;52:435s–465s.

33. Urma V, Tejani N, Weiss RR, Chatterjee S, Halitsky V. Sinusoidal fetal heart rate patterns in severe Rh disease. *Obstet Gynecol* 1980;55:666–669.

34. Oxorn H. Multiple pregnancy. In: Oxorn H, ed. *Human Labor and Birth*. 4th ed. New York: Appleton-Century-Crofts; 1980; 275–279.

35. Zipursky A. The universal prevention of Rh immunization. *Clin Obstet Gynecol* 1971;14:869–884.

36. Caspi B, Lancet M, Kessler I. Sinusoidal pattern of uterine contractions in abruptio placentae. *Int J Gynaecol Obstet* 1980;17: 615–616.

37. Young BK, Katz M, Wilson SJ. Sinusoidal fetal heart rate. I. Clinical significance. *Am J Obstet Gynecol Surg* 1979;34:561–572.

38. Bryan EM, Chaimongkol B, Harris DA. α-Thalassaemic hydrops fetalis. *Arch Dis Child* 1981;56:476–480.

39. Mentzer WC, Collier E. Hydrops fetalis associated with erythrocyte G-6PD deficiency and maternal ingestion of fava beans and ascorbic acid. *J Pediatr* 1975;86:565–567.

40. Driscoll SG. Hydrops fetalis. *N Engl J Med* 1966;275: 1432–1434.

41. Rodis JF. Parvovirus in pregnancy. In: Lee RV, Garner PR, Barron WM, Coustan DR, eds. *Current Obstetric Medicine*. St. Louis: Mosby-Yearbook; 1995;159–181.

42. Steinfeld L, Chitkara U, Raucher H. Transplacental cardioversion of intrauterine supraventricular tachycardia with digitalis. *Lancet* 1980;2:393–394.

43. Saarikoski P. Placental transfer and fetal uptake of ³H-digoxin in humans. *Br J Obstet Gynaecol* 1976;83:879–884.

44. Harrigan JT, Kanpos JJ, Sikka A, Spisso KR, Natarajan N, Rosenfeld D, Leiman S, Korn D. Successful treatment of fetal congestive heart failure secondary to tachycardia. *N Engl J Med* 1981;304:1527–1529.

45. Weiner CP, Thompson MIB. Direct treatment of fetal supraventricular tachycardia after failed transplacental therapy. *Am J Obstet Gynecol* 1988;158:570–573.

46. Moriguchi Mitani G, Steinberg I, Liew EJ, Harriton EC, Elkayam U. The pharmacokinetics of antiarrhythmic agents in pregancy and lactation. *Clin Pharmacokinet* 1987;12:253–291.

47. Heaton FC, Vaughan R. Intrauterine supraventricular tachycardia: cardioversion with maternal digoxin. *Obstet Gynecol* 1982;60:749–752.

48. Wladimiroff JW, Stewart PA. Fetal therapy: treatment of fetal cardiac arrhythmias. *Br J Hosp Med* 1985;34:134–140.

49. Kleinman CS, Copel JA, Winstein EM, Sourtulli TV, Hobbins JC. In utero diagnosis and treatment of fetal supraventricular tachycardia. *Semin Perinatol* 1985;2:113–129.

50. Nagorshima M, Asai T, Suzuki C, Matsushima M, Ogawa A. Intrauterine supraventricular tachyarrhythmias and transplacental digitalization. *Arch Dis Child* 1986;61:996.

51. Wiggins JW, Bowes W, Clewell W. Echocardiographic diagnosis and intravenous digoxin management and fetal tachyarrhythmias and congestive heart failure. *Am J Dis Child* 1985;140:202–204.

52. Lingman G, Ludstrom N-R, Marsal K, Ohrlander IS. Fetal cardiac arrhythmia: clinical outcome in 113 cases. *Acta Obstet Gynecol Scand* 1986;65:263–267.

53. Manolis AS, Mark Estes NA. Supraventricular tachycardia: mechanisms and therapy. *Arch Lut Med* 1987;147:1706–1716.

54. Sorland S, Torp KH, Jenssen J. Hjerte-arytmier hos foster og nyfdt. En oversikt og omtale av 5 kasus. *T Nor Laegeforen* 1963;83:1654–1659.

55. Spinnato JA, Shaver DC, Flinn GS, Sibou BM, Watson DL. Fetal supraventricular tachycardia in utero therapy with digoxin and quinidine. *Obstet Gynecol* 1984;64:730–735.

56. Ito S, Magee L, Smallhorn J. Drug therapy for fetal arrhythmias. *Clin Perinatol* 1994;21:543–572.

57. Pinsky WW, Rayburn WF, Evans MI. Pharmacologic therapy for fetal arrhythmias. *Clin Obstet Gynecol* 1991;34:304–309.

58. Guntheroth WG, Cyr DR, Mack LA. Hydrops from reciprocating atrioventricular tachycardia in a 27-week fetus requiring quinidine for conversion. *Obstet Gynecol* 1985;66(suppl):29.

59. Kileen AA, Bowen LD. Fetal supraventricular tachycardia treated with high dose quinidine: toxicity associated with marked elevation of the metabolite, 3(S)-3-hydroxy quinidine. *Obstet Gynecol* 1987;70:445–448.

60. Dumesic DA, Silverman WH, Tobious S, Yolbur MS. Transplacental cardioversion of fetal supraventricular tachycardia with procainamide. *N Engl J Med* 1982;307:1128–1131.

61. Given BD, Phillippe M, Sanders SP, Djou V. Procainamide cardioversion of fetal supraventricular tachyarrhythmia. *Am J Cardiol* 1984;53:1460–1461.

62. Wolff F, Breuher KH, Shleusher KH, Bolt A. Prenatal diagnosis and therapy of fetal heart rate anomalies: with a contribution on the placental transfer of verapamil. *J Perinatal Med* 1980;8:203–208.

63. Klein V, Repke J. Supraventricular tachycardia in pregnancy: cardioversion with verapamil. *Obstet Gynecol* 1984;63:165–185.

64. Mills M. Treatment of fetal supraventricular tachycardia with flecainide acetate after digoxin failure. *Am J Obstet Gynecol* 1992;166:1863. Letter.

65. Kofinas AD, Simon NV, Sagel H, et al. Treatment of fetal supraventricular tachycardia with flecainide acetate after digoxin failure. *Am J Obstet Gynecol* 1991;165:630–631.

66. Perry JC, Ayres NA, Carpenter RJ Jr. Fetal supraventricular tachycardia treated with flecainide acetate. *J Pediatr* 1991;118:303–305.

67. Allan LD, Chita SK, Sharland GK, et al. Flecainide in the treatment of fetal tachycardias. *Br Heart J* 1991;65:46–48.

68. Blanch G, Walkinshaw SA, Walsh K. Cardioversion of fetal arrhythmia with adenosine. *Lancet* 1991;344:1646. Letter.

69. Hallak M, Neerhof MG, Perry R, et al. Fetal supraventricular tachycardia and hydrops fetalis: combined intensive, direct, and transplacental therapy. *Obstet Gynecol* 1991;78:523–525.

70. Surp RJ, Castellanos A, Mallon SM. Mechanisms of spontaneous alteration between reciprocating tachycardia and atrial flutter: fibrillation in the Wolff–Parkinson–White syndrome. *Circulation* 1977;56:409–416.

71. Campbell RWF, Smith RA, Gallagher JJ. Atrial fibrillation in the preexcitation syndrome. *Am J Cardiol* 1977;40:514–520.

72. Kleinman CB, Daunerstein RC, Jafe CC. Fetal echocardiography; a tool for evaluation of in utero cardiac arrhythmias and monitoring of in utero therapy: analysis of 71 patients. *Am J Cardiol* 1983;51:237–243.

73. Huhta JC, Strasburger JF, Carpenter RJ, Reiter A, Abinader E. Pulsed Doppler fetal echocardiography. *J Clin Ultrasound* 1985;13:247–254.

74. Copel JA, Buyon JP, Kleinman CS. Successful in utero treatment of fetal heart block. *Am J Obstet Gynecol* 1994;170:281. Abstract.

75. Ishimaru S, Izaki S, Kitamura K, Morita Y. Neonatal lupus erythematosus: dissolution of atrioventricular block after administration of corticosteroids to the pregnant mother. *Dermatologia* 1994;189:92–94.

76. Carpenter RJ, Strasburger JF, Garson A Jr, Smith R, Deter RL, Engelhardt HT Jr. Fetal ventricular pacing for hydrops secondary to complete atrioventricular block. *J Am College Cardiol* 1986;8:1434–1436.

77. Holsgreve W, Curry CJR, Golbus MS, Callen PW, Filly RA, Smith JC. Investigation of non-immune hydrops fetalis. *Am J Obstet Gynecol* 1984;150:805–812.

78. DeVore GR, Siassi B, Platt LD. Fetal echocardiography. IV. M-mode assessment of ventricular site and contractility during the second and third trimesters of pregnancy in the normal fetus. *Am J Obstet Gynecol* 1984;150:981–988.

79. Groues AM, Allan CD, Rosenthal E. Outcome of isolated congenital complete heart block diagnosed in utero. *Heart* 1996;75:190–194.

80. Urig MA, Clewell WH, Ellio JP. Twin–twin transfusion syndrome. *Am J Obstet Gynecol* 1990;163:1522–1526.

81. Pinette MG, Pan Y, Pinette SG, Stubblefield PG. Treatment of twin–twin transfusion syndrome. *Obstet Gynecol* 1993;82:841–846.

82. Elliot JP, Sawyer AT, Radin TG, Strong RE. Large-volume therapeutic amniocentesis in the treatment of hydramnios. *Obstet Gynecol* 1994;84:1025–1027.

83. DeLia J, Kuhlmann R, Harstad T, Cruikshank D. Twin–twin transfusion syndrome treated by fetoscopic neodymium: YAG laser occlusion of chorioangiopagus. *Am J Obstet Gynecol* 1993;168:308. Abstract.

84. Barton JR, Thorpe AM, Shaver DC, Hager WD, Sibai BM. Nonimmune hydrops fetalis associated with maternal infection with syphilis. *Am J Obstet Gynecol* 1992:167:56–58.

46

DOPPLER ULTRASOUND IN PREGNANCY

HAROLD SCHULMAN, FACOG, MD

INTRODUCTION

The cardiovascular changes in pregnancy are based on the new hormonal milieu and the development of the uteroplacental circulation. Doppler ultrasound technology has progressed to the point of permitting clinicians to observe the evolution of the uterine and umbilical circulation in pregnancy. Normal development of these circulatory beds virtually guarantees that the fetus will be adequately nourished and the mother will not experience severe hypertensive sequelae.

Another application of Doppler ultrasound is in the study of the velocity flow patterns of individual fetal or maternal vessels to obtain more finite information about organ flow or estimates of cardiac output. This chapter reviews the work that has been done to explore the theoretical and clinical applications of this technology.

THEORY

The Doppler principle is well known. Briefly, it states that returning sound waves have altered frequency return proportional to the movement or velocity of the object from which they are reflected. This is the Doppler shift. Since the frequency of the origination signal is regulated and the returning signal can be captured, the remaining components of the equation are to process the signal and knowledge of the constant velocity of the sound waves in the medium under study. The solution to the processing of the signal was spectral analysis, a technique that summarizes the returning signals in the frequency domain. This allows a larger number of waveforms to be captured, which then can be displayed in the time

domain on an oscilloscope screen. The display is that of amplitude versus time, in which case the amplitude reflects the number of returning signals at that moment. Since the returning signals are created by the moving erythrocytes, the magnitude of the frequencies depends on the velocity of red cells and the mass of red cells present. The faster the blood is moving, the greater the amplitude; conversely, if the velocity stops, there will be no frequency return (no Doppler shift). In theory, density of red cell mass could also be an important variable, but anemia and polycythemia are not of significance in small blood vessels, where most of the resistance to velocity flow is generated.

Velocity is a component of volume flow. Flow is equal to vessel area times velocity. Hence, if the vessel can be visualized, the diameter measured, and the angle of incidence known, the volume flow can be calculated (Fig. 46.1). It is necessary to know the angle of incidence of the sonar signal because the returning signals were altered by the vector force of the velocity.

It is to be emphasized that Doppler reflects flow velocity and can be viewed as volume flow only indirectly. Velocity is altered primarily by the resistance beyond the point of measurement. The waveforms are complex and are a manifestation of many of the physical phenomena that occur in blood vessels (e.g., elasticity, pressure, turbulence, and vessel length).

It is also necessary to be aware of the differences between pulsed Doppler and continuous wave systems. The continuous wave systems provide better signals at lower energy levels. Continuous wave Doppler does not focus on one vessel but will return signals from all vessels crossed. The pulsed systems can be range-gated with real-time ultrasound, offering the advantage of studying specific vessels.

Cardiac Problems in Pregnancy, Third Edition
Edited by Uri Elkayam, MD, and Norbert Gleicher, MD
Copyright © 1998 by Wiley-Liss, Inc. ISBN 0-471-16358-9

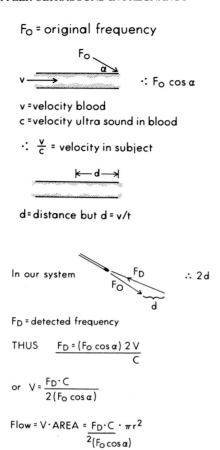

Figure 46.1 Doppler shift and the calculation of volume flow in a blood vessel. The sound waves are reflected by the moving red blood cells.

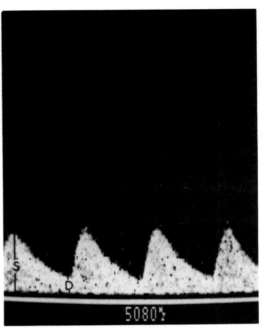

Figure 46.2 Umbilical artery velocity waveforms: time frame, 1.6 seconds. Frequency amplitude is relative and depends on the angle of insonation. The S/D ratio is calculated as shown.

The U.S. Food and Drug Administration established a safety limit of 94 mW/cm^2 for ultrasound use in pregnancy. Current instrumentation informs the user of the energy outputs in a typical examination.

Color flow Doppler echocardiography is useful for accurate identification of fetal and maternal vessels. The physical basis of color is simply frequency, and direction of the signal. Most commonly a spectrum of red to yellow represents flow toward the transducer, and blue is used for flow away from the transducer.[1]

UMBILICAL ARTERIES AND VEIN

McCallum et al, in 1978, were the first to publish photographs of the umbilical artery waveform.[2] This waveform is relatively simple when compared to the typical arterial velocity waveform seen in the body below the level of the heart. Since the waveform is triangular, a simple calculation is practical, the systolic/diastolic (S/D) ratio[3] (Fig. 46.2). The ratio calculation solves the problem of the dependence of the am-

plitude of the waveform on the angle of insonation. Because the calculation is the same for both systole and diastole, it is now angle independent. Given this theoretical judgment, it is still wise to obtain several waveforms from different screens. This is particularly true of pulsed Doppler, where sampling volume influences the magnitude of the velocity flow wave more than it does in continuous wave Doppler. The most popular calculation used is the pulsatility index PI: (systole − diastole)/mean of area under waveform[4,5] (Fig. 46.3). In theory PI encompasses all components of the waveform, but it is also subject to the most calculation errors. It must be used for complicated waveforms, however. Since equipment has improved, particularly with color, it is now possible to be confident about angle ranges; thus newer indices suggestive of quantitative flow are being used to measure the area under the waveform, the timed velocity integral, and to make absolute measurements of maximum flow velocity. Maximum or peak velocity is particularly useful in small vessels, where it will reflect flow rather than resistance (Fig. 46.4).

Another calculation used is the resistance index: systole minus diastole divided by systole. This measure avoids the problem of infinity that arises in the S/D ratio, but it has several disadvantages. A resistance index of "one" means that there is no flow at end diastole. This is a very serious medical situation, and yet the number "one" doesn't usually have this connotation. Statistical differences may be lost when dealing with two decimal places for numbers less than "one."

Pulsatility Index (PI)

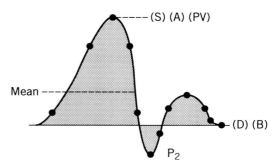

Figure 46.4   Arterial waveform as seen below the neck. During diastole there is transient reverse flow. Exceptions include the renal arteries, the uterine arteries in pregnancy, and new small arterioles.

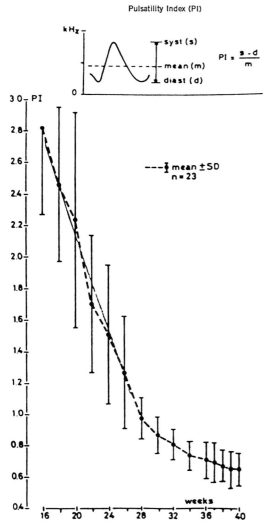

Figure 46.3   Pulsatility index of umbilical arteries. (Reproduced from Reuwer et al, *Eur J Obstet Gynecol Reprod Biol* 1984;18: 199–205, with permission of Elsevier Science Publishers.)

The technique for obtaining good signals with continuous wave Doppler is relatively easy.[6] It is similar to office Doppler auscultation of the fetus for confirmation of life. A 4 MHz probe is used, and the equipment provides an audio-

visual display of the vessel being insonated. Four major signals are obtained from the fetus (Fig. 46.5), and they can be easily differentiated by pattern recognition. We suggest that the umbilical signals be obtained from at least three different sites to ensure that approximately 12 waveforms are measured and averaged. Using this approach we found an average interobserver error of 6% and a maximum error of 16%. Sources of error include fetal tachycardia (> 160 beats/min) or bradycardia, and the presence of fetal breathing that produces a sinus arrhythmia. The sonographer should obtain the largest and densest waveform. Small or snowy patterns should not be used.

With the aid of color flow, the umbilical arteries can be detected as early as 6–8 weeks of gestation. The Doppler flow velocity profile shows only the systolic or ventricular component. By 20 weeks, all fetuses should have end-diastolic flow.[7] As pregnancy progresses, there is increasing end-diastolic flow velocity with lesser changes in systolic peak velocity (Fig. 46.6). A mature umbilical artery flow velocity waveform is usually present by 28–30 weeks, but some fetuses (e.g., twins) may show delayed maturation.

For clinical management, we use an S/D ratio of less than 3.0 at 30 weeks as a cutoff point for the detection of fetal disease.[8] This number was based on a receiver–operator curve calculation for maximum sensitivity and specificity for growth retardation in hypertensive women. Before 30 weeks the standard deviations are so high that a level of more than

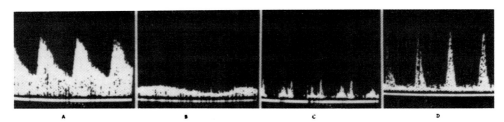

Figure 46.5   Four major signals obtained from the fetus when using the continuous wave Doppler instrumentation: (*A*) umbilical artery, (*B*) umbilical vein, (*C*) fetal heart, and (*D*) fetal aorta.

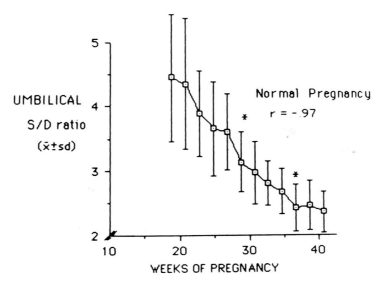

Figure 46.6 S/D ratio of umbilical arteries from the 18th gestational week onward. Note the similarity to pulsatility index. Statistical turning points at 28 and 35 weeks represent subsets in which the ratio drops to less than 3.

3 standard deviations is necessary for predicting fetal disease.

A persistently elevated S/D ratio is predictive of intrauterine growth retardation.[9-11] Since being small for gestational age is a fetal condition that encompasses multiple etiologies, velocimetry is uniquely useful for identifying the fetus whose growth impairment is secondary to placental or uterine flow disturbances. Morphometric ultrasound separates small fetuses into symmetrical and asymmetrical patterns. Asymmetrical growth is caused by reduced nutrition, and usually there will be flow disturbances: umbilical, uterine, or cardiac. When small fetuses are divided into normal versus abnormal umbilical flow, most of the perinatal morbidity and mortality arise in the disturbed flow group (Table 46.1).

Mortality happens primarily in fetuses with absent or reversed end-diastolic flow velocity[12,13] (Fig. 46.7). This represents the most severe form of reduction of flow velocity. In this situation, animal and human investigations suggest that two mechanisms may be operative. Persistent embolization

of the fetal umbilical artery circulation can produce reverse flow, perhaps comparable to intravascular coagulation. Also to be considered is increased venous pressure or hypervolemia, which arises clinically when there is compression of the umbilical vein, or when fetal heart failure secondary to right and left heart failure results in demands for more oxygen. The presence of reverse flow may signal a clinical emergency because most of these fetuses will die within 2 weeks.[14-16]

Most abnormal umbilical flow velocity waveforms represent failure to develop an adequate placental vasculature tree. The primary and secondary branches of the umbilical circulation are in place after the first trimester. For the next 3 months there is active proliferation of tertiary branches. Quantitative histology of the placenta shows that growth-retarded fetuses with abnormal flow velocity have half as many tertiary arterioles.[10]

Table 46.1 shows some of the consequences of reduced flow velocity. These consequences are growth retardation, mortality and morbidity, and the need for cesarean section.

TABLE 46.1 Perinatal Events in Fetuses Small for Gestational Age

S/D Ratio	Abnormal FHR	Events					
		PIH	CS	CS, FD	NICU	PPV	PNM
Normal (%)	8.3	16.7	16.7	8.3	16.7	0	0
Abnormal (%)	63*	50*	74*	53**	83.8*	31.6*	14.3

*p < 0.01.
**p < 0.05.

Abbreviations: FHR, ante- or peripartum fetal heart rate; PIH, pregnancy-induced hypertension; CS, cesarean section; CS, FD, cesarean section due to fetal distress; NICU, neonatal intensive care unit; PPV, positive pressure ventilation; PNM, perinatal mortality.

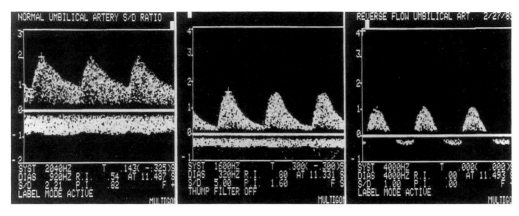

Figure 46.7 Normal mature flow velocity wave from the umbilical cord and vein (left), reduced arterial flow velocity (middle); and absent reverse flow velocity (right).

Interestingly, reduced flow velocity is also associated with maternal hypertension, and fetal trisomies and anomalies. Eighty percent of the flow velocity waveform is a reflection of the resistance beyond the point of measurement, but 20% can be a forward flow effect (i.e., reduced cardiac output, arrhythmia, and bradycardia). Measurements made when there is congenital heart disease, tachycardia, or bradycardia are difficult to interpret, and reports should reflect this.

In most cases of reduced umbilical blood flow, the middle cerebral artery is dilated, implying fetal hypoxia. At end stage disease, the umbilical and renal arteries and the aorta undergo further vasoconstriction. The middle cerebral arteries lose their autonomic reactivity and return to normal resistance indices.[17] The heart now becomes hypoxic, as manifested by a loss of fetal heart rate variability coupled with late decelerations.[18] Study of the venous system shows tricuspid regurgitation, and reverse flow in the vena cava, ductus venosus, and pulsating umbilical veins[19,20] (Fig. 46.8).

In twin pregnancy, there is a 25% incidence of growth retardation, usually secondary to placentation problems. Umbilical Doppler shows the twin with abnormal placentation.[21–23] In current clinical practice, surveillance of twins is driven by the concept of discordancy of fetal size. There is no standard definition of discordance.[24] Differences in size could be genetic, or they could be due to placentation or vascular problems. Doppler helps to solve these concerns because it distinguishes among these entities.[25] If both fetuses have normal umbilical flows, the difference in size should be genetic, and therefore not of clinical significance until delivery. If one or both fetuses have abnormal flow velocities, there is a risk of having the same consequences seen in the singleton fetus. Widely disparate values between the fetuses may indicate a vascular communication or fistula between monozygotic fetuses. A condition called TRAP (**t**win **r**eversal of **a**rterial **p**erfusion) arises when there is a twin pregnancy with acardius amorphous. In this circumstance color

flow confirms that there is a reversal of flow (e.g., arterial blood away from the placenta and venous flow to the placenta).

In many medical conditions, umbilical artery flow velocity will identify a fetus that is at risk.[26] In other words, in the presence of a medical or obstetrical disease, the finding of normal umbilical artery flow velocity puts the fetus in a low risk category. This classification is documented in lupus erythematosus, sickle cell disease, hypertension, previous fetal death, oligohydramnios (not postdates), and polyhydramnios. The role of Doppler in *diabetes* remains unsettled, but this disease may be a marker of the fetus at risk for hypoxia or death.[27–30]

An unexplained clinical problem is the mechanism of hypoxia in the postdate pregnancy.[31–33] Doppler and fetal heart

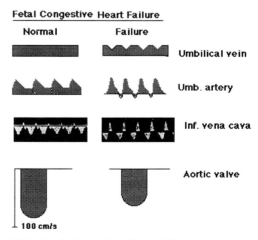

Figure 46.8 Evolution of fetal heart failure as demonstrated by Doppler flow velocity. When there is heart failure, there may be pulsations in the umbilical veins, reverse flow in the vena cava, and reduced left heart velocity time integral (see Ref. 55).

rate studies suggest that there is some cerebral dilatation and umbilical artery resistance when these fetuses are in difficulty. Since the changes in the Doppler are subtle, the ratio of cerebral to umbilical flow velocity may reflect this change. It should be more than one (i.e., the cerebral higher than the umbilical).[34]

FETAL CEREBRAL VESSELS

The circle of Willis is an easy landmark to identify with B-scan imaging. Color flow makes it easy to see the common carotid plus the anterior, middle, and posterior cerebral arteries.[35–38] Study of these vessels yields important information when there is fetal disease. In some growth-retarded fetuses, the cerebral vessels are dilated. Usually, these are fetuses with reduced umbilical artery flow velocity. This generality implies that the fetus with mild hypoxia will dilate its cerebral vessels as a compensatory response, thus explaining the so-called brain-sparing effect seen in asymmetrical growth retardation. These changes occur early and may be present for weeks to months before birth; some data suggest that they may persist into the early neonatal period. Sometimes, giving oxygen to the mother will cause the vessels to constrict and return to the normal values for that particular gestational age.[39] Study of the middle cerebrals is essential for the understanding of fetal hypoxia, particularly in the early third trimester, when the discriminatory zone between normal and abnormal is large.[40]

The anterior fontanell of the neonatal skull affords access to the cerebral circulation. Studies of this region suggested that severe hypoxia is accompanied by increased resistance to flow velocity. In premature babies with respiratory problems, severe fluctuations in flow velocity are associated with cerebral hemorrhage.[41]

FETAL AORTA AND OTHER ARTERIES

The fetal aorta is of interest for several reasons. The umbilical artery flow primarily reflects the status of the placenta, and in theory the aorta should give better information about the fetus. The thoracic aorta gives information about forward flow to the body and the placenta. During hypoxia there is peripheral vasoconstriction, and the aorta might reveal these changes. Also, since the aorta is a large vessel, it is easily identified and insonated by means of duplex Doppler.

The results of multiple studies have not been as rewarding as investigators had hoped, principally because there is only a small amount of diastolic flow, and calculations become more open to debate. The usual indices work poorly because the diastolic end points are low and the signals are fuzzy. Results of quantitative series suggest that normal flow

ranges from 190 to 285 mL/kg/min, with a median value of 215 mg/kg/min. Normal aortic velocity flow is 22 cm/s, with a range of 15–30/cm/s.[42,43]

Marsal's group has suggested that the best way to report the aortic flow velocity waveform is similar to that used in the umbilical artery, namely, normal, reduced end diastole, absent end diastole, and reverse diastole.[44] In the growth-retarded fetus, the aortic flow velocity wave becomes abnormal. As the fetus deteriorates, the aortic flow velocity wave undergoes the expected changes from mildly abnormal to loss of end-diastolic flow; terminally, as vasoconstriction increases, there is reverse flow.

Newer indices that require precise angle measurement may be useful in the aorta. Mean flow velocity decreases in growth retardation and in some postdate pregnancies. It may increase in hypervolemic states, such as Rh sensitization and diabetes. Changes in resistance indices using systole and diastole occur after large changes in blood flow ($\approx 30\%$).[45] Therefore mean velocity, peak velocity, and timed velocity integral may be more useful for smaller changes, such as the effects of drugs.

The fetal renal arteries are of interest because in chronic hypoxia there is reduced amniotic fluid, and neonatal renal failure.[46,47] The fetal renals do not have diastolic flow until approximately 35 weeks of gestation. As mentioned earlier, this makes measurements problematical. Some authors have suggested that PI calculations can be used to detect changes in association with hypoxia and declining amniotic fluid volume. The differences from normal, however, are too small to permit the use of this approach.

Doppler can help identify fetal anomalies and tumors. Thirty percent of fetuses with abnormal fetal karyotypes will have absent end-diastolic velocity in the umbilical artery. *Vasa previa* can be seen with color flow. *Chorioangioma* is a placental tumor that appears as an increased echogenic mass within the placenta. When a large umbilical vessel communicates with the tumor, there may be fetal heart failure secondary to a large fistula effect. The fistula manifests itself by a shunting effect on the umbilical circulation, namely, absent end-diastolic velocity. *Lung* tumors, such as teratomas, and maldevelopments, such as dysplasias, are diagnosed with color flow mapping of the communicating vessels.

Fetal heart *arrhythmias* can be diagnosed from the combined study of the aorta and the inferior vena cava.[48] The vena cava reflects atrial function, and the aorta ventricular action. When these waveforms are superimposed, deductions are made about the type of arrhythmia present.[48]

The *ductus arteriosus* delivers blood from the right ventricle to the descending aorta. Maintenance of flow is regulated by prostaglandins. Since we now use antiprostaglandins to treat premature labor, the effect on the ductus may be of interest. When indomethacin is used for premature labor, there is a reduction in ductus flow, but it quickly reverses when the drug is withdrawn.[49] This effect arises primarily after 32 weeks. Ductus arteriosus flow also changes when there are changes in fetal behavioral states (i.e., waking and sleeping).

Newer technology, such as digital ultrasound, visualizes smaller fetal vessels such as femoral, ulnar, radial, and pulmonary arteries. Study of these vessels may be useful in selective circumstances.

FETAL VENOUS SYSTEM

The venous system is characterized by low pressure and easily distended walls. The lower extremity venous flow is affected by the presence of valves and muscular action. Abdominal venous flow in the fetus is unique because of the umbilical vein, the ductus venosus, and its sphincterlike structure.[50,51]

The umbilical vein normally has continuous flow that may modulate in concert with fetal respirations. These changes happen by changes in intrathoracic and intraabdominal pressure. The blood from the umbilical vein empties into the ductus venosus, where it is joined by branches of the hepatic and splenic circulation. A complex frenulum is at the junction of the ductus venosus and inferior vena cava. This frenulum-like structure in the vena cava has separate openings for the ductus, hepatic veins, and flow from the lower body.

Since the fetus exists in water and is relatively weightless, the effects of hydrostatic pressure on the venous system are probably minimal. Multiple patterns of velocity flow are seen. The inferior vena cava waveform reflects the cardiac cycle and gives the typical atrial contraction, and ventricular systolic–diastolic peaks. The ductus venosus shows a systolic–diastolic peak, but its tributaries (the umbilical, right hepatic, and splenic veins) are generally monophasic.[52] Tributaries of the inferior vena cava reflect the cardiac cycle (Fig. 46.9).

The venous system is an extremely valuable marker of fetal health. The triphasic waveform is a reflection of the cardiac cycle. In fetal heart failure there is tricuspid insufficiency that causes reduced forward flow and increased regurgitation.[53,54] The venous system reflects the regurgitation by displaying large atrial waveforms. As heart failure progresses, the regurgitation moves through the sphincter of the ductus venosus into the umbilical vein. Pulsations in the umbilical vein that are synchronous with the arterial pulses are an indicator of severe fetal jeopardy. In hydrops fetalis, fetal venous flow gives a differential diagnosis. For example, if the waveforms are normal, the cause of the hydrops is metabolic or hydrostatic. If the waveforms show tricuspid insufficiency, the cause of the hydrops is cardiac, and the fetal prognosis is grim.[55]

THE FETAL HEART

Flow velocity in the fetal heart shows that blood speed is slowest through the tricuspid and mitral valves, and more

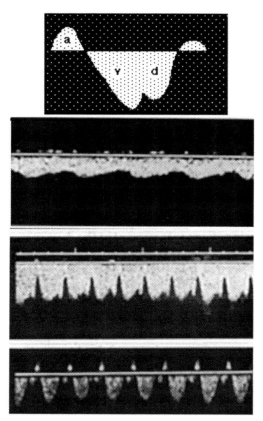

Figure 46.9 Venous velocity flow. Top panel: venous waveform in the inferior vena cava (a, atrial contraction; v, ventricular systole; d, ventricular diastole). Second panel: umbilical vein pulsations secondary to fetal breathing. Third panel: ductus venosus, showing v and d pulses. Bottom panel: inferior vena cava with a, v, and d pulses.

rapid in the pulmonic and aortic arteries. Velocity through the ascending aorta is greatest because of the lower resistance in the cerebral circulation. In fetal growth retardation, there is redistribution of flow, with the result that left-sided velocity increases because of the dilated cerebral circulation, and the right-sided flow decreases because of peripheral vasoconstriction in the descending aorta and its branches.[53,54]

CLINICAL ASSESSMENT OF THE AT-RISK FETUS

The growth-retarded fetus with reduced umbilical flow velocity redistributes its blood flow. This is shown initially by dilated cerebrals, increased left heart flow, and normal or decreased right heart output. During this period the fetal heart rate pattern is still normal. As hypoxia progresses, aortic and renal flow decrease, and fetal heart rate variation diminishes. When hypoxia worsens, the cerebrals lose their autonomic reactivity and return to the previous state; therefore the measurement indices get larger. At this time, left heart flow

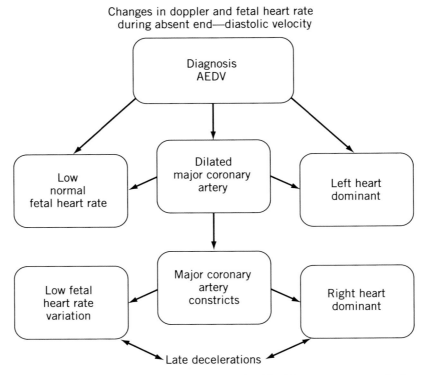

Changes in doppler and fetal heart rate
during absent end—diastolic velocity

Figure 46.10   Fetal circulatory dynamics and computerized fetal heart rate response. In the growth-retarded fetus with absent end-diastolic velocity (AEDV), there will be low normal fetal heart variation and left heart dominance secondary to a dilated cerebral circulation. With time (4–14 days), hypoxia worsens, and there is loss of cerebral autonomic reactivity, followed by cardiac depression and late decelerations. (See Refs. 17 and 32).

decreases, and tricuspid insufficiency appears and is transmitted into the venous system. The fetal heart beat interval will now show diminished variation, and late decelerations will appear in the heart rate pattern (Fig. 46.10). The preterminal flow pattern shows reverse diastolic flow in the umbilical artery, aorta, vena cava, and umbilical vein pulsations.

In the growth-retarded fetus that appears normal, one must first determine the state of the umbilical and uterine circulation. Next it must be learned whether the fetus is hypoxemic. This is determined by the middle cerebral Doppler. The fetus with significant reduction of umbilical flow (i.e., absent end-diastolic velocity) should have dilated cerebrals. It it does not, it is critically ill, or not hypoxic. If it is not hypoxic, it may have congenital heart disease, with the reduced peripheral flow being a result of reduced forward flow, not increased resistance. Careful evaluation of the heart then becomes imperative.

An important clinical question is whether use of Doppler ultrasound affects perinatal outcome.[56] In 12 randomized controlled trials of Doppler ultrasonography, a meta-analysis showed a significant reduction in the Doppler group in the number of antenatal admissions (44%; 95% confidence interval, 28–57%), inductions of labor (20%; 95% confidence

interval, 10–28%), and cesarean sections for fetal distress (52%; 95% confidence interval, 24–69%); moreover, the clinical action guided by Doppler ultrasonography reduced the odds of perinatal death by 38% (95% confidence interval, 15–55%). The reduction in perinatal deaths was also observed in five mortality subgroups: stillbirths, neonatal deaths, deaths of normally formed babies, normally formed stillbirths, and deaths of normally formed neonates. Post hoc analyses revealed a statistically significant reduction in elective delivery, intrapartum fetal distress, and hypoxic encephalopathy in the Doppler group. Conclusion: There is now compelling evidence that women with high risk pregnancies, including preeclampsia and suspected intrauterine growth retardation, should have access to Doppler ultrasonographic study of umbilical artery waveforms.[52]

UTERINE ARTERIES

With color flow, it is easy to visualize the uterine artery. With a transvaginal probe, the vessels are seen next to the uterus. Transabdominally, during pregnancy, they can be traced from the internal iliac directly into the uterus. Iliac vessels maintain low end-diastolic flow, but normal pregnant uterine arteries have large end-diastolic velocity.

During the secretory phase of the normal menstrual cycle, the uterine artery resistance index drops from 0.88 to 0.84. This change begins just before ovulation. Pregnancy does not produce significant Doppler changes in the main uterine branches until there is a well-developed intervillous circulation. Approximately 4 weeks after implantation, there are low resistance vessels at the site of the future placenta. Decreases in resistance occur in the feeding radial arteries as the pregnancy progresses.

The uterine artery generates a waveform more complex than seen in the umbilical vessels. It changes from a high resistance vessel showing one or more diastolic notches into a low resistance vessel with no diastolic notches.[57] The changes in end-diastolic velocity may be primarily regulated by the intervillous space flow. When there is a strong uterine contraction at term, uterine artery end-diastolic flow is blocked, but there is no reappearance of the notch. Disappearance of the notch will happen first in the uterine artery that is directly beneath the placenta. If the notch has not been lost by 24–26 weeks (see Fig. 46.11), most women will develop a hypertensive complication of pregnancy. The uterine artery does not return to its prepregnant level for 4–6 weeks after delivery.[58]

The calculation of quantitative uterine blood flow requires direct visualization of the vessel, and measurement of the diameter[59] (Fig. 46.12). Transvaginal ultrasound and color flow give access to the main branch of the artery in the first trimester, and transabdominal color studies provide access for continuation of these measurements. Estimated flow rates from these studies are 100–330 mL/min from early to late gestation.[60]

Impaired uterine artery flow velocity is identified by a persistent abnormal index, a persistent notch, and a significant difference between the indices in the two vessels. The upper limit of the S/D ratio is approximately 2.6, and the difference between the vessels should not exceed 1. Adverse outcomes associated with an abnormal uterine artery flow velocity include preeclampsia, as well as fetal growth retardation and its sequelae.[61] If the fetus has normal umbilical flow, the growth delay will be mild and the risk of fetal distress slightly above normal; the most common indication for intervention is maternal, not fetal. The most significant abnormality of the waveform with an abnormal outcome is the diastolic notch. The persistence of the notch, which is a manifestation of unaltered vascular tone or spasm, is analogous to the vascular response seen in the angiotensin infusion test. In other words, the normal adaptation of pregnancy has not occurred. Since most abnormal uterine artery waveforms are associated with unilateral implantation of the placenta, we hypothesized that normal pregnancy changes require both uterine arteries to be involved in the development of the placenta.[62,63] We were reminded of the kidney, where one-sided flow reduction is also associated with hypertension.

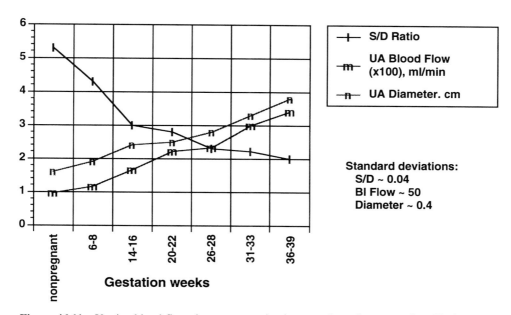

Figure 46.11 Uterine blood flow shows progressive increase throughout gestation. Uterine artery resistance shows precipitous change from early pregnancy to 14–16 weeks. (See Refs. 57 and 59.)

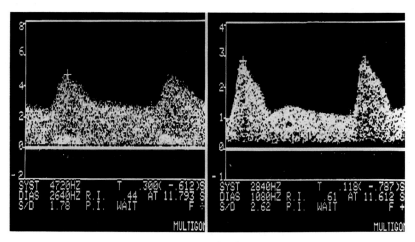

Figure 46.12

MATERNAL VESSELS

Cardiac output in the mother can be estimated by indirect Doppler assessment of the ascending aorta.[64] These devices are now used by anesthesiologists.

The retinal arteries are useful to assess the effect of drugs on the central circulation.[65] Transcranial Doppler has shown reversible vasospasm when there have been seizures.[66] In women with some forms of hypertension, magnesium sulfate dilates these vessels. The maternal renal arteries show no change in preeclampsia.

Doppler estimation of venous flow is standard for the evaluation of thrombophlebitis. The technique searches for obstruction to flow. Recall that if there is no flow, there is no separation of sound wave return, as expected in accordance with the Doppler principle.

HYPERTENSION

The prevailing theories for pregnancy-induced hypertension focus on uterine ischemia and endothelial disease. The term "uterine ischemia" should be replaced by "placental ischemia." Doppler investigations show that hypertension of pregnancy is associated with reduced uterine or umbilical flow or both. We proposed a classification based on these findings and found it to be clinically useful for anticipating outcome (Table 46.2).[68] The severest outcomes arise in the presence of abnormal uterine and umbilical flow velocity.[69] Abnormal uterine flow velocity alone presents primarily as maternal disease, but there can be mild fetal growth retardation. A maternal hypertension syndrome will develop when the fetus has absent end-diastolic velocity in the umbilical arteries (excluding trisomies), regardless of the status of uterine flow. Preeclampsia with normal flow happens predominantly after 36 weeks.

The uteroplacental vessels can be used to screen for hypertensive diseases in pregnancy in at-risk population.[70–72] When screening is done at 24 weeks, there is a sensitivity of 76%, specificity of 97% and positive predictive value of 44%.

Endothelial dysfunction is present in many cases of preeclampsia. Prostacyclin is reduced in pregnant sera in preeclampsia. Controlled studies based on Doppler velocimetry have shown that prophylactic aspirin can reduce the inci-

TABLE 46.2   Clinical Correlates in Hypertension of Pregnancy and Doppler Results

Correlate	Doppler Results			
	Normal Velocimetry	Abnormal Uterine	Abnormal Umbilical	Both Abnormal
Uric acid	Normal	Normal	Elevated	Elevated
Proteinuria	24%	75%	71%	86%
Thrombocytopenia	Rare	13%	26%	Rate
Gestational age at delivery	Normal	36 weeks	36 weeks	33 weeks
Intrauterine growth retardation	Normal	17%	29%	51%
Cesarean section due to fetal distress	Normal	Normal	39%	62%

Source: Adapted from Ducey et al.[68]

dence of hypertensive sequelae.[73] When similar studies were done in the United States using nulliparity rather than Doppler as the entrance criterion, no benefit was shown.

CONCLUSION

Doppler ultrasound has revealed much about the pathophysiology of pregnancy. This knowledge should lead to improved management of complicated pregnancies by identifying the compromised fetus. Clinical discussions can then be more accurately conducted in terms of disease states, rather than relying on current management schemes, which are discussed primarily in terms of test results.

REFERENCES

1. Burns PN. Hemodynamics (ch. 3) and Doppler examination (ch. 4). In: Taylor KJW, Burns PN, Wells PNT, eds. *Clinical Applications of Doppler Ultrasound* 2nd ed. New York: Raven Press; 1995;35–98.

2. McCallum WD, Williams CS, Napel S, Daigle RE. Fetal blood velocity waveforms. *Am J Obstet Gynecol* 1978;132:425–429.

3. Stuart B, Drumm J, Dingman NM. Fetal blood velocity waveforms in normal pregnancy. *Br J Obstet Gynaecol* 1980;87: 780–785.

4. Gosling RG, Dunbar G, King DH, Newman DL, Side CD, Woodcock JP. The quantitative analysis of occlusive peripheral arterial disease by a non-invasive technique. *Angiology* 1971;22:52–55.

5. Reuwer PJHM, Nuyen WC, Beijer HJM, Heethaar RM, Bruinse HW, Stoutenbeek P, Haspels AA. Characteristic flow velocities of the umbilical arteries associated by Doppler ultrasound. *Eur J Obstet Gynecol Reprod Biol* 1984;17:397–408.

6. Schulman H, Fleischer A, Stern W, Farmakides G, Jagani N, Blattner P. Umbilical velocity waveforms in human pregnancy. *Am J Obstet Gynecol* 1984;148:985–990.

7. Guzman ER, Schulman H, Karmel B, Higgins P. Umbilical artery Doppler velocimetry in pregnancies of less than 21 weeks' duration. *J Ultrasound Med* 1990;9:655–659.

8. Fleischer A, Schulman H, Farmakides G, Bracero L. Umbilical artery velocity waveforms and intrauterine growth retardation. *Am J Obstet Gynecol* 1985;151:502–505.

9. Trudinger BJ, Giles WB, Cook CM. Uteroplacental blood flow velocity–time waveforms in normal and complicated pregnancy. *Br J Obstet Gynaecol* 1985;92:39–45.

10. Giles WB, Trudinger BJ, Baird PJ. Fetal umbilical artery flow velocity waveforms and placental resistance: pathological correlation. *Br J Obstet Gynaecol* 1985;92:31–38.

11. Arduini D, Rizzo G, Romanini C, Mancuso S. Fetal blood flow velocity waveforms as predictors of growth retardation. *Obstet Gynecol* 1987;70:7–10.

12. Rochelson BL, Schulman H, Fleischer A, Farmakides GF, Bracero L, Ducey J, Winter D, Penny B. The clinical signifi-

13. Rochelson B, Schulman H, Farmakides G, Ducey J, Fleischer A, Penny B, Winter D. The significance of absent end-diastolic velocity in umbilical artery velocity waveforms. *Am J Obstet Gynecol* 1987;156:1213–1218.

14. Farine D, Ryan G, Kelly EN, Morrow RJ, Laskin C, Knox-Richie JW. Absent end-diastolic flow velocity waveforms in the umbilical artery — the subsequent pregnancy. *Am J Obstet Gynecol* 1993;168:637–640.

15. Karsdorp VHM, Van-Vugt JMG, Van-Geijn HP, Kostense PJ, Arduini D, Montenegro N, Todros R. Clinical significance of absent or reversed end diastolic velocity waveforms in umbilical artery. *Lancet* 1994;344:1664–1668.

16. Forouzan I. Absence of end-diastolic flow velocity in the umbilical artery: a review. *Obstet Gynecol Survey* 1995;50: 219–227.

17. Arduini D, Rizzo G, Romanini C. The development of abnormal heart rate patterns after absent end-diastolic velocity in umbilical artery: analysis of risk factors. *Am J Obstet Gynecol* 1993;168:43–50.

18. Weiner Z, Farmakides G, Schulman H, Penny B. Central and peripheral hemodynamic changes in fetuses with absent end-diastolic velocity in umbilical artery: correlation with computerized fetal heart rate pattern. *Am J Obstet Gynecol* 1994; 170:509–515.

19. Nakai Y, Miyazaki Y, Matsuoka Y, Matsumoto M, Imanaka M, Ogita S. Pulsatile umbilical venous flow and its clinical significance. *Br J Obstet Gynaecol* 1992;99:977–980.

20. Hecher K, Campbell S, Doyle P, Harrington K, Nicolaides K. Assessment of fetal compromise by Doppler ultrasound investigation of the fetal circulation: arterial, intracardiac, and venous blood flow velocity studies. *Circulation* 1995;91:129–138.

21. Farmakides G, Schulman H, Saldana LR, Bracero L, Fleischer A, Rochelson B. Surveillance of twin pregnancy with umbilical arterial velocimetry. *Am J Obstet Gynecol* 1985;153:789–792.

22. Pretorius DH, Manchester D, Barkin S, Parker S, Nelson TR. Doppler ultrasound of twin transfusion syndrome. *J Ultrasound Med* 1988;7:117–124.

23. Giles WB, Trudinger BJ, Cook CM, Connelly AJ. Doppler umbilical artery studies in the twin–twin transfusion syndrome. *Obstet Gynecol* 1990;76:1097–1099.

24. Blickstein I. The definition, diagnosis, and management of growth-discordant twins: an international census survey. *Acta Genet Med Gemellol* 1991;40:345–351.

25. Hecher K, Ville Y, Nicolaides KH. Fetal arterial Doppler studies in twin–twin transfusion syndrome. *J Ultrasound Med* 1995;14:101–108.

26. Fleischer A, Schulman H, Farmakides G, Bracero L, Rochelson B, Koenigsberg M. Uterine artery Doppler velocimetry in pregnant women with hypertension. *Am J Obstet Gynecol* 1986; 154:806–813.

27. Bracero L, Schulman H, Fleischer A, Farmakides G, Rochelson B. Umbilical artery velocimetry in diabetes and pregnancy. *Obstet Gynecol* 1986;68:654–658.

28. Rochelson B, Coury A, Schulman H, Dery C, Klotz M, Shmoys S. Doppler umbilical artery velocimetry in fetuses with polyhydramnios. *Am J Perinatol* 1990;7:340–342.

29. Guzman E, Schulman H, Bracero L, Rochelson B, Farmakides G, Coury A. Uterine–umbilical artery Doppler velocimetry in pregnant women with systemic lupus erythematosus. *J Ultrasound Med* 1992;11:275–281.

30. Trudinger BJ, Cook CM. Umbilical and uterine artery flow velocity waveforms in pregnancy associated with major fetal abnormality. *Br J Obstet Gynaecol* 1985;92:666–670.

31. Arduini D, Rizzo G, Romanini C, Mancuso S. Doppler assessment of fetal blood flow velocity waveforms during acute maternal oxygen administration as predictor of fetal outcome in post-term pregnancy. *Am J Perinatol* 1990;7:258–262.

32. Weiner Z, Farmakides G, Schulman H, Kellner L, Plancher S, Maulik D. Computerized analysis of fetal heart rate variation in postterm pregnancy: prediction of intrapartum fetal distress and fetal acidosis. *Am J Obstet Gynecol* 1994;171:1132–1138.

33. Battaglia C, Artini PG, Ballestri M, Bonucchi D, Galli PA, Bencini S, Genazzani AP. Hemodynamic, hematological and hemorrheological evaluation of post-term pregnancy. *Acta Obstet Gynecol Scand* 1995;74:336–340.

34. Arias F. Accuracy of the middle-cerebral-to-umbilical-artery resistance index ratio in the prediction of neonatal outcome in patients at high risk for fetal and neonatal complications. *Am J Obstet Gynecol* 1994;171:1541–1545.

35. Wladimiroff JW, Tonge HM, Stewart PA. Doppler ultrasound assessment of cerebral blood flow in the human fetus. *Br J Obstet Gynaecol* 1986;93:471–475.

36. Van-Bel F, Van deBor M, Stijnen T, Ruys JH. Decreased cerebrovascular resistance in small for gestational age infants. *Eur J Obstet Gynecol Reprod Biol* 1986;23:137–144.

37. Wladimiroff JW, Wijngaard JAGW, Degani S, Noordam MJ, Van Eyck J, Tonge HM. Cerebral and umbilical arterial blood flow velocity waveforms in normal and growth-retarded pregnancies. *Obstet Gynecol* 1987;69:705–709.

38. Woo JSK, Liang ST, Lo RLS, Chan FY. Middle cerebral artery Doppler flow velocity waveforms. *Obstet Gynecol* 1987;70:613–616.

39. Arduini D, Rizzo G, Mancuso S, Romanini C. Short-term effects of maternal oxygen administration on blood flow velocity waveforms in healthy and growth-retarded fetuses. *Am J Obstet Gynecol* 1988;159:1077–1080.

40. Mari G, Deter RL. Middle cerebral artery flow velocity waveforms in normal and small-for-gestational-age fetuses. *Am J Obstet Gynecol* 1992;166:1262–1270.

41. Perlman JM, Goodman S, Kreusser KL, Volpe J. Reduction in intraventricular hemorrhage by elimination of fluctuating cerebral blood flow velocity in premature infants with respiratory distress syndrome. *N Engl J Med* 1985;312:1353–1357.

42. Soothill PW, Nicolaides KH, Bilardo CM, Campbell S. Relation of fetal hypoxia in growth retardation to mean blood velocity in the fetal aorta. *Lancet* 1986;2:1118–1119.

43. Steiner H, Schaffer H, Spitzer D, Batka M, Graf AH, Staudach A. The relationship between peak velocity in the fetal descending aorta and hematocrit in rhesus isoimmunization. *Obstet Gynecol* 1995;85:659–662.

44. Laurin J, Marsal K, Persson PH, Lingman G. Ultrasound measurement of fetal blood flow in predicting fetal outcome. *Br J Obstet Gynaecol* 1987;94:940–948.

45. Gill RW, Kosoff G, Warren PS, Garret WJ. Umbilical venous flow in normal and complicated pregnancy. *Ultrasound Med Biol* 1984;10:349–363.

46. Arduini D, Rizzo G. Fetal renal artery velocity waveforms and amniotic fluid volume in growth-retarded and post-term fetuses. *Obstet Gynecol* 1991;77:370–373.

47. Mari G, Kirshon B, Abuhamad A. Fetal renal artery flow velocity waveforms in normal pregnancies and pregnancies complicated by polyhydramnios and oligohydramnios. *Obstet Gynecol* 1993;81:560–564.

48. Chan FY, Woo SK, Ghosh A, Tang M, Lam C. Prenatal diagnosis of congenital fetal arrhythmias by simultaneous pulsed Doppler velocimetry of the fetal abdominal aorta and inferior vena cava. *Obstet Gynecol* 1990;76(2):200–205.

49. Kirshon B, Mari G, Moise KJ Jr, Wasserstrum N. Effect of indomethacin on the fetal ductus arteriosus during treatment of symptomatic polyhydramnios. *J Reprod Med Obstet Gynecol* 1990;35(5):529–532.

50. Kiserud T, Eik-Nes SH, Blaas HGK, Hellevik LR. Ultrasonographic velocimetry of the fetal ductus venosus. *Lancet* 1991;338:1412–1414.

51. Huisman TWA, Gittenberger-deGroot AC, Wladimiroff JW. Recognition of a fetal subdiaphragmatic venous vestibulum essential for fetal venous Doppler assessment. *Pediatr Res* 1992;32:338–341.

52. Mari G, Uerpairojkit B, Copel J. Abdominal venous system. *Am J Obstet Gynecol* 1995;86:729–733.

53. Reed KL, Anderson CF, Shenker L. Changes in intracardiac Doppler blood flow velocities in fetuses with absent umbilical artery diastolic flow. *Am J Obstet Gynecol* 1987;157:774–779.

54. Rizzo G, Arduini D, Romanini C, Mancuso S. Doppler echocardiographic assessment of atrioventricular velocity waveforms in normal and small-for-gestational-age fetuses. *Br J Obstet Gynaecol* 1988;95:65–69.

55. Tulzer G, Gudmundson S, Wood DC, Cohen AW, Weiner S, Huhta JC. Doppler in non-immune hydrops fetalis. *Ultrasound Obstet Gynecol* 1994;4:279–283.

56. Alfirevic Z, Neilson JP. Doppler ultrasonography in high-risk pregnancies: systematic review with meta-analysis. *Am J Obstet Gynecol* 1995;172:1379–1387.

57. Schulman H, Fleischer A, Farmakides G, Bracero L, Rochelson B, Grunfeld L. Development of uterine artery compliance in pregnancy as detected by Doppler ultrasound. *Am J Obstet Gynecol* 1986;155:1031–1036.

58. Tekay A, Jouppila P. A longitudinal Doppler ultrasonographic assessment of the alterations in peripheral vascular resistance of uterine arteries and ultrasonographic findings of the involuting uterus during the puerperium. *Am J Obstet Gynecol* 1993;168:190–198.

59. Thaler I, Manor D, Itskovitz J, Rottem S, Levit N, Timor-Tritsch I, Brandes JM. Changes in uterine blood flow during human pregnancy. *Am J Obstet Gynecol* 1990;162:121–125.

60. Palmer SK, Zamudio S, Coffin C, Parker S, Stamm E, Moore LG. Quantitative estimation of human uterine artery blood flow and pelvic blood flow redistribution in pregnancy. *Obstet Gynecol* 1992;80:1000–1006.

61. Tyrrell SN, Bates J, Lilford RJ. Prediction of onset of preeclampsia in patient with pregnancy-induced hypertension by continuous-wave Doppler ultrasound. *Lancet* 1987;2:1328–1329.

62. Schulman H, Ducey J, Farmakides G, Guzman E, Winter D, Penny B. Uterine artery Doppler velocimetry: the significance of divergent systolic/diastolic ratios. *Am J Obstet Gynecol* 1987;157:1539–1542.

63. Kofinas AD, Penry M, Swain M, Hatjis CG. Effect of placental laterality on uterine artery resistance and development of preeclampsia and intrauterine growth retardation. *Am J Obstet Gynecol* 1989;161:1536–1539.

64. Easterling TR, Watts DH, Schmucker BC, Benedetti TJ. Measurement of cardiac output during pregnancy: validation of Doppler technique and clinical observations in preeclampsia. *Obstet Gynecol* 1987;69:845–850.

65. Mackenzie F, DeVermette R, Nimrod C, Ancl C, Dabrowski A, Jackson B. Doppler examination of both the ophthalmic and central retinal arteries in pregnancy—methodologic concerns. *J Matern Fetal Invest* 1995;5:88–91.

66. Vliegen JHR, Muskens E, Keunen RWM, Smith SJ, Godfried WH, Gerretsen G. Abnormal cerebral hemodynamics in pregnancy-related hypertensive encephalopathy. *Eur J Obstet Gynecol Reprod Biol* 1993;49:198–200.

67. Belfort MA, Moise KJ Jr. Effect of magnesium sulfate on maternal brain blood flow in preeclampsia: a randomized, placebo-controlled study. *Am J Obstet Gynecol* 1992;167:661–666.

68. Ducey J, Schulman H, Farmakides G, Bracero L. A classification of hypertension in pregnancy based on Doppler velocimetry. *Am J Obstet Gynecol* 1987;157:680–685.

69. Trudinger BJ, Cook CM. Doppler umbilical and uterine flow waveforms in severe pregnancy-induced hypertension. *Br J Obstet Gynaecol* 1990;97:142–148.

70. Fay RA, Ellwood D, Bewley S, Campbell S. Doppler investigation of uteroplacental blood flow resistance in the second trimester: a screening study for pre-eclampsia and intrauterine growth retardation. *Br J Obstet Gynaecol* 1992;99:527–528.

71. Soothill PW, Khullar V, Campbell S, Nicolaides KH. Prediction of the severity of preeclampsia by utero-placental Doppler studies. *J Obstet Gynecol* 1993;13:99–102.

72. Erkkola RU, Pirhonen JP. Uterine and umbilical flow velocity waveforms in normotensive and hypertensive subjects during the angiotensin II sensitivity test. *Am J Obstet Gynecol* 1992;166:910–916.

73. McParland P, Pearce JM, Chamberlain GVP. Doppler ultrasound and aspirin in recognition and prevention of pregnancy-induced hypertension. *Lancet* 1990;335:1552–1555.

47

FETAL ECHOCARDIOGRAPHY

Greggory R. DeVore, MD

INTRODUCTION

During the past 10 years, examination of the fetal cardiovascular system with diagnostic ultrasound has evolved from an academic exercise to a clinical tool that has wide application. This chapter describes the current use of fetal echocardiography in the diagnosis and management of congenital heart disease, pericardial effusion, and antenatal arrhythmias.

CONGENITAL HEART DISEASE

Background

Following birth, the most common congenital malformations involve the cardiovascular system, with an incidence varying between 7.6 and 8.8 per thousand live births (Table 47.1).[1,2] However, the number of fetuses with congenital heart disease (CHD) may be higher. In an autopsy series of 412 consecutive spontaneous abortuses between 8 and 28 weeks of gestation, 10 were noted to have CHD for an incidence of 2.4%.[3] In another study in which the incidence of cardiac malformations was determined in spontaneous abortions occurring after fewer than 24 weeks of gestation, 15.4% had CHD.[4] Given the increased incidence of CHD in spontaneous abortuses compared to live births, the number of fetuses with potentially diagnosable CHD during the second trimester may be greater than that reported for term live births.

The impact of CHD is underscored when one considers that of the 9200 infant deaths due to congenital anomalies in the United States in 1980, 31.7% were attributed to cardiovascular malformations, 11.37% to neural tube defects, and 7.09% to chromosomal anomalies.[5] Of the infants who died

as the result of CHD, 40% succumbed within the first 7 days of life.[6] Unlike chromosomal and neural tube defects, in which there are external morphological markers suggesting an abnormality, CHD often is not identified until the infant becomes cyanotic or develops congestive heart failure.[7,8]

Since the introduction of fetal echocardiography in 1980, most major malformations have been detected in utero. Table 47.2 lists those reported in the international literature.[9–90]

Screening Examination

Of the 3 million women in the United States who give birth each year, over 75% undergo fetal ultrasonic evaluation.[91] Because the majority of pregnant women are scanned by radiologists obstetricians, and/or their technicians, the burden for prenatal diagnosis is with an individual who often is not trained in cardiovascular imaging. A recent report of the Routine Antenatal Diagnostic Imaging with Ultrasound Study (RADIUS) stated that midtrimester identification of fetuses with congenital heart defects was significantly lower (0%) if the screening examination was performed at a nontertiary center instead of at a tertiary center (23%).[92] In a recent study from Norway in which the four-chamber view was examined to detect congenital heart defects, 26% of complex heart defects were identified during the second-trimester examination.[93] However, 0% of noncomplex heart defects were identified.[93] To facilitate evaluation of the "normal" fetus for cardiovascular anomalies, a rational, easy-to-perform screening examination would be ideal. For this purpose, the inflow four-chamber view of the heart has been suggested.[94]

Thus the most important consideration for the sonographer contemplating screening for CHD is the frequency with which the four-chamber view can be imaged. A study from

Cardiac Problems in Pregnancy, Third Edition
Edited by Uri Elkayam, MD, and Norbert Gleicher, MD
Copyright © 1998 by Wiley-Liss, Inc. ISBN 0-471-16358-9

TABLE 47.1 Incidence of Congenital Malformations

Malformation	Rate per 1000 Live Births
CARDIOVASCULAR SYSTEM	
Ventricular septal defect	1.963
Patent ductus arteriosus	1.840
Atrial septal defect	0.833
Anomalies of heart valves	0.698
Transposition of great vessels	0.381
Stenosis of pulmonary artery	0.378
Coarctation of aorta	0.333
Other anomalies of aorta	0.300
Tetralogy of Fallot	0.276
Anomalies of great veins	0.183
Ostium atrioventriculare commune	0.180
Common truncus	0.090
Fibroelastosis cordis	0.042
	7.496
NEURAL TUBE DEFECTS	
Anencephaly	0.716
Spina bifida	0.573
Encephalocele	0.546
	1.835
CHROMOSOMAL ABNORMALITIES	
Trisomy 21	0.953
Other	0.204
	1.157

TABLE 47.2 Congenital Malformations Diagnosed In Utero in the International Literature[9-90]

Absence of aortic valve
Acardia aortic stenosis
Atrial hemangioma
Bicuspid aortic valve
Coarctation of aorta
Double-outlet right ventricle
Dextrocardia
Ebstein's anomaly
Ectopic cordis
Endocardial cushion defect
Endocardial fibroelastosis
Hypoplastic left ventricle
Hypoplastic right ventricle
Mitral atresia
Pulmonary atresia
Ostium primum defect
Pericardial hemangioma
Pericardial teratoma
Rhabdomyoma
Single ventricle
Single atrium
Tetralogy of Fallot
Thoracopagus (single heart)
Tricuspid atresia
Transposition
Truncus arteriosus
Ventricular septal defect

our group found that the four-chamber and outflow tracts were identified in 90.7% of 643 second-trimester examinations.[95] In 1994 Tegnander et al published similar findings and reported that as the gestational age increased from 16 weeks to 21 weeks, the incidence of nonvisualization of the four-chamber view decreased from 8% to 2%.[96]

In an earlier study, Allan et al reported that the number of prenatally detected cardiovascular malformations increased from 3 in 1982 to 22 in 1985.[97] The 22 fetuses represented 66% of all cardiac detects diagnosed by their group. Of those referred because of abnormalities suspected on the basis of a four-chamber view, 80% demonstrated a congenital anomaly. Detected anomalies included hypoplastic left ventricle, mitral, pulmonary, or tricuspid atresia, and double-outlet right ventricle. These investigators concluded that the number of malformations detected in utero would be equivalent to 60% (2/1000) of infants in whom CHD is diagnosed during the first year of life (3/1000).

Fetal Circulation To appreciate the significance of the four-chamber screening examination, one must understand fetal circulation. Unlike the pediatric or adult patient in whom blood is delivered to the body and head by the left ventricle, the fetus requires both ventricles to meet its systemic requirements. Initially, oxygenated blood flowing from the ductus venosus and hepatic view enters the right atrium, and most of it then traverses the foramen ovale to the lower pressured left atrium. During ventricular diastole, blood from the left atrium enters the left ventricle where, during ventricular systole, it is ejected through the aortic valve into the ascending aorta and is distributed to the fetal heart, head, and upper extremities (Fig. 47.1).

Blood from the right atrium flows through the tricuspid valve into the right ventricle. During ventricular systole it is ejected through the pulmonary valve into the pulmonary arteries and the ductus arteriosus. The latter supplies blood to the descending aorta for distribution to the trunk and placenta.

Therefore, as the result of fetal circulation, the right and left ventricles function as a parallel system that is dependent on the patency of the foramen ovale and the ductus arteriosus. A partial or complete obstruction to blood flow at the level of the inflow (mitral and tricuspid valves) or outflow (aortic and pulmonic) tracts will result in redistribution of blood within the cardiac chambers. This is manifest as disproportion between the right and left atrial and ventricular chambers. This important observation is the basis for the fetal cardiovascular screening examination.

HEAD

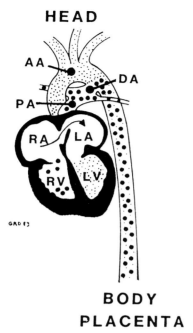

AA

DA

PA

RA LA

RV LV

GAD 13

BODY
PLACENTA

Figure 47.1 Distribution of fetal blood pumped from the right and left ventricles. A portion of oxygenated blood entering the right atrium (RA) traverses the foramen ovale (arrow), entering the left atrium (LA) and subsequently the left ventricle (LV). Blood from the left ventricle is pumped primarily to the fetal head and upper extremities via the arch of the aorta (AA). Blood from the right ventricle (RV) is pumped through the pulmonary artery (PA) and ductus arteriosus (DA) to the fetal body and placenta. (Reproduced from DeVore,[15] with permission of John Wiley & Sons, Inc.)

Real-Time Imaging

Four-Chamber View Initially, the transducer is directed parallel to the spine or aorta. Once either of these structures has been identified, the transducer is rotated 90°, thus imaging the fetal trunk transversely. The easiest method for identifying atrial and ventricular anatomy is to locate the fetal spine and mentally draw a line to the opposite anterior chest wall. The ventricle lying beneath the intersection of this line and the anterior chest wall is the right ventricle. The left ventricle, on the same side of the fetal trunk as the stomach, is inferior and to the left of the right ventricle (Fig. 47.2). Table 47.3 lists the differences in shape and location between the right and left ventricles in the normal fetus. A recent study reported the normal axis of the fetal heart as 45° (± 20°).[98] When left axis deviation of the fetal heart occurred (< 75°), 76% of the fetuses had structural heart defects.[98]

The interventricular and interatrial septa should be examined next. The interventricular septum separates the ventricular chambers. It is thickest at the apex of the heart, and then tapers as it approaches the insertion of the atrioventricular valves. During ventricular systole, the septum becomes shorter and thicker.

The interatrial septum is a thin, membranous-like structure that can be seen as a continuation of the interventricular septum. Approximately half the distance from the interventricular/interatrial junction, an interruption of the interatrial septum occurs. This is the foramen ovale, which can be seen to move within the left atrial chamber (Fig. 47.2).

Opening and closing of the mitral and tricuspid valves should be identified next. Normally the tricuspid valve is inserted lower on the interventricular septum than the mitral valve. Occasionally a prominent papillary muscle is visible within the right or left ventricular chambers. In the normal four-chamber view, the right and left atria and ventricular chambers have similar shapes and sizes, as do the right and left ventricular walls.

Outflow Tract Examination Evaluation of the aortic and pulmonic outflow tracts can be accomplished in one of two ways.[99] The first approach is used when the axis of the four-chamber view is perpendicular to the ultrasound beam (Fig. 47.3). From this view, the transducer is rotated approximately 30° until the characteristic left ventricular inflow and outflow tracts are imaged (Fig. 47.4). This view should demonstrate anatomical continuity of the left atria and ventricle with the corresponding outflow tract. The left ventricular outflow tract, however, must be further examined to confirm that the brachiocephalic, common carotid, and left subclavian arteries originate from the arch of the aorta. When this view has been obtained, the transducer is rocked to identify the pulmonary artery as it exits the right ventricle (Fig. 47.4).

The second approach is used when the axis of the four-chamber view is tangential or parallel to the ultrasound beam, with the fetus in the supine position (Fig. 47.5). Following imaging of the four-chamber view, the transducer is rotated 90°.[99] The ultrasound beam is directed laterally from the spine, so that the short axis of the outflow tracts comes into view. When the proper image has been obtained, the aorta is circular, located in the center, with the pulmonic outflow tract draping over it (Fig. 47.5). At this point, the right ventricular outflow tract should be examined carefully to confirm the bifurcation of the right pulmonary artery medially and the single ductus arteriosus laterally (Figs. 47.5 and 47.6).

Identification of Structural Anomalies When the sonographer understands the imaging relationships just presented, five questions should be asked during each examination of the heart:

1. Is the fetus in an optimal position to image cardiac anatomy? When the fetus is in the spine-up position, it is extremely difficult to image the four chambers and outflow tracts. Optimal cardiovascular imaging occurs when the spine is between the 3 and 9 o'clock positions in a nonobese patient.

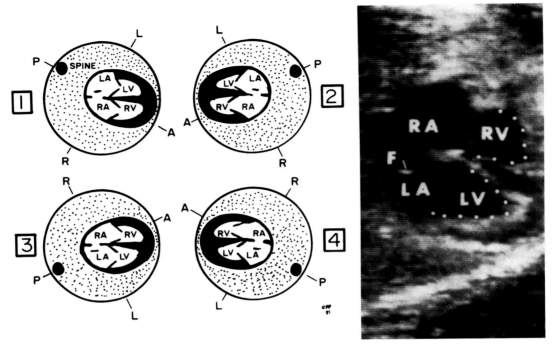

Figure 47.2   Orientation of the four-chamber view of the fetal heart in relation to the fetal spine. The right ventricle lies beneath the anterior chest wall (A), and the left ventricle (LV) is nearer the spine. The valve of the foramen ovale (F) is on the left side of the interatrial septum, within the left atrium (LA). Optimal imaging occurs with the spine at the 10, 2, 8, and 4 o'clock positions, as shown in diagrams 1–4, respectively. RA, right atrium; P, posterior; R, right; L, left. (Reproduced from DeVore,[15] with permission of John Wiley & Sons, Inc.)

2. Is the heart located in the left side of the chest? Fetuses with dextrocardia have a higher incidence of CHD than those with levocardia (Fig. 47.7).

3. Is there evidence of alteration of normal anatomy? Such an anomaly might be a cardiac tumor or ventricular or atrial septal defect (Fig. 47.8).

4. Do the ventricular chambers appear to be of similar size and shape in the four-chamber view, or is disproportion present? Ventricular disproportion might be an indicator of atrioventricular and/or semilunar valvular disease, as well as abnormalities of the aortic arch (Fig. 47.9).

5. Do the aortic and pulmonic outflow tracts at the level of the semilunar valves appear to be normal in size, or is disproportion present? A dilated aortic root with a diminished or absent pulmonary outflow tract is a marker for tetralogy of Fallot or truncus arteriosus.

If the answer to any of these questions suggests an abnormality, a comprehensive consultative echocardiographic examination should be undertaken to elucidate the nature of the suspected defect. To this end, M-mode, pulsed, and color Doppler examinations of the heart are useful.

TABLE 47.3   Identification of Right and Left Ventricles from the Four-Chamber View

Characteristic	Right Ventricle	Left Ventricle
Position within thorax	Beneath anterior chest wall	Left side of thorax, above spine, same side of trunk as stomach
Geometrical shape	Conical	Ellipsoid
Flap of foramen ovale		Present within left atrium
Insertion of AV valve leaflets on interventricular septum	Tricuspid valve is inserted lower than mitral	Mitral is inserted higher than tricuspid valve

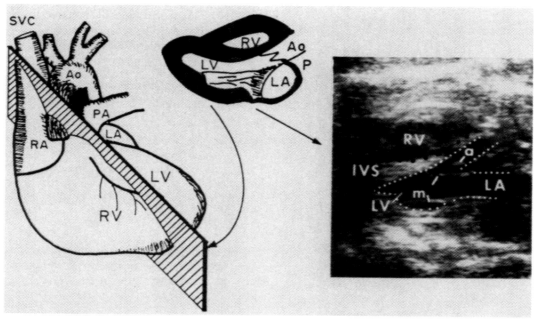

Figure 47.3 Fetal left parasternal view. THe schematic illustrates the plane through the fetal heart from which the corresponding real-time image was taken. The left ventricular (LV) inflow and outflow tracts are indicated by white dots; the right ventricle (RV) and right atrium (RA) are outlined by the black dots. Ao, aortic outflow tract; a, aortic valve; m, mitral valve; IVS, interventricular septum; LA, left atrium; PA, pulmonary artery; SVC, superior vena cava; P, posterior. (Reproduced from DeVore,[15] with permission of John Wiley & Sons, Inc.)

Consultative Examination

Real-Time Measurements Measurements of atrial and ventricular chamber dimensions as well as the outflow tracts have been reported in normal fetuses (Figs. 47.10 and 47.11).[100,101] A rule of thumb is that the diameters of the atrial and ventricular chambers are equal, and the same is true of the aortic and pulmonary arteries.

M-Mode Measurements While quantitation of ventricular and aortic dimensions has been obtained from real-time images, the sampling rate from real-time imaging is lower, which sometimes hinders identification of the endocardium. This difficulty is overcome with M-mode echocardiography because of the increased sampling rate plus the ability to simultaneously identify multiple cardiac cycles. The following structures can be measured using M-mode echocardiography: ventricular chamber dimensions, thickness of the ventricular walls and interventricular septum, tricuspid and mitral valve opening excursion, and aortic root and valve dimensions.

Measurements Obtained from the Four-Chamber View

Recording of the M Mode Utilizing real-time ultrasound, the M-mode cursor is directed perpendicular to the interventricular septum at the level of the atrioventricular valves (Fig. 47.12). Although other investigators have reported obtaining M-mode measurements at a level just below the mitral and tricuspid valves, it is felt that the recording should include opening and closing of the atrioventricular valves for three reasons[102]:

1. These points provide an internal marker for the proper orientation of the M-mode beam. If the ultrasound beam is not perpendicular to the interventricular septum but crosses it tangentially, for example, only one valve may be recorded. If the beam is not in the center of both chambers, the opening excursion of the valves will be abnormal even though both valves are recorded.

2. The widest diameter of the ventricular chambers is at the level of the atrioventricular valves.

3. Imaging the atrioventricular valves allows an accurate determination of ventricular diastole.

Measurements Figures 47.12 and 47.13 illustrate the schematic and an M-mode recording. The points in Figure 47.13 are identified, and M-mode measurements and their corresponding derived values computed. Although a number of

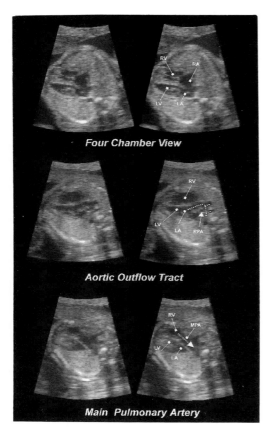

Four Chamber View

Aortic Outflow Tract

Main Pulmonary Artery

Figure 47.4 Identification of the aortic and pulmonary outflow tracts. After identifying the four-chamber View (upper panel) the transducer is rotated 30°, directing the ultrasound beam from the right shoulder to the left hip of the fetus. When this has been done, the aortic outflow tract is identified (middle panel). This view contains the ascending aorta (dotted lines) and a portion of the arch (dotted) from which originate arteries to the fetal head and upper extremities. The right pulmonary artery (RPA) can be observed perpendicular and posterior to the ascending aorta. When this view has been obtained, the transducer is rocked laterally, demonstrating the main pulmonary artery (lower panel). The direction of the main pulmonary artery is perpendicular to the ascending aorta. RV, right ventricle; LV, left ventricle; RA, right atrium; LA, Left atrium; MPA, main pulmonary artery; RPA, right pulmonary artery.

measurements and calculated values can be computed from computer analysis, the following can be obtained without the assistance of the computer program.[102]

Ventricular Chamber Dimensions at End Diastole   The advantage of M-mode measurements at end diastole is that an electrocardiogram, which often cannot be recorded from the fetus through the maternal abdominal wall, is not required for determination of end diastole. This is because closure of the atrioventricular valve leaflets represents the mechanical

equivalent of end diastole. Therefore, by drawing a line through the ventricles, perpendicular to the interventricular septum at the point of closure of the mitral and tricuspid valve leaflets, the following dimensions are obtainable.

1. Biventricular outer dimension (BOD): measures the transverse dimension across both ventricles from epicardium to epicardium.
2. Biventricular inner dimension (BID): measures the transverse dimension across both ventricles from the endocardium of the right ventricle to the endocardium of the left ventricle.
3. Right ventricular internal dimension (RVID): measured from the endocardium of the right ventricular wall to the endocardium of the interventricular septum.
4. Left ventricular internal dimension (LVID): measured from the endocardium of the left ventricular wall to the endocardium of the interventricular septum.

Ventricular Chamber Dimensions at End Systole   The BOD, BID, RVID, and LVID can also be measured at end systole, which is the point of maximal inward excursion of the right and left ventricular walls.

Atrioventricular Valve Opening Excursion   Measurement of the opening excursion of the mitral and tricuspid valve leaflets (E–E′) is important for assessment of valve hypoplasia or dilation. In the fetus with normal opening valve excursion, the tricuspid to mitral valve E–E′ ratio is 1:1 (range 0.83–1.15). If an M-mode recording is obtained and this ratio is greater or less than the range above, the M-mode may have been obtained tangentially to the interventricular septum, or pathology may be present.

Interventricular Septal and Ventricular Wall Thickness at End Diastole   Measurements of the thickness of the interventricular septum and the right and left ventricular walls are important in the evaluation of cardiovascular diseases that result in wall hypertrophy. Fetuses with complete heart block, pulmonary stenosis, and diabetic cardiomyopathy exhibit wall hypertrophy.

Right-to-Left Relationships   Table 47.4 lists the mean, 5%, and 95% confidence limits for the right-to-left ratios for ventricular internal chamber dimensions, tricuspid and mitral valve opening excursion, and ventricular wall thickness.

Measurements Obtained from the Aortic Root

Aortic Root Dimension   The aortic root dimension is measured at the level of the aortic valve, perpendicular to the aortic root (Figs. 47.14 and 47.15). This convention is used because the aortic valve provides a standard reference plane,

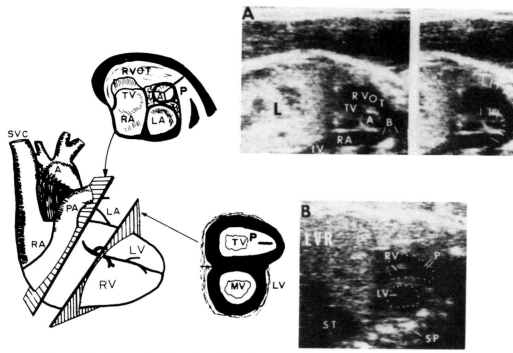

Figure 47.5   Short-axis views through the fetal heart at the level of the aortic and pulmonic outflow tracts. Schematic illustrates the planes through the fetal heart from which the images were obtained: (*A*) right ventricular outflow tract (RVOT) draping over the aorta (A) and bifurcating (B) into the right and left pulmonary arteries (white lines); (*B*) short-axis view at the level of the tricuspid and mitral valves. RV, right ventricle; LV, left ventricle; P, pulmonary outflow tract; TV, tricuspid valve; RA, right atrium; LA, left atrium; L and LVR, liver; IV, inferior vena cava; ST, stomach; SP, spine; SVC, superior vena cava. (Reproduced from DeVore,[15] with permission of John Wiley & Sons, Inc.)

which prevents measurement of an image inadvertently obtained by directing the M-mode beam tangential to the aortic root.[103]

Confidence Limits for Cardiac Measurements   Investigators have attempted to compare cardiac dimensions from the real-time and M-mode images with gestational age and estimated fetal weight.[104,105] Both of the latter were derived from regression analysis of the biparietal diameter and/or abdominal circumference. These approaches have two problems, however. First, real-time measurements of the fetal heart have a significantly smaller correlation than M-mode measurements.[102] Second, when fetal age and weight are derived from the biparietal diameter and/or abdominal circumference, they have their own standard error of the estimate.[102,104–106] Therefore, our group compares M-mode measurements against the following measured fetal biometric parameters: biparietal diameter, head circumference, abdominal circumference, and femur length (Fig. 47.16). Morphometric measurements (biparietal diameter, head circumference, abdominal circumference, and femur length) are

associated with correlation coefficients of greater than 0.90 for ventricular chamber dimensions and atrioventricular valve opening excursion, 0.78 for ventricular wall thickness, and 0.79 for aortic root dimensions and aortic valve excursion.[102,107,108] The benefit of multiple options is that the abdominal circumference or femur length curves can be used to evaluate ventricular and aortic dimensions when a fetus with hydrocephaly is examined.

Use of M-Mode Quantitation

CASE 1   A 23-year-old woman (G_2, P_1) underwent ultrasound evaluation and amniocentesis at 16 weeks of gestation because she had previously given birth to a child with a neural tube defect. During the real-time examination of the fetal heart, ventricular disproportion was noted. The patient returned 4 weeks later for a second ultrasound exam in which ventricular disproportion was again noted and the diagnosis of a hypoplastic left ventricle was entertained by the referring physician. Consultative echocardiography confirmed the real-time findings of ventricular disproportion. However,

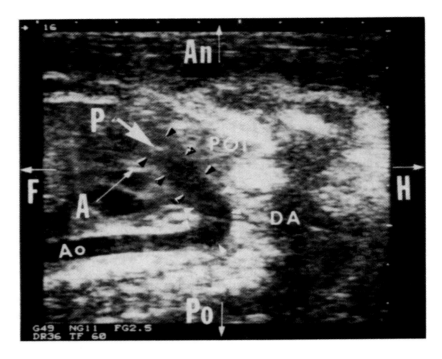

Figure 47.6 Imaging the ductus arteriosus (DA). The transducer is directed parallel to the spine. The DA can be followed from the pulmonary valve (P) to the descending aorta (Ao). Unlike the arch of the aorta, which looks like a cane, the ductal–aortic image has the appearance of a hockey stick. POT, pulmonary outflow tract; A, aortic valve; AN, anterior chest wall; Po, posterior; F, fetal feet; H, fetal head. Black arrows outline the pulmonary outflow tract; white arrows outline the DA. (Reproduced from DeVore,[15] with permission of John Wiley & Sons, Inc.)

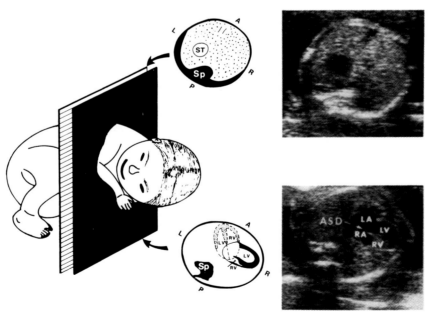

Figure 47.7 Evaluation of the four-chamber view. Schematic illustrates the orientation of the transducer perpendicular to the long axis of the trunk for identification of the fetal stomach (ST) (hatched) and four-chamber view of the heart (solid). In the normal fetus, the right ventricle (RV) lies directly under the anterior chest wall and the left ventricle (LV) within the left-posterior chest cavity. In this fetus, the heart was shifted to the right. Ventricular disproportion was noted, as well as an atrial septal defect (ASD). SP, spine; RA, right atrium; LA, left atrium; LV, left ventricle; RV, right ventricle; L, left; R, right; A, anterior; P, posterior. (Reproduced from DeVore et al.,[90] with permission of John Wiley & Sons, Inc.)

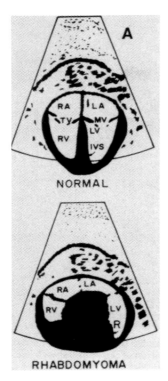
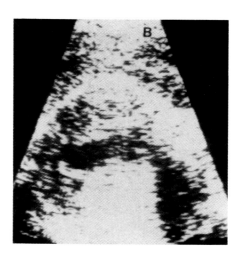

Figure 47.8 Interventricular septal rhabdomyoma. (*A*) Schematic illustrating the normal four-chamber view (top) and the four-chamber view with the interventricular septal tumor (bottom). (*B*) Corresponding four-chamber view of the rhabdomyoma. RA, right atrium; LA, left atrium; TV, tricuspid valve; MV, mitral valve; RV, right ventricle; LV, left ventricle; IVS, interventricular septum; R, rhabdomyoma. (Reproduced from DeVore, *Semin Ultrasound Comput Tomogr Med* 1984;5:229, with permission of Grune & Stratton, Inc.)

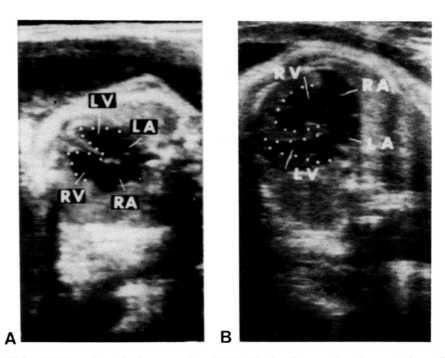

Figure 47.9 (*A*) Normal ventricular proportion. (*B*) Ventricular disproportion demonstrating a dilated right ventricle (RV) and a small left ventricle (LV). LA, left atrium; RA, right atrium. White dots outline the ventricular chambers. (Reproduced from DeVore, *Semin Ultrasound Comput Tomogr Med* 1984;5:229, with permission of Grune & Stratton, Inc.)

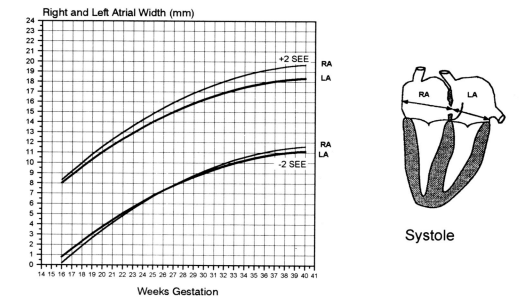

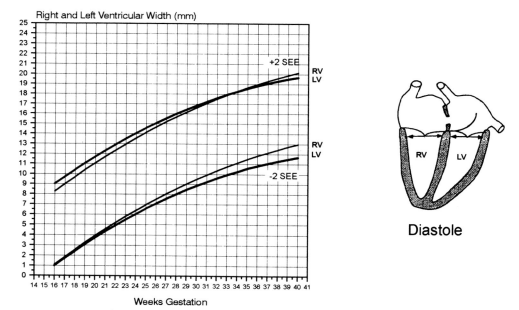

Figure 47.10 Real-time measurements of the width of the atrial and ventricular chambers. (Adapted from Tan et al.[101])

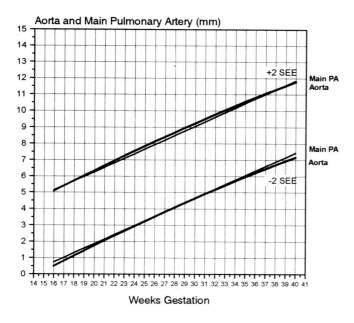

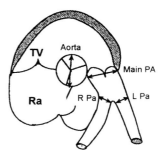

Short Axis of The Outflow Tracts

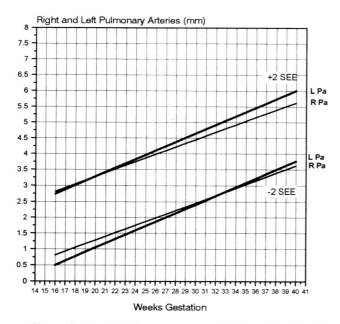

Figure 47.11 Real-time measurements of the outflow tracts from the short-axis view. (Adapted from Tan et al.[101])

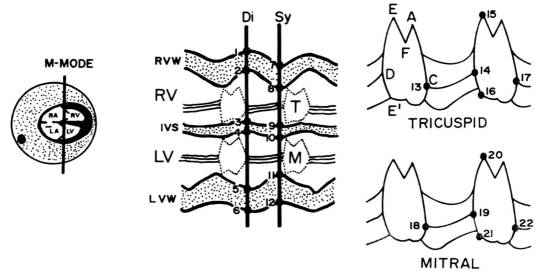

Figure 47.12   Schematic of the M-mode from which measurements are computed. The M-mode is recorded perpendicular to the interventricular septum, at the level of the mitral and tricuspid valves; numbers indicate the sequence in which the indicated points are digitized and the measurements subsequently computed. RA, right atrium; RV, right ventricle; LA, left atrium; LV, left ventricle; RVW, right ventricular wall; IVS, interventricular septum; LVW, left ventricular wall; T, tricuspid valve; M, mitral valve; D, beginning of diastole; E-E', maximal excursion of leaflets in early diastole; A, atrial systole; C, closure of leaflet at end diastole. (Reproduced from DeVore et al,[102] with permission of the American Gynecological and Obstetrical Society.)

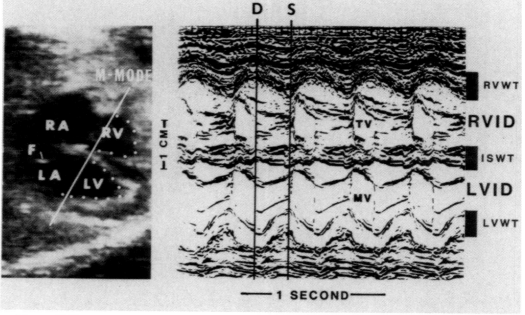

Figure 47.13   M-mode recording. The M mode is obtained by placing the cursor perpendicular to the interventricular septum, at the level of the atrioventricular valves. RA, right atrium; LA, left atrium; RV, right ventricle; LV, left ventricle; TV, tricuspid valve; MV, mitral valve; RVWT, right ventricular wall thickness; RVID, right ventricular internal dimension; ISWT, interventricular septal wall thickness; LVID, left ventricular internal dimension; LVWT, left ventricular wall thickness. (Reproduced from DeVore et al,[102] with permission of the American Gynecological and Obstetrical Society.)

TABLE 47.4   Right/Left Ventricular Ratios

	5%	Mean	95%	SD
Internal dimension—diastole	0.80	0.98	1.15	0.08
Tricuspid/mitral valve excursion	0.83	0.99	1.15	0.08
Wall thickness/diastole	0.58	1.12	1.65	0.27

Source: DeVore et al. [102]

M-mode measurements demonstrated the left ventricle and aortic root to be at the 5th percentile (Fig. 47.17). The experience of the consultant indicated a diagnosis of coarctation of the aorta.[89] The patient chose to continue the pregnancy. Serial M-mode measurements demonstrated growth of the left ventricle and aortic root as pregnancy progressed. Following birth, coarctation was confirmed by echocardiography and cardiac catheterization.

CASE 2   A 23-year-old woman (G₁) was referred for echocardiographic evaluation at 19 weeks of gestation because of first-trimester exposure to phenobarbital and diphenylhydantoin for control of a seizure disorder. Real-

time examination of the fetal heart demonstrated ventricular disproportion: The right ventricle was larger than the left ventricle. M-mode quantitation of the ventricular chambers and aortic root dimension demonstrated the left ventricle and aortic root dimension to be below the 5th and 95th percentile. These findings were compatible with a hypoplastic left ventricle (Fig. 47.18). The pregnancy was terminated, and autopsy confirmed the in utero findings.

CASE 3   A 24-year-old woman (G₁) underwent a routine ultrasound examination at 19 weeks of gestation. A routine real-time screening examination suggested an enlarged aortic root. A consultative echocardiographic examination

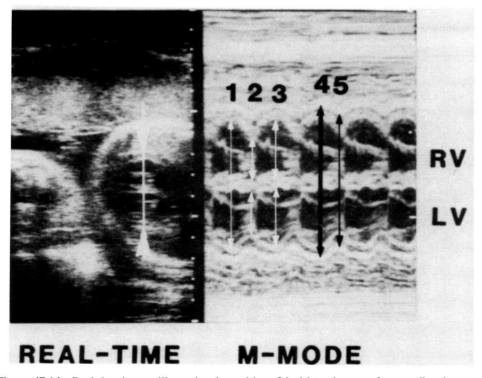

Figure 47.14   Real-time images illustrating the position of the M-mode cursor for recording the aortic root dimension and valve excursion. Schematics illustrate the planes through the heart from which the real-time views were obtained. SVC, superior vena cava; RA, right atrium; A and Ao, aorta; PA, pulmonary artery; LA, left atrium; LV, left ventricle; RV, right ventricle; M, mitral valve; TV, tricuspid valve; IVS, interventricular septum; RVOT, right ventricular outflow tract. (Reproduced from De-Vore et al,[103] with permission of the American Gynecological and Obstetrical Society.)

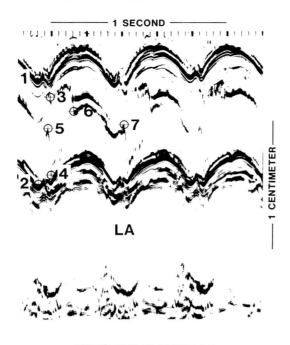

AORTIC ROOT DIMENSION 1-2
AORTIC VALVE EXCURSION 3-4
LEFT VENTRICULAR EJECTION TIME 5-6
HEART RATE 5-7

Figure 47.15 M mode of aortic valve and root; numbers indicate M-mode measurements. LA, left atrium. (Reproduced from DeVore et al,[103] with permission of the American Gynecological and Obstetrical Society.)

demonstrated a dilated aortic root that straddled a ventricular septal defect (Fig. 47.19). A diminished pulmonic outflow tract was also observed. After consultation with a pediatric cardiologist, the patient chose to terminate the pregnancy. Autopsy confirmed the in utero findings of tetralogy of Fallot.

Doppler Color Flow Mapping (DCFM)

The fetal sonographer has faced notable difficulties in the identification and complete elucidation of structural defects associated with intracardiac or great vessel flow disturbances. Unlike the angiographic examination in the adult or pediatric patient from whom detailed information concerning intracardiac blood flow is available, fetal sonography has been limited primarily to images derived from real-time and M-mode echocardiography for which flow information is not available.

Real-time DCFM has been utilized by adult and pediatric cardiologists to detect intracardiac and great vessel flow disturbance and to diagnose structural malformations of the heart.[109–112] Studies from our group have demonstrated the diagnostic potential of DCFM to diagnose simple as well as complex malformations in the fetus.[113–116] In this modality, moreover, the Doppler shift resulting from blood flow within the cardiac chambers and great vessels is displayed in color during the real-time examination. Currently, the conventional format displays blood flowing toward the transducer

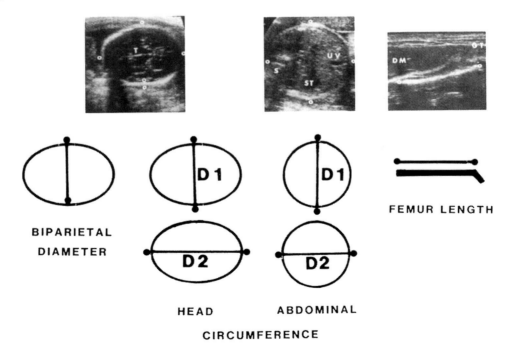

Figure 47.16 Fetal growth measurements: T, thalamus; UV, umbilical vein; ST, stomach; DM, distal metathesis; GT, greater trochanter. Schematic illustrates where the linear measurements were obtained from which the biparietal diameter, head and abdominal circumferences, and femur length were measured or derived: D1, diameter 1; D2, diameter 2.

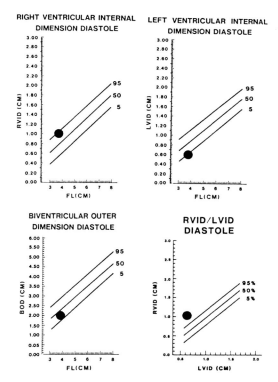

Figure 47.17 M-mode measurements in a fetus with coarctation of the aorta at 20 weeks of gestation. BOD, biventricular outer dimension at end diastole; RVID, right ventricular internal end diastole; LVID, left ventricular internal dimension at end diastole; FL, femur length.

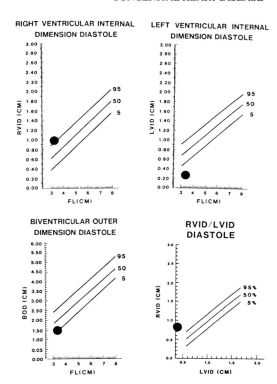

Figure 47.18 M-mode measurements in a fetus with a hypoplastic left ventricle at 19 weeks of gestation. BOD, biventricular outer dimension at end diastole; RVID, right ventricular internal end diastole; LVID, left ventricular internal dimension at end diastole; FL, femur length.

as red-orange and blood flow away as blue. If blood flow velocity exceeds the Nyquist limit, a reversal of color occurs. Turbulent flow is depicted as a mosaic pattern.

Four-Chamber View

Inflow Tracts Unlike real-time imaging of the four-chamber and left parasternal long-axis views, in which the ultrasound beam is directed perpendicular to the interventricular septum, DCFM is best displayed when the transducer is directed parallel or tangential to the interventricular septum. During ventricular diastole, DCFM displays blood flowing into each ventricle, the two being separated by the interventricular septum (Fig. 47.20).

Aortic and Pulmonary Outflow Tracts During ventricular systole, blood flows parallel to the interventricular septum as it empties into the ascending aorta (Fig. 47.21). In addition to the M-mode and four-chamber view approaches discussed in connection with real-time imaging, there is a third approach to identifying the outflow tracts: the use of color Doppler.[117] After the four-chamber view has been identified, the ultrasound beam is directed directly cephalad, without ro-

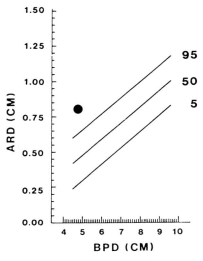

Figure 47.19 M-mode measurement of the aortic root diameter in a fetus at 19 weeks of gestation demonstrating aortic root dilation. ARD, aortic root dimension; BPD, biparietal diameter.

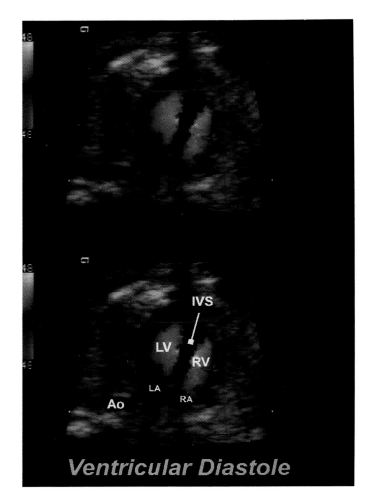

Figure 47.20 Real-time color Doppler of the four-chamber view during ventricular diastole; red represents the flow of blood into the ventricular chambers. The color enhances the identification of the interventricular septum (IVS). Ao, aorta; RV, right ventricle; LV, left ventricle; RA, right atrium; LA, left atrium. (See color plates.)

tating the transducer, to identify the main pulmonary artery, the left pulmonary artery, the ductus arteriosus, and the transverse arch of the aorta (Fig. 47.22).

Examination of the Interventricular and Interatrial Septa
With the ultrasound beam perpendicular to the interventricular and interatrial septa, flow is observed (1) at the base of the left ventricle at the level of the aortic outflow tract and (2) at the level of the interatrial septum as blood flows from the right atrial chamber to the left atrial chamber through the foramen ovale (Fig. 47.23).

CASE 4 The patient underwent genetic amniocentesis for advanced maternal age. The ultrasound results were inter-

preted to be normal. However, the karyotype demonstrated a balanced translocation. A consultative ultrasound examination, requested at 19 weeks of gestation, demonstrated tetralogy of Fallot. This abnormality was confirmed following birth (Fig. 47.24).

CASE 5 A patient was referred for diagnostic ultrasound at 26 weeks of gestation to examine the fetus because of a family history of congenital heart disease. The four-chamber view of the heart was normal, with no evidence of ventricular disproportion, ventricular wall hypertrophy, or abnormal contraction of the ventricular walls. Examination of the aortic outflow tract demonstrated normal flow along the interventricular septum as blood exited the left ventricle. Howev-

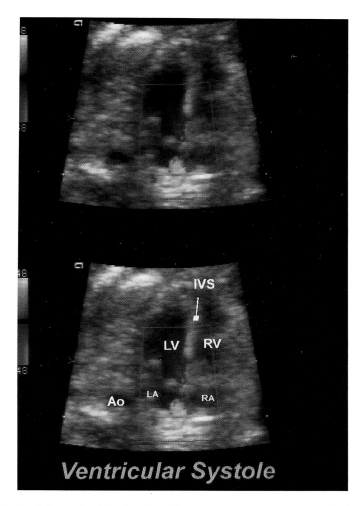

Figure 47.21   Real-time color Doppler of the four-chamber view during ventricular systole; blue represents the flow of blood along the interventricular septum of the left ventricle. In the normal heart, blood is not observed along the right interventricular septum during systole. Ao, aorta; RV, right ventricle; LV, left ventricle; RA, right atrium; LA, left atrium; IVS, interventricular septum. (See color plates.)

er, distal to the aortic valve, turbulent flow with aliasing was observed with color Doppler (Fig. 47.25). Pulsed Doppler confirmed the presence of a stenotic jet that was more rapid than 1.5 m/s. Examination of the transverse aortic arch demonstrated turbulent flow with aliasing (Fig. 47.25). Evaluation of the full aortic arch demonstrated a similar flow pattern, which extended from the aortic valve to the descending aorta. Following delivery the pathology was confirmed.

Further Considerations

Once the prenatal diagnosis of congenital heart disease is confirmed, strong consideration should be given to further ultrasound assessment of the fetus for noncardiovascular malformations. Recent studies have suggested that the latter occur with a frequency of 25–30% and include such malformations as hydrocephaly, microcephaly, holoprosencephaly, renal agenesis, renal dysgenesis, hydronephrosis, esophageal atresia, duodenal atresia, diaphragmatic hernia, gastroschesis, omphalocele, and skeletal dysplasias.[118]

Since the incidence of abnormal chromosomes is approximately 10–15% for all categories of CHD, an amniocentesis or a fetal umbilical cord blood sample should be performed to obtain cells for karyotyping.[28,119] This practice gives the obstetrician the opportunity to reconsider whether a cesarean section should be done for obstetrical indications if, for

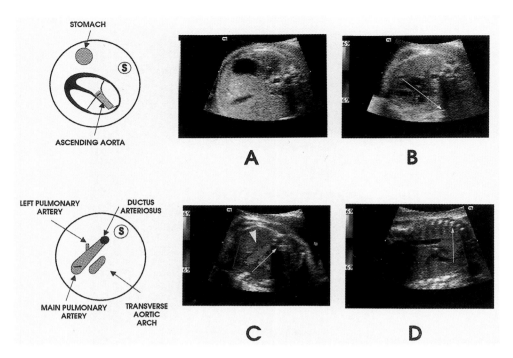

Figure 47.22 Identification of the outflow tracts. Upper schematic: the four-chamber view, with the left side of the fetus proximal to the ultrasound beam and the spine (S) at the 2 o'clock position. (*A*) Position of the fetal stomach within the left side of the abdomen. (*B*) By directing the transducer beam cephalad to the four-chamber view, the origin of the ascending aorta (small arrow) can be identified as it exits the left ventricle. Lower schematic: the orientation of the outflow tracts identified by directing the transducer beam in a transverse plane through the chest further cephalad to the four-chamber view. (*D*) The vessels identified are perpendicular to the ascending aorta; they include the main pulmonary artery, branching of the left pulmonary artery (arrowhead), ductus arteriosus, and transverse aortic arch (arrow). (*E*) Image of the aortic arch obtained in a left sagittal plane; arrow identifies the direction of the ascending aorta in which the transverse aortic arch is imaged perpendicular to this plane. (From DeVore.[117]) (See color plates.)

example, a lethal trisomy is found to be associated with a repairable cardiac lesion.

Although a number of newborn intensive care units are available in most major metropolitan centers, one must strongly consider delivery of the fetus at a center that offers full cardiovascular services. This is especially important for complex cardiovascular lesions and for those involving hypoplasia of the aortic or pulmonic outflow tracts, in which new and innovative surgical procedures might be considered.[120]

DIAGNOSIS OF A PERICARDIAL EFFUSION

Fetal hydrops is generally a global manifestation of hypoalbuminemia and/or disease intrinsic to the cardiovascular system. Hydrops can be determined ultrasonically by demonstrating ascites, scalp edema, or pleural effusions. A significant amount of fluid must be present in these potential spaces, however, before abnormalities can be seen with the ultrasound. The presence of a pericardial effusion appears to be an earlier indicator of fluid accumulation than the foregoing parameters.[121] It has been the author's experience that the effusion often develops before there is gross evidence of hydrops in fetuses with Rh-hemolytic anemia, congenital malformations of the heart, or supraventricular tachyarrhythmias. It must be emphasized, however, that an echo-free space around the heart can be misleading if the following characteristics, as seen on real-time and M-mode examination, are not properly appreciated.

Normal Anatomy

In the four-chamber view, the pericardium is apposed to the epicardium of the ventricles, thus creating a bright echo encircling the right and left ventricular walls. Lying beneath the

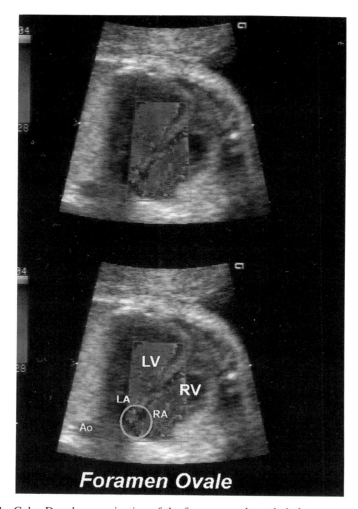

Figure 47.23   Color Doppler examination of the foramen ovale; red circle represents the flow of blood through the foramen ovale. In this image, the baseline of the color velocity was moved to the top of the velocity bar so that only one color is present in the image. This view makes it easy to see where blood is flowing but does not accurately indicate velocity. This technique is important for viewing areas of low flow, such as the foramen ovale, and for removing the aliasing effect observed in low flow states. (See color plates.)

epicardium is the muscular myocardium. Lining the ventricular chambers is the endocardium, which also can appear as a bright echo (Fig. 47.26). Thus, the following are important points to consider.

1. It is normal to see separation of the pericardium and epicardium at the antrio-ventricular junction during ventricular systole (Fig. 47.26).
2. Because refraction of returning echoes from the ventricular chambers due to their curvature can occur, the myocardium may appear to be completely filled with echoes or may demonstrate varying degrees of echo

dropout (Fig. 47.26). This is the most difficult problem for the novice because echo dropout can be misinterpreted as representing fluid, when indeed it does not. To assist in identification of such relationships, the M-mode recording is often necessary (Fig. 47.27).

Abnormal Anatomy

For diagnosis of a pathological effusion, there must be a clear separation between the pericardium and epicardium, as manifested by two bright echoes interspersed by an echo-free space (Fig. 47.26). This separation must be evident both in

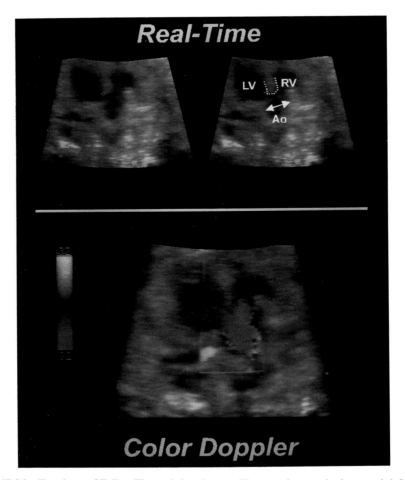

Figure 47.24   Tetralogy of Fallot. The real-time images illustrate the ventricular septal defect (dotted line), overriding the aorta. The color Doppler illustrates flow along both the right and left interventricular septum, exiting the aorta. LV, left ventricle; RV, right ventricle. (See color plates.)

diastole and systole, and/or the effusion must extend from the atrioventricular junction toward the apex of the heart. When hydrops occurs (ascites, pleural effusion), the pericardial effusion can extend beyond the atrioventricular junction, partially collapsing the atrial wall. The effusion is usually unilateral; in severe cases, however, it can be bilateral, with the heart contracting with a "rocking motion" within the fluid-filled cavity. Fetuses with severe pleural effusions might not demonstrate evidence of a pericardial effusion because the pericardium is compressed against the epicardium by the pleural fluid.

In a recent study the use of color Doppler ultrasound was described to identify a pericardial effusion.[121] Color Doppler is useful because it identifies fluid motion, whether the medium be blood or pericardial fluid. This new technique will greatly assist in the confirmation of a pericardial effusion when the real-time examination leads to suspicion of this anomaly (Fig. 47.28).

ANTENATAL DIAGNOSIS AND TREATMENT OF ARRHYTHMIAS

The incidence of cardiac arrhythmias in the newborn has been estimated to be 1%.[122] While the obstetrician can identify a fetal cardiac arrhythmia that occurs during labor by recording the electrocardiogram with the scalp electrode, diagnosis during the antenatal period is more difficult. Traditionally, clinicians have utilized the fetal heart rate monitor in an attempt to elucidate the underlying problem. Only ventricular rate is obtained, however, whereas diagnosis of a fetal arrhythmia requires assessment of atrial and ventricular rates, as well as the atrial–ventricular timing relationship.

Until recently, fetal arrhythmias during the antepartum period could only be inferred. The use of M-mode echocardiography, however, permits the evaluation of atrial and ventricular systole, as well as the timing relationship between the two. Table 47.5 lists the frequency of occurrence of fetal ar-

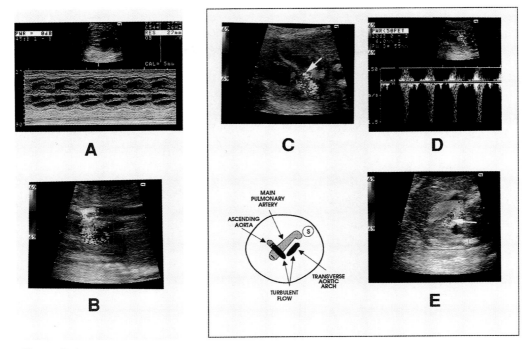

Figure 47.25   Aortic stenosis. (*A*) M-mode recording from the four-chamber view, which demonstrates normal ventricular wall contractility, with no evidence of ventricular disproportion. (*B*) The aortic arch demonstrates disturbed flow in the ascending aorta. (*C*) Blood exiting the left ventricle. The disturbed flow can be observed to originate at the aortic valve (arrow). (*D*) Pulsed Doppler of the aortic outflow tract, demonstrating increased flow across the valve. (*E*) Transverse plane in which disturbed flow is observed in the transverse aortic arch. (From DeVore.[117]) (See color plates.)

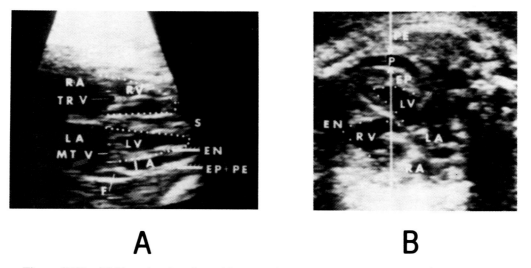

Figure 47.26   (*A*) Four-chamber view with a normal amount of pericardial fluid seen during systole at the atrioventricular junction (F). Artifact from dropout of echoes is seen in the myocardium of the left ventricular posterior wall (A). (*B*) Pericardial effusion, which extends from the atrioventricular junction to the apex of the heart (P). The fluid separates the pericardium (PE) from the epicardium (EP). The endocardium of both ventricles is outlined by the white dots. RA, right atrium; RV, right ventricle; LA, left atrium; LV, left ventricle; TR V, tricuspid valve; MT V, mitral valve; S, interventricular septum. (Reproduced from DeVore,[109] with permission of Grune & Stratton, Inc.)

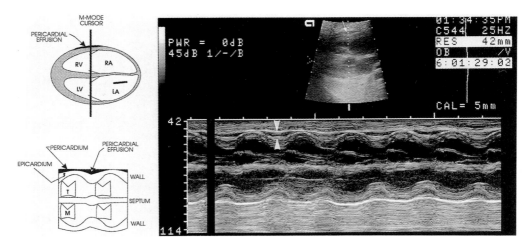

Figure 47.27   Schematic illustrates the four-chamber view from which the M-mode recording is obtained; ultrasound recording demonstrates the separation of the pericardium and the epicardium (arrowheads). (See color plates.)

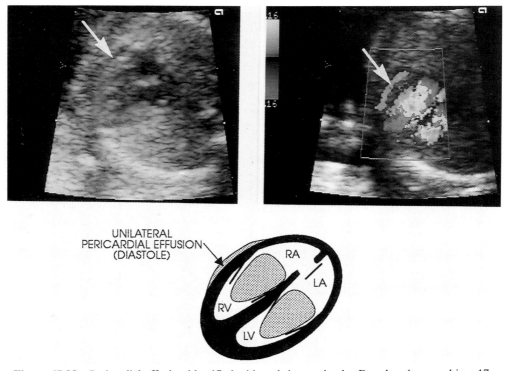

Figure 47.28   Pericardial effusion identified with real-time and color Doppler ultrasound in a 17-week fetus. The real-time image suggests separation of the pericardium from the epicardium (white arrow) along the right ventricular wall. The color Doppler image illustrates the pericardial space to be filled with color Doppler (red) (white arrow) with aliasing observed within the ventricles during diastole. RV, right ventricle; RA, right atrium; LV, left ventricle; LA, left atrium. (From DeVore and Horenstein.[121]) (See color plates.)

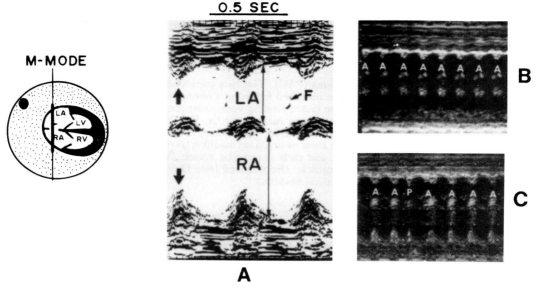

Figure 47.29 M-mode evaluation of atrial arrhythmias. The easiest method for evaluation of atrial arrhythmias simply requires the M-mode cursor to be placed perpendicular to the interatrial septum. (*A*) Hard-copy recording of normal atrial wall motion (single arrowheads). (*B*) Video recording of the same arrhythmia with atrial systole manifest by inward motion of the atrial walls (A). (*C*) Premature atrial contractions (P), which are seen to occur early, followed by a pause. LA, left atrium; LV, left ventricle; RA, right atrium; RV, right ventricle; F, foramen ovale. (Reproduced from DeVore, *Clin Obstet Gynecol* 1984;27:359–377, with permission of J.B. Lippincott Co.)

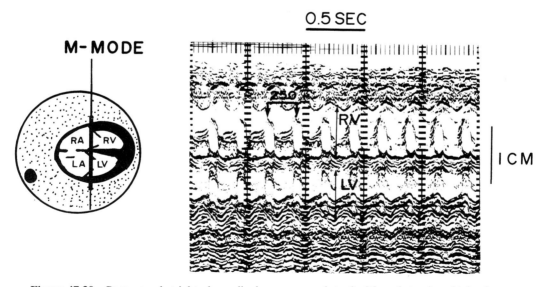

Figure 47.30 Paroxysmal atrial tachycardia; bar corresponds to the M-mode tracing obtained perpendicular to the interventricular septum. The rate is fixed at 250 beats per minute. RA, right atrium; LA, left atrium; RV, right ventricle; LV, left ventricle. (Reproduced from DeVore et al,[124] with permission of the American Gynecological and Obstetrical Society.)

TABLE 47.5 Fetal Arrhythmias in 58 of 71 Patients Studied

Arrhythmia	Number of Patients
SUSTAINED	
Atrial flutter	2
Supraventricular tachycardia	2
Complex arrhythmia	1
Complete heart block	2
Supraventricular ectopic beats	2
Sinus bradycardia	_1_
	10
SELF-LIMITED	
Supraventricular ectopic beats	32
Ventricular ectopic beats	2
Sinus bradycardia	6
Sinus pauses	_8_
	48

Source: DeVore et al.[107]

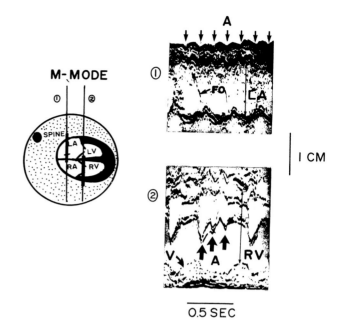

Figure 47.31 Atrial flutter. Bars correspond to (1) the M-mode tracing obtained perpendicular to the interatrial septum. A, atrial contraction (350/beats/min); FO, foramen ovale; LA, left atrium and (2) the M-mode tracing obtained at the level of the atrioventricular valves perpendicular to the interventricular septum. A, atrial contraction reflected by motion of the tricuspid valve leaflets; V, ventricular response consisting of a 2:1 to 3:1 block. LA, left atrium; RA, right atrium; RV, right ventricle; LV, left ventricle. (Reproduced from DeVore et al,[124] with permission of the American Gynecological and Obstetrical Society.)

rhythmias detected by M-mode echocardiography in a large series.[123] The most frequently encountered arrhythmia is the premature atrial contraction. Initially, investigators attempted to identify atrial systole by the A wave of the mitral or tricuspid valve leaflet excursion. However, this has proved to be confusing to many because the A wave is not always easy to identify.

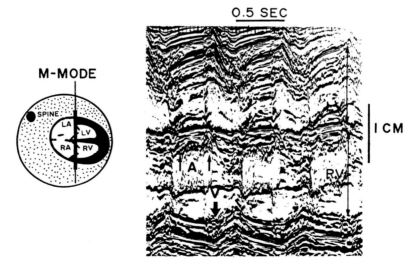

Figure 47.32 Fixed 2:1 atrioventricular block; bar corresponds to the M-mode tracing when the cursor is directed through both atrioventricular valves perpendicular to the interventricular septum. A, atrial systole (162 beats/min); V, ventricular systole (81 beats/min); LA, left atrium; RA, right atrium; LV, left ventricle; RV, right ventricle. (Reproduced from DeVore et al,[124] with permission of the American Gynecological and Obstetrical Society.)

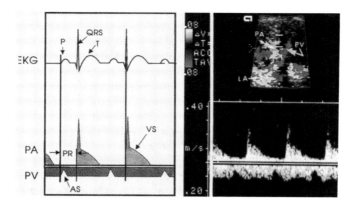

Figure 47.33 Schematic compares an electrocardiogram with the pulsed Doppler waveforms recorded from the pulmonary artery (PA) and pulmonary vein (PV) from the lung parenchyma. The real-time Doppler color image demonstrates a pulmonary vein entering the left atrium (LA) and a branch of the pulmonary artery within the lung. The left side of the fetus is at the top of the image. P, P wave of the atrial depolarization; QRS and T, electrical depolarization and repolarization of the ventricle; A, atrial systole recorded from the pulmonary veins; VS, ventricular systole recorded from the pulmonary artery; PR, interval from the onset of atrial systole to the onset of ventricular systole. (*B*) Color and pulsed Doppler recording from the lung parenchyma. (From DeVore and Horenstein.[121]) (See color plates.)

By placing the M-mode cursor perpendicular to the interatrial septum, one can record atrial activity and immediately determine whether premature atrial systoles are occurring (Fig. 47.29).[124] This can be accomplished with ultrasound equipment currently available to the obstetrician or radiologist.

Directing the M-mode cursor through atrial and ventricular walls, makes it possible to ascertain the timing relationship of atrial and ventricular systole and to determine the ventricular response. This method is important in searching for second- or third-degree atrioventricular block, atrial flutter, atrial fibrillation, or paroxysmal atrial tachycardia (Figs. 47.30–47.32).[124]

Pulsed and color Doppler can be utilized to identify fetal cardiac rhythm. In 1989 Chan et al reported that when the Doppler sample volume is placed simultaneously in the de-

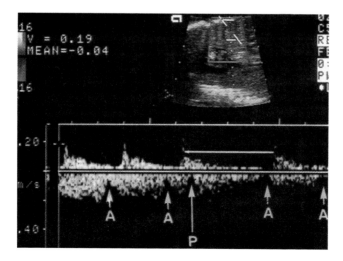

Figure 47.34 Color and pulsed Doppler recording from the lung parenchyma illustrating normal atrial contractions (A) interrupted by a premature atrial contraction (P) that is not conducted to the ventricles. This results in prolongation of ventricular systole (solid white line). (From DeVore and Horenstein.[121]) (See color plates.)

TABLE 47.6 Antepartum Evaluation and Treatment of the Fetus with an Arrhythmia

Arrhythmia	Further Ultrasound Examination	Treatment
Supraventricular		
Paroxysmal atrial tachycardia Atrial flutter Atrial fibrillation	Evaluate for percardial effusion, congenital anomalies of cardiovascular and other organ systems; monitor fetal growth	Hospitalize mother; consider transplacental treatment
Premature atrial contractions	As for other supraventricular arrhythmias; reevaluate on a weekly basis for evidence of intermittent or sustained tachyarrhythmia	Stop all caffeine, smoking, alcohol
Ventricular: premature ventricular contractions	As for supraventricular arrhythmias	Treat as for supraventricular arrhythmias
Second-degree heart block	Look for evidence of premature atrial contractions that are not conducted; evaluate all organ systems for evidence of congenital anomalies and abnormal growth	Treat as for supraventricular arrhythmias
Third-degree heart block	Evaluate all organ systems for evidence of congenital anomalies and abnormal growth; examine the fetus on a 7- to 14-day basis for evidence of hydrops	Evaluate mother for presence of collagen vascular disease

scending aorta and inferior vena cava, atrial (inferior vena cava) and ventricular (aorta) systole can be identified.[125] A similar relationship can be observed by placing the pulsed Doppler waveform within the left ventricle and recording the mitral waveform (atrial systole) and the aortic waveform (ventricular systole). While useful, these approaches may be difficult to implement because of fetal position. A third approach is to place the pulsed Doppler within the lung parenchyma and simultaneously record the pulmonary vein and artery.[126] Figure 47.33 illustrates this technique, and Figure 47.34 is an example of a recording of a premature atrial contraction.

Table 47.6 outlines the antepartum assessment and treatment for various arrhythmias. If the fetus demonstrates supraventricular tachycardia and an attempt intrauterine treatment is considered, the mother should be hospitalized and carefully monitored. Oral or intravenous pharmacological cardioversion should be performed in conjunction with a cardiologist, who can assist in choosing the proper medication for the fetus and can also evaluate the mother for drug toxicity.[127,128]

REFERENCES

1. Hoffman JI, Christianson R. Congenital heart disease in a cohort of 19,502 births with long term follow-up. *Am J Cardiol* 1978;42:641–647.

2. Lian ZH, Zack MM, Erickson JD. Paternal age and the occurrence of birth defects. *Am J Hum Genet* 1986;39:648–660.

3. Ursell PC, Byrne JM, Strobino BA. Significance of cardiac defects in the developing fetus: a study of spontaneous abortuses. *Circulation* 1985;72:1232–1236.

4. Gerlis LM. Cardiac malformations in spontaneous abortions. *Int J Cardiol* 1985;7:29–35.

5. Vital Statistics of the United States 1980. *Mortality.* Washington, DC: US Department of Health and Human Resources. 1985;2(sect 2):50.

6. Vital Statistics of the United States 1980. *Mortality.* Washington, DC: US Department of Health and Human Resources. 1985;2(sect 2):50–51.

7. Emmanouilides GC, Allen HD, Riemenschneider TA, Gutgesell HP, eds. *Moss and Adams, Heart Disease in Infants, Children, and Adolescents.* 5th ed. Baltimore: Williams & Wilkins, 1995.

8. Rowe RD, Freedom RM, Mehriz A, eds. *The Neonate with Congenital Heart Disease.* 2nd ed. Philadelphia: WB Saunders; 1981.

9. Morville P, Planche C, Mauran P, Santerne B. Endocardial fibroelastosis: prenatal manifestation of aortic valve stenosis. *Helv Paediatr Acta* 1986;41:69–75.

10. Allan LD, Campbell S, Tynan M. The feasibility of fetal echocardiography in the prediction of congenital heart disease. *Ultrasound Med Biol* 1983;2(suppl):565–568.

11. Presbitero P, Todros T, Pavone G, De Filippi G. Fetal echocardiography: diagnosis of congenital cardiomyopathies in a population at risk. *Gazz Ital Cardiol* 1985;15:590–596.

12. Allan LD, Crawford DC, Anderson RH, Tynan M. Spectrum of congenital heart disease detected echocardiographically in prenatal life. *Br Heart J* 1985;54:523–526.

13. Stewart PA, Wladimiroff JW, Becker AE. Early prenatal detection of double outlet right ventricle by echocardiography. *Br Heart J* 1985;54:340–342.

14. Huhta JC, Strasburger JF, Carpenter RJ, Reiter A, Abinader E. Pulsed Doppler fetal echocardiography. *J Clin Ultrasound* 1985;13:247–254.

15. DeVore GR. The prenatal diagnosis of congenital heart disease: a practical approach for the fetal sonographer. *J Clin Ultrasound* 1985;13:229–245.

16. Silverman NH, Golbus MS. Echocardiographic techniques for assessing normal and abnormal fetal cardiac anatomy. *J Am College Cardiol* 1985;5:20S–29S.

17. Wladimiroff JW, Stewart PA, Tonge HM. The role of diagnostic ultrasound in the study of fetal cardiac abnormalities. *Ultrasound Med Biol* 1984;10:457–463.

18. Takahashi M, Shimada H, Hirama N, Katagiri S, Kimura K, Morikawa Y, Osano M. Detection of the cardiac anomalies before birth by cross sectional echocardiography. *J Cardiogr* 1981;11:661–669.

19. Stewart PA, Becker AE, Wladimiroff JW, Essed CE. Left atrial isomerism associated with asplenia: prenatal echocardiographic detection of complex congenital cardiac malformations. *J Am College Cardiol* 1984;4:1015–1020.

20. Dalton ME, Newton ER, Cetrulo CL. Discordant anencephaly in a set of triplets. *Acta Genet Med Gemellol* 1984;33:71–73.

21. Stewart PA, Wladimiroff JW, Essed CE. Prenatal ultrasound diagnosis of congenital heart disease associated with intrauterine growth retardation. A report of two cases. *Prenatal Diagn* 1983;3:279–285.

22. Barkin SZ, Pretorius DH, Beckett MK, Manchester DK, Nelson TR, Manco Johnson ML. Severe polyhydramnios: incidence of anomalies. *Am J Roentgenol* 1987;148:155–159.

23. Bernstein D, Finkbeiner WE, Soifer S, Teitel D. Perinatal myocardial infarction: a case report and review of the literature. *Pediatr Cardiol* 1986;6:313–317.

24. Lu CC, Hsieh FJ, Chen HY, Lee TY, Lue HC, How SW. Prenatal diagnosis of congenital heart disease by real time sonography: a case report. *Taiwan I Hsueh Hui Tsa Chih* 1985; 84:735–741.

25. Crawford DC, Chapman MG, Allan LD. Echocardiography in the investigation of anterior abdominal wall defects in the fetus. *Br J Obstet Gynaecol* 1985;92:1034–106.

26. Kleinman CS, Donnerstein RL, DeVore GR, Jaffe CC, Lynch DC, Berkowitz RL, Talner NS, Hobbins JC. Fetal echocardiography for evaluation of in utero congestive heart failure. *N Engl J Med* 1982;306:568–575.

27. Allan LD, Crawford DC, Anderson RH, Tynan MJ. Echocardiographic and anatomical correlations in fetal congenital heart disease. *Br Heart J* 1984;52:542–548.

28. Wladimiroff JW, Stewart PA, Sachs ES, Niermeijer MF. Prenatal diagnosis and management of congenital heart defect: significance of associated fetal anomalies and prenatal chromosome studies. *Am J Med Genet* 1985;21:285–290.

29. Sanders SP, Chin AJ, Parness IA, Benacerraf B, Greene MF, Epstein MF, Colan SD, Frigoletto FD. Prenatal diagnosis of congenital heart defects in thoracoabdominally conjoined twins. *N Engl J Med* 1985;313:370–374.

30. Sohn DJ, Shenker L, Reed KL, Valdes Cruz LM, Sobonya R, Anderson C. Prenatal ultrasound diagnosis of hypoplastic left heart syndrome in utero associated with hydrops fetalis. *Am Heart J* 1982;104:1368–1372.

31. Mandorla S, Narducci PL, Migliozzi L, Pagliacci M, Cucchia G. Fetal echocardiography: prenatal diagnosis of hypoplastic left heart syndrome. *Gazz Ital Cardiol* 1984;14:517–520.

32. Rikitake N, Takechi T, Suzuki K, Matsunaga S, Yoshioka F, Kato H. Fetal echocardiography: structural evaluation of the fetal heart and prenatal diagnosis of congenital heart disease. *J Cardiogr* 1981;11:1319–1327.

33. Zanke S. Prenatal ultrasound diagnosis of acardius. *Ultraschall Med* 1986;7:172–175.

34. Leithiser RE Jr, Fyfe D, Weatherby E III, Sade R, Garvin AJ. Prenatal sonographic diagnosis of atrial hemangioma. *Am J Roentgenol* 1986;147:1207–1208.

35. Intody Z, Hajdu K, Fantoli L, Arato G, Laszlo J. Ultrasound in the prenatal diagnosis of heart and lung abnormalities: Down's syndrome. *Zentralbl Gynaekol* 1986;108:1006–1010

36. Hoadley SD, Wallace RL, Miller JF, Murgo JP. Prenatal diagnosis of multiple cardiac tumors presenting as an arrhythmia. *J Clin Ultrasound* 1986;14:639–643.

37. Gibson JY, D'Cruz CA, Patel RB, Palmer SM. Acardiac anomaly: review of the subject with case report and emphasis on practical sonography. *J Clin Ultrasound* 1986;14:541–545.

38. Schaffer RM, Cabbad M, Minkoff H, Schiller M, Haller JO, Shapiro AJ. Sonographic diagnosis of fetal cardiac rhabdomyoma. *J Ultrasound Med* 1986;5:531–553.

39. Allan LD, Crawford DC, Tynan MJ. Pulmonary atresia in prenatal life. *J Am College Cardiol* 1986;8:1131–1136.

40. Boxer RA, Seidman S, Singh S, LaCorte MA, Pek H, Goldman MA, Parnell V Jr. Congenital intracardiac rhabdomyoma: prenatal detection by echocardiography, perinatal management, and surgical treatment. *Am J Perinatol* 1986;3:303–305.

41. Ben Ami M, Shalev E, Romano S, Zuckerman H. Midtrimester diagnosis of endocardial fibroelastosis and atrial septal defect: a case report. *Am J Obstet Gynecol* 1986;155: 662–663.

42. Journel H, Roussey M, Plais MH, Milon J, Almange C, Le Marec B. Prenatal diagnosis of familial tuberous sclerosis following detection of cardiac rhabdomyoma by ultrasound. *Prenatal Diagn* 1986;6:283–289.

43. Brown J, Gunn TR, Mora JD, Mok PM. The prenatal ultrasonographic diagnosis of cardiomegaly due to tricuspid incompetence. *Pediatr Radiol* 1986;16:440.

44. DeVore GR, Sarti DA, Siassi B, Horenstein J, Platt LD. Prenatal diagnosis of cardiovascular malformations in the fetus with situs inversus viscerum during the second trimester of pregnancy. *J Clin Ultrasound* 1986;14:454–457.

45. Hata T, Hata K, Murao F, Kitao M. Antenatal diagnosis of congenital heart diseases and fetal arrhythmias. *Nippon Sanka Fujinka Gakkai Zasshi* 1986;38:678–684.

46. Muhlhaus K, Beisler G. Acardius prenatal diagnosis and pregnancy in two twin pregnancies. *Z Geburtshilfe Perinatol* 1986;190:98–103.

47. Muller L, de Jong G, Falck V, Hewlett R, Hunter J, Shires J. Antenatal ultrasonographic findings in tuberous sclerosis. Report of two cases. *S Afr Med J* 1986;69:633–638.

48. De Rochambeau B, Coicaud C, Bernard M, Noel M, Dumont M. Ectopia cordis: early echographic diagnosis in utero. *J Gynecol Obstet Biol Reprod (Paris)* 1986;15:99–103.

49. Allan LD, Crawford DC, Sheridan R, Chapman MG. Aetiology of nonimmune hydrops: the value of echocardiography. *Br J Obstet Gynaecol* 1986;93:223–225.

50. Andrade JL, Somerville J, Serino W, Carvalho AC, Mitre N, Tebexreni AS, Campos O, Atik E, Pieretti F, Martinez EE, et al. Two-dimensional echocardiographic study in the fetus of mothers with congenital heart diseases. *Arq Bras Cardiol* 1985;45:7–10.

51. Yurac C, Romero G. Five-year experience in the echographic diagnosis of structural abnormalities of the fetus. *Rev Chil Obstet Ginecol* 1984;49:369–399.

52. Intody Z, Palffy I, Hajdu K, Hajdu Z, Torok M, Laszlo J. Prenatal diagnosis of thoracopagus in the 19th week of pregnancy. *Zentralbl Gynaekol* 1986;108:57–61.

53. Yagel S, Mandelberg A, Hurwitz A, Jlaser Y. Prenatal diagnosis of hypoplastic left ventricle. *Am J Perinatol* 1986;3:6–8.

54. Intody Z, Hajdu K, Fantoli L, Arato G, Laszlo J. Prenatal ultrasonic diagnosis of a developmental heart defect and Down syndrome. *Orv Hetil* 1985;126:3207–3209.

55. Todros T, Presbitero P, Pavone G, Gagliardi L. Echographic diagnosis of fetal abnormalities: cardiovascular system. *Minerva Ginecol* 1985;37:459–464.

56. Plais MH, Baril JY, Lebret M. Prenatal diagnosis of a cardiac tumor resembling Bourneville's tuberous sclerosis. *J Gynecol Obstet Biol Reprod(Paris)* 1985;14:759–762.

57. Birnbaum SE, McGahan JP, Janos GG, Meyers M. Fetal tachycardia and intramyocardial tumors. *J Am College Cardiol* 1985;6:1358–1361.

58. Yagel S, Sherer D, Hurwitz A. Significance of ultrasonic prenatal diagnosis of ventricular septal defect. *J Clin Ultrasound* 1985;13:588–590.

59. Presbitero P, Todros T, Pavone G, De Filippi G. Fetal echocardiography: diagnosis of congenital cardiomyopathies in a population at risk. *Gazz Ital Cardiol* 1985;15:590–596.

60. Kragt H, Aarnoudse JG, Meyboom EJ, Laurini JL. Prenatal ultrasonic diagnosis and management of ectopia cordis. *Eur J Obstet Gynecol Reprod Biol* 1985;20:177–180.

61. Mortera C, Torrenta M, Alegre M, Barri PN, Carrera JM. Prenatal echocardiographic diagnosis of a case of atrioventricular septum defect. *Rev Esp Cardiol* 1985;38:288–290.

62. Walter HM. On diagnosis of acardius in pregnancy by ultrasound. *Geburtshilfe Frauenheilkd* 1982;42:551–553.

63. DeVore GR, Hakim S, Kleinman CS, Hobbins JC. The in utero diagnosis of an interventricular septal cardiac rhabdomyoma by means of real time directed, M mode echocardiography. *Am J Obstet Gynecol* 1982;143:967–969.

64. Harrison MR, Filly RA, Stanger P, de Lorimier AA. Prenatal diagnosis and management of omphalocele and ectopia cordis. *J Pediatr Surg* 1982;17:64–66.

65. Pizzuto F, Colloridi V, Tulli A, Gallo P, Pachi A, Reale A. Diagnosis of fetal heart abnormalities by echocardiography and its significance in the obstetric and fetal management. *Cardiologia* 1985;30:25–32.

66. Saitoh M, Yokota H, Tsunoda H, Kawagoe K. Early antepartum diagnosis of conjoined thoracopagus twins. *Nippon Sanka Fujinka Gakkai Zasshi* 1985;37:1046–1049.

67. Van Groeninghen JC, Franssen AM, Willemsen WN, Hijhuis JG, Puts JJ. An acardiac acephalic monster. *Eur J Obstet Gynecol Reprod Biol* 1985;19:317–325.

68. Dennis MA, Appareti K, Manco Johnson ML, Clewell W, Wiggins J. The echocardiographic diagnosis of multiple fetal cardiac tumors. *J Ultrasound Med* 1985;4:327–329.

69. Di Lollo L, Castellani R, Maiorana A. Ultrasonic patterns of a cardiac rhabdomyoma detected in utero. *J Perinatal Med* 1984;12:339–342.

70. Wexler S, Baruch A, Ekstein N, Libal Y, Yedwab G, Ornoy A. An acardiac acephalic anomaly detected on sonography. *Acta Obstet Gynecol Scand* 1985;64:93–94.

71. Radunovic N, Markovic A, Lazarevic B. Fetal echocardiography in the second half of pregnancy. *Srp Arh Celok Lek* 1984;112:703–708.

72. Grote W, Rehder H, Weisner D, Wiedemann HE. Prenatal diagnosis of a probable hereditary syndrome with holoprosencephaly, hydrocephaly, octodactyly, and cardiac malformations. *Eur J Pediatr* 1984;143:155–157.

73. Rydnert J, Holmgren G, Sigurd J. Intrauterine diagnosis of an acardiac monster. *Acta Obstet Gynecol Scand* 1984;63:569–570.

74. Bieber FR, Mostoufi Zadeh M, Birnholz JC, Driscoll SG. Amniotic band sequence associated with ectopia cordis in one twin. *J Pediatr* 1984;105:817–819.

75. Arena J, Nogues A, Sunol MA, Tovar JA. Omphalocsite monster (acardius acephalus). Apropos of a case. *Chir Pediatr* 1982;23:283–286.

76. Todros T, Presbitero P, Montemurro D, Levis F. Prenatal diagnosis of ectopia cordis. *J Ultrasound Med* 1984;3:429–431.

77. Riggs T, Sholl JS, Ilbawi M, Gardner T. In utero diagnosis of pericardial tumor with successful surgical repair. *Pediatr Cardiol* 1984;5:23–25.

78. Bovicelli L, Picchio FM, Pilu G, Baccarani G, Orsini LF, Rizzo N, Alampi G, Benenati PM, Hobbins JC. Prenatal diagnosis of endocardial fibroelastosis. *Prenatal Diagn* 1984;4:67–72.

79. Piela A, Kuzniar J, Skret A. Fetal echocardiography. IV. Prenatal diagnosis of fetal heart defects. *Ginekol Pol* 1983;54:719–722.

80. Bierman FZ, Yeh MN, Swersky S, Martin E, Wigger JH, Fox H. Absence of the aortic valve: antenatal and postnatal two dimensional and Doppler echocardiographic features. *J Am College Cardiol* 1984;3:833–837.

81. Pesonen E, Haavisto H, Ammala P, Teramo K. Intrauterine hydrops caused by premature closure of the foramen ovale. *Arch Dis Child* 1983;58:1015–1016.

82. Stewart PA, Tonge HM, Wladimiroff JW. Arrhythmia and structural abnormalities of the fetal heart. *Br Heart J* 1983;50:550–554.

83. Crawford DC, Garrett C, Tynan M, Neville BG, Allan LD. Cardiac rhabdomyomata as a marker for the antenatal detection of tuberous sclerosis. *J Med Genet* 1983;20:303–304.

84. Issel EP, Hahmann K, Musil A. Antepartal diagnosis of an acardius in a triplet pregnacy using ultrasound. *Zentralbl Gynaekol* 1983;105:874–881.

85. Platt LD, DeVore GR, Bieniarz A, Benner P, Rao R. Antenatal diagnosis of acephalus acardia: a proposed management scheme. *Am J Obstet Gynecol* 1983;146:857–859.

86. De Geeter B, Kretz JG, Nisand I, Eisenmann B, Kieny MT, Kieny R. Intrapericardial teratoma in a newborn infant: use of fetal echocardiography. *Ann Thorac Surg* 1983;35:664–666.

87. Mercer LJ, Petres RE, Smeltzer JS. Ultrasonic diagnosis of ectopia cordis. *Obstet Gynecol* 1983;61:523–525.

88. DeVore GR, Steiger RM, Larson EJ. Fetal echocardiography: the prenatal diagnosis of a ventricular septal defect in a 14-week fetus with pulmonary artery hypoplasia. *Obstet Gynecol* 1987;69:494–497.

89. DeVore GR, Siassi B, Platt LD. Ventricular disproportion: the prenatal manifestation of coarctation of the aorta. *J Perinatol* 1986;6:225–273.

90. DeVore GR, Siassi B, Platt LD. Fetal echocardiography: the prenatal diagnosis of tricuspid atresia (type 1C) during the second trimester of pregnancy. *J Clin Ultrasound* 1987;15:317–324.

91. Ewigman BG, Crane JP, Frigoletto FD, LeFevre ML, Bain RP, McNellis DA. A randomized trial of prenatal ultrasound screening: impact on perinatal outcome. *N Engl J Med* 1993;329:931–937.

92. Crane JP, LeFevre ML, Winborn RC, et al. A randomized trial of prenatal ultrasonographic screening: Impact on the detection, management, and outcome of anomalous fetuses. *Am J Obstet Gynecol* 1994;171:392–399.

93. Tegnander E, Eik-Nes SH, Linker D. Prenatal detection of heart defects at the routine fetal examination at 18 weeks in a non-selected population. *Ultrasound Obstet Gynecol* 1995;5:372–380.

94. DeVore GR. The prenatal diagnosis of congenital heart disease: a practical approach for the fetal sonographer. *J Clin Ultrasound* 1985;13:229–245.

95. DeVore GR, Medearis AL, Bear MB, Horenstein J, Platt LD. Fetal echocardiography: factors that influence imaging of the fetal heart during the second trimester of pregnancy. *J Ultrasound Med* 1993;12:659–663.

96. Tegnander E, Eik-Nes SH, Linker DT. Incorporating the four-chamber view of the fetal heart into the second-trimester routine fetal examination. *Ultrasound Obstet Gynecol* 1994;4:24–28.

97. Allan LD, Crawford DC, Chita SK, Tynan MJ. Prenatal screening for congenital heart disease. *Br Med J* 1986;292:1711–1719.

98. Smith RS, Comstock CH, Kirk JS, Lee W. Ultrasonographic left cardiac axis deviation: a marker for fetal anomalies. *Obstet Gynecol* 1995;85:187–191.

99. DeVore GR. The aortic and pulmonary outflow tract screening examination in the human fetus. *J Ultrasound Med* 1992;11:345–348.

100. Comstock CH, Riggs T, Lee W, Kirk J. Pulmonary to aorta diameter ratio in the normal and abnormal fetal heart. *Am J Obstet Gynecol* 1991;165:1038–1044.

101. Tan J, Silverman N, Hofman JIE, Villegas M, Schmidt KG. Cardiac dimensions determined by cross-sectional echocardiography in the normal human fetus from 18 weeks to term. *Am J Cardiol* 1992;70:1459–1467.

102. DeVore GR, Siassi B, Platt LD. Fetal echocardiography. IV. M-mode assessment of ventricular size and contractility during the second and third trimesters of pregnancy in the normal fetus. *Am J Obstet Gynecol* 1984;150:981–988.

103. DeVore GR, Siassi B, Platt LD. Fetal echocardiography. V. M-mode measurements of the aortic root dimension and aortic valve excursion in the second and third trimesters in the normal human fetus. *Am J Obstet Gynecol* 1985;152:543–550.

104. Sahn DJ, Lange LW, Allen HD, Goldberg SJ, Anderson C, Giles H, Kaber K. Quantitative real-time cross-sectional echocardiography in the developing human fetus and newborn. *Circulation* 1980;62:588–597.

105. Allan LD, Joseph MC, Boyed EC, Campbell S, Tynan M. M-mode echocardiography in the developing human fetus. *Br Heart J* 1982;47:573.

106. St John Sutton MG, Gewitz MH, Shah B, Cohen A, Reichek N, Gabbe S, Huff DS. Quantitative assessment of growth and function of the cardiac chambers in the normal human fetus: a prospective longitudinal echocardiographic study. *Circulation* 1984;69:645–654.

107. Devore GR, Siassi B, Platt LD. The use of the abdominal circumference as a means of assessing M-mode ventricular dimensions during the second and third trimesters of pregnancy in the normal fetus. *J Ultrasound Med* 1985;4:175–182.

108. DeVore GR, Siassi B, Platt LD. The use of the femur length as a means of assessing M-mode ventricular dimensions during the second and third trimesters of pregnancy in the normal fetus. *J Clin Ultrasound* 1985;13:619–625.

109. Suzuki Y, Kambaraa H, Kadota K, Tamaki S, Yamazato A, Nohara R, Osakada G, Kawai C. Detection of intracardiac shunt flow in atrial septal defect using a real-time two-dimensational color-coded Doppler flow imaging system and comparison with contrast two-dimensional echocardiography. *Am J Cardiol* 985;56:347–350.   ·

110. Miyatake K, Okamoto M, Kinoshita N, Park YD, Nagata S, Izumi S, Fusejima K, Sakakibara H, Nimura Y. Clinical applications of a new type of real-time two-dimensional Doppler flow imaging system. *Am J Cardiol* 1984;54:857–868.

111. Switzer DF, Nanda NC. Doppler color flow mapping. *Ultrasound Med Biol* 1985;11:403–410.

112. Swensson RE, Sahn DJ, Valdes-Cruz LM. Color flow Doppler mapping in congenital heart disease. *Echocardiography* 1985;2:545–550.

113. DeVore GR, Horenstein J, Siassi B, Platt LD. Doppler color flow mapping: its use in the prenatal diagnosis of congenital heart disease in the human fetus. *Echocardiography* 1985;2:545–550.

114. DeVore GR, Horenstein J, Siassi B, Platt LD. Fetal echocardiography. VII. Doppler color flow mapping: a new technique for the diagnosis of congenital heart disease. *Am J Obstet Gynecol* 1987;156:1054–1064.

115. DeVore GR, Alfi O. The association between an abnormal nuchal skin fold, trisomy 21, and ultrasound abnormalities

identified during the second trimester of pregnancy. *Ultrasound Obstet Gynecol* 1993;3:387–394.

116. DeVore GR, Alfi O. The use of color Doppler ultrasound to identify fetuses at increased risk for trisomy 21: an alternative for high-risk patients who decline genetic amniocentesis. *Obstet Gynecol* 1995;85:378–386.

117. DeVore GR. Color Doppler examination of the outflow tracts of the fetal heart: a technique for identification of cardiovascular malformations. *Ultrasound Obstet Gynecol* 1994;4: 463–471.

118. Copel JA, Pilu G, Kleinman CS. Congenital heart disease and extracardiac anomalies: associations and indications for fetal echocardiography. *Am J Obstet Gynecol* 1986;154: 1121–1132.

119. Berg KA, Boughman JA, Astemborski JA, Ferencz C. Implications for prenatal cytogenetic analysis from the Baltimore–Washington study of live-born infants with confirmed congenital heart defects. *Am J Hum Genet* 1986;39(suppl): A50.

120. Chang AC, Huhta JC, Yoon GY, Wood DC, Tulzer G, Cohen A, Mennuti M, Norwood WI. Diagnosis, transport, and outcome in fetuses with left ventricular outflow tract obstruction. *J Thorac Cardiovasc Surg* 1991;102:841–848.

121. DeVore GR, Horenstein J. Color Doppler identification of a pericardial effusion in the fetus. *Ultrasound Obstet Gynecol* 1994;4:115–120.

122. Southall DP, Johnson AM, Shinebourne EA. Frequency and outcome of disorders of cardiac rhythm and conduction in a population of newborn infants. *Pediatrics* 1981;68:581.

123. Kleinman CS, Hobbins JC, Jaffe CC, DeVore GR, Weinstein EV, Lynch DC, Talner NS, Berkowitz RC. Echocardiographic studies of the human fetus: prenatal diagnosis of congenital heart disease and cardiac dysrhythmias. *Pediatrics* 1980;65: 1059.

124. DeVore GR, Siassi B, Platt LD. Fetal echocardiography. III. The diagnosis of cardiac arrhythmias using real-time directed M-mode ultrasound. *Am J Obstet Gynecol* 1983;146:792.

125. Chan FY, Woo SK, Ghosh A, et al. Prenatal diagnosis of congenital fetal arrhythmias by simultaneous pulsed Doppler velocimetry of the fetal abdominal aorta and inferior vena cava. *Obstet Gynecol* 1989;76:200.

126. DeVore GR, Horenstein J. Simultaneous Doppler recording of the pulmonary artery and vein: a new technique for the evaluation of a fetal arrhythmia. *J Ultrasound Med* 1993;669–671.

127. Kleinman CS, Copel JA, Weinstein EM, Santulli TV Jr, Hobbins JC. Treatment of supraventricular tachyarrhythmias. *J Clin Ultrasound* 1985;13:265–273.

128. Kleinman CS, Donnerstein RL, Jaffe CC, DeVore GR, Weinstein EM, Lynch DC, Talner NS, Berkowitz RL, Hobbins JC. Fetal echocardiography: a tool for evaluation of in utero cardiac arrhythmias and monitoring of in utero therapy: analysis of 71 patients. *Am J Cardiol* 1983;51:237–243.

48

PRENATAL SCREENING FOR CONGENITAL HEART DISEASE

MICHAEL D. BORK, DO, AND JAMES F. X. EGAN, MD

INTRODUCTION

Congenital anomalies were the leading cause of infant death in the United States in 1992, accounting for 21.5% of infant deaths.[1] Congenital heart defects are the most common congenital anomalies, occurring in 7.4 of every thousand live births. They are almost 10 times more common than open neural tube defects and 6.5 times more likely to be encountered than chromosomal abnormalities (Table 48.1).[2] Cardiovascular defects account for more than 50% of the perinatal deaths resulting from congenital malformations.[3] Even excluding patent ductus arteriosus, which represents 48% of congenital heart defects and is a normal finding antenatally, structural cardiac defects occur in 3.8 per thousand live births. This corrected rate is still 3.3 times more common than trisomies 21, 18, and 13 combined and 4.8 times more likely to occur than an open neural tube defect.

With their high prevalence and mortality, congenital heart defects must be a major focus of antenatal diagnosis. Most congenital heart defects are structural and should therefore lend themselves to prenatal diagnosis by ultrasound. Antenatal ultrasound examination was performed in 57.8% of all pregnancies in the United States in 1993.[4] Despite its widespread use, obstetrical ultrasound has not achieved its full potential in detecting congenital heart defects. For example, complex cardiac defects involve more than one cardiac abnormality and should be apparent to the alert sonographer. However, complex cardiac defects were one of the most commonly missed lesions in the RADIUS (Routine Antenatal Diagnostic Imaging with Ultrasound) study, with only 5 of 19 (27%) being detected.[5] Of the complex cardiac lesions diag-

nosed antenatally, 5 of 11 (45%) were detected at tertiary centers while none of the 8 (0%) were seen at nontertiary centers.[6] This lack of sensitivity has been interpreted as either innate inability of the method to detect these lesions, given our current level of skill and technology, or lack of expertise and focus in our use of screening techniques.

The detection of any "common" abnormality requires a screening technique. The maternal serum "triple screen" for the detection of a group of pregnancies at high-risk for neural tube and ventral wall defects, or for aneuploidy, has found wide acceptance in the obstetrical community. There is no blood or chemical test for fetal cardiac anomalies. Obstetrical ultrasound is the best screening method. Both the American College of Obstetrics and Gynecology and the American Institute of Ultrasound in Medicine suggest the inclusion of a four-chamber view of the fetal heart in the antenatal ultrasound examination.[7,8] Screening with a four-chamber view will yield 16–92% sensitivity. Kirk et al reported that the addition of the proximal left outflow tract to the four-chamber view improved their prospective screening of fetuses for congenital heart defects after 14 weeks of gestation from 47% to 78%.[9] More views of the fetal heart may provide even greater sensitivity.

INDICATIONS FOR SCREENING

Most congenital heart defects are found in fetuses of mothers who have no risk factors. A case could therefore be made for performing a detailed cardiac examination on every fetus undergoing an ultrasound. This practice is not currently felt

Cardiac Problems in Pregnancy, Third Edition
Edited by Uri Elkayam, MD, and Norbert Gleicher, MD
Copyright © 1998 by Wiley-Liss, Inc. ISBN 0-471-16358-9

TABLE 48.1   Birth Prevalence of Congenital Malformations in 1,802,810 Newborns in the United States in 1987

Birth Defect	Rate/10,000	Relative Risk[a]
Cardiovascular	73.88	9.8
Chromosomal	11.82	1.5
Open neural tube defects	7.93	1

[a]Open neural tube defects were used as the reference.

Source: Edmonds and Levy.[2]

to be cost effective. Rather, to best utilize available health care resources and personnel, pregnancies at greatest risk for congenital heart defects should undergo fetal echocardiography. Indications for fetal echocardiography are listed in Table 48.2

Patients whose risk for having a fetus with congenital heart disease exceeds that of the general population (i.e., a risk > 8/1000) should be offered a targeted obstetrical ultrasound examination. If the results suggest a fetal cardiac abnormality, fetal echocardiography must be performed. Table 48.3 summarizes the results of reviews of seven series[10–16] of the more common referral indications for fetal echocardiography. An abnormal screening ultrasound, suspicion of fetal congenital heart disease, and chromosomal abnormalities were the referral diagnoses most likely to result in an antenatal diagnosis of congenital heart disease.

SCREENING TECHNIQUES

Early Pregnancy: Transvaginal Fetal Echocardiography

Until recently, the prenatal diagnosis of fetal cardiac anomalies was limited to the second and third trimesters. The de-

TABLE 48.2   Indications for Fetal Echocardiography

Referral ultrasound suspicious for congenital heart defect (CHD)
Referal ultrasound with known extracardiac anomaly
Family history of CHD (first-degree relative)
Known fetal aneuploidy
Increased risk of fetal aneuploidy (based on age or abnormal biochemical screen)
Fetal arrhythmia
Maternal insulin-dependent diabetes mellitus
Nonimmune hydrops fetalis
Polyhydramnios
Genetic syndromes associated with CHD (e.g., Noonan's syndrome, Holt–Oram syndrome)
Maternal infections (e.g., rubella virus, coxsackie virus)
Medications or cardiac teratogens (e.g., lithium, anticonvulsants, isotretinoin, alcohol)
Severe intrauterine growth retardation
Other (e.g., maternal phenylketonuria, connective tissue disease)

TABLE 48.3   Prenatal Detection Rates of Congenital Heart Defects (CHD) by Fetal Echocardiography Based on Indication

Indication	Number of Cases		Sensitivity (%)
	Total	CHD Detected	
Ultrasound suspicion of CHD	256	110	43
Abnormal chromosomes	197	31	15.7
Abnormal obstetric sonogram	772	114	14.8
Maternal diabetes	782	23	2.9
Maternal lithium	46	1	2.2
Family with CHD	2993	50	1.7

velopment of high frequency, high resolution transvaginal ultrasound probes has enabled assessment of fetal anatomy in the late first and early second trimesters of pregnancy. Several investigators have reported their experiences with the use of transvaginal ultrasound from 10 to 16 weeks of gestation.[17–21] In the initial report of a first-trimester diagnosis of congenital heart disease, Gembruch et al described a fetus with an atrioventricular canal defect, atrioventricular valve insufficiency, and complete heart block at 11 weeks of gestation.[19] Dolkart and Reimers, who obtained normative data from transvaginal fetal echocardiography performed on 52 patients between 10 and 14.9 weeks gestation, suggested that virtually all standard fetal echocardiographic views can be obtained by 13 weeks of gestation.[22] Achiron et al screened 660 fetuses at low risk for congenital heart defects between 13 and 15 weeks of gestation and were able to obtain a four-chamber view in all 660 (100%) and an "extended cardiac examination" (i.e., four-chamber view, left and right ventricular outflow tracts, aortic and ductal arches) in 644 (97.6%).[23] Only three of the six fetuses born with congenital heart defects in this series were detected by early transvaginal echocardiography, however.

The time required for transvaginal fetal echocardiography was problematic in several studies. Using only 10 minutes of scanning time per exam, Johnson et al studied 270 low risk women between 8 and 14 weeks of gestation; they obtained a four-chamber view in just over 70% of cases between 12 and 14 weeks.[24] However, these investigators were able to perform a complete cardiac evaluation, which they defined as a four-chamber view and outflow tracts, in only 31% of 12-week and 46% of 14-week fetuses. In the largest series to date, Bronshtein et al performed 12,793 transvaginal ultrasound examinations between 12 and 16 weeks of gestation on patients at low or high risk for congenital heart defects.[18] A complete cardiac examination was obtained in 80% of these patients at time of an initial 30-minute scanning session and in 95% after two sessions. Congenital heart defects were detected prenatally in 47 fetuses in this group. In 36 (77%) the diagnosis was made using the four-chamber view alone. The detection rate was 3.1% (29/9340) in Bronshtein's low risk patients and 5.2% in the high risk patients.

The primary advantage of transvaginal diagnosis of congenital heart disease is the early knowledge that the fetus has either a cardiac defect or, more likely, that the fetal heart appears normal. If an abnormality is seen, the patient and her provider have time for consultation before making decisions regarding further testing or the continuation of the pregnancy. If the exam is normal, a family at high risk for producing offspring with congenital heart disease are reassured at least to this extent. Prompted by the increased risk of chromosomal abnormalities in a fetus with congenital heart disease, earlier ultrasound detection may lead to earlier karyotype analysis. Amniocentesis or chorionic villus sampling could be performed. Such measures also allow more time for consultation, discussion of expected course, prognosis, antenatal management options, and critical decisions regarding the pregnancy. If the patient plans to continue the pregnancy, she will have time to prepare for the emotional and socioeconomic implications of bearing a child with a damaged heart. In most cases the exam will be normal and, since most major cardiac defects can be excluded, there should be decreased maternal and family anxiety.

The disadvantages of early transvaginal echocardiographic screening include the small size of the first-trimester fetal heart (which makes resolution more difficult than in later gestation), problems related to fetal position, the relatively long operator's learning curve for transvaginal ultrasonography, and technical factors (e.g., limited transducer arc, relatively narrow focal range of the vaginal probe). Additionally, the later development of certain lesions, such as outflow tract obstructions, coarctation, and hypoplastic left or right heart, warrants a follow-up transabdominal examination at 22–28 weeks of gestation to rule out lesions that may not be discernible until the late second or third trimester. Finally, Allan has argued that early transvaginal scanning may be very time-consuming, as it was in Bronshtein's report, where 20% of the patients had to be recalled because optimal views of the fetal heart were not obtained within 30 minutes.[25]

In summary, transvaginal echocardiographic screening in a low risk population can be successfully performed in a majority of patients after 13 weeks of gestation. This measure will detect some major structural cardiac defects. The suspicion of a cardiac defect on first-trimester or early second-trimester screening warrants a detailed ultrasonographic evaluation for associated fetal structural abnormalities. When CHD is diagnosed, fetal karotyping should be offered to assist in the subsequent management of the pregnancy.[26] In patients considered to be at high risk for congenital heart

defects, reevaluation by transabdominal fetal echocardiography by 22 weeks of gestation is indicated.

The Four-Chamber View

The four-chamber view is the most important screening tool in the detection of congenital heart defects. As noted earlier, both the American College of Obstetrics and Gynecology and the American Institute of Ultrasound in Medicine recommend that a four-chamber view of the fetal heart be obtained as part of a routine fetal anatomic survey.[7,8] Numerous investigators have documented the utility of the four-chamber view as a screening tool both in high and low risk populations (Table 48.4).[6,15,27–36]

The wide range (16–92%) in reported sensitivities for use of the four-chamber view reflects differences in patient populations, the experience of the individual sonographer, and gestational age at time of ultrasound. The 92% sensitivity reported by Copel et al may be explained by the retrospective nature of the study and the high skill level of the examiners in a prenatal echocardiography center.[15] No other large series has been able to reproduce these results. Bromley et al, in a combined high and low risk population, reported a sensitivity for the four-chamber view of 63%.[32] In studies that used only the four-chamber view as a screening tool in low risk populations, the reported sensitivities ranged from 16 to 64%.

The majority of studies suggest that the standard four-chamber view of the fetal heart has the potential to diagnose 50–60% of major structural cardiac defects in a low risk population. The lesions that are missed are generally associated with the outflow tracts (i.e., aorta and pulmonary artery), since these are not seen in the four-chamber view. A systematic approach to the four-chamber view is outlined as follows.

TABLE 48.4 Use of the Four-Chamber View as a Screening Tool in Detecting Congenital Heart Defects

Ref: First Author (year)	Sensitivity (%)	Specificity (%)
Copel[15] (1987)	92	
Rosendahl[27] (1989)	36	100
Brocks and Bang[28] (1991)	60	100
Bromley[32] (1992)	63	
Achiron[32] (1992)	48	99.9
Vergani[34] (1992)	81	100
Sharland[29] (1992)	77	99
Chitty[30] (1992)	64	100
Shirley[31] (1992)	56	100
Tegnander[35] (1994)	43	
Wigton[36] (1993)	33	
RADIUS[6] (1994)	16	

Systematic Approach to the Four-Chamber View

1. *Fetal Lie, Position, and Situs* Fetal lie is determined by the presenting part and the position of the fetal spine. Once the fetal right and left sides are known, situs is determined by the locations of the stomach and the apex of the fetal heart, both of which are normally on the fetal left side. This is important because congenital heart disease is found in up to 40% of fetuses with abdominal situs abnormalities.

2. *Standard Four-Chamber View* This is the most important step. It must be performed carefully and should be repeated until a representative view is obtained. This view is seen in a transverse plane just above the level of the diaphragm (Fig. 48.1). The majority of the fetal heart should lie within the left hemithorax, and the apex of the heart should lie at an angle of approximately 43° to a line that bisects the fetal spine and sternum.[37,38] An abnormal cardiac axis alone may be a marker for an underlying cardiac or extracardiac anomaly. (Evaluation of the fetal cardiac axis is discussed in detail later in this chapter).

3. *Fetal Heart Size* The fetal heart should occupy approximately one-third of the fetal thorax.

4. *Ventricles* The ventricles should be approximately equal in size, with a 1:1 ratio until after 32 weeks of gestation, at which time the right ventricle assumes more of the cardiac output and is slightly larger than the left ventricle. Morphologically, the wall of the right ventricle appears trabeculated, or slightly irregular, and the moderator band blunts the apex of the ventricle so that it adopts a U shape. The left ventricle is more V-shaped. The "inlet" portion of the interventricular septum, which includes the tricuspid and mitral valves, should be assessed for defects.

5. *Atria* The left atrium is the most posterior chamber in the thoracic cavity. The flap of the foramen ovale should be seen opening into the left atrium, documenting right-to-left flow. Additionally, pulmonary veins may be seen entering the left atrium, giving an irregular appearance to the surface of the left atrium, although this feature is often difficult to ascertain. The right atrium can be identified by following its connection with the suprahepatic portion of the inferior vena cava or the inferior segment of the superior vena cava.

6. *Atrioventricular Valves* The tricuspid (right) and mitral (left) valves separate the atria from the ventricles. The leaflets of the tricuspid valve insert slightly lower

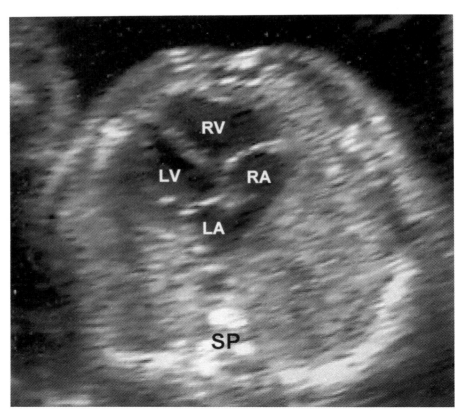

Figure 48.1 Standard four-chamber view of the fetal heart.

on the interventricular septum (i.e., are more apically displaced) than are the mitral valve leaflets. Patency of the atrioventricular valves may be seen by the movement of the valve leaflets with real-time imaging.

7. *Cardiac Rate and Rhythm* Finally, the cardiac rate and rhythm should be noted, with 1:1 conduction between the atria and the ventricles. This may be seen on a two-dimensional ultrasound image and, if any questions arise, may be documented by M-mode.

8. *Limitations of the Four-Chamber View* Remember that the cardiac outflow tracts and the anterior, or outflow portion, of the interventricular septum are *not* seen on the four chamber view.

There is a definite learning curve for sonographers attempting to evaluate the fetal heart in the four-chamber view. Tegnander et al, who reported that their ability to obtain a standard four-chamber view increased from 93% (2773/2993) in the initial 12 months of their study to 96% (4150/4329) in the last 16 months, speculated that this small increase represented a "learning effect."[35] Allan et al, after teaching referring obstetricians and sonographers how to properly obtain and interpret a four-chamber view, noted that the number of patients with congenital heart disease who were referred for echocardiography based on an abnormality of the four-chamber view increased from 31% (4/13) in 1983 to 69% (22/32) in 1985.[39] In a prospective cohort study by Vergani et al, the introduction of a policy of attempting to obtain a four-chamber view in all patients undergoing routine antenatal ultrasound examinations increased the detection of congenital heart disease from 43% to 81%.[34] These investigators reported that visualization of the four-chamber view increased from 20% prior to this policy to 95% afterward.

The importance of operator expertise is highlighted by the RADIUS study, in which the four-chamber view of the heart served as the standard screening tool for congenital heart defects. Across all gestational ages, the RADIUS study had an overall sensitivity for detecting congenital heart defects of only 12/75 (16%).[6] The type of ultrasound facility clearly influenced the ability to detect congenital heart disease. In tertiary centers, congenital heart defects were detected in 5/22 (22.7%) fetuses prior to 24 weeks, while in nontertiary care centers the detection rate was nil (0/16). While both these sensitivities are well below most reported fetal echocardiography series, the results do suggest greater skill at the tertiary centers.

The influence of gestational age on the detection of congenital anomalies is emphasized by Goncalves et al, who found that anomalies of all organ systems were more readily detected later in pregnancy.[40] These investigators reported that the sensitivity of prenatal ultrasonography in detecting all congenital anomalies in a series of 6616 fetuses was 52% (244/468). The sensitivity of the exam increased with increasing gestational age. Before 20 weeks of gestation, the detection rate of any anomaly was 47%, whereas between 20 and 23 weeks it was 59% and after 24 weeks it was 68%. Experience from the RADIUS and other studies suggests that such an increase in sensitivity applies as well for fetal cardiac anomalies.

The ability of transvaginal ultrasound to document a four chamber view in the late first and early second trimesters was discussed earlier in this chapter. As the fetus grows, a standard four chamber view of the fetal heart is more easily imaged. Shultz et al prospectively evaluated 520 consecutive fetuses between 13 and 39 weeks of gestation to determine the frequency of obtaining a satisfactory four-chamber view by transabdominal ultrasonography.[41] The four-chamber view was obtained in 95% (272/283) of cases after 19 weeks. The ability to document a four-chamber view increased progressively from 40% (6/15) at 14 weeks to 95% at 19 weeks. Interestingly, factors such as amniotic fluid volume, type of ultrasound equipment, and skill of the examiner did not significantly affect the ability to obtain this view in Schultz's study. Other investigators have reported similar results. Egan et al were able to obtain an adequate four-chamber view within a 10-minute window during level I and level II ultrasound exams in 95% (288/312) of fetuses between 15 and 36 weeks of gestation, with 100% detectability after 24 weeks.[42] Copel et al suggested that the four-chamber view of the fetal heart could be obtained in 95% of fetuses between 18 and 40 weeks.[15] In 7322 consecutive routine ultrasound examinations between 16 and 22 weeks of gestation, Tegnander and colleagues prospectively examined their ability to obtain a four-chamber view in the course of a normal 30-minute exam.[35] All exams were performed by nurse-midwives specially trained in ultrasound. At 16 weeks of gestation, an adequate four-chamber view was seen in 91.5% (393/425) of fetuses scanned; at 26 weeks 98.1% (153/156) adequate views were reported. Maternal obesity, unfavorable fetal position (i.e., spine anterior), and poor resolution (3.5 MHz vs. 5 MHz transducer) were the main reasons for not being able to obtain the four-chamber view in this series.

Lesions that are likely to be, or might be, detected utilizing a standard four-chamber view are listed in Table 48.5. Although the four-chamber view of the fetal heart is the current standard in screening for congenital heart defects, a number of cardiac defects will be missed by this view.[43] These include great vessel lesions (tetralogy of Fallot, transposition of the great vessels, coarctation of the aorta, truncus arteriosus), isolated ventricular and atrial septal defects, minor valve abnormalities (e.g., bicuspid valves), anomalous venous return, and patent ductus arteriosus. However, when lesions that are not directly visualized on a four-chamber view cause problems that distort the four-chamber view, such as aortic atresia leading to hypoplastic left heart, identification of these lesions may be improved.

TABLE 48.5   Lesions That May Be Detectable by Means of a Four-Chamber View

Lesions Likely to Be Detected by a Standard Four-Chamber View

Hypoplastic right or left ventricle	Single ventricle
Large VSD or ASD	Dextrocardia
Valve atresia/stenosis	Situs inversus
Atrioventricular canal defect	Ectopia cordis
Pericardial effusion	Ebstein's anomaly
Endocardial fibroelastosis	Cardiac tumors

Lesions Possibly Detected by Four-Chamber View

Small VSD or ASD	Tetralogy of Fallot
Coarctation of the aorta	Truncus arteriosus
Double-outlet right ventricle	Valve insufficiency
Transposition of the great vessels	Cardiac hypertrophy

Abbreviations: VSD, ventricular septal defect; ASD, atrial septal defect.

The Addition of Outflow Tract Views to the Standard Four-Chamber View

The addition of one or more of the outflow tracts will enhance the sensitivity of detection of congenital heart defects.[36] The aortic root, or "five-chamber," view will improve the sensitivity over that of a four-chamber view of the fetal heart in detecting congenital heart defects. Kirk et al reported a series of 6244 fetuses greater than 14 weeks gestation, scanned in a single unit over a 28-month period.[9] Attempts were made to obtain a four-chamber and aortic root view in each case. A four-chamber view was obtained in 5967 fetuses (96%), and in 5111 cases (82%) both the four-chamber view and the aortic root view could be obtained. The four-chamber view was able to detect 24 (47%) of the 51 fetuses with congenital heart defects. The addition of the aortic root view to the four-chamber view increased the sensitivity of detection of congenital heart defects from 47% to 78%.

Evaluation of both outflow tracts will further enhance the detection of congenital heart defects. Achiron et al compared the standard four-chamber view with the use of the four-chamber view plus outflow tracts in the detection of congenital heart defects between 18 and 24 weeks.[33] In their series, 23 infants were born with congenital heart defects out of a group of 5400 pregnancies at low risk for congenital heart defects. The four-chamber view alone was able to detect 11/23 (48%) of the fetuses with congenital heart defects. By adding views of the outflow tracts, the investigators increased the sensitivity to 78%. In a series by Wigton et al, 11 of 33 fetuses (33%) with confirmed congenital heart defects were detected by use of the four-chamber view alone during a standard obstetrical ultrasound examination between 14 and 41 weeks.[36] The rate of detection increased to 42% when views of the outflow tracts were added. Bromley et al, using the four-chamber view alone, identified congenital heart defects

in 42 (63%) of 67 fetuses with congenital heart defects at greater than 18 weeks of gestation.[32] When outflow tract views were added, 57/69 (83%) fetuses were identified as having structural heart abnormalities.

The Association Between an Abnormal Fetal Cardiac Axis and Congenital Heart Defects

Normal fetal cardiac axis and position were first described by Comstock.[44] In a series of 183 normal fetuses between the gestational ages of 13 and 40 weeks, the mean axis of the fetal heart was at a 45° angle to the left of an anteroposterior line bisecting the fetal chest and spine. The range was 22°–75° and 2 standard deviations included 25°–65°. In the four-chamber view, the heart was noted to lie predominantly in the left anterior quadrant of the chest. Although Comstock reported an association between an abnormal cardiac axis, and/or position, and intrathoracic defects (e.g., diaphragmatic hernia), no specific relationship was found between an abnormal cardiac axis and intrinsic cardiac defects.

Since Comstock's initial report, several investigators have reported on the use of fetal cardiac axis measurements as a marker for either congenital heart defects or other fetal anomalies. Shipp et al retrospectively measured cardiac axis using a protractor and an image of the four-chamber view of the heart in 75 fetuses with congenital heart defects.[38] When these measurements were compared to a control group of 75 normal fetuses, the mean cardiac axis (±2 SD) for the control group was found to be 43° ±14°. The mean cardiac axis (±2 SD) in the group of fetuses with congenital heart defects was 56° ±13° (range 30°–90°). Using these norms, it was found that 33/75 (44%) fetuses with congenital heart defects had an abnormal cardiac axis measurement. The authors concluded that the presence of a cardiac axis exceeding 57° was associated with a substantial risk of congenital heart defects.

Smith and colleagues attempted to determine whether a relationship existed between left cardiac axis deviation and fetal anomalies.[45] For the purposes of their study, "left cardiac axis deviation" was defined as a measurement greater than 75° to the left of a line bisecting the midportion of the fetal chest and spine. In a population of approximately 41,500 fetuses undergoing second- and third-trimester scanning, 57 fetuses were found to have a cardiac axis measurement of greater than 75°. Of the 34 fetuses in this group who had postnatal follow-up, 21/34 (62%) had congenital heart defects and 26/34 (76%) had either congenital heart defects or another major extracardiac anomaly. Of the 21 abnormal hearts identified, 8/21 (38%) were conotruncal lesions (tetralogy of Fallot, double-outlet right ventricle, transposition of the great vessels). We would not expect lesions of this type to be identified by a four-chamber view because the outflow tracts are not seen. Smith et al concluded that fetal cardiac axis should be routinely evaluated as part of the four-chamber view and that the finding of an abnormal fetal cardiac axis warrants echocardiography and a detailed fetal anatomic survey.

At our own institution, we retrospectively reviewed 81 fetuses with congenital heart defects.[46] We found an abnormal cardiac axis in association with 51/81 (63%) of all fetuses with congenital heart defects. Cardiac axis norms were established by a prospective evaluation of 200 fetuses having no antenatal or neonatal evidence of congenital heart defects. The mean axis (± 2 SD) in this study was $43°$ ($\pm 16°$). An abnormal cardiac axis was defined as more than 2 standard deviations above or below the mean axis ($< 27°$ or $> 59°$). Table 48.6 summarizes reported sensitivities for fetal cardiac axis measurements as markers for congenital heart defects.

In contrast to Shipp[38] and Smith,[45] who specifically studied left cardiac axis deviation, the study by Bork and Egan was unique in that both an abnormal left and right cardiac axis were examined.[46] Of the cases of congenital heart defects associated with an abnormal cardiac axis measurement, 8.6% (7/81) had evidence of mesocardia ($< 27°$; range 5–25°) and 54% (44/81) had levorotation of the cardiac axis ($> 59°$; range 60–334°). In this study, an abnormal fetal cardiac axis was also found to be strongly associated with several structural cardiac defects not always detected by the standard four-chamber view (e.g., coarctation of the aorta, atrial septal defect). Table 48.7 lists the types of cardiac defect identified and the number associated with an abnormal cardiac axis in this study.

We prospectively evaluated the utility of an abnormal fetal cardiac axis measurement to antenatally detect congenital heart disease.[47] In 500 fetuses referred for noncardiac indications, the sensitivity of an abnormal cardiac axis measurement as a marker for congenital heart defects was 55% (6/11). The specificity, and positive and negative predictive values, were 95.1, 20, and 98.9% respectively. We also developed an on-screen method of fetal cardiac axis measurement using electronic calipers (detailed later in this chapter), which simplifies the cumbersome manual protractor method used in earlier studies.

TABLE 48.6   Reported Sensitivities for an Abnormal Fetal Cardiac Axis Measurement as a Marker for Congenital Heart Defects (CHD)

Ref: First Author (year)	Ratio of Abnormal Axes Found to All Cases of CHD	Sensitivity (%)	Mean (deg) ±2 SD (normal)
Shipp[38] (1995)	33/75	44	43 ± 14 (29–57)
Smith[45] (1995)	21/34	62	45 ± 20 (25–65)
Bork[46] (1995)	51/81	63	43 ± 16 (27–59)

TABLE 48.7   Cardiac Anomalies Associated with an Abnormal Axis

Lesion	Ratio of Abnormal Axes Found to All Cases[a]	Sensitivity (%)
Ventricular septal defect	8/20	40
Tetralogy of Fallot	7/15	47
Hypoplastic left heart	8/8	100
Complex lesions	6/7	86
Atrioventricular canal defect	4/7	57
Atrial septal defect	4/6	67
Dextrocardia/situs inversus	5/5	100
Truncus arteriosus	2/4	50
Double-outlet right ventricle	2/2	100
Coarctation of the aorta	2/2	100
Hypoplastic right heart	1/1	100
Ebstein's anomaly	1/1	100
Hypertrophic cardiomyopathy	1/1	100
Cardiac rhabdomyoma	0/1	0
Pentalogy of Cantrell	0/1	0

[a]Of 81 fetuses examined, 51 anomalies were detected, for an overall average of 63%.
Source: Bork et al.[46]

The determination of fetal cardiac axis may be a valuable tool in identifying fetuses at risk for cardiac and extracardiac anomalies. When the studies detailed in Table 48.6 were combined, the sensitivity of cardiac axis alone in detecting congenital heart defects was found to be 55% (105/190). An attempt to obtain a cardiac axis measurement focuses the sonographer on the standard four-chamber view of the fetal heart, which may, of itself, increase the detection of congenital heart defects and situs or thoracic abnormalities. We feel that the determination of fetal cardiac axis should be included as an integral component of the standard four-chamber view. The finding of an abnormal cardiac axis should prompt referral for a targeted anatomic survey and fetal echocardiography.

On-Screen Determination of Fetal Cardiac Axis

Studies by Shipp, Smith, and Bork have documented the value of fetal cardiac axis measurement. Following the initial report on fetal cardiac axis measurement by Comstock, the determination of fetal cardiac axis was performed by manual protractor measurements or visual estimates, both of which were done off-line and were sometimes cumbersome. While many new obstetrical ultrasound devices come equipped with a software package that includes angle determination, older equipment lacks this on-line capability. We have developed an ultrasound method using multiple electronic calipers for on-screen measurement of fetal cardiac axis.[37]

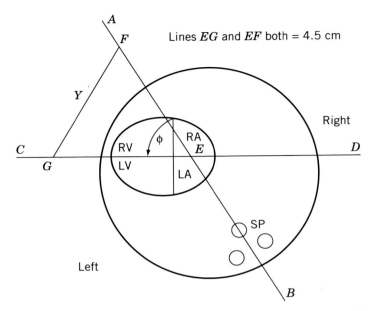

Figure 48.2   On-screen method of fetal cardiac axis determination: measurement of the cardiac axis from the four-chamber view.

The convenience of this on-screen method may enhance its routine use during fetal anatomic surveys.

On-Screen Method of Fetal Cardiac Axis Determination (Fig. 48.2)

1. A standard four-chamber view is obtained.
2. On-screen calipers are used to bisect the fetal thorax by traversing the fetal spine and midportion of the anterior abdominal wall (segment *AB*).
3. A second line (segment *CD*) is drawn through the interventricular septum.
4. The intersection of these two lines is designated point *E*.
5. Starting at point *E*, calipers are used to superimpose 4.5 cm lines (*EF* and *EG*) along each of the previously described lines (*AB* and *CD*).
6. The distance between points *F* and *G* is measured with calipers.
7. Using the following trigonometric formula:

$$\phi = 2 \left[\arcsin \left(\frac{FG}{9} \right) \right] \frac{180}{\pi}.$$

Table 48.8 was created to convert *FG* to the cardiac axis, in degrees.

To perform these on-screen measurements, an existing ultrasound device should have at least three and preferably five sets of calipers. This method is adaptable to many current ultrasound devices. Table 48.8 could be programmed into any ultrasound software package to allow on-screen measurements to be instantaneously converted to the corresponding angle in degrees. As a rule of thumb, if the *FG* segment measurement is 2 cm or less, or 4.5 cm or more, the cardiac axis is abnormal.

THE USE OF COLOR FLOW DOPPLER IN SCREENING FOR CHD

Screening for fetal cardiac anomalies relies almost entirely on two-dimensional ultrasound. Color flow Doppler images were essential to the correct anatomical diagnosis in 29% of 779 fetal echocardiograms reported by Copel et al.[48] Color flow and pulsed Doppler were not components of the basic echocardiogram but were added to the study if abnormal findings were encountered. They were considered to be essential to specific aspects of the diagnosis of 13 lesions that were first detected by two-dimensional scanning. Devore and Alfi reported an increase in their detection rate of fetal cardiovascular abnormalities from 12% to 60% with the use of color flow Doppler in a population at increased risk for trisomy 21.[49] The controls were historical, however, and a newer ultrasound device, with improved two-dimensional resolution, was used in the second phase of the study. Currently, there is little evidence suggesting that the addition of color flow Doppler to routine fetal cardiac screening would improve the detection rate for congenital cardiac defects.

TABLE 48.8   Conversion Table for On-Screen Axis Determination

FG (cm)	Axis (deg)	FG (cm)	Axis (deg)
0.1	1	4.6	61
0.2	3	4.7	63
0.3	4	4.8	64
0.4	5	4.9	66
0.5	6	5	67
0.6	8	5.1	69
0.7	9	5.2	71
0.8	10	5.3	72
0.9	11	5.4	74
1	13	5.5	75
1.1	14	5.6	77
1.2	15	5.7	79
1.3	17	5.8	80
1.4	18	5.9	82
1.5	19	6	84
1.6	20	6.1	85
1.7	22	6.2	87
1.8	23	6.3	89
1.9	24	6.4	91
2	26	6.5	92
2.1	27	6.6	94
2.2	28	6.7	96
2.3	30	6.8	98
2.4	31	6.9	100
2.5	32	7	102
2.6	34	7.1	104
2.7	35	7.2	106
2.8	36	7.3	108
2.9	38	7.4	111
3	39	7.5	113
3.1	40	7.6	115
3.2	42	7.7	118
3.3	43	7.8	120
3.4	44	7.9	123
3.5	46	8	125
3.6	47	8.1	128
3.7	49	8.2	131
3.8	50	8.3	135
3.9	51	8.4	138
4	53	8.5	142
4.1	54	8.6	146
4.2	56	8.7	150
4.3	57	8.8	156
4.4	59	8.9	163
4.5	60	9	180

THE FUTURE OF SCREENING FOR CHD

In the absence of antenatal blood or chemical tests to screen for congenital heart defects, we must rely on improving the ability and expertise of ultrasonographers to detect structur-al cardiac abnormalities. This must be accomplished by expanding the application of the four-chamber view to cardiac axis and outflow tracts. The addition of the aortic outflow tract to the four-chamber view alone increased the sensitivity from 47% to 78% in Kirk's study.[9] With the further addition of both outflow tracts, the sensitivity improved from 33–63% to 42–83% in series from Bromley,[32] Achiron,[33] and Wigton.[36] Measurement of cardiac axis in a prospective series gave a sensitivity of 55%.[47] Two studies address the practicality of expanding obstetrical ultrasound examinations to include the aortic root or a full fetal echocardiogram in a reasonable time period. Blake et al studied the likelihood of obtaining a five-step fetal echocardiogram, which included a four-chamber view along with the outflow tracts, cardiac inflow, aortic and ductal arches, and long and short axes of the great vessels, in 60 study fetuses having gestational ages between 18 and 42 weeks.[50] They documented all five views in every case, averaged 10 minutes per fetal cardiac exam, and obtained results that were not dependent on gestational age. In an attempt to determine how often a five-view fetal echocardiogram could be obtained in any 10-minute window during the exam, Egan et al studied 312 patients who presented for level I or II obstetrical ultrasound exams from 15 to 36 weeks of gestation.[42] The views were: (1) the four-chamber view, (2) the five-chamber or long-axis view of the left ventricle, (3) the proximal right outflow tract, (4) the distal left outflow tract, and (5) the ductal arch. These investigators were able to obtain a four-chamber view in 96% of the exams, any two views in 88% of the fetuses, and all five views in 34% of the exams during the 10-minute window. There was no difference in the percentage of views imaged by sonographers, maternal-fetal medicine fellows, or attending physicians from the participating institutions. Factors that enhanced the ability to obtain the views were a depth of field between 2 and 7 cm, fetal spine posterior, and a gestational age greater than 19 weeks.

SUMMARY

Because fetal cardiac defects are the most common congenital anomalies, surveillance for these abnormalities must be enhanced. Ultrasound is the most efficacious method of screening for these defects. The four-chamber view must be obtained whenever possible, and measurement of cardiac axis may improve the efficacy of this view. As "centers of excellence" in ultrasound develop, a five-view fetal echocardiogram may become an integral component of every second- and third-trimester ultrasound examination. Any suspicious cardiac finding should be further evaluated with a full fetal echocardiogram including two-dimensional, color Dop-pler, M-mode, and pulsed Doppler techniques.

REFERENCES

1. *MMWR* 1994;43:905–909.

2. Edmonds LD, Levy MJ. Temporal trends in the prevalence of congenital malformations at birth based on the Birth Defects Monitoring Program, United States, 1979–87. *MMWR* 1990; 39:19–23.

3. Iyasu S, Lynberg MC, Rowley D, Saftlas AF, Atrash HK. Surveillance of postneonatal mortality, United States, 1980–1987. *MMWR* 1991;40:43–55.

4. Wegman ME. Annual summary of vital statistics—1993. *Pediatrics* 1994;94:792–803.

5. Ewigman BG, Crane JP, Frigoletto FD, LeFevre ML, Bain RP, McNellis D, et al. Effect of prenatal ultrasound and perinatal outcome. *N Engl J Med* 1993;329:812–817.

6. Crane JP, Lefevre ML, Windborn RC, Evans JK, Ewigman BG, Bain RP, Frigoletto FD, McNellis D. The RADIUS Study Group: a randomized trial of prenatal ultrasonographic screening impact on the detection, management and outcome of anomalous fetuses. *Am J Obstet Gynecol* 1994;171:392–399.

7. American College of Obstetricians and Gynecologists. *Ultrasonography in Pregnancy.* ACOG Technical Bulletin 1987. Washington, DC: ACOG;1993.

8. American Institute of Ultrasound in Medicine. *Guidelines for the Performance of the Antepartum Obstetrical Ultrasound Examination.* Rockville, MD: AIUM;1993.

9. Kirk JS, Riggs TW, Comstock CH, Lee W, Yang S, Weinhouse E. Prenatal screening for cardiac anomalies: the value of routine addition of the aortic root to the four-chamber view. *Obstet Gynecol* 1994;84:427–431.

10. Cooper MJ, Enderlin MA, Dyson DC, Roge CL, Tarnoff H. Fetal echocardiography: retrospective review of clinical experience and review of indications. *Obstet Gynecol* 1995;86: 577–582.

11. Schmidt KG, de Araujo LMD, Silverman NH. Evaluation of structural and functional abnormalities of the fetal heart by echocardiography. *Am J Cardiac Imaging* 1988;2:57–76.

12. Wheller JJ, Reiss R, Allen HD Clinical experience with fetal echocardiography. *Am J Dis Child* 1988;63:1137–1145.

13. Martin GR, Ruckman RN. Fetal echocardiography: a large clinical experience and follow-up. *J Am Soc Echocardiogr* 1990; 3:4–8.

14. Smythe JF, Copel JA, Kleinman CS. Outcome of prenatally detected cardiac malformations. *Am J Cardiol* 1992;69: 1471–1474.

15. Copel JA, Pilu G, Green J, Hobbins JC, Kleinman CS. Fetal echocardiographic screening for congenital heart disease: the importance of the four-chamber view. *Am J Obstet Gynecol* 1987;157:648–655.

16. Allan LD, Crawford DC, Chita SK, Anderson RH, Tynan MJ. Familial recurrence of congenital heart disease in a prospective series of mothers referred for fetal echocardiography. *Am J Cardiol* 1986;58:334–347.

17. Achiron R, Rotstein Z, Lipitz S, Mashiach S, Hegesh J. First trimester diagnosis of fetal congenital heart disease by transvaginal ultrasonography. *Obstet Gynecol* 1994;84:69–74.

18. Bronshtein M, Zimmer EZ, Gerlis LM, Lorber A, Drugan A. Early ultrasound diagnosis of fetal congenital heart defects in high-risk and low-risk pregnancies. *Obstet Gynecol* 1993;82: 225–229.

19. Gembruch U, Knopfle G, Chatterjee M, Bald R, Hansmann M. First trimester diagnosis of fetal congenital heart disease by transvaginal two-dimensional and Doppler echocardiography. *Obstet Gynecol* 1990;75:496–498.

20. Bronshtein M, Zimmer EZ, Milo S, Ho SY, Lorber A, Gerlis LM. Fetal cardiac abnormalities detected by transvaginal sonography at 12–16 weeks' gestation. *Obstet Gynecol* 1991; 78:374–378.

21. Bronshtein M, Siegler E, Eshcoli Z, Zimmer EZ. Transvaginal ultrasound measurements of the fetal heart at 11 to 17 weeks of gestation. *Am J Perinatol* 1992;9:38–42.

22. Dolkart LA, Reimers FT. Transvaginal fetal echocardiography in early pregnancy: normative data. *Am J Obstet Gynecol* 1991;165:688–691.

23. Achiron R, Weissman A, Rotstein Z, Lipitz S, Mashiach S, Hegesh J. Transvaginal echocardiographic examination of the fetal heart between 13 and 15 weeks' gestation in a low-risk population. *J Ultrasound Med* 1994;13:783–793.

24. Johnson P, Sharland G, Maxwell D, Allan L. The role of transvaginal sonography in the early detection of congenital heart disease. *Ultrasound Obstet Gynecol* 1992;2:248–251.

25. Allan LD. Fetal congenital heart disease: diagnosis and management. *Curr Opin Obstet Gynecol* 1994;6:45–49.

26. Copel JA, Cullen M, Green J, Mohoney MJ, Hobbins JC, Kleinman CS. The frequency of aneuploidy in prenatally diagnosed congenital heart disease: an indication for fetal karyotyping. *Am J Obstet Gynecol* 1988;158:409–413.

27. Rosendahl H, Kivinen S. Antenatal detection of congenital malformations by routine ultrasonography. *Obstet Gynecol* 1989;73:947–950.

28. Brocks V, Bang J. Routine examination by ultrasound for the detection of fetal malformations in a low risk population. *Fetal Diagn Ther* 1991;6:37–45.

29. Sharland GK, Allan LD. Screening for congenital heart disease prenatally—results of a 2 1/2 year study in the southeast Thames region. *Br J Obstet Gynaecol* 1992;99:220–225.

30. Chitty LS, Hunt GH, Moore J, Lobb MO. Effectiveness of routine ultrasonography in detecting fetal structural abnormalities in a low risk population. *Br Med J* 1992;303:1165–1169.

31. Shirley IM, Bottomley F, Robinson VP. Routine radiographic screening for fetal abnormalities by ultrasound in an unselected low risk population. *Br J Radiol* 1992;65:564–569.

32. Bromley B, Estroff JA, Sanders SP, Parad R, Roberts D, Frigoletto FD, Bencerraf BR. Fetal echocardiography: accuracy and limitations in a population at high risk and low risk for heart defects. *Am J Obstet Gynecol* 1992;166:1473–1481.

33. Achiron R, Glaser J, Gelernter I, Hegesh J, Yagel S. Extended fetal echocardiographic examination for detecting cardiac malformations in low risk pregnancies. *Br Med J* 1992;304: 671–674.

34. Vergani P, Mariani S, Ghidini A, Schiavina R, Cavallore M, Locatelli A, Strobell N, Cerruti P. Screening for congenital heart

disease with the four chamber view of the fetal heart. *Am J Obstet Gynecol* 1992;167:1000–1003.

35. Tegnander E, Eik-Nes SH, Linker DT. Incorporating the 4 chamber view of the fetal heart into the routine ultrasound examination. *Ultrasound Obstet Gynecol* 1994;4:24–28.

36. Wigton TR, Sabbagha RE, Tamura RK, Cohen L, Minogue JP, Strasburger JF. Sonographic diagnosis of congenital heart disease; comparison between the four chamber view and multiple cardiac views. *Obstet Gynecol* 1993;82:219–224.

37. Bork MD, Egan JFX, Diana DJ, Scorza WE, Fabbri EL, Feeney LD, Campbell WA. A new method for on-screen determination of fetal cardiac axis. *Am J Obstet Gynecol* 1995;173:1192–1195.

38. Shipp TD, Bromley B, Hornberger LK, Nadel A, Benacerraf BR. Levorotation of the fetal cardiac axis: a clue for the presence of congenital heart disease. *Obstet Gynecol* 1995;85:97–102.

39. Allan LD, Crawford DC, Chita SK, Tynan MJ. Prenatal screening for CHD. *Br Med J* 1986;292:1717.

40. Goncalves LF, Jeanty P, Piper JM. The accuracy of prenatal ultrasonography in detecting congenital anomalies. *Am J Obstet Gynecol* 1994;171:1606–1612.

41. Schultz SM, Pretorius DH, Budorick NE. Four chamber view of the fetal heart: demonstration related to menstrual age. *J Ultrasound Med* 1994;13:285–289.

42. Egan JFX, Cutney C, Scorza WE, Cusick W, Smulian JC, Vintzileos AM. The feasibility of obtaining a five view fetal echocardiogram within 10 minutes during a level of I or II ultrasound between 16–36 weeks. *Am J Obstet Gynecol* 1994;170:367. Abstract 331.

43. McGahan J. Sonography of the fetal heart: findings on the four-chamber view. *Am J Radiol* 1991;156:547–552.

44. Comstock CH. Normal fetal heart axis and position. *Obstet Gynecol* 1987;70:255–259.

45. Smith RS, Comstock CH, Kirk JS, Lee W. Ultrasonographic left cardiac axis deviation: a marker for fetal anomalies. *Obstet Gynecol* 1995;85:187–191.

46. Bork MD, Egan JFX, Diana DJ, Scorza WE, McLean DM, Campbell WA. Fetal cardiac axis: a useful screening tool for congenital heart disease? *Am J Obstet Gynecol* 1995;172:355. Abstract 344.

47. Bork MD, Egan JFX, Borgida AF, Hardardottir H, Fabbri EL, Feeney LD, Smeltzer JS, Campbell WA. Sonographically measured fetal cardiac axis as a marker for congenital heart disease. *Am J Obstet Gynecol* 1996;174:418. Abstract 394.

48. Copel JA, Morotti R, Hobbins JC, Kleinman CS. The antenatal diagnosis of congenital heart disease using fetal echocardiography: is color flow mapping necessary? *Obstet Gynecol* 1991;78:1–8.

49. DeVore GR, Alfi O. The use of color Doppler ultrasound to identify fetuses at increased risk for trisomy 21: an alternative for high-risk patients who decline genetic amniocentesis. *Obstet Gynecol* 1995;85:378–386.

50. Blake DM, Mastrogiannis D, Reece EA. Is a five-step approach to fetal echocardiography feasible throughout pregnancy? *Am J Perinatol* 1995;12:290–293.

49

GENETIC CAUSES OF CARDIAC DISEASES

Harold Chen, MD

INTRODUCTION

Genetic factors play a role in most congenital heart defects, in certain cardiomyopathies, and in cardiac diseases as components of systemic disorders. Genetic causes of cardiac diseases are generally classified into chromosomal, single-gene, and multifactorial disorders. In Mendelian disorders (e.g., Apert syndrome) and chromosome disorders (e.g., Down syndrome), genetic effects are readily apparent. However, in most congenital heart defects, the role of genetic factors is less obvious, and its discernment requires the specialized knowledge of clinical geneticists, cardiologists, and other scientists. This knowledge notwithstanding, many of the fundamental genetic mechanisms remain obscure.

Whenever the clinician suspects a genetic component in a disease, a carefully obtained family history is a critical tool in arriving in a diagnosis. Relevant information includes name, sex, date of birth, age at the onset of disease, medical data, ethnic background, and other essential information such as twinning and consanguinity. This information, collected on family members in multiple generations, can be summarized concisely in a pedigree,[1,2] and in this form it will help determine the inheritance pattern of a particular genetic disorder in the family. A family history of multiple spontaneous abortions or stillbirths may suggest a segregating structural chromosomal abnormality. Ethnic background may be important in certain genetic disorders (e.g., sickle cell anemia in blacks, Tay–Sachs disease in Ashkenazic Jews). Parental ages are also important: An advanced maternal age is associated with an increased risk of having a child with a chromosomal anomaly (e.g., trisomy 21); advanced paternal age may suggest an autosomal dominant new mutation (e.g., Apert syndrome).

Certain familial diseases do not conform readily to traditional inheritance, either Mendelian or multifactorial. These instances are better explained as novel phenomena at the cellular, chromosomal, and DNA levels.[3] Uniparental disomy is the derivation of both copies of a chromosome pair from one parent. In genomic imprinting, regions of some chromosomes show differential gene inactivation depending on the parent of origin. A germ-line mosaicism may produce repeatedly abnormal offspring from a parent whose somatic cells are normal. Unstable mutations of DNA segments in diseases like the fragile X syndrome result in variable expression and in generations "skipped" by the disease. Inheritance of mitochondrial genes, called cytoplasmic or mitochondrial inheritance, is through mothers only.

Fetal echocardiography is a well-established technique for the prenatal detection of congenital heart defects. Cardiac evaluation should be pursued when a fetus is suspected to have extracardiac anomalies such as hydrocephalus, microcephaly, holoprosencephaly, agenesis of the corpus callosum, Meckel–Gruber syndrome, esophageal atresia, duodenal atresia, diaphragmatic hernia, omphalocele, or renal dysplasia.[4] Prenatal diagnosis of a congenital cardiovascular malformation by fetal echocardiography influences the management of pregnancy, labor, and delivery, and of postnatal care.[5,6] Fetal echocardiography series have revealed strong associations of chromosomal abnormalities with congenital cardiovascular malformations. The risk of aneuploidy associated with fetal cardiac anomalies is much greater than that associated with elevated maternal age.[7] Amniocentesis and cytogenetic analysis are considered appropriate in a fetus with echo-diagnosed congenital cardiovascular malformations,[8,9] especially with certain associated extracardiac anomalies.[10,11]

Cardiac Problems in Pregnancy, Third Edition
Edited by Uri Elkayam, MD, and Norbert Gleicher, MD
Copyright © 1998 by Wiley-Liss, Inc. ISBN 0-471-16358-9

The study of congenital heart diseases is starting to benefit from the major advances provided by the advent of molecular biology methods.[12] Genes that are responsible for congenital heart diseases can now be identified. For example, the molecular basis of certain heritable cardiac and vascular diseases was recently determined by means of linkage analysis and positional cloning and the identification of candidate protein.[13] Examples include β-myosin heavy chain gene mutations in familial hypertrophic cardiomyopathy, fibrillin mutations in Marfan syndrome, elastin mutations in Williams syndrome, and microdeletions in chromosome band 22q11 in DiGeorge syndrome, velocardiofacial syndrome, and nonsyndromic conotruncal malformations. These exciting discoveries have provided a springboard for studies better to characterize how mutations in extracellular matrix, contractile, and membrane proteins lead to a disease phenotype. Discovering the genes and their protein products implicated in cardiac morphogenesis will change our understanding of these cardiac malformations.[12]

MULTIFACTORIAL INHERITANCE[14,15]

The genetic contribution to disease varies; some disorders are entirely environmental, while others are primarily genetic. Although many common disorders have an appreciable genetic contribution, they do not follow a simple Mendelian inheritance pattern. Polygenic or multifactorial inheritance describes the etiologies of many such disorders.

The recurrence risk for a multifactorial disorder within a family is generally low, with first-degree relatives at greater risk. The rate at which relatives of the proband have been affected can be calculated from family studies. The empiric recurrence risk can then be calculated and applied to genetic counseling.

Congenital Heart Defects

Congenital heart defects are the most common congenital abnormality with prevalence of 8 per thousand live births.[16,17] Congenital heart defects per thousand live births in developed western industrialized countries occur from about 3–5 times to about 12 times.[18] They account for almost half the perinatal and infant deaths caused by congenital malformations.[19] Since our knowledge of congenital heart defects in the developmental stage of life is limited, embryologic phenomena were described and abnormal embryologic events that could contribute to the morphogenesis of congenital heart defects were suggested.[20]

The advent of echocardiography with Doppler color flow evaluation suggests a higher estimate, since this technology allows us to accurately diagnose cardiac lesions in patients who are asymptomatic or without overt clinical findings. However, in infants who die before term, there is an even higher incidence of congenital heart defects with excess complex cardiac lesions.[21] In experienced hands, fetal echocardiography can show most congenital heart lesions at 18–20 weeks of gestation.[22]

Most patients with congenital heart defects have no recognizable genetic syndromes. The recurrence risk is determined empirically. A family that has one affected child has a higher risk of recurrence of congenital heart defects than the general population (Table 49.1).[15,23–25] The recurrence risk is almost tripled if two siblings are affected.[23] A further em-

TABLE 49.1 Recurrence Risks for Sibs and Offspring

Congenital Heart Defect	Recurrence Risk[25] each Subsequent Child (%)	Recurrence Risk[23] (%)		Recurrence Risk in Fetus (%)[15,23,24]	
		If 1 Affected Sib	If 2 Affected Sibs	Mother Affected	Father Affected
Ventricular septal defect	5	3	10	6–10	2
Atrial septal defect	3	2.5	8	4–4.5	1.5
Patent ductus arteriosus	4	3	10	3.5–4	2.5
Pulmonic stenosis	3	2	6	4–6.5	2
Aortic stenosis	2	2	6	13–18	3
Tetralogy of Fallot	3	2.5	8	2.5	1.5
Transposition of great vessels	2	1.5	5		
Coarctation of aorta	2	2	6	4	2
Atrioventricular canal				14	1
Endocardial cushion defect		3	10		
Fibroelastosis		4	12		
Hypoplastic left heart		2	6		
Tricuspid atresia		1	3		
Ebstein's anomaly		1	3		
Truncus arteriosus		1	3		
Pulmonary atresia		1	3		

pirical finding is the higher risk of recurrence of congenital heart defects in the fetus when the mother is affected than when the father is affected.[15,24,26]

Multifactorial inheritance is the most common cause of congenital heart defects.[27] The essential factors of cardiovascular maldevelopment include a genetic predisposition to react adversely to one or more environmental triggers, a genetic predisposition to one or more forms of maldevelopment, and exposure to an environmental influence at a vulnerable period of embryogenesis.[28] As already noted, the risk for a fetal congenital heart defect is observed to be higher in the case of an affected mother than in the case of other first-degree relatives.[15] One possible explanation for this discrepancy is that in some cases congenital heart defects are transmitted by means of cytoplasmic (mitochondrial) inheritance.[24] The congenital heart defect might represent a susceptibility to one or more teratogens that act on the heart. The susceptibility would be enhanced if both mother and fetus shared the trait.[15]

A rational approach for the prevention of a multifactorial disorder is the modification of known environmental triggers in genetically susceptible individuals. For example, modifying diet and smoking habits for individuals at risk for coronary heart disease and supplementing folic acid for those at risk for neural tube defects are effective interventions. This approach is currently unavailable for most multifactorial disorders, however, since the triggers are unknown.

Recent advances in cardiac catheterization techniques and the surgical management of complex congenital defects continue to be the focus of attention of cardiologists and surgeons.[29,30] The refinements in these techniques have initiated a new era in the clinical management of congenital heart diseases in childhood.

The observation that most congenital heart defects are sporadic is based on earlier surveys of the incidence of familial heart disease, in which 8% of defects were thought to be due to chromosomal or single gene defects, 2% due to environmental factors, and 90% "multifactorial."[3] "Multifactorial" implies that cardiac malformations are caused by the combined effects of one or more alleles at a number of loci interacting with stochastic and/or environmental factors. Such a complex multivariable model has limited the generation of testable hypotheses and the focus on single genes crucial in causing congenital heart defects. The additive multifactorial model does not adequately account for the risks in all forms of isolated congenital heart defects of unknown etiology.[31]

Recent clinical investigations have clearly shown genetic etiologies for congenital heart defects. The advent of molecular genetics has shown the feasibility of investigating genetic defects in congenital heart defects: (1) detection of chromosomal microdeletions and small translocations by high resolution chromosomal analysis and fluorescence in situ hybridization, (2) delineation of the genetic defects of fa-

milial heart disease through linkage analysis and reverse genetics, and (3) advances in animal genetics and embryo manipulation that permit detailed studies of animal models of congenital heart defects.[32]

CHROMOSOME DISORDERS

Chromosomal abnormality is the second most common cause of congenital heart defects, after multifactorial inheritance. About 10–13% of newborns with congenital heart defects (CHD) have chromosomal abnormalities.[33,34] Factoring in fetal losses, it is estimated that a threefold increase in chromosome aneuploidies exists among fetuses with CHD.[8] In spontaneous abortuses and stillborn fetuses with CHD, chromosomal abnormalities have been confirmed in 19% of the cases and are suspected in up to 36%.[35] Most of these abnormalities are associated with such extreme maldevelopment of multiple organ systems that fetal death occurs in utero. For example, monosomy X is frequently associated with congenital heart defects that cause the fetus to die in utero. However, monosomy X is not always lethal, and a slight increase in the survival of these infants could affect the incidence of newborn congenital heart defects.[21]

Congenital heart defects are extremely common in patients with autosomal aneuploidies such as trisomy 18 and trisomy 13. Besides complete trisomies, other chromosomal anomalies such as duplications, deletions, and mosaic trisomies are associated with an increased risk of congenital heart defects.[36]

Specific patterns of CHD observed in certain chromosomal disorders suggest that genetic factors play a role in determining cardiac development.[34] Despite the specificity of these patterns, there is a considerable degree of variability and overlap among the different aneuploid states.[37] The exact etiologic relationships between the imbalance of chromosomal material and abnormal development of any embryologic structure, such as the heart, are not yet fully understood.[38]

Technical and basic scientific advances are improving the diagnosis and basic understanding of cardiac diseases. The development of fluorescent in situ hybridization (FISH) technique has allowed for the identification of specific chromosomes and chromosomal segments involved in pathology. Fluorochrome-labeled probes for sequences unique to individual chromosomes are commercially available, and these include probes for chromosomes 13, 18, 21, X, and Y, and chromosome-specific regions such as the DiGeorge critical region. High resolution banding techniques are combined with probes for single-copy chromosomal DNA, and FISH to detect subtle structural rearrangements such as submicroscopic chromosome duplications and deletions.[39] Most clinical cytogenetic laboratories currently apply FISH to the diagnosis of microdeletion syndromes, the identification of marker chromosomes, and the interphase analysis of aneuploidy.

Autosomal Trisomy and Tetrasomy Syndromes
(Table 49.2)[2,36,40–87]

Trisomy 13 (Patau) Syndrome[2]   This classic trisomy syndrome has also been known as the Patau syndrome. The prognosis is poor, with most babies dying during early infancy. For those who survive, failure to thrive, apneic episodes, hypotonia, deafness, seizures (hypsarrhythmia), and severe psychomotor retardation are likely to be present.

Characteristic craniofacial features are microcephaly, trigonocephaly, ocular hypertelorism, anophthalmia/microphthalmia, coloboma of iris or retina, a broad, flat nose, choanal atresia, hare lip/cleft palate, micro/retrognathia, low-set/malformed ears, glabellar hemangioma, and punched-out scalp lesions. Other ocular lesions include cloudy corneas, cataracts, retinal dysplasia, glaucoma, and hyperplastic vitreous bodies. The holoprosencephaly–arrhinencephaly spectrum is the most common malformation of the central nervous system. Other CNS malformations include cerebellar hypoplasia, agenesis of corpus callosum, hydrocephaly, and meningomyelocele.

Urogenital anomalies include multicystic kidneys, dysplastic kidneys, duplication of the kidneys/ureter, unilateral renal agenesis, hydronephrosis, urethral stenosis, persistent urachus, abnormal fallopian tubes, duplicated labia minora, hypoplastic ovaries, bicornuate uterus, abnormal scrotum, and cryptorchidism. Postaxial polydactyly, camptodactyly, long hyperconvex fingernails, nail hypoplasia, talipes equinovarus, cervical ribs, and absent 12th thoracic ribs are characteristic musculoskeletal features. Various other anomalies are found in the gastrointestinal tract (colonic malrotation, Meckel's diverticulum, single umbilical artery, omphalocele, and umbilical hernia) and in the muscles (hypoplasia, absence, supernumerary, and variations). Characteristic dermatoglyphic findings include simian creases, t′ or t″, thenar and interdigital patterns, an increased frequency of arches and radial loops, and a fibular S-shaped hallucal arch.

Congenital heart defects are very common. The cardiac lesions are ventricular septal defect, secundum atrial septal defect, patent ductus arteriosus, bicuspid aortic valve, bicuspid pulmonary valve, a double-outlet right ventricle, tetralogy of Fallot, transposition of the great arteries, and dextrocardia. Cardiac surgery cannot be justified in patients with trisomy 13, since the principal mode of death was apnea in about 88% of patients irrespective of the presence of a cranial abnormality.[88]

Prenatal ultrasound findings in 33 consecutive fetuses with trisomy 13 were reviewed by Lehman et al.[89] Thirty fetuses (91%) had one or more abnormalities: holoprosencephaly (38%) or other central nervous system anomalies (58%), facial anomalies (48%), renal (11%) and cardiac (48%) defects, growth retardation (48%), and echogenic chordae tendineae (30%). Other findings not generally associated with trisomy 13 but present in the series included a large cisterna magna (18%), mild cerebral ventricular dilatation (9%), nuchal thickening or cystic hygroma (21%), and a hypoplastic left heart (21%). In a series of seven fetuses with trisomy 13, all displayed prenatal ultrasonographic findings of single or multiple cardiac defects, the majority representing double-outlet right ventricle and hypoplastic left ventricle, followed by ventricular septal defect, and tetralogy of Fallot.[90]

Trisomy 18 (Edwards) Syndrome[2]   Trisomy 18 syndrome, also known as Edwards syndrome, is the second most common multiple malformation syndrome in man. Although the prognosis is poor, long survival is possible. For those who survive beyond infancy, severe psychomotor and growth retardation are invariably present.

Typical craniofacial features include microcephaly, elongated skull, prominent occiput, ocular hypertelorism, epicanthal folds, microphthalmia, iris coloboma, micro/retrognathia, and low-set/malformed ears. There may be hypotonia, followed by hypertonia, jitteriness, apnea, and seizures. The most common CNS malformations are a small brain and cerebellar hypoplasia. Other CNS malformations include meningoencephalocele, anencephaly, hydrocephaly, holoprosencephaly, Arnold–Chiari malformation, hypoplasia/agenesis of the corpus callosum, and defective falx cerebri. Genitourinary anomalies are common; they include cystic kidneys, double ureters, hydronephrosis, hydroureters, horseshoe kidneys, unilateral renal agenesis, cryptorchidism and micropenis in the male, and hypoplasia of labia and ovaries, bifid uterus, and clitoral hypertrophy in the female. Furthermore, malrotation of the intestine, Meckel's diverticulum, esophageal atresia with or without tracheoesophageal fistula, diaphragmatic eventration, prune belly anomaly, pyloric stenosis, imperforate anus, umbilical, inguinal, and diaphragmatic hernias may be present.

An abnormal finger-grasping pattern (clenched hands with the index finger overriding the middle finger and the fifth finger overriding the fourth finger) and rocker-bottom feet are characteristics. Nails are hypoplastic. The great toes are often dorsiflexed. The neck and the sternum are both short. The pelvis is characteristically narrowed. Increased numbers of simple arches on the fingertips are diagnostic. Simian creases and t′ or t″ may be present.

Cardiac anomalies in trisomy 18 are extremely common. They occur as follows: ventricular septal defect (most common), tetralogy of Fallot, double-outlet right ventricle, and congenital polyvalvular nodular dysplasia. In a series of 15 autopsied cases with trisomy 18 and dup(18q) syndrome, the types of congenital heart defect were polyvalvular disease (100%), ventricular septal defect (87%), high takeoff of the right coronary ostium (80%), patent ductus arteriosus (73%),

TABLE 49.2   Cardiac Lesions and Noncardiac Manifestations of Autosomal Trisomy and Tetrasomy Syndromes[2,36]

Autosomal Trisomy and Tetrasomy Syndromes	Cardiac Lesions[a]	Noncardiac Manifestations
Trisomy 1p[40]	VSD	Intrauterine growth retardation, microcephaly, downward slanting palpebral fissures, ptosis, depressed nasal bridge, anteverted nostrils, cleft lip/palate, malformed ears, micrognathia, hypoplastic phalanges, hernias, cryptorchidism
Trisomy 1q[41]	TA, AA, COA, PDA, VSD, ASD, PS	Severe psychomotor/growth retardation, hirsutism, hypertelorism, microphthalmia, low-set/malformed ears, beaked nose, micrognathia, hypoplastic/aplastic thymus, omphalocele, renal anomalies, hand/finger deformities
Trisomy 2p[42]	AS, DOV, PDA, TGV	Neural tube defects, bronchopulmonary hypoplasia, diaphragmatic hernia, neuroblastoma
Trisomy 2q[43]	TOF, AS, COA, VSD	Mental retardation, frontonasal dysplasia, arrhinencephaly, microcephaly, hypertelorism, small narrow palpebral fissures, short nose, anteverted nares, long philtrum, thin upper lip, everted lower lip, kyphoscoliosis, pectus excavatum
Trisomy 3p[44]	VSD, ASD, PDA, DORV, TOF	Psychomotor retardation, brachycephaly, frontal bossing, hypertelorism, full cheek, short prominent philtrum, micro/retrognathia, short neck
Trisomy 3q[45]	VSD, COA, ASD, TOF, AVC	Psychomotor retardation, abnormal head shape, hypertrichosis, ocular anomalies, anteverted nares, long philtrum, maxillary prognathism, cleft palate, micrognathia, malformed auricles, short/webbed neck, clinodactyly, talipes, phenotype overlapped with de Lange phenotype
Trisomy 4[46]	ASD, VSD, TA, APAV, MVA	Mostly mosaic, holoprosencephaly facies spectrum, anal atresia, oligosyndactyly, cystic hygroma, skeletal abnormalities
Trisomy 4p[47]	ASD, COA	Mental retardation, low frontal hairline, microphthalmia, deep-set eyes, short nose, depressed nasal bridge, full cheeks, small/pointed chin, duplication of thumbs, vertebral anomalies
Trisomy 4q[48]	COA, ASD, PS, TA, TOF, TCA	Psychomotor retardation, congenital hypotonia, abnormal auricles, depressed nasal bridge, short neck, renal malformations especially renal hypoplasia, cryptorchidism, bifid/hypoplastic thumb
Trisomy 5p[49]	PDA, TGV	Psychomotor retardation, hypotonia, macrocephaly, hydrocephalus, prominent occiput, hypertelorism, upslanting palpebral fissures, epicanthal folds, depressed nasal bridge, long philtrum, micro/retrognathia, low-set/dysplastic ears
Trisomy 5q[50]	ASD, VSD, CD	Psychomotor/growth retardation, microcephaly, epicanthal folds, hypertelorism, large eyes, antimongoloid slanting of palpebral fissures, large upper lip, carplike mouth, dental caries, low-set/dysplastic ears, brachydactyly, clinodactyly, hernias
Trisomy 6p[51]	ASD, VSD, PDA	Psychomotor/growth retardation, prominent forehead, large fontanelle, wide sagittal suture, blepharophimosis, strabismus, low-set/malformed ears, small kidneys, proteinuria
Trisomy 6q[52]	PS, VSD, COA	Psychomotor/growth retardation, brachycephaly, flat face, down-slanting palpebral fissures, low-set ears, neck webbing, joint contractures, scoliosis
Trisomy 7p[53]	ASD, AVC, PDA, COA, PS, VSD, TOF	Psychomotor retardation, microbrachycephaly, wide cranial sutures/fontanel, hypertelorism, large low-set ears, micrognathia, choanal atresia/stenosis, hyperextensible joints/dislocation, joint contractures
Trisomy 7q[54]	VSD, ASD, PDA, PS, TGA, TA, COA, DC	Microcephaly, wide-open fontanels, frontal/parietal bossing, hypertelorism, epicanthal folds, small/up-slanting palpebral fissures, small nose, depressed nasal bridge, large/malformed ears, short neck, cleft palate, kyphoscoliosis, club feet, hip dislocation
Trisomy 8[55]	VSD, PDA, ASD, TA, COA, RAA, VR, TAPVR	Mostly are mosaics; psychomotor retardation, long face, prominent forehead, "pear-shaped" nose, thick, everted lower lip, slender trunk, long limbs, deep plantar/palmar furrows, skeletal and urogenital anomalies
San Luis Valley *rec*(8)[56]	TOF, DORV, TA, VSD, PS, ASD, HLH	Coloboma, abnormal face, prominent calcanei
Trisomy 8p[57]	OPD, COA, VSD, MA, PAPVR	Hypotonia, feeding difficulties, developmental delay, prominent forehead, high arched palate, large mouth, thin upper lip, malformed/low-set ears, broad nasal bridge, dental/skeletal anomalies, joint laxity

(Continued)

TABLE 49.2   *(Continued)*

Autosomal Trisomy and Tetrasomy Syndromes	Cardiac Lesions[a]	Noncardiac Manifestations
Tetrasomy 8p, mosaic[58]	VSD, PDA, ASD	Motor/developmental delay, expressive language delay, hydrocephalus, absent corpus callosum, dysmorphic facies, hemivertebrae, abnormal ribs, fused vertebrae
Trisomy 8q[56]	VSD, TOF, DORV, PS, ASD, AVC	Mental retardation, prominent forehead, hypertelorism, micrognathia, genital hypoplasia, long thorax, joint contractures
Trisomy 9[59,60]	VSD, PDA, PLSVC, ASD, DORV, ECFE, PA, COA	Microcephaly, narrow temples, hypertelorism, microphthalmia, enophthalmos, deep-set eyes, narrow/up-slanted palpebral fissures, prominent nose with bulbous tip, micro/retrognathia, low-set/malformed ears, short neck, skeletal/renal anomalies, hypoplastic male genitalia
Tetrasomy 9p[61]	PLSVC, PDA, VSD, ASD, PS	Low birth weight, psychomotor retardation, brachycephaly, large fontanel, hydrocephalus, hypertelorism, short palpebral fissures, beaked nose, cleft lip/palate, low-set/malformed ears, micro/retrognathia, skeletal anomalies
Trisomy 9q[62]	VSD, TOF, DAA	Failure to thrive, microcephaly, dolichocephaly, bulging forehead, epicanthal folds, narrow palpebral fissures, deep-set eyes, beaked nose, small mouth, upper lip over lower lip, retro/micrognathia, long fingers, stiff joints
Trisomy 10, mosaic[63]	CD	Growth/mental retardation, high forehead, hypertelorism, up-slanted palpebral fissures, blepharophimosis, retrognathia, dysplastic large ears, long slender trunk, plantar/palmar furrows, cryptorchidism
Trisomy 10p[64]	ASD, PDA, COA	Narrow face, broad nasal bridge, cleft lip/palate, small chin, large low-set ears, clinodactyly, scoliosis, osteoporosis, club feet, hyperflexed limbs, pulmonary/renal anomalies
Trisomy 10q[65]	ECCD, VSD, PA, TOF, DC	Psychomotor/growth retardation, microcephaly, hypotonia, high forehead, flat face, fine/arched eyebrows, narrow/antimongoloid slant of palpebral fissures, hypertelorism, short nose, bow-shaped mouth, short neck, kyphoscoliosis
Trisomy 11q[66]	VSD, PDA, ECCD, HRV, PA, TA, COA, ASD	Postnatal growth deficiency, mental deficiency, microcephaly, retro/micrognathia, low-set ears, short nose, long philtrum, retracted lower lip, epicanthus, short neck, flexion contractures of limbs, hypoplastic genitalia, anal atresia/stenosis
Trisomy 12p[67]	DORV, MA, VSD	Mental retardation, turricephaly, high bulging forehead, short nose, large mouth, low-set ears, flat face, corpulent body, hypotonia
Tetrasomy 12p, mosaic (Pallister–Killian)[68]	VSD, COA, PDA, ASD, AS, HC	Diaphragmatic hernia, rhizomelic micromelia, mental retardation, coarse facies, oligohydramnios
Trisomy 12q[69]	VSD, PDA, COA	Psychomotor retardation, dolichocephaly, brachycephaly, wide-spaced eyes, flat nasal bridge, downturned mouth angles, low-set/poorly formed ears, small chin, short neck, loose skin, wide-spaced nipples, skeletal anomalies
Trisomy 13 (Patau) (text)	VSD, ASD, PDA, BAV, BPV, RORV, TOF, TGV, DC, HLH	Severe psychomotor retardation, microcephaly, trigonocephaly, hypertelorism, anophthalmia/microphthalmia, coloboma, flat nose, choanal atresia, harelip/cleft palate, micro/retrognathia, low-set/malformed ears, glabella hemangioma, punched-out scalp lesions, ocular anomaly, holoprosencephaly–arrhinencephaly spectrum, urogenital/GI/skeletal anomalies including postaxial polydactyly
Trisomy 13q[70]	VSD, PDA, TGV	Mental retardation, microcephaly, trigonocephaly, hemangioma, thick converging eyebrows, long philtrum, malformed ears, umbilical hernia, limb anomalies
Trisomy 14, mosaic[71]	ASD, VSD, TOF, PDA, PS, AVC	Psychomotor/growth retardation, prominent forehead, hypertelorism, narrow palpebral fissures, broad nose, low-set/dysplastic ears, large mouth, micrognathia, cleft palate, short neck, body/facial asymmetry, abnormal skin pigmentation
Trisomy 14q[72]	TOF, VR, TA, COA, VSD	Psychomotor/growth retardation, hypotonia, spasticity, seizures, microcephaly, wide cranial sutures, hypertelorism, downward slant of palpebral fissures, abnormally placed ears, hypogenitalism, cryptorchidism, sparse hair
Trisomy 15q[73]	PS, VSD, PDA	Psychomotor/growth retardation, microcephaly, hypotonia, facial asymmetry, down-slanting palpebral fissures, ptosis, prominent nose, long philtrum, downturned mouth, midline crease in lower lip, micrognathia, short neck, pectus, scoliosis, cryptorchidism

TABLE 49.2 *(Continued)*

Autosomal Trisomy and Tetrasomy Syndromes	Cardiac Lesions[a]	Noncardiac Manifestations
Trisomy 16, mosiac[74]	VSD, ASD, PDA, COA, AVC, DORV, DC	Intrauterine growth retardation, dolichocephaly, hypertelorism, low-set/malformed ears, respiratory distress, musculoskeletal anomalies
Trisomy 16p[75]	ASD, TOF	Psychomotor retardation, microcephaly, hypertelorism, narrow/up-slanting palpebral fissures, scant eyelashes/brows, round tip of nose, anteverted nares, prominent glabella, long philtrum, micro/retrognathia, thin lip, long philtrum, cleft palate, ear/digital anomalies
Trisomy 16q[76]	ASD, VSD, PDA	Psychomotor/growth retardation, hypotonia, abnormal shape of skull, prominent forehead, small/antimongoloid slant of palpebral fissures, micrognathia, periorbital edema, low-set/dysplastic ears, limb anomalies
Trisomy 17p[77]	PDA, VSD, AA	Intrauterine growth retardation, psychomotor retardation, microcephaly, hirsutism, antimongoloid slant of palpebral fissures, hypertelorism, long philtrum, thin upper lip, micrognathia, malformed/low-set ears, wide-spaced nipples, renal anomalies, clinodactyly, flexion contractures
Trisomy 17q[78]	ASD, SAS, SV, MA, TGV	Facial asymmetry, hypertelorism, frontal bossing, temporal narrowness, broad nasal bridge, epicanthal folds, wide mouth, thin upper lip, micrognathia, webbed neck, low-set/posteriorly rotated ears, polydactyly, flexion contractures, hypotonia
Trisomy 18 (text)	VSD, BAV, BPV, AMV, PDA, TOF, DORV, COA, MA, HLV, AVC, TA, AA, PS	Severe psychomotor retardation, microcephaly, elongated skull, prominent occiput, hypertelorism, microphthalmia, iris coloboma, micro/retrognathia, low-set/malformed ears, CNS/GI/GU anomalies, short sternum, abnormal finger grasping pattern, rocker-bottom feet
Tetrasomy 18p[79]	ASD	Mental retardation, microcephaly, crowded facial structures, low-set ears, high-arched palate, contractures of fingers, spasticity
Trisomy 18q[80]	VSD, ASD, PDA, AS	Psychomotor/growth retardation, hypertonicity, microcephaly, short/slanting palpebral fissures, low-set/malformed ears, high-arched palate, micrognathia, short neck with redundant folds, limited hip abduction, overlapping fingers, prominent calcaneus, club feet
Isochromosome 18q[81]	DORV, VSD, BPV, MA	Abnormal head shape, low-set/malformed ears, short/webbed neck, wide-spaced nipples, GI/GU/skeletal anomalies
Trisomy 19q[82]	TOF, ASD, PDA, PS	Low birth weight, short stature, microcephaly, seizures, apnea, ptosis, low-set/posteriorly rotated ears, limb/GU anomalies
Trisomy 20p[83]	VSD, TOF, PDA	Psychomotor retardation, coarse hair, round face, prominent cheeks, retrognathia, epicanthal folds, up-slanting palpebral fissures, short nose with upturned tip, large nostrils, dental/renal/vertebral anomalies
Trisomy 20q[84]	TA, SV, MVA	Brachycephaly, epicanthal folds, anteverted nostrils, chin dimple, low-set/posteriorly rotated ears, microphthalmia, short neck, clinodactyly, camptodactyly, large toes
Trisomy 21 (text)	ECCD (AVC), VSD, ASD, TOF, PDA, PS, COA, AS, TGV	Psychomotor retardation, brachy/microcephaly, sloping forehead, up-slanting palpebral fissures, epicanthal folds, strabismus, Brushfield spots, blephalitis, ectropion, flat nasal bridge, short nose, protruding tongue, small ears with over-folded helix, abundant skin in the back of neck, diastasis recti, short hands/fingers, clinodactyly of 5th fingers, simian creases, increased atd angle, hypotonia, hyperextensible joints
Trisomy 22[85]	PS, VSD, PDA, TCA, AVC	Intrauterine growth retardation, microcephaly, hypertelorism, epicanthal folds, broad flat nasal bridge, micrognathia, microtia, cleft palate, anorectal/renal anomalies, hypoplastic distal digits, thumb anomalies
Inv Dup(22) (cat eye)[86]	TAPVR, ASD, VSD, PLSVC, AIVC, PDA, EC	Ocular coloboma, anal atresia, preauricular skin tags/pigs, microtia, hypertelorism, microphthalmia, down-slanting palpebral fissures, renal/biliary/GI anomalies
Trisomy 22q[87]	TAPVR	Phenotypic overlap with cat eye syndrome

[a]For abbreviations, see chapter appendix.

common brachiocephalic trunk (47%), coarctation of the aorta (20%), mitral atresia with hypoplastic left ventricle (7%), and patent foramen ovale (93%).[91] In another series of 16 fetuses with trisomy 18, all had prenatal ultrasound findings of single or multiple cardiac anomalies, and the majority presented with a ventricular septal defect, double-outlet right ventricle, or complete atrioventricular septal defect.[90]

Trisomy 21 (Down) Syndrome[2]   Trisomy 21 syndrome, also known as Down syndrome (DS), is the most common and the first described human chromosome disorder. DS occurs in approximately 1 in 800 live births. The most common cytogenetic type is primary trisomy 21 (93%), which results from nondisjunction arising at the time of the first or second maternal or paternal meiotic division. About 5% of cases are translocations and about 2% are mosaic.

In 1984 maternal serum α-fetoprotein (MSAFP), a biochemical marker, was observed to be reduced in pregnancies affected with Down syndrome.[92] In 1988 maternal serum unconjugated estriol (uE3), a steroid produced by the fetoplacental unit, was found to be about 25–30% lower in pregnancies affected with Down syndrome.[93] In the same year, maternal serum human chorionic gonadotropin (hCG), a placental hormone, was noted to be about twice the normal level in pregnancies affected with Down syndrome.[94] These markers, combined with MSAFP and maternal age, were proposed as a screening test to increase the sensitivity of Down syndrome detection[95] and were prospectively studied.[96] Triple-marker screening has been noted to be an effective

means of identifying fetal Down syndrome (amniocentesis was recommended for 6.1% of women screened with 75% the rate of detection for Down syndrome) and other chromosome abnormalities, especially trisomy 18 syndrome.[97] Using FISH for chromosome 21–specific probes to interphase nuclei, rapid prenatal diagnosis of trisomy 21 can be made from uncultured amniotic fluid (Fig. 49.1). It is predicted that the future antenatal diagnosis of fetal chromosome aneuploidy (e.g., trisomy 21) will be made by using fetal cells isolated from the maternal peripheral blood.[98]

Craniofacial features of Down syndrome are distinctive: a small brachycephalic head with a sloping forehead and a flat occiput, epicanthal folds, upward slant of the palpebral fissures, strabismus, speckling of the iris (Brushfield spots), conjunctivitis, blepharitis, ectropion, flat nasal bridge, a short nose, a protruding tongue, and small ears with an overfolded helix. Abundant skin is usually present on the back of the neck. Diastasis recti is common. The hands are short, with short fingers and incurved fifth fingers. Dermatoglyphic findings are characteristic, including simian creases and t′ and other patterns. Degrees of mental retardation range from moderate to severe. Children with Down syndrome have many potential life-threatening complications such as intestinal obstruction, leukemia, and congenital heart defects.

Congenital heart defects are common (40–50%)[99]; they are frequently seen in hospitalized DS patients (62%)[100] and are the main cause of death in this aneuploidy in the first two years of life.[101] The most frequent congenital heart defects are endocardial cushion defect (43%), ventricular septal de-

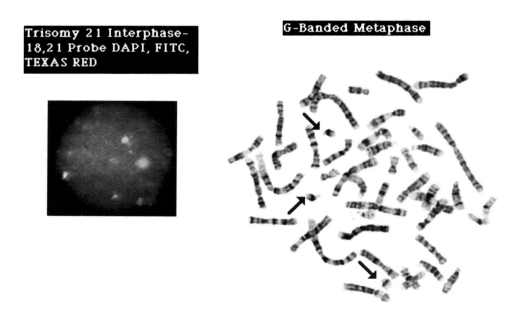

Figure 49.1   Interphase FISH analysis using probes for chromosomes 21 and 18 reveals three green (for chromonsome 21) and two red (for chromosome 18) signals (left half of the picture). This is compatible with trisomy 21 which is shown on the right half of the picture (G-banded metaphase). (See color plates.)

fect (32%), secundum atrial septal defect (10%), tetralogy of Fallot (6%), and isolated patent ductus arteriosus (4%).[102] Thirty percent of patients have multiple cardiac defects. The most common associated lesions are patent ductus arteriosus (16%) and pulmonic stenosis (9%). About 70% of all endocardial cushion defects are associated with Down syndrome.[34]

The presence of an extra copy of the proximal part of 21q22.3 appears to result in the typical physical phenotype: mental retardation, characteristic facial features, hand anomalies, and congenital heart defects.[37] Molecular analysis revealed that the 21q22.1–22.3 region appears to contain the gene(s) responsible for the congenital heart disease observed in Down syndrome.[103] the new gene (DSCR1), identified from region 21q22.1–q22.2, is highly expressed in the brain and the heart and is a candidate for involvement in the pathogenesis of Down syndrome, in particular mental retardation and/or cardiac defects.[104]

Autosomal Deletion Syndromes (Table 49.3)[2,36,105–133]

Monosomy 22q Syndrome Deletions and microdeletions involving chromosome 22 (22q11.2) have been demonstrated in patients with velocardiofacial (Shprintzen) syndrome,[134] DiGeorge syndrome,[135] conotruncal anomaly face syndrome,[136] conotruncal congenital heart anomalies,[137] absent pulmonary valve syndrome,[138] and Opitz GBBB syndrome.[139]

Velocardiofacial syndrome, which has McKusick Catalog number MIM (for Mendelian inheritance in man), 192430, is an autosomal dominant disorder characterized by cleft palate, cardiac defects consistent with a conotruncal classification (vascular ring, interrupted aortic arch, hypoplastic pulmonary arteries, hemitruncus, tetralogy of Fallot, and ventricular septal defect), learning disabilities, and a typical facial appearance.[140] DiGeorge syndrome (MIM 188400), a developmental field defect of the third and fourth pharyngeal pouches, is characterized by the association of conotruncal cardiac malformations, hypoplastic or absent thymus and parathyroids, and facial dysmorphism.[141] The conotruncal anomaly face syndrome is characterized by a variety of cardiac outflow tract defects such as tetralogy of Fallot, double-outlet right ventricle, and truncus arteriosus and distinct facies (hypertelorism, lateral displacement of the inner canthi, a flat nasal bridge, narrow palpebral fissures, a nasal voice, and minor ear anomalies).[136] However, substantial overlapping of clinical features subsequently was recognized among velocardiofacial syndrome, DiGeorge syndrome, and conotruncal anomaly face syndrome.

Using probes and cosmids from the DiGeorge critical region to perform DNA dosage analysis and fluorescence in situ hybridization, Hall recognized deletions of 22q11 among 83% of DiGeorge Syndrome patients, 68% of Shprintzen syndrome patients, and 29% of sporadic non-syndromic conotruncal patients.[142] FISH of metaphase chromosomes

using cosmid probes from the DiGeorge chromosomal region has been an efficient method for the detection of 22q11 deletions in at-risk patients, families, and pregnancies.[143]

The acronym CATCH-22 (**c**ardiac defects, **a**bnormal facies, **t**hymic hypoplasia, **c**left palate, and **h**ypocalcemia on chromosome **22**) was coined to encompass the various clinical presentations.[144] The cardiac defects implied in CATCH-22 are interrupted aortic arch (particularly type B), persistent truncus arteriosus, tetralogy of Fallot, patent ductus arteriosus, double-outlet right ventricle, transposition of the great arteries, aortic coarctation, and ventricular septal defect. Recently, nine families with at least two members affected by congenital heart defects were reported.[145] Five families had deletions of the DiGeorge critical region, demonstrating that deletions within 22q11 are likely to be an important cause of a familial congenital heart defect.[145,146]

The genetic basis of cardiac morphogenesis is poorly understood; the conotruncal cardiac defects of CATCH-22 syndrome may result from an altered interaction between neural crest cells[147] and elements of the phalangeal arches. New genes isolated recently within 22q11.2 may ultimately be shown to play a role in the expression of some phenotypic features observed in association with deletions of 22q11.[148] It appears that a very important gene or genes on conotruncal development of the heart lie in the 22q11 region.[142]

Sex Chromosome Anomalies (Table 49.4)[149–151]

Turner Syndrome[2,152] About 45–60% of the cases are 45,X. Others are 45,X/46,XX and other mosaicisms or X chromosome structural aberrations (such as isochromosome and X/autosome translocation). A missing X chromosome produces a distinctive phenotype, often called "Turner stigmata" (streak gonads or gonadal dysgenesis, short stature, and other somatic anomalies).

The approximate incidence of Turner syndrome is 1 in 2500 live female births.[153] About 1% of all conceptions have Turner syndrome, 98–99% of which abort spontaneously.

The birth weight is usually lower than normal. The height is short throughout life. Most patients have normal or near normal intelligence. Nevertheless, deficiencies in space–form perception and visual motor deficits are frequently present.[154]

Craniofacial features include antimongoloid slant of the eyes, receding chin, highly arched palate, and low-set ears. The neck is short, with either redundant skin on the nape or a webbed appearance. Cystic hygroma of the neck is present in many 45,X abortuses. Posterior hairline is low.

The chest appears shieldlike. Although some patients have distally displaced nipples, the appearance of wide-set nipples in most patients is an optical illusion.[155] Renal anomalies are also frequent: The most common anomaly is a horseshoe or ectopic kidney, followed by ureteral duplication or absent kidney.

Although ovaries contain primordial follicles during the

TABLE 49.3   Cardiac Lesions and Noncardiac Manifestations of Autosomal Deletion Syndromes[2,36]

Autosomal Deletion Syndrome	Cardiac Lesions[a]	Noncardiac Manifestations
Monosomy 1p[105]	VSD, TOF, PS, CM	Microcephaly, large fontanel, small palpebral fissures, cleft lip/palate, depressed nasal bridge, low-set ears, growth failure, mental retardation
Monosomy 1q[106]	PTA, VSD	Psychomotor/growth retardation, microcephaly, asgenesis of corpus callosum, round face, "cupid's bow," downturned corners of mouth, smooth philtrum, short nose, epicanthal folds, low-set ears, micrognathia, genital anomalies, neural tube defects, abnormal hands and feet
Monosomy 2q[107]	PS, COA, ASD, TAPVR, VSD	Psychomotor/growth retardation, hypoplastic midface, small nose, long philtrum, narrow vermillion border, microphthalmia, cleft palate, limb anomalies (syndactlyly, ectrodactyly
Monosomy 3p[108]	VSD, ASD	Psychomotor retardation, microcephaly, blepharoptosis, epicanthal folds, hypertelorism, ptosis, prominent nose, long philtrum, downturned mouth, micrognathia, ear anomalies, abnormal muscle tone, polydactyly, rocker-bottom feet, umbilical hernia, cryptorchidism, urinary tract anomalies
Monosomy 3q[109]	VSD	Growth/developmental delay, microcephaly, telecanthus, broad nasal bridge, blepharophimosis, ptosis, large malformed ears, prominent, beaked nasal tip, abnormal fingers/toes, equinovarus foot deformity
Monosomy 4p (Wolf–Hirschhorn)[110]	ASD, VSD, PS, AA, PDA, DC, TOF, TA	Psychomotor/growth retardation, microcephaly, triangular-shaped nasal root/ flat facial profile resembling a Greek warrior helmet, large/simple ears, micrognathia, cleft lip/palate, hip dislocations, hypospadias, cryptorchidism, hypoplastic scrotum, micropenis, talipes equinovarus
Monosomy 4q[111]	VSD, ASD, PDA, PA, PS, TA, TOF, COA	Psychomotor/growth retardation, hypotonia, abnormal skull shape, hypertelorism, short/upturned nose, depressed nasal bridge, cleft palate, Pierre–Robin anomaly, malformed ears, genital/digital anomalies
Monosomy 5p (cri-du-chat)[112]	VSD, ASD, PDA	Mental retardation, microcephaly, "catlike" cry secondary to larynx hypoplasia, failure to thrive, round/moon-shaped facies, epicanthal folds, hypertelorism, antimongoloid slant of eyes, micro/retrognathia, large ears, preauricular tags, small hands/feet, hip dislocation, urogenital anomalies
Monosomy 6p[113]	ASD, VSD, PDA	Mental retardation, microcephaly, abnormal skull sutures, flat/broad nasal bridge, eye/ear abnormalities, pectus excavatum, short neck with excess skin folds, palatal/genital abnormalities
Monosomy 6q[114]	ASD, VSD, PDA, DV, DORV, AVC, CTA	Psychomotor/growth retardation, microcephaly, round face, hypertelorism, short palpebral fissures, epicanthus, broad nasal tip, long philtrum, thin lips, micrognathia, high arched/cleft palate, malformed ears
Monosomy 7p[115]	TOF, VSD, PDA, PA	Psychomotor retardation, craniostenosis, abnormal skull shape, flat nasal bridge, low-set malformed ears, urogenital/digital anomalies
Monosomy 7q[116]	VSD, TA, ASD, RAA, PLSVC, PS, PDA, AS, APV, HPA	Psychomotor retardation, hypotonia, microcephaly, holoprosencephaly, prominent forehead, hypotelorism, micrognathia, broad nasal bridge, male genital anomalies, absent adrenal gland, caudal regression
Monosomy 8p[117]	AVC, PS, VSD	Psychomotor/growth retardation, microcephaly, epicanthal folds, malformed ears, short neck, increased internipple distance
Monosomy 8q[118]	VSD, PDA	Psychomotor/growth retardation, prominent forehead, wide nasal bridge, hypertelorism, eye abnormalities, small nose, "carp-shaped" mouth, micrognathia, abnormal ears, digital anomalies, craniostenosis
Monosomy 9p[119]	VSD, PDA, PS	Trigonocephaly, upward-slanting palpebral fissures, long philtrum, stunted nasal tip, short/webbed neck, dolichomesophalangy, excess digital whorls
Monosomy 9q[120]	VSD, PDA	Developmental delay, malformed ears, unusually shaped nares
Monosomy 10p[121]	PS, ASD, BAV, PDA, VSD, TA	Psychomotor/growth retardation, frontal bossing, hypertelorism, epicanthal folds, down-slanted/short palpebral fissures, ptosis, depressed nasal bridge, micrognathia, abnormal philtrum, ear anomalies, short neck, wide-spaced nipples, renal anomalies, cryptorchidism
Monosomy 10q[122]	TOF, TA, DORV, DAA, PDA, AS, VSD	Psychomotor retardation, absence of corpus callosum, facial/urogenital anomalies, limb defects
Monosomy 11p[123]	HCM	Aniridia–Wilms' tumor association, glaucoma, cataracts, megacornea, nystagmus, ptosis, catalase deficiency, mental retardation

TABLE 49.3 *(Continued)*

Autosomal Deletion Syndrome	Cardiac Lesions[a]	Noncardiac Manifestations
Monosomy 11q[124]	VSD, HLV, TGV, PS, SV, TA, TOF, MA	Intrauterine growth retardation, microcephaly, trigonocephaly, epicanthal folds, up-slanting palpebral fissures, hypertelorism, ptosis, iris coloboma, depressed nasal bridge, short/bulbous nose, everted lips, cleft lip/palate, micro/retrognathia, low-set/dysplastic ears, thrombocytopenia
Monosomy 12p[125]	HRV, VSD, COA	Psychomotor/growth retardation, hypotonia, microcephaly, narrow forehead, long nose, retrognathia, large/low-set ears
Monosomy 13q[126]	ASD, VSD, TOF, PDA, TA, COA	Psychomotor/growth retardation, CNS malformations, retinoblastoma, minor dysmorphic facies, GI/renal/limb/digital anomalies
Monosomy 14q[127]	ASD, ASD, PAPVR, BAV	Psychomotor/growth retardation, microcephaly, small palpebral fissures, bushy eyebrows, small upturned nose, carplike mouth, micrognathia, abnormal ears, skeletal anomalies
Monosomy 17p (Smith–Magenis)[128]	VSD, ASD	Psychomotor/growth retardation, brachycephaly, midface hypoplasia, prognathism, hoarse voice, hearing loss, speech delay, behavior problems
Monosomy 17q[129]	ASD	Developmental delay, round face, up-slanted palpebral fissures, low-set ears, long philtrum, micrognathia, skeletal anomalies (symphalangism)
Monosomy 18p[130]	VSD, TOF, PDA, COA, AVC, TAV	Mental retardation, short stature, microcephaly, holoprosencephaly, round face, hypertelorism, ptosis, strabismus, epicanthal folds, broad nose, large ears, carp-shaped mouth, micro/retrognathia, short/webbed neck, micropenis, cryptorchidism
Monosomy 18q[131]	ASD, PS, PDA, VSD	Psychomotor/growth retardation, microcephaly, midfacial hypoplasia, deep-set eyes, short nose, cheek dimples, absent columella, carplike mouth, prognathism, abnormal ears, atretic ear canals, cleft lip/palate, hypoplastic genitalia, skeletal anomalies, absent/decreased IgA
Monosomy 20p[132]	PS, PDA, VSD, TOF, LSVC	Chronic cholestasis due to intrahepatic bilary hypoplasia (Allergille syndrome), psychomotor/growth retardation, hearing loss, hypotonia, prominent forehead, hypertelorism, down-slanting palpebral fissures, deep-set eyes, micrognathia, palatal/vertebral arch/skeletal anomalies
Monosomy 21[133]	COA, PDA	Intrauterine growth retardation, antimongoloid slant of palpebral fissures, broad nasal bridge, large nose, large pinnae, micrognathia, cleft lip/palate, flexed overlapping fingers, kyphoscoliosis, short thorax, narrow pelvis, hypertonicity, foot deformities
Monosomy 22q (text)	VR, IAA, HPA, HT, TOF, VSD, APV	Include syndromes of Shprintzen, DiGeorge, conotruncal anomaly face, conotruncal congenital heart anomalies, absent pulmonary valve, and Opitz GBBB

[a]For abbreviations, see chapter appendix.

prenatal and perinatal period, they are replaced by yellowish-white streaks that contain no follicles by the time of puberty. Inadequate secretion of ovarian steroids (estrogens and androgens) leads to sexual infantilism: infantile external genitalia, sparse and fine pubic hair, underdeveloped axillary hair, underdeveloped breasts, and relatively small uterus and vagina. Primary amenorrhea is the rule. However, spontaneous menstruation occurs in about 5% of patients; some of these women can even give birth. The presence of a Y chromosome in 45,X/46,XY individuals predisposes to gonadoblastoma formation in the gonadal streaks, with a broad spectrum of clinical manifestation from typical Turner syndrome stigmata to a normal male phenotype.

Kyphoscoliosis, cubitus valgus, short fourth metacarpals, and nail hypoplasia may be present. Lymphedema is often present in the dorsum of the hands and feet during the newborn period. Pigmented nevi are commonly present. Patients may be particularly prone to develop thyroid autoantibodies and other concomitant autoimmune disorders.

The occurrence of cardiovascular anomalies in patients with Turner syndrome is well recognized.[156] Indeed, 80–95% of those exhibiting turner syndrome have various cardiovascular anomalies, the most common one being coarctation of the aorta. Other cardiac anomalies include bicuspid aortic valve, aortic stenosis, and hypoplastic left heart syndrome. The most serious complication, fortunately an uncommon one, is aortic dissection, secondary to coarctation of the aorta, aortic valve abnormalities, and hypertension. Telangiectasia of the small intestine may be present and may lead to gastrointestinal bleeding. Other rare vascular malformations include lymphangiectasia, hemangiomas, and venous ectasias.

TABLE 49.4   Cardiac Lesions and Noncardiac Manifestations of Sex Chromosome and Polyploidy Syndromes

Syndrome	Cardiac Lesions[a]	Noncardiac Manifestations
Fragile X (text)	ARD, MVP	Mental retardation, abnormal behavior, long face, large/prominent ears, prognathism, macroorchidism, hyperextensible finger joints, pectus carinatum, high-arched palate, flat feet
Klinefelter (47,XXY and variants)[149]	MVP, TOF	Tall stature, inadequate sexual development at puberty, sterility, gynecomastia, occasional hypospadias, skeletal abnormalities (decreased upper/lower body segment ratio, long arm span, radioulnar synostosis, coxa valga, clinodactyly, pes planus), venous thromboembolic disease
Penta X (49, XXXXX)[150]	VSD, PDA, COA	Psychomotor/growth retardation, microcephaly, hypertelorism, epicanthal folds, up-slanting palpebral fissures, low nasal bridge, flat nose, micrognathia, dental anomalies, dislocated hips, elbows, wrists, radioulnar synostosis, clinodactyly, ovarian dysgenesis
Tretraploidy (92, XXXX; 92, XXYY)[151]	TOF, HRV, VSD	Psychomotor/growth retardation, microcephaly, prominent/narrow forehead, microphthalmia, iris coloboma, hypertelorism, beaked nose, short philtrum, bifid uvula, micrognathia, low-set/malformed ears, preauricular tags, CNS malformations, hypoplastic lungs, genitourinary/skeletal anomalies, spina bifida
Triploidy (text)	VSD, ASD, PDA, TA	Lethal, prematurity, low birth weight, large hydatidiform placenta, "cracked eggshell" feeling of skull, enlarged posterior fontanel, hypertelorism, epicanthal folds, anophthalmia/microphthalmia, coloboma, cataracts, cleft lip/palate, micrognathia, low-set/malformed ears, short neck, CNS malformations, urogenital anomalies, cutaneous syndactyly between 3rd and 4th digits
Turner (45,X) (text)	COA, BAV, AS, HLH, AD, VSD, ASD, DC	Short stature, antimongoloid slanting eyes, receding chin, high-arched palate, low-set ears, short/webbed neck, cystic hygroma, low posterior hairline, shield chest, increased internipple distance, renal anomalies, streak gonads, sexual infantilism, primary amenorrhea, sterility, lymphedema of hands/feet, cubitus valgus, short 4th metacarpals, nail hypoplasia, telangiectasia of small intestine, lymphangiectasia, hemangioma

[a]For abbreviations, see chapter appendix.

There is a significant difference in the prevalence of cardiovascular malformations between 45,X and mosaic monosomy X (38% to 11%), primarily because there is a significant difference in the prevalence of aortic valve abnormalities and aortic coarctation.[157] Pulmonary valve abnormalities are seen only in females with mosaic monosomy X, but the prevalence is low (3%).

Embryos and fetuses affected with Turner syndrome are frequently recognized in utero, particularly when the pregnancy is complicated or prenatal ultrasonography is performed. The presence of fetal edema or hydrops, particularly associated with a septated nuchal mass (cystic hygroma), suggests the diagnosis of Turner syndrome, and amniocentesis or chorionic villus sampling is indicated to confirm Turner syndrome or other chromosomal abnormality.

Fragile X Syndrome   The fragile X (Martin–Bell) syndrome is the most common cause of inherited mental retardation. It is observed in approximately one in 1200 males and one is 2500 females. Males with the fragile X syndrome usually have mental retardation, abnormal behavior, and certain physical characteristics, which include long face, large/prominent ears, prognathism, macroorchidism, hyperextensible finger joints, pectus carinatum, a high-arched palate,

flat feet, and cardiac defects. The females are usually less severely affected.

Recently, a fragile X gene (*FMR1*) has been characterized and found to contain a tandemly repeated trinucleotide sequence (CGG) near its 5′ end. The ranges of the numbers of repeats in the normal, carrier, and affected individuals are 6–50 (normal), 50–200 (premutation), and more than 200 (full mutation), respectively.

Males and females carrying premutations are not affected. Male carriers, called "normal transmitting" males, pass the mutation, relatively unchanged in size, to all their daughters, who are at risk of having affected offspring. Most but not all of the males who carry the full mutation are affected; approximately one-third of the females who carry the full mutation have normal intelligence, one-third are borderline in intelligence, and one-third are mentally retarded.

Patients with the fragile X syndrome have cardiac defects similar to those seen in other disorders of connective tissue such as Marfan syndrome and Ehlers–Danlos syndrome. An aortic root dilatation is present in 52% of patients with fragile X syndrome, and 22% have mitral valve prolapse.[158]

The standard laboratory test used in the past to identify individuals affected with the fragile X syndrome was a search for the fragile site at band Xq27.3 by means of chromosome analysis. Although such studies may occasionally be useful, the current method of choice is direct DNA analysis to identify affected individuals, supplemented by carrier testing of their unaffected relatives.[159] Prenatal testing of a fetus is indicated following a positive carrier test in the mother. When the mother is a known carrier, DNA testing should be offered to determine whether the fetus inherited the normal or mutant *FMR1* gene. Testing by means of chorionic villus sampling must be interpreted with caution, since the methylation status of the *FMR1* gene is incomplete in chorionic villi in the first trimester and follow-up amniocentesis and fetal blood sampling may be needed.[160]

Polyploidy Syndromes

Triploidy Syndrome[2]   Triploidy is one of the major chromosomal abnormalities in spontaneous abortions (10–20%). It is only rarely encountered in human live births.[161] Pure triploidy has the karyotype 69,XXX, 69,XXY, or 69,XYY. Patients with triploidy syndrome seldom survive more than several months. Those who live beyond the neonatal period into childhood and early adolescence are diploid/triploid mosaics.

The infants are born prematurely, with low birth weight. A large and hydatidiform placenta is characteristic. Craniofacial features are the following: "cracked eggshell" feeling on palpation of skull, enlarged posterior fontaneles, hypertelorism, epicanthal folds, anophthalmia/microphthalmia, vertically ovoid corneae with colobomata, cataracts, facial asymmetry, cleft lip/palate, macroglossia, micrognathia, low-set and malformed ears, and short neck. CNS manifestations include mental retardation, hypotonia, absent corpus callosum, holoprosencephaly, partial aplasia of the falx cerebri, hydrocephaly, Arnold–Chiari malformation, encephalocele, and meningomyelocele. Urogenital anomalies include cryptorchidism, aplastic or bifid scrotum, microphallus, hypospadias, hypoplasia of gonads, dysplastic seminiferous tubules, dysplastic or cystic kidneys, and hydronephrosis. Cutaneous syndactyly between the third and fourth fingers is characteristic. Long fingers with bulbous tips, talipes equinovarus, hallucal hypoplasia, malimplantation of toes, and partial aplasia of the sternum also may be present.

Most diploid/triploid mosaic infants present a milder but clinically recognizable malformation pattern: mental and growth retardation, facial or body asymmetry, malformed or apparently low-set ears, syndactyly of the third and fourth fingers, and ambiguous genitalia in genetic males. Longer survival of these children is due to absence of severe cardiac, renal, and brain anomalies.

Congenital heart defects are commonly present.[162] They include ventricular septal defect (most common), atrial septal defect, patent ductus arteriosus, and truncus arteriosus. Ectopia cordis in a triploid fetus was detected by transvaginal color Doppler ultrasonography and chorionic villus sam-

pling in the first trimester.[163] Using FISH of chromosome-specific probe to interphase nuclei, 14 cases of triploidy were rapidly diagnosed from uncultured amniotic fluid cells.[164]

SINGLE-GENE DISORDERS (Table 49.5[166–201])

A single mutant gene is responsible for 5–10% of congenital heart defects.[202] Single-gene (Mendelian) disorders occur in approximately 1% of all live births. Single-gene disorders are caused by a single mutant gene that is transmitted to the offspring in one of the following ways: autosomal dominant, autosomal recessive, X-linked dominant, and X-linked recessive.

Connective Tissue Disorders/Skeletal Dysplasias Affecting the Heart

Marfan Syndrome[203,204]   Marfan syndrome (MIM 154700) is an autosomal dominant connective tissue disorder with wide variability in clinical expression. It is extremely pleiotropic in that most organ systems and tissues are affected. About 60–80% of patients have an affected parent; new mutations account for the remainder of cases.

The patient is usually tall and thin. The limbs are disproportionately long compared with the trunk (dolichostenomelia). The ratio of upper segment to lower segment is reduced. Arachnodactyly is a very common feature. The following simple maneuvers may be of help in demonstrating the presence of arachnodactyly: the thumb sign (it is positive if the thumb, when completely opposed within the clenched hand, projects beyond the ulnar border); the wrist sign (it is positive if the distal phalanges of the first and fifth digits of one hand overlap when wrapped around the opposite wrist).

Scoliosis is present in about 40–60% of cases. Other musculoskeletal abnormalities include pectus excavatum/carinatum, joint laxity, and inguinal hernias. Hypotonia is frequent.

Subluxation of the lens (ectopia lentis, predominantly dislocated upward) is present in about 50–80% of cases. Other ocular complications include myopia, glaucoma, and retinal detachment. Abnormal palatal growth causes a high, narrow palate, with crowding of the incisors.

The extent of cardiovascular involvement in Marfan syndrome is often underestimated. In addition to auscultation, echocardiography permits noninvasive detection of the cardiovascular structural changes and their functional consequences. Almost all affected persons have mitral valve prolapse, and 40–80% show aortic root enlargement or both on echocardiography, despite normal auscultatory findings on cardiac examination.[205–207] The most common cardiovascular complications are aortic dilatation, aortic aneurysms, aortic dissection, and aortic valve insufficiency, all of which are related to degeneration of the aortic media. Dissection of the ascending aorta is the leading cause of morbidity and mor-

TABLE 49.5 **Genetics (Autosomal and X Chromosome Dominance, and Recessivity), Cardiac Lesions and Noncardiac Manifestations of Single-Gene Disorders/Syndromes**

Disorder/Syndrome (MIM number)	Genetics	Cardiac Lesions[a]	Noncardiac Manifestations
Connective Tissue Disorders/Skeletal Dysplasias Affecting the Heart			
Apert (acrocephalosyndactyly) (101200)[166]	AD	VSD, TOF, COA	Craniostenosis, acrocephaly, high/prominent/steep forehead, hypoplastic midfaces, mandibular prognathism, wide-set eyes, shallow orbits, proptosis, antimongoloid slants, strabismus, optic atrophy, keratoconus, ectopia lentis, congenital glaucoma, depressed nasal bridge, beaked nose, malocclusion/supernumerary/teeth, high-arched/cleft palate, syndactyly, stubby/deformed big toes
Beals (congenital contractural arachnodactyly) (121050)[167]	AD	ARD, MVP, MR	Flexion joint contractures of fingers/elbows/knees, arachnodactyly, kyphoscoliosis, osteopenia, pectus excavatum/carinatum, asthenic/Marfanoid habitus, hypotonia, "crumpled" ears, high palate, retrognathia
Beemer–Langer (short rib-polydactyly) (269860)[168]	AR	PDA, VSD, ASD, AA, COA, TGV	Hydrops, ascites, median cleft of upper lip, narrow chest, short ribs, short/bowed limbs with or without polydactyly
Carpenter (acrocephalopoly-syndactyly) (201000)[166]	AD	PDA, VSD, ASD, PS, TGV	Craniostenosis, acro/oxybrachycephaly, polysyndactyly, short stature, short hands, broad thumbs, other skeletal changes, obesity, mental deficiency, flat/broad face, exophthalmos, epicanthal folds, low-set/malformed ears, high-arched palate, micrognathia
Cutis laxa (123700; 219100)[169]	AR, AD	PPAS, ARD, CP, AOA, MVP	Growth retardation, pulmonary emphysema, wide cranial sutures/fontanel, hypertelorism, epicanthal folds, hooked nose, long upper lip, short columella, long ear lobes, ectropion of lids, blue sclerae, microcornea, macular colobomas, micrognathia, laxity of vocal cord, loose and pendulous skin folds, senile appearance, GI/bladder diverticulum, gastric/rectum/uterus prolapse, redundant vagina, congenital hip dislocation, hyperextensible joints, hypotonia
Ehlers–Danlos (types I–XI) (130000, 130010, 130020, 305200, 225350, 130060, 225410, 130080, 304150, 225310)[170]	AR, AD, XR	MVP, TVP, ARD, DA, VSD, PS, ASD, TOF, AAA, ARR	Skin fragility, hyperextensible but not lax skin, joint hypermobility, epicanthal folds, flat nasal bridge, lop/stretchable ears, eyes (myopia, microcornea, blue sclerae, ocular fragility, everted upper eyelids), periodontitis, skin scars, ureteropelvic anomalies, emphysema, pneumothorax, diverticuli of GI/GU, arterial/bowel/uterine rupture, hernias, hypotonia, cardiopulmonary complications in infancy
Ellis–van Creveld (chondro-ectodermal dysplasia) (225500)[171]	AR	SA, ASD	Disproportionate short-limbed dwarfism, polydactyly, dysplastic fingernails, abnormal frenula between upper lip and alveolar process
Frontonasal dysplasia (136760, 305645)[172]	AD,XR	TOF, AS	Hypertelorism, prominent forehead, wide nasal bridge, clefting nasal tip (bifid nose), cleft upper lip, widow's peak, cranium bifidum occultum, arrhinencephaly
Homocystinuria (cystathionine synthetase deficiency) (236200)[173]	AR	AT, VT, CT, MI	Psychomotor retardation, seizures, tall stature, muscle weakness, livedo reticularis, sparse fair hair, malar flushing, progressive downward dislocation of ocular lens, pectus deformities, scoliosis, genu valgum, pes planus, osteoporosis, thromboembolic episodes
Larsen (150250, 245600, 245650)[174]	AD, AR	ARD, AR	Multiple joint dislocation (elbows, hips, knees, wrists), flat facies, prominent forehead, hypertelorism, depressed nasal bridge, cleft palate, long nontapering fingers, multiple carpal ossification centers, club feet
Lethal multiple pterygium (253290)[175]	AR	HH, ASD	Multiple pterygium, hydrops, cystic hygroma, spinal/bone fusions, hypoplastic lungs
Marfan (154700) (text)	AD	MVP, MI, ARD, AA, AI, AD	Dolichostenomelia, arachnodactyly, musculoskeletal abnormalities (scoliosis, pectus, joint laxity, inguinal hernias, hypotonia), ocular anomalies (ectopia lentis, myopia, glaucoma, retinal detachment)
Osteogenesis imperfecta (166200; 166210, 259400; 259200; 166220)[176]	AR, AD	MVP, MR, ARD, ARC, CP	Multiple bone fractures from minimal trauma; type I (blue sclerae, bone fragility, little or no deformity, hearing loss); type II (severe bone deformity, extreme bone fragility, blue sclerae, perinatal death); type III (progressive bone deformity, normal sclerae, severe bone fragility, severe short stature, rare hearing loss, with or without

TABLE 49.5   *(Continued)*

Disorder/Syndrome (MIM number)	Genetics	Cardiac Lesions[a]	Noncardiac Manifestations
			dentinogenesis imperfecta); type IV (normal sclerae, bone fragility, variable short stature, mild bone deformity, rare hearing loss, dentinogenesis imperfecta)
Pena–Shokeir (208150)[177]	AR	HH	Fetal akinesia sequence, camptodactyly, multiple ankyloses, hypertelorism, epicanthal folds, depressed nasal tip, micro/retrognathia, high-arched/cleft palate, low-set/malformed ears, pulmonary hypoplasia, multiple pterygia, ankylosis, club feet, fractures from osteopenia
Pseudoxanthoma elasticum (177850, 264800)[178]	AD, AR	ARC, A, AAC, RCM, MVP, MI, CI	Xanthoma-like skin lesions, impaired vision, angioid streaks of retina, hemorrhage (GI, retina, kidneys, bladder, uterus, nose, joints, subarachnoid space), abdominal pain, systemic hypertension
Spondylothoracic dysostosis Jarcho–Levin) (277300)[179]	AR	DC, ASD, VSD, OA, PA	Severe costospinal anomalies, short neck/trunk, urogenital/anal anomalies, respiratory insufficiency
Stickler (arthroophthalmyopathy (108300)[180]	AD	MVP	Progressive myopia resulting in retinal detachment/blindness, hearing deficits, cleft palate, Pierre–Robin anomaly, premature degenerative changes in joints with epiphyseal/vertebral anbormalities

Other Single-Gene Disorders Affecting the Heart and the Cardiac Rhythm

Aarskog–Scott (305400)[181]	XD	VSD, PS, COA, AS, AI	Short stature, fetal face, hypertelorism, down-slanting eyes, short stubby nose, anteverted nostril, widow's peak, syndactyly, inguinal hernia, cryptorchidism, shawl scrotum, short hands/feet
Adams–Oliver (100300)[182]	AD	ASD, MVP, VSD, TOF, PA	Aplasia cutis congenita, terminal digital anomalies, microcephaly, epilepsy, mental retardation, arrhinencephaly, hydrocephaly, bronchial/renal anomalies
Alagille (arteriohepatic) (118450)[183]	AD	PS, ASD, VSD, COA, TOF	Peculiar facies (broad forehead, pointed mandible, bulbous nasal tip), chronic cholestasis, posterior embryotoxon, vertebral defects, psychomotor/growth retardation, skeletal/renal anomalies
Asymmetric crying face (125520)[184]	AD	TOF, VSD	Unilateral hypoplasia of depressor anguli oris muscle causing unilateral partial facial paresis and asymmetric crying facies
Bardet–Biedl (209900)[185]	AR	DCM	Polydactyly, obesity (usually trunk), pigmentary retinopathy, mental retardation, hypogonadism, hypogenitalism, renal involvement
Beckwith–Wiedemann (130650)[186]	AD	ASD, VSD, HLH, PDA, TOF, COA, PS	Congenital overgrowth, macroglossia, abdominal wall defect (omphalocele, hernia), nephromegaly, hypoglycemia, hemihypertrophy, developmental delay, polydactyly, neoplasia
Cardiofacio-cutaneous (115150)[187]	AD	PS, ASD	Relative macrocephaly, stunted growth, ectodermal dysplasia, characteristic facies (hypoplastic supraorbital ridges, epicanthal folds, downward-slant eyes), psychomotor retardation, sparse curly hair, ichthyosis, keratosis pilaris, palmoplantar keratoderma
Faciocardiorenal (Eastman–Bixler) (227280)[188]	AR	SECFE, CD	Face (plagiocephaly, broad nasal root, malar hypoplasia, stiff outstanding pinnae, hypoplastic philtrum, thin vermillion), mental retardation, horseshoe kidneys
Fryns (229850)[189]	AR	AAA, VSD, ASD, PLSVC	Abnormal facies, cleft lip/palate, small thorax, wide-spaced/hypoplastic nipples, distal limb/nail hypoplasia, diaphragmatic hernia, pulmonary hypoplasia, GI/urorenal anomalies, CNS malformations
Generalized arterial calcification (208000)[190]	AR	CAO, MI	Mineralized internal elastica lamina of small-to-large arteries, narrowing of arterial lumen
Holt–Oram (heart–hand) (142900) (text)	AD	ASD, VSD, NVP, ODA, AVC, LPRI, SB, NER	Upper limb anomalies (absent/hypoplastic/dysplastic thumbs/carpals/metacarpals/radius)
Ivemark (cardiosplenic) (208530)[191]	AR	TGV, PS, PA, TAPVR, AVC, CV, DC, BSVC, ACS	Spleen agenesis, situs inversus, thoracic isomerism, GI (hiatal hernia, incomplete rotation of intestine, volvulus, imperforate anus, diaphragmatic hernia, agenesis of gallbladder), GU (renal dysplasia, cystic kidneys), endocrine (unilateral absence of adrenal gland) anomalies

(Continued)

TABLE 49.5 (Continued)

Disorder/Syndrome (MIM number)	Genetics	Cardiac Lesions[a]	Noncardiac Manifestations
Kaufman–McKusick (236700)[192]	AR	ASD, VSD	Hydrometrocolpos, polydactyly, GI/GU anomalies
LEOPARD (151100) (text)	AD	CD, PS, AS, ECFE, HCM	Lentigines, ocular hypertelorism, anomalies of genitalia, growth retardation, sensorineural deafness, chest pain, dyspnea, syncope, palpitations
Meckel–Gruber (249000)[193]	AR	VSD, ASD, COA, PDA	Occipital encephalocele, multicystic kidneys, fibrocystic liver, polydactyly, cleft lip/palate, urinary tract anomalies, ambiguous genitals, club feet
Neurofibromatosis (NF1, von Recklinghausen) (162200) (text)	AD	CM, PS	Café-au-lait macules, neurofibromas, axillary/inguinal freckling, optic glioma, Lisch nodules, distinctive osseous lesions (sphenoid dysplasia, pseudarthrosis)
Noonan (163950) (text)	AD	PS, ASD, HCM, VSD, PDA, PAS, MVP, EC, SV	Short stature, mild mental retardation, epicanthal folds, down-slanting palpebral fissures, ptosis, hypertelorism, strabismus, low-set/posteriorly rotated ears, neck webbing, low posterior hairline, renal anomalies, cryptorchidism, skeletal deformities
Opitz GBBB (145410)[194]	AD	VSD, PDA, ASD, COA, VR, PLSVC, TOF	Hypertelorism, hypospadias, laryngotracheoesophageal defects, stridor, swallowing dysfunction, imperforate anus, urinary/CNS anomalies
PHAVER (261575)[195]	AD	VSD, ASD, HAA, DORV, PA	Limb pterygia, vertebral/radial defect, ear anomalies, meningomyelocele
Robinow (180700)[196]	AD, AR	RVOO	Mesomelic brachymelia, fetal face (frontal bossing, hypertelorism, wide palpebral fissures, short upturned broad nose with anteverted nares, long philtrum, small chin), hemivertebrae, genital hypoplasia
Rutledge lethal multiple congenital anomaly (268670)[197]	AR	HLH, COA, ASD	Polydactyly, sex reversal, renal hypoplasia, unilobular lung, cerebral, laryngeal and gallbladder hypoplasia
Simpson–Golabi–Behmel (312870)[198]	XR	VSD, CD	Overgrowth, coarse facies, dysplastic changes in several tissues, mild intellectual impairment
Smith–Lemli–Opitz (270400)[199]	AR	PDA, VSD, TOF, ARSA, ASD	Failure to thrive, mental retardation, prominent occiput, syndactyly, genital anomalies, reduced plasma cholesterol, increased plasma 7-dehydrocholesterol
Steinfeld (184705)[200]	AD	PT	Holoprosencephaly, micrognathia, cleft lip/palate, absent nose, dysplastic ears, radial deficiency, renal/vertebral/rib anomalies, absent gallbladder
Thrombocytopenia/absent asbsent radius (TAR) (274000)[201]	AD	ASD, TOF, DC	Bilateral radial aplasia, hypoplastic carpals/phalanges/ulnas, abnormal humeri, phocomelia, thrombocytopenia
Treacher Collins (154500)[166]	AD	VSD, PDA, ASD	Abnormal pinnae, atretic external auditory canals, middle ear ossicle anomalies, hearing loss, hypoplastic facial bones, downward slant of eyes, coloboma of lower eyelids, paucity of lid lashes medial to defect
Tuberous sclerosis (191000) (text)	AD	CRM, ECFE, AS, PS, CD, CP	Skin (adenoma sebaceum, hypopigmented and shagreen patches, café-au-lait spots), retinal hamartomas, poliosis, leukotrichia, fibroma (gum, palate, tongue, pharynx, larynx, sub/periungual), deep pits in tooth enamel, CNS (seizures, hypsarrhythmia, mental retardation), renal (cystic kidneys), lung (lymphangiomyomatosis, dyspnea, hemoptysis, pneumothorax), rhabdomyosarcomas
Romano–Ward (long QT) (192500) (text)	AD	PQTI, IT, VA, VF	Stress-induced/emotional syncope, family history of unexplained sudden death

[a]For abbreviations, see chapter appendix.

tality, accounting for 95% of deaths in untreated individuals in one large series.[208] Mitral valve prolapse and insufficiency may occur in more than 80% of young patients. Severe mitral regurgitation is the most common cause of cardiac decompensation in children. Cardiovascular disease is the most common cause of death (93%) in patients with Marfan syndrome.[209]

Some progress has been made in understanding the variability and pleiotropy at the molecular level.[210] Marfan syndrome is characterized by mutations of the fibrillin-1 (*FBN1*) gene and by abnormal patterns of synthesis, secretion, and matrix deposition of the fibrillin protein.[211,212] Fibrillin, a large glycoprotein (350 kDa), is a major building block of microfibrils, which represent the structural component of the suspensory ligament of the lens and serve as the substrate for elastin in the aorta and other elastic tissues.[213]

The mutations in the fibrillin gene that is located on chromosome 15q21 underlie the basis of classic Marfan syndrome.[214] Different fibrillin mutations are responsible for the genetic heterogeneity of Marfan syndrome. The phenotypic variability in the presence of the same fibrillin mutation suggests the importance of other, yet-to-be-identified factors that affect penetrance of the syndrome.[210] These findings suggest that identifying a given mutation may be of limited value in establishing the phenotype and clinical course of family members with the Marfan genotype.[13]

The requirement of a major manifestation of Marfan syndrome for the clinical diagnosis, even when there is an unequivocal family history, complemented by molecular analysis for those with atypical disease, should help optimize the assessment of cardiovascular risk in families in which the Marfan phenotype is segregated. Direct clinical application of molecular studies has resulted in successful efforts at presymptomatic and prenatal diagnosis.[215]

Other Single Gene Disorders Affecting the Heart and the Cardiac Rhythm

Holt–Oram (Heart–Hand) Syndromes   Holt–Oram syndrome (MIM 142900) is the prototypical heart–hand syndrome. It is an autosomal dominant disorder, characterized by various limb anomalies and congenital heart defects. Limb anomalies include absent, hypoplastic, or triphalangeal thumbs associated with absent, hypoplastic, or dysplastic carpals and metacarpals.[216] Hypoplastic, dysplastic, or synostosed radius may be present.

Upper limb malformations can also occur in patients with congenital heart disease in many multifactorial, chromosomal, genetic, or teratogenic syndromes.[217] Upper limb malformations are the most common skeletal abnormalities observed in patients with congenital heart defects. Recognition of upper limb malformations helps to identify the accompanying cardiac disease and aids in diagnosis so that appropriate therapeutic interventions and genetic counseling can be made.

The most common cardiac defects seen in patients with Holt–Oram syndrome are atrial septal defect and ventricular septal defect. Other cardiac lesions include mitral valve prolapse, patent ductus arteriosus, atrioventricular canal defect, long PR interval, sinus bradycardia, and nodal escape rhythm.[218]

Recently, the Holt–Oram syndrome gene defect was mapped to the long arm of human chromosome 12q2 in several families.[218,219] The role of this disease locus in the pathogenesis of related conditions such as heart–hand syndrome type III (cardiac conduction disease accompanied by skeletal malformations) or familial atrial septal defects is unknown.

LEOPARD Syndrome   LEOPARD syndrome (MIM 15110) is an autosomal dominant disorder, characterized by lentigines, electrocardiographic conduction abnormalities, ocular hypertelorism, pulmonic stenosis, anomalies of genitalia, growth retardation, and sensorineural deafness.[220] Clinical manifestations include chest pain, dyspnea, near syncope, syncope, and palpitations.

Cardiac abnormalities consist of not only anatomic malformations but also of electrocardiographic conduction defects.[221] Pulmonary valve stenosis is the most common cardiac lesion, followed by aortic stenosis, endocardial fibroelastosis, and hypertrophic cardiomyopathy.[222] The cardiac defects appear early in childhood and usually run a progressive course. The electrocardiographic conduction defects include prolonged P-R interval, left anterior hemiblock, widening of the QRS, and complete heart block. The effects of these conduction defects are widely variable, ranging from normal to sudden death.

Neurofibromatosis   Neurofibromatosis (NF), an autosomal dominant disorder characterized by café-au-lait spots and neurofibromatous tumors of the skin, is associated with many, variable, pleiotropic manifestations that may result in disfigurement and functional impairment.[223] It affects about 100,000 Americans. One baby in every 3000–4000 is born with NF. It is one of the most common mutations known in man, with the estimate as high as 10^{-4} mutations per gamete per generation. At least 50% of index cases represent new mutations.

Genetic heterogeneity exists in NF. Two major types of the disorder can be identified.

Classical or Peripheral NF (von Recklinghausen disease or NF1) (MIM 162200)   This is the most common (85–90%) and classical type, as originally described by von Recklinghausen. The discovery of two patients with NF1 and balanced translocations involving the long arm of chromosome 17 (17q11.2) suggested that the gene for NF1 might reside at 17q11.2,[224] precisely where *NF1* had been mapped by linkage analysis. The gene for NF1 is large, spanning approximately 300 kilobases of DNA on chromosome 17q11.2.[225] Neurofibromin, the protein product of the *NF1*, has been identified. The role of neurofibromin (guanosine triphosphatase activating protein) as a tumor suppressor gene product suggests a more general function of this protein in cells.

Central or Acoustic NF (NF2) (MIM 10100) This is a rare autosomal dominant trait. The most recent diagnostic criteria proposed for NF2 are bilateral acoustic neuromas or a first-degree relative with NF2 and either a unilateral eighth nerve mass or two of the following: meningioma, glioma, schwannoma, neurofibroma, and juvenile posterior subcapsular lenticular opacity.[226] The locus for the disease is near the center of the long arm of chromosome 22 (22q11.1-22q13.1).[227]

In 1987 a National Institutes of Health Consensus Development Conference Statement[226] identified the following diagnostic criteria for NF1:

1. Six or more café-au-lait macules, the greatest diameter of which is more than 5 mm in prepubertal patients and more than 15 mm in postpubertal patients.
2. Two or more neurofibromas of any type, or one plexiform neurofibroma.
3. Freckling in the axillary or inguinal region.
4. Optic glioma
5. Two or more Lisch nodules.
6. A distinctive osseous lesion such as sphenoid dysplasia or pseudarthrosis.
7. A first-degree relative with NF1 according to the preceding criteria.

Most of the patients with NF1 have café-au-lait spots, which are called by the French term for coffee (café) with milk (lait) because of their light tan color. The spots are usually present at birth but continue to increase in number and size during the first decade. Six or more café-au-lait spots exceeding 1.5 cm at the broadest diameter are pathognomonic for NF1. Five spots with a diameter of at least 0.5 cm should be considered diagnostic until proven otherwise. These criteria should not be considered as definitively diagnostic of NF1, but other features of NF1 should be sought.

Hyperpigmented patches may be associated with underlying plexiform neurofibromas, which are congenital in origin and may lead to extensive localized hypertrophy. Axillary freckles (smaller pigmented spots) are a helpful diagnostic criterion for NF1.

A plexiform neurofibroma may involve the eyelid, producing buphthalmos and asymmetric facial hypertrophy. Nonplexiform cutaneous neurofibromas may be variable in number (few to numerous), size (pea, grapefruit, or larger),

and shape (sessile, polypoid, or pedunculated). Neurofibromas of the areolae occur frequently in postpubertal females. Pruritus can be a prominent symptom. Osseous lesions (hemihypertrophy, spinal deformities, and congenital tibial pseudarthrosis) may be characteristic.

Neurofibromas are benign histologically but may result in functional compromise and cosmetic disfigurement. They may involve viscera, such as bowel, bladder, and liver, causing bleeding and obstruction. Lisch nodules (pigmented iris hamartomas) are characteristic and are present in 97% of postpubertal patients. Malignant tumors are known to occur. These include neurofibrosarcomas, malignant schwannomas, Wilms' tumor, rhabdomyosarcoma, and leukemias.

Although the occurrence of congenital heart defects may not be increased in patients with NF1, there are numerous reports of NF1 associated with cardiomyopathy.[223] In addition, the entire arterial tree, from the proximal aorta to the small arteries, may show involvement by the NF1 mutation.[228–230] Pulmonary stenosis has been seen in NF1 patients.[231]

Noonan Syndrome Noonan syndrome is an autosomal dominant disorder (MIM 163950) with highly variable expression. It is characterized by short stature, mild mental retardation, a unique facial appearance (epicanthal folds, down-slanting palpebral fissures, ptosis of eyelids, hypertelorism, strabismus, low-set, posteriorly rotated ears with thick helix), webbing of the neck, low posterior hairline, renal anomalies, cryptorchidism, skeletal deformities, and congenital heart defects. The incidence is estimated to be 1 in 2500 to 1 in 1000 individuals.[232] Noonan syndrome is likely to be the second most common syndrome with congenital heart defects after Down syndrome.[233]

About 50% of patients with Noonan syndrome[232,234] have congenital heart defects. The most common cardiac lesion is valvular pulmonic stenosis (60%), followed by atrial septal defect and eccentric hypertrophic cardiomyopathy (20%). Other cardiac lesions include ventricular septal defect, patent ductus arteriosus, pulmonary artery branch stenosis, mitral valve prolapse, Ebstein's anomaly, and single ventricle.

Tuberous Sclerosis[2] Tuberous sclerosis (TS) (MIM 191100) is inherited in an autosomal dominant fashion with high penetrance but variable expression and a high mutation rate.

Adenoma sebaceum usually develops at 2–8 years of age, with lesions becoming more numerous at puberty. These lesions are small reddish-brown papules with a characteristic butterfly distribution over the nose, nasolabial folds, and cheek areas. Histologically, they are angiofibromas rather than adenomas. About 86% of persons with TS have adenoma sebaceum.

Retinal hamartomas (phakomas) are characteristics of TS and are seen in about 50% of cases. Poliosis (premature graying of the hair) and leukotrichia (white hair) are common and are seen in eyebrows, eyelashes, and scalp. Oral fibromatous tumors are usually seen on gum and palate and rarely on tongue, pharynx, and larynx. Deep pits in tooth enamel, not found in normal individuals, occur in a larger number of cases of TS.

CNS signs and symptoms are the most outstanding presenting features: seizures, EEG abnormalities (nonspecific or hypsarrhythmia), mental retardation (60–85%), or schizophrenia and other disturbances in personality. Renal findings include enlarged cystic kidneys, flank pain, episodic hematuria, hemorrhage, and progressive renal failure.

Cutaneous lesions are the most common clinical signs of TS. In addition to adenoma sebaceum, the cutaneous lesions include hypopigmented patches, shagreen patches, café-au-lait spots, and subungual fibromata.

Hypopigmented patches are the early diagnostic signs of TS and may occur in 15–85% of cases. They are described as "mountain ash leaf" and may be observed, especially with the help of ultraviolet light, in the trunk or limbs. They are nonspecific for TS and may be noted also in other clinical conditions, such as nonpigmented nevi, vitiligo, and albinism.

Shagreen patches are slightly raised, flesh-colored, leathery plaques, commonly seen in the lumbosacral region. These patches are common (20–70%) and are highly characteristic of TS.

Subungual (or periungual) fibromas are diagnostic signs for TS and occur in about 17% of cases. Café-au-lait spots are also present occasionally and are less numerous than in neurofibromatosis. Pedunculated fibromas are typically located in the neck and axilla.

Pulmonary involvement is rare. Pulmonary lymphangiomyomatosis is currently considered to be a forme fruste of TS. The symptom may include dyspnea (most common), hemoptysis, pneumothorax, and cor pulmonale.

Computed tomography is the most sensitive and reliable radiographic method for diagnosis of TS. CT is often diagnostic if there are calcified (paraventricular) subependymal nodules encroaching on the lateral ventricle and calcified cortical or cerebellar nodules.

A routine urinalysis may reveal albuminuria or hematuria. Fluorescein angiography of the fundus should be performed to rule out retinal phakomas. Intravenous pyelograms, sonograms, angiograms, and CT may be indicated for the renal lesions. Echocardiograms can be diagnostic for cardiac lesions. EEGs are frequently abnormal.

About two-thirds of patients have cardiac rhabdomyoma.[235] These hamartomas are usually multiple, but their size and number tend to regress with age.[236] At least 50% of patients with cardiac rhabdomyoma have other evidence of tuberous sclerosis.[237] Most patients with these cardiac hamartomas remain asymptomatic; those who manifest cardiac dysfunction usually present soon after birth with cardiac failure.[238] Other cardiac lesions include endocardial fibro-

elastosis, aortic stenosis, pulmonary stenosis, arrhythmias, and sarcomas (including rhabdomyosarcomas). Ultrasonography or echocardiography can diagnose rhabdomyoma in utero.

Romano-Ward (Long QT) Syndrome Romano-Ward (long QT) syndrome (MIM 192500) is an autosomal dominant disorder characterized by stress-induced syncope, malignant ventricular arrhythmias, and ventricular fibrillation, and sudden death.[239,240] Characteristic ECG findings include an prolonged QT interval and inverted T waves. Clinical history of stress-induced or emotional syncope, a peculiar form of ventricular tachyarrhythmia known as *torsades de pointes,* a family history of unexplained sudden death, and low heart rate for age are among the diagnostic criteria for the long QT syndrome. Linkage analysis mapped the locus for this gene to 11p15.5[241] and 4q25-27.[242]

When prolonged QT interval in ECG and sudden death are associated with sensorineural deafness, the term "cardioauditory syndrome of Jervell and Lange-Nielsen" (MIM 220400) is applied.[243]

HEREDITARY METABOLIC CARDIOMYOPATHIES[244–247] (Table 49.6[248–270])

Hypertrophic and Dilated Cariomyopathies

Cardiomyopathies, a heterogeneous group of cardiac diseases designating primary myocardial disease of unknown etiology, are an important cause of morbidity and mortality (heart failure) affecting children and adults. The cardiomyopathies are also a major indication for cardiac transplantation.[271]

The term "idiopathic cardiomyopathy" is often used to describe primary myocardial disease of unknown causes and pathogenesis. Using clinical examination, chest radiography, electrocardiography, echocardiography, and hemodynamic studies, one can exclude congenital heart anomalies or acquired disease and help classify cardiomyopathies into dilated, hypertropic, and restrictive types.[272,273] Recent advances in molecular genetics and the application of these techniques to cardiovascular disease have significantly improved our understanding of the molecular basis of cardiomyopathies.[274] Localization and identification of disease genes of several inherited cardiomyopathies may afford new insights into the pathogenesis and classification of cardiomyopathies.[247]

Familial Hypertrophic Cardiomyopathy Hypertrophic cardiomyopathy is characterized by unexplained left ventricular hypertrophy predominantly in the interventricular septum, with or without right ventricular hypertrophy. The onset of symptoms occurs mostly in early adulthood, with

TABLE 49.6 Genetics (Autosomal and X Chromosome Dominance, and Recessivity), Cardiac Lesions and Noncardiac Manifestations of Hereditary Metabolic Cardiomyopathies

Disorder/Syndrome (MIM number)	Genetics	Cardiac Lesions[a]	Noncardiac Manifestations
Neuromuscular Disorders			
Becker muscular dystrophy (310200)[248]	XR	DCM	Mild functional disability (difficulty with running or climbing steps, cramps on exercise), proximal muscle weakness, prominence of calves, waddling gait, lordosis
Duchenne muscular dystrophy (310200) (text)	XR	DCM, CD	Progressive proximal muscle weakness by 3–5 years, Gower's sign, hyperlordosis, pseudohypertrophy especially of calves/thigh/buttock, confined to wheel chair by age 12
Emery–Dreifuss muscular dystrophy (310300)[249]	XR	CM, CD	Difficulty with walking/running, rigidity of neck or spine, early contractures of Achilles tendons, elbows, postcervical muscles; slowly progressive muscle wasting and weakness with predominant humeroperoneal distribution in the early stages
Friedreich ataxia (229300)[250]	AR	HCM, CD	Loss of deep tendon reflexes, limb ataxia, Babinski sign, cerebellar dysarthria, muscle wasting, nystagmus, optic atrophy, deafness, pes cavus
Limb–girdle muscular dystrophy (159000, 253600)[251]	AD, AR	DCM	Progressive myopathies mainly affecting muscles of hip/girdle and eventual involvement of distal muscles, difficulty with gait, running or climbing steps; cramps on exercise, abnormal gait, lordotic posture, deformities after loss of ambulation
Myotonic muscular dystrophy (160900) (text)	AD	DCM, CD	Myotonia, myopathic facies, ptosis, frontal balding in males, "tent-shaped" mouth, cataracts, muscle wasting in distal extremities/head/neck, infertility
Glycogen Storage Diseases			
Acid maltase deficiency (Pompe) (232300) (text)	AR	CM	Infantile form (fatal, macroglossia, failure to thrive, generalized hypotonia, progressive muscle weakness including respiratory muscle), childhood/juvenile/adult forms (milder)
Lysosomal glycogen storage disease with normal acid maltase (153360, 232330)[252]	XD, AD	HCM, AVNB	Myopathy, mental retardation, increasesd serum creatine kinase
Branching enzyme deficiency (232500)[253]	AR	DCM	Failure to thrive, hepatosplenomegaly, ascites, liver cirrhosis
Debrancher enzyme deficiency (232400)[254]	AR	AI, MR	Hepatomegaly, growth retardation, fasting hypoglycemia, seizures, benign course with tendency to remit spontaneously by puberty
Phosphorylase *b* kinase deficiency[255]	AR	DCM, HCM	Four variants: benign infantile hepatomegaly (XR); hepatomegaly, failure to thrive, hypotonia, mild weakness (AR); myopathy alone; fatal infantile dilated or hypertrophic cardiomyopathy
Disorders of Lipid Metabolism			
Carnitine palmitoyl transferase II deficiency (255110)[256]	AR	CM, CD	Infantile form (hypoketotic hypoglycemia); lethal neonatal form (nonketotic hypoglycemia, liver failure, dysmorphic features, sudden death)
Primary systemic carnitine deficiency (212140)[257]	AR, AD	HCM	Muscle weakness, motor delay, failure to thrive, anemia, hypoketotic hypoglycemic coma
Mitochondrial (Mt) Diseases Caused by Defects in Nuclear DNA			
Complex I deficiency, fatal form[258]	Mt	CM	Severe lactic acidosis, psychomotor delay, generalized hypotonia, weakness
Complex III deficiency[259]	Mt	CM	Myopathy, encephalopathy
Complex IV (cytochrome *c* oxidase) deficiency[260]	Mt	HCM	Myopathy (severe generalized weakness at or soon after birth, respiratory distress, lactic acidosis), brain dysfunction (Leigh syndrome,

TABLE 49.6   *(Continued)*

Disorder/Syndrome (MIM number)	Genetics	Cardiac Lesions[a]	Noncardiac Manifestations
			myoclonic epilepsy with ragged red fibers, Menkes disease), progressive external ophthalmoplegia (ocular myopathy or Kearns–Sayre syndrome)
Complex V deficiency[261]	Mt	HCM	Congenital lactic acidosis, respiratory distress, 3-methylglutaconic aciduria
Combined deficiency of respiratory chain enzymes[262]	Mt	HCM	Myopathy, progressive muscular hypotonia, severe lactic acidosis, Sengers syndrome (complex I/IV defects, congenital hypotonia, easy fatiguability, cataracts, lactic acidosis)
Mitochondrial Diseases Caused by Defects in Mitochondrial DNA			
Kearns–Sayre syndrome (text)	Mt, AD	HB, DCM	Progressive external ophthlmoplegia, atypical pigmentary retinopathy, cerebellar ataxia, elevated cerebrospinal fluid protein, cranial nerve involvement, stunted growth, hearing loss, proximal muscular weakness, "ragged red" myopathy
Mitochondrial DNA point mutations[263]	Mt	CM	Myopathy
Leigh syndrome (subacute necrotizing encephalo-myelopathy)[264]	Mt, AR, XR	HCM	Devastating encephalopathy of infancy or early childhood, lactic acidosis
Other Metabolic Cardiomyopathies			
GM1 gangliosidosis (β-galactosidase deficiency) (230500, 230600, 230650)[265]	AR	CM, MI, ECFE	Infantile form (developmental arrest, progressive neurologic deterioration and generalized spasticity, sensorimotor/psychointellectual dysfunctions, macular cherry-red sponts, facial dysmorphism, hepatosplenomegaly, coarse facies, generalized skeletal dysplasia)
Fabry disease (α-galactosidase deficiency 301500)[266]	XR	CAVB, CI, CM, MVP	Angiokeratoma, excruciating pain, acroparesthesias, hypohydrosis, transient ischemic attacks of brain, strokes, renal failure
Galactosialidosis (combined deficiency of β-galac-tosidase and neuraminidase) (256540)[267]	AR	CM	Early infantile type (fetal hydrops/ascites, psychomotor retardation, coarse facies, macular cherry-red spot, visceromegaly, inguinal hernias, telangiectasias, skeletal changes); late infantile type; juvenile/adult type
3-Methylglutaconic aciduria, type II (302060)[268]	XR	CM	Myopathy, neutropenia, recurrent infections, inconsistent mental retardation
Sandhoff (GM2 gangliosidosis, type II; hexosaminidase A and B deficiency) (268800)[269]	AR	CM, ECFE	Phenotype similar to Tay–Sachs disease (hyperacusis, dementia, seizures, cherry-red spot of macula, blindness, macrocephaly)
Mucolipidoses (252500; 252600)[270]	AR	HCM, AI, AVP	ML II (I-cell disease) (psychomotor retardation, short stature, hernias, congenital hip dislocation, thoracic deformity, hyperplastic gums, coarse facies, joint stiffness, severe dysostosis multiplex); ML III (pseudo-Hurler polydystrophy) (similar to Hurler phenotype without urinary excretion of mucopolysaccharides)
Mucopolysaccharidoses (252800; 309900; 252900; 253000; 253200; 253220; 253230) (text)	AR, XR	AI, MR, MI, CAD, CM, ECFE	Coarse facies, corneal clouding, mixed/sensorineural deafness, dysostosis multiplex (platyspondyly, genu valgum, odontoid hypoplasia/aplasia, atlantoaxial subluxation, lumbar gibbus, macrocephaly, J-shaped sella, oar-shaped ribs, oval/hook-shaped vertebral bodies, short tubular bones), short stature, mental retardation in some forms, stiff joints, claw hands, nerve/tendon entrapment

[a]For abbreviations, see chapter appendix.

functional limitation caused by congestive symptoms of exertional dyspnea or fatigue, chest pain, lightheadedness, palpitation, or syncope.[275] This primary cardiac abnormality, characterized by myocardial hypertrophy and myocyte and myofibrillar disarray, is an important cause of sudden death in adolescents and young adults.[13] Stillbirth, fetal distress with aspiration of amniotic sac content, ischemic bowel disease, and cerebral atrophy and sclerosis may be underappreciated features of hypertrophic cardiomyopathy in childhood, and patients with hypertrophic cardiomyopathy may be liable to die from certain types of septic shock, such as acute meningococcemia.[276]

Fifty-five percent of hypertrophic cardiomyopathy is familial, and the condition is commonly inherited as an autosomal dominant disorder (MIM 192600).[277] The clinical phenotype is heterogeneous, ranging from normal to sudden cardiac death. This disorder is the first familial primary myocardial disease for which the gene (*CMH1*) was identified (β-myosin heavy chain gene, FHC-1, located in 14q11-12).[278,279] The genetics of familial hypertrophic cardiomyopathy is also heterogeneous: three other loci (*CMH2* on chromosome 1q3, *CMH3* on chromosome 15q2, and *CMH4* on chromosome 11p13-q13) have been identified.[280–282]

Familial Dilated Cardiomyopathy

Dilated cardiomyopathy (DCM) is characterized by a marked ventricular dilatation, impaired myocardial contractility, progressive congestive heart failure, and a poor prognosis. The cause of DCM is often unknown. However, DCM was familial in 20% of cases,[283] suggesting an autosomal dominant disorder (MIM 115200) with incomplete penetrance. In addition, autosomal recessive[284] and X-linked inheritance[285] have been observed. A gene defect that causes conduction system disease and dilated cardiomyopathy has been mapped to chromosome 1p1-1q1.[286] Familial dilated cardiomyopathy was mapped to chromosome 9 (9q13-q22) by linkage analysis.[287]

Neuromuscular Disorders

Duchenne Muscular Dystrophy

DMD (MIM 310200) is an X-linked recessive disorder manifesting as progressively deteriorating musculoskeletal systems. Elucidation of the molecular defect in DMD was based on the identification of several X-autosome translocations in affected females.[288,289] The gene for dystrophin was cloned.[290] and its protein product (dystrophin) determined.[291] The majority of mutations are deletions (60%) and duplications (6%).[292] In most cases dystrophin is totally absent.[291]

The affected boy is usually normal for the first 1–2 years, develops progressive proximal muscle weakness by the age of 3–5 years, is confined to a wheelchair by the age of 12, and is not likely to survive beyond 20. Gower sign and pseudohypertrophy of the calves are characteristic. In the preclinical and early stages, the serum creatine kinase is greatly elevated.

Dilated cardiomyopathy along with congestive cardiac failure and significant arrhythmias usually occur toward the later stages of the disease.

Myotonic Muscular Dystrophy

Myotonic muscular dystrophy (DM) (MIM 160900) is the most prevalent form of muscular dystrophy in adults and is inherited in an autosomal dominant fashion. Congenital myotonic dystrophy syndrome occurs only when the child inherits the disease from the mother.[293] Recently, the myotonin protein kinase gene on chromosome 19q13 was identified as the gene responsible for DM. The molecular basis of DM was found to be expansion of the unstable triplet repeat CTG.[294]

Clinical manifestations include myotonia, myopathic facies, ptosis, frontal balding in males, cataracts, muscle wasting in the distal extremities, head, and neck, infertility, and cardiac myopathy. The most severe congenital form is exclusively maternally transmitted. It is associated with muscular hypoplasia, mental retardation, and high neonatal mortality. Infants who survive the neonatal period invariably exhibit the classic form of the disease (myotonic and muscle weakness) with the onset in early adult life and adolescence. The phenomenon of anticipation (more severe symptoms and earlier age of the onset in successive generations)[293] is often strikingly manifested in a family producing a congenitally affected child.

There is a high incidence of serious cardiac involvement (dilated cardiomyopathy). Electrocardiographic evidence of conduction defects (first-degree atrioventricular block and intraventricular conduction defects) is present approximately 75% of patients.[295] Sudden death remains the single most common cause of death.

Glycogen Storage Diseases[245]

Based on echocardiography, cardiomyopathies seen in glycogen storage diseases can be subdivided into dilated cardiomyopathies (e.g., debrancher deficiency, branching enzyme deficiency, phosphorylase *b* kinase deficiency) and hypertrophic cardiomyopathies (e.g., acid maltase deficiency, phosphorylase *b* kinase deficiency). The genes for most of the housekeeping enzymes and tissue-specific isozymes whose defects cause glycogenoses have been isolated, sequenced, and localized on different chromosomes.[245]

Acid Maltase Deficiency (Pompe Disease)

Pompe disease (MIM 232300), the infantile form of acid maltase deficiency (glycogenosis type II), is an autosomal recessive disorder.[296] The most severe infantile form is a generalized and invariably fatal condition characterized by massive cardiomegaly, macroglossia, failure to thrive, generalized hypotonia, and progressive muscle weakness (including respiratory muscle). In the childhood form, the cardiomyopathy is rare and usually mild. In the juvenile and adult forms, involvement of skeletal muscles dominates the clinical picture.

Serum creatine kinase levels are invariably elevated, and muscle biopsy shows severe vacuolar myopathy and glycogen storage. Biochemical studies show deficiency of acid α-glucosidase in muscle, lymphocytes, fibroblasts, or urine. Prenatal diagnosis has been made by determining acid α-glucosidase in cultured amniocytes and chorionic villus biopsies. The gene has been mapped to 17q23, and several mutations have been identified that prevent mRNA expression.[297]

Disorders of Lipid Metabolism

Mitochondrial β-oxidation of fatty acids is the major source of energy for the heart. Inborn errors of myocardial fatty acid oxidation are important causes of inherited cardiomyopathy, skeletal myopathy, metabolic disturbances, and sudden death in childhood. Oxidation defects involving long-chain fatty acids are more likely to cause cardiomyopathy than those involving medium-chain or short-chain fatty acids. Cardiomyopathy may be caused by abnormalities in carnitine transport into cell (primary systemic carnitine deficiency), carnitine–acylcarnitine shuttling (carnitine palmitoyltransferase II defects), and several mitochondrial enzymes involved in fatty acid β-oxidation (long-chain acyl–coenzyme A dehydrogenase and long-chain 3-hydroxyacyl–coenzyme A dehydrogenase deficiencies).

Mitochondrial Diseases Caused by Defects in Nuclear DNA

Mitochondrial respiratory chain enzyme deficiency is the major cause of congenital lactic acidosis.[298] The respiratory chain catalyzes the oxidation of fuel molecules by oxgyen with a concomitant energy transduction into ATP. During the oxidation process, electrons are transferred to oxygen via four multienzyme complexes.

Mitochondrial Diseases Caused by Defects in Mitochondrial DNA: Kearns–Sayre Syndrome

Kearns–Sayre syndrome is characterized by a triad of progressive external ophthalmoplegia, atypical pigmentary retinopathy, and at least one of the following: heart block, cerebellar ataxia, or cerebrospinal fluid protein concentration above 100 mg/dL.[299] Additional features are other cranial nerve involvement, stunted growth, hearing loss, and proximal muscular weakness.

The cardiac conduction system is typically involved; a heart block can develop early in the course of the disease. Timely placement of a pacemaker can be lifesaving. Single, large-scale mitochondrial DNA was shown to be deleted in all tissues including the heart.[299] Rarely, the patients can have dilated cardiomyopathy.[300]

Other Metabolic Cardiomyopathies

Mucopolysaccharidoses[2]   The mucopolysaccharidoses (MPS) are lysosomal storage diseases produced by a deficiency of specific lysosomal enzymes involved in the degradation of acid mucopolysaccharides (AMPS) (glycosaminoglycans).

The elucidation of the biochemical defects in the MPS has provided a firm basis for the classification of these diseases according to the mutant gene products (deficient enzymes). Such classification reveals that phenotypic variation exists not only among different types of MPS but also within certain types of MPS. All MPS are autosomal recessive disorders, except the Hunter syndrome (MPS II, MIM 309900), which is an X-linked recessive disorder. Prenatal diagnosis is possible for all the MPS by enzyme assays on cultured amniocytes.

Genetic heterogeneity is demonstrated by the four forms of Sanfilippo syndrome (MPS III, MIM 252900) and two forms of Morquio syndrome (MPS IV, MIM 253000) in which one cannot clinically distinguish the precise forms of the syndrome. Multiple phenotypic effects are produced by each MPS (pleiotropy). Variability in severity resulting from allelic mutation of the same lysosomal enzyme is demonstrated by MPS I (Hurler/Scheie compound, MIM 252800), MPS II, and MPS VI (Maroteaux–Lamy syndrome, MIM 253200). Homozygosity for the different alleles results in varying clinical severity. Some individuals are presumably compound heterozygotes (an individual carrying two different alleles at a locus is said to be a genetic compound).

Progressive clinical deterioration usually follows the first year of apparently normal growth. Short stature is characteristic of all types of MPS, except Scheie syndrome. Mental retardation is noted in MPS I-H, MPS II-severe, MPS III, MPS VII (Sly syndrome, MIM 253220), and MPS VIII (Differante syndrome, MIM 253230). Seizures occasionally occur in patients with MPS III.

Coarse facial features are characteristic of all types of MPS. Corneal clouding occurs to some degree in most cases of MPS, except Hunter syndrome (occasionally in the late stage and in severe cases) and Sanfilippo syndrome. Glaucoma occurs in several MPS (e.g., MPS I). Pigmentary degeneration of the retina is present in MPS I, II, and III, but not in MPS IV and VI. Deafness of mixed or sensorineural type is frequent in all types.

Severe scoliosis in Morquio syndrome may produce cardiopulmonary complications. Deposition of AMPS may obstruct the upper airway, producing respiratory insufficiency and cor pulmonale. Accumulation of undegraded AMPS causes hepatosplenomegaly in most cases.

Focal nodular thickening of the skin over the scapulae occurs in Hunter syndrome. Hirsutism is a feature of most MPS, especially of Sanfilippo syndrome. Dentinal cysts occur in most types, except Morquio syndrome, in which the teeth are widely spaced with thin enamel.

Dysostosis multiplex is seen in all types of MPS. Platyspondyly and genu valgum are characteristic features. Odontoid hypoplasia or aplasia with atlantoaxial subluxation is frequently seen in the Morquio syndrome and occasionally in the Hurler syndrome, and in the severe form of the Maroteaux–Lamy syndrome. Lumbar gibbus deformity is seen in MPS-IH, MPS IV, and MPS VII. Consequences of the secondary collagenosis include stiff joints and claw hands (mild in Sanfilippo syndrome; absent in Morquio syndrome), nerve entrapment (e.g., carpal tunnel syndrome), and tendon entrapment (e.g., trigger finger).

Characteristic radiographic features are macrocephaly, J-shaped sella, thick clavicle, oar-shaped ribs, wide clavicle, plump scapulae, oval- and hook-shaped vertebral bodies, wide iliac flare, dysplasia of capital femoral epiphyses, coxa valga, short tubular bones with metaphyseal widening, epiphyseal dysplasia, proximal tapering of second to fifth metacarpal bones, and osteoporotic bone changes, with coarsely laced trabeculation.

Arteriosclerosis develops in most MPS as a result of deposition of AMPS in the arterial smooth muscle cells. Involvement of the heart valves produces stenosis and regurgitation. Aortic and mitral regurgitations are observed in Hurler syndrome, Hurler/Scheie compound, Hunter syndrome, and Maroteaux–Lamy syndrome. In Scheie and Morquio syndromes, only aortic regurgitation is observed. In Hurler syndrome, patients also have coronary artery disease and cardiomyopathy.

Echocardiography may show thickening of the septum and the left ventricular posterior wall; a reduction in QRS voltage may be demonstrated by electrocardiography.[301] Children may present with acute cardiomyopathy with or without endocardial fibroelastosis as the initial manifestation before 1 year of age.[302–305]

Despite some success in treating MPS patients by bone marrow transplantation, prenatal diagnosis continues to be important because of lack of evidence that the transplantation can arrest the long-term neurological deterioration in affected patients. Recent advances in the prenatal diagnosis of MPS include first-trimester diagnosis by chorionic villus sampling, the possibility of early amniocentesis, the introduction of more sensitive assay techniques, the recognition of further clinical heterogeneity in the MPS, the use of DNA analysis for detecting mutations, and the possibility of preimplantation diagnosis of early embryos after in vitro fertilization.[306]

MALFORMATION SYNDROMES (Table 49.7[307–329])

Malformation Syndromes Associated with Congenital Heart Defects

Congenital heart defects (CHDs) are common in malformation syndromes.[162] Approximately 70% of spontaneous abortuses and stillborn fetuses[35] and 25% of children with a CHD have extracardiac malformations.[330] A substantial proportion of these children will have malformation syndromes conveying a significant recurrence risk. Certain cardiac defects may be characteristic for a syndrome, but none is pathognomonic. Presence of cardiac defects should prompt clinicians to search for extracardiac abnormalities and identification of syndromes.

Kartagener Syndrome

Kartagener syndrome (MIM 244400) is an autosomal recessive disorder, characterized by a triad of sinusitis, bronchiectasis, and situs inversus.[331] The patients also are infertile. Cardiac lesions are mostly situs inversus with dextrocardia but may include rare transposition of the great arteries and other complex defects.

Abnormal cilia are considered to be the underlying cause of the anomalies in Kartagener syndrome.[332] Electron microscopy of cilia and sperm shows absence of dynein arms, which contain almost all the ATPase activity necessary for motility of cilia.[333] Ciliary immotility causes abnormalities in mucocilliary transport, accounting for diffuse bronchiectasis and sinusitis. About half the patients with immotile cilia syndrome have situs inversus (Kartagener syndrome).[334] Human cytoplasmic dynein heavy chain has been mapped to 14qter by FISH.[335]

Williams Syndrome

Williams syndrome (MIM 194050) is an autosomal dominant disorder, characterized by infantile hypercalcemia, dysmorphic facial features (elfin faces), hoarse voice, mental retardation, gregarious disposition, vascular pathology identical to that found in supravalvular aortic stenosis, hypertension, premature aging of skin and graying of hair, lax joints early in life following by joint contractures later in life, and diverticulosis of the bladder and colon.[336] All patients with Williams syndrome have supravalvular aortic stenosis, pulmonic stenosis, or peripheral pulmonary artery stenosis.

Supravalvular aortic stenosis can be an isolated or autosomal dominant trait associated with severe narrowing of large elastic arteries, including the aorta and the pulmonary, coronary, and carotid arteries. Supravalvular aortic stenosis can also appear as one of the features of Williams syndrome. In a family described by Ewart et al,[337] a family member with severe supravalvular aortic stenosis had characteristics that satisfied the diagnostic index for Williams syndrome. These findings suggest that the two syndromes are allelic disorders whose phenotypic differences are the result of other undefined factors.

Recently, the supravalvular stenosis gene was mapped to the long arm of chromosome 7.[337] The finding that several DNA markers on the long arm of chromosome 7 were linked

TABLE 49.7 Genetics (Sporadic, Autosomal and X-Linked Recessive/Dominant), Cardiac Lesions and Noncardiac Manifestations of Malformation Syndromes

Disorder/Syndrome (MIM number)	Genetics	Cardiac Lesions[a]	Noncardiac Manifestations
Acardius acephalus[307]	S	AC	A bizarre fetal malformation occurring only in twins or triplets; 3 main types (paracephalus, acephalic, and amorphous)
Antley–Bixler (207410)[308]	S, AR	ASD, ECFE	Craniosynostosis, severe midface hypoplasia, proptosis, choanal atresia/stenosis, frontal bossing, dysplastic ears, depressed nasal bridge, radiohumeral synostosis, long-bone fractures, femoral bowing, urogenital anomalies
Arthrogryposis multiplex congenita (108110)[309]	S, AD	PDA, VSD, COA, AS	Congenital contractures of hands/feet and feet
Baller–Gerold (218600)[310]	S, AR	VSD, TOF, SAS, PA	Craniostenosis, preaxial reduction defects (radial aplasia), anal/urogenital/CNS/vertebral defects
Cantrell pentalogy (313850)[311]	S, XR	TOF, TCA, VSD, AVC, ECC	Midline supraumbilical abdominal wall defect, lower sternum cleft, deficient anterior diaphragm, defective diaphragmatic pericardium
Charge association (214800)[312]	S, AR	TOF, AVC, VR, IAA	Coloboma of eye, choanal atresia, postnatal growth or mental retardation, hypoplastic genitalia, ear abnormality
Cranio cerebello cardiac (220210)[313]	S, AR	VSD, ASD, AVC, TOF	High/prominent forehead, hypoplastic vermis, posterior fossa cyst, hydrocephalus, psychomotor/growth retardation
De Lange (122470)[314]	S, AD	VSD, TOF, PDA, DORV	Distinctive face (low anterior hairline, synophrys, anteverted nares, maxillary prognathism, long philtrum, "carp" mouth), psychomotor/growth retardation, upper limb anomalies
Femoral hypoplasia—unusual facies (134780)[315]	S, AD	VSD, PS, TA, PDA	Femoral hypoplasia, unusual facies (up-slanting palpebral fissures, short nose with broad tip, long philtrum, thin upper lip, micrognathia, cleft palate)
Goldenhar (164210)[316]	S, AD, AR	TOF, VSD, DORV, PA, TGV, AAA	Epibulbar dermoids, lipodermoids, uper eyelid colobomas, Duane's syndrome, dacryocystitis, stenotic lacrimal duct, anophthalmos, microphthalmia, microcornea, cataract, auricular defects, hearing loss, hemifacial microsomia, vertebral anomalies, pulmonary malformations, rare CNS manifestations
Holzgreve (236110)[317]	S, AR	HLHS, AAA, AVC, TOF	Potter sequence (bilateral renal agenesis), cleft palate, polydactyly, skeletal defects
Hydrolethalus (236680)[318]	AR	VSD, AVC, TA, DAA, HLH	Lethal entity, hydrocephalus, micrognathia, polydactyly, polyhydramnios, stillborn, occipital bone defect, cleft lip/palate, abnormal nose, small/deep-set eyes, malformed/low-set ears, abnormal larynx/trachea, defective lobulation of lungs, urogenital anomalies, short limbs, club feet
Hypoplastic left heart (241550)[319]	S, AR	HLHS	Extracardiac anomalies (skeletal, respiratory, CNS, urogenital)
Kartagener (244400) (text)	AR	DC, TGV	Sinusitis, bronchiectasis, situs inversus, abnormal cilia (absent dynein arms)
Klippel–Feil (148900, 214300)[320]	S, AD, AR	VSD, TAPVR, TGA, TOF, ASD, PDA	Cervical fusion, short neck, ear anomaly, cleft palate, micrognathia, urogenital anomalies, hearing impairment
Microphthalmia with linear skin defects (309801)[321]	XR	OCM	Variable eye abnormalities (microphthalmia, corneal opacity, orbital cyst, iris coloboma, glaucoma, retinal detachment), irregular linear areas of erythematous skin hypoplasia involving the head and neck
Microgastria–limb reduction complex with congenital heart disease (156810)[322]	AD	ASD, VSD, PDA, TAPVR, TA, ECCD, TVA	Microgastria, limb reduction defects
Opitz "C" trigonocephaly (211750)[323]	S, AR	VSD, PDA, PS, SAS, TIF, TA, AA, PLSVC	Trigonocephaly, mental retardation, craniosynostosis, unusual face (metopic prominence, upward slant of eyes, epicanthal folds, hypoplastic nasal root and nose, ear anomaly, wide alveolar ridges, multiple frenula), lung/genitourinary anomalies

(Continued)

TABLE 49.7 *(Continued)*

Disorder/Syndrome (MIM number)	Genetics	Cardiac Lesions[a]	Noncardiac Manifestations
Pallister–Hall (146510)[324]	S, AD	PDA, VSD, ECCD, MVD, AVD, COA	Hypothalamic hamartoblastoma, craniofacial anomalies, renal defects, postaxial polydactyly, imperforate anus, endocrine dysfunction
Poland anomaly (173800)[325]	S, AD	COA, VSD	Unilateral defect of pectoralis muscle, abnormality of an ipsilateral limb (syndactyly, brachydactyly, polydactyly, hypoplasia of arm and hand, absence of metacarpals and phalanges)
Pseudotrisomy 13 (264480)[326]	S, AR	ASD, VSD, AVC, DC, TA	Holoprosencephaly, hydrocephaly, microcephaly, micro/anophthalmia, hypoplastic nose, cleft lip/palate, polydactyly
Rubenstein–Taybi (180849)[327]	S, AD	PS, PDA, ASD, VSD, MR	Broad thumbs and big toes, characteristic facies, mental retardation, keloid formation, large foramen magnum, vertebral/sternal anomalies
Russell–Silver (180849) (180860, 312780)[328]	S, AD, XR	TOF, VSD	Low birth weight, short stature, asymmetry, characteristic craniofacial features (relatively large cranium, triangular face, frontal bossing, downturned corners of mouth, micrognathia, cleft/high-arched palate, low-set/malformed ears), syndactyly, clinodactyly of 5th fingers
VACTERL association (192350)[329]	S, AD	VSD	Veterbral malformastions, imperforate anus, tracheoesophageal anomalies, renal/limb defects
Williams (194050) (text)	S, AD	SVAS, PS, PPAS	Infantile hypercalcemia, elfin facies, hoarse voice, mental retardation, gregarious disposition, hypertension, premature aging of skin, graying of hair, lax joints followed by joint contractures, diverticulosis of bladder/colon

[a]For abbreviations, see chapter appendix.

to supravalvular aortic stenosis in two families indicates that a gene for supravalvular aortic stenosis is located in the same chromosomal subunit as elastin, a candidate gene for the disease gene. Furthermore, the observation that the elastin gene was disrupted by a translocation associated with supravalvular aortic stenosis suggests that mutations in the elastin gene can cause supravalvular stenosis.[338]

Recently, it was demonstrated that patients with Williams syndrome show allelic loss of elastin (ELN), exhibiting a submicroscopic deletion, at 7q11.23, detectable by fluorescence in situ hybridization (Fig. 49.2).[339] Hemizygosity is the cause of vascular abnormalities in these patients. Ninety-six percent of a series of 235 patients with classic Williams syndrome revealed molecular cytogenetic deletions.

SUMMARY

A brief review of the genetic causes of cardiac diseases was attempted in multifactorial, chromosomal, and single-gene disorders, and malformation syndromes. A total of 51 complete and partial autosomal trisomies and tetrasomies, 30 partial autosomal monosomies, 4 sex chromosome anomalies, 2 polyploidy syndromes, 45 single-gene disorders, 30 hereditary metabolic cardiomyopathies, and 25 malformation syndromes were presented in tabular form for easy reference.

Certain syndromes are described in more detail in the text because they are classical or known to be associated with a specific pattern of cardiac malformations. This review is by no means exhaustive.

The references quoted are skewed toward recent or review articles instead of the original descriptions of the disorders. For karyotypic designation, readers are encouraged to refer to the International System for Human Cytogenetic Nomenclature.[340] For single-gene disorders, McKusick Catalogue numbers (MIM, Medelian inheritance in man) are provided.

Wherever possible, the current status of the molecular basis of the syndromes relevant to cardiogenesis is given. The molecular basis of some forms of heritable cardiac disease is presented: β-myosin heavy chain gene mutations in familial hypertrophic cardiomyopathy, fibrillin mutations and Marfan syndrome, elastin mutations and supravalvular aortic stenosis and Williams syndrome, and microdeletions in 22q11 in DiGeorge syndrome, velocardiofacial syndrome, and nonsyndromic patients with conotruncal malformations. Prenatal diagnosis is currently available in many genetic disorders, and an attempt was made in this chapter to provide current progress in this area. To keep up to date with the latest developments in the field of prental diagnosis, a current awareness service is provided in each section of the journal of *Prental Diagnosis,* with an excellent bibliography of newly published material.[341]

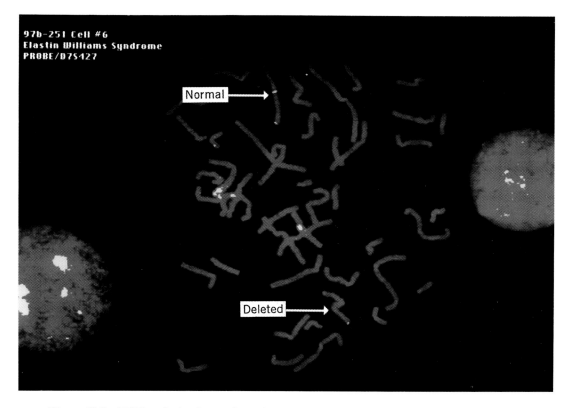

Figure 49.2   FISH analysis of metaphase chromosomes with Elastin Williams syndrome chromosome region (ELN) probe shows the deletion in that region of the chromosome 7.

ACKNOWLEDGMENT

I am grateful to the following individuals for their reading and helpful comments on the chapter: Alexander Asamoah, Edwin Brown, Eudice Fontenot, Ed Gustavson, Ernest Kiel, Davis Lewis, Leonard and Miriam Prouty, and Susonne Ursin. Figures 49.1 is kindly furnished by PSI, Ltd.

REFERENCES

1. Chen H. Genetic disorders. In: Liu PI, ed. *Blue Book of Diagnostic Tests.* Saunders Blue Books Series. Philadelphia: WB Saunders; 1986;421–462.

2. Chen H. *Medical Genetics Handbook.* St. Louis: Warren H. Green; 1988.

3. Nora JJ. Causes of congenital heart diseases: old and new modes, mechanisms, and models. *Am Heart J* 1993;125: 1409–1419.

4. Copel JA, Pilu G, Kleinman CS. Congenital heart disease and extracardiac anomalies: associations and indications for fetal echocardiography. *Am J Obstet Gynecol* 1986;154: 1121–1132.

5. DeVore GR. The prenatal diagnosis of congenital heart disease—a practical approach for the fetal sonographer. *J Clin Ultrasound* 1985;13:229–245.

6. Smythe JF, Copel JA, Kleinman CS. Outcome of prenatally detected cardiac malformations. *Am J Cardiol* 1992;69: 1471–1474.

7. Paladini D, Calabro R, Palmieri S, D'Andrea T. Prenatal diagnosis of congenital heart disease and fetal karyotyping. *Obstet Gynecol* 1993;81:679–682.

8. Berg KA, Clark EB, Astemborski JA, Boughman JA. Prenatal detection of cardiovascular malformations by echocardiography: an indication for cytogenetic evaluation. *Am J Obstet Gynecol* 1988;159:477–481.

9. Copel JA, Cullen M, Green JJ, Mahoney MJ, Hobbins JC, Kleinmen CS. The frequency of aneuploidy in prenatally diagnosed congenital heart disease: an indication for fetal karyotyping. *Am J Obstet Gynecol* 1988;158:409–413.

10. Fogel M, Copel JA, Cullen MT, Hobbins JC, Kleinman CS. Congenital heart disease and fetal thoracoabdominal anomalies: association in utero and the importance of cytogenetic analysis. *Am J Perinatol* 1991;8:411–416.

11. Allan LD, Sharland GK. Prognosis in fetal tetralogy of Fallot. *Pediatr Cardiol* 1992;13:1–4.

12. Bouvagnet P, Sauer U, Debrus S, Genz T, Alonso S, Berger G, de Meeus A, Bühlmeier K, Demaille J. Deciphering the molecular genetics of congenital heart disease. *Herz* 1994;19:119–125.

13. Anderson PA. Cardiovascular molecular genetics. *Curr Opin Cardiol* 1994;9:78–90.

14. Kingston HM. ABC of clinical genetics. Genetics of common disorders. *Br Med J* 1989;298:949–952.

15. Pitkin RM, Perloff JK, Koos BJ, Beall MH. Pregnancy and congenital heart disease. *Ann Intern Med* 1990;112:445–454.

16. Mitchell SC, Korones SB, Berendes HW. Congenital heart disease in 56,109 births. Incidence and natural history. *Circulation* 1971;43:323–331.

17. Hoffman JIE. Congenital heart diseases: incidence and inheritance. *Pediatr Clin North Am* 1990;37:25–43.

18. Hoffman JIE. Incidence of congenital heart disease. I. Postnatal incidence. *Pediatr Cardiol* 1995;16:103–113.

19. Fyler DC, Buckley LP, Hellenbrand WE, Cohn HE. Report of the New England Regional Infant Cardiac Program. *Pediatrics* 1980;65:375–461.

20. Angelini P. Embryology and congenital heart disease. *Texas Heart Inst J* 1995;22:1–12.

21. Hoffman JIE. Incidence of congenital heart disease. II. Prenatal incidence. *Pediatr Cardiol* 1995;16:155–165.

22. Bromley B, Estroff JA, Sanders SP, Parad R, Roberts D, Frigoletto FD, Benacerraf BR. Fetal echocardiography: accuracy and limitations in a population at high and low risk for heart defects. *Am J Obstet Gynecol* 1992;166:1473–1481.

23. Nora JJ, Nora AH. Update on counseling the family with a first-degree relative with a congenital heart defect. *Am J Med Genet* 1988;29:137–142.

24. Nora JJ, Nora AH. Maternal transmission of congenital heart diseases: new recurrence risk figures and the questions of cytoplasmic inheritance and vulnerability to teratogens. *Am J Cardiol* 1987;59:459–463.

25. Nadler HL, Burton BK. Genetics. In: Quilligan EJ, Kretchmer N, eds. *Fetal and Maternal Medicine.* New York: John Wiley & Sons; 1980;59–107.

26. Whittemore R, Hobbins JC, Engle MA. Pregnancy and its outcome in women with and without surgical treatment of congenital heart disease. *Am J Cardiol* 1982;50:641–651.

27. Nora JJ. Multifactorial inheritance hypothesis for the etiology of congenital heart diseases. The genetic–environmental interaction. *Circulation* 1968;38:604–617.

28. Nora JJ. Genetics and the cardiovascular system. In: Cheng TO, ed. *The International Textbook of Cardiology.* New York: Pergamon Press; 1986;460–475.

29. Armstrong BE. Congenital cardiovascular disease and cardiac surgery in childhood. I. Cyanotic congenital heart defects. *Curr Opin Cardiol* 1995;10:58–67.

30. Armstrong BE. Congenital cardiovascular disease and cardiac surgery in childhood. 2. Acyanotic congenital heart defects and interventional techniques. *Curr Opin Cardiol* 1995;10:68–77.

31. Boughman JA, Berg KA, Astemborski JA, Clark EB, McCarter RJ, Rubin JD, Ferencz C. Familial risks of congenital heart defect assessed in a population-based epidemiologic study. *Am J Med Genet* 1987;26:839–849.

32. Payne RM, Johnson MC, Grant JW, Strauss AW. Toward a molecular understanding of congenital heart disease. *Circulation* 1995;91:494–504.

33. Hoffman JIE, Christianson R. Congenital heart disease in a cohort of 19,502 births with long-term follow-up. *Am J Cardiol* 1978;42:641–647.

34. Ferencz C, Neill CA, Boughman JA, Rubin JD, Brenner JI, Perry LW. Congenital cardiac malformations associated with chromosome abnormality: an epidemiologic study. *J Pediatr* 1989;114:79–86.

35. Chinn A, Fitzsimmons J, Shephard TH, Fantel AG. Congenital heart disease among spontaneous abortuses and stillborn fetuses: prevalence and associations. *Teratology* 1989;40:475–482.

36. Pierpont MEM, Gorlin RJ, Moller JH. Chromosomal abnormalities. In: Pierpont MEM, Moller JH, eds. *The Genetics of Cardiovascular Disease.* Boston: Martinus Nijhoff Publishing; 1987;69–94.

37. Epstein CJ. The consequences of chromosome imbalance. *Am J Med Genet* 1990(suppl);7:31–37.

38. Roskes EJ, Boughman JA, Schwartz S, Cohen MM. Congenital cardiovascular malformations (CCVM) and structural chromosome abnormalities: a report of 9 cases and literature review. *Clin Genet* 1990;38:198–210.

39. Adinolfi M, Crolla J. Nonisotopic in situ hybridization. Clinical cytogenetics and gene mapping applications. *Adv Hum Genet* 1994;22:187–255.

40. Elejalde BR, Opitz JM, de Elejalde MM, Gilbert EF, Abellera M, Meisner L, Lebel RR, Hartigan JM. Tandem dup(1p) within the short arm of chromosome 1 in a child with ambiguous genitalia and multiple congenital anomalies. *Am J Med Genet* 1984;17:723–730.

41. Chen H, Kusyk CJ, Tuck-Muller CM, Martinez JE, Dorand RD, Wertelecki W. Confirmation of proximal 1q duplication using fluorescence in situ hybridization. *Am J Med Genet* 1994;50:28–31.

42. Lurie IW, IIyina HG, Gurevich DB, Rumyantseva NV, Naumchik IV, Castellan C, Hoeller A, Schinzel A. Trisomy 2p: analysis of unusual phenotypic findings. *Am J Med Genet* 1995;55:229–236.

43. Chen H, Rightmire D, Zapata C, Fowler M, Hogan G, Wolfson J, Muenke M. Frontonasal dysplasia and arrhinencephaly resulting from unbalanced segregation of a maternal t(2;7)(q31;q36). *Dysmorph Clin Genet* 1992;6:99–106.

44. Braga S, Schmidt A. Clinical and cytogenetic spectrum of duplication 3p. *Eur J Pediatr* 1982;138:195–197.

45. Wilson GN, Dasouki M, Barr M Jr. Further delineation of the dup(3q) syndrome. *Am J Med Genet* 1985;22:117–123.

46. Van Allen MI, Ritchie S, Toi A, Fong K, Winsor E. Trisomy 4 in a fetus with cyclopia and other anomalies. *Am J Med Genet* 1993;46:193–197.

47. Crane J, Sujansky E, Smith A. 4p trisomy syndrome: report of 4 additional cases and segregation analysis of 21 families with different translocations. *Am J Med Genet* 1979;4:219–229.

48. Zollino M, Zampino G, Torrioli G, Pomponi MG, Neri G. Further contribution to the description of phenotypes associated with partial 4q duplication. *Am J Med Genet* 1995;57:69–73.

49. Fujita M, Flori E, Lemaire F, Casanova R, Astruc D. A new case of "complete" trisomy 5p with isochromosome 5p associated with a de novo translocation t(5;8)(q11;p23). *Clin Genet* 1994;45:305–307.

50. Rodewald A, Zankl M, Gley E-O, Zang KD. Partial trisomy 5q: three different phenotypes depending on different duplication segments. *Hum Genet* 1980;55:191–198.

51. Wauters JG, Bossuyt PJ, Roelen L, van Roy B, Dumon J. Application of fluorescence *in situ* hybridization for early prenatal diagnosis of partial trisomy 6p/monosomy 6q due to a familial pericentric inversion. *Clin Genet* 1993;44:262–269.

52. Pivnick EK, Qumsiyeh MB, Tharapel AT, Summitt JB, Wilroy RS. Partial duplication of the long arm of chromosome 6: a clinically recognisable syndrome. *J Med Genet* 1990;27:523–526.

53. Talley JD, Dooley KJ, Tuboku-Metzger A, Burgess GH, Wilcox WD, Click LA, Blackston RD. The cardiovascular abnormalities associated with duplicated segments of chromosome 7. *Clin Cardiol* 1989;12:227–232.

54. Lurie IW, Schwartz MF, Schwartz S, Cohen MM. Trisomy 7p resulting from isochromosome formation and whole-arm translocation. *Am J Med Genet* 1995;55:62–66.

55. Riccardi VM. Trisomy 8: an international study of 70 patients. *Birth Defects* 1977;8:171–184.

56. Gelb BD, Towbin JA, McCabe ERB, Sujansky E. San Luis Valley recombinant chromosome 8 and tetralogy of Fallot: a review of chromosome 8 anomalies and congenital heart disease. *Am J Med Genet* 1991;40:471–476.

57. Feldman GL, Weiss L, Phelan MC, Schroer RJ. Van Dyke DL. Inverted duplication of 8p: ten new patients and review of the literature. *Am J Med Genet* 1993;47:482–486.

58. Newton D, Hammond L, Wiley J, Kushnick T. Mosaic tetrasomy 8p. *Am J Med Genet* 1993;46:513–516.

59. Arnold GL, Kirby RS, Stern TP, Sawyer JR. Trisomy 9: review and report of two new cases. *Am J Med Genet* 1995;56:252–257.

60. Tarani L, Colloridi F, Raguso G, Rizzuti A, Bruni L, Tozzi MC, Palermo D, Panero A, Vignetti P. Trisomy 9 mosaicism syndrome. A case report and review of the literature. *Ann Génét* 1994;37:14–20.

61. Jalal SM, Kukolich MK, Garcia M, Benjamin TR, Day DW. Tetrasomy 9p: an emerging syndrome. *Clin Genet* 1991;39:60–64.

62. Stalker HJ, Aymé S, Delneste D, Scarpelli H, Vekemans M, der Kaloustian VM. Duplication of 9q12-q33: a case report and implications for the dup(9q) syndrome. *Am J Med Genet* 1993;45:456–459.

63. de France HF, Beemer FA, Senders RC, Schaminée-Main SCE. Trisomy 10 mosaicism in a newborn; delineation of the syndrome. *Clin Genet* 1985;27:92–96.

64. Wiktor A, Feldman GL, Kratkoczki P, Ditmars DM Jr, Van Dyke DL. 10p duplication characterized by fluorescence in situ hybridization. *Am J Med Genet* 1994;52:315–318.

65. Klep-de Pater JM, Bijlsma JB, de France HF, Leschot NJ, Duijndam-Van den Berge M, van Hemel JO. Partial trisomy 10q: a recognizable syndrome. *Hum Genet* 1979;46:29–40.

66. Pihko H, Therman E, Uchida IA. Partial 11q trisomy syndrome. *Hum Genet* 1981;58:129–134.

67. Tenconi R, Giorgi PL, Tarantino E, Formica A. Trisomy 12p due to an adjacent 1 segregation of a maternal reciprocal translocation t(12;18)(p11;q23). *Ann Génét* 1978;21:229–233.

68. Schinzel A. Tetrasomy 12p (Pallister–Killian syndrome). *J Med Genet* 1991;28:122–125.

69. Pratt NR, Bulugahapitiya DTD. Partial trisomy 12q: a clinically recognisable syndrome. Genetic risks associated with translocations of chromosome 12q. *J Med Genet* 1983;20:86–89.

70. Schinzel A, Hayashi K, Schmid W. Further delineation of the clinical picture of trisomy for the distal segment of chromosome 13. *Hum Genet* 1976;32:1–12.

71. Fujimoto A, Allanson J, Crowe CA, Lipson MH, Johnson VP. Natural history of mosaic trisomy 14 syndrome. *Am J Med Genet* 1992;44:189–196.

72. Atkin JF, Patil S. Duplication of the distal segment of 14q. *Am J Med Genet* 1983;16:357–366.

73. Schnatterly P, Bono KL, Robinow M, Wyandt HE, Kardon N, Kelly TE. Distal 15q trisomy: phenotypic comparison of nine cases in an extended family. *Am J Hum Genet* 1984;36:444–451.

74. Devi AS, Velinov M, Kamath MV, Eisenfield L, Neu R, Ciarleglio L, Greenstein R, Benn P. Variable clinical expression of mosaic trisomy 16 in the newborn infant. *Am J Med Genet* 1993;47:294–298.

75. Pletcher BA, Sanz MM, Schlessel JS, Kunaporn S, McKenna C, Bialer MG, Alonso ML, Zaslav A, Brown WT, Ray JH. Postnatal confirmation of prenatally diagnosed trisomy 16 mosaicism in two phenotypically abnormal liveborns. *Prenatal Diagn* 1994;14:933–940.

76. Savary JB, Vasseur F, Manouvrier S, Daudignon A, Lemaire O, Thieuleux M, Poher M, Lequien P, Deminatti MM. Trisomy 16q23−>qter arising from a maternal t(13;16)(p12;q23): case report and evidence of the reciprocal balanced maternal rearrangement by the Ag-NOR technique. *Hum Genet* 1991;88:115–118.

77. Schrander-Stumpel C, Schrander J, Fryns JP, Hamers G. Trisomy 17p due to a t(8;17)(p23;p11.2)pat translocation. Case report and review of the literature. *Clin Genet* 1990;37:148–152.

78. Bridge J, Sanger W, Mosher G, Buehler B, Hearty C, Olney A, Fordyce R. Partial duplication of distal 17q. *Am J Med Genet* 1985;22:229–235.

79. Park VM, Gustashaw KM, Bilenker RM, Golden WL. Diagnosis of tetrasomy 18p using in situ hybridization of a DNA probe to metaphase chromosomes. *Am J Med Genet* 1991;41:180–183.

80. Mewar R, Kline AD, Harrison W, Rojas K, Greenberg F, Overhauser J. Clinical and molecular evaluation of four patients with partial duplications of the long arm of chromosome 18. *Am J Hum Genet* 1993;53:1269–1278.

81. Van Essen AJ, Schoots CJF, van Lingen RA, Mourits MJE, Tuberlings JHAM, Leegte B. Isochromosome 18q in a girl with holoprosencephaly, DiGeorge anomaly, and streak ovaries. *Am J Med Genet* 1993;47:85–88.

82. Valerio D, Lavorgna F, Scalona M, Conte A. A new case of partial trisomy 19q(q13.2−>qter) owing to an unusual maternal translocation. *J Med Genet* 1993;30:697–699.

83. Chen H, Hoffman WH, Tyrkus M, Al Saadi A, Bawle E. Partial trisomy 20p syndrome and maternal mosaicism. *Ann Génét* 1983;26:21–25.

84. Sax CM, Bodurtha JN, Brown JA. Case report: partial trisomy 20q (20q13.13−>qter). *Clin Genet* 1986;30:462–465.

85. Bacino CA, Schreck R, Fischel-Ghodsian N, Pepkowitz S, Prezant TR, Graham JM Jr. Clinical and molecular studies in full trisomy 22: further delineation of the phenotype and review of the literature. *Am J Med Genet* 1995;56:359–365.

86. Schinzel A, Schmid W, Fraccaro M, Tiepolo L, Zuffardi O, Opitz JM, Lindsten J, Zetterqvist P, Enell H, Baccichetti C, Tenconi R, Pagon RA. The "cat eye syndrome": dicentric small marker chromosome probably derived from a no. 22 (tetrasomy 22pter−>q11) associated with a characteristic phenotype. Report of 11 patients and delineation of the clinical picture. *Hum Genet* 1981;57:148–158.

87. Knoll JHM, Asamoah A, Pletcher BA, Wagstaff J. Interstitial duplication of proximal 22q: phenotypic overlap with cat eye syndrome. *Am J Med Genet* 1995;55:221–224.

88. Wyllie JP, Wright MJ, Burn JM, Hunter S. Natural history of trisomy 13. *Arch Dis Child* 1994;71:343–345.

89. Lehman CD, Nyberg DA, Winter TC III, Kapur RP, Resta RG, Luthy DA. Trisomy 13 syndrome: prenatal US findings in a review of 33 cases. *Radiology* 1995;194:217–222.

90. Wladimiroff JW, Stewart PA, Reuss A, Sachs ES. Cardiac and extracardiac anomalies as indicators for trisomies 13 and 18: a prenatal ultrasound study. *Prenatal Diagn* 1989;9:515–520.

91. Matsuoka R, Misugi K, Goto A, Gilbert EF, Ando M. Congenital heart anomalies in the trisomy 18 syndrome, with reference to congenital polyvalvular disease. *Am J Med Genet* 1983;14:657–668.

92. Merkatz IR, Nitowsky HM, Macri JN, Johnson WE. An association between low maternal serum α-fetoprotein and fetal chromosomal abnormalities. *Am J Obstet Gynecol* 1984;148:886–894.

93. Canick JA, Knight GJ, Palomaki GE, Haddow JE, Cuckle HS, Wald NJ. Low second trimester maternal serum unconjugated oestriol in pregnancies with Down's syndrome. *Br J Obstet Gynaecol* 1988;95:330–333.

94. Bogart MH, Pandian MR, Jones OW. Abnormal maternal serum chorionic gonadotropin levels in pregnancies with fetal chromosome abnormalities. *Prenatal Diagn* 1987;7:623–630.

95. Wald NJ, Cuckle HS, Densem JW, et al. Maternal serum screening for Down's syndrome in early pregnancy. *Br Med J* 1988;297:883–887.

96. Burton BK, Prins GS, Verp MS. A prospective trial of prenatal screening for Down syndrome by means of maternal serum α-fetoprotein, human chorionic gonadotropin, and unconjugated estriol. *Am J Obstet Gynecol* 1993;169:526–530.

97. Bradley LA, Horwitz JA, Downman AC, Ponting NR, Peterson LM. Triple marker screening for fetal Down syndrome. *Int Pediatr* 1994;9:168–174.

98. Bianchi DW, Mahr A, Zickwolf GK, Houseal TW, Flint AF, Klinger KW. Detection of fetal cells with 47,XY,+21 karyotype in maternal peripheral blood. *Hum Genet* 1992;90:368–370.

99. Rowe RD, Uchida IA. Cardiac malformation in mongolism: a prospective study of 184 mongoloid children. *Am J Med* 1961;31:726–735.

100. Greenwood RD, Nadas AS. The clinical course of cardiac disease in Down's syndrome. *Pediatrics* 1976;58:893–897.

101. Marino B. Congenital heart disease in patients with Down's syndrome: anatomic and genetic aspects. *Biomed Pharmacother* 1993;47:197–200.

102. Park SC, Mathews RA, Zuberbuhler JR, Rowe RD, Neches WH, Lenox CC. Down syndrome with congenital heart malformation. *Am J Dis Child* 1977;131:29–33.

103. Korenberg JR, Bradley C, Disteche CM. Down syndrome: molecular mapping of the congenital heart disease and duodenal stenosis. *Am J Hum Genet* 1992;50:294–302.

104. Fuentes J-J, Pritchard MA, Planas AM, Bosch A, Ferrer I, Estivill X. A new human gene from the Down syndrome critical region encodes a proline-rich protein highly expressed in fetal brain and heart. *Hum Mol Genet* 1995;4:1935–1944.

105. Keppler-Noreuil KM, Carroll AJ, Finley WH, Rutledge SL. Chromosome 1p terminal deletion: report of new findings and confirmation of two characteristic phenotypes. *J Med Genet* 1995;32:619–622.

106. Meinecke P, Vögtel D. A specific syndrome due to deletion of the distal long arm of chromosome 1. *Am J Med Genet* 1987;28:371–376.

107. Kreuz FR, Wittwer BH. Del(2q)—cause of the wrinkly skin syndrome? *Clin Genet* 1993;43:132–138.

108. Nienhaus H, Mau U, Zang KD. Infant with del(3)(p25-pter): karyotype–phenotype correlation and review of previously reported cases. *Am J Med Genet* 1992;44:573–575.

109. Alvarado M, Bocian M, Walker AP. Interstitial deletion of the long arm of chromosome 3: case report, review, and definition of a phenotype. *Am J Med Genet* 1987;27:781–786.

110. Estabrooks LL, Lamb AN, Aylsworth AS, Callanan NP, Rao KW. Molecular characterisation of chromosome 4p deletions resulting in Wolf–Hirschhorn syndrome. *J Med Genet* 1994;31:103–107.

111. Lin AE, Garver KL, Diggans G, Clemens M, Wenger SL, Steele MW, Jones MC, Israel J. Interstitial and terminal deletions of the long arm of chromosome 4: further delineation of phenotypes. *Am J Med Genet* 1988;31:533–548.

112. Niebuhr E. The cri du chat syndrome. Epidemiology, cytogenetic, and clinical features. *Hum Genet* 1978;44:227–275.

113. Palmer CG, Bader P, Slovak ML, Comings DE, Pettenati MJ. Partial deletion of chromosome 6p: delineation of the syndrome. *Am J Med Genet* 1991;39:155–160.

114. Valtat G, Galliano D, Mettey R, Toutain A, Moraine C. Monosomy 6q: report on four new cases. *Clin Genet* 1992;41:159–166.

115. Chotai KA, Brueton LA, van Herwerden L, Garrett C, Hinkel GK, Schinzel A, Mueller RF, Speleman F, Winter RM. Six cases of 7p deletion: clinical, cytogenetic, and molecular studies. *Am J Med Genet* 1994;51:270–276.

116. Finley BE, Seguin JH, Bennett TL, Ardinger R, Burlbaw J, Levitch L, Keifer C, Fasztor L. Terminal deletion of 7q presenting in utero with a truncus arteriosus and nonimmune hydrops. *Am J Med Genet* 1993;47:221–222.

117. Marino B, Reale A, Giannotti A, Digilio MC, Dallapiccola B. Nonrandom association of atrioventricular canal and del (8p) syndrome. *Am J Med Genet* 1992;42:424–427.

118. Donahue ML, Ryan RM. Interstitial deletion of 8q21→22 associated with minor anomalies, congenital heart defect, and Dandy–Walker variant. *Am J Med Genet* 1995;56:97–100.

119. Huret JL, Leonard C, Forestier B, Rethoré MO, Lejeune J. Eleven new cases of del(9p) and features from 80 cases. *J Med Genet* 1988;25:741–749.

120. Farrell SA, Siegel-Bartelt J, Teshma I. Patients with deletions of 9q22q34 do not define a syndrome: three case reports and a literature review. *Clin Genet* 1991;40:207–214.

121. Hon E, Chapman C, Gunn TR. Family with partial monosomy 10p and trisomy 10p. *Am J Med Genet* 1995;56:136–140.

122. Lobo S, Cervenka J, London A, Pierpont MEM. Interstitial deletion of 10q: clinical features and literature review. *Am J Med Genet* 1992;43:701–703.

123. Gilgenkrantz S, Vigneron C, Gregoire MJ, Pernot C, Raspiller A. Association of del(11)(p15.1p12), aniridia, catalase deficiency, and cardiomyopathy. *Am J Med Genet* 1982;13:39–49.

124. Hustinx R, Verloes A, Grattagliano B, Herens C, Jamar M, Soyeur D, Schaaps JP, Koulischer L. Monosomy 11q: report of two familial cases and review of the literature. *Am J Med Genet* 1993;47:312–317.

125. Fryns JP, Kleczkowska A, van den Berghe H. Interstitial deletion of the short arm of chromosome 12. Report of a new patient and review of the literature. *Ann Génét* 1990;33:43–45.

126. Brown S, Gersen S, Anyane-Yeboa K, Warburton D. Preliminary definition of a "critical region" of chromosome 13 in q32: report of 14 cases with 13q deletions and review of the literature. *Am J Med Genet* 1993;45:52–59.

127. Gorski JL, Uhlmann WR, Glover TW. A child with multiple congenital anomalies and karyotype 46,XY,del(14)(q31q32.2): further delineation of chromosome 14 interstitial deletion syndrome. *Am J Med Genet* 1990;37:471–474.

128. Smith ACM, McGavran L, Robinson J, Waldstein G, Macfarlane J, Zonona J, Reiss J, Lahr M, Allen L, Magenis E. Interstitial deletion of (17)(p11.2p11.2) in nine patients. *Am J Med Genet* 1986;24:393–414.

129. Khalifa MM, MacLeod PM, Duncan AMV. Additional case of *de novo* interstitial deletion del(17)(q21.3q23) and expansion of the phenotype. *Clin Genet* 1993;44:258–261.

130. Movahhedian HR, Kane HA, Borgaonkar D, McDermott M, Septimus S. Heart disease associated with deletion of the short arm of chromosome 18. *Del Med J* 1991;63:285–289.

131. Lurie IW, Lazjuk GI. Partial monosomies 18: review of cytogenetical and phenotypical variants. *Hum Genet* 1972;15:203–222.

132. Anad F, Burn J, Matthews D, Cross I, Davison BCC, Mueller R, Sands M, Lillington DM, Eastham E. Alagille syndrome and deletion of 20p. *J Med Genet* 1990;27:729–737.

133. Wisniewski K, Dambaska M, Jenkins EC, Sklower S, Brown WT. Monosomy 21 syndrome: further delineation including clinical, neuropathological, cytogenetic and biochemical studies. *Clin Genet* 1983;23:102–110.

134. Goldberg R, Motzkin B, Marion R, Scambler PJ, Shprintzen RJ. Velo-cardio-facial syndrome: a review of 120 patients. *Am J Med Genet* 1993;45:313–319.

135. Driscoll DA, Budarf ML, Emanuel BS. A genetic etiology for DiGeorge syndrome: consistent deletions and microdeletions of 22q11. *Am J Hum Genet* 1992;50:924–933.

136. Matsuoka R, Takao A, Kimura M, Imamura S, Kondo CI, Joh-o K, Ikeda K, Nishibatake M, Ando M, Momma K. Confirmation that the conotruncal anomaly face syndrome is associated with a deletion within 22q11.2. *Am J Med Genet* 1994;53:285–289.

137. Goldmuntz E, Driscoll D, Budarf ML, Zackai EH, McDonald-McGinn DM, Biegel JA, Emanuel BS. Microdeletions of chromosomal region 22q11 in patients with congenital conotruncal cardiac defects. *J Med Genet* 1993;807–812.

138. Johnson MC, Strauss AW, Dowton SB, Spray TL, Huddleston CB, Wood MK, Slaugh RA, Watson MS. Deletion within chromosome 22 is common in patients with absent pulmonary valve syndrome. *Am J Cardiol* 1995;76:66–69.

139. McDonald-McGinn DM, Driscoll DA, Bason L, Christensen K, Lynch D, Sullivan K, Canning D, Zavod W, Quinn N, Rome J, Paris Y, Weinberg P, Clark BJ III, Emanuel BS, Zackai EH. Autosomal dominant "Opitz" GBBB syndrome due to a 22q11.2 deletion. *Am J Med Genet* 1995;59:103–113.

140. Lipson AH, Yuille D, Angel M, Thompson PG, Vandervoord JG, Beckenham EJ. Velocardiofacial (Shprintzen) syndrome: an important syndrome for the dysmorphologist to recognize. *J Med Genet* 1991;28:596–604.

141. Lammar EJ, Opitz JM. The DiGeorge anomaly as a developmental field defect. *Am J Med Genet* 1986;2(suppl):113–127.

142. Hall JG. CATCH 22. *J Med Genet* 1993;30:801–302.

143. Van Hemel JO, Schaap C, van Opstal D, Mulder MP, Niermeijer MF, Meijers JHC. Recurrence of DiGeorge syndrome: prenatal detection by FISH of a molecular 22q11 deletion. *J Med Genet* 1995;32:657–658.

144. Wilson DJ, Burn J, Scambler P, Goodship J. DiGeorge syndrome: part of CATCH-22. *J Med Genet* 1993;30:852–856.

145. Wilson DI, Goodship JA, Burn J, Cross IE, Scambler PJ. Deletions within chromosome 22q11 in familial congenital heart disease. *Lancet* 1992;340:573–575.

146. Scambler PJ. Deletions of human chromosome 22 and associated birth defects. *Curr Opin Genet Dev* 1993;3:432–437.

147. Kirby ML, Waldo KL. Role of neural crest in congenital heart disease. *Circulation* 1990;82:332–340.

148. Aubry M, Demczuck S, Desmaze C, Aikem M, Auris A, Julien J-P, Rouleau GA. Isolation of a zinc finger gene consistently deleted in DiGeorge syndrome. *Hum Mol Genet* 1993;2:1583–1587.

149. Meschede D, Nekarda T, Kececioglu D, Löser H, Vogt J, Miny P, Horst J. Congenital heart disease in the 48,XXYY syndrome. *Clin Genet* 1995;48:100–102.

150. Kassai R, Hamada I, Furuta H, Cho K, Abe K, Deng HX, Niikawa N. Penta X syndrome: a case report with review of the literature. *Am J Med Genet* 1991;40:51–56.

151. Pajares IL, Delicardo A, de Bustamante AD, Pellicer A, Pinel I, Pardo M, Martin M. Tetraploidy in a liveborn infant. *J Med Genet* 1990;27:782–783.

152. Hall JG, Gilchrist DM. Turner syndrome and its variants. *Pediatr Clin North Am* 1990;37:1421–1440.

153. Hook EB, Warburton D. The distribution of chromosomal genotypes associated with Turner's syndrome: livebirth prevalence rates and evidence for diminished fetal mortality and severity in genotypes associated with structural X abnormalities or mosaicism. *Hum Genet* 1983;64:24–27.

154. Chen H, Faigenbaum D, Weiss H. Psychosocial aspects of patients with the Ullrich–Turner syndrome. *Am J Med Genet* 1981;8:191–203.

155. Chen H, Espiritu C, Casquejo C, Boriboon K, Woolley P Jr. Internipple distance in normal children from birth to 14 years, and in children with Turner's, Noonan's, Down's and other aneuploidies. *Growth* 1974;38:421–436.

156. Subramaniam PN. Turner's syndrome and cardiovascular anomalies: a case report and review of the literature. *Am J Med Sci* 1989;297:260–262.

157. Gøtzsche C-O, Krag-Olsen B, Nielsen J, Sørensen KE, Kristensen BO. Prevlance of cardiovascular malformations and association with karyotypes in Turner's syndrome. *Arch Dis Child* 1994;71:433–436.

158. Sreeram N, Wren C, Bhate M, Robertson P, Hunter S. Cardiac abnormalities in the fragile X syndrome. *Br Heart J* 1989;61:289–291.

159. Park V, Howard-Peebles P, Sherman S, Taylor A, Wulfsberg E. Policy statement: American College of Medical Genetics. Fragile X syndrome: diagnostic and carrier testing. *Am J Med Genet* 1994;53:380–381.

160. Strain L, Porteous MEM, Gosden CM, Ellis PM, Neilson JP, Bonthron DT. Prenatal diagnosis of fragile X syndrome: management of the male fetus with a premutation. *Prenatal Diagn* 1994;14:469–474.

161. Saadi AA, Juliar JF, Harm J, Brough AJ, Perrin EV, Chen H. Triploidy syndrome. A report on two live-born (69,XXY) and one still-born (69,XXX) infants. *Clin Genet* 1976;9:43–50.

162. Lin AE. Congenital heart defects in malformation syndromes. *Clin Perinatol* 1990;17:641–673.

163. Sepulveda M, Weiner E, Bower S, Flack NJ, Bennett PR, Fisk NN. Ectopia cordis in a triploid fetus: first-trimester diagnosis using transvaginal color Doppler ultrasonography and chorionic villus sampling. *J Clin Ultrasound* 1994;22:573–575.

164. Gersen SL, Carelli MP, Klinger KW, Ward BE. Rapid prenatal diagnosis of 14 cases of triploidy using FISH with multiple probes. *Prenatal Diagn* 1995;15:1–5.

165. Goldstein JL, Brown MS. Genetics and cardiovascular disease. In: Braunwald E, ed. *Heart Disease. A Textbook of Cardiovascular Medicine.* 3rd ed. Philadelphia: WB Saunders; 1988;1617–1649.

166. Nora JJ, Nora AH. The evolution of specific genetic and environmental counseling in congenital heart diseases. *Circulation* 1978;57:205–213.

167. Anderson RA, Koch S, Camerini-Otero RD. Cardiovascular findings in congenital contractural arachnodactyly: report of an affected kindred. *Am J Med Genet* 1984;18:265–271.

168. Chen H, Mirkin D, Yang S. De novo 17q paracentric inversion mosaicism in a patient with Beemer–Langer type short rib–polydactyly syndrome with special consideration to the classification of short rib polydactyly syndromes. *Am J Med Genet* 1994;53:165–171.

169. Beighton PH. The dominant and recessive forms of cutis laxa. *J Med Genet* 1972;9:216–221.

170. Leier CV, Call TD, Fulkerson PK, Wooley CF. The spectrum of cardiac defects in the Ehlers–Danlos syndrome, types I and III. *Ann Intern Med* 1980;92:171–178.

171. Giknis FL. Single atrium and the Ellis–van Creveld syndrome. *J Pediatr* 1963;62:558–564.

172. Meinecke P, Blunck W. Frontonasal dysplasia, congenital heart defect and short stature: a further observation. *J Med Genet* 1989;26:408–409.

173. Rees MM, Rodgers GM. Homocysteinemia: association of a metabolic disorder with vascular disease and thrombosis. *Thromb Res* 1993;71:337–359.

174. Chen H, Chang C-H, Perrin E, Perrin J. A lethal, Larsen-like multiple joint dislocation syndrome. *Am J Med Genet* 1982;13:149–161.

175. Chen H, Immken L, Lachman R, Yang S, Rimoin DL, Rightmire D, Eteson D, Stewart F, Beemer FA, Opitz JM, Gilbert EF, Langer LO, Shapiro LR, Duncan PA. Syndrome of multiple pterygia, camptodactyly, facial anomalies, hypoplastic lungs and heart, cystic hygroma, and skeletal anomalies: delineation of a new entity and review of lethal forms of multiple pterygium syndrome. *Am J Med Genet* 1984;17:809–826.

176. Pyeritz RE, Levin LS. Aortic root dilatation and valvular dysfunction in osteogenesis imperfecta. *Circulation* 1981;64:311.

177. Chen H, Blumberg B, Immken L, Lachman R, Rightmire D, Fowler M, Bachman R, Beemer FA. The Pena–Shokeir syndrome: report of five cases and further delineation of the syndrome. *Am J Med Genet* 1983;16:213–224.

178. McKusick VA. *Heritable Disorders of Connective Tissue.* St. Louis: CV Mosby; 1972;486–493.

179. Simpson JM, Cook A, Fagg NLK, MacLachlan NA, Sharland GK. Congenital heart disease in spondylothoracic dysostosis: two familial cases. *J Med Genet* 1995;32:633–635.

180. Liberfarb RM, Goldblatt A. Prevalence of mitral-valve prolapse in the Stickler syndrome. *Am J Med Genet* 1986;24:387–392.

181. Fernandez I, Tsukahara M, Mito H, Yoshii H, Uchida M, Matsuo K, Kajii T. Congenital heart defects in Aarskog syndrome. *Am J Med Genet* 1994;50:318–322.

182. Zapata HH, Sletten LJ, Pierpont MEM. Congenital cardiac malformations in Adams–Oliver syndrome. *Clin Genet* 1995;47:80–84.

183. Alagille D, Estrada A, Hadchouel M, Gautier M, Odievre M, Dommergues JP. Syndromic paucity of interlobular bile ducts (Alagille syndrome or arteriohepatic dysplasia): review of 80 cases. *J Pediatr* 1987;110:195–200.

184. Miller M, Hall JG. Familial asymmetric crying facies: its occurrence secondary to hypoplasia of the anguli oris depressor muscles. *Am J Dis Child* 1979;133:743–746.

185. Elbedour K, Zucker N, Zalzstein E, Barki Y, Carmi R. Cardiac abnormalities in the Bardet–Biedl syndrome: echocardiographic studies of 22 patients. *Am J Med Genet* 1994;52:164–169.

186. Cohen MM Jr. A comprehensive and critical assessment of overgrowth and overgrowth syndromes. *Adv Hum Genet* 1989;18:262–274.

187. Reynolds JF, Neri G, Herrmann JP, Blumberg B, Coldwell JG, Miles PV, Opitz JM. New multiple congenital anomalies/mental retardation syndrome with cardio-facio-cutaneous involvement—the CFC syndrome. *Am J Med Genet* 1986;25:413–427.

188. Eastman JR, Bixler D. Facio-cardio-renal syndrome: a newly delineated recessive disorder. *Clin Genet* 1977;11:424–430.

189. Moerman P, Fryns JP, van den Berghe K, Devlieger H, Lauweryns JM. The syndrome of diaphragmatic hernia, abnormal face and distal limb anomalies (Fryns syndrome): report of two sibs with further delineation of this multiple congenital anomaly (MCA) syndrome. *Am J Med Genet* 1988;31:805–814.

190. Chen H, Fowler M, Yu CW. Generalized arterial calcification of infancy in twins. *Birth Defects* 1982;18(3B):67–80.

191. Ruttenberg HD. Corrected transposition (L-transposition) of the great arteries and splenic syndromes. In: FH Adams, GC Emmanouilides, Riemenschneider TA, eds. *Moss' Heart Disease in Infants, Children, and Adolescents.* 3rd ed. Baltimore: Williams & Wilkins; 1983;333–350.

192. Goecke T, Dopler R, Huenges R, Conzelman W, Feller A, Majewski F. Hydrometrocolpos, postaxial polydactyly, congenital heart disease, and anomalies of the gastrointestinal and genitourinary tracts: a rare autosomal syndrome. *Eur J Pediatr* 1981;136:297–305.

193. Hsia YE, Bratu M, Herbordt A. Genetics of the Meckel syndrome. *Pediatrics* 1971;48:237–247.

194. Opitz JM. G syndrome (hypertelorism with esophageal abnormality and hypospadias, or hypospadias–dysphagia, or "Opitz–Frias" or "Opitz–G" syndrome). Perspective in 1987 and bibliography. *Am J Med Genet* 1987;28:275–285.

195. Powell CM, Chandra RS, Saasl HM. PHAVER syndrome: an autosomal recessive syndrome of limb ptergia, congenital heart anomalies, vertebral defects, ear anomalies, and radial defects. *Am J Med Genet* 1993;47:807–811.

196. Atalay S, Ege B, Imamoğlu A, Suskan E, Öcal B, Gümüs H. Congenital heart disease and Robinow syndrome. *Clin Dysmorphol* 1993;2:208–210.

197. Rutledge JC, Friedman JM, Harrod MJE, Currarino G, Wright CG, Pinckney L, Chen H. A "new" lethal multiple congenital anomaly syndrome: joint contractures, cerebellar hypoplasia, renal hypoplasia, urogenital anomalies, tongue cysts, shortness of limbs, eye abnormalities, defects of the heart, gall-

bladder agenesis, and ear malformations. *Am J Med Genet* 1984;19:255–264.

198. König R, Fuchs S, Kern C, Langenbeck U. Simpson–Golabi–Behmel syndrome with severe cardiac arrhythmias. *Am J Med Genet* 1991;38:244–247.

199. Opitz JM, Penchaszadeh VB, Holt MC, Spano LM. Smith–Lemli–Opitz (RSH) syndrome bibliography. *Am J Med Genet* 1987;28:745–750.

200. Nöthen MM, Knöpfle G, Födisch HJ, Zerres K. Steinfeld syndrome: report of a second family and further delineation of a rare autosomal dominant disorder. *Am J Med Genet* 1993;46:467–470.

201. Hays RM, Bartoshesky LE, Feingold M. New features of thrombocytopenia and absent radius syndrome. *Birth Defects* 1982;18(3B):115–121.

202. Nora JJ, Berg K, Nora AH. *Cardiovascular Diseases: Genetics, Epidemiology and Prevention.* New York: Oxford University Press; 1991;53–134.

203. Godfrey M. The Marfan syndrome. In: Beighton P, ed. *McKusick's Heritable Disorders of Connective Tissue.* 5th ed. St. Louis: CV Mosby; 1993; ch. 3.

204. Pyeritz RE. Marfan syndrome: Current and future clinical and genetic management of cardiovascular manifestations. *Semin Thorac Cardiovasc Surg* 1993;5:11–16.

205. Brown OR, DeMots H, Kloster FE, Roberts A, Menashe VD, Beals RK. Arotic root dilatation and mitral valve prolapse in Marfan's syndrome. *Circulation* 1975;52:651–657.

206. Pyeritz RE, McKusick VA. The Marfan syndrome: diagnosis and management. *N Engl J Med* 1979;300:772–777.

207. Geva T, Hegesh J, Frand M. The clinical course and echocardiographic features of Marfan's syndrome in childhood. *Am J Dis Child* 1987;141:1179–1182.

208. Murdoch JL, Walker BA, Halpern BL, Kuzma JW, McKusick VA. Life expectancy and causes of death in the Marfan syndrome. *N Engl J Med* 1972;286:804–808.

209. Roberts WC, Honig HS. The spectrum of cardiovascular disease in the Marfan syndrome: a clinico-morphologic study of 18 necropsy patients and comparison to 151 previously reported necropsy patients. *Am Heart J* 1982;104:115–135.

210. Dietz HC, Pyeritz RE, Puffenberger EG, Kendzior RJ Jr, Corson GM, Maslen CL, Sakai LY, Francomano CA, Cutting GR. Marfan phenotype variability in a family segregating a missense mutation in the epidermal growth factor–like motif of the fibrillin gene. *J Clin Invest* 1992;89:1674–1680.

211. Pereira L, Levran O, Ramirez F, Lynch JR, Sykes B, Pyeritz RE, Dietz HC. A molecular approach to the stratification of cardiovascular risk in families with Marfan's syndrome. *N Engl J Med* 1994;331:148–153.

212. Aoyama T, Francke U, Gasner C, Furthmayr H. Fibrillin abnormalities and prognosis in Marfan syndrome and related disorders. *Am J Med Genet* 1995;58:169–176.

213. Sakai LY, Keene DR, Engvall E. Fibrillin, a new 350-kD glycoprotein, is a component of extracellular microfibrils. *J Cell Biol* 1986;103:2499–2509.

214. Kainulainen K, Sakai LY, Child A, Pope FM, Puhakka L, Ryhanen L, Palotie A, Kaitila I, Peltonene L. Two mutations in

Marfan syndrome resulting in truncated fibrillin polypeptides. *Proc Natl Acad Sci USA* 1992;89:5917–5921.

215. Dietz HC, Ramirez F, Sakai LY. Marfan's syndrome and other microfibrillar diseases. *Adv Hum Genet* 1994;22:153–186.

216. Smith AT, Sack GH Jr, Taylor GJ. Holt–Oram syndrome. *J Pediatr* 1979;95:538–543.

217. Lin AE, Perloff JK. Upper limb malformations associated with congenital heart disease. *Am J Cardiol* 1985;55:1576–1583.

218. Terrett JA, Newbury-Ecob R, Cross GS, Fenton I, Raeburn JA, Yound ID, Brook JD. Holt–Oram syndrome is a genetically heterogeneous disease with one locus mapping to human chromosome 12q. *Nature Genet* 1994;6:401–404.

219. Basson CT, Cowley GS, Solomon SD, Weissman B, Poznanski AK, Traill TA, Seidman JG, Seidman CE. The clinical and genetic spectrum of the Holt–Oram syndrome (heart–hand syndrome). *N Engl J Med* 1994;330:889–891.

220. Gorlin RJ, Anderson RC, Blaw M. Multiple lentigenes syndrome. Complex comprising multiple lentigenes, electrocardiographic conduction abnormalities, ocular hypertelorism, pulmonary stenosis, abnormalities of genitalia, retardation of growth, sensorineural deafness, and autosomal dominant hereditary pattern. *Am J Dis Child* 1969;117:652–662.

221. Somerville J, Bonham-Carter RE. The heart in lentiginosis. *Br Heart J* 1972;41:205.

222. St John Sutton MG, Tajik AJ, Giuliani ER, Gordon H, Su WPD. Hypertrophic obstructive cardiomyopathy and lentiginosis: a little known neural ectodermal syndrome. *Am J Cardiol* 1981;47:214–217.

223. Riccardi VM. Type 1 neurofibromatosis and the pediatric patient. *Curr Probl Pediatr* 1992;22:66–106.

224. Ledbetter DH, Rich DC, O'Connell P, Leppert M, Carey JC. Precise localization of *NF1* to 17q11.2 by balanced translocation. *Am J Hum Genet* 1989;44:20–24.

225. Marchuk DA, Saulino AM, Tavakkol R, Swaroop M, Wallace MR, Andersen LB, Mitchell AL, Gutmann DH, Boguski M, Collins FS. cDNA cloning of the type 1 neurofibromatosis gene: complete sequence of the NF1 gene product. *Genomics* 1991;11:931–940.

226. National Institutes of Health Consensus Development Conference Statement. *Neurofibromatosis* 1987;6:1–7.

227. Wertelecki W, Rouleau GA, Superneau DW, Forehand LW, Williams JP, Haines JL, Gusella JF. Neurofibromatosis. 2. Clinical and DNA linkage studies of a large kindred. *N Engl J Med* 1988;319:278–283.

228. Halpern M, Currarino G. Vascular lesions causing hypertension in neurofibromatosis. *N Engl J Med* 1965;273:248–252.

229. Salyer WR, Salyer DC. The vascular lesions in neurofibromatosis. *Angiology* 1974;25:510–519.

230. Donaldson MC, Ellison LH, Ramsby GR. Hypertension from isolated thoracic aortic coarctation associated with neurofibromatosis. *J Pediatr Surg* 1985;20:169–171.

231. Neiman HL, Mena E, Holt JF, Stern AM, Perry BL. Neurofibromatosis and congenital heart disease. *Am J Roentgenol* 1974;122:146–149.

232. Mendez HMM, Opitz JM. Noonan syndrome: a review. *Am J Med Genet* 1985;21:493–506.

233. Patton MA. Noonan syndrome: a review. *Growth Genet Hormone* 1994;10:1–3.

234. Nora JJ, Nora AN, Sinha AK, Spanglei RD, Lubs HA. The Ullrich–Noonan syndrome (Turner phenotype). *Am J Dis Child* 1974;127:48–55.

235. Gibbs JL. The heart and tuberous sclerosis. An echocardiographic and electrocardiographic study. *Br Heart J* 1985;54:596–599.

236. Smith HC, Watson GH, Palel RG, Super M. Cardiac rhabdomyomata in tuberous sclerosis: their course and diagnostic value. *Arch Dis Child* 1989;64:196–200.

237. Fenoglio JJ, McAllister HA, Ferrans VJ. Cardiac rhabdomyoma: a clinicopathologic and electron microscopic study. *Am J Cardiol* 1976;38:241–251.

238. Shaher RM, Mintzer J, Farina M, Alley R, Bishop M. Clinical presentation of rhabdomyoma of the heart in infancy and childhood. *Am J Cardiol* 1972;30:95–103.

239. Romano C. Congenital cardiac arrhythmia. *Lancet* 1965;1:658–659.

240. Ward OC. A new familial cardiac syndrome in children. *J Indian Med Assoc* 1964;54:103–106.

241. Keating M, Atkinson D, Dunn C, Timothy K, Vincent GM, Leppert M. Linkage of a cardiac arrhythmia, the long QT syndrome, and the Harvey *ras*-1 gene. *Science* 1991;252:704–706.

242. Schott J-J, Charpentier F, Peltier S, Foley P, Drouin E, Bouchour J-B, Donnelly P, Vergnaud G, Bachner L, Moisan J-P, Le Marec H, Pascal O. Mapping of a gene for long QT syndrome to chromosome 4q25-27. *Am J Hum Genet* 1995;57:1114–1122.

243. Jervell A, Lange-Nielsen F. Congenital deaf-mutism, functional heart disease with prolongation of Q-T interval and sudden death. *Am Heart J* 1957;54:59–68.

244. Mares A Jr, Roberts R. The techniques of molecular biology and their application to the cardiomyopathies. *Adv Intern Med* 1994;39:395–434.

245. Servidei S, Bertini E, DiMauro S. Hereditary metabolic cardiomyopathies. *Adv Pediatr* 1994;41:1–32.

246. Kelly DP, Strauss AW. Inherited cardiomyopathies. *N Engl J Med* 1994;330:913–919.

247. Schwartz K, Carrier L, Guicheney P, Komajda M. Molecular basis of familial cardiomyopathies. *Circulation* 1995;91:532–540.

248. Baumbach LL, Chamberlain JS, Ward PA, Farwell NJ, Caskey CT. Molecular and clinical correlation of deletion leading to Duchenne and Becker muscular dystrophies. *Neurology* 1989;39:465–474.

249. Yates JRW. Workshop report. European Workshop on Emery–Dreifuss Muscular Dystrophy 1991. *Neuromusc Disord* 1991;1:393–396.

250. Ackroyd RS, Finnegan JA, Green SH. Friedreich's ataxia: a clinical review with neurophysiological and echocardiographic findings. *Arch Dis Child* 1984;59:217–221.

251. Mascarenhas DAN, Spodick DH, Chad DA, Gilchrist J, Townes PL, DeGirolami U, Mudge GH, Maki DW, Bishop RL. Cardiomyopathy of limb–girdle muscular dystrophy. *J Am College Cardiol* 1994;24:1328–1333.

252. Tachi N, Tachi M, Sasaki K, Tomita H, Wakai S, Annaka S, Minami R, Tsuui S, Sugie H. Glycogen storage disease with normal acid maltase: skeletal and cardiac muscles. *Pediatr Neurol* 1989;5:60–63.

253. Servidei S, Riepe RE, Langston C, Tani LY, Bricker JT, Crisp-Lindgren N, Travers H, Armstrong D, DiMauro S. Severe cardiopathy in branching enzyme deficiency. *J Pediatr* 1987;11:51–56.

254. Moses SW, Wandemann KL, Myroz A, Frydman M. Cardiac involvement in glycogen storage disease type III. *Eur J Pediatr* 1989;148:764–766.

255. DiMauro S, Servidei S. Disorders of carbohydrate metabolism: glycogen storage disease. In: Rosenberg RN, Prusiner SB, DiMauro S, et al, eds. *The Molecular and Genetic Basis of Neurological Disease.* Boston: Butterworth-Heinemann; 1993;93–119.

256. Demaugre F, Bonnefont J-P, Colonna M, Cepanec C, Leroux J-P, Saudusbray J-M. Infantile form of carnitine palmitoyltransferase II deficiency with hepatomuscular symptoms and sudden death. *J Clin Invest* 1991;87:859–864.

257. Bautista J, Rafel E, Martinez A, Sainz I, Herrera J, Segura L, Chinchon I. Familial hypertrophic cardiomyopathy and muscle carnitine deficiency. *Muscle Nerve* 1990;13:192–194.

258. Hoppel CL, Kerr DS, Dohms B, Dahms B. Roessman U. Deficiency of the reduced nicotinamide adenine dinucleotide dehydrogenase component of complex I of mitochondrial electron transport. *J Clin Invest* 1987;80:71–77.

259. Papadimitriou A, Neustein HB, DiMauro S, Stanton R, Bresolin N. Histocytoid cardiomyopathy of infancy: deficiency of reducible cytochrome *b* in heart mitochondria. *Pediatr Res* 1985;18:1023–1028.

260. Zeviani M, Van Dyke DH, Servidei S, Bauserman SC, Bonilla E, Beaumont ET, Sharda J, VanderLaan K, DiMauro S. Myopathy and fatal cardiomyopathy due to cytochrome *c* oxidase deficiency. *Arch Neurol* 1986;43:1198–1202.

261. Holme E, Greter J, Jacobson C-E, Larsson N-G, Lindstedt S, Nilsson KO, Oldfors A, Tulinius M. Mitochondrial ATP-synthase deficiency in a child with 3-methylglutaconic aciduria. *Pediatr Res* 1992;32:731–735.

262. Sengers RCA, ter Haar BGA, Trijbels JMF, Willems JL, Daniels WO, Stadhouders AM. Congenital cataract and mitochondrial myopathy of skeletal and heart muscle associated with lactic acidosis after exercise. *J Pediatr* 1975;86:873–880.

263. Zeviani M, Gellera C, Antozzi C, Rimoldi M, Morandi L, Villani F, Tiranti V, DiDonato S. Maternally inherited myopathy and cardiomyopathy: association with mutation in mitochondrial DNA tRNA^Leu(UUR). *Lancet* 1991;338:143–147.

264. Rutledge JC, Haas JE, Monnat R, Milstein JM. Hypertrophic cardiomyopathy is a component of subacute necrotizing encephalomyelopathy. *J Pediatr* 1982;101:706–710.

265. Hadley RN, Hagstrom JWC. Cardiac lesions in a patient with familial neurovisceral lipidosis (generalized gangliosidosis). *Am J Clin Pathol* 1971;55:237–240.

266. Desnick RJ, Blieden LC, Sharp HL, Hofschire PJ, Moller JH. Cardiac valvular anomalies in Fabry disease: clinical, morphologic, and biochemical studies. *Circulation* 1976;54:818–825.

267. Sewell AC, Pontz BF, Weitzel D, Humburg C. Clinical heterogeneity in infantile galactosialidosis. *Eur J Pediatr* 1987;146:528–531.

268. Gibson KM, Sherwood WG, Hoffman GF, Stumpf DA, Dianzani I, Schutgens RBH, Barth PG, Weismann U, Bachmann C, Schrynemackers-Pitance P, Verloes A, Narisawa K, Mino M, Ohya N, Kelley RI. Phenotypic heterogeneity in the syndromes of 3-methylglutaconic aciduria. *J Pediatr* 1991;118:885–890.

269. Blieden LC, Desnick RJ, Carter JB, Krivit W, Moller JH, Sharp HL. Cardiac involvement in Sandhoff's disease. Inborn error of glycosphingolipid metabolism. *Am J Cardiol* 1974;34:83–88.

270. Kornfeld S, Sly WS. I-cell disease and pseudo-Hurler polydystrophy: disorders of lysosomal enzyme phosphorylation and localization. In: Scriver CR, Beaudet AL, Sly WS, Valle D, eds. *The Metabolic and Molecular Bases of Inherited Disease.* 7th ed. New York: McGraw-Hill; 1995;2495–2508.

271. Manolio TA, Baughman KL, Rodeheffer R, Pearson TA, Bristow JD, Michels W, Abelmann WH, Harlan WR. Prevalence and etiology of idiopathy dilated cardiomyopathy (Summary of a National Heart, Lung, and Blood Institute Workshop). *Am J Cardiol* 1992;69:1458–1466.

272. Gravanis MB, Ansari AA. Idiopathic cardiomyopathies. A review of pathologic studies and mechanisms of pathogenesis. *Arch Pathol Lab Med* 1987;111:915–929.

273. Report of the WHO/ISFC Task Force on the Definition and Classification of Cardiomyopathies. *Br Heart J* 1980;44:672–673.

274. Marian AJ, Roberts R. Molecular basis of hypertrophic and dilated cardiomyopathy. *Texas Heart Inst J* 1994;21:6–15.

275. Maron BJ. Hypertrophic cardiomyopathy. *Curr Probl Cardiol* 1993;18:643–704.

276. Landing BH, Recalde AL, Lawrence TYK, Shankle WR. Cardiomyopathy in childhood and adult life, with emphasis on hypertrophic cardiomyopathy. *Pathol Res Pract* 1994;190:737–749.

277. Maron BJ, Nichols PF III, Pickle LW, Wesley YE, Mulvihill JJ. Patterns of inheritance in hypertrophic cardiomyopathy: assessment by M-mode and two-dimensional echocardiography. *Am J Cardiol* 1984;1087–1094.

278. Jarcho JA, McKenna W, Pare JAP, Solomon SD, Holcombe RF, Dickie S, Levi T, Donis-Keller H, Seidman JG, Seidman CE. Mapping a gene for familial hypertrophic cardiomyopathy to chromosome 14q1. *N Engl J Med* 1989;321:1372–1378.

279. Geisterfer-Lawrance AAT, Kass S, Tanigawa G, Vosberg H-P, McKenna W, Seidman CE, Seidman JG. A molecular basis for familial hypertrophic cardiomyopathy: a β-cardiac myosin heavy chain gene missense mutation. *Cell* 1990;62:999–1006.

280. Watkins H, MacRae C, Thierfelder L, Chou Y-H, Frenneaux M, McKenna W, Seidman JG, Seidman CE. A disease locus for familial hypertrophic cardiomyopathy mags to chromosome 1q3. *Nature Genet* 1993;3:333–337.

281. Thierfelder L, MacRae C, Watkins H, Tomfohde J, Williams M, McKenna W, Bohm K, Noeske G, Schlepper M, Bowcock A, Vosberg H-P, Seidman JG, Seidman C. A familial hypertrophic cardiomyopathy locus maps to chromosome 15q2. *Proc Natl Acad Sci USA* 1993;90:6270–6274.

282. Carrier L, Hengstenberg C, Beckmann JS, Guicheney P, Dufour C, Bercovici J, Dausse E, Berebbi-Bertrand I, Wisnewsky C, Pulvenis D, Fetler L, Vignal A, Weissenbach J, Hillaire D, Feingold J, Bouhour J-B, Hagege A, Desnos M, Isnard R, Dubourg O, Komajda M, Schwartz K. Mapping of a novel gene for familial hypertrophic cardiomyopathy to chromosome 11. *Nature Genet* 1993;4:311–313.

283. Michels VV, Moll PP, Miller FA, Tajik AJ, Chu JS, Driscoll DJ, Burnett JC, Rodeheffer RJ, Chesebro JH, Tazelaar HD. The frequency of familial dilated cardiomyopathy in a series of patients with idiopathic dilated cardiomyopathy. *N Engl J Med* 1992;326:77–82.

284. Emanuel R, Withers R, O'Brien K. Dominant and recessive modes of inheritance in idiopathic cardiomyopathy. *Lancet* 1971;2:1065–1067.

285. Berko BA, Swift M. X-linked dilated cardiomyopathy. *N Engl J Med* 1987;316:1186–1191.

286. Kass S, MacRae C, Graber HL, Sparks EA, McNamara D, Boudoulas H, Basson CT, Baker PB III, Cody RJ, Fishman MC, Cox N, Kong A, Wooley CF, Seidman JG, Seidman CE. A gene defect that causes conduction system disease and dilated cardiomyopathy maps to chromosome 1p1–1q1. *Nature Genet* 1994;7:546–551.

287. Krajinovic M, Pinamonti B, Sinagra G, Vatta M, Severini GM, Milasin J, Falaschi A, Camerini F, Giacca M, Mestroni L, and the Heart Muscle Disease Study Group. Linkage of familial dilated cardiomyopathy to chromosome 9. *Am J Hum Genet* 1995;57:846–852.

288. Jacobs PA, Hunt PA, Mayer M, Bart RD. Duchenne muscular dystrophy (DMD) in a female with an X/autosome translocation: further evidence that the DMD locus is at Xp21. *Am J Hum Genet* 1981;33:513–518.

289. Zatz M, Vianna-Morgante AM, Campos P, Diament AJ. Translocation (X;6) in a female with Duchenne muscular dystrophy: implications for the localisation of the DMD locus. *J Med Genet* 1981;18:442–447.

290. Koenig M, Hoffman EP, Bertelson CJ, Monaco AP, Feener C, Kunkel LM. Complete cloning of the Duchenne muscular dystrophy (DMD) cDNA and preliminary genomic organization of the DMD gene in normal and affected individuals. *Cell* 1987;50:509–517.

291. Hoffman EP, Brown RH Jr, Kunkel LM. Dystrophin: the protein product of the Duchenne muscular dystrophy locus. *Cell* 1987;51:919–928.

292. Passo-Bueno MR, Bakker E, Kneppers ALJ, Takata RI, Rapaport D, den Dunnen JT, Zatz M, van Ommen GJB. Different mosaicism frequencies for proximal and distal Duchenne muscular dystrophy (DMD) mutations indicate difference in etiology and recurrence risk. *Am J Hum Genet* 1992;51:1150–1155.

293. Höweler CJ, Busch HFM, Geraedts JPM, Niermeijer MF, Staal A. Anticipation in myotonic dystrophy: fact or fiction? *Brain* 1989;112:779–797.

294. Brook JD, McCurrach ME, Harley HG, Buckler AJ, Church D, Aburatani H, Hunter K, Stanton VP, Thirion J-P, Hudson T, Sohn R, Zemelman B, Snell RG, Rundle SA, Crow S, Davies J, Shelbourne P, Buxton J, Jones C, Juvonen V, Johnson K, Harper PS, Shaw DJ, Housman DE. Molecular basis of myotonic dystrophy: expansion of a trinucleotide (CTG) repeat at the 3' end of a transcript encoding a protein kinase family member. *Cell* 1992;68:799–808.

295. Zoghbi WA, Pacifico A, Epstein HF, Ashizawa T, Armstrong R, Perryman B, Quinones MA. Prevalence of cardiac abnormalities in a large kindred with myotonic dystrophy. *J Am College Cardiol* 1989;13(suppl A):89A. Abstract.

296. Engel AG, Seybold ME, Lambert EH, Gomez MR. Acid maltase deficiency: comparison of infantile, childhood, and adult types. *Neurology* 1970;20:382.

297. Zhong N, Martiniuk F, Tzall S, Hirschhorn R. Identification of a missense mutation in one allele of a patient with Pompe disease, and use of endonuclease digestion of PCR-amplified RNA to demonstrate lack of mRNA expression from the second allele. *Am J Hum Genet* 1991;49:635–645.

298. Wallace DC. Diseases of the mitochondrial DNA. *Annu Rev Biochem* 1992;61:1175–1212.

299. DiMauro S. Mitochondrial encephalomyopathies. In: Rosenberg RN, Prusiner SB, DiMauro S, et al, eds. *The Molecular and Genetic Basis of Neurological Disease.* Boston: Butterworth-Heinemann; 1993;665–694.

300. Tveskov C, Angelo-Nielson K. Kearns–Sayre syndrome and dilated cardiomyopathy. *Neurology* 1990;40:553–554.

301. Nelson J, Shields MD, Mulholland HC. Cardiovascular studies in the mucopolysaccharidoses. *J Med Genet* 1990;27:94–100.

302. Miller G, Partridge A. Mucopolysaccharidosis type VI presenting in infancy with endocardial fibroelastosis and heart failure. *Pediatr Cardiol* 1983;4:61–62.

303. Fong LV, Menahem S, Wraith JE, Chow CW. Endocardial fibroelastosis in mucopolysaccharidosis type VI. *Clin Cardiol* 1987;10;362–364.

304. Donaldson MDC, Pennock CA, Berry PJ, Duncan AW, Cawdery JE, Leonard JV. Hurler syndrome with cardiomyopathy in infancy. *J Pediatr* 1989;114:430–432.

305. Hayflick S, Rowe S, Kavanaugh-McHugh A, Olson JL, Valle D. Acute infantile cardiomyopathy as a presenting feature of mucopolysaccharidosis VI. *J Pediatr* 1992;120:269–272.

306. Fensom AH, Benson PF. Recent advances in the prenatal diagnosis of the mucopolysaccharidoses. *Prenatal Diagn* 1994;14:1–12.

307. Chen H, Gonzalez E, Hand AM, Cuestas R. The acardius acephalus and monozygotic twinning. *Schumpert Med Q* 1983;1:195–199.

308. Hassell S, Butler MG. Antley–Bixler syndrome: report of a patient and review of literature. *Clin Genet* 1994;46:372–376.

309. Hall JG, Reed SD, Greene G. The distal arthrogryposes: delineation of new entities—review and nosologic discussion. *Am J Med Genet* 1982;11:185–239.

310. Lin AE, McPherson E, Nwokoro NA, Clemens M, Losken HW, Mulvihill JJ. Further delineation of the Baller–Gerold syndrome. *Am J Med Genet* 1993;45:519–524.

311. Carmi R, Boughman JA. Pentalogy of Cantrell and associated midline anomalies: a possible ventral midline developmental field. *Am J Med Genet* 1992;42:90–95.

312. Wyse RK, Al-Mahdawi S, Burn J, Blake K. Congenital heart disease in CHARGE association. *Pediatr Cardiol* 1993;14:75–81.

313. Marles SL, Chodirker BN, Greenberg CR, Chudley AE. Evidence for Ritscher–Schinzel syndrome in Canadian native Indians. *Am J Med Genet* 1995;56:343–350.

314. Ptacek LJ, Opitz JM, Smith DW, Gerritsen T, Waisman HA. The Cornelia de Lange syndrome. *J Pediatr* 1963;63:1000–1020.

315. Daentl DL, Smith DW, Scott CI, Hall BD, Gooding CA. Femoral hypoplasia–unusual facies syndrome. *J Pediatr* 1975;107–111.

316. Kumar A, Friedman JM, Taylor GP, Paterson MWH. Pattern of cardiac malformation in oculoauriculovertebral spectrum. *Am J Med Genet* 1993;46:423–426.

317. Thomas IT, Honore GM, Jewett T, Velvis H, Garber P, Ruiz C. Holzgreve syndrome: recurrence in sibs. *Am J Med Genet* 1993;45:767–769.

318. Salonen R, Herva R. Hydrolethalus syndrome. *J Med Genet* 1990;27:756–759.

319. Bailey LL, Gundry SR. Hypoplastic left heart syndrome. *Pediatr Clin North Am* 1990;37:137–150.

320. Gunderson CH, Greenspan RH, Glaser GH, Lubs HA. The Klippel–Feil syndrome: genetic and clinical reevaluation of cervical fusion. *Medicine* 1967;46:491–512.

321. Bird LM, Krous HF, Eichenfield LF, Swalwell CI, Jones MC. Female infant with oncocytic cardiomyopathy and microphthalmia with linear skin defects (MLS). A clue to the pathogenesis of oncocytic cardiomyopathy? *Am J Med Genet* 1994;53:141–148.

322. Lurie IW, Magee CA, Sun CCJ, Ferencz C. "Microgastria–limb reduction" complex with congenital heart disease and twinning. *Clin Dysmorphol* 1995;4:150–155.

323. Glickstein J, Karasik J, Caride DG, Marion RW. "C" trigonocephaly syndrome: report of a child with agenesis of the corpus callosum and tetralogy of Fallot, and review. *Am J Med Genet* 1995;56:215–218.

324. Hall JG, Pallister PD, Clarren SK, Beckwith JB, Wiglesworth FW, Fraser FC, Cho S, Benke PJ, Reed SD. Congenital hypothalamic hamartoblastoma, hypopituitarism, imperforate anus, and postaxial polydactyly—a new syndrome? I. Clinical, causal, and pathogenetic considerations. *Am J Med Genet* 1980;7:47–74.

325. Ireland DCR, Takayama N, Flatt AE. Poland's syndrome. A review of forty-three cases. *J Bone Joint Surg (Am)* 1976;58:52–58.

326. Cohen MM Jr, Gorlin RJ. Pseudo–trisomy 13 syndrome. *Am J Med Genet* 1991;39:332–335.

327. Kanjilal D, Basir MA, Verma RS, Rajegowda BK, Lala R, Nagaraj A. New dysmorphic features in Rubinstein–Taybi syndrome. *J Med Genet* 1992;29:669–670.

328. Patton MA. Russell–Silver syndrome. *J Med Genet* 1988;25:557–560.

329. Quan L, Smith DW. The VATER association: vertebral defects, anal atresia, trancheoesophagel fistula with esophageal atresia, radial dysplasia. *Birth Defects* 1972;8(2):75–78.

330. Greenwood RD, Rosenthal A, Parisi L, Flyer DC, Nadas AS. Extracardiac abnormalities in infants with congenital heart disease. *Pediatrics* 1975;55:485–492.

331. Miller RD, Divertie MB. Kartagener's syndrome. *Chest* 1972;62:130–135.

332. Rossman CM, Forrest JB, Ruffin RE, Newhouse MT. Immotile cilia syndrome in persons with and without Kartagener's syndrome. *Am Rev Respir Dis* 1980;121:1011–1016.

333. Gibbons IR, Rowe AJ. Dynein: a protein with adenosine triphosphatase activity from cilia. *Science* 1965;149:424–426.

334. Turner JAP, Corkey CWB, Lee JYC, Levison H, Sturgess J. Clinical expressions of immotile cilia syndrome. *Pediatrics* 1981;67:805–810.

335. Narayan D, Desai T, Banks A, Patanjali SR, Ravikumar TS, Ward DC. Localization of the human cytoplasmic dynein heavy chain (DNECL) to 14qter by fluorescence in situ hybridization. *Genomics* 1994;22:660–661.

336. Morris CA, Demsey SA, Leonard CO, Dilts C, Blackburn BL. Natural history of Williams syndrome: physical characteristics. *J Pediatr* 1988;113:318–326.

337. Ewart AK, Morris CA, Ensing GJ, Loker J, Moore C, Leppert M, Keating M. A human vascular disorder, supravalvar aortic stenosis maps to chromosome 7. *Proc Natl Acad Sci USA* 1993;90:3226–3230.

338. Curran ME, Atkinson DL, Ewart AK, Morris CA, Leppert MF, Keating MT. The elastin gene is disrupted by a translocation associated with supravalvar aortic stenosis. *Cell* 1993;73:159–168.

339. Lowery MC, Morris CA, Ewart A, Brothman LJ, Zhu XL, Leonard CO, Carey JC, Keating M, Brothman AR. Strong correlation of elastin deletions, detected by FISH, with Williams syndrome: evaluation of 235 patients. *Am J Hum Genet* 1995;57:49–53.

340. ISCN (1995). *An International System for Human Cytogenetic Nomenclature.* Mitelman F, ed: Basel: S Karger; 1995.

341. Current awareness in prenatal diagnosis. *Prenatal Diagn* 1995;15:783–790.

APPENDIX TO CHAPTER 49

Abbreviations of Cardiac Lesions Used in Tables 49.2–49.7

A	atherosclerosis
AA	aortic atresia/hypoplasia
AAA	aortic arch abnormality
AC	acardia

cate and sequentially crucial developmental processes. Other factors, such as population-specific infection rates, socioeconomic conditions, and racial and genetic differences, may also affect the incidence and severity of congenital infections and cardiac malformations.[7–11] In spite of the many limiting factors for investigation of etiologies and the uncertainty of congenital damage even when maternal infection can be documented, the pathophysiology of infectious agent cardiac malformation is probably not significantly different from other organ structural congenital malformations. Figure 50.1 outlines the wide range of possible maternal, placental, fetal, and neonatal disease effects for infectious agents. Fetal viremia can affect the vascular tree and the vascular endothelial lining, potentially causing sequential "downstream" organ damage.[12,13] Endocardial cushions and lining damaged as a result of an insult by an infectious agent may produce valvular defects and endocardial fibroelastosis.[14,15] Therefore, the ability to associate suspected pathogens with specific lesions is at best severely limited and difficult to scientifically prove.

Rubella is the only infectious agent for which specific congenital cardiac anomalies have been identified. Precise patterns and lesions of expected cardiac congenital anomalies from other infectious agents remain uncertain, partially because of the widely varying effects of such early cellular and tissue insults and the difficulty in proving causality.[16,17]

Advances in ultrasound imaging and a growing body of sonographer experience have made it possible to identify fetal and neonatal cardiac anomalies with increasing accuracy. It is accepted that once a cardiac malformation has been identified, awareness of the increased incidence of chromosomal abnormalities that accompany a cardiac structural defect should prompt serious consideration for further prenatal diagnosis. Investigation of maternal history and prenatal course may assist in identifying a possible infectious cause for such an abnormality. When a cardiac structural anomaly is identified in utero, diagnosis of congenital infections can be performed through amniocentesis or cordocentesis. These techniques yield amniotic fluid, fetal blood, and other cells for the identification of cultures and infectious agents spe-

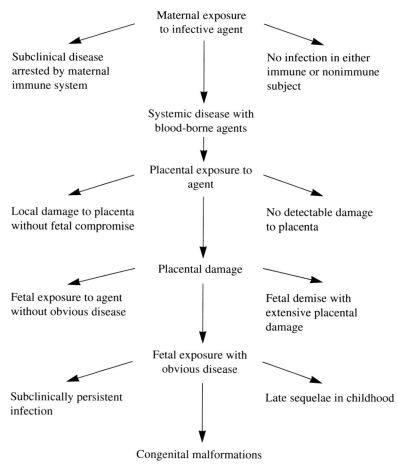

Figure 50.1 Routes of congenital infection associated with malformations.

cific to various antibodies. Laboratory methods used in such investigations include polymerase chain reaction DNA amplification, radioimmunoassay (RIA), immuno-fluorescence assay (IFA), and latex agglutination (LA).[3]

INFECTIOUS AGENTS ASSOCIATED WITH CONGENITAL CARDIAC ANOMALIES

Congenital Rubella Infection

Rubella remains the single infectious agent for which ensuing cardiac malformations have been clearly demonstrated. The cardiovascular anomalies associated with rubella infection are patent ductus arteriosus, pulmonary artery branch stenosis, pulmonary vein stenosis, ventricular septal defect, atrial septal defect, coarctation of the aortic isthmus, and tetralogy of Fallot. Cardiovascular anomalies occur in at least two-thirds of severely affected fetuses.[18] These lesions may also be accompanied by other vascular abnormalities.[19] Myocarditis also may accompany congenital rubella infection. The subsequent physiologic dysfunction may increase the clinical severity of fetal or neonatal infection and compound the anatomical abnormality's effect.[2] Rubella virus isolation has been performed from amniotic fluid, and rubella-specific IgM antibody is present in the infected neonate. Since as a rule the fetus does not develop IgM before 18–21 weeks of gestation, the role of fetal serum antibody detection to confirm infection is limited by gestational age.[20]

Congenital Cytomegalovirus (CMV) Infection

Intrauterine infection by CMV may be the most ubiquitous and unpredictable of fetal and neonatal infections. Maternal susceptibility and subsequent fetal infection rates indicate that a primary maternal infection may lead to a wide range of neonatal clinical findings.[21] Affected infants usually demonstrate neurologic and growth abnormalities. However, cardiac malformations have been reported to occur sporadically in severely affected infants with multiorgan involvement.[22] This virus has been detected in amniotic fluid by culture, in chorionic villi by polymerase chain reaction amplification of CMV-specific DNA, and in maternal and fetal sera by CMV-specific IgM.[23–25]

Congenital Mumps Infection

The association between the mumps virus and endocardial fibroelastosis (EFE) remains unclear and controversial. This viral agent has been cultured from fetal and placental tissue and appears to usually not cause any increased risk of congenital anomalies. Injection of mumps virus into chick embryos produces thickening of the endocardium in a fashion similar to that seen in EFE.[26] Evidence associating EFE in neonates is based on a comparison of infected children and normal controls for skin test reactivity to the mumps virus. This type of skin testing has been inconsistently interpretable and thus, this association is questionable.[27]

Congenital Enteroviruses

The congenital enteroviruses comprise several subgroups, including polio viruses, Coxsackie virus groups A and B, and echoviruses. Coxsackieviruses A and B have been isolated from fetal and placental tissues and are known to be capable of inducing myocarditis. Usually these viruses have not been associated with any increase in congenital anomalies. One study identified an increased incidence of cardiovascular malformations in the presence of infections with more than one coxsackievirus.[28] The most common malformations associated with this group of viruses are patent ductus arteriosus and ventricular and atrial septal defects.

Congenital Rubeola Infection

Recent outbreaks of rubeola (measles) have involved young children as well as women of reproductive age. Occasional case reports have indicated an increased risk of congenital anomalies in neonates born to women who were infected during pregnancy. A single study reported an increased incidence of infants with cardiac anomalies.[29] The virus cannot be confirmed as a teratogen on the basis of this study, however, because the work appears to have been inadequately controlled.

Congenital Human Immunodeficiency Virus Infection

The increase in infection by HIV among women of reproductive age and their fetuses has been dramatic over the past decade. The maternal, placental, fetal, and neonatal factors influencing the rate of transmission and infection were well summarized in a review in an AIDS journal.[30] Postnatal cardiomyopathy has been noted in infected children.[31,32] No studies have been published to date linking infection by this group of viruses with fetal congenital cardiac anomalies.

CONCLUSION

This chapter has presented the infectious agents known to be linked with congenital cardiac anomalies. Obviously many other organisms, bacterial as well as viral, present threats to developing fetal tissues and subsequent neonatal growth. It is possible that with improvements in laboratory testing, diagnostic ultrasound capabilities, and specific epidemiologic surveillance, other infectious agents may be linked with such potentially severe malformations. The lack of a treatment for any of the preceding disease states that might prevent or minimize the clinical severity for the infected child is indeed a frustrating medical reality. As is usually the case in medicine, our ability to identify and diagnose precedes our capability to treat or correct an infection and its sequelae.

REFERENCES

1. Swan C, Tostevin AL, Moore B, Mayo H, Black GHB. Congenital defects in infants following infectious diseases during pregnancy. *Med J Aust* 1943;2:201–210.

2. Rosenberg HS. Cardiovascular effects of congenital infections. *Am J Cardiovascular Pathol* 1987;1(2):147–156.

3. Valente P, Sever JL. *In utero* diagnosis of congenital infections by direct fetal sampling. *Isr J Med Sci* 1994;30:414–420.

4. Overall JC. Intrauterine virus infections and congenital heart disease. *Am Heart J* 1972;84:823–833.

5. McKeown T, Record RG. Malformations in a population observed for 5 years after birth. In: Wolstenholme GEW, O'Connor CM, eds. *Ciba Foundation Symposium on Congenital Malformations*. Boston: Little, Brown; 1960;5.

6. Kerrebijn KF. Incidence in infants and mortality from congenital malformations of the circulatory system. *Acta Paediatr Scand* 1966;55:316–320.

7. Witte JJ, Karchmer AW, Case G, Hermann KL, Abrotyn E, Kassanoff I, Neill JS. Epidemiology of rubella. *Am J Dis Child* 1969;118:107–111.

8. Honeyman MC, Menser MA. Ethnicity is a significant factor in the epidemiology of Rubella and Hodgkin's disease. *Nature* 1974;251:441–442.

9. Honeyman MC, Dorman DC, Menser MA, Forest JM, Guinan JJ, Clark P. HLA antigens in congenital rubella and the role of antigens 1 and 8 in the epidemiology of natural rubella. *Tissue Antigens* 1975;5:12–18.

10. Schweitzer IL, Mosley JW, Ashcaval M, Edwards VM, Overby IB. Factors influencing neonatal infection by hepatitis B virus. *Gastroenterology* 1973;65:277–283.

11. Schweitzer IL, Dunn AGE, Peters RL, Spears RL. Viral hepatitis B in neonates and infants. *Am J Med* 1973;55:762–771.

12. Singer MC, Rudolph AJ, Rosenberg HS, Rawls WE, Bonivk M. Pathology of the congenital rubella syndrome. *J Pediatr* 1967;71:665–675.

13. Campbell PE. Vascular abnormalities following maternal rubella. *Br Heart J* 1965;27:134–138.

14. Neda K, Nishida Y, Oshima K, Shephard TH. Congenital rubella syndrome: correlation of gestational age at time of maternal rubella with type of defect. *J Pediatr* 1979;94:763–765.

15. Aase JM, Noren GR, Reddy DV, St. Geme JW Jr. Mumps-virus infection in pregnant women and the immunologic response of their offspring. *N Engl J Med* 1972;286:1379–1382.

16. Hanshaw JB, Dudgeon JAL. Congenital heart disease. In: *Viral Diseases of the Fetus and Newborn*. Philadelphia: WB Saunders; 1978.

17. Brown GC, Krunas RS. Relationship of congenital anomalies and maternal infection with selected enteroviruses. *Am J Epidemiol* 1972;95:207–217.

18. Catalano LW, Sever JL. The role of viruses as causes of congenital defects. *Annu Rev Microbiol* 1971;25:255–282.

19. Menser MA, Dorman DC, Reye RDK, Reid RR. Renal-artery stenosis in the rubella syndrome. *Lancet* 1966;1:790–792.

20. Daffos F, Forestier F, Capella-Pavlovsky M. Prenatal management of 746 pregnancies at risk for congenital toxoplasmosis. *N Engl J Med* 1988;318:271–275.

21. Fowler KB, Stagno S, Pass RF, Britt WJ, Boll TJ, Alford CA. The outcome of congenital cytomegalovirus infection in relation to maternal antibody status. *N Engl J Med* 1992;326(10): 663–667.

22. Ahltors K, Ivarsson SA, Johnsson T, Svanbergh L. Primary and secondary maternal cytomegalovirus infections and their relation to congenital infection. *Acta Paediatr Scand* 1982;71: 109–113.

23. Weiner CP, Grose C. Prenatal diagnosis of congenital cytomegalovirus infection by virus isolation from amniotic fluid. *Am J Obstet Gynecol* 190:163:1253–1255.

24. Hogge WA, Buffonet GJ, Hogge JS. Prenatal diagnosis of cytomegalovirus (CMV) infection: a preliminary report. *Prenatal Diagn* 1993;13:131–136.

25. Goff E, Griffith BP, Booss J. Delayed amplification of cytomegalovirus infection in the placenta and maternal tissues during late gestation. *Am J Obstet Gynecol* 1987;156: 1265–1270.

26. St. Geme JW Jr, Peralta H, Farias E, Davis CWC, Noren GR. Experimental gestational mumps virus infection and endocardial fibroelastosis. *Pediatrics* 1966;38:309.

27. Guntheroth WG. Endocardial fibroelastosis and mumps. *Pediatrics* 1966;38:309.

28. Brown GC, Karunas RS. Relationship of congenital anomalies and maternal infection with selected enteroviruses. *Am J Epidemiol* 1972;95:207–217.

29. Jesperseu CS, Littaner J, Sagild R. Measles as a cause of fetal defects. *Acta Paediatr Scand* 1977;66:367–372.

30. Mofenson LM, Wright PF, Fast PE. Summary of the working group of perinatal intervention. *AIDS Res Hum Retroviruses* 1992;8(8):1435–1438.

31. Joshi VV. Pathologic findings associated with HIV infection in children. In: Pizzo PA, Wilfert CM, eds. *Pediatric AIDS: The Challenge of HIV Infection in Infants, Children and Adolescents*. Baltimore: Williams & Wilkins; 1991;125–134.

32. Roldan E. Pathology of the heart in acquired immunodeficiency syndrome. *Arch Pathol Lab Med* 1987;III:943–946.

51

METABOLIC CAUSES OF CONGENITAL CARDIAC ABNORMALITIES

NINA L. GOTTEINER, MD

INTRODUCTION

Fetal cardiac development occurs from the third through the eighth week of organogenesis. During this time the fetal heart is vulnerable to metabolic abnormalities that may be present as a result of maternal disease or ingested teratogens. The fetal heart may be affected later in gestation as well. Cardiac effects from metabolic abnormalities depend on the type of teratogen, its concentration in the fetus, the specific time of exposure, and the fetal genotype.

DIABETES MELLITUS (SEE ALSO CHAPTER 41)

The incidence of insulin-dependent diabetes mellitus varies between 1 and 5.6 cases per thousand pregnancies.[1–6] In addition, there are approximately 7.5–40 gestational diabetics (i.e., women of White class A,[7] who develop glucose intolerance during pregnancy but revert to normal postpartum) per thousand pregnancies.[4,5] Overall, approximately 1–4% of all pregnancies are complicated by diabetes mellitus. Table 51.1 presents White's classification of diabetes mellitus in pregnancy;[7] it is the system most commonly used to correlate severity of this disease with both fetal and maternal morbidity.

Rates of congenital malformations are two to four times higher in infants of diabetic mothers compared to the general population (5–17% vs. 2–4%, respectively).[4,8–17] Since malformation rates are not higher in infants whose fathers are diabetic, an abnormal intrauterine environment rather than a genetic predisposition is postulated as an etiologic fac-

tor.[17,18] Congenital malformations are the most common cause of perinatal death in infants of diabetic mothers.[4,19–23]

Cardiac malformations are three to five times more likely to occur in infants of diabetic mothers, and they account for approximately 33% of all congenital abnormalities in this group.[6,20–34] Ventricular septal defect is the most common cardiac defect reported, with a relative risk of 18 (95% confidence interval, 3.9–83) compared to the general population. The incidence of transposition of the great vessels is also increased compared to the general population (relative risk 27, with a confidence interval 3.5–209). Other cardiac malformations seen among infants of diabetic mothers include coarctation of the aorta, double-outlet right ventricle, truncus arteriosus, single ventricle, atrial septal defect, hypoplastic left ventricle, and situs inversus.[26,33,34] Specific cardiac anomalies diagnosed in 130 infants of diabetic mothers with significant odds ratios are listed in Table 51.2. It is important to note that fetal ultrasonic evaluation solely utilizing the standard four-chamber cardiac view will not detect conotruncal defects such as transposition of the great vessels, double-outlet right ventricle, and truncus arteriosus.[35]

The incidence of congenital anomalies correlates with the degree of diabetic control and maternal hyperglycemia.[24] Fetal anomaly rates were no higher than expected for the general population in the presence of gestational diabetes without glucose abnormalities in the first trimester.[5,18] Glycosylated hemoglobin or hemoglobin A1C provides a measurement of mean glucose levels for a specific individual during the preceding 4–6 weeks.[36,37] Fetal anomalies generally occur in the presence of elevated hemoglobin A1C.[38–43] Attempts to maintain normoglycemia during the entire preg-

Cardiac Problems in Pregnancy, Third Edition
Edited by Uri Elkayam, MD, and Norbert Gleicher, MD
Copyright © 1998 by Wiley-Liss, Inc. ISBN 0-471-16358-9

713

TABLE 51.1 Classification of Diabetes in Pregnancy

Class	Description
A	Gestational or chemical diabetic; asymptomatic
B	Overt diabetes, onset after age 20, duration < 10 years
C	Overt diabetes, onset before age 20, duration 10–20 years
D	Overt diabetes, onset before age 10, duration > 20 years; benign retinopathy
E[a]	Calcified pelvic vessels
F	Nephropathy (proteinuria, azotemia)
R	Malignant (proliferative) retinopathy (retinitis proliferans)

[a]This classification is generally not used in current practice.
Source: White.[7]

nancy have resulted in a decrease in congenital malformations.[38,44–46] The general recommendation is for detailed fetal echocardiographic imaging in all pregnancies with initial hemoglobin A1C values above the upper limit of normal of 6.1%.[43]

The fetal heart continues to be sensitive to maternal glucose metabolism in the third trimester.[47] Elevated levels of insulin result in macrosomia and visceromegaly, including cardiac hypertrophy.[48–51] Echocardiographic evaluation of the fetus of a diabetic mother may reveal ventricular hypertrophy with wall thickness measuring greater than 5 mm. Doppler flow indices may indicate an impairment in diastolic function.[35,52–57] Though cardiac hypertrophy may be present in approximately 30% of infants of diabetic mothers, only 10% (or less) display cardiac dysfunction.[58–59] Symptomatic neonates may present with pulmonary edema, a systolic murmur, or hypotension. Cardiac hypertrophy usually resolves within the first 6 months of postnatal life.[48,58,60]

Several pathogenetic mechanisms, such as hyperglycemia, hypoglycemia, ketosis, abnormal insulin levels, and placental insufficiency, have been purported to cause the increased incidence of congenital abnormalities seen in infants of diabetic mothers. Animal models show a direct effect of hyperglycemia.[61–67] Though insulin itself does not cross the placenta,[68] it may play a secondary role in cardiac malformations. This suggestion is based on one result of a rabbit model that used insulin to induce hypoglycemic convulsions: namely, a high incidence of ectopia cordis.[69] Though the etiology of cardiac abnormalities in infants of diabetic mothers remains unclear, meticulous monitoring and good control of maternal glucose levels will result in a decreased incidence of cardiac problems.[38]

TABLE 51.2 Cardiovascular Abnormalities in Infants of Diabetic Mothers

Cardiac Anomaly	Types of Diabetes (number of cases)		Odds Ratio (for IDDM)
	IDDM	Gestational	
VSD	10	23	3.46 (1.06–11.25)[a]
TOF	5	7	6.17 (1.39–27.37)[a]
DORV	3	2	21.33 (3.34–136.26)[a]
Truncus arteriosus	2	1	12.81 (1.43–114.64)[a]
ASD	2	11	2.16 (0.26–18.28)
ECD	2	6	1.99 (0.24–16.87)
D-TGV	2	6	3.10 (0.37–26.20)
HLH	2	5	3.67 (0.43–32.05)
Coarctation	2	6	2.97 (0.35–25.17)
Heterotaxy	2	1	3.67 (0.43–32.05)
Aortic stenosis	1	6	2.89 (0.16–53.65)
Tricuspid atresia	1	4	3.32 (0.18–61.71)
Pulmonary stenosis	1	8	1.03 (0.06–19.15)
L-TGV	0	2	
Patent ductus arteriosus	0	4	
Ebstein's anomaly	0	1	
Bicuspid aortic valve	0	1	
Single ventricle	0	1	
	35	95	

[a]Significant associations.

Abbreviations: IDDM, insulin-dependent diabetes prior to pregnancy; VSD, ventricular septal defect; TOF, tetralogy of Fallot; DORV, double-outlet right ventricle; ASD, atrial septal defect; ECD, endocardial cushion defect; TGV, transposition of the great vessels (D, D loop; L, L loop); HLH, hypoplastic left heart.
Source: Ferencz et al.[34]

PHENYLKETONURIA AND HYPERPHENYLALANINEMIA

Phenylketonuria (PKU) is an autosomal recessive inborn error of phenylalanine metabolism resulting in a defect in phenylalanine hydroxylase, the enzyme that converts phenylalanine to tyrosine.[70] Accumulation of phenylalanine results in mental retardation. Prevention of this complication requires strict adherence to a phenylalanine-restricted diet.[71,72] As increasing numbers of women with PKU and hyperphenylalaninemia are becoming pregnant, adverse fetal effects such as low birth weight, microcephaly, and cardiac congenital malformations are becoming evident in this group of patients.[73–77] Of 397 children born to mothers with either PKU or hyperphenylalaninemia, 31 (7.8%) had documented congenital cardiac malformations, while an additional 25 (6%) infants either were suspected of having a cardiac anomaly based on clinical presentation (murmur or cyanosis) or had an unspecified cardiac anomaly.[77] The specific lesions are listed in Table 51.3. Tetralogy of Fallot and hypoplastic left heart syndrome were two anomalies that occurred at rates much higher than expected for the general population.[73,77] The overall incidence of congenital heart disease in these infants correlated with maternal serum phenylalanine levels, with no cardiac defects detected in those with first-trimester maternal phenylalanine levels less than 10 mg/dL. Similar findings were reported with respect to birth weight and microcephaly. These results underscore the importance of preconception counseling and strict adherence to the phenylalanine-restricted diet in this population during pregnancy to improve fetal outcome.

TABLE 51.3   Cardiac Defects Versus Maternal Phenylalanine Levels

First-Trimester Maternal Phenylalanine Level (mg/DL)	Cardiac Defect (number of cases)
< 10	None
10–15	PS (1), TGV (1)
15–20	HLH (2), TOF (4), PDA (1), complex (3)
20–25	HLH (4), TOF (1), PDA (2), VSD (2), complex (2)
25–30	Co (1), HLH (2), complex (1)
> 30	HLH (1), PS (1), complex (2)

Abbreviations: PS, pulmonary stenosis; TGV, transposition of the great vessels; HLH, hypoplastic left heart complex; TOF, tetralogy of Fallot; PDA, patent ductus arteriosus; VSD, ventricular septal defect; Co, coarctation of the aorta; complex, greater than one lesion [PDA, ASD (2), PDA, VSD (1), PDA, ASD, VSD, Co (1), PDA, Co (1), VSD, Co (1), pulmonary atresia, common atrium, anomalous pulmonary venous return (1), VSD, anomalous left coronary artery (1)].
Source: Pierpont et al.[77]

THYROID HORMONE

The incidence of hyperthyroidism is approximately 1–2 cases per thousand pregnancies, with Graves' disease the most common diagnosis.[78] Neonatal thyrotoxicosis, due to transplacental passage of maternal thyroid-stimulating hormone receptor antibodies, usually manifests itself in the first few days of life and lasts 2–3 months.[79,80] Propylthiouracil (PTU), which is commonly used to treat this disorder, appears to cross the placenta less readily than other agents such as methimazole.[81] Five of 26 (19%) children born to women receiving PTU or methimazole during pregnancy had congenital anomalies, including one infant (4%) with aortic atresia.[82]

Hyperthyroidism can also be associated with abnormalities of glucose metabolism, which in turn can be associated with an increase in congenital cardiac anomalies, as described earlier.

STEROID HORMONES

Cushing's syndrome may be exacerbated by pregnancy and may result in an increased incidence of prematurity and stillbirth.[83–85] No increase in cardiac malformations has been reported to date in infants of this small group of patients.

Perinatal outcome is complicated by chronic, medication-dependent asthma. In a study of 81 pregnancies in asthmatics requiring chronic medication, there was a significant increase in gestational diabetes (12.9%) and insulin-requiring diabetes (9.7%) in 31 women who were steroid dependent compared to controls (1.5 and 0%, respectively). Infants born to asthmatics requiring chronic medication (steroid or non-steroid therapy) were noted to have an increased incidence of prematurity (54.8%) and birth weight less than 2500 g (45.2%) compared to controls (14 and 14%, respectively). There was no evidence of cardiac anomalies in this group of infants.[86]

ESTROGENS

To date, prenatal use of estrogens has not been shown to cause cardiac malformations; however, there have been reports of neonatal cardiac anomalies in a small subgroup of patients receiving this therapy.[87–90]

ETHANOL

Fetal alcohol syndrome comprises intrauterine and postnatal growth retardation, microcephaly, motor and mental retardation, small palpebral fissures, hypoplastic philtrim, antevert-

TABLE 51.4 Cardiac Defects in Fetal Alcohol Syndrome

	Cases	
Description	Number	Percent
VSD	15	20
VSD (complex)	6	8
TOF	4	5
ASD	3	4
PPS	2	3
DORV	1	1
PDA	1	1

Abbreviations: VSD, ventricular septal defect; VSD (complex), VSD associated with subpulmonic and subaortic obstruction (1), aortic regurgitation (1), coarctation (1), hypoplastic left heart (1), secundum atrial septal defect (1), and dextrocardia (1); TOF, tetralogy of Fallot; ASD, atrial septal defect; PPS, peripheral pulmonic stenosis; DORV, double-outlet right ventricle; PDA, patent ductus arteriosus.
Source: Sanders et al.[95]

ed nostrils, and midfacial hypoplasia.[91–93] The exact prevalence of fetal alcohol syndrome is unknown, but estimates range from 1 to 5 infants per thousand live births. An abnormality resulting in glycosolated hemoglobin, which is distinct from hemoglobin A1C and is formed in a reaction between acetaldehyde and dihydroxyacetone phosphate, is found in the blood of alcoholics.[94] An assay yielding a measure of maternal glycosylated hemoglobin is useful in determining the level of alcohol consumption in the preceding 4–8 weeks. Specific cardiac abnormalities identified in 76 patients with documented features of this syndrome are listed in Table 51.4.[95] Ventricular septal defects were the most common cardiac defect identified in this series. Earlier reports found atrial septal defects to be most prevalent.[96–98]

COCAINE

Cocaine crosses the placenta and can be measured in the urine of newborns. Based on results of animal studies, maternal cocaine ingestion is thought to induce uterine artery vasoconstriction and impair fetal placental perfusion.[99] Cocaine use during pregnancy is associated with increased rates of intrauterine growth retardation, fetal death, and stillbirth.[100,101] Cocaine, unlike many other agents, is thought to affect organs after the period of organogenesis (first 10 weeks after conception) by episodic restriction of blood flow and oxygen due to fetal vasoconstriction.[102] The fetus is therefore vulnerable to maternal cocaine ingestion throughout the entire pregnancy. Reported malformations include central nervous system anomalies, intestinal atresia, limb defects, and urinary tract anomalies.[103–106] Abnormalities in fetal blood flow and oxygen have also been proposed as an etiology for cardiac anomalies.[107,108] Cardiac malformations appear to be increased in this population of infants.[107–110] In a

review of 554 neonates exposed to cocaine in utero, a relative risk of 3.7 was found for congenital heart disease (95% confidence interval, 1.4–9.4). Cardiac anomalies in this group included ventricular septal defects, atrial septal defects, single ventricle, congenital heart block, peripheral pulmonic stenosis, and patent ductus arteriosus.[107] ST-segment changes, higher blood pressure, and lower cardiac output have all been reported in newborns with positive urine screens for cocaine.[111,112]

VITAMIN DEFICIENCIES

To date all the studies assessing the effect of dietary deficiencies on cardiac development have been performed in animals. Vitamin A deficiency in gravid rats resulted in aortic arch abnormalities and retarded myocardial differentiation or "spongy" myocardium in the offspring.[113] Riboflavin-deficient rats produced offspring with anomalies of the interventricular septum and aortic arch.[114] Vitamin B_{12} deficiency has been shown to produce abnormalities in the liver, spleen, and heart of rat offspring.[115] The cardiac defects seen in the vitamin-B_{12}-deficient rats were similar to those detected in the group deficient in vitamin A. Dextrocardia was found in the offspring of a group of vitamin-E-deficient rats.[116]

SUMMARY

Various maternal metabolic abnormalities are associated with congenital cardiac abnormalities. Though the exact mechanisms of their teratogenicity are not known, the fetus is most vulnerable to their effects in the first trimester, when organogenesis is occurring. The data regarding improved outcome with good control of maternal glucose in diabetics and phenylalanine levels in PKU and hyperphenylalaninemia patients are very encouraging. Efforts to minimize maternal metabolic abnormalities in pregnancy regardless of the cause appear to have a great impact on improving fetal outcome.

REFERENCES

1. White P. Pregnancy and diabetes: medical aspects. *Med Clin North Am* 1965;49:1015–1024.

2. North AF Jr, Mazumdar S, Logrillu VM. Birth weight, gestational age and perinatal deaths in 5471 infants of diabetic mothers. *J Pediatr* 1977;90:444–447.

3. Niswander KR, Gordon M. *The Collaborative Perinatal Study of the National Institute of Neurological Disease and Stroke. The Women and Their Pregnancies.* Philadelphia: WB Saunders; 1972;239–245.

4. Chung CS, Myrianthopoulos NC. Factors affecting risks of congenital malformations. II. Effects of maternal diabetes. *Birth Defects* 1975;11:23–37.

5. Moore PR. Diabetes in pregnancy. In: Creasy RK, Resnick R, eds. *Maternal and Fetal Medicine*. Philadelphia: WB Saunders; 1994;934–978.

6. Ferencz C, Loffredo CA, Rubin JD, Magee CA. Maternal medical, anthropometric, and reproductive characteristics: In: Anderson RH, ed. *Perspectives in Pediatric Cardiology; vol 4; Epidemiology of Congenital Heart Disease: The Baltimore–Washington Infant Study, 1981–1989*. Mount Kisco, NY: Future, 1993;170.

7. White P. Pregnancy and diabetes: In: Marble A, White P, Bradley RF, Krall LP, eds. *Joslin Diabetes Mellitus*. 11th ed. Philadelphia: Lea & Febiger; 1971.

8. Mills JL. Malformations in infants of diabetic mothers. *Teratology* 1982;25:385–394.

9. Reece EA, Hobbins JC. Diabetic embryopathy: pathogenesis, prenatal diagnosis and prevention. *Obstet Gynecol Survey* 1986;41;325–335.

10. White P. Diabetes mellitus in pregnancy. *Clin Perinatol* 1974;1:331–347.

11. Navarette VN, Torres IH, Rivera IR, Shor UP, Gracia PN. Maternal carbohydrate disorder and congenital malformations. *Diabetes* 1967;16:127–130.

12. Molsted-Pedersen L, Tygstrup I, Pedersen J. Congenital malformations in newborn infants of diabetic women: correlation with maternal diabetic vascular complications. *Lancet* 1964;1:1124–1126.

13. Kucera J. Rate and type of congenital anomalies among offspring of diabetic women. *J. Reprod Med* 1971;7:61–70.

14. Comess NJ, Bennett PH, Burch TA, Miller M. Congenital anomalies and diabetes in the Pima Indians of Arizona. *Diabetes* 1969;18:471–477.

15. Kitzmiller JL, Cloherty JP, Younger MD, Tabatabail A, Rothchild SB, Sosenko I, Ebstein MF, Singh S, Neff RK. Diabetic pregnancy and perinatal morbidity. *Am J Obstet Gynecol* 1978;131:565–580.

16. Boughman JA, Neill CA, Ferencz C, Loffredo CA. The genetics of congenital heart disease: In: Anderson RH, ed. *Perspectives in Pediatric Cardiology; vol 4; Epidemiology of Congenital Heart Disease: The Baltimore–Washington Infant Study 1981–1989*. Mount Kisco, NY: Futura; 1993;128.

17. Mitchell SC, Sellman AH, Westphal MC, Park J. Etiologic correlates in a study of congenital heart disease in 56,109 births. *Am J Cardiol* 1971;28:653–657.

18. Soler NG, Walsh CH, Malins JM. Congenital malformations in infants of diabetic mothers. *Q J Med* 1976;45:303–313.

19. Dundon S, Murphy A, Ratery J, Drury MI. Infants of diabetic mothers. *J Ir Med Assoc* 1974;67:371–375.

20. Driscoll SG, Bernirschke K, Curtis GW. Neonatal deaths among infants off diabetic mothers. *Am J Dis Child* 1960;100:818–835.

21. Gabbe SG, Nestman JH, Freeman RK, Anderson GV, Lowensohn RI. Management and outcome off class A diabetes. *Am J Obstet Gynecol* 1977;127:465–469.

22. Gabbe SG, Nestman JH, Freeman RK, Goebelsmann UT, Lowensohn RI, Nochimson P, Cetrulo C, Quilligan EJ. Management and outcome of pregnancy in diabetes mellitus, classes B to R. *Am J Obstet Gynecol* 1977;129:723–728.

23. Gabbe SG. Congenital malformations in infants of diabetic mothers. *Obstet Gynecol Survey* 1977;32:125–132.

24. Miller E, Hare JW, Cloherty JP, Dunn PJ, Gleason RE, Soeldner JS, Kitzmiller JL. Elevated maternal hemoglobin A1c in early pregnancy and major congenital anomalies in infants of diabetic mothers. *N Engl J Med* 1981;304:1331–1334.

25. Cousins L. The California Diabetes in Pregnancy Program: A statewide collaborative programme for the preconception and prenatal care of diabetic women. *Bailleres Clin Obstet Gynaecol* 1991;5:443–459.

26. Becerra JE, Khoury MJ, Cordero JF, et al. DM during pregnancy and the risks for specific birth defects: a case control study. *Pediatrics* 1990;85:1–9.

27. Albert T, Landon M, Wheller J et al. Prenatal detection of fetal anomalies in pregnancy complicated by insulin-dependent diabetes mellitus. *Am J Obstet Gynecol* 1994;170 (pt 2): 327. Abstract.

28. Miller HC. The effect of diabetic and prediabetic pregnancies on the fetus and newborn infant. *J Pediatr* 1946;28:455–461.

29. Rowland TW, Hubbell JP, Nadas AS. Congenital heart disease in infants of diabetic mothers. *J Pediatr* 1973;83:815–820.

30. Day RE, Insley J. Maternal diabetes and congenital malformations. Survey of 205 cases. *Arch Dis Child* 1976;51:935–938.

31. Levin SE, Kanarek KS. The incidence of congenital heart disease in Johannesburg. A 5-year study of liveborn infants at the Queen Victoria Maternity Hospital. *S Afr Med J* 1973;47:1855–1858.

32. Rubin A, Murphy DP. The frequency of congenital malformations in the offspring of nondiabetic and diabetic individuals. *J Pediatr* 1958;53:579–585.

33. Rowe RD, Mehrizi A. *The Neonate with Congenital Heart Disease*. Philadelphia: WB Saunders; 1968; 411.

34. Ferencz C, Rubin JD, McCarter RJ, Clark EB. Maternal diabetes and cardiovascular malformations: predominance of double outlet right ventricle and truncus arteriosus. *Teratology* 1990;41:319–326.

35. Kleinman CS. Diabetes in the fetal heart: application of fetal echocardiography. In: Reece EA, Hobbins DR eds. *Diabetes Mellitus in Pregnancy: Principles and Practice*. New York: Churchill Livingstone; 1988; 363–373.

36. Bunn HF, Haney DN, Kamin S, Gabbay KH, Gallop PM. The biosynthesis of human hemoglobin A1C; slow glycosylation of hemoglobin in vivo. *J Clin Invest* 1976;56:1652–1659.

37. Koenig RJ, Peterson CM, Jones RL, Saudek C, Lehrman M, Cerami A. Correlation of glucose regulation and hemoglobin A1C in diabetes mellitus. *N Engl J Med* 1976;295:417–420.

38. Kitzmiller JL, Gavin LA, Gin GD, et al. Preconception care of diabetes: glycemic control prevents congenital anomalies. *JAMA* 1991;265:731–736.

39. Molsted-Pedersen L, Pedersen JF. Congenital malformations in diabetic pregnancies. *Acta Paediatr Scand* 1985;320:79–82.

40. Ylinen K, Aula P, Stenman UH, et al. Risk of minor and major fetal malformations in diabetics with high hemoglobin A1c values in early pregnancy. *Br Med J* 1984;289:345–346.

41. Greene MF, Hare JW, Cloherty JP, Benacerraf BR. First trimester hemoglobin A1c and risk for major malformation and spontaneous abortion in diabetic pregnancy. *Teratology* 1989;39:225–231.

42. Leslie RDG, Pyke DA, John PM, White JM. Haemoglobin A1c in diabetic pregnancy. *Lancet* 1978;2:958–959.

43. Sheilds LE, Gan EA, Murphy HF, Sahn DJ, Moore TR. The prognostic value of hemoglobin A1c in predicting fetal heart disease in diabetic pregnancies. *Obstet Gynecol* 1993;81(6): 954–957.

44. Drury MI. Diabetes mellitus and pregnancy: the 9-month experiment. *Postgrad Med J* 1979;55 (suppl 2):36–39.

45. Karlsson K, Kjellmer I. The outcome of diabetic pregnancies in relation to the mother's blood sugar level. *Am J Obstet Gynecol* 1972;112:23–220.

46. Mills JL. A controlled prospective study of glycemic control and malformations. The Diabetes in Early Pregnancy study (DIEP). *Diabetes* 1987;36(suppl I): 5A.

47. Pedersen J. *Diabetes and Pregnancy: Blood Sugar and Newborn Infants.* Copenhagen: Danish Science; 1952.

48. Breitweser JA, Meyer RA, Sperling MA, et al. Cardiac septal hypertrophy in hyperinsulinemic infants. *J Pediatr* 1980;96: 535–539.

49. Miller HV, Wilson HM. Macrosomia, cardiac hypertrophy, erythroblastosis and hyperplasia of the island of Langerhans in infants born to diabetic mothers. *J Pediatr* 1943;23:251–266.

50. Wolfe RR, Way GC. Cardiomyopathies in infants of diabetic mothers. *Johns Hopkins Med J* 1977;140:170–180.

51. Hurwitz D, Irving FC. Diabetes and pregnancy. *Am J Med Sci* 1937;194:85–92.

52. Gutgesell HP, Spear MF, Rosenberg HS, Characterization of the cardiomyopathy in infants of diabetic mothers. *Circulation* 1980;61:441–450.

53. Rizzo G, Arduini D, Romanini C. Cardiac function in fetuses of type I diabetic mothers. *Am J Obstet Gynecol* 1991;164: 837–843.

54. Rizzo G, Arduini D, Romanini C. Accelerated cardiac growth and abnormal cardiac flow in fetuses of type I diabetic mothers. *Obstet Gynecol* 1992;80 (3 pt 1): 369–376.

55. Veille JC, Hanson R, Sivakoff M, Hoen H, Ben-Ami M. Fetal cardiac size in normal, intrauterine growth retarded, and diabetic pregnancies. *Am J Perinatol* 1993;10(4):275–279.

56. Weber HS, Botti JJ, Baylen BG. Sequential longitudinal evaluation of cardiac growth and ventricular diastolic filling in fetuses of well controlled diabetic mothers. *Pediatr Cardiol* 1994;15(4):184–189.

57. Rizzo G, Pietropolli A, Capponi A, Cacciatore C, Arduini D, Romanini C. Analysis of factors influencing ventricular filling patterns in fetuses of type I diabetic mothers. *J Perinat Med* 1994;22(2):149–157.

58. Way GL, Wolfe RR, Eshaghpour E, et al. The natural history of hypertrophic cardiomyopathy in infants of diabetic mothers. *J Pediatr* 1979;95:1020–1025.

59. Walther FJ, Siassi B, King J, Wu PYK. Cardiac output in infants of insulin-dependent diabetic mothers. *J Pediatr* 1985;107:109–114.

60. Gutgesell HP, Mullins CE, Gillette PC, Speer M, Rudolph AJ, McNamara DG. Transient hypertrophic subaortic stenosis in infants of diabetic mothers. *J Pediatr* 1976;89:120–125.

61. Cockroft DL, Coppola PT. Teratogenic effect of excess glucose on head-fold rat embryos in culture. *Teratology* 1977; 16:141–146.

62. Sadler TW. Effects of maternal diabetes on early embryogenesis. II. Hyperglycemmia induced exencephaly. *Teratology* 1980;21:349–356.

63. Cockroft DL, Freinkel N, Phillips LS, Shambaugh GE. Metabolic factors affecting organogenesis in diabetic pregnancy. *Clin Res* 1981;29:577A. Abstract.

64. Eriksson UJ. Congenital malformations in diabetic animal models: A review. *Diabetes Res* 1984;1:57–66.

65. Deuchar EM. Embryonic malformations in rats resulting from maternal diabetes: preliminary observations. *J Embryol Exp Morphol* 1977;41:93–99.

66. Ornoy A, Cohen AM. Teratogenic effects of sucrose diet in diabetic and non-diabetic rats. *Isr J Med Sci* 1985;16:789–791.

67. Sadler TW. Effects of maternal diabetes on early embryogenesis. I. The teratogenic potential of diabetic serum. *Teratology* 1980;21:339–347.

68. Adam PAJ, Teramo K, Raiha N et al. Human fetal insulin metabolism early in gestation: response to acute elevation of the fetal glucose concentration and placental transfer of human insulin. *Diabetes* 1969;18:409–413.

69. Chomette G. Entwicklungsstorungen nach insulin Schock beim trachtiger Kaninchen. *Beitr Pathol Anat* 1955;115: 439–451.

70. Scriver CR, Clow C. Phenylketonuria: epitome of human biochemical genetics, first of two parts. *N Engl J Med* 1980; 303:1336–1342.

71. Koch R, Azen C, Friedman EG, Williamson ML. Paired comparisons between early treated PKU children and their matched sibling controls on intelligence and school achievement test results at eight years of age. *J Inherited Metab Dis* 1984;7:86–90.

72. MacCready RA. Admissions of phenylketonuric patients to residential institutions before and after screening programs of the newborn infant. *J Pediatr* 1974;85:383–385.

73. Lenke RR, Levy HL. Maternal phenylketonuria and hyperphenylalaninemia: an international survey of the outcome of untreated and treated pregnancies. *N Engl J Med* 1980;303: 1202–1208.

74. Verkerk PH, Van Sprosen FJ, Smit GPA, Cornel MC, Kuipers JRG, Verloove-Vanhorick SP. Prevalence of congenital heart disease in patients with phenylketonuria. *J Pediatr* 1991; 2(119):282–283.

75. Platt LD, Kock R, Azen C, Hanley WB, Levy HL, Matalon R, Rouse B, de la Cruz F, Walla CA. Maternal phenylketonuria collaborative study, obstetric aspects and outcome: the first 6 years. *Am J Obstet Gynecol* 1992;166:1150–1162.

76. Koch R, Levy HL, Matalon R, Rouse B, Hanley W, Azen C. The North American Collaborative Study of Maternal Phenylketonuria—status report 1993. *Am J Dis Child* 1993;147:1224–1230.

77. Pierpont MA, Sletten LJ, Firkins Smith C, Berry H, Berry SA, Fisch RO. Congenital cardiac malformations in offspring of mothers with phenylketonuria and hyperphenylalaninemia. *Int Pediatr* 1995;10(3):242–249.

78. Burrow GN. Thyroid diseases: In: Burrow GN, Ferris T, eds. *Medical Complications During Pregnancy*. Philadelphia: WB Saunders; 1975.

79. Matsuura N, Konishi J, Fujieda K, et al. TSH-receptor antibodies in mothers with Graves' disease and outcome in their offspring. *Lancet* 1988;1:14–17.

80. Mandel SH, Hanna CE, LaFranchi SH, Tamaki H, Amino N, Miyai K. Thyroid function in infants born to mothers with Graves' disease. *J Pediatr* 1990;117:169–170.

81. Marchant B, Brownlie BEW, Hart DM, Horton PW, Alexander WD. The placental transfer of propylthiouracil, methimazole and carbimazole. *J Clin Endocrinol Metab* 1977;45:1187–1193.

82. Mujtaba Q, Burrow GN. Treatment of hyperthyroidism in pregnancy with propylthiouracil and methimazole. *Obstet Gynecol* 1975;46:282–286.

83. Gimes EM, Fayez JA, Miller GL. Cushing's syndrome and pregnancy. *Obstet Gynecol* 1973;42:550–556.

84. Guilhaume B, Sanson ML, Billaud L, Bertagna X, Laudat MH, Luton JP. Cushing's syndrome and pregnancy: aetiologies and prognosis in twenty-two patients. *Eur J Med* 1992;1(2):83–89.

85. Buescher MA, McClamrock HD, Adashi EY. Cushing syndrome in pregnancy. *Obstet Gynecol* 1992;79(1):130–137.

86. Perlow JH et al. Severity of asthma and perinatal outcome. *Am J Obstet Gynecol* 1992;167(4 pt 1):936–967.

87. Heinonen OP, Slone D, Monson RR, Hook EB, Shapiro S. Cardiovascular birth defects and antenatal exposure to female sex hormones. *N Engl J Med* 1977;296:76–70.

88. Wiseman RA, Dodds-Smith IC. Cardiovascular birth defects and antenatal exposure to female sex hormones: a reevaluation of some base data. *Teratology* 1984;30:359–370.

89. Hook EB. Cardiovascular birth defects and prenatal exposure to female sex hormones: a reevaluation of data reanalysis from a large prospective study. *Teratology* 1992;46:261–266.

90. Levy EP, Cohen A, Fraser FC. Hormone treatment during pregnancy and congenital heart defects. *Lancet* 1973;1:611–614.

91. Lemoine P, Harousseau H, Borteyru J-P, Menuet J-C. Les enfants de parents alcooliques: anomalies observeés. *Quest Med* 1968;25:476–481.

92. Ulleland CN. The offspring of alcoholic mothers. *Ann Acad Sci New York* 1972;197:167–169.

93. Jones KL, Smith DW, Ulleland CN, Streissguth AP. Pattern of malformation in offspring of chronic alcoholic mothers. *Lancet* 1973;1:1267–1271.

94. Hoberman HD. Synthesis of 5-deoxy-D-xylulose-1-phosphate by human erythrocytes. *Biochem Biophys Res Commun* 1979;90:757–763.

95. Sanders GGS, Smith DF, MacLeod PM. Cardiac malformations in the fetal alcohol syndrome. *J Pediatr* 1981;98:771–773.

96. Veghely PV, Oxztovics M, Kardos G, Leisztner L, Szaszovsky E, Igali S, Imrei J. The fetal alcohol syndrome: symptoms and pathogenesis. *Acta Paediatr Acad Sci Hung* 1978;19:171–181.

97. Clarren SK, Smith DW. The fetal alcohol syndrome. *N Engl J Med* 1978;298:1063–1067.

98. Loser H, Majewski M. Type and frequency of cardiac defects in embryofetal alcohol syndrome: report of 16 cases. *Br Heart J* 1977;39:1374–1379.

99. Woods JR, Plessinger NA, Clark KE. The effect of cocaine on uterine blood flow and fetal oxygenation. *JAMA* 1987;257:957–961.

100. Chasnoff IJ, Griffith D, MacGregor S, et al. Temporal patterns of cocaine use in pregnancy. *JAMA* 1989;261:1741–1744.

101. Slutsker L. Risks associated with cocaine use during pregnancy. *Obstet Gynecol* 1992;79:778–779.

102. Jones KL. Developmental pathogenesis of defects associated with prenatal cocaine exposure: fetal vascular disruption. *Clin Perinatol* 1991;18:139–146.

103. Chasnoff IJ, Bussey ME, Savich R, et al. Perinatal cerebral infarction in neonatal cocaine use. *J Pediatr* 1986;108:456–459.

104. Hoyme HE, Jones KL, Dixon SD, et al. Prenatal cocaine exposure and fetal vascular disruption. *Pediatrics* 1990;85:743–747.

105. Hoyme HE, Jones KL, Van Allen MI, et al. Vascular pathogenesis in transverse limb-reduction defects. *J Pediatr* 1982;101:839–842.

106. Chasnoff IJ, Chisum GM, Kaplan WE. Maternal cocaine use in genital urinary tract malformations. *Teratology* 1988;37:201–204.

107. Lipshultz SE, Frassica JJ, Orav EJ. Cardiovascular abnormalities in infants prenatally exposed to cocaine. *J Pediatr* 1991;118:44–51.

108. Shepard TH, Fantel AG, Kapur RP. Fetal coronary thrombosis as a cause of single ventricular heart. *Teratology* 1991;43:117–170.

109. Little BB, Snell LM, Klein VR, et al. Cocaine abuse during pregnancy: maternal and fetal implications. *Obstet Gynecol* 1989;73:157–160.

110. Bingol N, Fuchs M, Diaz V. Teratogenicity of cocaine in humans. *J Pediatr* 1987;110:93–96.

111. Mehta SK, Finkelhor RS, Anderson RL, et al. Transient myocardial ischemia in infants prenatally exposed to cocaine. *J Pediatr* 1993;122:945–949.

112. Van de Bor M, Walther S, Ebrahimi M. Decreased cardiac output in infants of mothers who abuse cocaine. *Pediatrics* 1990;85:31–32.

113. Wilson JG, Warkany J. Aortic arch and cardiac anomalies in offspring of vitamin A deficient rats. *Am J Anat* 1949;85:113–155.

114. Nelson MM, Baird CDC, Wright HV, Evans HM. Multiple congenital abnormalities in the rat resulting from riboflavin deficiency induced by the antimetabolite galactoflavin. *J. Nutr* 1956;58:125–134.

115. Jones CC, Brown SO, Richardson LR, Sinclair JG. Tissue abnormalities in newborn rats from vitamin B12 deficient mothers. *Proc Soc Exp Biol Med* 1955;90:135–140.

116. Cheng DW, Thomas BH. Relationship of time of therapy to tertatogenicity in maternal avitaminosis E. *Proc Iowa Acad Sci* 1953;60:290–299.

52

ENVIRONMENTAL CAUSES OF CONGENITAL HEART ABNORMALITIES

LOUIS BUTTINO, JR., MD, and NORBERT GLEICHER, MD

INTRODUCTION

The incidence of some congenital anomalies such as ventricular septal defect (VSD) is increasing. The explanation for this is unknown. In fact, the etiology of the majority of birth defects is unknown. Drug exposure and environmental toxins probably are known causes of approximately only 2% of all congenital defects.[1,2]

An extremely difficult task in the evaluation of environmental exposures is the ascertainment of cause and effect. Controlling for all other factors to study the effect of a single agent is nearly impossible. There are 90,000 chemicals in commercial use in the United States and not many more than 3000 have actually been tested for teratogenicity or toxicity.[1] Fewer than a half a dozen have been shown to have a *possible* association with birth defects. Medication use is widespread among pregnant women and thus can also impact on the incidence of birth defects. At least 40% of pregnant women, perhaps as many as 90%, appear to be exposed to at least one drug during pregnancy, with many being exposed to multiple medications.[3] In fact, it has been suggested that 60–75% of pregnant women use from three to ten medications during pregnancy.[1] This obviously makes it extremely difficult to single out the effect of any specific drug. A possible relationship could exist between a genetic predisposition to certain congenital anomalies and the prenatal exposure to certain agents, which would then trigger expression of the anomaly. Thus under these circumstances, a birth defect cannot be attributed with certainty to any specific, single agent, and to call such an agent an independent variable could be inaccurate. Errors of this type may have medicolegal implications.

The association of a single agent with a specific congenital anomaly can, however, be obvious if the background incidence of the anomaly is rare and the abnormality is of significant impact, as was the case, for example, with thalidomide. However, if the defect itself is common, such as a ventricular septal defect, and an agent causes only a slight increase in incidence, an association may be extremely difficult to detect or prove. Other factors may also impede the identification of environmental exposure as a cause of congenital anomalies. Tikkanen and Heinnonen, who discussed some of these difficulties in 1991,[4] stated that "even a high relative risk would be difficult to detect if only a small proportion (e.g., 5%) of the population were exposed and the exposure classification system were 60% sensitive and 80% specific." The variation in timing, duration, and amount of exposure obviously can compound the process of determining a specific risk for environmental exposure. Moreover, recall bias will affect the accuracy of most epidemiologic studies on teratogen exposure since, by necessity, they are mostly retrospective. Also, the completeness of a mother's history may very well be influenced by whether her offspring is in the study or control population.

Exposure to a potential environmental toxin can have an effect on the incidence of some congenital anomalies even if these are not restricted to pregnancy. In fact, maternal or paternal exposure remote from an affected pregnancy may have an impact on the genetic integrity of the oocyte or the sperm that is later expressed in a child.

Cardiac Problems in Pregnancy, Third Edition
Edited by Uri Elkayam, MD, and Norbert Gleicher, MD
Copyright © 1998 by Wiley-Liss, Inc. ISBN 0-471-16358-9

Prospectively controlled studies on humans are almost impossible. The complexity and expense involved, as well as the ethical issues represented by the potential risk to offspring if there is true toxicity of the substance under study, are largely prohibitive. Much information on the teratogenicity of environmental agents is therefore obtained through animal studies. However, as the thalidomide tragedy clearly proved, extrapolation of animal information to humans is extremely risky. Only the widest possible animal exposure, with consistent results, will allow the prediction of human risks with some confidence. Major epidemiologic studies, involving large patient numbers and adequate controls for confounding factors, remain the mainstem of accurate assessment of environmental toxins on humans.

If we accept the limitations pointed out above, environmental exposure can be classified as behavioral (medications, personal habits, etc.), occupational, and ambient (passive exposure to toxins in air, water, etc.).

BEHAVIORAL EXPOSURE

Many studies commented on the relationship between female hormones and congenital heart defects.[5–7] There is some difference of opinion as to the status of these substances as teratogens, however. Some reports appeared to associate exposure to oral contraceptives or female sex hormones with congenital heart disease (CHD).[5] But more recently, researchers have been rather unimpressed with such an association. Rothman et al[6] suggested a small positive association between estrogen and progesterone exposure and cardiac malformation, the prevalence ratio estimate of exposed to nonexposed being 1.5. In contrast to earlier reports, no association was evident, however, between hormone exposure and truncocanal or any other specific class of defect, an observation that casts doubt on a causal relationship between hormone exposure and cardiovascular malformations. Even the reported relative risk of 1.5 is suspect because of potential recall bias in this study. In a reevaluation of the data from the Boston Collaborative Perinatal Project, Wiseman and Dodds-Smith[7] also failed to support the original claim of an association between the exposure to female sex hormones during pregnancy and the occurrence of cardiac malformations. It therefore appears safe to conclude that if prenatal exposure to female sex hormones has any effect on the incidence of congenital heart disease, it is at most minimal.

The data on diphenylhydantoin also are inconclusive. Although Hanson[8] reported an overall increased incidence of congenital anomalies, including those of the heart, after maternal ingestion of diphenylhydantoin, his study was weakened by extensive confounding data. Other authors have concluded that the incidence of congenital heart disease in offspring of mothers who took diphenylhydantoin was no greater than that due to background.[9] Again, although at least

10% of children from women on diphenylhydantoin demonstrate at least some stigmata of the Dilantin syndrome,[8] it would be inaccurate to list the medication as a cardiac teratogen.

There is also little evidence to indicate that prenatal exposure to β-adrenergic agents is associated with congenital heart disease in humans. However, there is some evidence of such a positive association in chick embryos.[10] Additionally, dextroamphetamine has been associated with congenital heart disease in both chick embryos and human offspring.[11,12] Nora et al[12] found a significant association between congenital heart disease and maternal dextroamphetamine usage. Since the administration of dextroamphetamine is followed by an increase in blood pressure,[13] the mechanism may be through β-adrenergic-type activity. Therefore, some caution is needed when β-mimetics are prescribed in the first trimester. In any event, regardless of the strength of any association with congenital heart disease, there really are no appropriate clinical scenarios for the prescription of dextroamphetamine in the first trimester.

Isotretinoin has been associated with a significant incidence of congenital heart disease, especially transposition of the great vessels, truncus arteriosus, and other anomalies of the aorta.[14,15] It is postulated that these anomalies are mediated by a deficiency of branchial arch mesenchyme and, although isotretinoin also has been associated with numerous other anomalies and therefore probably should be avoided throughout pregnancy, exposure approximately 2.5 weeks postconception is particularly critical for congenital heart disease.

There is also sufficient evidence in the literature to support the claim that lithium is a cardiac teratogen.[16–18] A French review estimates that 7.8% of lithium-exposed embryos develop congenital cardiac abnormalities.[16] The most common anomaly involves a defective tricuspid valve, in combination with atrialization of the right ventricle, known as Ebstein's anomaly. When caring for patients on lithium therapy, physicians must weigh the risk of congenital heart disease against the severity of the maternal condition. Moreover, the availability of an alternative therapy should always be considered when deciding on the appropriate treatment during the first trimester of pregnancy.

Consumption of alcohol during pregnancy is associated with a wide array of negative outcomes. Because of the widespread use of alcohol, the potential magnitude of birth defects stemming from ethanol exposure is significant. Fetal alcohol syndrome (FAS) is the name given to the constellation of anomalies that can occur in the offspring of women who drink alcohol. There are four main components of the fetal alcohol syndrome[19]: central nervous system dysfunction, growth deficiency, a characteristic facies, and variable minor and major anomalies. Cardiac anomalies are frequently present. The most common heart defect associated with alcohol consumption is atrial septal defect, but others reported include tetrology of Fallot, pulmonary stenosis, mitral stenosis, caval anomalies, and idiopathic hypertrophic subaortic stenosis.[15]

Like other components of the fetal alcohol syndrome, the severity of cardiac defects varies. The final form of congenital heart disease depends on timing, dosage, and duration of alcohol exposure. The incidence of full-blown fetal alcohol syndrome is 1–2 per thousand live births, and the incidence of partial expression is 3–5 per thousand live births.[19] The typical pattern of cardiac defects is seen in approximately 29% of fetal alcohol syndrome cases, but in severe cases of fetal alcohol syndrome there is a 50% incidence.[19] Clarren and Smith[19] interpret some evidence to suggest that the consumption of 84 mL of absolute alcohol per day represents a definitive risk to the fetus. Others are uncomfortable with such a generous cutoff, and the customary recommendation is to avoid alcohol consumption if at all possible during all of pregnancy. If abstinence is not possible, no more than two alcoholic beverages (one 12 oz. beer, one 6 oz. glass of wine, or one drink mixed with 1 oz. of 86 proof liquor equals one beverage) should be consumed daily.

Contrary to frequently voiced opinion in the public, there is no evidence that tobacco or caffeine causes an increase in congenital heart disease.[20]

OCCUPATIONAL EXPOSURE

Since women make up an ever-increasing portion of the workforce, there is a clear need to identify occupational risks for pregnancy. Unfortunately, there is little information to date on specific agents to which pregnant women may be exposed to while working.

Multiple studies have looked at the risk of prenatal exposure to anesthetic agents.[21–24] Some of these reviews failed to associate congenital heart disease with exposure to anesthetic gases.[21] In a national study on operating room personnel, however, a 10% incidence of congenital heart disease in offspring of members of the American Society of Anesthesiologists was noted, versus a 0% rate in offspring of members of the American Academy of Pediatrics.[22] In another study,[23] evaluating many outcome variables among pregnant women in anesthetic practice, the authors studied approximately 8000 pregnancies. The only significant difference noted related to congenital malformations of the heart and great vessels in the offspring of anesthesiologists, who demonstrated an incidence of 13.8 per thousand live births, versus 3.6 per thousand live births in other physician specialists. These reports suggest that prenatal exposure to anesthetic gases represents a true risk. Aggressive programs to minimize leaks of anesthetic agents and the utilization of efficient gas scavenging systems should reduce occupational exposure and its associated adverse perinatal effects to an absolute minimum.

Occupations that expose the pregnant woman to organic solvents also appear to increase the risk of congenital heart disease. Two Finnish studies demonstrated a weak association between first-trimester exposure to organic solvents and congenital heart disease, but a much stronger association, with relative odds ratio of 1.5 and 1.8, respectively, for ventricular septal defect.[21,25]

The analysis of data from the Collaborative Perinatal Project associated an increased incidence of congenital heart disease with the following conditions: work in metal or related industries, bartending, library work, textile industries, and having been a nurse's aide.[26] None of these exposure risks have been adequately studied, and no definite conclusions concerning the actual risk of these occupational exposures is therefore possible.

AMBIENT EXPOSURE

The actual environment in which we live (i.e., air, water) may contain some substances that pose a significant risk to pregnancy in general and for congenital heart disease specifically. Performing valid studies on any one agent in our environment is, of course, an impossible task. There are, however, scattered reports in the literature: Goldberg et al[27] reported a threefold increase in risk for congenital heart disease in offspring of parents exposed to drinking water contaminated with trichloroethylene, dichloroethylene, and chromium. In another study on the quality of drinking water, Zierler et al[28] found significant problems with respect to mercury, arsenic, and lead. Mercury and lead were associated with an increased relative odds ratio for patent ductus arteriosus. Arsenic was associated with a threefold increase in the incidence of coarctation of the aorta. Interestingly, in this same study, exposure to selenium appeared to decrease the incidence of conotruncal defects of the heart.

SUMMARY

Although there is evidence in the literature to support claims that several environmental agents are developmental toxins, such data are convincing for only a very few. The vast majority of agents have not been specifically tested, and no increased association has been identified with a majority of those tested. The potential for risk, however, is always present. There are variations in the background incidence of congenital heart disease that will affect the accuracy of all epidemiologic studies on developmental toxicity. Also to be considered, moreover, are such findings as differences in the incidence of patent ductus arteriosus based on gender.[18] There is some evidence, as well, to support a seasonal variation in the incidence of ventricular septal defect and of other anomalies.[18] Additional confounding variables, such as population density or the prevalence of certain viruses, may translate into a seasonal variation for some cardiac defects.

Other difficulties for the study of environmental toxicity include the low incidence of any specific lesion, the infrequent exposure to agents in question, and the hypothesis that most congenital heart disease is multifactorial in origin.[29] Additionally, differences in dosage, timing, and duration of exposure, placentation, metabolism, and genetic vulnerability will influence the occurrence or the extent of developmental toxicity.

REFERENCES

1. Mattison DR, Jelovsek FR. Risk assessment for developmental toxicity: effects of drugs and chemical on the fetus. In: Reece EA, Hobbus JC, Mahoney MJ, Petrie RH, eds. *Medicine of the Fetus and Mother.* Philadelphia. JB Lippincott; 1992;328–341.

2. Brent RL. The complexities of solving the problem of human malformations. In: Sever JL, Brent RL, eds. *Teratogen Update: Environmentally Induced Birth Defect Risks.* New York: Alan R. Liss; 1986;189–97.

3. Koren G, Bologa M, Long D, Feldman Y, Shear NH. Perception of teratogenic risk by pregnant women exposed to drugs and chemicals during the first trimester. *Am J Obstet Gynecol* 1989;160:1190–1194.

4. Tikkanen J, Heinnonen OP. Maternal exposure to chemical and physical factors during pregnancy and cardiovascular malformations in the offspring. *Teratology* 1991;43:591–600.

5. Heinnonen OP, Slone D, Monson RR, Hook EB, Shapiro S. Cardiovascular birth defects and antenatal exposure to female sex hormones. *N Engl J Med* 1977;296:67–70.

6. Rothman K, Fyler DC, Goldblatt A, Kreidbehg MB. Exogenous hormones and other drug exposures of children with congenital heart disease. *Am J Epidemiol* 1979;109:433–439.

7. Wiseman RA, Dodds-Smith IC. Cardiovascular birth defects and antenatal exposure to female sex hormones: a reevaluation of some base data. *Teratology* 1984;30:359–370.

8. Hanson JW. Fetal hydantoin effects. In: Sever JL, Brent RL, eds. *Teratogen Update: Environmentally Induced Birth Defect Risks.* New York: Alan R. Liss; 1986;29–33.

9. Friis ML, Hauge M. Congenital heart defects in live born children of epileptic patients. *Arch Neurol* 1985;42:374–376.

10. Hodach RL, Hodach AE, Fallon JF, Folts JD, Bruyere HJ, Gilbert EF. The role of β-adrenergic activity in the production of cardiac and aortic arch abnormalities in chick embryos. *Teratology* 1975;12:33–45.

11. Cameron RH, Kolesari GL, Kalbfleisch JH. Pharmacology of dextroamphetamine-induced cardiovascular malformations in the chick embryo. *Teratology* 1983;27:253–259.

12. Nora JJ, Vargo TA, Nora AA, et al. Dexamphetamine: a possible environmental trigger in cardiovascular malformations. *Lancet* 1970;1:1290–1291.

13. Cameron RH, Kolesari GL. Dextroamphetamine: embryonic cardiovascular sensitivity. *Teratology* 1982;25:25A.

14. Rosa FW, Wilk AL, Kelsey FO. Vitamin A congeners. In: Sever JL, Brent RL, eds. *Teratogen Update: Environmentally Induced Birth Defect Risks.* New York: Alan R. Liss; 1986;61–70.

15. Ruckman RN. Cardiovascular defects associated with alcohol, retinoic acid, and other agents. *Ann New York Acad Sci* 1990;588:281–288.

16. Mignot G, Devic M, Dumont M. Lithium et grossesse. *J Gynecol Obstet Biol Reprod* 1978;7:1303–1307.

17. Weinstein MR, Goldfield MD. Cardiovascular malformations with lithium use during pregnancy. *Am J Psychiatr* 1975;132:529–531.

18. Zierler S. Maternal drugs and congenital heart disease. *Obstet Gynecol* 1985;65:155–165.

19. Clarren SK, Smith DW. The fetal alcohol syndrome. *N Engl J Med* 1978;298:1063–1067.

20. Kurppa K, Holmberg PC, Kuosma E, Saxen L. Coffee consumption during pregnancy and congenital malformations: a nationwide case-control study. *Am J Public Health* 1983;73:1397–1397.

21. Tikkanen J, Heinnonen, OP. Risk factors for ventricular septal defects in Finland. *Public Health* 1991;105:99–112.

22. Occupational disease among operating room personnel: a national study. *Anesthesiology* 1974;41:321–340.

23. Pharoah POD, Alberman B, Doyle P. Outcome of pregnancy among women in anesthetic practice. *Lancet* 1977;1:34–36.

24. Cohen EN, Gift HC, Brown BW, Greenfield W, Wu ML, Jones TW, Whitcher CE, Driscoll EJ, Brodsky JB. Occupational disease in dentistry and chronic exposure to trace anesthetic gases. *Am J Dent Assoc* 1980;101:21–31.

25. Tikkahen J, Heinnonen OP. Cardiovascular malformations and organic solvent exposure during pregnancy in Finland. *Am J Ind Med* 1988;14:1–8.

26. Occupational exposures and selected congenital defects 12/01/78–1/31/80. Cincinnati, Oh: NIOSH Final Report. Grant no. 1ROIOH00803-01.

27. Goldberg ST, Lebowitz MD, Graver EJ, Hicks S. An association of human congenital cardiac malformations and drinking water contaminants. *J Am College Cardiol* 1990;16:155–164.

28. Zierler S, Theodore M, Cohen H, Rothman KJ. Chemical quality of maternal drinking water and congenital heart disease. *Int J Epidemiol* 1988;17:589–594.

29. Nora JJ, Nora AH. The evolution of specific genetic and environmental counselling in congenital heart disease. *Circulation* 1978;57:205–213.

53

MANAGEMENT OF THE PREGNANCY COMPLICATED BY FETAL CONGENITAL HEART DEFECTS

WILLIAM CUSICK, MD, BARBARA K. BURTON, MD, AND LOUIS BUTTINO, JR., MD

INTRODUCTION

The diagnosis of congenital heart disease in a fetus is usually just the beginning of a long and difficult journey for parents and child. Close surveillance and consultations with geneticists, neonatalogists, pediatric cardiologists, and pediatric cardiac surgeons will usually become necessary. Serial evaluation of the fetus, to refine/confirm the diagnosis and to examine any change in the clinical status of the fetus, will become routine. Prognosis and treatment options are presented to the parents in every possible detail. Only patients who are fully informed will be appropriately prepared to deal with the many decisions that will arise concerning the affected pregnancy and, possibly, future childbearing as well.

Congenital birth defects affect 2–4% of all infants. Cardiac defects, affecting an estimated 0.8% of all infants,[1] represent one of the most common groups of congenital defects. The development of high resolution ultrasound imaging has assisted the trained sonologist in identifying a substantial number of fetuses with congenital heart defects. Consequently, it is imperative that the clinician be familiar with the evaluation, antenatal management, and prognosis of fetuses with prenatally diagnosed cardiac defects. Furthermore, familiarity with the genetics of congenital heart disease will allow the caregiver to provide the parents of such affected children with an estimate of recurrence risk for future offspring. This chapter offers a framework for the management of a pregnancy complicated by prenatally diagnosed fetal congenital heart defects.

DIAGNOSIS

Once a cardiac defect has been diagnosed, in addition to a characterization of the anatomical defects of the fetal heart, a meticulous survey of the complete fetal anatomy is essential. Smythe et al found major extracardiac abnormalities in 32% of fetuses with prenatally diagnosed heart defects.[2] Similarly, Respondek et al reported associated anomalies in 42% of fetuses with prenatally diagnosed congenital heart lesions.[3] The documentation of associated noncardiac anomalies may provide supportive evidence for the presence of a possible genetic syndrome. Many multiple malformation syndromes are associated with abnormalities of the heart structure (Table 53.1). Conversely, in fetuses with extracardiac malformations, a significant percentage of fetuses will also suffer from concomitant cardiac defects.[4] When counseling parents about an affected fetus, the clinician must take into account the potential impact of these associated findings on neonatal survival.

Congenital heart defects are frequently present in fetuses with karyotypic abnormalities. Between 40 and 50% of fetuses with trisomy 21 and over 90% of fetuses with trisomies 13 and 18 will possess structural cardiac disease.[5] Alternatively, 17–38% of fetuses with heart defects diagnosed prenatally have an underlying abnormality in their chromosomal complement.[2,3,6–8] In the presence of other fetal anatomical defects or growth impairment, the likelihood for karyotypic abnormalities is further increased. For example, Smythe reported a 15% incidence of aneuploidy in fetuses with iso-

Cardiac Problems in Pregnancy, Third Edition
Edited by Uri Elkayam, MD, and Norbert Gleicher, MD
Copyright © 1998 by Wiley-Liss, Inc. ISBN 0-471-16358-9

TABLE 53.1 Multiple Malformation Syndromes Commonly Associated with Cardiac Defects

Disorder	Most Common Cardiac Lesions	Other Findings that May Be Seen on Ultrasound
MAJOR CHROMOSOME ANOMALIES		
Trisomy 21	VSD or AV canal, ASD	Short femur, short humerus, echogenic bowel, renal pyelectasis, nuchal thickening, cystic hygroma, duodenal atresia, ventriculomegaly
Trisomy 18	VSD, PS	IUGR, CNS anomalies, renal anomalies, choroid plexus cysts, omphalocele, many others
Trisomy 13	VSD, dextrocardia	Oral clefts, polydactyly, holoprosencephaly, many others
XO Turner syndrome	Coarctation of aorta, AS, ASD	Cystic hygroma
Triploidy	VSD, ASD	IUGR
MICRODELETION SYNDROMES		
DiGeorge/velocardiofacial syndromes (del 22q11)	Truncus, TOF, interrupted aortic arch	None
Williams syndrome (del 7q11.23)	Supravalvular AS	Usually none
SINGLE-GENE DISORDERS		
Noonan syndrome	PS, cardiomyopathy	Cystic hygroma, renal anomalies
Holt–Oram syndrome	ASD, VSD	Thumb anomalies; occasional radial aplasia
Thrombocytopenia–absent radius (TAR) syndrome	ASD, TOF	Absent radii
Tuberous sclerosis	Cardiac rhabdomyoma	None
Cornelia de Lange syndrome	VSD	IUGR, microcephaly, limb defect
SYNDROMES WITH COMPLEX OR UNCERTAIN INHERITANCE		
VATER association	VSD	Vertebral anomalies, renal or radial defects, esophageal atresia
CHARGE association	TOF, DORV, VSD	Ear anomalies; occasional IUGR
Ivemark syndrome (asplenia/polysplenia sequences)	Complex lesions, dextrocardia	Abnormal visceral situs
NONGENETIC SYNDROMES		
Fetal alcohol syndrome	VSD, ASD	IUGR, microcephaly
Retinoic acid embryopathy	Truncus, TOF, TGV	CNS malformations, facial clefts, small or absent ears
Congenital rubella syndrome	Peripheral PS	IUGR, microcephaly
Maternal PKU syndrome	TOF, trucus, TGV	IUGR, microcephaly

Abbreviations: AS, aortic stenosis; ASD, atrial septal defect; AV, atrioventricular; CHARGE, coloforma, heart disease, arrested growth or development, genital hypoplasia, ear abnormalities association; CNS, central nervous system; DOVR, double-outlet right ventricle; IUGR, intrauterine growth retardation; PKU, phenylketonuria; PS, pulmonic stenosis; TGV, transposition of great vessels; TOF, tetralogy of Fallot; Truncus, truncus arteriosus; VATER, vertebral anomalies, anal atresia, tracheoesophageal fistula, and renal and radial dysplasia; VSD, ventricular septal defect.

lated cardiac defects versus a 28% incidence in fetuses with associated extracardiac malformations.[2] It is therefore recommended that fetal karyotypic analysis be offered to all women carrying fetuses with congenital heart defects.[6]

Consultation with a pediatric cardiologist who is experienced in fetal echocardiography can provide parents with important information related to the specific anatomical defect(s) present. Early referral will allow the patients to discuss neonatal management, palliative and corrective surgical options, long-term survival, and quality of life. The services of a pediatric cardiologist are not available at all hospitals. Consequently, when severe fetal cardiac defects are present it may be necessary to arrange for delivery at a re-

ferral hospital, experienced in managing newborns with congenital heart defects.

MANAGEMENT

After all available information has been compiled, a thoughtful discussion regarding pregnancy management should be undertaken with the parents. When defects are detected in the early and mid-second trimester, parents should be informed of the availability of pregnancy termination. In Sharland's series, 50% of 442 women with prenatally diagnosed fetal congenital heart defects opted for pregnancy termination.[9] In continuing pregnancies, plans for follow-up care and antenatal assessment should be outlined. In the third trimester, ongoing antepartum assessment, hospital of delivery, intrapartum fetal surveillance, and possible cesarean section for fetal indications should be discussed.

Serial ultrasound evaluations of the fetus with congenital heart defects serve several important functions. The ultrasonic appearance of certain cardiac lesions may evolve throughout gestation. Severe aortic stenosis, for example, may progress to a picture of a hypoplastic left ventricle. Fluid accumulation in the fetus, detected by ultrasound monitoring, and manifested by fetal hydrops in its most severe form, represents an ominous finding with a dismal prognosis.[10] Sharland et al[9] reported a single survivor in 28 fetuses with sonographically detected hydrops secondary to cardiac failure. Furthermore, the repeated reassessment of the fetal anatomy by ultrasound may reveal previously undetected anomalies that impact on neonatal survival. Finally, serial ultrasound examinations will allow for the monitoring of fetal growth.

Because of the 10–25% incidence of intrauterine fetal death in fetuses with congenital heart defects, some clinicians institute routine antepartum testing in the third trimester. It is unlikely that any benefit would be derived from the testing of fetuses with lethal anomalies such as trisomy 18 and hypoplastic left ventricle. In fetuses with potentially correctable defects (e.g., tetralogy of Fallot), the impact of such testing on fetal survival is presently unknown. Although universal testing of fetuses with congenital heart defects may decrease the rate of intrauterine death, the ultimate impact, if any, on neonatal survival is uncertain. In addition, the benefits of immediate delivery for fetal indications of an affected infant with uncertain potential for survival must be weighed against the maternal risks of cesarean section.

The intrapartum management of fetuses with severe, congenital defects has remained somewhat controversial. A nonaggressive approach, including no fetal heart rate monitoring and the avoidance of cesarean section for fetal indications, has been advocated by some clinicians in circumstances in which the likelihood for neonatal survival is small. Although this path will minimize the operative risk to the mother, the psychological repercussions of an intrapartum death may be grave. Spinnato et al[11] recently reported on an approach designed to avoid intrapartum fetal death: namely, the aggressive intrapartum management of fetuses with severe, lethal anomalies. These authors implemented fetal heart rate monitoring and instituted conservative measures (change of position, maternal oxygen administration, amnioinfusion), designed to optimize the fetal condition even in the presence of fetal heart abnormalities. Cesarean section for fetal reasons was thus avoided. Three of the patients, successfully managed using such an approach, found comfort in live birth. A fourth patient, who experienced an intrapartum fetal death, found this experience to be very stressful.

Intrapartum management decisions should therefore be individualized and must incorporate all relevant information regarding the specific anomaly and the potential for neonatal survival. The complexity of such situations requires that the principles of intrapartum management be agreed on with the patient prior to the onset of labor. On occasion, advice from medical ethicists and/or hospital ethics committees should be requested.

PROGNOSIS

The likelihood for prenatal detection of an abnormality of the fetal heart increases with the severity of the abnormality and the presence of concomitant chromosomal or structural abnormalities. Accordingly, the outcome of neonates with prenatally diagnosed congenital heart defects is worse than that of the infants diagnosed neonatally. Crawford et al[12] reported a 17% one-year survival in infants with congenital heart defects diagnosed antenatally, versus an 81% survival in infants diagnosed after birth. Four reports exist describing the outcome of fetuses with prenatally detected congenital heart defects (Table 53.2).[2,3,9,13] Almost 50% of reported patients

TABLE 53.2   Fetal Congenital Heart Defects and Pregnancy Outcome

Ref: First Author (year)	Number of Cases	Outcomes			
		Termination	Intrauterine Death	Newborn Death	Infant Survived
Smyth[2] (1992)	170	77	15	43	35
Sharland[9] (1991)	442	220	57	118	47
Callan[13] (1991)	21	3	6	10	2
Respondek[3] (1994)	100	26	5	24	45
	773	326 (45.5%)	83 (11.3%)	195 (6.6%)	129 (17.6%)

TABLE 53.3   Cardiac Malformations and Outcomes in Continuing Pregnancies

Diagnosis	Number of Cases	Outcomes		
		Intrauterine Death	Death After Birth/Surgery	Infant Survived
Hypoplastic left ventricle	41	4	19	18 (43.9%)
Mitral atresia; double-outlet right ventricle	13	4	9	0
Aortic stenosis	30	10	19	1 (3.3%)
Coarctation	24	6	9	9 (37.5%)
Interrupted aortic arch	2	0	2	0
Tricuspid valve abnormality	39	10	21	8 (20.5%)
Pulmonary atresia/stenosis	30	4	12	14 (46.7%)
Tetralogy of Fallot	31	4	17	10 (32.3%)
Absent pulmonic valve	5	2	3	0
AV–septal/canal defect	58	10	27	21 (36.2%)
Ventricular septal defect	36	4	14	18 (50%)
Truncus arteriosus	7	0	6	1 (14.3%)
Transposition	12	0	3	9 (75%)
Cardiomyopathy	13	6	2	5 (38.5)
Tumor	5	4	0	1 (20%)
Aortic valve atresia	11	4	6	1 (9.1%)
Atrial isomerism	5	0	4	1 (20%)
Atrial septal defect	2	0	0	2 (100%)
Other	25	5	12	8 (32%)
	389	77	185	127

Source: Modified from Smythe et al,[2] Respondek et al,[3] Sharland et al.[9]

opted for pregnancy termination. Of the continuing pregnancies, 23.4% (78/333) were complicated by intrauterine fetal death.

The prognosis for any given neonate is strongly dependent on the specific cardiac lesion, the severity of the anatomical defect, and the potential for corrective surgery.[10] Table 53.3 summarizes the survival rates for the more common cardiac defects diagnosed prenatally. When counseling patients in the second trimester, it is important to remember that these neonatal survival percentages may represent best estimates, for fetuses with more severe anomalies are more likely to be terminated or to die in utero.[2] Thus, the prognosis for an affected fetus in the second trimester may be worse than that of a fetus surviving to term.

As stated earlier, the development of fetal hydrops portends a poor prognosis in fetuses with congenital heart defects. Fetuses with congenital heart defects as a feature of an underlying karyotypic abnormality are less likely to survive than are euploid fetuses.[3] The prognosis, however, ultimately depends on the chromosomal abnormality present. The most common severe chromosomal abnormalities, *trisomy 13, trisomy 18,* and *triploidy,* are associated with minimal potential for prolonged neonatal survival. Other antenatal findings associated with a decreased potential for neonatal survival include the presence of extracardiac abnormalities and concomitant intrauterine growth retardation.[3] Ultimately, the prognosis for any given fetus can be established only after a comprehensive examination in the neonatal period.

GENETIC COUNSELING

Accurate genetic counseling for affected families depends on having a definitive diagnosis of the affected family member, a complete prenatal history, and a family history. Once a defect has been identified in utero, the counseling process should be initiated. When families are first confronted with the devastating news of a potentially serious birth defect, the focus of counseling should be on prognosis and options for the current pregnancy, with definitive genetic counseling regarding future pregnancies to be deferred until after pregnancy termination or delivery. At this later date, when a definitive diagnosis has been established, the parents are likely to be emotionally receptive to a discussion of the future.

A noncardiac chromosome analysis and careful ultrasound examination of the fetus to detect other noncardiac anomalies is of clinical importance, as noted earlier. The nature of a cardiac anomaly is rarely helpful in suggesting a specific multiple malformation syndrome but there can be exceptions. For example, up to 75% of fetuses and infants with a complete atrioventricular canal have Down syndrome.[14] Cardiac *rhabdomyomas,* which occasionally present prenatally as an isolated finding, are most often a manifestation of *tuberous sclerosis.*[15] In the case of most malformation syndromes, however, the most common cardiac lesions observed are those most commonly seen in the general population.

If parents choose pregnancy termination following the diagnosis of a cardiac defect in utero, and a fetal sample for chromosome analysis has not been obtained by amniocentesis, placental biopsy, or umbilical blood sampling, a karyotype should be obtained following delivery. This can be done from a sample of fetal blood, skin, or umbilical cord. Certain circumstances may warrant specialized testing for microdeletions, using fluorescence in situ hybridization (FISH). For example, many infants with the *DiGeorge* sequence of anomalies (conotruncal cardiac defects or aortic arch anomalies, hypoparathyroidism, thymic hypoplasia) and the *velocardiofacial syndrome* (cleft palate or velopharyngeal incompetence, unusual facies, developmental disabilities, and conotruncal defects) have deletions of a specific region of chromosome 22 that is not commonly detected with routine chromosome analysis. Since the cardiac defect may be the only abnormality noted in fetuses or newborns with these disorders, microdeletion testing is indicated whenever conotruncal or aortic arch abnormalities are diagnosed.[16] The importance of an autopsy should be stressed to the family as well. This procedure is critical not only for confirmation of the cardiac findings detected by ultrasonography but also for the detection of other organic anomalies that might have significance for genetic counseling. After the results of the chromosome analysis and autopsy have become available, a meeting should be scheduled with the family to review the findings and to discuss the recurrence risks for future pregnancies.

Parents who choose termination of a wanted pregnancy, following the diagnosis of a fetal abnormality, experience profound grief, comparable to that associated with prenatal loss at term. Therefore, counseling should focus not only on the medical issues but on the emotional ones as well. A referral to appropriate local support groups may be helpful to many families.

Parents should always be counseled that the absence of other detectable abnormalities by ultrasound examination, even combined with normal karyotypic finding, does not rule out the presence of a multiple malformation syndrome, which could have important prognostic and genetic implications. In many cases, the other features of the multiple malformation syndromes in which cardiac defects are prominent, such as dysmorphic facial features and developmental disabilities, are not readily detectable by ultrasonography. Definitive genetic counseling should therefore be deferred until after delivery, when the nature of the cardiac defect can be confirmed.

Genetic counseling can begin during pregnancy as long as the parents understand that it is based on assumptions that cannot be confirmed until after delivery. Some issues, however, can often be definitively addressed even during pregnancy and even in the absence of final diagnosis. For example, many parents confronted with the news of a birth defect in their infant will experience feelings of guilt and will imagine that the defect could have been predicted or prevented in some way. They may have specific concerns related to certain drug or occupational exposures or to some aspect of their personal medical history or family history. In many cases, there will be no possible relationship to the defect identified, and these concerns can be dispelled. Parents can be made aware that congenital heart defects are relatively common and that the vast majority are neither predictable or preventable.

During the initial encounter with an affected family, a detailed family history should be obtained. Attention should be paid to other individuals with congenital heart disease or other birth defects, fetal loss or perinatal death, and consanguinity. In some cases, other abnormalities that at first glance appear unrelated may turn out to be of great significance. For example, a history of thumb or radial anomalies in the parent of the fetus with a cardiac defect would suggest the possibility of the *Holt–Oram syndrome,* a highly variable autosomal dominant disorder involving abnormalities of the heart, thumbs, and upper extremities.

On establishment of a definitive diagnosis following the birth of an infant with a cardiac defect, more definitive genetic counseling can be provided. Most cases of isolated congenital heart defects have a multifactorial basis, implying that both genetic and environmental factors play a role. The environmental factors can rarely be specifically identified, except in the case of fetuses exposed to known cardioteratogens, such as lithium, retinoic acid, or maternal diabetes mellitus. Parents of a single affected child with an isolated cardiac defect face an increased risk of recurrence in future pregnancies compared with couples in the general population. Empiric recurrence risk data are available for most of the common lesions and are summarized in Table 53.4. Affected individuals also face an increased risk for their own offspring, and the risk is often higher if it is the mother, as opposed to the father, who is affected.[17]

In counseling parents of their increased risk of recurrence, it is important to put the risk in context by comparing it with the general population risk of congenital heart disease, which is close to 1%. Words like *high* or *low* should be avoided in describing risk, since the perception of a given risk as high or low varies widely among individuals. In counseling parents of their recurrence risk, it should also be pointed out that when there is a recurrence, the defect in the second child is not always the same as that observed in the first. Although there is a general tendency for defects appearing in the same family to be similar in nature, this is not universally the case, and even when the same type of defect recurs, variations in severity are commonly noted.

In addition to recurrence risks, reproductive options

TABLE 53.4   Recurrence Risk for Common Congenital Heart Defects

		Recurrence Risk (%)	
Defect	Incidence	1 Child Affected	1 Parent Affected
VSD	1 in 400	3.0	2–10[a]
PDA	1 in 800	3.0	2–4[a]
ASD	1 in 1,000	2.5	2–5[a]
TOF	1 in 1,000	2.5	3.0
PS	1 in 1,000	2.0	2–6[a]
Coarctation of aorta	1 in 2,000	2.0	2.4[a]
AS	1 in 2,000	2.0	3–18[a]
TGV	1 in 2,000	2.0	NA
AV canal	1 in 2,500	3.0	1–14[a]
TA	1 in 5,000	1.0	NA
HLH	1 in 10,000	2.0	NA
PA	1 in 10,000	1.0	NA
Ebstein's anomaly	1 in 20,000	1.0	NA
Truncus	1 in 30,000	1.0	NA

[a]The higher recurrence risk is applicable when the affected parent is the mother; NA, data not available.

Abbreviations: ASD, atrial septal defect; AS, aortic stenosis; AV, atrioventricular; HLH, hypoplastic left heart; PA, pulmonary atresia; PDA, patent ductus arteriosus; PS, pulmonary stenosis; TA, tricuspid atresia; TGV, transposition of great vessels; TOF, tetralogy of Fallot; Truncus, truncus arteriosus; VSD, ventricular septal defect.

should be addressed. Sometimes parents may view the demands of caring for an affected child as an impediment to future childbearing, regardless the magnitude of the risk of recurrence. Couples should be discouraged from undergoing sterilization procedures immediately after the birth of an affected child or after a pregnancy termination, since their perspective on childbearing may change over time. Prenatal diagnosis, with selective pregnancy termination, should be discussed as an option for couples who desire additional children, although the limitations of ultrasonography and fetal echocardiography in detecting congenital heart defects should be clearly outlined. Adoption is an additional alternative that should be addressed in counseling couples who express concern about the possibility of recurrence. Other reproductive options, such as artificial insemination by male donor or in vitro fertilization with ovum donation, useful options in reducing the risk of single-gene disorders, are not useful in the context of multifactorial conditions, which most isolated cardiac defects represent.

If there is more than a single affected individual in a family with congenital heart disease, the recurrence risks listed in Table 54.4 do not apply. With a history of two affected first-degree relatives, recurrence risks are two to three times higher than they are in families with a single affected individual. If three or more affected individuals are identified, the diagnosis and mode of inheritance should be carefully reassessed. Although there are "high risk" families with isolated nonsyndromic congenital heart defects in which multifactorial inheritance still applies, there is now increasing evidence that some isolated cardiac defects may be transmit-

ted in a single-gene fashion.[18] Caution should therefore be exercised in counseling such high risk families. In addition, it should be noted that the associated findings, observed in some of the genetically determined multiple malformation syndromes, can be subtle. For example, most patients with Noonan syndrome, a common disorder frequently associated with pulmonic stenosis, have normal intelligence and no other life-threatening structural defects. The dysmorphic features associated with the condition, including altered facial features and a broad or webbed neck, may be disregarded as representing familial characteristics. Another example of a disorder that can be easily overlooked is the velocardiofacial syndrome, an often underdiagnosed disorder associated with conotruncal cardiac defects, mildly dysmorphic facial features, learning disabilities or psychiatric problems, and palatal defects, ranging from cleft palate to hypernasal speech. Not all features are present in every affected individual. It would therefore be possible to have an infant with significant cardiac disease born to a mother who has only mildly dysmorphic facial features and hypernasal speech.

REFERENCES

1. Hoffman JIE, Christianson R. Congenital heart disease in a cohort of 19,502 births with long-term follow-up. *Am J Cardiol* 1978;42:641.

2. Smythe JF, Copel JA, Kleinman CS. Outcome of prenatally detected cardiac malformations. *Am J Cardiol* 1992;69: 1471–1474.

3. Respondek ML, Binotto CN, Smith S, Donnenfeld DR, Weil SR, Huhta JC. Extracardiac anomalies, aneuploidy and growth retardation in 100 consecutive fetal congenital heart defects. *Ultrasound Obstet Gynecol* 1994;4:272–278.

4. Copel JA, Pilu G, Kleinman CS. Congenital heart disease and anomalies: associations and indications for fetal echocardiography. *Am J Obstet Gynecol* 1986;154:118–132.

5. Nora JJ, Nora AH. Chromosomal anomalies. In: Nora JJ, Nora AH, eds. *Genetics and Counseling in Cardiovascular Diseases.* Springfield, IL: Charles C. Thomas; 1978; 63.

6. Wladimiroff JW, Stewart PA, Sachs ES, Niermeijer MF. Prenatal diagnosis and management of congenital heart defect: significance of associated fetal anomalies and prenatal chromosome studies. *Am J Med Genet* 1985;21:285.

7. Copel JA, Cullen M, Green JJ, Mahoney MJ, Hobbins JC, Kleinman CS. The frequency of aneuploidy in prenatally diagnosed congenital heart disease: an indication for fetal karyotyping. *Am J Obstet Gynecol* 1998;158:409–413.

8. Bromley B, Estroff JA, Sanders SP, Parad R, Roberts D, Frigoletto FD, Benacerraf BR. Fetal echocardiography: accuracy and limitations in a population at high and low risk for heart defects. *Am J Obstet Gynecol* 1992;166:1473–1481.

9. Sharland GK, Lockhart SM, Chita SK, Allan LD. Factors influencing the outcome of congenital heart disease detected prenatally. *Arch Dis Child* 1991;66:284.

10. Baumann P, Copel JA, Kleinman CS. Management of the fetus with cardiac disease. *Ultrasound Q* 1991;10:57–78.

11. Spinnato JA, Cook VD, Cook CR, Voss DH. Aggressive intrapartum management of lethal fetal anomalies: beyond fetal beneficence. *Obstet Gynecol* 1995;85:8992.

12. Crawford DC, Chita SK, Allan LD. Prenatal detection of congenital heart disease: factors affecting obstetric management and survival. *Am J Obstet Gynecol* 1998;159:352–356.

13. Callan NA, Maggio M, Steger S, Kan JS. Fetal echocardiography: indications for referral, prenatal diagnoses, and outcomes. *Am J Perinatol* 1991;8:390–394.

14. Chin AJ, Keane JF, Norwood WI, Castenada AR. Repair of complete common atrioventricular canal in infancy. *J Thorac Cardiovasc Surg* 982;84:437–445.

15. Journel H, Roussey M, Plais MH, Milon J, Almange C, LeMarec B. Prenatal diagnosis of familial tuberous sclerosis following detection of cardiac rhabdomyoma by ultrasound. *Prenatal Diagn* 1986;6:283–289.

16. Goldmuntz E, Driscoll D, Biedarf ML, Zackai EH, McDonald-McGinn DM, Biegel JA, Emanuel BS. Microdeletions of chromosomal region 22q11 in patients with congenital conotruncal cardiac defects. *J Med Genet* 1993;30:807–812.

17. Nora JJ, Nora AH. Maternal transmission of congenital heart diseases: new recurrence risk figures and the questions of cytoplasmic inheritance and vulnerability to teratogens. *Am J Cardiol* 1987;59:459–463.

18. Payne RM, Johnson MC, Grant JW, Strauss AW. Toward a molecular understanding of congenital heart disease. *Circulation* 1995;91:494–504.

54

RECOGNITION AND MANAGEMENT OF CONGENITAL HEART DISEASE IN THE NEONATE

TERRENCE DILLON, MD

INTRODUCTION

Although congenital heart disease (CHD) is one of the leading causes of death in the first year of life, its incidence has remained stable at 1%[1] for decades. Moreover, 25% of cases present in the newborn period,[2] making early identification critical for long-term survival, since even the most serious forms of CHD, such as transposition of the great vessels (d-TGV)[3,4] and hypoplastic left heart syndrome (HLHS),[5] are now amenable to surgical repair with excellent results. The purpose of this chapter is not to describe in detail each form of CHD that presents in the neonatal period but to develop an approach that will allow early recognition of CHD to be followed by prompt transport to a tertiary center for sophisticated diagnostic evaluation, optimal medical management, and surgery. The approach to these infants will follow the traditional pathways: history (including family, prenatal, and perinatal), physical examination, diagnostic evaluation, and medical management.

HISTORY

The family and maternal history should be reviewed for CHD and other birth defects, as well as for diabetes, collagen vascular disease, or other inherited disease. The incidence of CHD increases from 1% to a range of 2–4% if a sibling has CHD, with the risk varying according to the type of CHD in the index case.[6] The risk increases to 10% if two previous children have CHD and to nearly 50% if three siblings have CHD. If CHD is present in one of the parents without a recognizable syndrome or other family history of CHD, the overall risk of transmission has been estimated to be 10%. Whether the sex of the parent with CHD alters the risk for CHD in offspring remains controversial Whittemore et al[7] suggested no sexual difference for transmission of CHD, whereas eight studies reviewed by Nora and Nora[8] demonstrated a substantially higher risk if the mother was the affected parent. The history of a previous spontaneous abortion or stillbirth is important because the incidence of chromosomal abnormalities and CHD is significantly higher in this group.[9] Infants born to diabetic mothers have a five-fold increase in CHD, with ventricular septal defect and dextro-transposition of the great vessels most common. Infants born to mothers with collagen vascular disease are at significant risk for developing complete heart block.[10]

The maternal health during the pregnancy must also be reviewed. Rubella during the first trimester will frequently result in patent ductus arteriosus and branch pulmonary artery stenosis. Other maternal viral infections can result in neonatal myocarditis. A maternal drug history should also be obtained. A mother with a seizure disorder may be taking a drug that is teratogenic to the heart (e.g., diphenylhydantoin, valproic acid, trimethadione). Because Coumadin is teratogenic, women of childbearing age rarely have mechanical valve prostheses inserted. If, however, anticoagulation is necessary during pregnancy, heparin is most commonly used.[11] Lithium and retinoic acid also increase the risk of CHD, with the fetus at greatest risk during the period of organogenesis from 2 to 10 weeks after conception.

The social history is also important. The older the mother at conception, the greater the risk for fetal abnormalities. Pre-

Cardiac Problems in Pregnancy, Third Edition
Edited by Uri Elkayam, MD, and Norbert Gleicher, MD
Copyright © 1998 by Wiley-Liss, Inc. ISBN 0-471-16358-9

natal care, however, does not appear to play a major role in the incidence of CHD, since most CHD is already determined by the time of the first prenatal visit. The ingestion of alcohol can result in fetal alcohol syndrome, with an increased risk of CHD.[12] The recreational use of cocaine is also associated with an increased incidence of CHD,[13] along with a variety of other congenital anomalies.

The perinatal history should also be reviewed. Abnormal fetal heart rate patterns and low Apgar scores suggest perinatal asphyxia. The presence of maternal fever may be a harbinger of neonatal sepsis, including group B streptococcal sepsis. The presence of meconium-stained amniotic fluid may be associated with meconium aspiration. Each of these clinical situations can result in persistent pulmonary hypertension, hypoxia, and myocardial dysfunction, which in turn can masquerade as a severe primary cardiac abnormality.[14]

PHYSICAL EXAMINATION

General Appearance

The general appearance of the infant is extremely important. Is the infant moving spontaneously or very quiet? Does the infant appear anxious and fretful? Are the color and breathing pattern normal? Is the skin pink and well perfused, as in the normal newborn, or pale, gray, mottled, and diaphoretic, suggesting a low cardiac output [e.g., critical aortic stenosis (AS), HLHS, severe coarctation, myocarditis, or sepsis]? Remembering that light source and skin pigmentation must be taken into account, does the infant appear to be cyanotic? If so, is the cyanosis peripheral or central? Peripheral cyanosis involves primarily the extremities and results from a spectrum of etiologies including vasomotor instability of the newborn, cold stress, polycythemia, hypovolemia, hypoglycemia, and sepsis. The oxygen saturation and P_{O_2} are normal. Central cyanosis involves the tongue, lips, conjunctivae, and mucous membranes and implies at least 3–5 g of desaturated hemoglobin. Infants with higher hemoglobin levels (i.e., as in polycythemia) appear centrally cyanotic at higher oxygen saturations, whereas anemic infants may appear only mildly cyanotic despite a much greater decrease in oxygen saturation. For example, a term newborn (TNB) with a hemoglobin of 20g/dL would appear cyanotic at an oxygen saturation of 85%, whereas an anemic TNB with a hemoglobin of 10g/dL would not appear cyanotic until the oxygen saturation had fallen to 70%.

Central cyanosis typically results from one of four conditions:

1. *Primary pulmonary disease,* with intrapulmonary and intracardiac right-to-left shunting [i.e., persistent pulmonary hypertension of the newborn (PPHNB)] or inadequate ventilation due to structural abnormalities (choanal atresia, diaphragmatic hernia). The breathing pattern is one of tachypnea, dyspnea, retractions, and nasal flaring, with vigorous but labored respirations.

2. *Primary cardiac disease* due to inadequate ACTUAL pulmonary blood flow, resulting from obstruction to pulmonary blood flow and secondary intracardiac right-to-left shunting [i.e., pulmonary atresia with intact septum or severe tetralogy of Fallot (TOF)] or due to inadequate EFFECTIVE pulmonary blood flow, where fully saturated blood is returned to the pulmonary circulation and significantly desaturated blood is returned to the systemic circulation (d-TGV). These infants are often only mildly tachypneic in response to the cyanosis but not truly dyspneic until the persistent hypoxemia has resulted in a significant metabolic acidosis. Typically the infant with cyanotic CHD becomes more cyanotic with crying, while the infant with primary pulmonary disease becomes less cyanotic with crying, because in the second case, ventilation is increased.

3. *Primary CNS abnormality* with hypoventilation, due most commonly to a depressed respiratory center secondary to maternal oversedation, neonatal asphyxia, or intracranial hemorrhage. These infants have a weak, irregular breathing pattern, often associated with a weak sucking reflex, convulsions, and generalized depression.

4. *Primary hematologic abnormality.* Methemoglobinemia is a rare cause of central cyanosis in the newborn period. Recognizable cyanosis occurs when 10–15% of the total hemoglobin is replaced by methemoglobin, which is unable to bind and transport oxygen normally. The *measured* (not calculated) oxygen saturation will be decreased despite a normal arterial P_{O_2} and normal response to the hyperoxia test. The breathing pattern and cardiac exam are normal and the prognosis for these infants is generally good.

Any unusual features in the appearance of the child should be noted. A number of chromosomal and genetic abnormalities are associated with a high incidence of CHD (see Table 54.1). Approximately 15% of newborns identified with CHD[15] and nearly 33% of fetuses stillborn or aborted spontaneously with CHD have a chromosomal abnormality.[9] A careful search for dysmorphic craniofacial, visceral, and skeletal features will alert the physician to seek a full genetics consultation.[16] It is especially important to identify the infant with Down syndrome, since the prognosis has improved markedly from both societal and surgical points of view.[17] Forty percent of infants with Down syndrome have CHD, with AV septal defect (AVSD) or ventricular septal defect (VSD) most common. Since these infants often have no murmur in the neonatal period but are at great risk to develop pul-

TABLE 54.1   Syndromes Associated with CHD Identified in the Newborn[a]

Syndrome	Frequency (%)	Common Abnormalities
Trisomy 21	40	AV septal defect, VSD
Turner syndrome	40	Aortic coarctation, bicuspid aortic valve
Trisomy 13	80	VSD
Trisomy 18	90	VSD, PDA, DORV
Williams syndrome	33	Supravalvar AS, branch PA stenosis
VACTERL syndrome	20	VSD, TOF
DiGeorge syndrome	80	Truncus, IAA, TOF
Noonan syndrome	40	PS, ASD
Tuberous sclerosis	50	Rhabdomyoma
Holt–Oram syndrome	20	ASD

[a]For abbreviations, see chapter appendix.

monary vascular disease early and become inoperable, an echocardiographic examination should be performed by an experienced pediatric echocardiographer during the first month.

Vital Signs

Birth weight is estimated to be less than 2.5 kg in 20% of infants with CHD[18]; VSD and AV septal defect are most commonly involved, and simple transposition only rarely. The reasons for the growth retardation in utero are not known, although clearly the genetic abnormalities must be partially responsible.

As noted before, respiratory pattern and rate are of critical importance. The respiratory rate should be less than 50 with no dyspnea in the TNB. The resting pulse in the TNB is 120–130 during the first week and increases to 150 during weeks 2–4. Less than 5% have resting heart rates of less than 100 or greater than 160 beats per minute in the first week on the standard ECG.[19] However, transient fluctuations in the pulse, to as high as 220 and to as low as 59, have been reported in healthy TNB infants in the first 3 days of life with 24-hour Holter monitoring.[20]

The blood pressure should be measured in the right arm and one leg. The blood pressure in the right arm should be 65–75 mmHg systolic and 35–45 mmHg diastolic when measured by Doppler. Blood pressures measured in the leg are generally slightly higher than those in the arm owing to technical factors. A systolic pressure in the arm that is 20 mmHg higher than in the leg suggests the possibility of aortic coarctation. However, the absence of any pressure gradient does not rule out coarctation, especially in the presence of a patent ductus arteriosus (PDA). On the other hand, hypotension suggests (1) cardiogenic shock related to severe left ventricular outflow tract (LVOT) obstruction, including critical AS, HLHS, and severe aortic coarctation, or severe left ventricular (LV) dysfunction secondary to neonatal sepsis or viral myocarditis, or (2) severe anemia with decreased oxygen de-

livery. On the other hand, the presence of a normal blood pressure does not necessarily imply a normal cardiac output. That is, the definition of shock is a compromised circulation, not hypotension which is *not* present in the early stages of shock.

The pulses in all four extremities should be felt, with the right brachial and either femoral pulse palpated simultaneously. The two pulses should be felt synchronously with equal intensity or pulse volume. If all pulses are weak, hypovolemia, severe obstruction of the left ventricular outflow tract (LVOT) or severe LV dysfunction with neonatal myocarditis or neonatal sepsis should be considered. If the femoral pulses alone are not felt or are only weakly palpable, aortic coarctation should be considered. If the pulses are bounding, lesions with significant aortic runoff should be considered: PDA, truncus arteriosus, systemic arteriovenous (AV) fistula (especially intracranial), and aortic–left ventricular tunnel.

Head

A cranial bruit should be listened for in any infant with signs of high output congestive heart failure (CHF) with bounding pulses, hyperactive precordium, and cardiomegaly on chest X-ray. An intracranial AV fistula is one of the very rare circumstances in a TNB in which increased venous return from the brain and elevated central venous pressure cause distension of the jugular veins. Occasionally these infants develop hydrops fetalis as a manifestation of in utero CHF.

Chest

Inspect the chest for any asymmetry. Although a precordial bulge is rare in the TNB, this sign is often related to marked cardiomegaly. Palpate the point of maximal impulse, which is normally in the fourth intercostal space in the left midclavicular line. If this point is displaced further to the left or downward, cardiomegaly is frequently present. If displaced medially and to the right, dextrocardia or even cardiac displacement due to a diaphragmatic hernia should be considered.

Following visual inspection, the chest should be palpated for excessive precordial activity and thrills. Because of the predominance of the right ventricle in utero[21] and its anterior location in the chest, an RV lift or heave is frequently palpated in the left parasternal region at birth. As the pulmonary vascular resistance falls normally, this sign generally disappears during the first day of life. However, typically, it is not possible to ascribe excessive precordial activity specifically to either the right or left ventricle. Precordial activity is increased with increased pulmonary blood flow, right ventricular hypertrophy (RVH) for whatever reason (e.g., CHD, PPHNB), significant AV valve insufficiency, or semilunar valve stenosis or insufficiency.

A thrill is a palpable murmur and is rare in the TNB. When a precordial thrill is present, the common etiologies include severe AV valve insufficiency or semilunar valve stenosis. A thrill in the suprasternal notch can often be palpated in significant AS, truncal valve stenosis, and coarctation of the aorta.

Auscultation begins with the first and second heart sounds. The first heart sound is produced by closure of the tricuspid and mitral valves; it is best heard at the apex and less frequently at the left lower sternal border. The first heart sound is almost always single, with the notable exception of Ebstein's anomaly of the tricuspid valve, in which there is delayed closure of that valve. The first heart sound increases in intensity with increased blood flow across either AV valve, AV valve stenosis, and increased cardiac output for whatever reason. In contrast, the first heart sound can be decreased in intensity with LV dysfunction (e.g., viral myocarditis or LVOT obstruction).

The second heart sound is produced by closure of the aortic and pulmonary valves and is heard best at the left upper sternal border. Because of the normal elevation in pulmonary vascular resistance at birth, the second heart sound typically remains single during the first day of life, but it is audibly split in 80% of normal TNB by 48 hours of age. With tachycardia and respiratory distress, splitting is often difficult to appreciate. If splitting is appreciated, however, the presence of two semilunar valves can be inferred, ruling out pulmonary atresia, aortic atresia, and truncus arteriosus. A widely split second heart sound is unusual but can occur with increased blood flow across the pulmonic valve, with mild pulmonic stenosis, or with right bundle branch block on electrocardiogram (ECG). A single loud second heart sound can relate to either pulmonic valve closure (e.g., pulmonary hypertension for whatever reason) or to aortic valve closure (d- or l-TGV due to the anterior location of the aortic valve).

Ejection clicks heard after 24 hours of life are always abnormal and relate to either semilunar valve stenosis (i.e., AS, PS, or truncal valve stenosis) or to vessel dilatation (the aor-

ta with neonatal Marfan syndrome and the main pulmonary artery with pulmonary hypertension). The presence of an ejection click even in the asymptomatic TNB implies underlying CHD and requires further evaluation, including echocardiographic examination (although up to 2% of TNB may have a bicuspid aortic valve without stenosis).[1]

The presence of a heart murmur in the TNB is common and frequently is not associated with CHD. Braudo and Rowe noted that 60% of infants examined frequently in the first 48 hours of life had a heart murmur.[22] The majority of these murmurs are physiologic: a small PDA in the first day of life that has not closed completely; physiologic branch pulmonary artery stenosis due to the relatively small size and acute angle takeoff of the branch pulmonary arteries in relation to the main pulmonary artery; functional systolic ejection murmurs at the left upper and lower sternal border similar to the functional murmurs heard in the older child (e.g., Still's murmur). These murmurs are typically grade I or II in intensity and resolve spontaneously.

Murmurs occur in systole, diastole, or continuously through parts of both systole and diastole. In addition to noting the timing of the murmur relative to the cardiac cycle, the clinician should mark the loudness of the murmur (i.e., grade I–VI), the location on the chest where the murmur is best heard, the radiation of the murmur, and the pitch of the murmur. The systolic murmur in the TNB is either ejection or pansystolic. The systolic ejection murmur occurs during ventricular ejection; it starts shortly after the first heart sound and results from turbulent blood flow exiting the heart. This turbulence is due to right or left ventricular outflow tract obstruction (i.e., PS, TOF, and AS) or to increased blood flow across a normal semilunar valve. The murmur due to semilunar valve stenosis is often heard on the first day of life.

The pansystolic murmur occurs throughout systole, starting with the first heart sound and often obscuring it, and ending with the second heart sound. These murmurs result from either AV valve insufficiency or a ventricular septal defect. The murmur of a VSD is not audible until the pulmonary vascular resistance (PVR) has fallen enough for turbulent left-to-right shunting to cause the murmur. The VSD murmur is seldom heard on the first or second day of life, especially in the large VSD, where the fall in PVR is delayed.

Diastolic murmurs are audible in all three phases of diastole: early, mid, and late. The early diastolic murmur is quite uncommon and results from semilunar valve insufficiency. The middiastolic murmur relates to increased flow across an AV valve, whereas the late diastolic murmur is quite rare and almost always results from mitral stenosis.

Continuous murmurs typically arise when there is an abnormal communication between the high pressure systemic arterial circulation and the low pressure systemic venous or pulmonary circulations (i.e., PDA, intracranial or systemic AV fistula, PA-VSD with collateral pulmonary blood flow). Less common causes for continuous murmurs include pulmonary arteriovenous fistulas and total anomalous pulmonary venous connection (TAPVC) to an unobstructed left vertical vein.

The location at which the murmur is best heard and its radiation are important in identifying the etiology of the murmur. A systolic ejection murmur at the left upper sternal border that radiates to the back almost always reflects right ventricular outflow tract (RVOT) obstruction (i.e., PS or TOF). A pansystolic murmur at the left lower sternal border in a sick TNB with PPHNB is almost certainly related to tricuspid incompetence. A continuous murmur in the left infraclavicular region almost always results from a PDA. The pitch of a murmur is also important. A high-pitched murmur usually occurs when there is turbulence due to blood flow from a high pressure to low pressure area (i.e. mitral or aortic incompetence).

In summary, listening for a heart murmur is important, although the presence or absence of a heart murmur does not rule in or rule out the presence of CHD. For example, the infant with d-TGV may have no murmur but severe cyanosis. The infant with severe perinatal asphyxia and no CHD may have a loud murmur related to tricuspid insufficiency due to pulmonary hypertension and/or papillary muscle ischemia. The significance of a murmur, then, is determined by the associated characteristics of the murmur as just discussed and by the accompanying historical, physical, and laboratory findings.

Auscultation of the lungs should reveal equal air entry bilaterally. The presence of wheezing, rales, and an expiratory grunt suggest pulmonary disease or severe congestive heart failure due either to LV inflow obstruction (e.g., TAPVC, mitral stenosis, cor triatriatum), severe LV dysfunction (e.g., myocarditis), or severe LVOT obstruction (e.g., critical AS).

Abdomen

The abdomen should be inspected for distension that might suggest ascites, which can result from circulatory congestion. The abdomen should then be palpated to determine the location and size of the liver. The liver span in infants is normally 6 cm, and the organ may be palpated 3 cm below the right costal margin. Hepatic enlargement is frequently associated with CHF, but hyperinflation should be ruled out as a possible cause for apparent hepatic enlargement. If the liver is pulsatile, severe tricuspid incompetence (Ebstein's anomaly) or an obstructive lesion of the right atrium (e.g., tricuspid atresia with a restrictive interatrial communication) should be considered.

Normally the liver is palpated in the right upper quadrant, and maximal precordial activity or the PMI is felt in the left chest (i.e., thoracic and abdominal concordance or situs solitus). If the chest and abdominal contents are completely reversed (situs inversus totalis), CHD is uncommon. If, on the other hand, there is discordance, with both liver and heart po-

sitioned primarily left of midline or both primarily right of midline, CHD is quite common. In addition, although a midline liver is difficult to determine with certainty on palpation, its presence as revealed on X-ray or ultrasound examination is frequently associated with severe CHD and visceral heterotaxia with asplenia or polysplenia.[23]

Extremities

Capillary refill, as a rough estimation of systemic perfusion and the presence of nailbed cyanosis, should be determined. The extremities are rarely edematous even with severe neonatal CHF unless the edema develops in utero (hydrops fetalis). Pulses should be palpated as discussed previously.

DIAGNOSTIC EVALUATION

Hyperoxia Test

The majority of cyanotic infants have either severe pulmonary disease or severe cardiac disease. The hyperoxia test can be quite helpful in differentiating the two.[24,25] Although arterial blood gases can be difficult to obtain in the sick newborn, oxygen saturations can now be obtained quite simply and noninvasively in almost every nursery. Initially the probe is placed on the right hand or right upper chest to maximize the reading even in the presence of right-to-left ductal shunting. If the oxygen saturation is less than 90%, the infant is placed in 100% oxygen for 10 minutes: if the oxygen saturation then increases significantly, a diagnosis of primary lung disease is suggested. If there is no response, primary cardiac disease is suggested or, less commonly, severe lung disease with PPHNB and right-to-left atrial and/or ductal shunting. Right-to-left atrial shunting can be determined by simple contrast echocardiography at the bedside. Right-to-left ductal shunting can be identified with the simultaneous measurement of the oxygen saturations in the right arm/hand and a lower extremity/foot. If the preductal saturation is greater than the postductal saturation, serious pulmonary or cardiac disease should be suspected.

If the infant is obviously sick, an umbilical artery catheter should be placed and arterial blood gases from the descending aorta in room air and 100% oxygen (for 10 min by endotracheal tube, head hood, or face mask) should be obtained. If the P_{O_2} is low in room air (< 50 torr) and increases significantly with oxygen administration (> 70 torr) as the ventilation–perfusion inequalities or diffusion gradient are overcome, primary lung disease is most likely and "critical life-threatening" cyanotic CHD is extremely unlikely. If, however, the cyanotic CHD is associated with increased pulmonary blood flow and good mixing of systemic and pulmonary venous blood, the P_{O_2} may well rise above 100 torr, as in the cases of TAPVC without obstruction to pulmonary venous return, tricuspid atresia without obstruction to pulmonary blood flow, and truncus arteriosus.[25]

If the P_{O_2} remains decreased with no response to oxygen, the infant has either severe cyanotic CHD or severe primary lung disease, probably with persistence of the fetal blood flow pathways. If a right radial blood gas is then obtained simultaneously with a descending aortic sample and if the P_{O_2} is higher in the former, right-to-left ductal shunting is strongly suggested, as already noted in regard to simultaneous oxygen saturation measurements. This situation is common in PPHNB and less common in CHD (e.g. IAA, severe aortic coarctation). The combination of an elevated P_{CO_2} and at least moderate respiratory distress suggests primary lung disease. A normal or low P_{CO_2} and an unlabored respiratory pattern suggest cyanotic CHD. The presence of a respiratory and/or metabolic acidosis can be determined by measurement of the pH and P_{CO_2}. The former again suggests primary pulmonary disease and the latter could be related to either CHD or primary pulmonary disease with prolonged hypoxia and/or decreased cardiac output. Although findings of the presence of a metabolic acidosis and the absence of any change in the P_{O_2} with oxygen administration do not necessarily differentiate cardiac from pulmonary disease, this combination clearly identifies a critically ill newborn, and emergency arrangements for referral to a tertiary center should be made, since the therapies for these two disease processes are quite different. The symptomatic cardiac infant may require a balloon atrial septostomy (for d-TGV), emergency surgery (for obstructed TAPVC below the diaphragm), or prostaglandin administration (for HLHS). The cyanotic pulmonary infant may require high frequency jet or oscillator ventilation or even cardiopulmonary bypass with extracorporeal membrane oxygenation.

In summary, despite the vagaries of the hyperoxia test[26] and rarely misleading information,[27] the hyperoxia test remains a very valuable tool for evaluating cyanotic newborns and differentiating cardiac and pulmonary disease (see Table 54.2).[28]

Chest Roentgenography

The chest radiograph remains a simple, noninvasive, and very valuable tool in the evaluation of the TNB with suspected heart or lung disease. Several details need to be worked out before a film can be properly interpreted. First the film is placed on the view box in the proper orientation utilizing either the "right" or "left" label placed on the film by the technician (Fig. 54.1) or the position of the patient's name on the radiograph, which is standardized for each institution. If the apex of the heart is used, cardiac and abdominal organ malpositions (e.g., dextrocardia) may well be overlooked. Next the quality of the film is assessed for both degree of penetration, which can alter the interpretation of the pulmonary vascular markings, and degree of inspiratory effort, which can alter the interpretation of heart size. Finally, the chest roentgenogram is inspected for thoracic and abdominal situs, cardiac size, shape, and contour, including the pulmonary arc configuration, the pulmonary vascular markings, and the presence of pulmonary parenchymal disease, aortic arch situs, and associated skeletal anomalies.

Thoracic and Abdominal Situs As already noted, discordance of thoracic and abdominal situs or a midline liver and stomach are strongly associated with CHD that is frequently complex (Fig. 54.2).

Cardiac Size The normal cardiothoracic ratio in the TNB is less than 0.60. A poor inspiratory effort or a prominent thymus can often indicate apparent cardiomegaly. Massive cardiomegaly in which the heart occupies almost the entire thorax suggests Ebstein's anomaly or HRHS with severe tricuspid incompetence, myocarditis (Fig. 54.3), or an intracranial AV malformation. On the other hand, a normal heart size can frequently be associated with severe CHD (d-TGV, obstructed TAPVC, HRHS with small RV), and other distinguishing radiographic and clinical signs must be employed to ensure that the abnormality is correctly identified.

TABLE 54.2 Hyperoxia Test

	Room Air				100% Oxygen			
Condition	P_{O_2}	P_{CO_2}	pH	O_2(sat)	P_{O_2}	P_{CO_2}	pH	O_2 (sat)
Cyanotic CHD, ↓ actual or effective pulmonary blood flow	↓↓	N	N, ↓	↓↓	NC	NC	NC	NC
Cyanotic CHD, ↑ pulmonary blood flow and common mixing	↓	N	N	↓	↑	NC	NC	↑
Pulmonary	↓	N, ↑	N, ↓	↓	↑	NC	NC	↑
Neurologic	↓	↑	↓	↓	↑	NC	NC	↑
Hematologic (methemoglobinemia)	N	N	N	↓	↑↑	NC	NC	NC

Abbreviations and symbols:, N, normal; NC, no change; ↑, increased; ↑↑, greatly increased; ↓, decreased; ↓↓, greatly decreased.

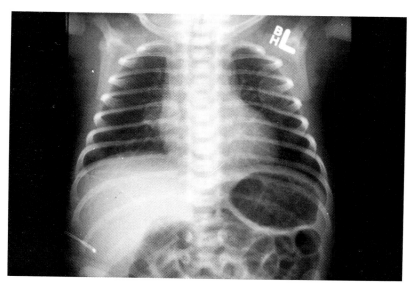

Figure 54.1   Normal chest roentgenogram demonstrating proper labeling of the film with "L" signifying the left side of the patient. The film also demonstrates situs solitus, with the apex of the heart and the stomach bubble to the patient's left and the liver to the patient's right.

Cardiac Shape and Contour   A large globular heart again suggests severe myocarditis with generalized chamber enlargement or Ebstein's anomaly with severe tricuspid incompetence. The boot-shaped heart with upturned apex and deficient or concave pulmonary arc suggests tetralogy of Fallot (Fig. 54.4). The deficient pulmonary arc suggests severe obstruction to PBF and hypoplastic pulmonary arteries. With d-TGV the mediastinum is narrowed as a result of the very anterior–posterior arrangement of the great vessels, and the heart appears egg-shaped ("egg on string" sign, Fig. 54.5). A widened mediastinum and increased pulmonary vascular markings can be seen with unobstructed TAPVC to a left vertical vein, where both the right SVC and the left vertical vein are enlarged, making up the lateral margins of the widened mediastinum ("snowman" sign). It is uncommon for this sign to be fully developed in the neonate.

Pulmonary Vascular Markings and Parenchymal Disease
Pulmonary vascular markings can be classified as normal, decreased as a result of decreased PBF (pulmonary atresia, severe TOF) or increased for other reasons: increased PBF (truncus arteriosus, d-TGV, unobstructed TAPVC) or obstructed pulmonary venous return (cor triatriatum, severe mitral stenosis, obstructed TAPVC below the diaphragm). CHD associated with increased PBF results in enlargement of the pulmonary arteries. Radiographically, the main pulmonary artery diameter is increased, resulting in a convex main pulmonary artery segment. The hila are prominent because the proximal right and left pulmonary arteries are enlarged. The

normally prominent thymus in the TNB can obscure these findings, but distinct enlargement of the more peripheral arteries will suggest a search for anomalies of this nature.

With pulmonary venous obstruction, the pulmonary vascular markings appear prominent but indistinct, leading to a ground glass or diffusely granular appearance that is not dissimilar from the radiographic pattern seen early in respiratory distress syndrome. Typically, however, the gestational age and other clinical characteristics will allow differentiation. This radiographic appearance is most commonly seen in the TNB with obvious cyanosis and moderate respiratory distress with obstructed TAPVC below the diaphragm (Fig. 54.6) and truly represents a medical emergency, since stabilization with the usual measures (prostaglandin E_1 infusion, intubation, oxygen, ventilation, and inotropic agents) is not always possible and surgery is necessary on an emergent basis.

The lung fields should then be examined for evidence of primary lung disease (e.g., pneumonia, meconium aspiration) or structural abnormalities (diaphragmatic hernia, lobar emphysema, pulmonary lymphangiectasia, vascular ring with hyperinflation).

Aortic Arch Situs   The normal left aortic arch ascends on the person's right and descends on the left. A right aortic arch (RAA) is often associated with CHD (Table 54.3). As the normal transverse aortic arch crosses the mediastinum, the trachea is deviated slightly to the patient's right. With tracheal visualization on plain film, the aortic arch situs can often be

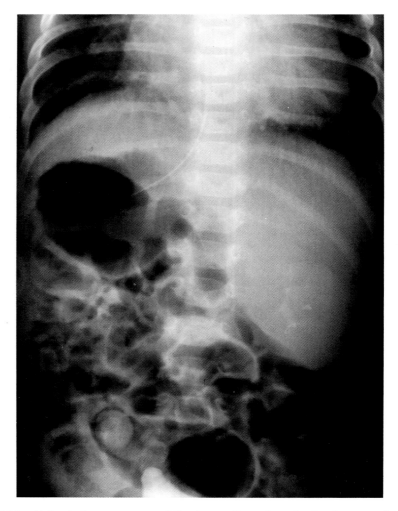

Figure 54.2 Abdominal roentgenogram following cardiac cathe-terization demonstrating levocardia with situs inversus abdominalis. This combination is almost always associated with CHD, and the cardiac silhouette appears considerably enlarged. Normal contrast opacification of both kidneys is also apparent following angiography.

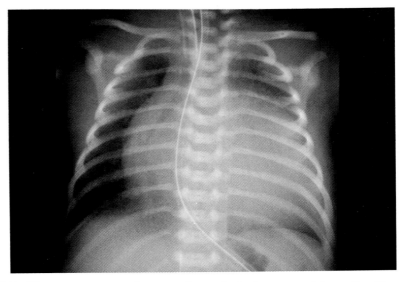

Figure 54.3 Chest roentgenogram demonstrating marked enlargement of the cardiac silhouette in a 1-day-old infant with acute viral myocarditis and severe CHF.

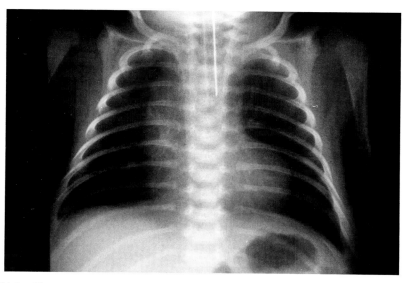

Figure 54.4 Chest roentgenogram demonstrating situs solitus with an upturned apex of the heart, decreased pulmonary vascular markings, and deficient pulmonary arc, suggesting hypoplasia of the pulmonary arteries in a 1-day-old infant with severe TOF.

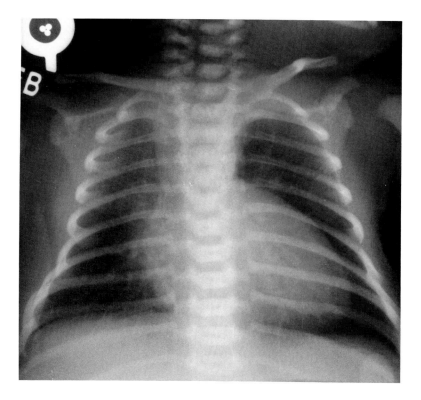

Figure 54.5 Chest roentgenogram demonstrating an "egg-shaped" heart with a narrowed mediastinum and increased pulmonary vascular markings in a 2-day-old infant with dextrotransposition of the great vessels.

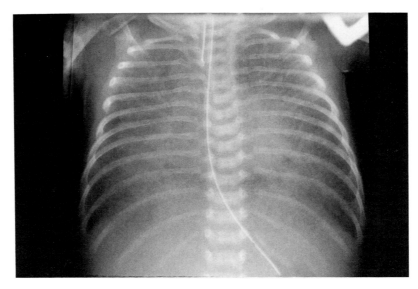

Figure 54.6 Chest roentgenogram revealing a heart of normal size (although difficult to see clearly) and severe pulmonary venous congestion in a 2-day-old infant with total anomalous pulmonary venous connection to the portal vein.

inferred. The aortic knob and the descending thoracic aorta cannot be visualized definitively on the plain film in most term newborns. If the arch situs remains in doubt, careful suprasternal notch ultrasound can determine the position of the descending aorta. A right aortic arch is especially common with truncus arteriosus and PA-VSD.

Associated Skeletal Abnormalities Infants with CHD have an increased incidence of skeletal abnormalities that are frequently apparent on the plain chest film.[29] The combination of 11 ribs and multiple sternal ossification centers is common in Down syndrome. Vertebral and less commonly rib anomalies are seen in the VACTERL syndrome.

Electrocardiogram

Since the advent of bedside echocardiography, the ECG is often overlooked despite its ready availability, low cost, and

TABLE 54.3 Incidence of RAA and CHD[a]

Type of CHD[b]	Incidence with RAA (%)
PA-VSD	50
Truncus arteriosus	30–50
TOF	25
DORV	15–20
Tricuspid atresia	5
d-TGV	2–3

[a]Incidence of this combination in the normal population of 0.04%.
[b]For abbreviations, see chapter appendix.

frequent great usefulness. As Friedman noted: "The ECG is less helpful in suggesting a diagnosis of heart disease in the premature and newborn infant than in the older child. However, specific observations may offer major clues to the presence of a cardiovascular anomaly."[30] The TNB ECG is quite distinct from that of the older infant and toddler. These remarkable changes occur during the transition from the fetal to neonatal circulation, resulting in a significant impact on both the axis and the major QRS vector. In utero the pulmonary vascular resistance is quite elevated, such that only 10% of the combined cardiac output enters the lungs, whereas the systemic vascular resistance is decreased owing to the low resistance placental circulation. This combination results in an RV/LV weight ratio of 1.25:1.00 at birth, with a rapid decrease to 0.67:1.00 at 1 month of age and 0.50:1.00 by 3–6 months as the PA pressure and PVR resistance fall and the SVR and cardiac output increase. With this brief overview of the transitional circulation, the TNB ECG can be interpreted in systematic fashion.

Pulse and Rhythm The normal mean pulse at birth is approximately 123 ± 30; it increases to 148 ± 30 by one week of age and gradually decreases in the ensuing weeks and months. The rhythm is sinus, with occasional premature atrial (PAC) and premature ventricular contractions (PVC). PACs occur not uncommonly during the first several days of life, whereas PVCs are less common at that time (Table 54.4). The incidence of both PACs and PVCs decreases significantly during the first year of life.[31,32] Although PACs will trigger supraventricular tachycardia (SVT) rarely, they are

TABLE 54.4   **Incidence of Premature Beats**

	Contractions (%)	
Age	PACs	PVCs
1–2 days (ECG)	1.2	0.3
1 day (Holter)	26	18
1 year (Holter)	3	Rare

not routinely treated. When PVCs are present, however, it is important to rule out structural heart disease: cardiac tumors (especially rhabdomyomas with tuberous sclerosis) and the long QT interval syndrome, which often presents with sinus bradycardia or 2:1 AV block in the TNB. The corrected QT interval is the QT interval (measured in a lead where the beginning of the QRS complex and the end of the T wave are easily visible) divided by the square root of the preceding RR interval; it should be less than 0.45. This syndrome, which can be familial, predisposes to life-threatening ventricular arrhythmias and may be associated with sensorineural deafness. The presenting manifestations are frequently sudden death, seizures, or syncope. The presence of the long QT interval syndrome is often overlooked, however, and more litigation results from this pediatric arrhythmia than from any other. In contrast, death due to isolated PVCs has never been reported in a healthy TNB.[33]

The most common serious rhythm disturbances in the TNB include SVT and atrial flutter (AF). The diagnostic features of SVT include a rate exceeding 230 beats per minute, abnormal or unidentifiable P waves that may be superim-

posed on the T waves, and a normal narrow QRS morphology with a very regular RR interval (Fig. 54.7). The arrhythmia usually starts and stops abruptly. The etiology for SVT in the neonate includes AV nodal reentrant, accessory AV connection (e.g., Wolff–Parkinson–White syndrome), and automatic atrial tachycardia due to an ectopic focus of increased automaticity. Underlying heart disease is not common, although Ebstein's anomaly, l-TGV, cardiac tumors, and myocarditis have all been associated with SVT. Treatment strategies depend primarily on the neonate's presenting signs, since severe cardiac compromise is more common in the TNB than in the older child. Unrecognized prolonged SVT (> 24 h) can produce a marked decrease in cardiac output and LV dysfunction, resulting in severe CHF. Rapid cardioversion should be undertaken:

1. Ice bag (crushed ice) to the face or facial immersion in cold water (5–15°C) for 15–20 seconds to initiate the diving reflex and increase parasympathetic tone.

2. Adenosine (50 μg/kg) by rapid intravenous push. The dose should be doubled every 60 seconds to a maximum of 250 μg/kg. The half-life is 10–15 seconds, and side effects are rare. A continuous rhythm strip should be recorded on hard copy to show any signs of an accessory connection, an ectopic atrial focus, or atrial flutter as the AV node is blocked temporarily (Fig. 54.8).

3. Rapid esophageal overdrive pacing if readily available.

4. Synchronous DC cardioversion with 0.25–1 J/kg. If the diving reflex is ineffective, an IV cannot be start-

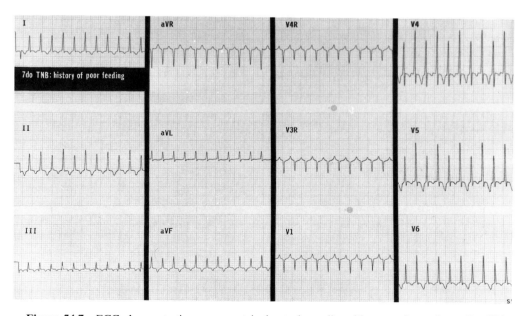

Figure 54.7   ECG demonstrating supraventricular tachycardia with a regular tachycardia (270 beats/min), narrow QRS complex, and inverted P waves in leads II, III, and aVF.

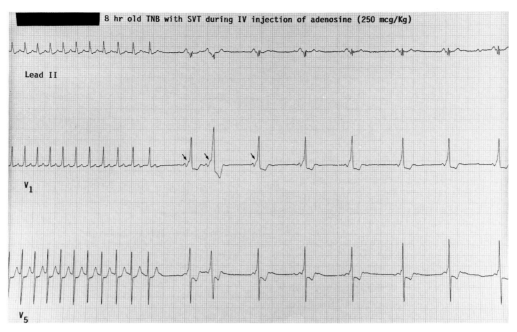

Figure 54.8   Simultaneous three-lead ECG rhythm strip demonstrating cardioversion of SVT to sinus rhythm following an intravenous injection of adenosine. With conversion, the typical findings of Wolff–Parkinson–White syndrome, including short PR interval, wide QRS complex, and prominent delta waves (arrows in lead V_1) are apparent as conduction through the AV node is temporarily blocked by the adenosine.

ed, and esophageal pacing is not available, one should not hesitate to go directly to electrical synchronous cardio-version. Verapamil should *never* be used in infants less than one year of age because of the propensity of this agent to cause profound hypotension, bradycardia, and cardiovascular collapse as a result of its negative inotropic effect and vasodilatation.

In the asymptomatic neonate, steps 1–3 should be carried out. If the SVT persists, IV digitalization can be initiated in a dosage of 20–50 μg/kg over 24 hours (1/2, 1/4, 1/4), depending on the gestational age of the infant. The mean time for cardioversion with digoxin is 7 hours. Maintenance therapy consists of oral digoxin in the absence of WPW at a dose of 10 μg/kg/day. Optimal treatment for SVT in the presence of WPW remains controversial, although digoxin, propranolol (2–4 mg/kg/day in four divided doses), and sotalol (4–6 mg/kg/day in two divided doses)[34] have all been used. Intravenous phenylephrine, edrophonium, and propranolol are very rarely used in the newborn. Phenylephrine exerts its effect by increasing the blood pressure and ultimately the vagal tone, but the neonate is frequently unable to tolerate an increase in afterload. Edrophonium is directly vagotonic, and extreme and prolonged sinus bradycardia may result following cardioversion. Intravenous propranolol can result in se-

vere sinus bradycardia and myocardial depression. If all the foregoing modes of therapy fail, intracardiac overdrive atrial pacing should be considered.

Atrial flutter is the second most common serious rhythm disturbance in the neonate. The diagnosis depends on the presence of sawtooth undulations in the baseline that are larger than normal P waves and are seen best in leads II, III, aVF, and V_1 (Fig. 54.9).[34] The atrial rate varies between 300 and 600. There are varying degrees of AV block, although 2:1 block is most common.

In any newborn with a regular pulse in the range of 180–200 and no obvious etiolgy (fever, severe anemia, hyperthyroidism) the diagnosis of atrial flutter with 2:1 block should be considered. A full 12-lead ECG should be obtained, since the monitor ECG is inadequate to rule out AF. Treatment consists of IV digoxin, sotalol, esophageal overdrive pacing, or synchronous DC cardioversion.[35,36] Recurrence is uncommon, and maintenance oral digoxin is used rarely.

Complete heart block (CHB), rare in the neonate, occurs in three situations:

1. Infant born to mother with collagen vascular disease, especially systemic lupus erythematosus (SLE),[10] with a fetal risk for CHB of 4% and an 8% recurrence risk[37]

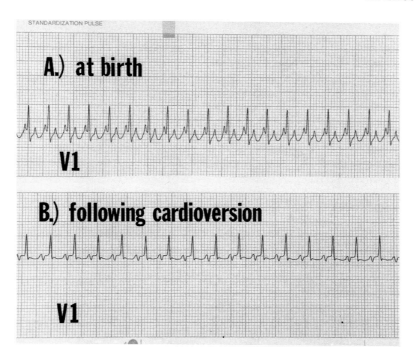

Figure 54.9   Two rhythm strips from lead V$_1$ in an hour-old newborn demonstrating atrial flutter with (*A*) 2:1 block and (*B*) sinus rhythm following dc cardioversion. (From Dillon et al,[34] with permission of WB Saunders Co.)

2. infant with complex CHD, frequently the visceral heterotaxy syndrome (most commonly left atrial isomerism presenting with hydrops fetalis and CHB

3. infant with no obvious etiology and no structural heart disease

The ECG typically reveals a slow ventricular rate with a narrow QRS complex and a faster atrial rate with no relationship between the P waves and QRS complexes (Fig. 54.10). Treatment is limited. Congestive heart failure is uncommon in the infant without CHD who has normal ventricular function and a ventricular rate exceeding 55, and the overall prognosis is good in childhood, although pacemaker therapy is presently recommended for the adult to prevent syncope and sudden death.[38] In the TNB if the rate is below 55 beats per minute, a ventricular demand pacemaker may be necessary, especially if signs of CHF develop. If CHD is present, the mortality and morbidity are significantly greater[39] and a pacemaker should be placed emergently in almost all cases. To date, efforts both to prevent the development of CHB and to treat effectively CHB in utero with or without hydrops fetalis and myocarditis have been limited to the very occasional anec-

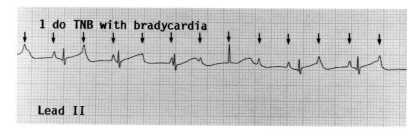

Figure 54.10   Lead II rhythm strip with 3° AV block in day-old infant born to SLE-antibody-positive mother. The atrial and ventricular rates are 180 and 80 beats per minute, respectively. The P waves are identified by the arrows. There is superimposition of a P wave on the fourth QRS complex, resulting in a taller QRS complex. There is no relationship between the P waves and the QRS complexes.

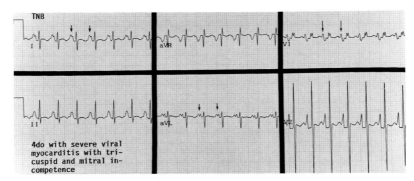

4do with severe viral myocarditis with tricuspid and mitral incompetence

Figure 54.11   Six-lead ECG demonstrating biatrial enlargement with notched or bifid P waves in leads I and aVL (small arrows), peaked P waves in leads II and V_2, and a negative terminal P wave in V_1 of 0.04 ms (tall arrows). This ECG was obtained from the 1-day-old infant with acute viral myocarditis whose chest roentgeno-gram is shown in Figure 53.3.

dotal success with steroids,[40–42] plasmaphoresis,[41] intravenous immunoglobulin,[42] transuterine transthoracic fetal ventricular pacing,[43] and the maternal administration of β-adrenergic agonists to increase the fetal heart rate.[44]

Intervals and Axis   The normal PR interval during the first week varies between 79 and 138 ms with a mean of 104 ms. The normal QRS interval varies between 25 and 69 ms with a mean of 49 ms. The normal frontal plane QRS axis in the first week varies between +92 and 187° with a mean of +135°. This rightward axis relates to the relative RV dominance in the TNB that is due to the normal fetal circulation. As a result, any axis of less than +90° or more than +210° strongly suggests a cardiac abnormality. If the axis is leftward (i.e., < +90°), underdevelopment of the right ventricle should be considered [e.g., HRHS with pulmonary atresia (PA) and intact ventricular septum, tricuspid atresia (TA), single ventricle]. Other causes of congenital left axis include any form of endocardial cushion defect and levotransposition or ventricular inversion. The endocardial cushion defect (AV septal defect) is the most common type of CHD in Down syndrome. With both partial and complete forms of endocardial cushion defect, the axis varies between 0 and −150° in greater than 95% of cases regardless of age and should be determined in all infants suspected of Down syndrome, even in the outlying nursery.

Right axis deviation, defined as an axis exceeding +200°, is not common in the TNB even in the presence of significant RVH.

Enlargement and Hypertrophy: Atrial and Ventricular
Atrial enlargement or hypertrophy should be diagnosed only with sinus P waves (i.e., a frontal P-wave axis of +30 to +90°). A P wave greater than 3 mm in any lead suggests right atrial hypertrophy (usually lead II or V_1). Left atrial enlargement is suggested by terminal inversion of the P wave in V_1 of 1 mm in depth and 40 ms in duration or a bifid P wave in lead II. Biatrial hypertrophy is suggested by a combination of the above or a prolonged P wave (≥80 ms), especially if the P wave is bifid (Fig. 54.11). The combination of cyanosis and RAH suggests an abnormality of the pulmonic and/or tricuspid valves: tricuspid atresia, Ebstein's anomaly, HRHS with PA and intact ventricular septum, critical PS, and TAPVC with or without obstruction.

Because of the normal RV dominance of the TNB (Fig. 54.12), RVH is often difficult to diagnose even in the presence of severe CHD (e.g., d-TGV). However, Table 54.5 lists a number of criteria for RVH, which are often associated with HLHS, coarctation of the aorta, critical PS, obstructed TAPVC (Fig. 54.13), and TOF. In contrast, the absence of the

TABLE 54.5   Ventricular Hypertrophy in the Term Newborn

RIGHT VENTRICULAR HYPERTROPHY
Q wave in V_{4R}–V_1
R in lead aVR > 7 mm
Positive T wave in V_1 after day 3
Pure R wave in V_1 > 10 mm
R in V_1 > 28 mm
S in V_6 > 13 mm
ST depression in V_{4R}–V_1
LEFT VENTRICULAR HYPERTROPHY
S in V_1 > 19 mm
R in V_6 > 11 mm
R/S ratio in V_1 < 0.5
Q in V_6 > 3 mm
S in a VR > 15 mm
COMBINED VENTRICULAR HYPERTROPHY
Direct signs of RVH and LVH from above
RVH plus Q in V_6 ≥ 2 mm
RVH plus R in V_6 > 5 mm
RVH plus inverted T wave in V_6
LVH plus R in V_1 > 15 mm

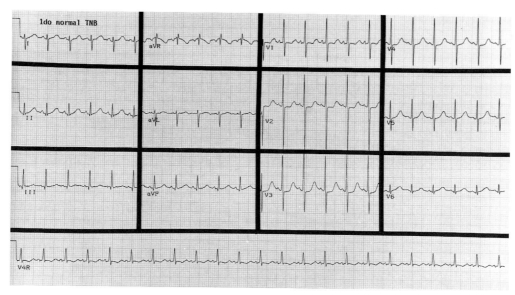

Figure 54.12 Twelve-lead ECG from a normal day-old term newborn with typical right axis deviation, prominent right-sided forces (V_1), and decreased left-sided forces (V_6).

normal RV dominance is an important sign that frequently suggests underdevelopment of the right ventricle as seen in TA, HRHS with PA, and single ventricle.

Changes in the ECG during the first 6 weeks of life mirror the hemodynamic changes in the neonatal transitional circulation. The very positive voltage in the right precordial leads transfers to the left precordial leads. In like manner, as

the PA pressure and PVR fall after birth, the positive T wave in V_{4R} and V_1 becomes negative by 3–4 days of age and remains negative until the preteen years.

In summary, although the ECG can often be helpful in the evaluation of CHD,[45] the absence of any abnormal finding does not rule out significant CHD, and the presence of an abnormal finding does not necessarily imply CHD (e.g., PPHNB).

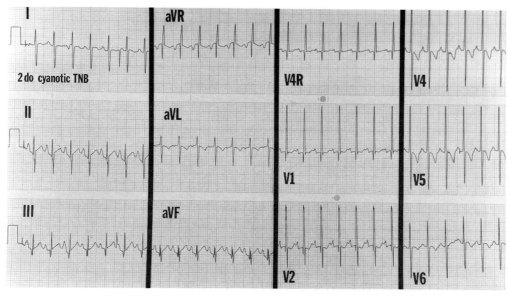

Figure 54.13 ECG from a cyanotic infant 2 days old, demonstrating right atrial enlargement (lead II) and right ventricular hypertrophy (qR in V_4R and V_1, tall R in V_1, and deep S in V_6).

Echocardiography

Echocardiography has changed the practice of pediatric cardiology profoundly, and nowhere has its impact been greater than in the newborn intensive care unit. A complete review of cardiac ultrasound is beyond the scope of this chapter, although several monographs are available that review the subject thoroughly.[34,46,47] However, it is important to have a solid understanding of what information can be provided by two-dimensional and Doppler echocardiography.

Two-dimensional echocardiography allows us to look at both the structure and function of the heart. The complete evaluation includes scanning directly over the heart (parasternal long and short axes), inferior to the heart (subcostal and apical), and superior to the heart (suprasternal notch). This thorough systematic approach will rarely overlook significant abnormalities. The two-dimensional study can answer the following questions definitively:

1. How many cardiac chambers are present (Fig. 54.14)?
2. Are the ventricles of normal size (Fig. 54.15) and are they contracting normally (Fig. 54.16)?
3. How many valves are present?
4. Do the valves appear normal (e.g., with respect to thickness and leaflet mobility), and are they in the proper location (Figs. 54.17 and 54.18)?
5. Are the septa intact (Fig. 54.19)? Is the foramen ovale patent?
6. Do the systemic and pulmonary veins drain normally (Fig. 54.20)?
7. Are the great vessels of normal size and normal orientation (Fig. 54.21)?
8. Does the aortic arch descend on the left, and is there evidence to suggest an aortic coarctation (Fig. 54.22) or PDA?

With this information in hand, one can proceed to the Doppler interrogation including color, pulsed, and continuous wave (CW) modalities. With color Doppler, a color is assigned to the direction and velocity of blood flow within the cardiovascular system. By convention, blood flow is red toward the transducer and blue away from the transducer. However, with disturbed or turbulent flow across stenotic valves, septal defects, or great vessel obstruction (e.g., aortic coarctation), higher Doppler velocities are generated, resulting in a hybrid or mosaic pattern of multiple colors. Therefore, color Doppler can identify both normal flow patterns (e.g., normal pulmonary venous drainage to the left atrium) and also abnormal flow patterns, indicating further interrogation with pulsed and continuous wave Doppler.

With pulsed Doppler, a single crystal is utilized to alternately transmit and receive the Doppler velocity signal. When this form of Doppler is combined with two-dimensional imaging, a specific localized area in the cardiovascular system can be interrogated. For example, one might look behind an AV valve for incompetence or near the insertion of the

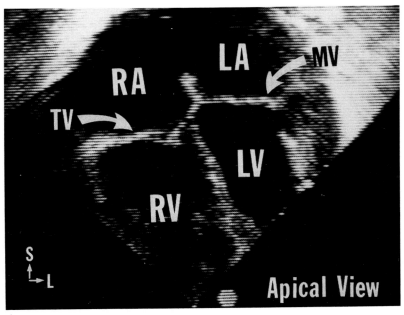

Figure 54.14 Apical four-chamber view. LA, left atrium; LV, left ventricle; MV, mitral valve; RA, right atrium; RV, right ventricle; TV, tricuspid valve; S, superior; L, left. (From Dillon et al,[34] with permission of WB Saunders Co.)

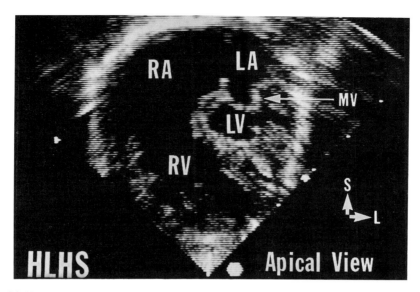

Figure 54.15 Hypoplastic left heart syndrome from apical view with stenotic and thickened mitral valve and small cavity left ventricle. LA, left atrium; RA, right atrium; LV, left ventricle; RV, right ventricle; MV, mitral valve; S, superior; L, left.

ductus arteriosus into the main pulmonary artery for ductal flow (Fig. 54.23). Since, however, pulsed Doppler is unable to interrogate adequately higher velocities across a stenotic or incompetent valve or a VSD to determine pressure gradients, the continuous wave Doppler technique is sometimes necessary.

The CW Doppler transducer contains two crystals, one continuously sampling ALL the various Doppler velocities along the Doppler beam, in contrast to pulsed Doppler that samples only a discrete area. With CW Doppler, very high velocities can be measured, and with use of the modified Bernoulli equation (the pressure gradient = 4 times the max-

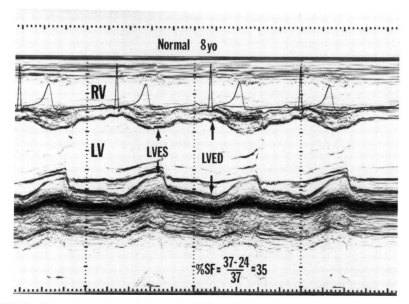

Figure 54.16 M-mode cut through the right (RV) and left (LV) ventricles. The percentage of the shortening fraction (%SF) is equal to the left ventricular end-diastolic dimension (LVED) minus the left ventricular end-systolic dimension (LVES) divided by the left ventricular end-diastolic dimension. (From Dillon et al,[34] with permission of WB Saunders Co.)

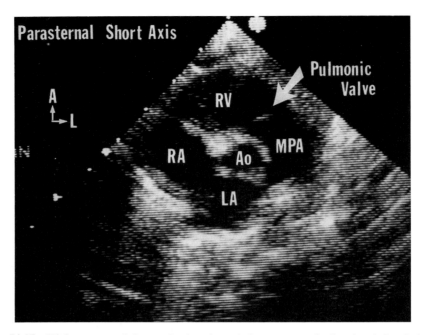

Figure 54.17   High parasternal short-axis view through the great vessels showing their relationship to one another. Ao, aorta; MPA, main pulmonary artery; RV, right ventricle; RA, right atrium; LA, left atrium; A, anterior; L, left. (From Dillon et al,[34] with permission of WB Saunders Co.)

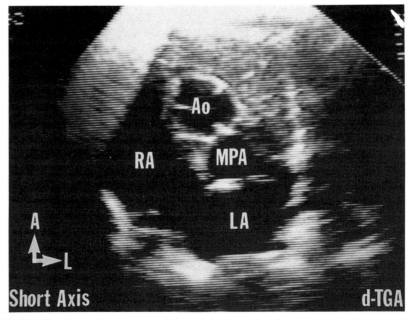

Figure 54.18   Simple or dextrotransposition of the great arteries (d-TGA) with the circle–circle arrangement of the great arteries in the parasternal short-axis view. Ao, aorta; MPA, main pulmonary artery; LA, left atrium; RA, right atrium; A, anterior; L, left. (From Dillon et al,[34] with permission of WB Saunders Co.)

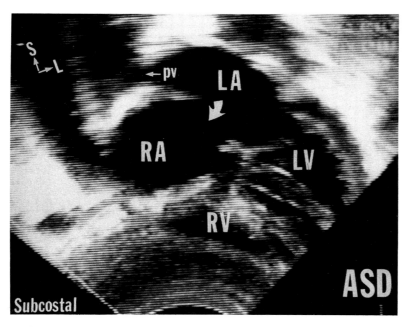

Figure 54.19   Secundum atrial septal defect (ASD) from subcostal imaging. LA, left atrium; LV, left ventricle; RA, right atrium; RV, right ventricle; pv, pulmonary vein; S, superior; L, left. (From Dillon et al,[34] with permission of WB Saunders Co.)

imum velocity squared), pressure gradients across stenotic or incompetent valves, coarctation of the aorta, and septal defects (Fig. 54.24) can be estimated. This technique can be extremely valuable in determining the PA systolic pressure in

PPHNB after tricuspid incompetence has been demonstrated by color Doppler (Fig. 54.25).

In summary, a complete echocardiographic examination can usually decipher the cardiac anatomy allowing differen-

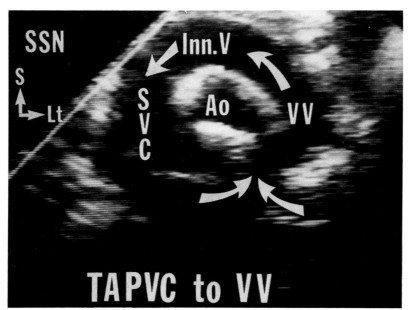

Figure 54.20   Total anomalous pulmonary venous connection (TAPVC) to a left vertical vein (VV) from the suprasternal notch view (SSN). Inn. V, innominate vein; SVC, superior vena cava; Ao, aorta; S, superior; L, left. (From Dillon et al,[34] with permission of WB Saunders Co.)

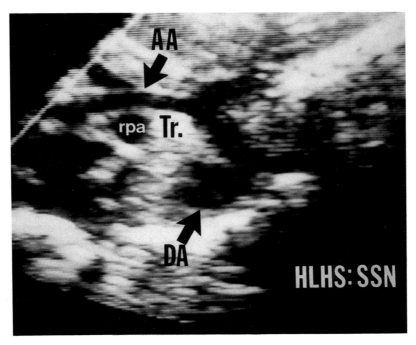

Figure 54.21 Hypoplastic left heart syndrome (HLHS) from the long-axis suprasternal notch view (SSN) demonstrating the hypoplastic ascending aorta (AA). DA, descending aorta; rpa, right pulmonary artery; Tr, trachea. (From Dillon et al,[34] with permission of WB Saunders Co.)

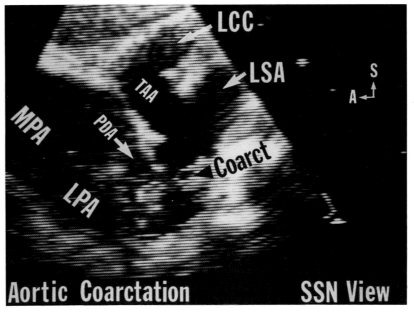

Figure 54.22 Coarctation of the aorta from the suprasternal notch view (SSN). LCC, left common carotid artery; LSA, left subclavian artery; TAA, transverse aortic arch; PDA, patent ductus arteriosus; MPA, main pulmonary artery; LPA, left pulmonary artery; S, superior; A, anterior. (From Dillon et al,[34] with permission of WB Saunders Co.)

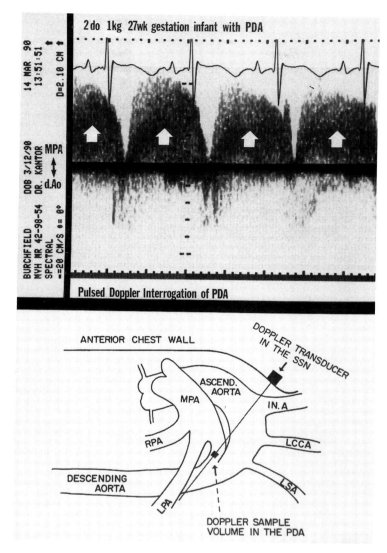

Figure 54.23   Pulsed Doppler interrogation of a patent ductus arteriosus (PDA) in a 2-day-old premature infant from the suprasternal notch (SSN). Upper panel: near continuous left-to-right shunting into the main pulmonary artery from the descending aorta. Lower panel: the Doppler approach to the PDA from the suprasternal notch. MPA, main pulmonary artery; RPA, right pulmonary artery; LPA, left pulmonary artery; IN.A, innominate artery; LCCA, left common carotid artery; LSA, left subclavian artery. (From Dillon et al,[34] with permission of WB Saunders Co.)

tiation of cardiac from pulmonary cyanosis (i.e., PPHNB). Now that high quality imaging and very accurate anatomic and hemodynamic information are available, newborns presenting with cyanotic CHD can receive surgery or interventional catheterization without first undergoing cardiac catheterization and angiography. If significant questions and uncertainties remain following a complete echocardiographic and Doppler examination, however, cardiac catheterization and angiography should be undertaken to determine optimal management.

MANAGEMENT

Medical management of symptomatic CHD presenting in the neonatal period consists primarily of maintaining oxygen delivery to the vital organs while transfer to a tertiary center is being arranged. Oxygen delivery to the tissues by the systemic circulation is determined by the systemic blood flow and the oxygen content of the blood. Oxygen content is primarily related to the product of the oxygen saturation of the hemoglobin and the oxygen-carrying capacity or Hb con-

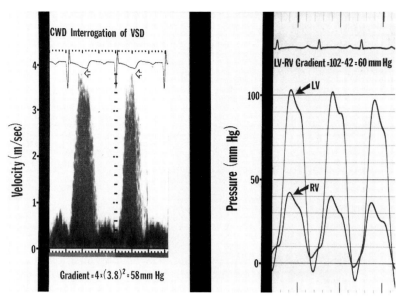

Figure 54.24   (Left) Continuous wave Doppler (CWD) interrogation of a ventricular septal defect (VSD) resulting in a maximum velocity of 3.8 m/s. With application of the Bernoulli equation, the left ventricular (LV)/right ventricular (RV) systolic gradient is estimated to be 58 mmHg. (Right) Simultaneous left and right ventricular pressure measurements at cardiac catheterization, demonstrating a similar gradient. (From Dillon et al,[34] with permission of WB Saunders Co.)

centration. In the TNB, the high percentage of fetal Hb will result in less oxygen delivery than in the adult, reflecting a leftward shift in the oxygen–hemoglobin dissociation curve (i.e., fetal Hb will release less oxygen than adult Hb at a given P_{O_2}).

Oxygen saturation can be increased by increasing the frac-

tion of inspired oxygen (fi_{O_2}) delivered to the neonate, placing the infant on a ventilator to overcome hypoventilation, and adding positive end-expiratory pressure (PEEP) to treat pulmonary edema or atelectasis. The use of these methods to increase oxygen delivery, however, must be tailored to the in-

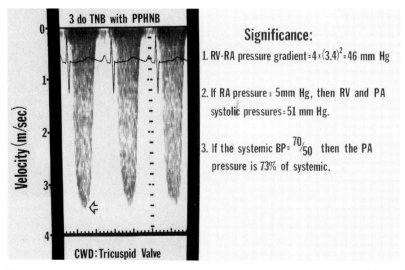

Figure 54.25   Continuous wave Doppler (CWD) of the tricuspid valve in a 3-day-old term newborn with persistent pulmonary hypertension of the newborn (PPHNB). RV, right ventricle; RA, right atrium; BP, blood pressure. (From Dillon et al,[34] with permission of WB Saunders Co.)

dividual cardiac lesion. For example, the use of excessive PEEP (> 8 cmH$_2$O) can compromise cardiac output by increasing intrathoracic pressure and right ventricular afterload. The fi$_{O_2}$ should be increased only when the end result will be increased oxygen delivery. Typically increasing the fi$_{O_2}$ will decrease the pulmonary vascular resistance and increase pulmonary blood flow. This would be problematic in situations of ductal-dependent systemic perfusion (e.g., HLHS, IAA, severe aortic coarctation). The resultant increase in pulmonary blood flow would be at the expense of systemic blood flow. For this reason, intubation, hypoventilation, and a low fi$_{O_2}$ are often utilized to maximize systemic perfusion in these ductal-dependent lesions. In regard to oxygen-carrying capacity, the Hb concentration should be maintained in the range of 15g/dL, especially in the cyanotic infant with a decreased oxygen saturation. However, overtransfusion (to a Hb of 18–20g/dL) may result in increased viscosity and decreased systemic perfusion.

The systemic perfusion or cardiac output is equal to the product of the heart rate and the stroke volume. Stroke volume is determined by preload, afterload, and myocardial contractility. Following birth, the neonatal myocardium is operating at near maximal capacity with a very high cardiac output,[48] thus limiting its ability to adapt to stress, given its small functional reserve capacity.[49] The neonatal myocardium has fewer myofilaments with which to increase contractility and has decreased ventricular compliance, resulting in a limited response to alterations in preload.[50] In addition, the neonatal heart is less able to tolerate increases in afterload.[51] Finally, the cardiac output is very much heart rate dependent, but since the resting neonatal heart rate is already high, there is again limited reserve. Heart rates greater than 180 beats per minute reduce diastolic filling time and coronary perfusion, resulting in increased oxygen consumption and energy expenditure. Heart rates less than 55 beats per minute also compromise cardiac output and oxygen delivery.

The neonate has limited oxygen delivery and adapts poorly to decreased oxygen saturation and decreased myocardial contractility. Therefore, to prevent the development of anaerobic metabolism, with resulting metabolic or lactic acidosis, every effort must be made to minimize oxygen consumption. If such acidosis develops and is not corrected quickly, the infant's ability to tolerate a diagnostic or interventional catheterization or surgery will be greatly reduced.

Medical management in the referring hospital, therefore, should include efforts to decrease oxygen consumption and increase oxygen delivery.[52] Decreasing oxygen consumption includes providing a neutral thermal environment, decreasing the work of breathing (e.g., by means of ventilator and muscle relaxants), decreasing body activity and anxiety (e.g., by means of morphine or fentanyl), avoiding unnecessary procedures, and ensuring that the child takes no oral nourishment, to avoid loss of energy to digestion and to prevent aspiration.

To increase oxygen delivery, one should increase the oxygen content (i.e., $\uparrow$fi$_{O_2} \rightarrow \uparrow_{O_2 \, sat}$) and increase oxygen carrying capacity (i.e., $\uparrow$Hb) as noted earlier. To maximize myocardial contractility, negative inotropic factors (hypoxia, acidosis, hypocalcemia, hypomagnesemia, hypoglycemia) should be diagnosed early and corrected quickly. Correction of acidosis is imperative, since acidosis depresses myocardial function and inhibits responsiveness to catecholamines. The usual dosage of sodium bicarbonate in milliequivalents is $0.2 \times$ wt (kg) $\times$ [27-serum sodium bicarbonate]. With severe acidosis, half of the calculated dose can be given intravenously over several minutes and the remainder over 30–60 minutes. If the acidosis is at least moderate, follow-up blood gases should be obtained every 15–30 minutes to guide further therapy. Early placement of an umbilical artery catheter (UAC) is vital for obtaining blood for rapid laboratory evaluation. Once in place, the UAC will obviate the need for repeated painful venipunctures, allow continuous blood pressure monitoring, and provide easy access for repeated blood gas determinations. If hypovolemia (decreased preload) is a consideration, an umbilical venous catheter can be advanced into the left or right atrium to measure filling pressures and determine whether volume expansion is indicated. In normal neonates, the mean right atrial pressure is 0–4 mmHg and the mean left atrial pressure is 3–6 mmHg. If volume expansion is not necessary, maintenance fluids should be started at 75–100 mL/kg/day with glucose added. On the other hand, if obvious pulmonary edema is present, furosemide (1 mg/kg/dose) should be administered intravenously and the maintenance fluids decreased accordingly.

Once the basic stabilization procedures have been carried out in the outlying hospital, the need for a continuous PGE$_1$ infusion may be difficult to decide with certainty. However, the physical examination, chest roentgenogram, electrocardiogram, and blood gases will often be helpful in making that determination. At times, however, even with the use of the physical examination and the ancillary laboratory procedures, the precise diagnosis may not be known in the referral hospital, and initiation of PGE$_1$ (0.05–0.10 μg/kg/min) on an empiric basis may be warranted in the infant with severe cyanosis or decreased systemic perfusion. The primary side effects of PGE$_1$ include apnea, fever, and cutaneous vasodilatation. Whenever PGE$_1$ is used, ventilation by face mask and subsequent intubation must be readily available (including during transport).

If poor perfusion and decreased cardiac output persist, continuous infusion inotropic support should be started. Dopamine is typically the first drug of choice. The dosage range is 1–20 μg/kg/min. At the lower range (< 5 μg/kg/min), dopamine dilates the renal arterial bed, increasing renal blood flow and promoting diuresis. As one increases the dosage (> 10 μg/kg/min) α-adrenergic vasoconstriction becomes dominant, resulting in increased systemic vascular resistance (including renal) and increased pulmonary vascular resistance (especially with hypoxic pulmonary vasoconstriction), nullifying any beneficial effect from increased cardiac output due to enhanced myocardial contractility. However, when high dose dopamine ($>$ 15 µg/kg/min) is necessary, the addition of a vasodilator (e.g., nitroprusside) should be considered if the heart is enlarged to counteract the undesirable effects of dopamine.

When the lower dose dopamine ($<$ 10 µg/kg/min) is ineffective in achieving the desired hemodynamic result, dobutamine is often added as a continuous infusion (1–15 µg/kg/min). Dobutamine has the advantage of decreasing systemic and pulmonary vascular resistance, in contrast to dopamine, while both increase myocardial contractility.

The remaining inotropes are used much less commonly. Digoxin cannot provide immediate improvement in myocardial contractility because it takes a number of hours to accomplish full digitalization. Isoproterenol is a pure β-adrenergic agonist, increasing heart rate and cardiac output while decreasing systemic vascular resistance. Unfortunately, the vasodilatation is not selective and the increased cardiac output redistributes blood flow to nonvital organs (e.g., skeletal muscle and skin) and actual oxygen delivery to vital organs is decreased. The primary use for isoproterenol (0.1–1.0 µg/kg/min) is to temporarily increase the heart rate in the neonate with 3° AV block or severe sinus bradycardia.

Epinephrine (0.1–1.0 µg/kg/min) is predominantly a β-adrenergic agonist at low dose, but at high dose it possesses potent α-adrenergic effects. This agent appears to have no particular advantage over dopamine and is definitely more arrhythmogenic. Norepinephrine also has very potent β-inotropic effects and α-vasoconstrictor properties. The latter effect results in a considerable increase in afterload that is prohibitive unless the norepinephrine is combined with an α-adrenergic blocker such as phentolamine or some other vasodilator. The standard mix is 4 mg of norepinephrine and 10 mg of phentolamine in 50 mL D_5W (40 µg of norepinephrine per milliliter concentration) with the dosage range 0.5–2.0 µg/kg/min based on the norepinephrine. This combination, which can increase cardiac output significantly without increasing afterload, has been used extensively in the postoperative cardiac intensive care unit.

Because cardiac reserve in the neonate is limited, manipulation of afterload should also be considered when the aforementioned therapy has not resulted in significant improvement. Although selective pulmonary vasodilatation has been attempted for a number of years to treat PPHNB, the use of afterload reduction or systemic vasodilation has been a much more recent advance.[53] The infants who would benefit most are those with severe primary myocardial disease: neonatal asphyxia, myocarditis, dilated congestive cardiomyopathy, or septic shock. Nitroprusside is used as a continuous infusion (0.5–8.0 µg/kg/min). Since this drug reduces both preload and afterload, continuous monitoring of the systemic blood pressure (UAC) and the ventricular filling pressure or

TABLE 54.6 Management of Critically Ill Newborn

MINIMIZE O_2 CONSUMPTION

Neutral thermal environment, decrease work of breathing, sedation, nothing by mouth, avoid unnecessary procedures

MAXIMIZE O_2 DELIVERY

Increase O_2 carrying capacity (i.e., Hb) and fi_{O_2} (unless contraindicated: HLHS)

Maximize myocardial contractility by correcting negative inotropic factors, by correcting hypovolemia by starting continuous inotropic infusion, by starting PGE_1 if ductal-dependent pulmonary or systemic circulation, by decreasing afterload if LV contractility and perfusion remain poor and heart enlarged

Maintain HR between 120 and 180 beats per minute

PROCEED QUICKLY WITH DIAGNOSTIC EVALUATION

History and physical examination, blood work with arterial blood gas, chest roentgenogram, hyperoxia test, ECG, echocardiogram if available

PREPARE FOR TRANSPORT

Intubation and ventilator with continuous O_2 saturation monitoring, UAC with continuous blood pressure measurement, ±UVC or peripheral IV, maintenance fluids and glucose, start necessary drips and check calculations

preload (UVC) is encouraged. The major adverse side effect associated with nitroprusside is the development of cyanide toxicity. Although such toxicity is quite uncommon, cyanide and thiocyanade levels should be followed, especially in the presence of hepatic or renal compromise.[54] Efficacy can be judged by improved perfusion, increased urine output, and increased ventricular contractility on follow-up echocardiography. If long-term afterload reduction is necessary, the nitroprusside can be weaned while starting oral captopril (0.1 to 0.5 mg/kg/dose every 8 h). Rarely hyperkalemia and renal toxicity have been reported in the neonate and should be monitored. Table 54.6 summarizes our approach to the critically ill newborn.

SUMMARY

The recognition and optimal management of critical congenital heart disease is of paramount importance, for interventional and surgical techniques have improved so dramatically in the last decade that successful palliation or correction can be provided in even the most serious forms of CHD presenting in the neonatal period: dextrotransposition of the great vessels,[3,4] hypoplastic left heart syndrome,[5] pulmonary atresia–ventricular septal defect,[55] complex interrupted aortic arch,[56,57] and critical aortic stenosis.[58] More children born with serious CHD are reaching adult life than ever before. However, a recent report from Britain revealed that 30% of infants dying with CHD in the first year of life were undiagnosed.[59] Thus, only with early recognition of the subtle signs of CHD, followed by definitive diagnosis and appropriate management, can the prospects for survival and a favorable long-term outlook be improved.

APPENDIX TO CHAPTER 54

Abbreviations and Acronyms

AF	atrial flutter
AS	aortic stenosis
ASD	atrial septal defect
AVSD	atrioventricular septal defect
AV	atrioventricular, arteriovenous
CHB	complete heart block
CHD	congenital heart disease
CHF	congestive heart failure
CVH	combined ventricular hypertrophy
CW	continuous wave
d-TGV	dextrotransposition of the great vessels
DORV	double-outlet right ventricle
ECG	electrocardiogram
fi_{O_2}	fraction of inspired oxygen concentration
Hb	hemoglobin
HLHS	hypoplastic left heart syndrome
HR	heart rate
HRHS	hypoplastic right heart syndrome
IAA	interrupted aortic arch
l-TGV	levotransposition of the great vessels
LV	left ventricle
LVH	left ventricular hypertrophy
LVOT	left ventricular outflow tract
PA	pulmonary atresia, pulmonary artery
PAC	premature atrial contraction
PA-VSD	pulmonary atresia–ventricular septal defect
PBF	pulmonary blood flow
PDA	patent ductus arteriosus
PEEP	positive end-expiratory pressure
PGE_1	prostaglandin E_1
PMI	point of maximal impulse
PPHNB	persistent pulmonary hypertension of the newborn
PS	pulmonic stenosis
PVC	premature ventricular contraction
PVR	pulmonary vascular resistance
RV	right ventricle
RVH	right ventricular hypertrophy
SLE	systemic lupus erythematosus
SVT	supraventricular tachycardia
TA	tricuspid atresia
TAPVC	total anomalous pulmonary venous connection
TNB	term newborn
TOF	tetralogy of Fallot
UAC	umbilical artery catheter
UVC	umbilical venous catheter
VACTERL	vertebral, anal, cardiac, tracheoesophageal, renal, and limb association
VSD	ventricular septal defect
WPW	Wolff–Parkinson–White syndrome

REFERENCES

1. Hoffman, JIE. Incidence of congenital heart disease. I. Postnatal incidence. *Pediatr Cardiol* 1995;16:103–113.
2. Fyler DC, Buckley LP, Hellenbrand WE, Cohn HE. Report of the New England Regional Infant Cardiac Program. *Pediatrics* 1980;65(suppl):375–461.
3. Mee RBB. Results of the arterial switch procedure for complete transposition with intact ventricular septum. *Cardiol Young* 1991;1:97–98.
4. Wernovsky G, Mayer JE Jr, Jonas RA, Hanley FL, Blackstone EH, Kirklin JW, Castaneda AR. Factors influencing early and late outcome of the arterial switch operation for transposition of the great arteries. *J Thorac Cardiovasc Surg* 1995;109:289–302.
5. Iannettoni MD, Bove EL, Mosca RS, Lupinetti FM, Dorostkar PC, Ludomirsky A, Crowley DC, Kulik TJ, Rosenthal A. Improving results with first-stage palliation for hypoplastic left heart syndrome. *J Thorac Cardiovasc Surg* 1994;107:934–940.
6. Allan LD, Crawford DC, Chita SK, Anderson RH, Tynan MJ. Familial recurrence of congenital heart disease in a prospective series of mothers referred for fetal echocardiography. *Am J Cardiol* 1986;58:334–337.
7. Whittemore R, Wells JA, Castellsaque X. A second-generation study of 427 probands with congenital heart defects and their 837 children. *J Am College Cardiol* 1994;23:1459–1467.
8. Nora JJ, Nora AH. Maternal transmission of congenital heart disease: new recurrence risk figures and the question of cytoplasmic inheritance and vulnerability to teratogens. *Am J Cardiol* 1987;59:459–463.
9. Chin NA, Fitzsimmons J, Shephard TH, Fantel AG. Congenital heart disease among spontaneous abortuses and stillborn fetuses: prevalence and association. *Teratology* 1989;40:475–482.
10. Lockshin MD, Bonsa E, Elkon K, et al. Neonatal lupus risk to newborns of mothers with SLE. *Arthritis Rheum* 1988;33:697–701.
11. Oakley CM. Anticoagulants in pregnancy: a review. *Br Heart J* 1995;74:107–111.
12. Sandor GGS, Smith DF, MacLeod PM. Cardiac malformations in the fetal alcohol syndrome. *J Pediatr* 1981;98:771–773.
13. Lipshulz SE, Frassica JJ, Orav EJ. Cardiovascular abnormalities in infants prenatally exposed to cocaine. *J Pediatr* 1991;118:44–51.
14. Kinsella JP, Abman SH. Recent developments in the pathophysiology and treatment of persistent pulmonary hypertension of the newborn. *J Pediatr* 1995;126:853–864.
15. Ferencz C, Neil CA, Boughman JA, Rubin JD, Brenner JI, Perry LW. Congenital cardiac malformations associated with chro-

mosomal abnormality: an epidemiologic study. *J Pediatr* 1989;114:79–86.

16. Aase JM, Dysmorphologic diagnosis for the pediatric practitioner. *Pediatr Clin North Am* 1992;39:135–156.

17. Weintraub RG, Brawn WJ, Venables AW, Mee RBB. Two-patch repair of complete AV septal defect in the first year of life. *J Thorac Cardiovasc Surg* 1990;99:320–326.

18. Anderson RC, Moller JH. Ten year and longer follow-up of 1,000 consecutive children with cardiac malformations. The University of Minnesota experience. In: Engle MA, Perloff JK, eds. *Congenital Heart Disease After Surgery.* Chicago: York Medical Books; 1983;49.

19. Davignon A, Rautaharju P, Boiselle E, Soumis F, Megelas M, Choquette A. Normal ECG standards for infants and children. *Pediatr Cardiol* 1980;1:123–131.

20. Southall DP, Richards J, Mitchell P, Brown DJ, Johnston PGB, Shinebourne EA. Study of cardiac rhythm in normal newborns. *Br Heart J* 1980;43:14–20.

21. Rudolph AM, Heymann MA. Circulatory changes during growth in the fetal lamb. *Circ Res* 1970;26:289–299.

22. Braudo M, Rowe RD. Auscultation of the heart—early neonatal period. *Am J Dis Child* 1961;101:575–587.

23. Van Praagh S, Santini F, Sanders SP. Cardiac malpositions with special emphasis on visceral heterotaxy (asplenia and polysplenia syndromes). In: Fyler DC, ed. *Nadas' Pediatric Cardiology.* St. Louis: Mosby-Year Book; 1992;589–608.

24. Shannon DC, Lusser M, Goldblatt A. The cyanotic infant—heart disease or lung disease? *N Engl J Med* 1972;287:951–953.

25. Jones RWA, Baumer JH, Joseph MC, Shinebourne EA. Arterial oxygen tension and response to oxygen breathing in differential diagnosis of congenital heart disease in infancy. *Arch Dis Child* 1976;51:667–673.

26. Yabek SM. Neonatal cyanosis: reappraisal of response to 100 percent oxygen breathing. *Am J Dis Child* 1984;138:880–884.

27. Batton DG, Maisels MJ, Fripp RR, Heald JI. Arterial hyperoxia in a newborn with transposition of the great vessels. *J Pediatr* 1982;100:300–302.

28. Warburton D, Rehan M, Shinebourne EA. Selective criteria for differential diagnosis of infants with symptoms of congenital heart disease. *Arch Dis Child* 1981;56:94–100.

29. Fellows KE, Rosenthal A. Extracardiac roentgenographic abnormalities in congenital heart disease. *Am J Radiol* 1972; 114:371–379.

30. Friedman WF. Congenital heart disease in infancy and childhood. In: Braunwald E, ed. *Heart Disease: A Textbook of Cardiovascular Medicine.* 4th ed. Philadelphia: WB Saunders; 1992;903.

31. Jones RWA, Sharp C, Rabb LR, Lambert BR, Chamberlain DA. 1028 neonatal electrocardiograms. *Arch Dis Child* 1979;54: 427–431.

32. Nagashima M, Matsushima M, Ogawa A, et al. Cardiac arrhythmias in healthy children revealed by a 24-hour ambulatory ECG monitoring. *Pediatr Cardiol* 1987;8:103–108.

33. Scagliotti D, Deal BJ. Benign cardiac arrhythmias in the newborn. In: Emmanoulides GC, Allen HD, Reimenschneider TA,

Gutgesell HP, eds. *Moss and Adams Heart Disease in Infants, Children, and Adolescents.* Baltimore: Williams & Wilkins; 1995;628–633.

34. Dillon T, Unger FM, Kerns L. Echocardiography. In: Tonkin ILD, ed. *Pediatric Cardiovascular Imaging.* Philadelphia: WB Saunders; 1992;49–82.

35. Maragnes P, Tipple M, Fournier A. Effectiveness of oral sotalol for treatment of pediatric arrhythmias. *Am J Cardiol* 1992;69: 751–754.

36. Mendelsohn A, Dick M II, Serwer GA. Natural history of isolated atrial flutter in infancy. *J Pediatr* 1992;119:386–391.

37. Julkunen WG, Kaaja R, Wallgren E, Teramo K. Isolated congenital heart block: fetal and infant outcome and familial incidence of heart block. *Obstet Gynecol* 1993;82:11–16.

38. Michaelsson M, Jonzon A, Riesenfeld T. Isolated congenital complete atrioventricular block in adult life: a prospective study. *Circulation* 1995;92:442–449.

39. Schmidt KG, Ulmer HE, Silverman NH, Kleinman CS, Copel JA. Perinatal outcome of fetal complete atrioventricular block: a multicenter experience. *J Am College Cardiol* 1991;17: 1360–1366.

40. Watson WG, Katz VL. Steroid therapy for hydrops associated with antibody-mediated congenital heart block. *Am J Obstet Gynecol* 1991;165:553–554.

41. Buyon JP, Swersky SH, Fox H, et al. Intrauterine therapy for presumptive myocarditis with acquired heart block due to systemic lupus erythematosus. *Arthritis Rheum* 1987;30:44–49.

42. Kaaja R, Julkunen H, Ammala P, Teppo AM, Kurki P. Congenital heart block: successful prophylactic treatment with intravenous gamma globulin and corticosteroid therapy. *Am J Obstet Gynecol* 1991;165:1333–1334.

43. Carpenter RJ, Strasburger JF, Garson A Jr, et al. Fetal ventricular pacing for hydrops secondary to complete atrioventricular block. *J Am College Cardiol* 1986;8:1434–1436.

44. Friedman AH, Copel JA, Kleinman CS. Fetal echocardiography and fetal cardiology: indications, diagnosis, and management. *Semin Perinatol* 1993;17:76–88.

45. Fowler RS, Finlay CD. The electrocardiogram of the neonate. In: Freedom RM, Benson LN, Smallhorn JF, eds. *Neonatal Heart Disease.* London: Springer-Verlag; 1992;91–100.

46. Snider AR, Serwer GA, Ritter SB. *Echocardiography in Pediatric Heart Disease.* 2nd ed. St. Louis Mosby-Year Book; 1997.

47. Silverman, NH. *Pediatric Echocardiography.* Baltimore: Williams & Wilkins; 1993.

48. Rudolph AM. Developmental considerations in neonatal heart failure. *Hosp Pract* 1985;20:53–70.

49. Romero TE, Friedman WF. Limited left ventricular response to volume overload in the neonatal period. A comparative study with the adult animal. *Pediatr Res* 1979;13:910–915.

50. Kirkpatrick SE, Pitlick PT, Nabiloff J, Friedman WF. Frank–Starling relationship as an important determinant of fetal cardiac output. *Am J Physiol* 1976;231:495–500.

51. Berman WJ, Christensen D. Effects of acute preload and afterload stress on myocardial function in newborn and adult sheep. *Biol Neonate* 1983;43:61–66.

52. Rudolph AM. General problems of severe heart disease in the newborn. *Modern Probl Paediatr* 1983;22:1–6.

53. Benitz WE, Malachowski N, Cohen RS, Stevenson DK, Akiagno RL, Sunshine P. Use of sodium nitroprusside in neonates: efficacy and safety. *J Pediatr* 1985;106:102–110.

54. Dillon TR, Janos GG, Meyer RA, Benzing G III, Kaplan S. Vasodilator therapy for congestive heart failure. *J Pediatr* 1980;96:623–629.

55. Reddy VM, Liddicoat JR, Hanley FL. Midline one-stage complete unifocalization and repair of pulmonary atresia with ventricular septal defect and major aortopulmonary collaterals. *J Thorac Cardiovasc Surg* 1995;109:832–845.

56. Jonas RA, Quaegebeur JM, Kirklin JW, Blackstone EH, Daicoff G. Outcomes in patients with interrupted aortic arch and ventricular septal defect. *J Thorac Cardiovasc Surg* 1994;107:1099–1113.

57. Sandhu SK, Beekman RH, Mosca RS, Bove EL. Single stage repair of aortic arch obstruction and associated intracardiac defects in the neonate. *Am J Cardiol* 1995;75:370–373.

58. Mosca RS, Iannettoni MD, Schwartz SM, Ludomirsky A, Beekman RH III, Lloyd T, Bove EL. Critical aortic stenosis in the neonate. *J Thorac Cardiovasc Surg* 1995;109:147–154.

59. Abu-Harb M, Hey E, Wren C. Death in infancy from unrecognized congenital heart disease. *Arch Dis Child* 1994;71:3–7.

INDEX